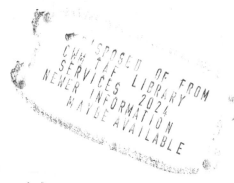

ADLER'S

Physiology

OF THE
Eye

Clinical Application

ADLER'S

Physiology
OF THE
Eye

Clinical Application

EDITED BY
WILLIAM M. HART, Jr., M.D., Ph.D.

Professor of Ophthalmology and Visual Sciences
Washington University School of Medicine
St. Louis, Missouri

NINTH EDITION

with 1342 illustrations

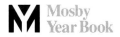

St. Louis Baltimore Boston Chicago London Philadelphia Sydney Toronto

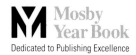

Mosby
Year Book
Dedicated to Publishing Excellence

Publisher: George S. Stamathis
Editor: Laurel Craven
Assistant Editor: Penny Rudolph
Project Supervisor: Barbara Merritt
Editing and Production: University Graphics
Designer: Elizabeth Fett

NINTH EDITION

Printed in the United States of America

Mosby-Year Book, Inc.
11830 Westline Industrial Drive
St. Louis, Missouri 63146

Library of Congress Cataloging in Publication Data

Adler's physiology of the eye : clinical application / edited by
  William M. Hart, Jr. — 9th ed.
    p.   cm.
  Includes bibliographical references and index.
  ISBN 0-8016-2107-0
  1. Eye—Physiology.   I. Hart, William M.   II. Adler, Francis
Heed, 1895-   .   III. Title: Physiology of the eye.
  [DNLM: 1. Eye—physiology.   WW 103 A238]
  RE67.A32   1992
  612.8'4—dc20
  DNLM/DLC
  for Library of Congress   92-12791
                                           CIP

  93 94 95 96 UG/MV 9 8 7 6 5 4 3 2

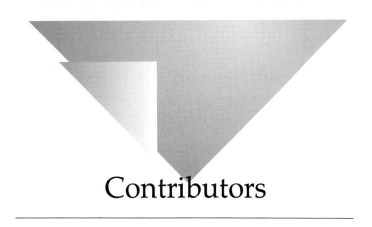

Contributors

ALBERT ALM, M.D.
Professor
Department of Ophthalmology
University Hospital
Uppsala, Sweden

DOUGLAS R. ANDERSON, M.D.
Professor of Ophthalmology
Bascom Palmer Eye Institute
University of Miami School of Medicine
Miami, Florida

ELIOT L. BERSON, M.D.
William F. Chatlos Professor of Ophthalmology
Harvard University Medical School;
Director, Berman-Gund Laboratory for the Study of
  Retinal Degenerations at the Massachusetts Eye
  and Ear Infirmary
Boston, Massachusetts

HAROLD BURTON, Ph.D.
Professor of Anatomy and Neurobiology
Washington University School of Medicine
St. Louis, Missouri

JOSEPH CAPRIOLI, M.D.
Associate Professor
Director, Glaucoma Services
Department of Ophthalmology
Yale University School of Medicine
New Haven, Connecticut

ADOLPH I. COHEN, Ph.D., D.Sc. (Hon.)
Professor of Anatomy and Neurobiology in
  Ophthalmology
Washington University School of Medicine
St. Louis, Missouri

NICHOLAS A. DELAMERE, M.D.
Department of Ophthalmology and Visual Sciences
Kentucky Lions Eye Research Institute
University of Louisville
Louisville, Kentucky

STEVEN E. FELDON, M.D.
Associate Professor of Ophthalmology and
  Neurological Surgery
University of Southern California
Los Angeles, California

JONATHAN CHARLES HORTON, M.D., Ph.D.
Assistant Professor of Ophthalmology and
  Neurosurgery
Neuro-Ophthalmology Unit
University of California, San Francisco
San Francisco, California

PAUL L. KAUFMAN, M.D.
Professor and Director of Glaucoma Services
Department of Ophthalmology
University of Wisconsin Medical School, Hospital
  and Clinics
Madison, Wisconsin

MICHAEL A. LEMP, M.D.
Professor and Chairman
Georgetown University
Washington, D.C.

CHRISTOPHER A. PATERSON, Ph.D., D.Sc.
Department of Ophthalmology and Visual Sciences
Kentucky Lions Eye Research Institute
University of Louisville
Louisville, Kentucky

JAY S. PEPOSE, M.D., Ph.D.
Associate Professor of Ophthalmology
Washington University School of Medicine
St. Louis, Missouri

HARRY A. QUIGLEY, M.D.
Professor of Ophthalmology
Johns Hopkins University
Wilmer Institute
Baltimore, Maryland

JOHN SAARI, Ph.D.
Professor
Departments of Ophthalmology and Biochemistry
University of Washington School of Medicine
Seattle, Washington

J. SEBAG, M.D.
Adjunct Associate Clinical Scientist
Eye Research Institute of Retina Foundation
Harvard Medical School
Boston, Massachusetts

STANLEY THOMPSON, M.D.
Professor
Department of Ophthalmology
University of Iowa
Iowa City, Iowa

LAWRENCE TYCHSEN, M.D.
Director, Pediatric Ophthalmology
Washington University School of Medicine
St. Louis, Missouri

JOHN L. UBELS, Ph.D.
Associate Professor
Department of Ophthalmology
University of Pittsburgh School of Medicine
Pittsburgh, Pennsylvania

GERALD WESTHEIMER, Ph.D., F.R.S.
Professor and Head of Division of Neurobiology
University of California
Berkeley, California

DARRELL E. WOLFLEY, M.D.
Professor
Department of Ophthalmology
Georgetown University Medical Center
Washington, D.C.

For
MARY PRIAL HART
My life's companion

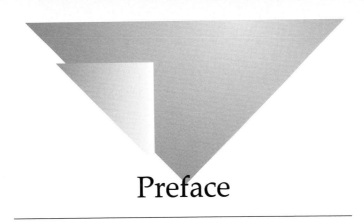

Preface

This edition is one of many periodic revisions of a text that serves as a general reference for students seeking a broad introduction to the world of visual function. The need for revisions has grown, as our understanding of visual physiology has been in a perpetually accelerating flux. Occasionally, new insights have been the result of unexpected revelations, but more often progress has been slow and steady, and limited by available resources. Much still depends on the development of new experimental technologies, the nature of which is difficult to anticipate.

Current changes appear to be taking place on multiple fronts, as reflected in the revised chapters herein. The complex microstructure and chemistry of the vitreous body can now be seen in sharp contrast to our previously poor understanding that regarded the vitreous as a relatively simple tissue whose sole functions were to maintain ocular shape and provide transparency. The molecular events defining the processes of visual receptor transduction and light adaptation are being ever more clearly defined; the biology of genetically determined variations in human color vision is being unraveled, greatly increasing our understanding of receptor function; and the microcircuitry of neural image processing in the retina and cerebral cortex is being slowly but surely opened to our inspection. Some of these developments are truly wonderful, generating a sense of awe at the marvelous complexity of the biology of vision and the ingenuity of those who study it.

As the volume of knowledge has expanded, so too has the need for multiple contributors. To the strengths of diversity and multiple forms of expertise, this trend has also created an additional editorial burden. Consistency of writing style is difficult to maintain, as reflected in the varied approaches taken by the several chapter authors. However, it is hoped that the freedom to choose individual forms of expression will have added to the text's value as a teaching and learning tool.

WILLIAM M. HART, JR.

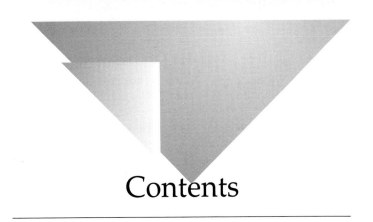

Contents

ADLER'S

Physiology
OF THE
Eye

Clinical Application

The Eyelids

WILLIAM M. HART, Jr., M.D., Ph.D.

The principal optical element of the eye is the anterior surface of the cornea, which is covered by a thin tear film. The eyelids function to maintain the integrity of the corneal surface and its thin layer of tears. The blinking action of the lids serves to spread the tear film across the cornea, forming a smooth surface of high optical quality. A loss of this blinking action will result in an immediate degradation in the health of the corneal surface.

The lids also serve to maintain proper position of the globe within the orbital contents. This supportive function, which is achieved by the elastic properties of the lids, is demonstrable by the slight retraction of the globe into the orbit with lid closure and a corresponding degree of forward motion of the globe during voluntary widening of the interpalpebral fissure.[11] Forcible retraction of the upper lid behind the margin of the bony orbit results in an increase in the volume of the orbital tissues, which in turn forces the globe forward against the elastic tether of the extraocular muscles, resulting in a transient increase in intraocular pressure.

The eyelids thus play an important role in maintaining the health of the ocular surface and the physical position of the eye within the orbit. They can also transiently affect the intraocular pressure, serve to regulate the amount of light allowed to enter the eye, and provide protection from airborne particles. The protective function of the eyelids derives from three principal components of lid function. These are (1) the sensory function of the cilia (lashes), (2) spontane-ous and reflex blinking, and (3) secretions of the glands of the lids.

ANATOMY OF THE EYELID

From anterior to posterior, the lids are comprised of five principal layers of tissue. These are the skin (Fig. 1-1), the orbicularis muscle (Fig. 1-3), the levator aponeurosis (Fig. 1-4), the tarsal layer, and the conjunctiva (Figs. 1-5 and 1-6). The skin of the lids is the thinnest of any area of the human body. This delicacy of the skin, coupled with the loose areolar tissue of the subcutaneous fascia, permits extremely rapid lid movement. Fine lanugo hairs, invisible except under magnification, are found in moderate numbers across the palpebral skin. The primary structural component of the lids, serving to maintain their general shape and to match their curvature to that of the globe, consists of a wide fibrous tarsal plate that is firmly attached to the medial and lateral palpebral ligaments and to the orbital septum. The orbital septum is a thin fascial membrane that connects the tarsal plate to the periosteum of the skull at the margin of the bony orbit. The tarsal plate is the fourth layer of the lid and is covered posteriorly by the palpebral conjunctiva, the fifth layer. The broad aponeurotic insertion of the levator palpebrae superioris muscle, the third layer of the lid, attaches to the superior and anterior surface of the tarsal plate as well as to the skin by means of a series of fine collagenous fibers that pierce the muscular layer of the lid just anterior to the tarsal plate. Thus the tarsal plate is covered ante-

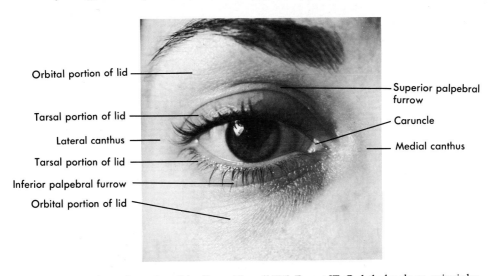

Orbital portion of lid

Tarsal portion of lid

Lateral canthus

Tarsal portion of lid

Inferior palpebral furrow

Orbital portion of lid

Superior palpebral furrow

Caruncle

Medial canthus

FIG. 1-1 External surface of eyelids. (From Newell FW, Ernest JT: Ophthalmology, principles and concepts, 4th ed, St Louis, CV Mosby, 1978.)

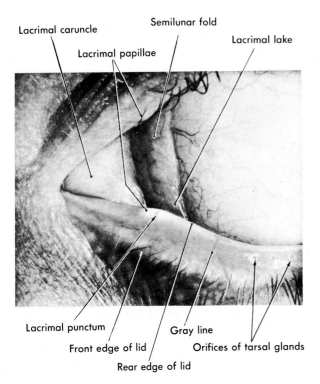

Lacrimal caruncle

Semilunar fold

Lacrimal papillae

Lacrimal lake

Lacrimal punctum

Front edge of lid

Rear edge of lid

Gray line

Orifices of tarsal glands

FIG. 1-2 Lacrimal portion of lid margin. (From Gibson HL: Med Radiogr Photogr 28:126, 1952.)

riorly by skin, orbicularis muscle, and levator tendon and posteriorly by conjunctiva (Fig. 1-6).

THE CILIA

The margins of the lids contain a series of cilia or lashes that are arranged in two rows in the upper lid totalling approximately 100 to 150, with about half that number in the lower lid The cilia are curved outward and away from the palpebral fissure. Each is a short, stout, cylindri-

cal hair arising from a typical follicle, which in turn is surrounded by a neural plexus with a very low threshold for tactile excitation. Each follicle has an associated group of sebaceous glands (the glands of Zeis), which empty into the hair follicle by short, wide ducts. Cells within the marginal layer at the base of these glands proliferate slowly. They are slowly pushed toward the center of the gland, filling with a granular material that results in the pro-

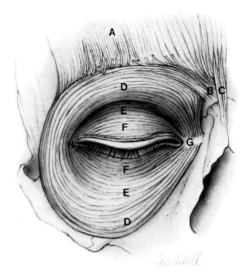

FIG. 1-3 Major components of orbicularis muscle and related musculature. A, frontalis muscle; B, superciliary corrugator muscle; C, procerus muscle; D, orbicularis muscle (orbital portion); E, orbicularis muscle (preseptal portion); F, orbicularis muscle (pretarsal portion); G, medial canthal tendon; H, lateral canthal tendon. (From Beard C: Ptosis, 3rd ed, St Louis, CV Mosby, 1981.)

duction of sebum as the cells degenerate. The sebaceous secretions are forced to the surface at the base of the lashes. Each cilium has a life of from 3 to 5 months, after which it is shed to be replaced by a new one. Cilia that are forcibly removed from their follicles are replaced by a new growth within approximately 2 months. Cilia that are cut off near the base, as is often done prior to surgical procedures on the eye, can be expected to regrow within a few weeks.

Cilia that have recently been shed are not infrequently found as foreign bodies, either within the conjunctival fornices or occasionally even occluding one of the lacrimal puncta. Congenital anomalies of eyelid anatomy and pathologic changes in the margins of the lid can cause the cilia to be misdirected toward rather than away from the palpebral fissure. If such cilia make contact with the corneal surface, they can result in a chronic superficial corneal abrasion. Cilia have also been found within the anterior chamber of the eye after penetrating injuries.

The eyebrows are curvilinear patches of short hairs in the skin just above the orbital margins. They are of limited physiologic importance, performing largely as tactile sensors for objects approaching from above. They are elevated by the frontalis muscle, depressed by the orbicularis muscle, and drawn toward one another by the corrugator supercilii muscles. Voluntary elevation of the brows results in a facial expression of surprise when the eyes are held stationary,

whereas extreme upward gaze is accompanied by elevation of the brows unrelated to facial expression. Upgaze involves, therefore, the simultaneous participation of upward rotation of the globes, elevation of the upper lids, and elevation of the brows. Paralysis of the seventh cranial (facial) nerve results in a brow that is lower than that on the unaffected side. Weakness of the levator superioris, innervated by the third cranial (oculomotor) nerve, results in a ptosis of the upper lid, accompanied by elevation of the brow as the frontalis muscle contracts in an attempt to raise the upper lid.

SECRETIONS OF THE EYELIDS

The chief secretion of the eyelids is sebum, an oily material secreted by the Meibomian glands, which are a series of large sebaceous glands embedded within the tarsal plates (Fig. 1-6). There are approximately thirty of these glands in each tarsus. They are oriented perpendicular to the lid margin, with their openings aligned in a single row posterior to the two rows of cilia (Fig. 1-2). When viewed from the posterior surface of the lid, the Meibomian glands appear as a series of light parallel stripes beneath the palpebral conjunctiva. Pressure on the glands will cause sebum to be excreted from the openings of the glands at the lid margins. This oily material forms a superficial layer over the precorneal tear film, serving to retard evaporation of the aque-

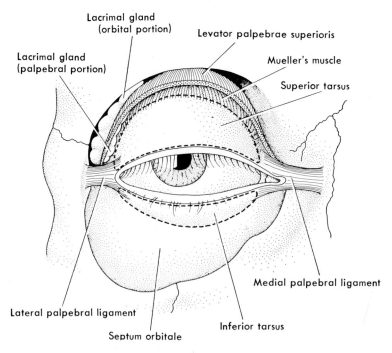

FIG. 1-4   Anterior dissection of orbit after removal of skin and orbicularis muscle. Upper portion of orbital septum has been removed. *Broken line,* Extent of superior and inferior tarsi. Note that entire front of orbit is closed in by firm, resistant tissues except for palpebral fissure, and this can be completely closed by lid and accessory muscles. Palpebral ligaments reinforce diaphragm. (Modified from Wolff.)

ous component of the tear fluid. It also forms a hydrophobic barrier at the margin of the eyelid, preventing spillage of tears at the lid margin. The lids also contain accessory lacrimal gland tissue, the glands of Krause and Wolfring.

EYELID MOVEMENT

The third protective element of eyelid function is the motor system controlling eyelid movement. The lids are relatively low in mass and are propelled by muscles that are large relative to lid size. The levator palpebrae superioris serves to elevate the upper lid, the orbicularis oculi serve to close the lids, and the smooth muscle fibers of Müller serve to modulate the position of the upper and lower eyelids when the eye is open. Both opening and closing movements of the lids may be voluntary or reflex. On opening of the eye, the upper lid is moved through a distance of approximately 10 mm as it is drawn up and back along the curvature of the globe, such that the upper portions of the lid are retracted behind the orbital rim. A fold of skin separating the palpebral from the orbital portion of the lid

marks the site of insertion of the levator into the skin of the lid and is the primary folding crease for this movement. Contraction of the levator is controlled by neural innervation from the third cranial (oculomotor) nerve. The tendon of this muscle is a broad, flat aponeurosis that inserts into the skin on the anterior surface of the upper lid from its free margin all the way up to the aforementioned skin fold. In addition, it inserts directly into the superior margin of the tarsal plate. A few fibers of the aponeurosis insert directly into the anterior surface of the tarsal plate (Fig. 1-6). To reach the skin of the lid, the fibers of the levator tendon pierce the layer of orbicularis muscle just anterior to the tarsal plate. The lid crease or superior palpebral furrow is absent in Asian races, among whom the levator tendon inserts only on the anterior surface of the tarsal plate and not in the skin.[18]

The smooth muscle of Müller participates in elevation of the upper lid, regulating the resting position of the upper lid while the eyes are open. Müller's muscle is a sheet of smooth muscle fibers arising from the undersurface of the levator

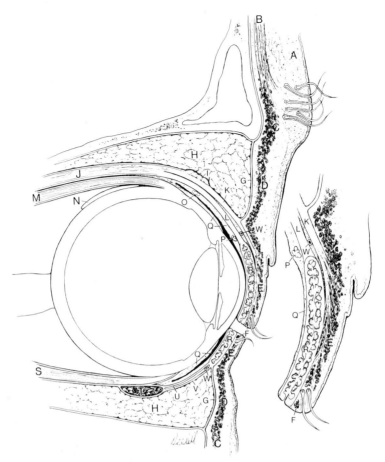

FIG. 1-5 Diagrammatic cross-section of lids, eye, and anterior orbit. A, skin; B, frontalis muscle; C, orbicularis (orbital portion); D, orbicularis (preseptal portion); E, orbicularis (pretarsal portion); F, orbicularis (marginal muscle of Riolan); G, orbital septum; H, orbital fat; I, superior transverse (check) ligament; J, levator muscle; K, levator aponeurosis; L, Müller's muscle; M, superior rectus muscle; N, superior oblique tendon; O, gland of Krause; P, gland of Wolfring; Q, conjunctiva; R, tarsus; S, inferior rectus muscle; T, inferior oblique muscle; U, inferior tarsal muscle; V, capsulopalpebral fascia; W, peripheral arterial arcade. (From Beard C: Ptosis, 3rd ed, CV Mosby, 1981.)

and inserting into the upper tarsal border (Fig. 1-5). Innervation to this smooth muscle arises from the sympathetic nervous system, which forms alpha-adrenergic synapses with the smooth muscle fibers. A similar smooth muscle component is found in the lower lid. This arises from a fascial extension of the inferior rectus sheath and inserts into the lower fornix of the conjunctiva as well as into the tarsal plate of the lower lid.

The action of the levator is closely synergistic with that of the superior rectus muscle.[3] When gaze is directed upward, the upper lid closely follows the movement of the globe. The levator and superior rectus muscles are encased within a common fascial sheath, and the two muscles are innervated by branches of the same (third) cranial nerve. This close relationship is reflected in the frequent association of congenital ptosis and paralysis of the superior rectus muscle, a fact that is especially important when surgery is planned for correction of congenital ptosis. Such patients do not have the normal Bell's phenomenon (upward rotation of the globe on forced closure of eyes) to aid in protection of the corneal surface during attempted eyelid closure.

The levator muscles of the two upper lids are innervated as yoke muscles. Yoke muscles are those that act together as a team. According to Hering's law of equal innervation, yoke muscles receive equal degrees of innervational input. When the levator on one side has been weak-

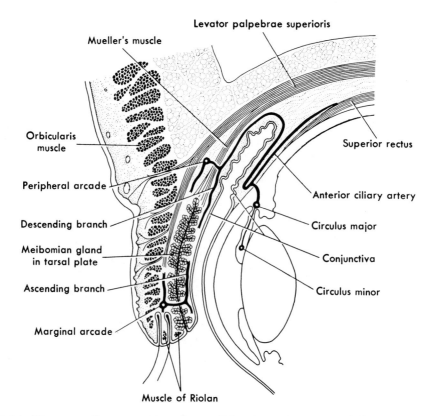

Mueller's muscle

Levator palpebrae superioris

Orbicularis
muscle

Peripheral arcade

Descending branch

Meibomian gland
in tarsal plate

Ascending branch

Marginal arcade

Superior rectus

Anterior ciliary artery

Circulus major

Conjunctiva

Circulus minor

Muscle of Riolan

FIG. 1-6 Diagrammatic cross-section of upper lid and anterior portion of globe, showing fibers of levator tendon passing between bundles of orbicularis muscle to insert in skin of lids. (Modified from Wolff.)

ened, the lid on the opposite, unaffected, side is frequently retracted, as an unconscious attempt to elevate the ptotic lid results in an excess of elevation of the normal partner. Similarly, abnormal retraction of one lid may result in a pseudoptosis of the opposite, uninvolved, eye. Occlusion of an eye with a pathologically retracted or ptotic lid often results in alleviation of the pseudoretraction or pseudoptosis of the uninvolved partner.[5]

While the upper lid synergistically follows movement of the globe during voluntary upgaze movements, forced closure of the eye will result in opposite movements of globe and lid. The globe turns upward as the eyelids are forced closed, a pattern referred to as *Bell's phenomenon.* Upward rotation of the globe with forced closure of the lids rotates the anteroposterior axis about 15 degrees above the horizontal.

This phenomenon is not found during reflex blink closure of the eyelids. Eye movements during a blink are much smaller. Rotational movements of approximately 1 to 2 degrees occur rapidly during the closing phase of a blink

and tend to turn the eye toward the primary direction of regard. With the eye in the primary position, very little rotational movement occurs with blinking. High-speed motion picture photography has revealed a simultaneous retraction of the globe of approximately 1 mm synchronous with closure of the lids.[17]

The common fascial sheath shared by the levator and the superior rectus muscle is an anatomic feature of importance when planning surgery on the superior rectus and levator muscles. A surgical recession of the rectus muscle insertion on the globe will result in some retraction of the upper lid unless the fascial attachments between the superior rectus and the levator are divided. Advancement or resection of the superior rectus tendon will result in a ptosis or drooping of the upper lid. The sympathetically innervated fibers of Müller's muscle arise from the undersurface of the levator muscle and insert into the upper border of the tarsal plate. Therefore a weakness of the levator muscle or an elongation of its tendon will result in a drooping of the upper lid that cannot be counteracted by the action of Müller's muscle. Therefore complete paralysis of the levator muscle results in complete closure of the upper lid. Sympathetic paralysis of the Müller's muscle, on the other hand, will result in a relatively minor degree of ptosis, one of the components of Horner's syndrome of oculo-sympathetic paralysis. This syndrome also results in sympathetic hypersensitivity to adrenergic pharmacologic agents. Weak solutions of epinephrine applied topically will result in a reversal of the ptosis of sympathetic paralysis. Such low doses of epinephrine do not have

an effect on the normally innervated smooth muscle. Conversely, in the treatment of pathologic lid retraction, a characteristic of thyroid eye disease, pharmacologic paralysis of Müller's muscle has been used to relieve the excessive ocular exposure produced by the excessive sympathetic tone.[6] (Although guanethidine has been used for this purpose in the past, it is no longer commercially available as an ophthalmic preparation.)

As shown in Figure 1-7, gradual downward rotation of the eyeball, as in pursuing a falling

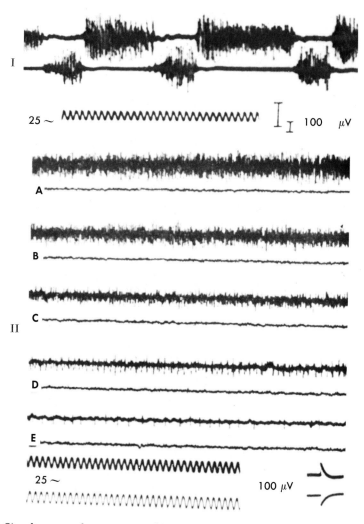

FIG. 1-7 **I,** Simultaneous electromyographic recording from levator muscle (upper trace) and orbicularis (lower trace) during repeated voluntary blinking. Note reciprocal activity in muscles, with absence of activity in levator muscle during active contraction of orbicularis. Compare with **II,** which shows activity during gradual lid descent. **II,** Recordings of same muscles as in **I**; **A,** high levels of levator activity with eyes looking straight ahead. Other strips show decreasing activity in levator as lids are gradually lowered in 10-degree steps. **E,** Only one motor unit still active with lids dropped 40 degrees from horizontal. Note lack of activity in orbicularis as upper lid is lowered. (From Björk A: Br J Ophthalmol 38:605, 1954.)

object of regard, will result in a synchronous downward movement of the upper lid margin, controlled by a progressive relaxation of tonus in the levator.[2] This motion of the lid is not controlled entirely by gravitational influences since it can be observed in the recumbent or even in the inverted position. This is presumably due to elastic influences in the subcutaneous tissue of the lid as well as to some tonus in the orbicularis muscle.

Voluntary vertical changes in the direction of gaze (so-called vertical saccades) are accompanied by similar abrupt vertical movements of the upper eyelid. Magnetic search coil recordings of lid position and electromyographic recordings of levator and orbicularis activity have revealed that bursts of levator activity accompany the vertical upward saccades of the upper lid on redirection of gaze in the upward direction.[3] The lid movement that accompanies a downward saccade is generated almost exclusively by passive elastic forces of the tissues during an abrupt lapse in levator activity.

CLOSURE

Closure of the eyelids is controlled by orbicularis oculi muscle (Fig. 1-3), which is innervated by the seventh cranial (facial) nerve (Fig. 1-8). Hoyt and Loeffler have reviewed the function of this muscle in detail.[9] The orbicularis is a broad, flat oval of subcutaneous muscle that underlies the skin of the lids and an area of surrounding face, including portions of the forehead, temple, and cheek. It is divided into two main anatomic portions: the palpebral and the orbital. The high-speed closure mechanisms of winking are controlled by the palpebral portion of the muscle that overlies the tarsus and orbital septum. Forcible closure of the eyelids (such as occurs involuntarily in benign essential blepharospasm) is characterized by participation of the orbital portion of the muscle along with other muscles of the brow region. The division of the orbicularis into palpebral and orbital portions is both physiologic and anatomic. The functions of the two can be differentiated physiologically by their chronaxie. (Chronaxie is a measure of the electrophysiologic irritability of a muscle. It is defined as the duration of time that a current of twice the galvanic threshold intensity must flow in order to elicit muscular excitation.) The chronaxie of the palpebral portion of the orbicularis is approximately half that of the orbital portion. Muscles that are specialized for rapid movement characteristically have chronaxie values that are lower than those muscles that exhibit slower but more forcible contractions.

Closure movements of the eyelid are broadly separable according to their speed and the participation of differing fiber bundles of the palpebral, orbital, and brow regions. These move-

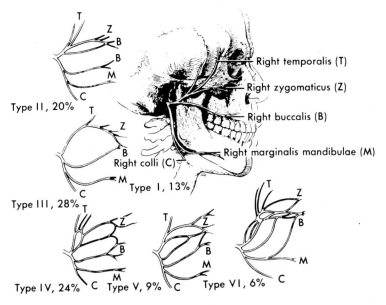

FIG. 1-8 Variations of branching pattern of facial nerve. Note relationship of temporal and zygomatic branches to zygoma and extreme degree of anastomosis that is possible. (From Davis RA, et al: Gynecol Obstet 102:385, 1956.)

ments are referred to as blinking, voluntary winking, and blepharospasm. Blinking is a high-speed closure movement of short duration that has both reflex and volitional origins.

REFLEX BLINKING

Reflex blinking is a rapid closure movement of short duration that is elicited by a variety of external stimuli, including strong lights, approaching objects, loud noises, and corneal, conjunctival, or ciliary touch. The three primary sensory modalities activated in reflex blinking include tactile, optic, and auditory sensations. Corneal and ciliary reflexes are tactile in origin. The dazzle reflex and the menace reflex (initiated by the perception of sudden motion in depth toward the eye) are examples of common, optically initiated, blink reflexes. The ophthalmic division of the fifth cranial nerve is the afferent pathway for the tactile corneal reflex, while the efferent pathway is that of the seventh cranial nerve. This reflex persists in the animal whose brainstem is transected below the thalamic level. Connections of this afferent arc at the cortical level are reflected in the conscious perception of pain associated with corneal touch and the strong reflex closure of the eyelids with which it is associated. This reflex may be abolished with cortical lesions in the rolandic area. Tumors in the vicinity of the cerebellopontine angle commonly cause loss of the corneal touch reflex. Loss of this very sensitive reflex is frequently the initial clinical manifestation of damage to branches of the fifth cranial nerve. The corneal reflex may be quantified with an instrument called an aesthesiometer. Common clinical practice is to use a twisted wisp of sterile cotton filaments to touch the cornea without any associated optic stimulus. Diminution of the tactile corneal reflex is common in contact lens wearers. This allows adaptation to otherwise uncomfortable corneal foreign bodies, such as contact lenses, but simultaneously increases the risk of unintended corneal damage.

The optic nerve is the afferent pathway for the blink reflexes of visual origin, the menace and dazzle reflexes. It appears that the optic blink reflexes may have well-developed subcortical reflex pathways in primates. There is a direct visual afferent subcortical input to the supraoptic nuclei and the superior colliculus, while the efferent pathway of the reflex is by way of association fibers to the facial nuclei. Some mesencephalic lesions may be characterized by loss of the dazzle reflex in the absence of other neurologic findings. The menace reflex appears to be more cortically dependent, requiring the presence not only of primary visual cortex, but also of associational connections to the rolandic area. Thus reflex blinking in response to visual threats may be lost while tactile and dazzle reflexes persist.

Reflex blink closure is a high-speed response to tactile and proprioceptive stimuli. Blepharospasm is a slow, sustained closure initiated by nociceptive stimuli.

SPONTANEOUS BLINKING

Spontaneous blinking, as the name implies, is blinking that occurs on a regular basis without an apparent external stimulus. There is a great deal of interspecies and interindividual variation in the rate of spontaneous blinking, but for a given individual this rate is fairly constant, as long as the external environment is stable. This spontaneous rate may change in response to changes in levels of visual activity, emotional states, and environmental conditions such as dryness or windiness.

The spontaneous blink rate is extremely low or absent in infants. While spontaneous blinking occurs in all vertebrates possessing eyelids and living in air, its rate varies considerably. Large, predatory animals such as jungle cats may blink at rates of less than 1 per minute, while some species of small monkey have blink rates of up to 45 times per minute. Spontaneous blinking is present despite blindness and does not depend on optic stimulation. Spontaneous blinking has been likened to a conditioned reflex because it is a stereotyped and repetitive response to apparently indifferent stimuli.[14]

High-speed motion picture photography of spontaneous blinking has shown that the lower lid remains nearly stationary, the majority of the motion being accomplished by dropping of the upper lid. Completion of the blinking closure is characterized by a narrowing of the palpebral fissure in a zipperlike motion, proceeding from the lateral canthus toward the medial side of the palpebral fissure. This traveling wave of closure moving from the lateral to medial serves to displace the marginal tear strip toward the lacrimal puncta.[1]

The spontaneous blink rate in human adults is approximately fifteen times per minute. The duration of each blink varies from 300 to 400 msec. The average time between blinks is 2.8 sec in men and just under 4 sec in women. Visual input is, of course, interrupted during the blink, which might be expected to cause problems of practical importance in such occupations as piloting of high-speed aircraft or controlling high-speed tools. This interruption of visual input, however, does not produce a conscious discontinuity of visual perception. Experimental obscuration of visual input of up to 3 msec duration may be barely detectable at photopic levels of adaptation, whereas complete darkening of the entire visual field for periods of 30 msec or more by means other than spontaneous blinking is easily detectable. Therefore the perception of continuity of visual images during a spontaneous blink is analogous to the same continuity experienced during saccadic movements of the eye, when vision is also suspended to a large degree (page 556).

Electrophysiologic characterization has revealed three main functional components of orbicularis muscle: (1) those responding in reflex and spontaneous blinking, (2) those responding in both blinking and sustained activity, and (3) those responding in sustained activity only.[8] There is considerable overlap in the anatomic distributions of these units. Most of those in the first group were found mainly in the pretarsal region, while those in second group were clustered primarily in the preseptal region. Those in the third group extended from the preseptal region into the orbital portion of the muscle. Porter and coworkers have reported that there are three distinct anatomic types characterized on the basis of oxidative enzyme profiles and mitochondrial content (primate studies).[15] These three muscle fiber types were designated as (1) slow twitch, (2) intermediate fast twitch, and (3) pale fast twitch. Slow twitch fibers have characteristics indicative of high aerobic oxidative capacity, implying a high resistance to fatigue. These comprised approximately 10% of the total fibers in the orbicularis. The remaining 90% of fibers were made up of intermediate fast twitch and pale fast twitch types. While slow twitch fibers have small, circular mitochondrial profiles and poorly developed internal membrane systems, the intermediate fast twitch and pale fast twitch fibers have more irregular mitochondrial profiles and highly developed internal membrane systems.

Motor units participating in blink movements (those predominantly in the palpebral portion) discharge brief bursts of electrical activity at high frequencies, up to 182 spikes per second in a single unit.[16] This frequency is close to the highest reported by Reid for extraocular muscle motoneurons of the cat. These properties allow for extremely rapid movements capable of responding intermittently at high frequencies. In the human, voluntary blinking has been recorded at a maximum frequency of 390 per minute.

The first electrophysiologic change detectable during a blink is a diminution of activity in the levator, which precedes onset of contraction of the pretarsal component of the orbicularis (Fig. 1-7). Following lid closure, the maintenance of a narrowed palpebral fissure at the conclusion of a blink depends on participation by motor units in the preseptal and orbital portions of the muscle, where the slow twitch fibers are predominantly located. Although an anticipatory relaxation of an antagonist is not an uncommon feature of muscle contractions in general, it may have unusual significance in the blink mechanism by allowing the orbicularis muscle to initiate its contraction from the start against a reduced resistance, thus minimizing the time needed to complete a blink movement.

Consciously initiated volitional closure of one eye is called voluntary winking. This is accomplished by simultaneous contraction of the palpebral and orbital portions of the orbicularis. It is an acquired skill. Most people have the ability to blink with one eye or the other, but are usually not capable of freely alternating the movement. Most people can wink freely with the left eye rather than with the right. This has been related to the predominance of right-handedness. It has been proposed that there is a greater development of uncrossed fibers from cortical areas for facial movement to ipsilateral subcortical centers on the left-hand side in right-handed persons.[19] While voluntary winking can be repeated at frequent intervals, its frequency does not approach that of blinking, there being a minimum period between winks of approximately 300 msec.

BLEPHAROSPASM

Simultaneous forcible contraction of both portions of the orbicularis and the muscles of the brow produces a tonic squeezing of the eyelids. This contraction invariably raises the intraocular pressure, making it a dangerous phenomenon during any surgical procedure in which the globe is open, such as in cataract extraction or corneal transplantation. Surgical specula are designed to hold the lids in an open position with minimal pressure being transmitted to the globe. However, even the best designs fail to prevent transmission of some force to the globe with active orbicularis contraction. The orbicularis must therefore be completely paralyzed by local anesthetic prior to surgical opening of the globe in the awake patient. Many surgeons consider it important to paralyze the orbicularis even during procedures under general anesthesia. Local anesthetic may be infiltrated around branches of the facial nerve in the subcutaneous tissue of the eyelids themselves or the trunks of the nerve may be anesthetized by infiltration of anesthetic in the vicinity of the stylomastoid foramen or along the *pes anserinus* immediately overlying the parotid region anterior to the ear.

Reflex blepharospasm is a frequent accompaniment of injury to the anterior segment of the eye. This can make examination of an inflamed eye particularly difficult. In addition to closing the eye, pain and reflex blepharospasm results in an upward rotation of the globe (Bell's phenomenon). Patients should be instructed to fix their attention on some visual object rather than being exhorted to open their eyes. In extreme situations it is occasionally necessary to paralyze the orbicularis by local anesthetic in order to complete an adequate examination.

Benign essential blepharospasm is an idiopathic disorder of neuromuscular control that results in bilateral, symmetrical, progressive, involuntary closure of both eyes.[10] Initially, this disease may be confused with xerophthalmia or other irritative phenomena, being characterized by increased frequency and duration of blinking. This condition progresses, however, over months or years to produce a prolonged, spastic contraction of the orbicularis, which occasionally causes an associated aching pain. This can result in a severe visual disability, with affected individuals being unable to engage in any visually dependent tasks such as reading or automobile driving. Benign essential blepharospasm is thought to belong to a group of cervico-facial dystonias including Meige's syndrome (dystonic movements of face, neck, and larynx), spastic torticollis, and spastic dysphonia. Temporary relief from benign essential blepharospasm has been successfully accomplished with the use of subcutaneously injected botulinum-A toxin.[10]

Myokymia, or fibrillary twitching of the eyelids, is a common complaint not related to the more severe dystonias. It may be aggravated by fatigue, thyrotoxicosis, or psychological stress. The focus of irritation is thought to be within the facial nerve fibers themselves.[7] When myokymia becomes more generalized and pronounced in the distribution of a single facial nerve, it produces a condition called hemifacial spasm. This is thought to be a peripheral neural phenomenon associated with damage to the extraaxial portion of the facial nerve. Most cases have no clear cause, but may be sometimes associated with compressive injury to the nerve within the cerebellopontine angle or in its intracanulicular course through the temporal bone.

Clinical disorders of importance producing weakness of the orbicularis muscle include myotonic dystrophy, progressive external ophthalmoplegia, and myasthenia gravis. Weakness of the orbicularis may result in ectropion, a flaccid falling away of the lower lid from the surface of the globe. This, in turn, results in epiphora and poor blink closure.

PATHWAYS FOR EYELID MOVEMENT

In the oculogyric centers of the frontal cortex are areas where stimulation produces a raising of one or both eyelids. This movement is generally greater on the contralateral side. Motor cortex stimulation in the prefrontal gyrus close to the representation for the thumb results in closure of the eyelids, usually bilaterally, but greater on the contralateral side (Figs. 1-9 and 1-10). Ablative lesions in this general region result in a paralysis of eyelid closure in monkeys. The fact that the cortical representation for lid movement is divorced from that for ocular movement is consistent with the fact that the extrinsic eye muscles are innervated by the third, fourth, and sixth cranial nerves, while the orbicularis muscle is supplied by the seventh cranial nerve, which also supplies the other muscles of the face (Fig. 1-11).

The subcortical pathways from frontal cortex to brainstem mediating eyelid movements have not been well characterized. Lesions in the region of the posterior commissure often result in a paralysis of upward gaze associated with changes in eyelid movement, either ptosis or lid retraction. Pathways mediating conjugate movements of the eyes and lids must be separate, since lesions in the pons or tectum may separately abolish movements of either the lids or the eyes (Fig. 1-11). In some nonhuman vertebrates, the centers for lid movement may continue to function following ablation of the primary visual cortex. This has been demonstrated in dogs and monkeys.[12,13]

In the monkey the motoneurons innervating the levator are located in a midline subnucleus of the third nerve nuclear complex. This is referred to as the caudal central subdivision of the third nerve nuclear complex and has been reported present only in carnivores and primates. It begins caudally at the level of the trochlear nucleus and extends rostrally to the mid-portion of the medial rectus motoneuron subgroup, where it is replaced by the Edinger-Westphal nuclei. Within the caudal central subdivision there is no apparent laterality in the distribution

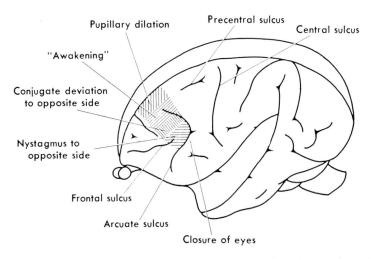

FIG. 1-9 Cortical subdivisions of frontal eye field and area yielding closure of eyes in monkey *(Macaca mulatta).* (According to WK Smith.)

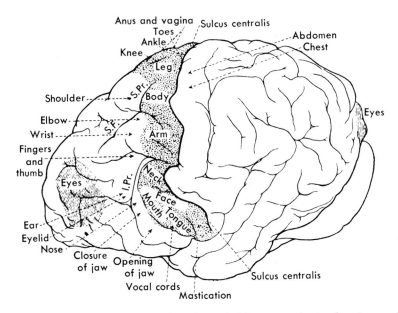

FIG. 1-10 Diagram of external cortical surface of chimpanzee brain showing position of motor centers. Electrical stimulation at parts indicated causes coordinated movements of corresponding muscle groups. (After Sherrington.)

of motoneurons. The caudal central subnucleus thus represents a final common pathway for bilaterally symmetrical levator movements. In the human nuclear third nerve palsies that involve lid function invariably produce bilaterally symmetrical ptosis. (See Porter et al.[15] regarding motoneuron anatomy.) Retrograde staining of motoneurons of the facial nucleus following injection of horseradish peroxidase into the pal-

pebral portion of the orbicularis oculi muscle of monkeys results in staining of neurons throughout the rostro-caudal extent of the ipsalateral facial nucleus. Injection into the upper lid retrogradely labeled neurons whose somas were largely confined to the dorsal nuclear subgroup. A few labeled neurons were also found within the contralateral facial nucleus, suggesting that there may be some decussating axons.

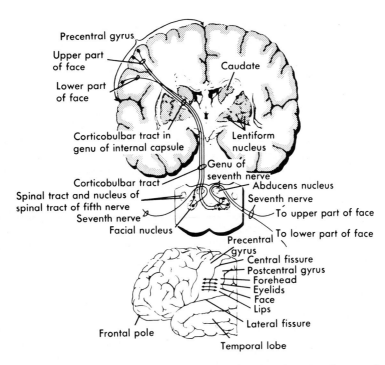

FIG. 1-11 Diagram of corticobulbar pathways serving facial nuclei. Note direct path through internal capsule and bilateral input for upper facial muscles. (From Crosby EC, DeJonge BR: Ann Otol Rhinol Laryngol 72:735, 1963.)

ASSOCIATED MOVEMENTS OF THE EYELIDS

Synchronous movements of the levator and superior rectus have been previously mentioned. As the direction of gaze is gradually directed upward from the horizontal, the upper lid moves synchronously with rotation of the globe. There is a converse relation between movements of the lids and globes when the eyes are closed. In a majority of persons the globes rotate upward with forcible lid closure. This is called Bell's phenomenon. Bell's phenomenon is absent in approximately 10% of normal people. Although the pathway mediating this phenomenon is unknown, it is thought to be different from that for voluntary upgaze since it may still be present in supranuclear paralyses of upgaze.

Other associated movements of lids and ocular or visual muscles occur in pathologic conditions. A curious phenomenon known as the pseudo-Graefe phenomenon occurs following recovery from paralysis of the third cranial nerve. A partial ptosis may persist following such injuries. This ptosis may persist with abduction of the eye, but disappear or even be replaced by excessive elevation of the lid when the eye is adducted. The cause of the phenomenon is thought to be aberrant regeneration or misdi-

rection of regenerating nerve fibers intended for the medial rectus muscle into the third nerve bundle innervating the levator. This conclusion, however, is only inferential as there have been no documented anatomic studies to support this conclusion. It is also possible that synaptic reorganization at the level of the third cranial nerve nucleus may be responsible for the aberrant regeneration phenomenon.

Jaw winking, or the Marcus Gunn phenomenon, is another unusual pathologic form of associated eyelid movement. It consists of a synchronous contracture of the levator muscle with chewing movements of the jaw. Apparently, pterygoid muscle function is involved in this motion, since the associated lid movement is best produced by horizontal chewing movements of the mandible. Pterygoid innervation is abnormally linked neurologically in some way with the levator muscle on the ipsilateral side. Although this associated movement has also been attributed to a misdirection phenomenon, this seems unlikely since the third nerve nucleus and the motor nucleus of the fifth nerve are so distinctly separated from one another. It may be significant that the cortical representation for eyelid elevation lies close to that for jaw movement. This anatomic association at the cortical level and the fact that the condition is congenital may indicate that the defect is located at the very highest levels of motor integration.

THE PALPEBRAL FISSURE

In normal adults the palpebral fissure is 8 to 11 mm wide (vertically) and 27 to 30 mm long (horizontally).[4] The maximum width of the fissure is just medial to its center, making it slightly almond-shaped. Without participation of the frontalis muscle the upper lid has a maximal excursion of about 15 mm, while frontalis action adds another 2 to 3 mm of upward movement. The amplitude of excursion of the lower lid from upgaze to down is approximately 5 mm. These values for the adult are fairly uniform, with little variation by sex or race.

In young children the palpebral fissure is somewhat shorter and wider, while in infants the fissures may be nearly circular in outline (Tables 1-1 to 1-5). The margin of the upper lid normally rests just below the level of the upper limbus, obscuring its margin from approximately 10 to 2 o'clock. The lower lid margin is somewhat more variable in position but usually lies less than 1 mm below the lower limbus. If the superior limbus is completely exposed, the palpebral fissure is pathologically widened. Bilaterally, symmetric exposure of this sort may have little significance, the eyeballs being equally prominent. Asymmetric widening of the palpebral fissure on one side generally is of pathologic significance, however. The width of the palpebral fissure is to a large degree determined by the size of the globe and its position within the orbit. A large eye within a shallow orbit will appear as a prominent globe with a wider fissure. Thus any process that results in proptosis or forward movement of the globe within the orbit will produce widening of the palpebral fissure on that side. Likewise, abnormal recession of the globe into the orbit will result in a distinct narrowing of the palpebral fissure. The width of the palpebral fissure may also vary as a function of the individual's psychologic state. The characteristic wide-eyed expression of surprise and fright may also be seen in chronic anxiety states.

The width of the palpebral fissure is determined in part by the level of tonic activity in the levator palpebrae superioris and the sympathetically innervated Müller's muscle, which raise the upper eyelids, and the orbicularis muscle, which closes the lids. With fatigue, the levator muscle loses its tonus, allowing the palpebral fissure to narrow.

To a large extent the apparent exophthalmos seen in thyroid eye disease is due to a widening of the palpebral fissures caused by a retraction of the upper eyelids. Exophthalmometry measurements in normal persons and in patients with thyroid eye disease yield remarkably similar values. Measurements ranging from 12 to 21 mm are obtained in normal subjects with a mean of 16 mm, while those with thyroid eye disease yield values ranging from 12 to 24 mm with a mean of 18 mm. Measurements of greater than 19 mm, however, were found in only about 5% of normals, while 32% of those with thyroid eye disease fell above this level. Notwithstanding this difference in distribution of measurements, the principal component in the apparent exophthalmos of thyroid eye disease is the degree of lid retraction. Thus measurement of the vertical palpebral fissure width may be a more important measure than exophthalmometry when evaluating patients with thyroid eye disease.

Widening of the palpebral fissure may be a result of excessive tonus of the sympathetically innervated Müller's muscle or excessive tonus of the levator. In the case of thyroid eye disease most of the evidence supports involvement of the sympathetic muscle of the lid. The fact that both upper and lower lids are involved in thyroid eye disease supports the conclusion that sympathetically innervated muscle is involved. This conclusion is also supported by the finding that the lid retraction of thyroid eye disease can be substantially diminished by the use of topical sympatholytic agents such as guanethidine.[6] An associated sign of the upper eyelid retraction resulting from sympathicotonia is lid lag, also referred to as *Von Graefe's sign*. In patients with a marked thyrotoxicosis the widening of the palpebral fissure and the delay of movement of the upper lid when shifting gaze from up to down cause a characteristic stark, staring expression. Retraction of the upper eyelid, referred to as *Collier's sign*, may be found in diseases affecting the pretectal region and especially the posterior commissure. Damage to the brainstem lower than this level will always result in ptosis rather than in lid retraction.

The general shape of the eyelids is maintained chiefly by the partial mechanical rigidity of the tarsal plates, which are molded to the surface of the globe by the overlying tension of the orbicularis oculi. The palpebral portion of the orbicularis is anchored at the medial palpebral ligament, which in turn affixes it to the nasal orbital margin. The domed curvature of the tarsus is determined by the pressure of the eyelid against the surface of the globe. Following enu-

TABLE 1-1 Distribution of Average Length of Palpebral Fissure According to Age Groups

| | Length of fissure (mm) | | | | | | | | | | | | | | | |
	18	19	20	21	22	23	24	25	26	27	28	29	30	31	32	33
Under 1 year	2	3	2	3												
Ages 1 to 10		5	2	9	19	31	20	24	47	14	4	2				
Ages 11 to 60						4	5	29	80	173	337	206	259	117	22	9
Over age 60	—	—	—	—	—	—	5	17	47	43	75	55	28	25	9	—
TOTAL	2	8	4	12	19	35	30	70	174	230	416	263	287	142	31	9

From Fox SA: Am J Ophthalmol 62:73, 1966.

TABLE 1-2 Average Width of Palpebral Fissure at Various Lengths in Various Age Groups

| | | Width of fissure (mm) | | | |
Number of patients	Length of fissure (mm)	Under 1 year	Ages 1 to 10	Ages 11 to 60	Over age 60
2	18	8			
8	19	8	8.7		
4	20	8.2	9		
12	21	8.5	9		
20	22		8.7		
34	23		8.5	8	
30	24		8.5	9	7.3
70	25		8.8	8.6	8.1
174	26		8.8	8.6	8.6
230	27		9	8.9	8.8
416	28		8.8	9	9
262	29		9	9.3	9.1
288	30			9.9	9.1
142	31			10.2	10.0
31	32			10.3	10.0
9	33			11.2	
TOTAL 1732					

From Fox SA: Am J Ophthalmol 62:73, 1966.

TABLE 1-3 Width of Palpebral Fissure in 1732 Normal Individuals

Width (mm)	Distribution (%)
7	3.3
8	22.0
9	29.2
10	32.5
11	10.0
12	2.1
13	0.9

From Fox SA: Am J Ophthalmol 62:73, 1966.

TABLE 1-4 Upward Excursion of Upper Lid in 1638 Normal Individuals

Upward movement (mm)	Distribution without frontalis action (%)	Distribution with frontalis action (%)
12	9.5	0.3
13	20.8	1.3
14	27.5	2.8
15	16.7	9.5
16	13.5	20.0
17	9.3	26.7
18	2.7	16.0
19		13.1
20		9.3
21		1.0

From Fox SA: Am J Ophthalmol 62:73, 1966.

TABLE 1.5   Upward Excursion of Lower Lid in 1638 Normal Individuals

Upward movement (mm)	Distribution (%)
3	1.7
4	21.1
5	36.8
6	26.0
7	13.0
8	1.4

From Fox SA: Am J Ophthalmol 62:73, 1966.

cleation of an eye, a prosthesis must be fitted within a few weeks or months in order to prevent a slow contraction of the unsupported lids.

The eyelid margins normally are held closely applied to the surface of the globe, so that rotational movements of the eye and opening and closing movements of the lid are accomplished with a smooth, continuous apposition, the lid margins never deviating from their closely held position against the surface. Eyelid disease frequently interferes with this normal function, causing the margins of the lids to lose their contact with the globe, turning either toward the eye (entropion) or away from the eye (ectropion). Ectropion of the lower lid is commonly caused by flaccid paralysis of the orbicularis muscle, as in the seventh nerve weakness of *Bell's palsy*. In senile ectropion the lower lid may sag away from the eye as the inferior portions of the orbicularis muscle lose tone. Surgical procedures for correction of this condition commonly involve tightening or shortening the band of orbicularis fibers overlying the tarsus of the lower lid.

Another common aging change is loss of the volume of orbital fat deep to the eye, which allows the globe to recede into the orbit. This produces a relative laxity of the eyelids. In some patients the pretarsal fascia holding the orbicularis over the tarsal plate becomes loose with age and in company with laxity of the lower lid the orbicularis can slide toward the lid margin, allowing the inferior edge of the tarsus to rotate forward. Thus contraction of the orbicularis can produce an inward rolling of the lower eyelid margin (entropion). Entropion may be initiated or aggravated by reflex or essential blepharospasm. Repair of entropion of this sort involves either shortening of the orbital septum at the inferior margin of the tarsus of the lower lid or

shortening and tightening of the orbicularis fibers over the lower portions of the tarsus.

Malposition and deformation of the eyelids are a frequent consequence of trauma and disease. Scarring of the lid can result in eversion or inversion of the lid margin. Cicatricial entropion and resulting trichiasis (contact between lashes and corneal surface) are characteristic of such diseases as late stage trachoma and ocular pemphigus.

THE EYELIDS DURING SLEEP

Muscle tonus of the eyelids during sleep is the exact converse of that found during waking. There is a tonic muscular activity in the orbicularis combined with a simultaneous inhibition of tonus in the levator. In a few normal persons, and as a common consequence of some diseases, some patients experience incomplete closure of their eyes during sleep, so-called lagophthalmos, and this often results in desiccation and excessive exposure of the lower portions of the cornea.

REFERENCES

1. Anantanarayana A: Note on the mechanism of eyelid closure in blinking, Proc All India Ophthalmol Soc 10:154, 1949.
2. Björk A: Electromyographic studies on coordination of antagonistic muscles in cases of abducens and facial palsy, Br J Ophthalmol 38:605, 1954.
3. Evinger C, Manning KA, Sibony PA: Eyelid movements; mechanisms and normal data, Invest Ophthalmol Vis Sci 32:387, 1991.
4. Fox SA: The palpebral fissure, Am J Ophthalmol 62:73, 1966.
5. Gay AJ, Salmon ML, Windsor CE: Hering's Law, the levators and their relationship in disease states, Arch Ophthalmol 77:157, 1967.
6. Gay AJ, Salmon ML, Wolkstein MA: Topical sympatholytic therapy for pathological lid retraction, Arch Ophthalmol 77:341, 1967.
7. Givner L, Jaffe N: Myokymia of the eyelids, Am J Ophthalmol 32:51, 1949.
8. Gordon G: Observations upon the movements of the eyelids, Br J Ophthalmol 35:339, 1951.
9. Hoyt WF, Loeffler JD: Neurology of the orbicularis oculi, in Smith, JL, ed: Neuro-Ophthalmology: Symposium of the University of Miami and the Bascom Palmer Eye Institute, vol 2, St Louis, CV Mosby, 1965.
10. Jordan D, Patrinely J, Anderson R, et al: Essential blepharospasm and related dystonias, Surv Ophthalmol 34:123, 1989.
11. Moses RA, et al: Proptosis and increase of intraocular pressure in voluntary lid fissure widening, Invest Ophthalmol Vis Sci 25:989, 1984.
12. Marquis D, Hilgard E: Conditioned lid responses to light in dogs after removal of the visual cortex, J Comp Psychol 22:157, 1936.

13. Marquis D, Hilgard E: Conditioned responses to light in monkeys after removal of the occipital lobes, Brain 60:1, 1937.

14. Martino G: The conditioned reflex of blinking, J Neurophysiol 2:173, 1939.

15. Porter JD, Burns LA, May PJ: Morphological substrate for eyelid movements: innervation and structure of primate levator palpebrae superioris and orbicularis muscles, J Comp Neurol 287:64, 1989.

16. Reid G: Rate of discharge of extraocular motoneurons, J Physiol (Lond) 110:217, 1949.

17. Riggs L, Kelly J, Manning K, et al: Blink-related eye movements, Invest Ophthalmol Vis Sci 28:334, 1987.

18. Sayoc B: Absence of superior palpebral fold in slit eyes, Am J Ophthalmol 42:298, 1956.

19. Suda K, Kitani K: Rinsho Ganka 9:222, 1955; quoted from Ophthalmic Literature 9:670, 1955.

The Lacrimal Apparatus

MICHAEL A. LEMP, M.D.
DARRELL E. WOLFLEY, M.D.

The exposed cornea and conjunctiva are covered by a complex liquid known as the pre-ocular tear film. This thin fluid layer is maintained by the interaction of the secretory, distributive, and excretory parts of the lacrimal system.[24] The tear film is essential in maintaining a normal, functioning ocular surface. The tear film serves to smooth out irregularities in the cornea, contributing to the smooth optical properties of the corneal surface; the tear film itself actually serves as the anterior refracting surface of the eye, providing the first interface between air and a liquid medium. The tear film also plays a role in regulating the hydration of the cornea by means of changes in the tonicity of the film secondary to evaporation from the tear layer.

It has been demonstrated by Mishima[37] that there is an osmotic gradient across the cornea that develops as a consequence of evaporation from the tear film; this determines also the movement of water from the aqueous through the cornea into the tear film. This flow has been estimated to be approximately 3 ml/cm^2/hr in studies in the rabbit.[38] In conditions in which excessive evaporation occurs, such as certain dry eye states[12,13] and obstructive Meibomian gland dysfunction of the lids,[46] there is an increase in the tonicity of the film that causes desiccation of the ocular surface. The tonicity of the tear film may be manipulated by the introduction of hyperosmotic solutions in order to accelerate fluid movement out of the cornea and into the tear film. This is sometimes useful in lessening corneal epithelial edema.

In addition, the tear film serves as the primary source of oxygen for the cornea.[24] Oxygen available from the atmosphere is dissolved within the tears and is available for uptake by corneal epithelial cells to support the normal aerobic metabolism of the corneal epithelium; a small amount of oxygen contained within the limbal vascular circulation may be available to the periphery of the cornea. Tears serve as a lubricant between the lids and the corneal surface. Tears contain at least three antibacterial substances, e.g., lysozyme, betalysin, and lactoferrin, that help to protect the surface against infection. The flushing action of the tears across the ocular surface helps to remove exfoliating cells, debris, and foreign bodies. In addition, tears contain a mucin network over the conjunctival surface that serves to entrap debris and foreign bodies further, aiding in their elimination. The tear film plays a role in the healing of central wounds of the avascular cornea, providing a pathway for white blood cells from the limbal and conjunctival circulation to reach the central cornea.

Tears are produced by a variety of glands located on and about the ocular surface and within the lid. The balance between production of tear film constituents and their distribution over the ocular surface and their elimination through the lacrimal drainage system is essential in maintaining a normal ocular surface. In conditions in which there is a significant decrease in tear production, particularly aqueous tear production, e.g., keratoconjunctivitis sicca, there is compromise of the normal ocular surface defense mechanisms, rendering the external eye more prone to infection. Conversely, the conditions that block the outflow of tears can also create a stagnant tear film, creating a situation more favorable for microbial colonization of the ocular surface.

Aqueous tear production decreases with advancing age. It does not cause symptoms in most patients until either a critical diminution in tear production is reached or other factors such as a concomitant lid infection occur. In Sjögren's syndrome there is not only a significant decrease in aqueous tear production but a chronic lymphocytic cell infiltration of the lacrimal and accessory lacrimal glands, and also inflammation of the ocular surface, probably immunogenically mediated. Patients with Sjögren's syndrome are not only more prone to infection of the ocular surface but demonstrate severe forms of ocular surface disease secondary to immune events at the ocular surface, e.g., scleritis, peripheral corneal ulcers, and rheumatoid nodules.

THE TEAR FILM— STRUCTURE AND FORMATION

The pre-ocular tear film enjoys an intimate relationship with the ocular surface. The tear film is approximately 7 to 10 μm in thickness. It is composed of three discrete layers first described by Wolff.[49] The outermost lipid layer is produced by the Meibomian glands in the upper and lower lids; a small portion may also be produced by the glands of Zeis and Moll. This layer has been demonstrated both by the observation of interference patterns and by direct testing of the tear film for lipid activity.[16,34] The thickness of this layer varies considerably, from 800 to over 2000 Å, depending primarily on its degree of compression by the lids.[22] As the space between the upper and lower lids is narrowed, the lipid layer is compressed. As its thickness exceeds 1,000 Å, interference patterns can be observed with the slit lamp biomicroscope. This layer serves to retard evaporation from the tear film, lubricates the action of the lids over the cornea and conjunctival surfaces, prevents contamination of the tear film by the more polar lipids of the skin of the lids, and thickens and stabilizes the tear film through interaction with the underlying aqueous layer.

The bulk of the tear film is made up of the aqueous layer, the product of the main and accessory lacrimal glands. The aqueous layer accounts for over 90% of the thickness of the tear film. It is reported that 95% of aqueous tears arise from the orbital and palpebral portions of the main lacrimal glands[3]; the remainder is produced by the accessory glands of Krause and Wolfring distributed along the upper cul-de-sac. There is considerable variation in the number of these accessory glands.[1] The relative importance of the main lacrimal gland in maintaining a normal film varies from individual to individual, depending upon the number and amount of accessory lacrimal gland tissue. Aqueous tears flow out of the ductal openings of the lacrimal glands and are either isotonic or slightly hypotonic.[3] Aqueous tears collect primarily in the forniceal spaces, in two strips or "rivers" adjacent to the upper and lower lids and in the thin pre-ocular tear film. The general movement of the tear film is from the outer reaches of the interpalpebral space toward the medial canthus. Most of this flow occurs along the lacrimal rivers and is driven by the muscular action of the orbicularis muscle of the eyelid. Tears reach the openings of the superior and inferior puncta through which they are drained into the canaliculi during the relaxation phase of the blink.[10,31] Some aqueous fluid is lost by evaporation from the surface and others by way of reabsorption through the conjunctival surface. There is considerable reabsorption of aqueous fluid along the mucosal passages of the canaliculi, lacrimal sac, and nasolacrimal ducts.[33]

Tear volume, in a relatively unstimulated state, ranges between 6 and 8 μl. Tear production in the so-called basal or resting stage has been reported to be about 1.2 μl per minute.[38] It has been suggested that all tear production is stimulus driven[27] as tear production decreases during sleep and general anesthesia.[4]

The innermost mucin layer of the tear film rests on the underlying corneal and conjunctival epithelium. This consists of hydrated glycoproteins. Recent evidence suggests that the mucin component of the tear film itself has a two-layer structure.[40] There is an innermost tightly bound component associated with epithelial cell surface that is thought to be a product of the secretion of the cells themselves, i.e., the glycocalyx. Just above this, there is a much thicker looser layer referred to as a "mucous blanket." This loosely attached outer mucin layer is thought to be the product of the goblet cells of the conjunctiva. These goblet cells are unicellular and distributed throughout the bulbar and palpebral conjunctiva; their topographical distribution is quite varied.[28] The cornea itself is free of goblet cells. Mucin produced by the goblet cells is discharged onto the ocular surface, distributed by

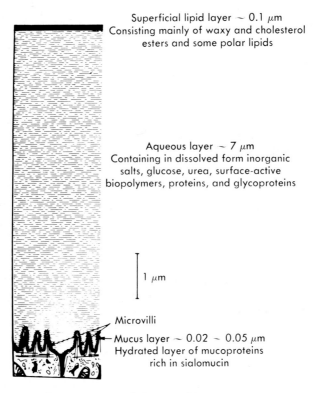

Superficial lipid layer ∼ 0.1 μm
Consisting mainly of waxy and cholesterol
esters and some polar lipids

Aqueous layer ∼ 7 μm
Containing in dissolved form inorganic
salts, glucose, urea, surface-active
biopolymers, proteins, and glycoproteins

1 μm

Microvilli

Mucus layer ∼ 0.02 ∼ 0.05 μm
Hydrated layer of mucoproteins
rich in sialomucin

FIG. 2-1 Structure and composition of the tear film. (From Holly FJ, Lemp MA: Surv Ophthalmol 22:69, 1977.)

the actions of the lids, and adsorbed. Tear mucin lipoproteins lower the tear surface tension from 70 dynes per cm to 40 dynes per cm.[23] It has been reported that the corneal surface epithelium is hydrophobic due to the lipid content of the epithelial cell walls and that mucin forms a loose adsorptive coating temporarily rendering the hydrophobic surface of the cornea and conjunctiva wettable by the overlying aqueous tears. Recent studies have questioned the hydrophobicity of the corneal epithelium and this remains a subject of dispute.[9]

The three-layer tear film is inherently unstable; the formation, maintenance, and rupture of the tear film results from a complex interaction between the lids, the tear film, and the ocular surface. Most of the volume of tears is in the lacrimal rivers, i.e., in the menisci visible adjacent to the upper and lower lid margins.

The cell walls of superficial corneal and conjunctival epithelial cells are composed of a complex structure of protein and lipid. In this structure the proteins are largely masked by the lipids. A glycoprotein is probably secreted by the cells, forming an outer glycocalyx. The relationship of this structure to the epithelial cell

wall is as yet not fully understood. As mentioned earlier, one theory of the wettability of the corneal surface involves the role of mucin produced by the goblet cells of the conjunctiva and spread by the action of the lids. In this theory mucin adsorbs into the corneal surface and is thought to be a critical factor in establishing a new, loosely absorbed layer that is wettable by the aqueous tears. In this theory conjunctival mucin transforms a low-energy corneal surface into one of higher energy via adsorption; in addition, mucin lowers the surface tension of tears. These actions are thought to be responsible for the wetting of the corneal surface. Other investigators, however, think that the cell membranes of the corneal surface cells are inherently wettable due to the structure of the glycocalyx, which creates a strong interaction between the strong end dipole of water and the polar cell surface.

THE TEAR FILM—
MAINTENANCE AND RUPTURE

The tear film is an unstable structure; if the action of the lids is not compromised, the tear film will "break," i.e., rupture, forming dry spots that will enlarge and form contiguous dry areas on the corneal and conjunctival surface. Indeed the break-up time, i.e., the interval from the last complete blink to the development of the first randomly distributed dry spot, is a clinical test that is used to measure the stability of the tear film.[29] When the upper lid moves downward over the ocular surface, it compresses the outermost lipid layer of the tear film, thickening this layer substantially. Even though this layer can be as much as 0.1 mm in thickness, it does not spill over onto the skin of the lids and thus keeps the underlying aqueous layer completely covered at all times. Despite this, rupture can occur between blinks, and several hypotheses have been advanced to explain the mechanisms of tear film rupture. One theory states that the innermost mucin layer becomes contaminated with the outer lipids to such an extent that this layer becomes hydrophobic.[23] As the tear film thins between blinks, the aqueous layer will rupture over such a hydrophobic location. It is thought that there is a diffusion of lipid molecules from the superficial layer across this very thin aqueous phase to the mucin layer, producing hydrophobic areas over which the aqueous tear film spontaneously ruptures.

A contrasting theory states that the key step in tear film rupture is instability and eventual rupture of the mucin layer; this is thought to be caused by van der Waals forces acting on the mucin layer. The overlying aqueous layer is then thought to rupture when it comes in contact with the hydrophobic epithelium.[44]

Yet another theory states that breakup may be caused by long-range intermolecular forces known as dispersion forces associated with coherent dipole-dipole interactions among mucin molecules.[32] Regardless of which of these theories is more reflective of actual events, it is clear that periodic reformation of the tear film via blinking is necessary for the maintenance of the normal preocular tear film.

PRODUCTION OF TEARS
Mucin production

Mucin is made up of an extremely heterogeneous group of hydrated O-linked oligosaccharides linked to protein. The bulk of mucin appears to be secreted by the goblet cells located in the apical surface layers of the conjunctiva. The proteineous portion of these glycoproteins appears to be synthesized in the endoplasmic reticulum, while the saccharide branches are added in the Golgi apparatus and the trans-Golgi network. These newly synthesized glycoproteins are condensed and stored in membrane-bound secretory granules at the apical side of the goblet cells. Little is known about the secretion of mucin in the conjunctiva, but in non-conjunctival epithelium it is known that goblet cells can be stimulated to produce mucin by a variety of agents, including parasympathetic agonists, histamines, chemical irritants, and prostaglandins.[6]

The so-called secondary mucus secreting system has been identified in non-goblet cells in the conjunctival epithelium.[14] This system of mucus secretion is thought to be located in vesicles seen in the apical sides of non-goblet cells of the conjunctiva. In certain allergic conditions such as vernal conjunctivitis and giant papillary conjunctivitis, the excessive mucus production is thought to be due to stimulation of the secondary mucus secreting system.[15]

Aqueous secretion

Aqueous tears are secreted by the main and accessory lacrimal glands. The main gland is a tubuloacinar exocrine gland composed of acini and ducts. The paraductal acinal cells surround the central lumen, which communicates with the ducts. In total, acini cells constitute approximately 80% of the main lacrimal gland substance. Aqueous tear secretion is a result of a complex pathway of molecular reactions resulting in the secretion of proteins, electrolytes, and fluids. Secretogogues interact with receptors on cell membranes of acinar and ductular cells.[36]

The lacrimal gland also contains myoepithelial cells that surround the acini in a basketlike pattern. It is thought that they probably act as a pump for the acini, squeezing out secreted fluid.[5] The relationship between the acini and ductular cells and secretogogues is only now becoming better elucidated. The main lacrimal gland is innervated by both parasympathetic and sympathetic nerve fibers. Parasympathetic fibers are in close contact with the acinar cells, duct cells, and blood vessels; sympathetic fibers appear to innervate blood vessels. Parasympathetic nerve supply exerts the principal neural control of electrolyte, water, and protein secretion. The stimulatory effect is mediated via neurotransmitters such as acetylcholine and probably other small peptides contained within the nerve endings, e.g., vasoactive intestinal peptide. Sympathetic axon terminals exert their effect via a beta 1-adrenergic agonist and probably serve to inhibit electrolyte and water secretion. Recently, other substances capable of exerting effects on lacrimal secretion include alpha-melanocyte stimulating hormone and adrenocorticotropic hormone, hormonal receptors

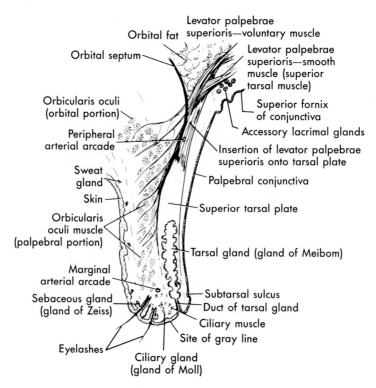

Levator palpebrae
superioris—voluntary muscle

Orbital fat

Orbital septum

Levator palpebrae
superioris—smooth
muscle (superior
tarsal muscle)

Orbicularis oculi
(orbital portion)

Superior fornix
of conjunctiva

Peripheral
arterial arcade

Accessory lacrimal glands

Insertion of levator palpebrae
superioris onto tarsal plate

Sweat
gland

Palpebral conjunctiva

Skin

Superior tarsal plate

Orbicularis
oculi muscle
(palpebral portion)

Tarsal gland (gland of Meibom)

Marginal
arterial arcade

Subtarsal sulcus

Sebaceous gland
(gland of Zeiss)

Duct of tarsal gland

Ciliary muscle

Site of gray line

Eyelashes

Ciliary gland
(gland of Moll)

FIG. 2-2   Structure of the upper eyelid as seen in vertical section. (From Snell RS, Lemp MA: Clinical anatomy of the eye, Boston, Blackwell Scientific Publications, 1989.)

having been demonstrated within the lacrimal glands.

The accessory lacrimal glands of Krause and Wolfring are small glands identical in structure to the main lacrimal gland. These glandular elements are quite variable in number and size and are located along the superior cul-de-sac primarily with an occasional gland found in the lower conjunctiva. They constitute about 10% of the mass of the main lacrimal gland. Originally, the main lacrimal gland was thought to function as a "reflex secreter" for tears, while the accessory glands functioned to produce "basal" tears. This distinction has now been largely discarded.[27] It is thought that all aqueous tear secretion is stimulus driven. Under normal conditions stimuli will produce a low level of aqueous tear production averaging about 1.2 μl per minute. Under conditions of stimulation, however, tear production can increase very rapidly. In conditions of very low-level stimulation, i.e., sleep and general anesthesia, tear production decreases to very low levels.

Lipid secretion

The superficial lipid layer of the tear film is a product of the Meibomian glands of the eyelids. These are sebaceous glands lying along the posterior edge of the lid margins. They number about 20 glands each in the upper and lower lids. The lipids secreted by these glands contain waxy esters, sterols, triacylglyceroles, cholesterol, a small amount of polar lipids, and free fatty acids. This secretion (meibum) has a lower melting temperature than the sebaceous secretion from the glands of the skin and forms a liquid at the temperature of the ocular surface.[2,41,47]

Meibomian glands consist of globules of secretory cells emptying into a single duct. Lipid-secreting cells undergo disintegration and are discharged from the center of the secretory alveolus into the ducts. The movement of lipid along the ducts to the surface is thought to be facilitated by the contraction of the orbicularis oculi muscle. Stimulation of meibum secretion is poorly understood. It may be at least partially under neural or hormonal control. As part of aging, the secretion of meibum frequently undergoes changes, resulting in a common clinical condition known as Meibomian gland dysfunction in which there is an abnormal secretion of meibum, which, in some cases, can decrease secondary to obstructive dysfunction of the Meibomian glands. This can give rise to in-

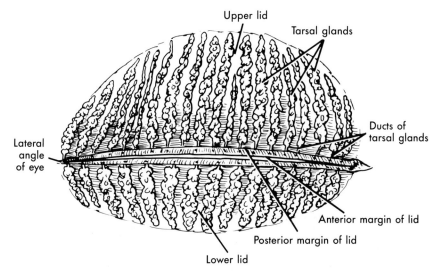

Upper lid

Tarsal glands

Lateral angle of eye

Ducts of tarsal glands

Anterior margin of lid

Posterior margin of lid

Lower lid

FIG. 2-3 Posterior view of Meibomian glands of the eyelids. (From Snell RS, Lemp MA: Clinical anatomy of the eye, Boston, Blackwell Scientific Publications, 1989.)

creased evaporation of the tear film, owing to disruption of the superficial lipid layer. Increased tear film osmolarity resulting from this evaporation can cause a syndrome like dry eye even in the presence of normal aqueous tear secretion.[46]

CLINICAL CORRELATIONS
Tear film abnormalities

Maintenance of a normal pre-ocular tear film is essential to protect the ocular surface. There are a number of clinical conditions in which there is a breakdown of one or more complex mechanisms responsible for the maintenance of pre-ocular tear film. With increasing age it is common for aqueous tear production to decrease. In many patients this decrease is sufficient to cause irritative symptoms and results in a discrete clinical condition, i.e., keratoconjunctivitis sicca.[8] Aqueous tear production is commonly measured using the Schirmer test in which a standardized strip of paper is inserted across the lid margin; the amount of wetting of the strip is then measured after 5 minutes.[50] This test is performed variously, either with or without topical anesthetic. In general, results of less than 5 ml of wetting in 5 minutes are considered abnormal.[30] In a subset of patients with keratoconjunctivitis sicca ocular changes are thought to be mediated by immunogenic mechanisms. These patients who have Sjögren's syndrome, consisting of dry eyes, dry mouth, and arthralgia, are thought to have an autoimmune process resulting in an infiltration of lymphocytic inflamma-

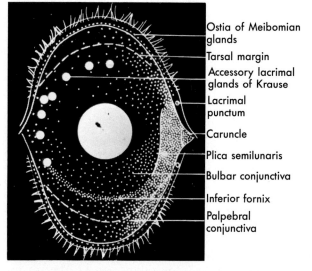

Ostia of Meibomian glands

Tarsal margin

Accessory lacrimal glands of Krause

Lacrimal punctum

Caruncle

Plica semilunaris

Bulbar conjunctiva

Inferior fornix

Palpebral conjunctiva

FIG. 2-4 Topographical distribution of conjunctival goblet cells. (From Kessing SV: Mucous gland system of the conjunctiva; a quantitative anatomical study, Acta Ophthalmol 95:1, 1968.)

tory cells in the main and accessory lacrimal glands[45] and in the ocular surface itself.[42]

A number of conditions result in increased evaporation from the tear film, including Meibomian gland dysfunction, neurotrophic keratitis, thyroid eye disease, contact lens wear, and the presence of an irregular corneal surface. All of these can give rise to dry eye symptoms. There is a relationship between systemic hormonal levels, e.g., estrogen, and the maintenance of a normal ocular surface. In cases of estrogen deficiency decreased hormonal levels may have an adverse effect on the ocular surface and aqueous tear production. In conditions in which there is chronic inflammatory disease of the conjunctiva, e.g., superficial cicatricial ocular pemphigoid and erythema multiforme, there is destruction of the mucin producing goblet cells of the conjunctiva in addition to cellular metaplasia, resulting in the production of keratinized stratified squamous epithelial surface cells. This results in marked areas of nonwetting in addition to conjunctival shrinkage.

It is clear that interruption of one or more of the complex mechanisms responsible for tear production and the establishment and maintenance of the tear film across the ocular surface can result in a variety of abnormalities. These abnormalities have a final common expression in the development of irritative symptoms and can lead to extensive desiccation of the ocular surface.

ELIMINATION OF TEARS

Approximately 25% of secreted tears is lost to the process of evaporation. The remaining 75% is pumped into the nasal cavity through the lacrimal drainage system. The tears secreted into the superotemporal fornix become part of the tear film of the lower eyelid through gravitational flow and the movement of the upper eyelid. In most age groups the lower canaliculus is responsible for the drainage of approximately 60% of the tear volume. However, when the lower canaliculus is abnormal, the upper canaliculus is capable of draining sufficient tears to avoid overflow tearing in approximately 90% of people. Capillary attraction plays a significant role in moving tears into the puncta and the vertical portion of the canaliculi. Blinking not only spreads the tears over the cornea, but also moves the tears toward the puncta. The firm fixation of the orbicularis muscle at the anterior and posterior insertions of the medial palpebral tendon results in a medial displacment of the upper and lower eyelid with each blink. With each blink, the upper and lower eyelid approximate first in the lateral canthal area and then proceed toward the medial canthal area. These two physiologic movements promote medial displacement of the tear film toward the lacrimal puncta.

There is a marked variation in the frequency of blinking that is, to a large extent, determined by the activity in which one is involved. Blinking is minimal when one is reading. It is apparent that maintaining a normal tear film and nor-

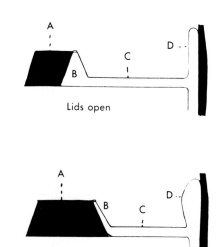

FIG. 2-5 Schematic drawing of lacrimal pump. (From Jones LT: Trans Am Acad Ophthal Otolaryng 66:506, 1962.)

mal rate of elimination of tears does not depend entirely on the blink mechanism or frequency. There is a definite increase in the rate of blinking in response to excessive tear formation.

As tears enter the lacrimal puncta, they are pumped through the canaliculi into the lacrimal sac by the blinking movements. In the adult human each of the canaliculi is made up of a 2 mm vertical segment that joins an 8 mm horizontal segment (Fig. 2-6). At the junction of the horizontal and vertical segments the canaliculi widen into an ampulla.[25] The longer horizontal sections join to form a common canaliculus in 98% of humans. The pretarsal orbicularis muscle intimately surrounds the horizontal portion of the canaliculus, causing the puncta to be displaced medially when the orbicularis muscle contracts. In this contracture the ampulla is closed and the horizontal segment is displaced medially, pumping tears into the lacrimal sac.[10]

An additional portion of the lacrimal pumping mechanism is created by the attachments of the preseptal and pretarsal orbicularis muscle at the medial palpebral tendon. The posterior insertion of the orbicularis muscle into the fascia surrounding the lacrimal sac causes lateral displacement of the lateral wall of the lacrimal sac when the orbicularis muscle is contracted. This creates a negative pressure within the lacrimal sac that draws the tears from the common canaliculus into the lacrimal sac. When the obicularis muscle relaxes, the sac collapses, driving the accumulated tears into the nasolacrimal duct. Thus, the lacrimal drainage system is

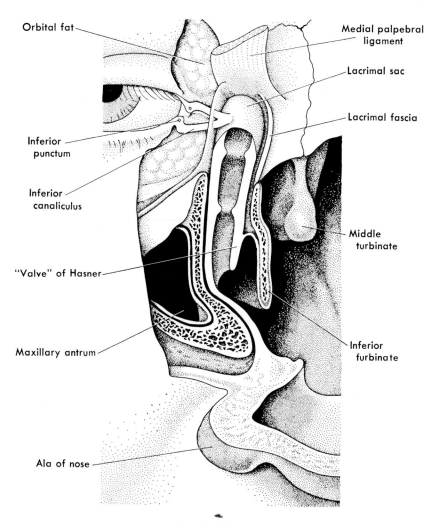

Orbital fat

Medial palpebral ligament

Lacrimal sac

Lacrimal fascia

Inferior punctum

Inferior canaliculus

Middle turbinate

"Valve" of Hasner

Maxillary antrum

Inferior turbinate

Ala of nose

FIG. 2-6 Lacrimal drainage system.

physiologically comprised of a canalicular pumping mechanism and a lacrimal sac siphoning mechanism. Technetium-99 scanning studies of lacrimal outflow have shown that the peak rate of lacrimal pumping into the sac, which occurs intermittently with each blink, is much more rapid than the continuous rate at which the sac empties into the nose.[18-21]

The membranous portion of the nasolacrimal duct plays little or no role in the active transport of tears from the sac into the nasolacrimal duct. Indeed, the variable folds or valves in the duct combine to create the greatest resistance to outflow of tears that is encountered throughout the entire lacrimal drainage system. However, these folds form a baffle that prevents air currents within the nose from invading the drainage system.

It is clinically convenient to think of the lac-

rimal drainage system as being comprised of an upper segment consisting of the lid margins, puncta, and canaliculi and a lower segment consisting of the lacrimal sac and nasolacrimal duct (Fig. 2-7). When one has eliminated hypersecretion of tears as a cause of epiphora, attention is turned to evaluation of the lacrimal drainage system. External examination of the eyelids and the lacrimal apparatus will determine the patency of the puncta and the apposition of the puncta to the globe. Poor orbicularis tone (eyelid laxity) can be evaluated by pulling the lower eyelid inferiorly and then releasing the eyelid to approximate the globe. The time required for the eyelid to approximate the globe is directly proportional to the age of the patient. A normal lower eyelid will always reapproximate the globe without a blink. The patency of the canaliculi can then be further evaluated by the in-

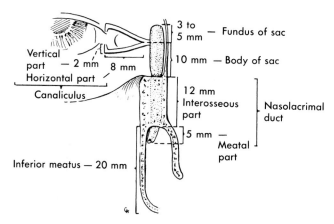

FIG. 2-7 Dimensions of lacrimal drainage system. (Modified from Wolff; from Jones LT: Trans Am Acad Ophthal Otolaryng 66:506, 1962.)

stillation of a topical anesthetic drop and the passage of a small Bowman's probe through the horizontal portion of the canaliculus. A normal canalicular system will reveal a "hard" stop as the probe reaches the bone of the lacrimal fossa. This should occur at a point 10 to 11 mm along the lacrimal probe. A "soft" stop or a tight passage are both indications of complete obstruction or stricture of the canaliculi. Further evaluation of the lacrimal drainage system involves physiologic testing.

THE JONES DYE TEST

In the fluorescein dye test of Jones one drop of 2% sodium fluorescein solution is instilled into the conjunctival sac.[25,26] The passage of this dye through the lacrimal drainage system is then determined by using nasal applicators to retrieve dye from the inferior meatus.[52] A normal lacrimal drainage system will pump this solution into the nose in 1 minute. However, many ophthalmologists had difficulty measuring the retrieval time with the test as described by Jones. Hecht described a modified dye test that has become more widely used than the dye test described by Jones.[51] Hecht recommended the instillation of three drops of 2% fluorescein solution into the inferior fornix with each drop placed several seconds apart. The patient is then encouraged to blink frequently, and the head is placed in a slightly face-down position (face 45° to the horizontal) for 5 minutes. The patient is then instructed to obstruct the left nostril and blow the right nostril into a clean tissue paper. The right nostril is then obstructed and the left nostril blown into a clean tissue paper. This test is always performed bilaterally, using the asymptomatic side as a control. Retrieval of dye is a normal finding. Due to the confusion of the test results as described by Jones, Hecht recommended that the test results be recorded as "dye retrieved" or "no dye retrieved." If there is no dye retrieved on the Jones #1 dye test, then a Jones #2 dye test is performed. The lacrimal sac is irrigated with saline solution or water. Retrieval of dye after the irrigation of the lacrimal sac is recorded as "dye retrieved" or "no dye retrieved."

Interpretation of results is relatively simple. Failure to retrieve dye on the Jones #1 dye test indicates that the lacrimal drainage system is not pumping solution in a normal fashion into the nose. However, the location of the obstruction or dysfunction cannot be determined from the Jones #1 dye test alone. The Jones #2 dye test will determine whether or not the dye solution reached the lacrimal sac. If the Jones #2 dye test reveals dye retrieved, then the dye was pumped through the canaliculi into the lacrimal sac but was not pumped from the lacrimal sac into the nose. Consequently, this is a physiologic obstruction of the nasolacrimal duct and must be managed with silicone intubation of the lacrimal drainage system or a dacryocystorhinostomy. However, if no dye is retrieved on the Jones #2 dye test, one of two possibilities exists. If the clear fluid was irrigated into the nose, the upper portion of the system above the lacrimal sac is dysfunctional. If the irrigation of fluid reveals complete reflux of the fluid through the opposite canaliculus, a complete obstruction of the canaliculus or lacrimal sac is the cause of the epiphora.

FLUORESCEIN DYE DISAPPEARANCE TEST

An accurate qualitative appraisal of the lacrimal drainage system can be obtained by observing the appearance and change of the tear film when a single drop of 2% fluorescein solution is instilled into the inferior fornix.[53] The intensity of the fluorescein color, as well as the rate of dilution of the fluorescein in the tear film, can be evaluated over a period of 3 to 5 minutes. With a normal tear drainage system, there will be minimal fluorescein dye remaining in the tear film after 5 minutes. This is a particularly useful test in dealing with unilateral epiphora, as the behavior of the fluorescein in the tear film can be compared between the symptomatic and asymptomatic eye. With a normal lacrimal drainage system, there will be minimal fluorescein remaining in the tear film after a 5-minute period. However, this test does not distinguish between pathology of the upper or lower segment of the lacrimal drainage system. It is a very useful test to substantiate findings from the Jones dye test.

DACRYOSCINTIGRAPHY

Technetium-99 scanning of the lacrimal drainage system has proven to be a very accurate qualitative and quantitative procedure.[17,43,48] However, the cost and the lack of availability have made this primarily a research tool that is not readily available to the clinician.

DACRYOCYSTOGRAPHY

Radiographic visualization of the lacrimal drainage system using a low-viscosity contrast medium was a popular and a relatively widely used procedure in years past. However, the previously described testing procedures have proven to be much more readily available.[7,35] In addition, the information obtained from dacryocystography can be obtained by the surgeon at the time of lacrimal drainage system surgery. Consequently, dacryocystography has been relegated to a test of only historical importance.

REFERENCES

1. Allansmith MR, Kajiyama G, Abelson M, et al: Plasma cell content of main and accessory lacrimal glands and conjunctiva, Am J Ophthalmol 82:819, 1976.
2. Andrews JS: The meibomian section, Internat Ophthalmol Clinics 13:1, 1973.
3. Bron AJ: Prospects for the dry eye, Trans Ophthalmol Soc UK 104:801, 1985.
4. Cross DA, Krupin T: Implications of the effects of general anesthesia on basal tear production, Anesth Analg 56:357, 1977.
5. Dartt DA: Signal transduction and control of lacrimal gland protein section: a review, Current Eye Res 8:619, 1989.
6. Dartt DA, Lemp MA, Marquardt RC: Physiology of tear production in the dry eye, New York, Springer Verlag, in press.
7. Demorest BH, Milder B: Dacryocystography, II, The pathologic lacrimal apparatus, Arch Ophthalmol 54:410, 1955.
8. De Roeth AF: Low flow of tears—the dry eye, Am J Ophthalmol 35:782, 1952.
9. Dilly PW, Mackie IA: Surface changes in the anaesthetic conjunctiva in man with special reference to the production of mucus from non-goblet cell source, Br J Ophthalmol 65:833, 1981.
10. Doane MG: Blinking and the mechanics of the lacrimal drainage system, Ophthalmol 88:844, 1981.
11. Reference deleted in proofs.
12. Gilbard JP, Farris RL: Tear osmolarity and ocular surface disease in keratoconjunctivitis sicca, Ophthalmol 97:1642, 1979.
13. Gilbard JP, Farris RL, Santamaria J: Osmolarity of tear microvolumes in keratoconjunctivitis sicca, Arch Ophthalmol 96:677, 1978.
14. Greiner JV, Weidman TA, Korb DR, et al: "Second" mucus secretory system of the human conjunctiva, Invest Ophthalmol Vis Sci 18(ARVO Suppl):123, 1979.
15. Greiner JV, Weidman TA, Korb DR, et al: Histochemical analysis of secretory vesicles in non-goblet conjunctival epithelial cells, Acta Ophthalmol 63:89, 1985.
16. Hamano H, Hori M, Kawabe H, et al: Biodifferential interference microscopic observations on anterior segment of the eye. First report. Observation of precorneal tear film, J Jpn CL Soc 21:229, 1979.
17. Heyman S, Katowitz JA, Smoger B: Dacryoscintography in children. Ophthalmol Surgery 16(11):703, 1985.
18. Hilditch TC, Kwok CS, Amanat LA: Lacrimal scintigraphy, I, Compartmental analysis of data, Br J Ophthalmol 67:713, 1983.
19. Hilditch TC, Kwok CS, Amanat LA: Lacrimal scintigraphy, III, Physiological aspects of lacrimal drainage, Br J Ophthalmol 67:729, 1983.
20. Hill JC, Bethell W, Smirinaul HJ: Lacrimal drainage—a dynamic evaluation, I, Mechanics of tear transport, Can J Ophthalmol 9:411, 1974.
21. Hill JC, Bethell W, Smirinaul HJ: Lacrimal drainage—a dynamic evaluation, II, Clinical aspects, Can J Ophthalmol 9:417, 1974.
22. Holly FJ: Tear film physiology and contact lens wear, I, Pertinent aspects of tear physiology, Amer J Optom Physiol Optics 58:324, 1981.
23. Holly FJ: Tear film formation and rupture: an update, in Holly FJ, ed: The preocular tear film in health, disease and contact lens wear. Lubbock, TX, The Dry Eye Institute, 1986, pp 634–645.
24. Holly FJ, Lemp MA: Tear physiology and dry eyes, Survey Ophthalmol 22:69, 1989.
25. Jones LT: The cure of epiphora due to canalicular disorders, trauma and surgical failures on the lacrimal passages, Trans Am Acad Ophthalmol Otolaryngol 66:506, 1962.
26. Jones LT, Marquis MM: Lacrimal function, Am J Ophthalmol 73:658, 1972.
27. Jordan A, Baum JL: Basic tear flow, does it exist? Ophthalmol 87:920, 1980.
28. Kessing SV: Mucous gland system of the conjunctiva, a quantitative anatomical study, Acta Ophthalmol 95:1, 1968.

29. Lemp MA: Breakup of the tear film, Intern Ophthalmol Clin 13(1):97, 1973.

30. Lemp MA: Recent developments in dry eye management, Ophthalmol 94:1299, 1987.

31. Lemp MA, Weiler HH: How do tears exist? Invest Ophthalmol Vis Sci 24:619, 1983.

32. Lin SP, Brenner H: Stability of the tear film, in Holly FJ, ed: The preocular tear film in health, disease and contact lens wear, Lubbock, TX, The Dry Eye Institute, 1986, pp 670–676.

33. Lutofsky S, Maurice DM: Absorption of tears by the nasolacrimal system, in Holly FJ, ed: The preocular tear film in health, disease and contact lens wear, Lubbock, TX, The Dry Eye Institute, 1986, pp 663–669.

34. McDonald JE: Surface phenomena of the tear films, Trans Am Ophthalmol Soc 66:905, 1965.

35. Milder B, Demorest BH: Dacryocystography, I, The normal lacrimal apparatus, Arch Ophthalmol 51:180, 1954.

36. Mircheff AK: Lacrimal fluid and electrolyte section: a review, Current Eye Res 8:607, 1989.

37. Mishima S: Some physiologic aspects of the precorneal tear film, Arch Ophthalmol 73:233, 1965.

38. Mishima S, Gasset A, Klyce S, et al: Determination of tear flow, Invest Ophthalmol 5:264, 1966.

39. Mishima S, Maurice DM: The effect of normal evaporations on the eye, Exp Eye Res 1:46, 1961.

40. Nichols BA, Chiappino ML, Dawson CR: Demonstration of mucus layer tear film by electron microscopy, Invest Ophthalmol Vis Sci 26:464, 1985.

41. Nicolaides N, Kataranta JK, Rawdah TN, et al: Meibomian gland studies: comparison of steer and human lipids, Invest Ophthalmol Vis Sci 20:522, 1981.

42. Pflugfelder SC, Hwang A, Feuer W, et al: Conjunctival cytologic features of primary Sjögren's syndrome, Ophthalmol 97:985, 1990.

43. Rabinovitch J, Hurwitz JJ, Ching-Sang H: Quantitative evaluation of canalicular flow using lacrimal scintillography, Orbit 3(4):263, 1984.

44. Ruckenstein E, Sharma A: A surface chemical explanation of tear film breakup and its implication, in Holly FJ, ed: The preocular tear film in health, disease and contact lens wear, Lubbock, TX, The Dry Eye Institute, 1986, pp 687–726.

45. Shearn MA: Sjögren's syndrome, in Smith CH Jr, ed: Major problems in internal medicine, vol 2, Philadelphia, WB Saunders, 1971.

46. Shields WJ, Mathers WD, Roberts J, et al: Criteria for the evaluation of lid margin in blepharitis, Invest Ophthalmol Vis Sci 31(4):483, 1990.

47. Tiffany JM: Individual variation in human meibomian lipid composition, Exp Eye Res 27:289, 1978.

48. White WL, Glover AT, et al: Relative canalicular tear flow as assessed by dacryoscintography, Ophthalmol 96:167, 1989.

49. Wolff E: Anatomy of the eye & orbit, 4th ed, New York, Blakiston, 1954, pp 207–209.

50. Wright P: Diagnosis and management of dry eye, Trans Ophthalmol Soc UK 91:119, 1971.

51. Wright MM, Bersani TA, et al: Efficacy of the primary dye test, Ophthalmol 96:481, 1989.

52. Zappia R, Milder B: Lacrimal drainage function, I, The Jones fluorescein test, Am J Opthalmol 74:154, 1972.

53. Zappia RJ, Milder B: Lacrimal drainage function, II, The fluorescein dye disappearance test, Am J Ophthalmol 74:160, 1972.

CHAPTER 3

The Cornea

JAY S. PEPOSE, M.D., Ph.D.

JOHN L. UBELS, Ph.D.

The cornea is the epitome of efficiently unified structure and function, providing the eye with a clear refractive interface, tensile strength, and protection from external factors. These diverse functions have been achieved with simplicity of design. The cornea is comprised of six concentric layers (Fig. 3-1): (1) an outer *epithelium* anchored to (2) an underlying *basement membrane,* (3) the acellular *Bowman's layer,* (4) the *corneal stroma* comprised of keratocytes, extracellular matrix, and ordered collagen lamellae, and (5) *Descemet's membrane* onto which adheres (6) the *corneal endothelium.* The corneal endothelium is a nonvascular, highly metabolic single cell layer forming the innermost aspect of the cornea bathed by the aqueous humor of the anterior chamber of the eye.

The many unique structural features of the cornea have evolved over time, affording clarity, a smooth transparent refractive surface, tectonic strength, impermeability, and protection. Corneal avascularity is essential for optical clarity but also demands that oxygen be derived predominantly from the oxygen in the tear film rather than from traversing red blood cells and that most nutritional requirements be fulfilled by the aqueous humor. Given the absence of blood vessels, protection from microbes and pathogens is provided by immunoglobins and other antimicrobial factors in the tear film, by blinking and epithelial cell desquamation, and by migrating Langerhans cells, macrophages, and immune effector cells derived from the limbal region (i.e., the interface between the cornea

and conjunctiva). The combination of tissue transparency and tensile strength is achieved by collagen fibrils of uniformly small diameter, maintained at close periodicity, which is highly dependent on the state of corneal hydration. The latter "pump" function is provided predominantly by the corneal endothelium, accomplishing ion transport and corneal deturgescence via a Na^+-K^+ ATPase. The cornea also protects the eye from both chemical and physical insults. A chemical barrier is produced by focal tight functions joining the superficial epithelial cells. The multilayered, non-keratinized epithelium has substantial mitotic wound healing ability and is normally firmly anchored to the basement membrane and, at specialized zones, to the stroma. Further protection is provided by a rich subepithelial nerve plexus with extensive free nerve endings interdigitating between corneal epithelial cells, thus achieving exquisite sensitivity without compromising tissue clarity. In this chapter we review the specialized anatomic, developmental, physiologic, and metabolic properties of the cornea in an effort to provide a framework for understanding normal corneal function as well as disease states.

OPTICAL CHARACTERISTICS

The cornea is the clear transparent tissue comprising the central one sixth of the outer tunic of the eye, in continuity with the surrounding white sclera. Measured externally, the cornea is oval-shaped, with average horizontal diameter 12.6 mm and 11.7 mm vertical diameter.

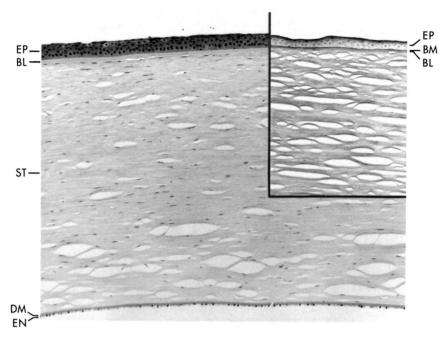

FIG. 3-1 Histologic section of a normal human cornea stained with periodic-acid Schiff reveals the outer epithelium (EP), basement membrane (BM), acellular Bowman's layer (BL), stroma (ST), Descemet's membrane (DM), and endothelial monolayer (EN). (Courtesy Dr. Morton E. Smith.)

The anterior surface of the cornea represents the major refractive component of the eye, contributing approximately 48 diopters of plus power toward the convergence of an image onto the retina. The central third of the cornea is of a generally spherical or toroidal contour,[12] with the radius of curvature of its outer aspect averaging 7.8 mm. The more peripheral portion of the cornea is flatter, radially asymmetric, and thicker (0.65 mm) than the central portion (0.52 mm).

The cornea transmits radiation from approximately 310 nm in the ultraviolet to 2500 nm in the infrared.[11] The cornea appears to be most sensitive to ultraviolet radiation at 270 nm,[183] and it is the corneal absorption of ultraviolet radiation that results in the photokeratitis and corneal pathology that develops after exposure to a welding arc.[9] Much of the potential ultraviolet damage to the cornea from overhead sunlight is avoided by shielding from the superior lid and the brow ridge and by reflection of 30 to 60% of overhead radiation according to Fresnel's law of specular reflection. In contrast, ultraviolet light reflected upward off snow or white sand may produce hazardous UV levels incident upon the cornea that may be amenable to either spatial or spectral means of filtering.[207]

ANATOMY AND DEVELOPMENT
The tear film

The tear film provides a clear refractive interface for the cornea, filling the depressions caused by the 0.5 μm high microprojections that emanate from the cell membrane of the outer epithelial cells. The tear film is 7 μm thick. It is comprised of a thin anterior lipid layer derived from Meibomian gland secretions that limit tear evaporation, a thick aqueous layer supplied predominantly by the lacrimal glands, and an inner layer of tear mucin provided by the differentiated conjunctival goblet cells.[142] Mucin aids in lowering tear surface tension, thereby facilitating the even spread of the preocular tear film, which occurs by blinking. Each of the layers of the tear film can be adversely influenced by pathologic clinical conditions such as blepharitis, acne rosacea, and meibomitis, causing lipid abnormalities in the outer oily layer, keratoconjunctivitis sicca, Sjögren's syndrome, familial dysautonomia, and other dry eye conditions associated with a decrease in the production of the aqueous layer, and by cicatricial pemphigoid, Stevens Johnson syndrome, and alkali burns, which reduce the number of mucin producing goblet cells.

The chemical composition of tears includes

over sixty polypeptides and proteins in addition to electrolytes, enzymes, lipids, metabolites, and mucin. Tear proteins include tear-specific prealbumin, IgA, IgG, secretory component, transferin, B-lysin, lysozyme, and lactoferrin.[67] Several of these components have antimicrobial effects, which are mentioned in Chapter 2. In addition, epidermal growth factor, a polypeptide first isolated from the submaxillary glands of male mice, has been found in both reflex and basal human tear secretions.[176] Epidermal growth factor has been reported to increase epithelial wound closure both in vivo and in vitro and also to stimulate epithelial cell proliferation and DNA synthesis.[198]

Anatomy of the epithelium

The outermost layer of the cornea is a stratified, non-keratinized, non-secretory epithelium five to seven cells thick. It consists of three types of cells; superficial cells are outermost and most differentiated. Wing cells lie beneath the superficial cells, while the innermost cells are known as basal cells, in which mitosis occurs (Figs. 3-2 and 3-3). As cell division occurs the daughter cells move toward the surface of the cornea while becoming more differentiated. Finally, they degenerate and are sloughed from the corneal surface. This process results in turnover of the entire epithelium every seven days.[88]

Superficial cells are terminally differentiated

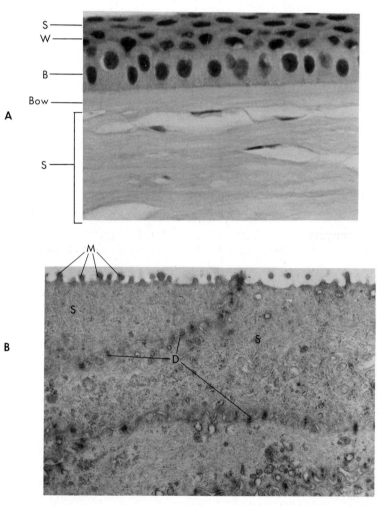

FIG. 3-2 **A,** Anterior layers of human cornea. S, surface epithelial cells; W, wing cells; B, basal epithelial cells; Bow, Bowman's layer; S, stroma. Basement membrane between basal epithelial cells and Bowman's layer is not visible by light microscopy. (Magnification × 700.) (Courtesy Dr. Martha G. Farber.) **B,** Surface epithelial cells of human cornea. S, surface epithelial cell; M, microvilli; D, desmosomes. (Magnification × 18,000.) (Courtesy Dr. Adolph I. Cohen.)

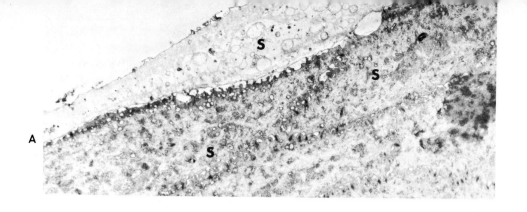

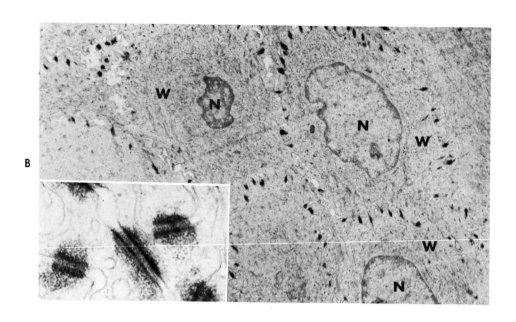

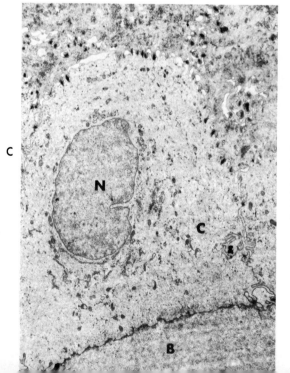

FIG. 3-3 **A**, Corneal epithelium, outer surface, shows surface cells, S, without nuclei. (Magnification × 3350.) **B**, Next layer deeper, wing cells, W, shows much rounder appearance of cells in which nuclei, N, can easily be seen. Note marked interdigitation of cell borders. (Magnification × 3840.) (Courtesy Dr. Jack Kayes.) **C**, Basal cell of corneal epithelium, C, shows nucleus, N, and Bowman's layer, B. (Magnification × 5950.)

and in a process of degeneration, as is evident from the relative paucity of cellular organelles and clumped chromatin in the nucleus. Staining with acridine orange also indicates that these cells have decreased levels of RNA.[66] When examined by scanning electron microscopy, the surface of the cornea is seen as an irregular array of polygonal cells. These cells can be divided into populations of small and large cells or dark and light cells. The smaller, light cells are younger cells that have recently reached the surface of the cornea while the larger, dark cells are mature cells that will be sloughed. The surface cells are covered with a dense coat of microvilli, and dark cells have fewer microvilli than light cells.[93,180] Adhering to these microvilli is a glycocalyx that interacts with the mucin layer of the tears to promote formation of a stable, smooth tear film on the corneal surface. Breaks in the epithelium, known as exfoliation holes, are also present. These represent areas where a cell is in

the process of peeling off the corneal surface, forming a hole through which the underlying superficial cell can be seen (Fig. 3-4). As discussed in more detail below, in spite of the fact that a portion of these cells are dying and will be sloughed these superficial cells form an essential barrier between the tears and the inner portions of the cornea.

The wing cells, named for their characteristic wing-shaped processes, form two to three layers of cells in an intermediate state of differentiation. A prominent characteristic of these cells is an abundance of intracellular tonofilaments made up of keratin subunits. Although the corneal epithelium is referred to as a non-keratinized epithelium, because it normally does not express the cornified cytoskeleton typical of epidermal cells, the cells are rich in a 64kD keratin that is specific to the corneal epithelium (Fig. 3-5). This situation changes in vitamin A deficiency when the corneal epithelium expresses

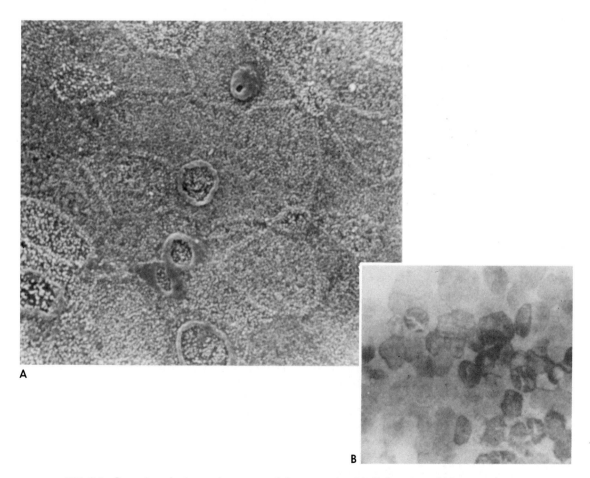

A

B

FIG. 3-4 Scanning electron microscopy of the corneal epithelial surface. **A**, Low power (× 190) showing light and dark cells. **B**, High power (× 2050) showing microvilli and exfoliation holes. (Courtesy Dr. Roswell Pfister. From Pfister RR, et al: Cornea 1:205, 1982.)

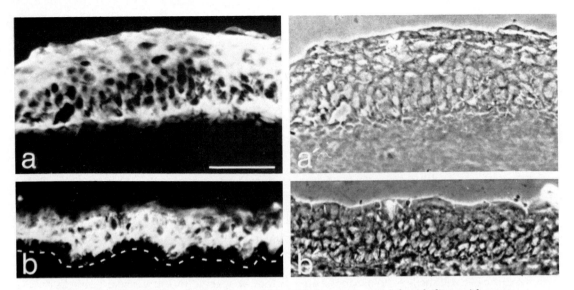

FIG. 3-5   **A**, Immunofluorescent staining of the 64 K keratin in corneal epithelium with mono-clonal antibody AE5. **B**, Immunofluorescent staining of suprabasal cells of the limbal epithe-lium with monoclonal antibody AE5. Note that the less differentiated basal stem cells do not stain for the 64 K keratin. Photos on right are phase contrast micrographs of the same sections. (Courtesy Dr. Tung-Tien Sun. From Schermer A, et al: J Cell Biol 103:49, 1986.)

keratins normally found only in the cornified epithelium, or epidermis, of the skin.[137,199,220]

The single layer of cuboidal basal cells, like the basal cell layer in other squamous epithelia, is the sole source of new cells within the corneal epithelium. No cell division occurs in wing cells or superficial cells. As expected, basal cells have a higher level of metabolic and synthetic activity than the more superficial cells and therefore have more prominent mitochondria and Golgi apparatus. They also contain significant stores of glycogen. The basal cells also contain tono-filaments and actin filaments.

The basement membrane and Bowman's layer

The basal cells of the epithelium rest on a base-ment membrane, or basal lamina, that is about 40 to 60 nm thick. This membrane is similar in structure and composition to the basal laminae of other squamous epithelia. It has been ana-lyzed histochemically and immunologically and contains type VII collagen, laminin, heparan sulfate proteoglycan, fibronectin, and fibrin.[130]

Bowman's layer, which among mammals is found only in primates, lies beneath the base-ment membrane and is about 12 μm thick. It ap-pears to be structureless by light microscopy but under the electron microscope it is revealed to be made of randomly arranged collagen fibrils. Bowman's layer is acellular and may be consid-ered to be a modified superficial layer of the stroma.

Cell adhesion in the epithelium

The maintenance of the well organized, stable epithelial structure described above requires ap-propriate cell-cell and cell-substrate adhesion. Accordingly, each cell type of the corneal epi-thelium possesses junctional structures suited to its position and function in the epithelial layer. The superficial cells are joined by numerous desmosomes. More important to the barrier function of these cells, however, are the tight junctional complexes that are found only be-tween the superficial cells of the epithelium. These junctions, or zonula occludens, com-pletely encircle the cells and represent an actual anastomosis of the lipid bilayer of the adjoining membranes.[162] In this way the superficial cells form a highly effective, semipermeable mem-brane on the surface of the cornea (Fig. 3-6, A).

Wing cells are attached to superficial cells and to one another by desmosomes. Numerous, large gap junctions are also present between the wing cells, allowing a high degree of intercellu-lar communication in this layer (Fig. 3-6, B).

The basal cells also have desmosomes and gap junctions, although they are smaller and fewer in number than in wing cells. Of greater interest in the basal layer are the hemidesmo-somes via which the basal cells, and thereby the entire epithelium, adhere to the basement mem-brane and stroma.[76,122] In the basal lamina the hemidesmosomes are linked to structures known as anchoring fibrils that pass through Bowman's layer into the stroma (Fig. 3-7). The

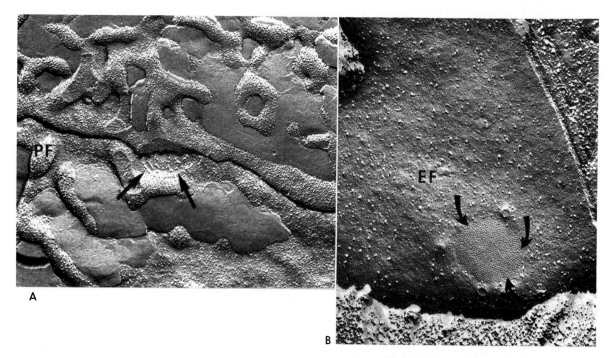

FIG. 3-6 Freeze-fracture electron micrographs of epithelial cell membranes. **A**, Tight junctions that consist of delicate particle strands are present between superficial epithelial cells (arrows) on P-face membranes. (Magnification × 60,000.) **B**, Lateral epithelial membranes of cells located deeper in the epithelium are joined by large gap junctional complexes (arrows and *) (Magnification × 80,000.) (Courtesy Dr. Barbara McLaughlin. From McLaughlin BJ, et al: Curr Eye Res 4:951, 1985.)

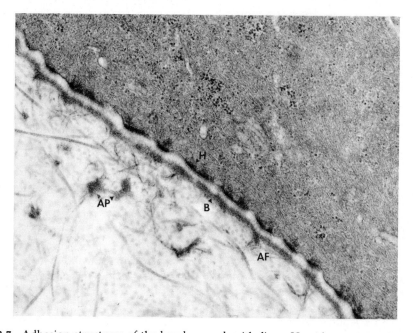

FIG. 3-7 Adhesion structures of the basal corneal epithelium. Hemidesmosomes (H), basement membrane (B), anchoring fibrils (AF), and anchoring plaques (AP). (Courtesy Dr. Ilene Gipson.)

anchoring fibrils penetrate as deeply as 2 μm into the stroma, branching intricately among the collagen fibrils and ending in structures known as anchoring plaques.[74,218] The anchoring fibrils are made of type VII collagen, while the components of the hemidesmosomes that have been identified are the bullous pemphigoid antigen[2] and integrin. It is likely that components of the basement membrane are involved in the linkage of anchoring fibrils to hemidesmosomes. In this regard the adhesion of the corneal epithelium to basement membrane and stroma is very similar to epidermal adhesion.

Clinical manifestations of abnormalities in epithelial structure

Various dystrophies (inherited diseases) and other abnormalities of the corneal epithelium, basement membrane, and Bowman's layer have been described. These diseases often present as deviations from normal corneal structure that interfere with the optical properties of the cornea. The reader is referred to textbooks of ophthalmology for detailed clinical descriptions of these conditions. Especially important are conditions such as epithelial basement membrane dystrophy, which leads to painful recurrent epithelial erosions, making the cornea susceptible to edema and infection. This is apparently due to abnormal adhesion of the epithelium and it has been demonstrated that basal cells in this condition have a decreased number of hemidesmosomes.

Reduplication of the basement membrane occurs in aging and diabetes.[1,121] This is associated with an increased incidence of epithelial erosions. This abnormality of epithelial adhesion may be due to a reduced depth of penetration of anchoring fibrils through the thickened basement membrane into the stroma.[74]

Stromal structure

Approximately 90% of the corneal thickness is constituted by the stroma.[118] The stroma is predominantly an extracellular matrix comprised of proteoglycans (i.e., glycosaminoglycans covalently attached to a protein core) and a lamellar arrangement of collagen fibrils running parallel to the corneal surface.[30] The collagen fibrils and extracellular matrix are maintained by flattened cells with scant cytoplasm called keratocytes lying between the collagen lamellae. Keratocytes in the same lamellar plane may form a syncytium by extending fine tapering processes in several directions, some of which may touch the processes of neighboring keratocytes to form tight junctions (Fig. 3-8). Finally, nerve axons and their surrounding Schwann cells are located in the anterior and middle aspect of the corneal stroma.

The normal corneal stroma is 71% collagen by dry weight, predominantly of the type I isotype, with lesser amounts of types III, V[170] and VI.[243] The collagen fibrils have a mean diameter of between 22.5 and 32 nm,[101,186] thickening toward the periphery. The fibrils have a macroperiodicity of approximately 64 nm (Fig. 3-9). The 300 or more collagen lamellae extend from limbus to limbus and may then wrap around the circumference of the cornea or fuse together to form larger fibrils. The orientation of the lamellae becomes more orthogonal to each other in the posterior stroma, with predominant orientations being inferior-superior and medial-lateral.[163] The interlamellar adhesive strength at 50% stromal depth is approximately 14.2 g-wt/mm of tissue width centrally and almost twice that in the far peripheral cornea. This predominantly reflects the force required to break the proteoglycan bonds between collagen lamellae centrally, as well as the tensile strength of interwoven collagen lamellae that increase in number toward the periphery.[209]

The structured organization of the collagen fibers may relate to the acidic glycosaminoglycan composition of proteoglycans in the surrounding matrix. In the central cornea, keratan sulfate is the major proteoglycan component and chondroitin (i.e., unsulfated form) is the minor.[14] The concentration of keratan sulfate falls toward the peripheral cornea and chondroitin sulfate increases. The highly negatively charged keratan sulfate molecules located at specific sites[203] around each collagen fiber maintain a precise spatial relationship between individual fibers. The larger, negatively charged chondroitin sulfate of the peripheral cornea would extend further into the interfiber space than chondroitin in the central cornea, accounting for the decreased number of fibers per unit area in the peripheral cornea.

The mucopolysaccharidoses are a group of inherited disorders of metabolism characterized by the accumulation of excess glycosaminoglycans in lysosomes. In these disorders deficiencies in lysosomal acid hydrolases (e.g., alpha-L-iduronidase or iduronate sulfatase) lead to keratan sulfate and dermatan sulfate accumulation in the cornea.[120] Normally the cornea is devoid of dermatan sulfate, which is present in corneal scars and in the sclera.[14] Patients with specific mucopolysaccharidoses, such as Hurler's, Hunter's, and Scheie's syndromes, present with corneal clouding early in life, but generally not at birth.

Corneal dystrophies are inherited disorders

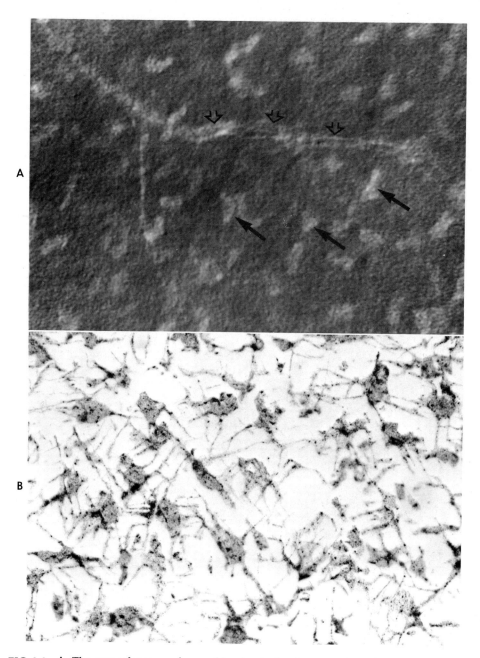

FIG. 3-8 A, The corneal stroma observed in vivo by tandem scanning microscopy (**A**) compared to conventional light micrograph of fixed, dead specimen stained with 1% gold chloride and cut en face (**B**). Note that in the in vivo image only the nuclei of the tissue fibrocytes are clearly identified (*A,* arrows). Nerves are also detected (open arrow) and can be followed throughout the cornea. In the conventional light micrograph the density of individual stromal fibrocytes appears comparable to that seen in vivo. Note also the thin, filipodial processes that appear to extend from one cell to another. (**A,** TSM, × 220; **B,** 1% AuCl × 450.) (Courtesy Dr. James V. Jester.)

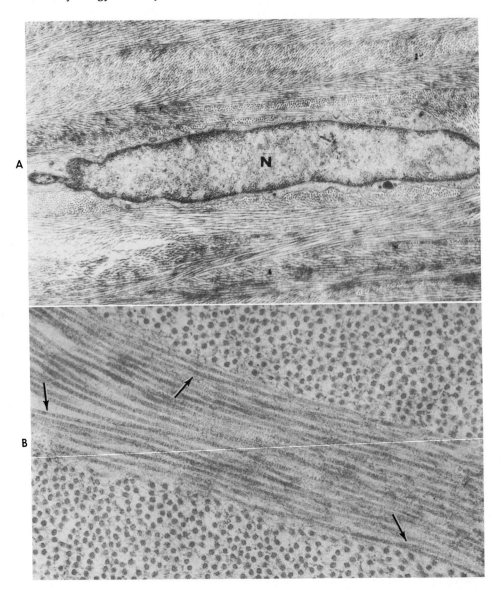

FIG. 3-9 **A**, Nucleus, N, of corneal stromal cell; layers of corneal stromal collagen are seen from various angles. (Magnification × 9000.) **B**, Higher magnification of stromal collagen, showing collagen fibrils cut on end and from side with their 640 A banding visible (arrows). (Magnification × 72,000.) (Courtesy Dr. Jack Kayes.)

that may also result from abnormal cellular metabolism. These conditions are usually bilateral, symmetrical, and lacking signs of inflammation or neovascularization.[196] Common stromal dystrophies include granular dystrophy, an autosomal dominant disorder in which microfibrillar deposits lead to corneal opacification. This process is thought to reflect altered phospholipid metabolism. Lattice dystrophy is a stromal disorder secondary to the localized accumulation of amyloid. Macular dystrophy is a heterogeneous recessive disease of two subtypes.[169,233]

Type 1 is characterized by a defect in the synthesis of keratan sulfate proteoglycan, leading to an absence of sulfated keratan sulfate in the cornea and serum.[47,126] These abnormalities in the corneal extracellular matrix are associated with more proximal spacing of collagen fibrils, which may account for corneal thinning observed clinically in these patients. In addition, in corneas with macular dystrophy, there are many regions where the normal collagen structure is disrupted and numerous lacunae are seen within the matrix.[187] The implication of these

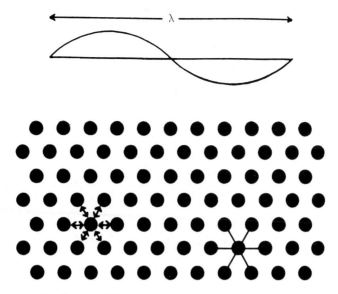

FIG. 3-10   Cross-sectional view of fibrils arranged in lattice. Size of wavelength shown above for comparison. Forces of repulsion and rigid links between fibrils shown schematically. (From Maurice D: The physics of corneal transparency, in Duke-Elder S, ed: Transparency of the cornea, Oxford, Blackwell Scientific Publications, 1960.)

latter findings with regard to corneal opacification in macular dystrophy is discussed below.

There are unique structural features inherent to the normal cornea that underlie its transparency and are perturbed by various conditions such as edema and scarring. When considered separately, the elements of the corneal stroma are not of uniform refractive index. The refractive index of dry collagen is 1.550 and of stromal ground substance 1.354, yet despite this disparity, the corneal stroma scatters less than 10% of normal incident light.[161] It was proposed by Maurice[161] that corneal transparency is a consequence of the crystalline lattice arrangement of collagen fibrils within stromal lamellae (Fig. 3-10) and that light scattered by individual fibrils of uniform diameter is canceled by destructive interference with scattered light from adjacent fibers. More recent studies indicate that significant light scattering occurs when the cornea contains fluctuations in refractive index that are distributed over distances larger than one half the wavelength of light (i.e., 2,000 Å).[56,79,80] Thus the opaqueness of the sclera is not the consequence of an absent lattice arrangement but of large variations in collagen fiber diameter so that neighboring regions have different refractive indexes. In contrast, the collagen fibrils in the corneal stroma are of uniformly small diameter (around 30 nm) and are closely spaced (64 nm). Bowman's layer of the cornea is also transparent, yet the axes of its collagen fibers

appear randomly oriented.[80] Similarly, other transparent structures, such as the corneal epithelium, endothelium, and the retina lack a lattice array. Studies using the electron microscope reveal that structural alterations occur with dimensions greater than 2000 Å in cases of corneal edema and pannus formation, consistent with a loss of transparency. Stromal edema expands the ground substance, greatly increasing the spacing between collagen fibrils, leading to large fluctuations in refractive index and consequent scattering of light. Furthermore, the uptake of stromal water associated with corneal edema may be accompanied by a loss of stromal glycosaminoglycans.[117]

Cellular anatomy of the corneal endothelium

The posterior surface of the cornea is covered by a single layer of cells known as the endothelium. This monolayer is formed by a regularly arranged array of polygonal cells, most of which are hexagonal in shape and cover the posterior surface of the cornea in the young human at about 3500 cells/mm². The cells are about 20 μm in diameter and 4 to 6 μm thick. By transmission electron microscopy it is evident that these cells, while essentially cuboidal in cross-section, adjoin one another in tortuous interdigitations, resulting in lateral borders with a length ten times the cell thickness.

The endothelial cells contain a large nucleus

that fills a significant portion of the cell, and as seen by scanning electron microscopy causes the apical membrane to bulge outward. The cells contain numerous mitochondria, a prominent endoplasmic reticulum, and Golgi apparatus. This is typical of cells that are metabolically active in transport, synthesis, and secretory functions (Fig. 3-11).

Endothelial cells are interconnected by tight junctions and gap junctions (Fig. 3-12). The apical tight junctional complexes, first demonstrated by transmission electron microscopy, have now been shown by freeze-fracture techniques to be macula occludens rather than zonula occludens in that they do not completely encircle the cells.[162] This results in the endothe-

lium forming a "leaky" barrier between the aqueous humor and the stroma, which, while impeding the free flow of water and solutes, does not form the more effective barrier seen in epithelia with zonular junctions. The gap junctions are numerous and are observed primarily on the lateral membranes of the cells, although some are also present at the junctions of the apico-lateral membranes. The gap junctions do not contribute to the endothelial barrier, but they function in intercellular communication. Fluorescent dye injected into a single endothelial cell quickly spreads to adjacent cells.[189] Unlike the basal cells of the corneal epithelium, the basal membranes of the endothelial cells have no specialized adhesion complexes.

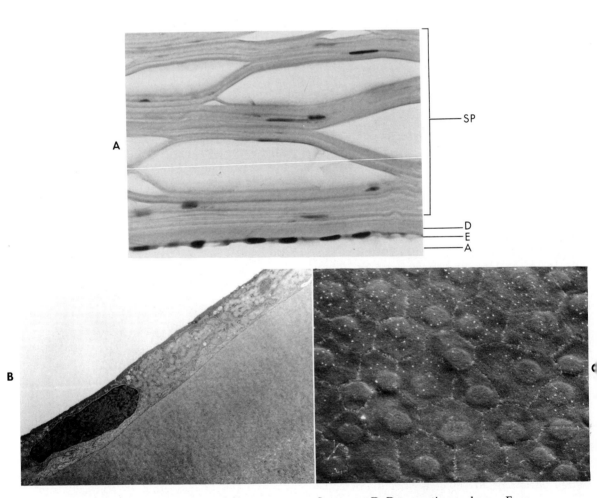

FIG. 3-11   A, Posterior layers of human cornea: S, stroma; D, Descemet's membrane; E, endothelial cell layer; A, space occupied by aqueous. Large open spaces in stroma are artifacts of histologic preparation. (Magnification × 1000.) (Courtesy Dr. Martha G. Farber.) **B,** Transmission electron micrograph of the human corneal endothelium. (Magnification × 3950.) (Courtesy Dr. Henry Edelhauser.) **C,** Scanning electron micrograph of human corneal endothelium. (Magnification × 1000.) (Courtesy Dr. Henry Edelhauser.)

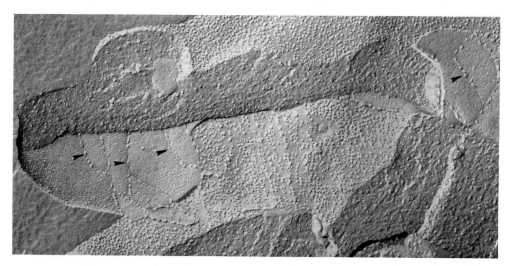

FIG. 3-12   Freeze-fracture electron micrograph of the rabbit corneal endothelial cell membrane demonstrating tight junctional strands (arrows). (Magnification $\times$ 8400.) (Courtesy Dr. Monica Stiemke.)

Endothelial morphometry

The development of the contact specular microscope and its adaptation for use in humans made feasible studies of endothelial functional morphology in vivo.[15,139] Using the original technology, analyses were limited to studies of cell density (number of cells/unit area), and detailed statistical studies were limited by the small number of cells visible in the narrow field of view. The wide-field specular microscope through which several hundred cells can be photographed in a single frame, and the introduction of computer software used to digitally analyze cell area and shape, have made detailed morphometry of the endothelium possible[134] (Fig. 3-13).

A stable corneal endothelium, in addition to having an adequate cell density to maintain corneal function, has cells of relatively uniform size and shape. The degree of uniformity of cell size is determined by measuring the areas of the apical membranes of a population of cells and calculating the coefficient of variation (CV) of cell size (standard deviation of mean cell area/mean cell area). The normal endothelium has a CV of about 0.25. An increase in this value means that cell size is variable and is known as polymegethism. This may be indicative of a stressed or unstable endothelium in which cell volume is not adequately regulated or in which the cytoskeleton is abnormal. Figure 3-14 shows that corneas with equal cell density may have widely varying degrees of polymegethism so that measurement of cell density alone is not an adequate measure of corneal endothelial stability.[236]

A mosaic of hexagonal structures, which is often found in nature, is geometrically and thermodynamically stable. The apical surfaces of the corneal endothelial cells form a mosaic that in the healthy, young cornea consists of 70 to 80% hexagonal cells. A decrease in hexagons with a concomitant increase in numbers of cells with more or fewer than six sides is known as pleomorphism and may also be a sign of endothelial stress.

The principles of polymegethism and pleomorphism can best be illustrated by a discussion of the effects of aging, disease, surgery, and contact lens wear on these parameters. At birth endothelial cell density is about 4000 cells/mm^2, but because these cells are amitotic the density decreases throughout life to about 2000 cells/mm^2 in the eighth to ninth decades of life (Fig. 3-15). This is still well above the minimum level of 400 to 700 cells/mm^2 required for maintenance of normal corneal function,[15] indicating that adequate cells are available for a lifetime of well over 100 years. Morphometric analysis has shown, however, that polymegethism and pleomorphism increase significantly with aging.[234] Corneal thickness does not increase with age, but these changes in endothelial morphology may render the aged cornea more vulnerable to the stress of intraocular disease or surgery.

The effects of surgery on endothelial morphology have also been documented. Initial studies using the clinical specular microscope documented the cell loss that occurs in the graft following penetrating keratoplasty (Fig. 3-16). The cell density in grafts is often less than 1000/

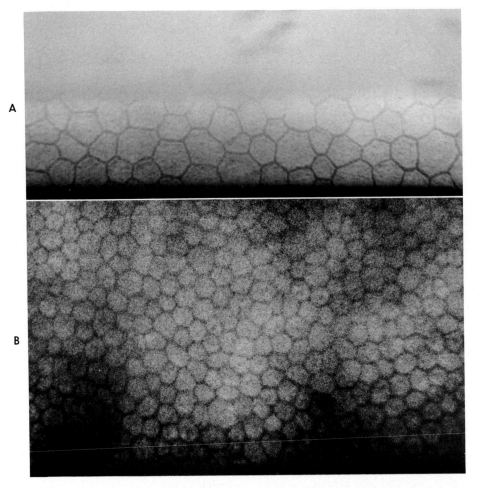

FIG. 3-13 Narrow (**A**) and wide-field (**B**) specular micrographs of the human endothelium. Note the regular mosaic of polygonal cells. (Courtesy Dr. Henry Edelhauser.)

mm^2 and in one study a clear cornea had a density of only 371 cells/mm^2.[16,190] Morphometric studies indicate that cell loss and increases in polymegethism and pleomorphism continue for six months following keratoplasty, after which the cornea stabilizes. Remodeling of the cornea continues after this point, until a normal hexagonal pattern of cell shape and normal CV are recovered by 2 years after surgery.[154]

Cataract surgery also causes an endothelial cell loss due to mechanical trauma to the cornea.[191] Increases in CV and decreases in numbers of hexagonal cells occur during the first four postoperative weeks as cells spread to replace lost cells. These changes are more pronounced in the superior cornea near the surgical incision than in the central cornea, and the changes are also greater after intracapsular extraction than after extracapsular procedures. Normal cell shape and CV are attained by 3

months after surgery, as the endothelium remodels itself with a more stable configuration[154,201] (Fig. 3-17).

Morphometric analysis of corneas of patients with keratoconus or diabetes has clearly shown that endothelial morphology may change without a decrease in cell density. Keratoconus corneas have a normal cell density but the coefficient of variation of cell size is significantly increased and the percentage of hexagonal cells drops from a normal 70% to 50%, showing that the stress placed on the cornea in this disease causes endothelial remodeling.[159] In type II diabetics of 10 years or longer duration, cell density is normal while CV is increased and the percentage of hexagonal cells decreases to 50%. Similar changes are seen in type I diabetes, and patients with disease of long duration also demonstrate a decrease in cell density.[202] The changes in endothelial morphology in the dia-

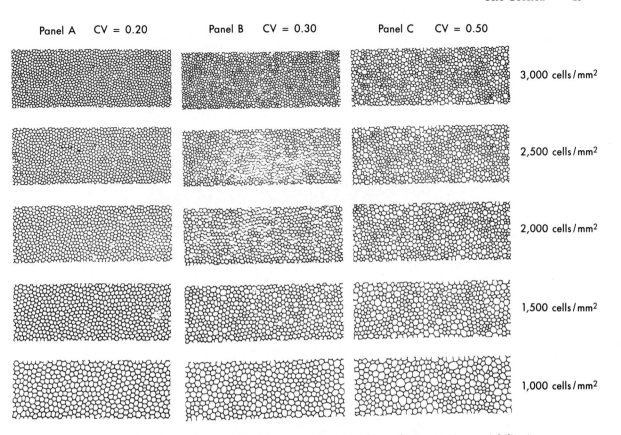

Panel A   CV = 0.20   Panel B   CV = 0.30   Panel C   CV = 0.50

3,000 cells/mm²

2,500 cells/mm²

2,000 cells/mm²

1,500 cells/mm²

1,000 cells/mm²

FIG. 3-14 Morphometric analysis of the corneal endothelium, demonstrating variability in cell density and coefficient of variation of cell size. Note that cell size can vary significantly with no change in cell density. (From Ref 236, courtesy Dr. Henry Edelhauser.)

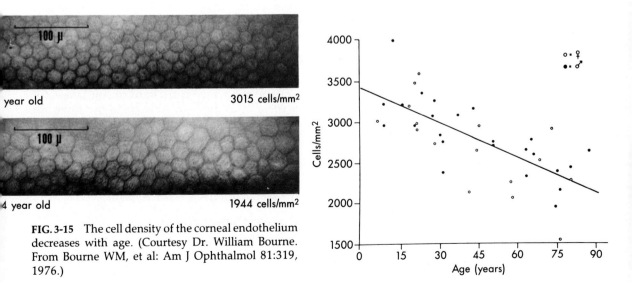

100 µ

year old   3015 cells/mm²

100 µ

4 year old   1944 cells/mm²

FIG. 3-15 The cell density of the corneal endothelium decreases with age. (Courtesy Dr. William Bourne. From Bourne WM, et al: Am J Ophthalmol 81:319, 1976.)

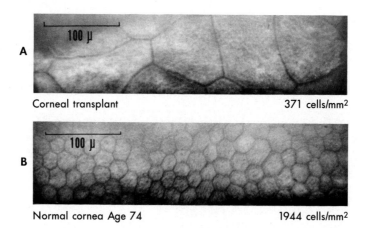

FIG. 3-16 Specular photomicrographs demonstrating the effect of penetrating keratoplasty on endothelial cell density. **A**, Normal endothelium, **B**, Graft endothelium. (Courtesy Dr. William Bourne. From Bourne, WM, et al: Am J Ophthalmol 81:319, 1976.)

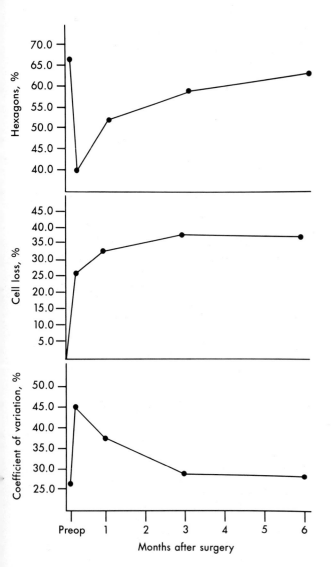

FIG. 3-17 Effect of intracapsular cataract extraction on the superior corneal endothelium. Cell loss continues for 1 month postoperatively, but a normal endothelial mosaic (hexagonality and coefficient of variation) is restored by 3 months. (Courtesy Dr. Richard Schultz. From Schultz RO, et al: Arch Ophthalmol 104:1164, 1986.)

betic are related to changes in cellular metabolism. In experimental models of diabetes these changes can be reversed or prevented by aldose reductase inhibitors,[164] indicating an involvement of the polyol pathway. It appears that cell volume regulation may be affected by osmotic effects of sugars like sorbitol or perhaps inhibition of the Na/K pump secondary to alterations in myoinositol metabolism. Given the endothelial changes that result from surgery, the diabetic patient may be at greater risk during surgery than the normal patient.

A particularly interesting change in endothelial morphology occurs during long-term contact lens wear (Fig. 3-18). Pleomorphism and polymegethism without cell loss are observed in patients who have worn hard or soft lenses for 6 years or more.[147] In contrast to the rapid remodeling of the endothelium that occurs after surgery, little recovery occurs for as long as 4 years after cessation of hard contact lens wear. Possible causes of endothelial changes accompanying contact lens wear will be discussed in the section on corneal metabolism.

Descemet's membrane

The corneal endothelium rests on a basement membrane, known as Descemet's membrane, which in the adult eye is 10 to 15 μm thick. This

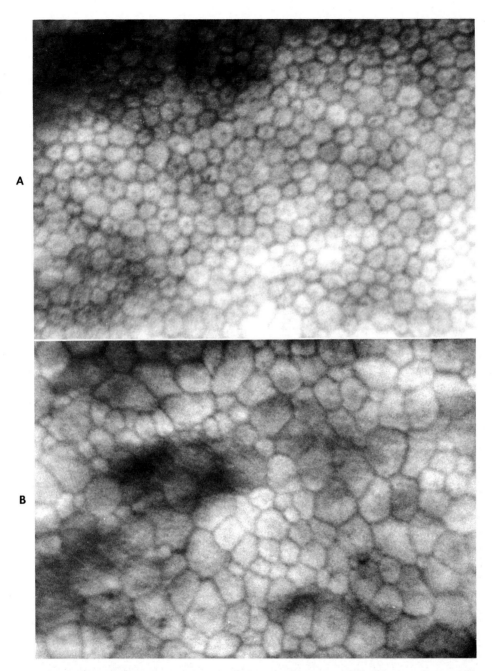

FIG. 3-18 Endothelial polymegethism and pleomorphism caused by 27 years of contact lens wear. **A**, 46-year-old non-contact lens wearer. Cell density = 3086 cells/mm^2; CV = 0.27; hexagonality = 63%. **B**, 46-year-old who has worn hard contact lenses for 27 years. Cell density = 1449 cells/mm^2; CV = 0.59; hexagonality = 22%. (Courtesy Dr. Scott MacRae.)

membrane is secreted by the endothelial cells and increases in thickness throughout life. The basement membrane components, type IV collagen, laminin, and fibronectin, are present in Descemet's membrane, and it has been suggested that the fibronectin functions in adhesion of endothelial cells to the membrane.[83,227] Descemet's membrane may remain intact in cases of severe corneal ulceration, forming a descemetocele after destruction of the epithelium and stroma. This shows that the membrane is highly resistant to proteolytic enzymes.

Fuchs' endothelial dystrophy is a disease of the endothelial cells in which an abnormal Descemet's membrane is secreted. Wartlike excrescences of collagenous material known as guttata form on the posterior surface of the membrane, causing thinning and enlargement of the overlying endothelial cells. In the specular microscope the guttata are seen as black, acellular areas because of the loss of specular reflection from these areas (Fig. 3-19). As the disease progresses, endothelial cell function is decreased, cells are lost, and the cornea decompensates.[227]

Corneal nerves

The cornea is richly supplied with sensory nerves. These are derived from the ciliary nerves that originate from the ophthalmic branch of the trigeminal nerve. The cornea is surrounded by a perilimbal nerve ring from which fibers penetrate the middle and anterior layers of the stroma, extending radially toward the center of the cornea. The nerve fibrils divide dichotomously and, emerging from the deeper layers of the cornea, penetrate Bowman's layer to form a subepithelial plexus. From the plexus axon terminals spread among the epithelial cells, innervating all layers of the epithelium with sensory receptors. Adrenergic sympathetic nerves that originate in the superior cervical ganglion also innervate the cornea. (Corneal nerves are discussed in greater detail in Chapter 4.)

The cornea is one of the most sensitive tissues of the body, and this sensitivity serves a protective function. Accordingly, most of the receptors in the cornea fall into the classification of nociceptors with simulation resulting in the perception of pain. The A-delta fibers and C fibers that supply the cornea are primarily polymodal fibers responding to mechanical, thermal, and chemical (low pH and hypertonic saline) stimuli. These receptors usually have the lowest threshold for mechanical stimulation. It is exquisitely painful when these nerves are stimulated by corneal abrasions, ulcers, or bullous keratopathy.

In addition to serving as sensory receptors, it is evident that corneal nerves also serve a trophic function. Patients with sensory denervation of the cornea due to stroke, diabetic neuropathy, or herpes simplex infections suffer a high incidence of epithelial erosions and ulcerations known as neurotrophic ulcers. This may in part be due to loss of foreign body sensations, which can lead to mechanical damage to the cornea. However, neuropeptides, including substance P and calcitonin gene-related peptide, are present in corneal nerves and appear to have a direct but poorly understood trophic effect on the epithelium. Retrobulbar or trigeminal injection of capsaicin depletes the nerves of these peptides, resulting in delayed epithelial wound healing.[68,222]

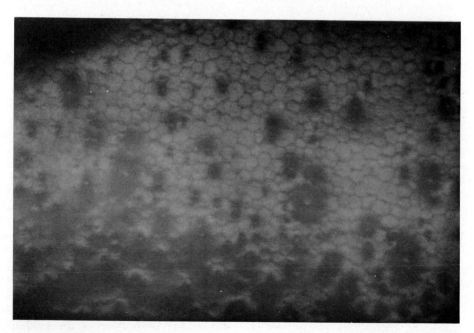

FIG. 3-19 Specular micrograph showing extensive (dark appearing) corneal guttata, which in areas are confluent.

The role of sympathetic nerves in the cornea is controversial. It has been suggested that they are involved in modulation of ion transport or mitotic activity.[24,129] Stimulation of the sympathetic nerves inhibits corneal epithelial wound healing.[179]

EMBRYOLOGY AND DEVELOPMENTAL ANOMALIES

Ocular development begins with an outpouching of the diencephalon. This protuberance, called the optic vesicle, communicates with the third ventricle of the brain via the optic stalk. The optic vesicle, as well as the entire embryo, is covered with a sheet of surface ectoderm. The ectodermal cells overlying the hollow optic vesicle thicken to form the lens placode.[244] The optic vesicle invaginates to form the optic cup, while the lens placode develops a pit. This pitted structure then itself invaginates to become the lens vesicle, which has an anatomic relationship with the optic vesicle resembling a ball in the pocket of a baseball glove. At 5 to 6 weeks of gestation, the lens vesicle detaches, and the adjacent surface ectoderm from which it has budded gives rise to the corneal epithelium, which is 1 to 2 cells thick with a gossamer underlying basement membrane. There is a loose, acellular layer destined to become corneal stroma comprised of collagen fibrils.[91] Early on, a population of mesodermal-derived cells accumulates circumferentially around the optic cup under surface ectoderm. However, cumulative evidence indicates that it is a later wave of neural crest-derived perilimbal mesenchymal cells that migrate between the lens and the acellular stroma at 6 weeks gestation, forming the corneal endothelium. Unlike vascular endothelium, the neural crest-derived corneal endothelium is factor VIII negative.[108] Neural crest cells from this primary wave also form the trabecular meshwork. A second wave of neural crest-derived mesenchymal cell invasion gives rise to corneal fibroblasts (keratocytes), and the crest cells from a third wave contribute to the anterior iris.

Between 6 to 8 weeks, there is development of eyelid folds, during which time the corneal epithelium is exposed to amniotic fluid. Between 8 weeks and 5 months, the lids meet and fuse, separating again around 6 months.[204] The corneal epithelium goes through many changes during this period. The number of epithelial cell layers increases from 1 to 2 at 8 weeks to 3 to 4 at 19 weeks, 4 to 5 at 27 weeks (around the time of lid separation), increasing to the adult level of 6 to 7 layers by 36 weeks gestation. The basal lamina is the first component of the epithelial adhesion complex to appear at 8 to 9 weeks. At 13 weeks, hemidesmosomes, anchoring fibrils, and type VII collagen have been observed. There is an increase in the number of hemidesmosomes following week 27, when the eyelids open, perhaps in some way associated with lid movement over the epithelium. At 13 weeks, in addition to anchoring fibrils and hemidesmosome formation, a palisade of fine filaments are observed extending perpendicular to the basal lamina into the anterior stroma. This may be a precursor to Bowman's layer, which is 3.8 μm in thickness at 19 weeks, thickening thereafter.[218] Concomitant with the developmental changes in the epithelial anchoring complex are varying patterns of keratin localization in the corneal epithelium during embryogenesis. A monoclonal antibody (AE5) to a basic 64-kilodalton keratin does not stain the single-layered corneal epithelium at 8 weeks of gestation. At 12 to 13 weeks, the superficial cells of the 3 to 4 layered epithelium become AE5 positive, providing an early sign of epithelial differentiation. At 30 weeks, the AE5 anti-keratin antibody elicits a suprabasal staining pattern, in contrast to the adult epithelium, which centrally is AE5 positive in all epithelial layers.[195]

Using immunofluorescence techniques, type I collagen has been detected in the epithelial basement membrane, stroma, and Descemet's membrane from 8 weeks gestation through postnatal life. Type III, but not type II, collagen is found in these same structures in early fetal life (between 8 and 20 weeks gestation), but can not be demonstrated at 27 weeks or thereafter. Type IV collagen is synthesized by epithelial and endothelial cells and is localized in the epithelial basement membrane as early as 8 weeks gestation and in Descemet's membrane at 9 weeks gestation and beyond. Bullous pemphigoid antigen, a component of the adult corneal epithelial basement membrane, was localized in the epithelial basement membrane starting at 10 to 15 weeks gestation. Staining for fibronectin is positive at 11 weeks gestation in Descemet's membrane and decreases thereafter, whereas the corneal stroma and epithelial basement membrane show staining in early fetal life up to 30 weeks gestation for both laminin and fibronectin.[6] At 10 to 12 weeks, keratan sulfate, a major component of the corneal extracellular matrix, has been immunologically localized in the stroma and endothelial layer.[108]

The corneal diameter enlarges from 4.2 mm at 16 weeks to between 9 and 10.5 mm at term. This fivefold increase in area and 2.3 fold increase in corneal diameter is accompanied by approximately a 2.3 fold decrease in endothelial cell density. At 16 weeks gestation there are

11.32 endothelial nuclei/100 microns and at term there are 5.61 nuclei/100 microns. There also appears to be a rapid decrease in cellular density following birth up to age 2, with a decline in endothelial cellularity from 6.09 nuclei/100 microns to 3.93 nuclei/100 microns (36% change). At the same time, the corneal diameter increases by a factor of 1.2 (from 9.8 mm at birth to 11.75 mm at age 2), while endothelial density declines by 1.55. This reflects an increase in endothelial cell size, which becomes stable by age 2. Following 2 years of age, endothelial cell loss occurs at an annual rate of approximately 0.56%.[167]

The important contribution of neural crest cells to the development of the anterior segment provides a framework for understanding a variety of congenital developmental anomalies.[5] Abnormal neural crest cell migration may result in sclerocornea, Peters' anomaly, Axenfeld's and Rieiger's anomalies and syndromes, as well as posterior embryotoxon and some forms of congenital glaucoma.[119,136] Abnormalities in crest cell terminal induction may underlie congenital hereditary endothelial dystrophy, posterior polymorphous dystrophy, and Fuchs' endothelial dystrophy. Descemet's membrane may give important clues regarding the nature and timing of some of these disorders. Descemet's membrane is composed of a 3 μm anterior banded layer that forms before birth (with a collagen periodicity of 110 μm) and a postnatal posterior nonbanded portion. Whereas the anterior banded portion appears stable with aging, the posterior nonbanded layer thickens with age after birth, increasing from approximately 2 μm at age 10 to 10 microns at age 80.[112] In some disorders, such as congenital hereditary endothelial dystrophy, the fetal anterior banded portion of Descemet's membrane is formed, thus indicating that fetal endothelium was initially present, and suggesting a defect in final differentiation of these neural crest-derived cells. This contrasts with sclerocornea and Peters' anomaly, where gross defects or attenuation of the fetal anterior portion of Descemet's membrane centrally suggest a fetal absence of endothelial cells more consistent with an arrest in neural crest cell migration.[5]

PHYSIOLOGY, CELL BIOLOGY, AND BIOCHEMISTRY
Maintenance of the corneal epithelium and its response to wounding

The corneal epithelium is maintained by a constant cycle of shedding of superficial cells and proliferation of cells in the basal layer. That mitosis is limited to the basal layer was well documented many years ago by observations of mitotic figures and tritiated thymidine labeling of proliferating cells.[64,88,89] The mitotic rate is about 10 to 15% per day but control of this mitotic activity is not well understood.

It is apparent that the epithelium is also maintained by a slow migration of basal cells toward the center of the cornea. Evidence for this centripetal cell migration first came from observation of corneal transplants, which showed that donor epithelium was slowly replaced by recipient epithelium and that pigmented cells from the recipient epithelium migrate toward the center of the graft.[124] It has also been demonstrated that India ink particles phagocytosed by basal cells of normal corneas migrate centripetally at about 123 μm per week.[20] The source of the new basal cells is the limbal epithelium, a band of cells 0.5 to 1 mm wide at the periphery of the cornea. The limbus contains stem cells, which differentiate into basal cells and migrate onto the cornea, constantly renewing the supply of basal cells. These stem cells are located in the basal layer of the limbus and do not express the 64K keratin typical of corneal epithelium[199]; as they migrate upward and onto the corneal basement membrane the cells begin to express the 64K keratin (see Fig. 3-5). These data support the hypothesis that the corneal epithelium is maintained by a balance of cell shedding, basal cell division, and renewal of basal cells by centripetal migration of new basal cells originating from the limbal stem cells (Fig. 3-20). A disease process or corneal stress that upsets this balance through an increase in cell loss or a decrease in mitosis or migration would lead to epithelial breakdown.[205,217]

The primary function of the corneal epithelium is to form a barrier to invasion of the eye by pathogens and to uptake of excess fluid by the stroma. Accidental or iatrogenic abrasion of the corneal epithelium demands a prompt healing response to re-cover the exposed basement membrane with cells. After abrasion, mitosis ceases and the cells at the wound edge retract, thicken, and lose their hemidesmosomal attachments to the basement membrane. The cells enlarge and the epithelial sheet begins to migrate by ameboid movement to cover the defect. The edges of the cell membranes ruffle and send out filopodia and lamellopodia toward the center of the wound[181] (Fig. 3-21). Staining with fluorescent probes reveals actin stress fibers oriented in the direction of migration[211] (Fig. 3-22). The leading edge of the migrating cells is only one cell thick, but the wound is actually covered by a multilayered sheet made up of both basal and squamous cells.[28] After wound closure, mitosis

X, Y, Z Hypothesis of corneal epithelial maintenance

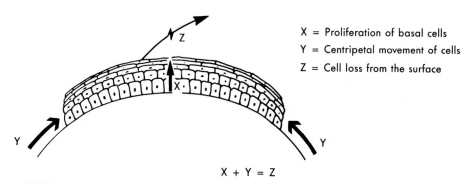

X = Proliferation of basal cells

Y = Centripetal movement of cells

Z = Cell loss from the surface

X + Y = Z

FIG. 3-20   The corneal epithelium is maintained by a balance among sloughing of cells from the corneal surface, cell division in the basal layer, and centripetal migration of cells from the limbus. (Courtesy Dr. Richard Thoft. From Thoft R, Friend J: Invest Ophthalmol Vis Sci 24:142, 1983.)

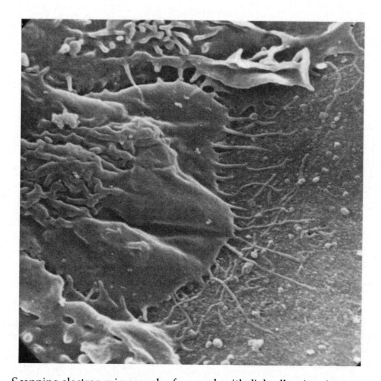

FIG. 3-21   Scanning electron micrograph of corneal epithelial cells migrating to cover an epithelial abrasion. (Courtesy Dr. Roswell Pfister. From Pfister RR: Invest Ophthalmol 14:648, 1975.)

resumes to restore the epithelium to its normal configuration.

The healing process occurs rapidly. An experimental epithelial wound 6 mm in diameter is closed within 48 hours and the rate of epithelial cell migration is 60 to 80 μm/hr[33,155,177] (Fig. 3-23). When the corneal epithelium is completely removed, the rate of cell migration from the limbus or conjunctiva is only 40 to 45 μm/ hr.[177] During corneal healing from conjunctiva, goblet cells also migrate onto the cornea. Following wound closure, a process of biochemical and morphologic transdifferentiation occurs with loss of goblet cells and establishment of a corneal epithelial phenotype.[216]

Several biochemical and synthetic events that are involved in cell migration have been identified. Migration requires energy, and one of

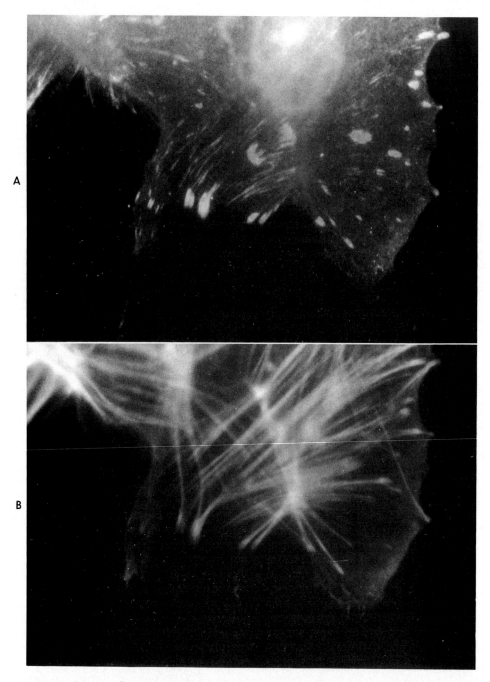

FIG. 3-22   Immunofluorescent staining of vinculin (**A**) and rhodamine phalloidin staining of actin stress fibers (**B**) of rat corneal epithelial cells migrating in vitro. (Courtesy Dr. H. Kaz Soong.)

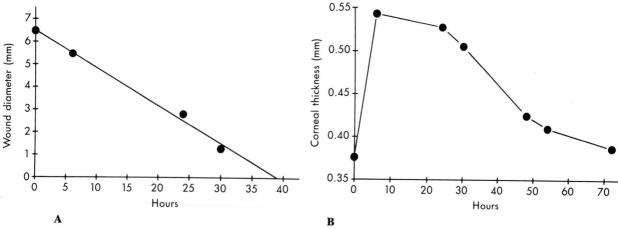

FIG. 3-23   Changes in corneal wound diameter (**A**) and thickness (**B**) during healing of a 6.5 mm diameter epithelial wound in the rabbit. The cell migration rate is 0.8 μm/hr. The cornea swells due to uptake of fluid from the tears and then returns to normal thickness as the barrier is reestablished.

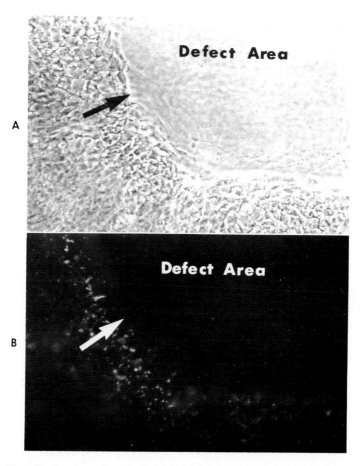

FIG. 3-24   Vinculin in corneal epithelial cells during in vivo wound healing in the rat. **A**, Phase contrast micrograph of the epithelial wound edge *(arrow)* and defect. **B**, Immunofluorescent staining of vinculin in cells near the wound edge. (Courtesy Dr. James Zieske. From Zieske JD, et al: J Cell Biol 109:571, 1989.)

the earliest changes that occurs during healing is a depletion of glycogen from the cells at the leading edge of migration.[138] Enlargement of the cells is apparently the result of an increase in cell water content, and the actual movement of the cells is calcium dependent, as calmodulin inhibitors stop migration by preventing microfilament assembly.[28,211] The processes that initiate migration are mediated by cyclic AMP. Treatment of corneas with cholera toxin, which increases cyclic AMP, causes more rapid cell migration, but the physiologic signal that mediates cyclic AMP levels and its effects on healing has not been identified.[115]

Migration of corneal epithelium during wound repair is accompanied by an increase in protein synthesis. In organ culture incorporation of radiolabeled leucine and glucosamine increases significantly during migration and then decreases upon wound closure.[73] The increase in protein synthesis in part represents an increase in proteins found in both stationary and migrating epithelium; however, a specific increase in synthesis of a 110kD protein has also been demonstrated. This protein has been identified as vinculin.[211,242,243] Vinculin is a cytoplasmic protein that links actin to talin, a cytoskeletal protein, at points on the cell membrane known as focal adhesion plaques,[69] which appear in cells near the migrating wound edge during healing (Figs. 3-22 and 3-24). Talin is in turn linked to integrin, thereby anchoring the cell to the substrate. It appears therefore that the increase in vinculin synthesis during wound healing promotes the adhesion of the epithelial cells to the basement membrane during the healing process in the absence of hemidesmosomes.

Following wound healing, the adhesion of the epithelium is reestablished by formation of new hemidesmosomes in the basal cell layer. The location of these hemidesmosomes corresponds precisely to the locations of anchoring fibrils in the basement membrane. When a corneal abrasion is limited to the epithelium and the basement membrane is not damaged, a normal epithelium with adhesion complexes is formed soon after healing. In experimental keratectomy wounds of the cornea where basement membrane is removed, the epithelium must lay down new basement membrane following healing, and development of normal adhesion complexes is delayed for more than 12 months.[75,77,122] These observations raise serious questions concerning stability of the regenerated epithelium following surgical procedures, such as laser keratectomy, which destroy the basement membrane.

Pharmacologic stimulation of corneal epithelial healing

Normally, a simple epithelial abrasion heals quickly without complication. In conditions such as basement membrane dystrophy, diabetes, persistent or recurrent epithelial defects, and severe injuries, such as alkali burns, healing is delayed or normal epithelial adhesion is not established. Several agents, including epidermal growth factor,[219] fibronectin,[173] vitamin A,[221] and citrate,[182] have been studied for their potential as topical drugs for promotion of corneal healing. Experimental work has in most cases produced a mixture of promising and contradictory results. Results of clinical trials have been inconclusive and as yet no drug has been identified that will consistently stimulate corneal epithelial healing and adhesion in humans.

Corneal epithelial electrophysiology and ion transport

In keeping with its function as a barrier the corneal epithelium is a "tight" epithelium with a relatively low ionic conductance through its apical cell membranes and a high resistance (12 to 16 kohm/cm^2) paracellular pathway. It generates a transepithelial potential of 25 to 35 mV due to passive diffusion of ions through these resistances.[131] The paracellular resistance and transepithelial potential are dependent on the existence of the apical tight junctions, as these values go to zero when the junctions are disrupted in a calcium free solution or by exposure of the corneal surface to digitonin.[232] When the resting membrane potential of the superficial cells is recorded by a microelectrode, a potential of about -30 mV is recorded. If the electrode is advanced into the wing cells, no change in potential is recorded. This is evidence that the superficial and wing cell layers form a functional syncytium by virtue of the large number of gap junctions connecting these cells. Upon entry of the electrode into a basal cell an additional voltage drop of about 10 to 20 mV is recorded, indicating that a reduced degree of electrical coupling exists between wing cells and basal cells.[127]

The potentials described above are maintained by epithelial transport of sodium and chloride ions (Fig. 3-25). Sodium is pumped from tears to stroma while chloride is transported into the tears. The inward flux of sodium is balanced by the chloride current so that the net flux of solute is zero. Sodium enters the corneal epithelial cells through channels in the apical membrane of the superficial cells, but the sodium permeability of this membrane is lower than that of other epithelia due to a lack of ame-

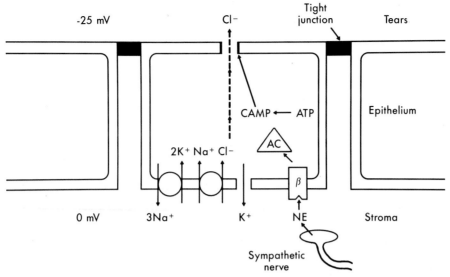

FIG. 3-25 Model of ion transport, ion channels, and sympathetic neural control of chloride channels in the corneal epithelium. The Na^+/K^+ pump in the basolateral membrane maintains the Na^+ gradient for Na/Cl co-transport. Chloride diffuses down its chemical gradient through apical channels, which are opened by cAMP. NE = Norepinephrine; β = adrenergic receptor; AC = adenylate cyclase. (Based on models proposed in Candia OA: Invest Ophthalmol Vis Sci 31 (Suppl): 440, 1990 and Klyce SD: J Physiol 321:49, 1981.)

lioride sensitive channels, which have a high sodium conductance. Sodium is then extruded into the stroma by the ouabain sensitive Na^+-K^+ ATPase located in the basolateral membranes of the cells.[41,131,238]

The maintenance of the inward sodium gradient from the stroma into the epithelial cells by the sodium pump serves as the driving force for transport of chloride into the tears. Chloride moves into the cells against an electrochemical gradient via a sodium-chloride co-transport mechanism[26] in which sodium moves down its electrochemical gradient, carrying with it the chloride ions. Once inside the cell, chloride diffuses into the tears through channels in the apical cell membrane. This transport of chloride accounts for 50% of the short-circuit current across the corneal epithelium; its essential coupling to sodium transport is evident from the fact that the chloride secretion is blocked when the sodium pump is inhibited by ouabain.

The presence of the sodium-potassium pump in the corneal epithelium would imply an outward potassium flux. A high conductance K^+ channel has been identified in the basolateral membrane.[190] Evidence also exists for an apical bicarbonate current.[26]

The transport processes of the corneal epithelium result in osmotic transport of water out of the cornea, and under certain experimental conditions this can promote dehydration of a swollen cornea. In vivo the importance of this transport in maintenance of normal corneal thickness and transparency is minimal compared to that of the corneal endothelium (as discussed below). In contrast to the endothelium, however, epithelial transport can be regulated, perhaps allowing the cornea to respond to stress.[131] Epithelial chloride transport is stimulated by catecholamines, which act via the second messenger cyclic AMP to increase the apical chloride conductance.[133] Release of catecholamines from sympathetic corneal nerves can be regulated by serotonergic nerves that end on sympathetic nerve terminals, and serotonin also stimulates chloride secretion by the cornea.[129,131] Based on these observations it has been suggested that sympathetic nerves can regulate epithelial ion transport (Fig. 3-25).

Stromal physiology

Stromal hydration (i.e., the water content of the stroma) is normally about 3.5 gm H_2O/gm dry weight and increases linearly with increasing corneal thickness. The relative resistance of the nonedematous epithelium, stroma, and endothelium to diffusion of electrolytes is 2000:1:10, thereby restricting electrolytes (and associated water) to the stromal compartment.[49,96,160] The corneal stroma has an inherent tendency to imbibe water and to swell. This property reflects the water-binding capacity of the proteoglycans in the extracellular matrix.[40,57,165] Stromal edema occurs in the ground substance, leading to increased spacing of collagen fibrils. In corneas of normal thickness the swelling pressure is approximately 55 mm Hg (i.e., 80 g/cm²). Swelling pressure is inversely related to corneal thickness. For example, a cornea of 150% normal thickness has a swelling pressure of only 15 mm Hg as compared to 55 mm Hg in the nonedematous cornea. Conversely, compression of the cornea by any means is associated with an increase in stromal swelling pressure.[65,95]

The swelling pressure of the stroma relates to the electrostatic repulsion of the negatively charged glycosaminoglycan polyelectrolytes (i.e., keratan sulfate, chondroitin, chondroitin sulfate). In addition, their macromolecular structure increases fluid viscosity and defines the colloidosmotic characteristics of the stroma. The actual concentration of Na^+ and K^+ is higher in the stroma than in the aqueous humor.[178] However, the ionic *activity*, which determines the osmotic and diffusional gradients for Na^+, is less in the stroma than the aqueous,[19] reflecting cationic binding by anionic sites on stromal glycosaminoglycans.[94] This binding decreases the effective osmolarity of Na^+ in the corneal stroma and favors movement of water from the stroma to the aqueous. As discussed in a later section, active dehydration of the cornea is a consequence of the osmotic gradient established by the corneal endothelial metabolic pump, compensating for the leakage of fluid from the aqueous and limbus into the stroma as a consequence of swelling pressure.

Water evaporates from the corneal surface at a rate of 2.5 µl/cm²/hour.[175] Evaporation accounts for a 5% thinning of the cornea during the day, compared with thickness measured at the time the eyelids open in the morning after nighttime closure.[151] In patients with compromised endothelial metabolic pump function, such as those in Fuchs' endothelial dystrophy, epithelial edema is worse in the morning when arising, due to lack of evaporation at night when the lids are closed. Localized areas of corneal drying and evaporation may result in focal corneal thinning, known as dellen. The persistence of dellen may reflect the decrease in stromal fluid flow facility[157] when stromal hydration is abnormal in addition to minimal lateral flow of water in the cornea.

The normal cornea maintains a constant thickness in the presence of intraocular pressures up to 50 mm Hg.[238] This is because the stromal swelling pressure is also in a similar range. However, in eyes with intraocular pressures above 50 mm Hg or in those with abnormal endothelial function, there will be resultant epithelial edema and increased stromal thickness. The relationship between intraocular pressure (IOP) and stromal swelling pressure (SP) is:

$$IP = IOP - SP,$$

where IP is stromal imbibition pressure. In rabbits in which the central corneal stroma was implanted with a saline filled cannula, the suction on the cannula necessary to prevent the stroma from drawing fluid from the tube is the imbibition pressure.[96] As discussed earlier, stromal swelling pressure decreases precipitously with increased corneal thickness. Thus, mild corneal edema (for example, in a marginally functioning corneal transplant) combined with slightly elevated intraocular pressure, can lead to high imbibition pressures and subsequent microbullous epithelial edema.

Stromal wound healing

Stromal wound healing involves the resynthesis and crosslinking of collagen, alterations in proteoglycan synthesis, and gradual wound remodeling leading to the restoration of tensile strength. Within hours, polymorphonuclear cells appear around areas of cellular necrosis in a penetrating corneal wound, followed thereafter by monocytes. Adjacent corneal cells are seen to undergo a process of transformation, leading to an accumulation of fibroblasts. Stromal keratocytes, which normally form a syncytium, may begin to lose their interconnections and go through morphologic changes, some undergoing hypertrophy, proliferation, and finally reformation of cellular processes and connecting gap junctions.[141] Activated corneal cells involved in stromal healing may transiently express fetal antigens,[82,149] and these scars may have a decrease in the concentration of sulfated epitopes of keratan sulfate and an increase in dermatan sulfate.[3,27] Following excimer laser keratectomy or mechanical keratectomy in monkeys,[82] fibrinogen is detected at 1 month in the underlying corneal stroma, but not in the overlying healed region, which contains newly synthesized type III collagen, poorly sulfated keratan sulfate, fibronectin, and laminin. Type VI collagen is present uniformly in both untreated and healed corneal stroma, suggesting that newly formed collagen may interdigitate with the old in corneal scars.[35]

Tensile strength in corneal wounds increases gradually up to the fourth postoperative year.[206] Incisions in avascular cornea far from the limbus heal more slowly then peripheral cornea wounds or in chronically inflamed corneas with neovascularization.[84] Studies of delayed corneal wound healing following radial keratotomy showed evidence of epithelial plugs in the incision site up to 47 months postoperatively, along with gaping keratotomy incisions and malapposed Bowman's layer.[36] The use of potent topical steroids may delay the early phases of corneal wound healing.

Endothelial physiology

As described above, the stroma tends to imbibe water due to the charge characteristics of the proteoglycans of the stromal ground substance. In spite of the swelling pressure of the stroma, it does not swell in vivo under normal conditions. Two factors contribute to the prevention of stromal swelling and the maintenance of its water content at 78% (3.8 mg water/mg dry weight): these are the barrier and pump functions of the endothelium. The barrier is incomplete compared to the epithelial barrier.

This is illustrated by comparing swelling rates of the cornea in vitro after removal of the endothelium or inhibition of the metabolic pump (see below). When the endothelium is disrupted, the cornea swells at 127 μm per hour, clearly demonstrating the importance of this cell layer as a barrier. When the metabolic pump is inhibited, the cornea swells at about 33 μm per hour and this swelling represents the movement of fluid and solutes from the aqueous humor into the stroma through the incomplete barrier of the intact cell layer[227] (Fig. 3-26). This normal leakage of fluid into the cornea serves a vital function; because of the avascularity of the cornea, this fluid is the source of nutrients including glucose and amino acids for the cornea.

The continual movement of water into the stroma would lead to stromal swelling and loss of transparency if mechanisms were not present to remove fluid from the stroma. Early studies of corneal hydration showed that maintenance of the normal corneal thickness and water content is temperature dependent. The cornea swells when cooled and returns to normal thickness when returned to its normal temperature[90] (Fig. 3-27). This phenomenon is known as temperature reversal and is clearly demonstrated by eye bank corneas, which swell during refrigeration and return to normal thickness and transparency after grafting. This temperature reversal clearly shows that the maintenance of corneal hydration is a metabolic, energy dependent process, and it was subsequently shown that 6 to 8 μl per hour of water is moved by the endothelium from stroma to aqueous humor.[38,158] It was initially suggested that water itself was actively transported by the cornea, leading to the use of terminology describing a corneal "fluid pump." It is now known that cell membranes contain transporters for ions, amino acids, and sugars, but no active transport mechanism that directly transports water molecules is known to exist.

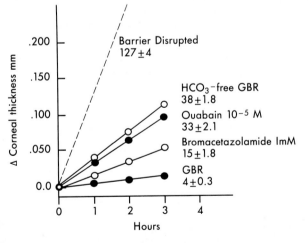

FIG. 3-26 Maintenance of corneal thickness requires an intact barrier and metabolic pump. Inhibition of the Na^+/K^+ ATPase with ouabain, inhibition of carbonic anhydrase with bromacetazolamide or lack of bicarbonate all result in swelling. Numbers indicate swelling rates in μm/hr. GBR = glutathione bicarbonate Ringer's solution. (Courtesy Dr. Henry Edelhauser. From Waring GO, et al: Ophthalmol 89:531, 1982.)

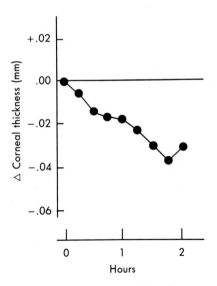

FIG. 3-27 Temperature reversal in a human cornea during in vitro perfusion. (Courtesy Dr. Henry Edelhauser.)

Rather, water moves osmotically down gradients set up by active transport of ions and therefore the term "metabolic pump" rather than "fluid pump" should be used. The concept has developed that normal corneal hydration represents a balance between the leak across the corneal endothelium and the extrusion of ions and fluid via the endothelial metabolic pump.

Endothelial ion transport

Several ion transport systems have been identified or postulated to exist in the corneal endothelium. Each of these mechanisms will be characterized and then placed into a unified model of the endothelial metabolic pump.

The enzyme Na^+/K^+ ATPase was shown to be present in cat cornea during the initial studies of this enzyme,[13] and it is now the most completely characterized of the endothelial ion transporters.[17,58,71,105,143,230] The sodium-potassium pump is located in the basolateral membrane of the endothelial cell and is present in normal humans at about 1.5×10^6 pump sites/cell and in rabbits at 3×10^6 pump sites/cell.[70,72,215] These values may be compared to levels of 4 to 5×10^6 sites/cell in the renal tubule and ventricular muscle. The activity of Na^+/K^+ ATPase is vital to maintenance of normal corneal hydration. Inhibition of the pump with the specific inhibitor, ouabain, stops sodium transport, causes corneal swelling, prevents temperature reversal, and eliminates the transendothelial potential difference. It also appears that the sodium pump can respond to increases in endothelial permeability since human corneas with guttata have pump site densities of 6×10^6 sites/cell, which suggests a greater capacity for the endothelial pump to counteract the leak across the barrier.[72] In contrast, the inflamed, edematous cornea has decreased endothelial pump sites in spite of increased permeability. These responses appear to be mediated by the cyclooxygenase pathway of the arachidonic acid cascade.[146]

The basolateral membrane of the endothelial cell also contains an amelioride sensitive sodium-hydrogen exchanger. It moves sodium into the cell and hydrogen ions outward.[111]

Bicarbonate is also essential to the maintenance of corneal thickness.[99] Removal of bicarbonate from the solution irrigating the endothelium of the isolated, perfused cornea results in corneal swelling[227] (Fig. 3-26), and a net flux of bicarbonate from stroma to aqueous humor has been demonstrated. This transport of bicarbonate is apparently responsible for the $-500 \ \mu V$ (aqueous humor negative to stroma) potential across the endothelium.[135] The bicarbonate transported by the endothelium is generated intracellularly via the action of carbonic anhydrase. Carbon dioxide diffuses into the cells from the extracellular space and combines with water in a reaction catalyzed by carbonic anhydrase to form carbonic acid. The carbonic acid readily dissociates into hydrogen and bicarbonate ions. Inhibition of this reaction by carbonic anhydrase inhibitors can result in corneal swelling in vitro.[106] The effect is not as great as that seen when Na^+/K^+ ATPase is inhibited,[227] and it is also interesting that systemic treatment with acetazolamide has no effect on corneal hydration. The transport of bicarbonate across the apical membrane of the cells is energy dependent[99,230] but the transporter is not well defined. Electrophysiologic evidence points to the existence of an electrogenic bicarbonate-sodium cotransport, which moves these ions out of the cell in a 2:1 ratio in a process that is inhibitable by stilbene.[111] This type of transport has not been identified in other cell types and evidence also exists to indicate that bicarbonate and sodium transport are not directly coupled.

Although the details of endothelial transport are not yet fully elucidated, the components of the system as described above can be assembled into a model that explains ion transport and osmotic water flow across the endothelium[111,135,227] (Fig. 3-28). The sodium-hydrogen exchanger acidifies the extracellular fluid, increasing the level of carbon dioxide that diffuses into the cell. Carbonic anhydrase converts carbon dioxide to hydrogen ion and bicarbonate, which are transported out of the cell by the basolateral sodium-hydrogen exchanger and the apical bicarbonate transport, respectively. As suggested above, sodium may accompany the bicarbonate with the stoichiometry favoring the anion, setting up the aqueous negative transendothelial potential. Central to the entire system is the sodium pump, which maintains the sodium gradient required for sodium-hydrogen exchange, thereby promoting bicarbonate production. Transport of sodium into the lateral space may also contribute to the transendothelial potential and, although given the apical location of the junctional complexes the path of least resistance for sodium movement is into the stroma, the negative potential of the aqueous homor may also result in movement of sodium ions from the lateral spaces into the aqueous humor. Potassium and sodium channels required for the function of this model have also been identified.[135,188] Although not shown in the model, chloride transport is also required for correct stoichiometry but this has not yet been adequately identified.

Essential to the function of an endothelial

Na$^+$ activity = 134 mEq/l

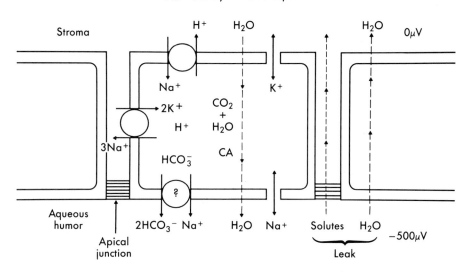

FIG. 3-28   Model of ion and water movements across the corneal endothelium. Activity of the metabolic pump sets up an osmotic gradient resulting in movement of fluid from the stroma to the aqueous humor balancing the leak of fluid from the aqueous humor into the stroma. CA = carbonic anhydrase. (Based on models proposed in Jentsch TJ, et al: Curr Eye Res 4:361, 1985 and Kuang K, et al: Exp Eye Res 50:487, 1990.)

metabolic pump capable of fluid transport is the existence of an osmotic gradient that favors the movement of water from the stroma to the aqueous humor. The sodium concentration of aqueous humor is 143 mEq/l, all of which is osmotically active. The sodium concentration of the stroma is more that 160 mEq/l, which would imply a gradient favoring inward movement of water. A large portion of this sodium is bound by the stromal ground substance, leaving an osmotically active sodium level of only 134 mEq/l in the stroma. This results in an osmotic pressure of 163.8 mm Hg drawing water out of the cornea.[213] The metabolic pump model described above, although incomplete, is clearly able to set up the ionic gradient required to counteract the leak of fluid into the cornea. It is evident that the bulk of water movement occurs through the cells, probably through glucose channels. Blockers of glucose transport, like phloretin, also block water movement across the endothelium.

Endothelial function and intraocular irrigating solutions

The pH and osmotic requirements of the corneal endothelium are well defined.[81,227] A pH range of 6.8 to 8.2 must be maintained to prevent corneal edema. When the corneal endothelium is exposed to an environment outside this range, cells swell and become vacuolated, junctional breakdown occurs, and corneal thickness increases. The cellular swelling that occurs suggests impaired metabolic pump function so that the corneal edema is due not only to increased leak as cells degenerate but also to decreased ion and water transport. These factors must be considered when irrigating solutions and drugs are introduced into the anterior chamber. Poorly buffered solutions such as 0.9% saline and lactated Ringer's solution or acidic drug formulations that overcome the buffering capacity of the aqueous humor may expose the cornea to extremes of pH and cause corneal edema[43,45] (Fig. 3-29). The osmotic tolerance of the endothelium is quite broad as it can maintain normal thickness over a range of 200 to 400 mOsm/kg; the optimal osmolality is that of the aqueous humor, 304 mOsm/kg.

Irrigation of the endothelium with 0.9% NaCl results in immediate and rapid swelling of the cornea due to a loss of pump and barrier.[43,227] This is clearly the result of a lack of ions essential to endothelial function. The absence of extracellular potassium inhibits the Na$^+$/K$^+$ ATPase. Bicarbonate is required for the endothelial transport system and absence of this ion also results in corneal swelling. The endothelial cells of

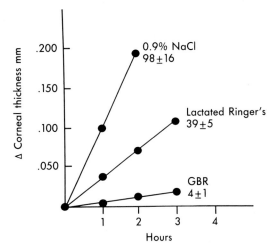

FIG. 3-29 Changes in corneal thickness of rabbit corneas perfused with three intraocular irrigating solutions. NaCl causes rapid swelling because it lacks calcium, bicarbonate, and other essential ions. Lactated Ringer's solution has a low pH. Glutathione bicarbonate Ringer's (GBR) solution resembles aqueous humor and maintains normal corneal thickness. (Courtesy Dr. Henry Edelhauser. From Edelhauser HF, et al: Am J Ophthalmol 93:327, 1982.)

these corneas are swollen and vacuolated, which again is evidence of impaired pump function (Fig. 3-30, *A*). As discussed below, normal saline also lacks other components of the aqueous humor known to be required for endothelial function.[45]

An intact endothelial barrier requires the presence of calcium, because this ion is always involved in the maintenance of junctional complexes. Irrigation of the endothelium with a calcium-free solution causes breakage of the apical junctions[227] (Fig. 3-30, *B*). The cells separate and round up, exposing large areas of Descemet's membrane, with a resultant increase of fluid uptake by the stroma. Replacement of calcium in the solution allows re-formation of the junctions. It must be pointed out that loss of intercellular junctions not only disrupts the barrier; the separation of the cells from one another also causes a loss of pump polarity so that the cells can no longer transport ions vectorially and set up the osmotic and ionic gradients required for movement of fluid into the aqueous humor.[231]

Glutathione, which is present in aqueous humor and endothelial cells, has been shown to promote maintenance of endothelial function in vitro.[38,100,194] This tripeptide is normally present in both its reduced (GSH) and oxidized (GSSG) forms. This balance appears to be important since oxidation of all glutathione by diamide re-

sults in breakage of cell junctions.[46] It is suggested that glutathione protects the cell membranes from free radical damage, thereby helping to maintain both the pump and the barrier of the endothelium.

These observations concerning the physiologic requirements of the corneal endothelium clearly illustrate that any irrigating solution introduced into the anterior chamber of the eye should closely resemble the aqueous humor in composition since the normal environment of the intraocular fluid provides for all of these requirements (Table 3-1). Even a short-term, 30-minute irrigation of the cat endothelium *in vivo* with a balanced salt solution deficient in bicarbonate and glutathione can cause a transient increase in polymegethism and pleomorphism.[78] Based on data presented above, these changes in endothelial cell morphology, as seen *enface*, are apparently the result of altered cell volume regulation and pump function. This lends support to the earlier argument that pleomorphism and polymorphism are indicative of a physiologically stressed endothelium.

The physiologic requirements of the corneal endothelium must also be considered when designing a corneal preservation medium.[200] The ionic composition of such a solution should be such that the endothelial monolayer is preserved intact for normal barrier function and so that the transporters will function effectively to promote temperature reversal if the cornea has been stored in the cold.

TABLE 3-1 The Composition of Aqueous Humor and Glutathione-Bicarbonate Ringer's Solution (GBR) (all concentrations in nmol/L)

	Aqueous humor	GBR
Sodium	162.9	160
Potassium	2.2–3.9	5
Calcium	1.8	1
Magnesium	1.1	1
Chloride	131.6	130
Bicarbonate	20.15	25
Phosphate	0.62	3
Lactate	2.5	—
Glucose	2.7–3.7	5
Ascorbate	1.06	
Glutathione	0.002	0.3
pH	7.38	7.2–7.4
Osmolarity (mOsm/kg)	304	305

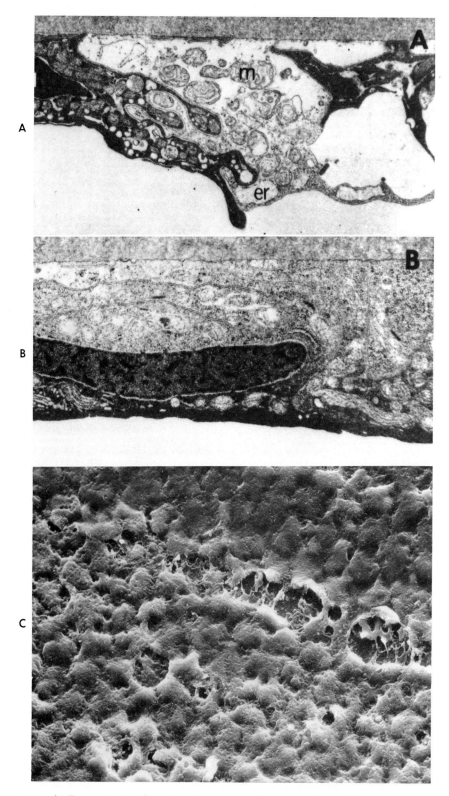

FIG. 3-30 A, Transmission electron micrograph of corneal endothelial cells perfused with 0.9% NaCl solution. Note cell swelling and vacuolization indicative of impaired pump function. **B,** Normal corneal endothelium. **C,** Scanning electron micrograph of a corneal endothelium perfused with a calcium-free solution. Note breakage of cell junctions. (Magnification × 1000.) (Courtesy Dr. Henry Edelhauser.)

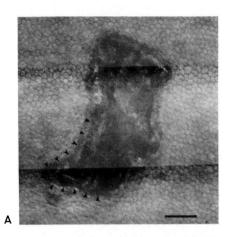
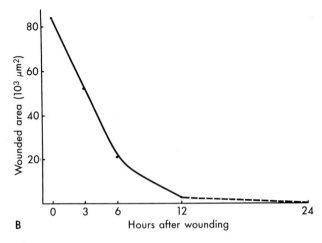

FIG. 3-31 **A**, Wide-field specular micrograph of a corneal endothelial wound. Bar $= 100\ \mu$m.
B, Changes in wound area during healing of a corneal endothelial wound. (From Ref 156,
courtesy Dr. John Ubels.)

Endothelial wound healing

Little or no mitosis occurs in the adult human
corneal endothelium. For this reason when endothelial cells are lost due to surgical trauma,
disease, or the aging process, the defect must be
covered by the spreading of cells from areas adjacent to the wound to cover the wounded area.
When a single cell is lost, as in aging, the cells
immediately surrounding the defect spread to
fill in the area left by the missing cell. Over time
this leads to the marked cell enlargement typical
of the aged cornea.[15]

When a large defect occurs as a result of surgical insult or a decompensation episode in keratoconus, more extensive cell migration occurs.
In experimental wounds cells as far as 250 μm
from the wound edge are involved in migration
toward the wound center. Cells near the wound
edge migrate at 80 to 100 μm per day in the initial stages of healing, elongating toward the center of the wound, and finally spreading as the
wound closes[152,156] (Fig. 3-31). This is followed
by remodeling into a more normal hexagonal
shape. In vivo the cells do not break contact
with one another during spreading and
migration[223] (Fig. 3-32). The pump and barrier of
the endothelium are reestablished upon restoration of the confluent monolayer, allowing the
cornea to return to normal thickness.[235]

The mechanisms of cell migration in the endothelium have not been extensively studied.
Actin stress fibers have been demonstrated oriented in the direction of cell spreading in cultured cells, and the formation of these fibers and
the cell movement can be stimulated by indomethacin.[113,114] The endothelium also contains
abundant EGF receptors. Although wound

healing can be stimulated by EGF in vitro, its
usefulness as a pharmacologic agent to promote
endothelial healing has not yet been established.

Corneal nutrition and metabolism

Corneal metabolism is dependent upon oxygen
derived predominantly from the atmosphere,[208]
with minor amounts supplied by the aqueous
humor and limbal vasculature.[98] The normal
amount of oxygen present in the aqueous
humor is low (around 40 mm Hg) in comparison
to tears (i.e., 155 mm Hg). During sleep or under
closed-eye conditions, oxygen is delivered to the
cornea via the highly vascularized superior palpebral conjunctivae,[103] albeit at reduced levels
(i.e., pO$_2$ 21% with eyelid open, 8% with eyelid
closed).[48] Following cataract removal (i.e., aphakia), oxygen tension may increase in the aqueous humor due to decreased oxygen metabolism
by the crystalline lens.[102] Thus, in the aphakic
eye, oxygen in the aqueous may supplement oxygen dissolved in the tears, better meeting corneal oxygen demands and allowing greater tolerance to hypoxic stress such as contact lens use.

The corneal epithelium consumes oxygen at
a rate approximately ten times faster than the
stroma.[193] Several investigators have presented
evidence suggesting that there may be a role for
intact corneal innervation in maintaining the
high metabolic rate of the epithelium.[102,225] Most
of the metabolic requirements for glucose, as
well as amino acids, vitamins, and other nutrients, are supplied to the cornea by the aqueous
humor (via the ciliary body), with lesser
amounts available in the tears or via limbal vessels. In addition, glucose can be derived from

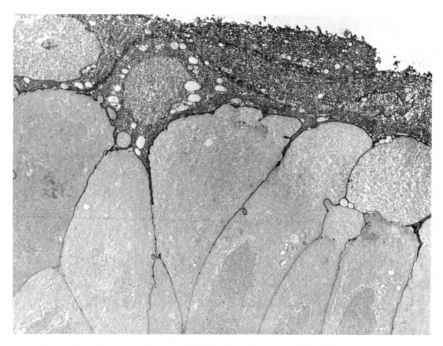

FIG. 3-32 Scanning electron micrograph of migrating corneal endothelial cells. (From Ref 223, courtesy Dr. Diane Van Horn Hatchell.)

glycogen stores in the corneal epithelium. Under both hypoxic and normoxic conditions, some glucose is diverted to the hexose monophosphate (HM) shunt (Fig. 3-33), regulating levels of nicotinamide adenosine dinucleotide phosphate (NADPH) and converting hexoses to pentoses, which are utilized in nucleic acid synthesis. In addition, glucose derived from the aqueous or from epithelial glycogen stores is converted to pyruvate by the anaerobic Embden-Meyerhof pathway (i.e., glycolysis), yielding 2 molecules of adenosine triphosphate (ATP) per glucose molecule. Under aerobic conditions, pyruvate is then oxidized in the tricarboxylic acid (TCA or Krebs or citric acid cycle) to yield water, carbon dioxide, and 36 molecules of ATP per cycle. Under hypoxic conditions, such as during contact lens use, increasing amounts of pyruvate are converted by lactate dehydrogenase to lactate, which diffuses from the epithelium into the stroma, osmotically inducing epithelial and stromal edema.[128] Epithelial edema leads to clinical symptoms such as halo and rainbow formation, increased glare sensitivity, and decreased contrast sensitivity. Because the anterior surface of the cornea is structurally fixed by Bowman's membrane and the anterior stroma, stromal corneal edema manifests in a posterior direction, with buckling of the posterior stroma and Descemet's membrane

giving rise to vertical striae.[140,185,228] Because of the barrier provided by the superficial epithelial cells, the dispersion of lactate into the tear film is precluded and the elimination of lactate is dependent upon slow diffusion across the stroma and endothelium into the aqueous humor. In addition to causing osmotic edema of the epithelium and stroma, metabolic acidosis consequent to lactate metabolism may result in structural and functional alterations in corneal endothelial cells.[239] In the absence of corneal edema, the oxygen permeability of the corneal stroma is somewhat less than 29×10^{-11} ml $O_2/cm^2/sec/mm$ Hg^{229}, a value less than that of most high water content soft contact lenses.[208]

The oxygen requirements of the cornea have important implications with regard to contact lens use. It has been shown that the cornea can maintain a deturgescent state with sustained oxygen levels as low as 25 mm Hg before edema is induced.[150] For small diameter hard polymethyl methacrylate lenses, which are impermeable to oxygen, good lens movement is essential to allow an exchange of tears under the lens with oxygenated tears from the periphery, which is accomplished by the action of the lid blink. For larger diameter soft lenses, especially those used on an extended wear basis, oxygen permeability must be sufficient for an adequate supply of oxygen to reach the cornea by diffusion through

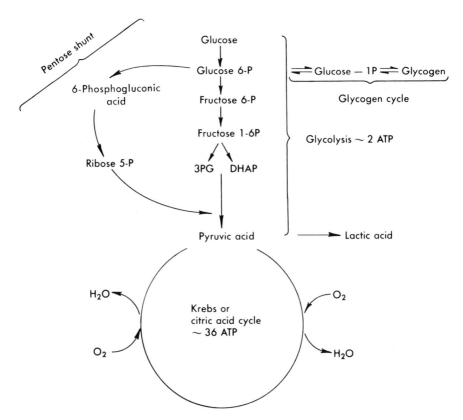

FIG. 3-33 Metabolism of glucose in cornea.

the lens itself, in addition to the lesser effect of the tear pump exchange with these lenses.

Extended wear contact lenses alter many aspects of epithelial metabolism. Their use has been associated with a decreased rate of mitosis[87,104] (possibly contributing to corneal epithelial thinning associated with long term use), reduced oxygen uptake[104] and glucose utilization,[123] and smaller numbers of intercellular desmosomes (thought to be secondary to prolonged epithelial edema).[10] The decrease in desmosomal connections between cells increases the likelihood of abrasions and erosions.[174] This, in concert with the reduced metabolic activity of the epithelium under hypoxic conditions, may compromise the epithelial barrier function and increase the likelihood of ulcerative microbial keratitis.[166]

CORNEAL NEOVASCULARIZATION

The human cornea is normally avascular and transparent. Corneal neovascularization, sometimes accompanied by lipid deposition, may result from a variety of diverse conditions. These include ocular surface disease such as acne rosacea[18] and staphylococcal hypersensitivity,[166] immunologic disorders such as corneal allograft rejection[110] and cicatricial pemphigoid,[63] and collagen vascular diseases with peripheral corneal ulceration and neovascularization.[62] Other causes of corneal inflammation may induce new blood vessel formation such as alkali or silver nitrate burns,[32] Cogan's syndrome,[29] herpetic, syphilitic, or zoster keratitis, as well as many other microbial infections. Hypoxia may play a role in some forms of corneal neovascularization reported with the use of soft contact lenses.[148,197] Corneal neovascularization has been associated with some dystrophic conditions, such as Peters' anomaly, and the influence of genetic factors is suggested by the high incidence of corneal neovascularization in specific inbred strains of mice.[53,171]

Corneal neovascularization is a result of sprouting from perilimbal vessels. New capillaries arise from the perilimbal capillaries[116] and parent venules[21] by focal degradation of the venular basement membrane, followed by movement of endothelial cells toward the angiogenic stimulus. The migrating vascular endothelial cells elongate and form a solid sprout, which later develops a lumen. Two sprouts join tips to form a loop, the outer surface of which is lined by pericytes, and blood flow begins.[59] The process is repeated by new sprouts emanating from the apex of the loop. The angiogenic process can therefore be conceptualized as three basic steps: (1) enzymatic degradation of the basement membrane, (2) endothelial cell movement, and (3) endothelial cell proliferation.[125]

The specific angiogenic factors leading to corneal neovascularization are likely to be multiple and diverse. Some factors, such as acidic fibroblast growth factor (FGF), basic FGF, and transforming growth factor-alpha appear to have a direct effect in inducing endothelial cell proliferation. Certain inflammatory cells or their products also appear to play a role in corneal vascularization. Klintworth and associates[7,214] have demonstrated that polymorphonuclear cell infiltrates may be important in corneal angiogenesis, although the underlying mechanisms remain elusive. The supernatants of stimulated lymphocytes[52-54,145,168] as well as lymphokines[8,51,240] and prostaglandins[60] in slow release polymers have been shown to induce corneal neovascularization in rabbits, and similar findings have been made in inbred strains of mice. These factors may be either chemotactic for endothelial cells (e.g., prostaglandins E_1 and E_2) or function by attracting and activating macrophages to secrete angiogenic growth factors. Alternatively, indirect acting angiogenic factors may cause release of vascular endothelial cell mitogens stored intracellularly or in the extracellular matrix[210,241] (e.g., basic FGF). Once corneal neovascularization starts, the process may be driven and amplified by the secretion of platelet-derived growth factor from vascular endothelial cells, which has potent angiogenic activity. Other factors that may modulate corneal neovascularization include heparin[125] and tissue levels of copper ions.[172]

A variety of approaches to the inhibition of corneal neovascularization have been investigated. Angiostatic steroids alone or in combination with heparin[61] or heparin substitutes[4] have been shown to inhibit corneal vascularization in rabbits. Systemic amiloride[109] has resulted in partial suppression of experimentally induced corneal neovascularization, perhaps by inhibiting plasminogen activators, whose activation would set off proteolysis of the extracellular matrix at the leading edge of new vessels. Pharmacologic modulators of collagen metabolism may lead to regression of new blood vessels by promoting basement membrane dissolution.[92] A variety of inhibitors of arachidonic acid metabolism have had varying effects in animal

models of corneal neovascularization.[37,42,55,97,226] Systemic immunosuppression with cytotoxic agents has been used to treat immunologically mediated disorders, such as cicatricial pemphigoid[63] and ocular manifestations of rheumatoid arthritis.[62] Finally, several investigators have treated corneal neovascularization using laser photocoagulation with an argon or tunable dye laser with or without use of a photoactivating substance.

CORNEAL PHARMACOLOGY
Factors affecting drug penetration

Many factors influence the degree of drug penetration through the cornea. The volume of the normal adult tear film is 7 to 9 μl and the maximum amount of fluid that the cul-de-sac can maintain is 20 to 30 μl. Thus, much of the 50 μl in the average drop of topical medication runs out of the eye immediately after instillation and the remainder is diluted in the preexisting tear film.[158] Reflex tearing due to irritating or hypertonic solutions will result in more rapid tear dilution. Increased protein concentration in tears bathing inflamed or infected eyes may also decrease the bioavailability of drugs that bind to protein.

Following topical drug administration, most of the drug enters the aqueous humor by corneal penetration.[39] The corneal epithelium provides an initial barrier to penetration with its tight junctions, thereby limiting adsorption of hydrophilic, ionized substances and favoring the penetration of lipid-soluble hydrophobic compounds. The drug-saturated epithelium may act as a reservoir to release drugs into the hydrophilic corneal stroma. Thus drugs that are delivered at a pH favoring their more lipid-soluble undissociated form will more readily enter the epithelium. At the pH of the corneal epithelium, more of the drug will dissociate into its water-soluble ionized form, facilitating penetration through the stroma. Loss of the corneal epithelium greatly enhances the penetration of hydrophilic, water-soluble pharmacologic agents, such as gentamicin, that normally traverse the epithelium via transcellular or paracellular routes.

The corneal stroma, comprised of collagen and extracellular matrix, allows diffusion of solutes of less than 500,000 molecular weight. The hydrophilic nature of the stroma results in a barrier to lipid-based drugs. Drug penetration through the corneal endothelium is determined mostly by molecular size.

Other means to increase drug penetration through the cornea include increasing the duration of contact of the drug with the ocular surface. This can be accomplished through mechanical means such as pressing on the lacrimal sac, or by use of viscous drops, suspensions or ointments, slow-release delivery systems, contact lenses, or porcine collagen corneal shields. The inclusion of surfactants and detergents, such as benzalkonium chloride or Tween 20 in topical ocular medications, or the preparation of drug-containing liposomes may also improve drug penetration through the outer epithelial barrier, in addition to the preservative effect inherent to these agents.[160]

Effects of preservatives

Preservatives, such as benzalkonium chloride, chlorhexidine digluconate, and thimerosal, must be used in opthalmic preparations to prevent bacterial growth. The antibacterial action of some of the preservatives, notably benzalkonium chloride, is based on the detergent property of the compound, which acts to break down bacterial cell walls. Thimerosal exerts its action via its mercuric content. These characteristics of a preservative also render the corneal epithelium and endothelium susceptible to damage when exposed to these agents.[22,23,144]

The effects of benzalkonium chloride on the epithelium have been studied extensively. Application of a drop containing 0.01% benzalkonium chloride to the cornea causes an immediate, measurable increase in the permeability of the cornea to fluorescein. This is the result of breakage of junctions between the superficial cells and sloughing of the outer cell layer (Fig. 3-34). With prolonged exposure to a preservative the sloughing of the second layer of superficial cells and possibly some wing cells may also occur. Electrophysiologic experiments have shown that this loss of superficial cells is accompanied by a decrease in the transepithelial voltage due to the loss of the high resistance barrier formed by the apical tight junctions. Benzalkonium chloride also inhibits corneal epithelial wound healing.

Other preservatives have similar but milder effects on the corneal epithelial surface. Thimerosal, however, has the added disadvantage of causing a hypersensitivity reaction in some patients. Preservatives can generally be used without major side effects; in fact, benzalkonium chloride enhances the corneal penetration of some drugs. Certain patients, especially those with a dry eye who use preserved artificial tears frequently, risk further damage to an already compromised corneal epithelium, increasing

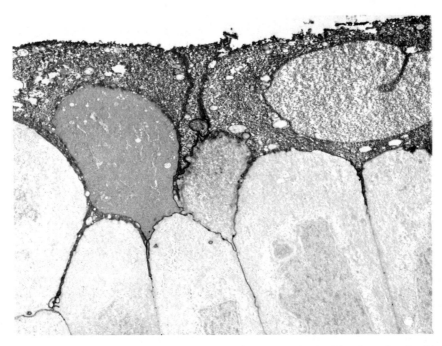

FIG. 3-34   Corneal epithelium damaged by 0.01% benzalkonium chloride and stained with ruthenium red. The dye penetrates the intercellular space due to disruption of the barrier formed by the superficial cells. (Courtesy Dr. Delores López Bernal.)

chances for corneal edema and ocular infection. They therefore benefit from the use of nonpreserved formulas.

The preservatives benzalkonium chloride, thimerosal, and chlorhexidine all cause endothelial cell degeneration and corneal edema in vitro.[85,86,225] Drugs or solutions containing preservatives should never be introduced directly into the anterior chamber of the eye.

REFERENCES

1. Alvarado J, Murphy C, Jester R: Age related changes in the basement membrane of the corneal epithelium, Invest Ophthalmol Vis Sci 24:1015, 1984.
2. Anhalt GJ, et al: Bullous pemphigoid autoantibodies are markers of corneal epithelial hemidesmosomes, Invest Ophthalmol Vis Sci 28:903, 1987.
3. Anseth A, Fransson LA: Studies on corneal polysaccharides, VI, Isolation of dermatan sulfate from corneal scar tissue, Exp Eye Res 8:302, 1969.
4. Avery RL, Connor TB Jr, Farazdaghi M: Systemic amiloride inhibits experimentally induced neovascularization, Arch Ophthalmol 108:1474, 1990.
5. Bahn CF, Falls HF, Varley GA, et al: Classification of corneal endothelial disorders based on neural crest origin, Ophthalmol 91:558, 1984.
6. Ben-Zvi A, Rodrigues MM, Krachmer JH, et al: Immunohistochemical characterization of extracellular matrix in the developing human cornea, Curr Eye Res 5:105, 1986.
7. BenEzra D: Possible mediation of vasculogenesis by products of the immune reaction, in Silverstein AM, O'Connor RG, eds: Immunology and immunopathology of the eye, New York, Masson, 1978, p 315.
8. BenEzra D, Hemo I, Maltzir G: In vivo angiogenic activity of interleukins, Arch Ophthalmol 108:573, 1990.
9. Bergmanson JPG: Corneal damage in photokeratitis— why is it so painful? Optom Vis Sci 67:407, 1990.
10. Bergmanson JPG, Chu LWF: Corneal response to rigid contact lens wear, Br J Ophthalmol 66:667, 1982.
11. Boettner EA, Wolter JR: Transmission of the ocular media, Invest Ophthalmol 6:776, 1962.
12. Bogan SJ, Waring GO, Ibrahim O, et al: Classification of normal corneal topography based on computer-assisted video keratography, Arch Ophthalmol 108:945, 1990.
13. Bonting S, Simon K, Hawkins N: Studies on sodium-potassium activated adenosine triphosphatase, I, Quantitative distribution in several tissues of the cat, Arch Biochem Biophys 95:416, 1961.
14. Borcherding MS, Blacik LJ, Sittig RA, et al: Proteoglycans and collagen fibre organization in human corneoscleral tissue, Exp Eye Res 21:59, 1975.
15. Bourne WM, Kaufman HE: Specular microscopy of the human corneal endothelium in vivo, Am J Ophthalmol 81:319, 1976.
16. Bourne WM, McCarey BE, Kaufman HE: Clinical specular microscopy, Trans Am Acad Ophthalmol Otolaryngol 81:OP-743, 1976.
17. Brown S, Hedbys B: The effect of ouabain on hydration of the cornea, Invest Ophthalmol 4:216, 1965.
18. Browning DJ, Proia AD: Ocular rosacea, Surv Ophthalmol 31:145, 1986.
19. Brubaker RF, Kupfer C: Microcryoscopic determination of the osmolality of interstitial fluid in the living rabbit cornea, Invest Ophthalmol 1:653, 1962.
20. Buck RC: Measurement of centripetal migration of normal corneal epithelial cells in the mouse, Invest Ophthalmol Vis Sci 26:1296, 1985.
21. Burger PC, Chandler DB, Klintworth GK: Corneal vascularization as studied by scanning electron microscopy of vascular casts, Lab Invest 48:169, 1983.
22. Burstein NL, Klyce SD: Electrophysiologic and morphologic effects of ophthalmic preparations on rabbit corneal endothelium, Invest Ophthalmol Vis Sci 16:899, 1977.
23. Burstein NL: Preservative alteration of corneal permeability in humans and rabbits, Invest Ophthalmol Vis Sci 25:1453, 1984.
24. Butterfield CC, Neufeld AH: Cyclic nucleotide and mitosis in the rabbit cornea following superior cervical ganglionectomy, Exp Eye Res 25:427, 1977.
25. Candia OA: The flux rates of the Na-Cl cotransport mechanism in the frog corneal epithelium, Curr Eye Res 4:333, 1985.
26. Candia OA: Forskolin-induced HCO_3^- current across the apical membrane of the corneal epithelium, Invest Ophthalmol Vis Sci 31 (Suppl): 440, 1990.
27. Cintron C, Covington HI, Kublin CL: Morphologic analysis of proteoglycans in rabbit corneal scars, Invest Ophthalmol Vis Sci 31:1789, 1990.
28. Cintron C, Kublin CL, Covington H: Quantitative studies of corneal epithelial wound healing in rabbits, Curr Eye Res 1:507, 1982.
29. Cobo LM, Haynes BF: Early corneal findings in Cogan's syndrome, Ophthalmol 91:903, 1984.
30. Cogan DG: Applied anatomy and physiology of the cornea, Trans Am Acad Ophthalmol 55:329, 1951.
31. Cogan DG, Kinsey VE: The cornea, V, Physiologic aspects, Arch Ophthalmol 28:661, 1942.
32. Collin HB, Kenyon KR, Rowsey JJ: Lymphatic vessels in chemically burned human corneas, Cornea 5:223, 1986.
33. Crosson CE, Klyce SD, Beuerman RW: Epithelial wound closure in the rabbit cornea, Invest Ophthalmol Vis Sci 27:464, 1986.
34. Dabezies OH: Contact lenses. The CLAO guide to basic science and clinical practice, Boston, Little, Brown. 1989.
35. Davison PF, Galbavy EJ: Connective tissue remodeling in corneal and scleral wounds, Invest Ophthalmol Vis Sci 27:1478, 1986.
36. Deg JK, Zavala EY, Binder PS: Delayed corneal wound healing following radial keratotomy, Ophthalmol 92:734, 1985.
37. Deutsch TA, Hughes WF: Suppressive effects of indomethacin on thermally induced neovascularization of rabbit corneas, Am J Ophthalmol 87:536, 1979.
38. Dikstein S, Maurice DM: The metabolic basis to the fluid pump in the cornea, J Physiol 221:29, 1972.
39. Doane MG, Jensen AD, Dohlman CH: Penetration routes of topically applied eye medications, Am J Ophthalmol 85:303, 1978.
40. Dohlman CH, Hedbys BO, Mishima S: The swelling pressure of the cornea, Invest Ophthalmol Vis Sci 1:158, 1962.
41. Donn A, Maurice DM, Mills NL: Studies in the living

cornea *in vitro*. II, The active transport of sodium across the epithelium, Arch Ophthalmol 62:748, 1959.

42. Duffin RM, Weissman BA, Glasser DB, et al: Flurbiprofen in the treatment of corneal neovascularization induced by contact lenses, Am J Ophthalmol 93:607, 1982.

43. Edelhauser HF, et al: Intraocular irrigating solutions, their effect on the corneal endothelium, Arch Ophthalmol 94:648, 1975.

44. Edelhauser HF, et al: The comparative toxicity of intraocular irrigating solutions on the corneal endothelium, Am J Ophthalmol 81:473, 1976.

45. Edelhauser HF, et al: Corneal edema and the intraocular use of epinephrine, Am J Ophthalmol 93:327, 1982.

46. Edelhauser HF, et al: The effect of thiol oxidation of glutathione with diamide on corneal endothelial function, junctional complexes and microfilaments, J Cell Biol 68:567, 1976.

47. Edward DP, Yue BYJJ, Sugar J, et al: Heterogeneity in macular corneal dystrophy, Arch Ophthalmol 106:1579, 1988.

48. Efron N, Carney LG: Oxygen levels beneath the closed eyelid, Invest Ophthalmol Vis Sci 18:93, 1979.

49. Elliott GF, Goodfellow JM, Woolgen AE: Swelling studies of bovine corneal stroma without bounding membranes, J Physiol 298:453, 1980.

50. Epstein RJ, Halkias A, Stulting RD, et al: Corneal opacities and anterior segment anomalies in DBA/2 mice, Cornea 5:95, 1986.

51. Epstein RJ, Hendricks RL, Stulting RD: Interleukin 2 induces corneal neovascularization in A/J mice, Cornea 9:318, 1990.

52. Epstein RJ, Hughes WF: Lymphocyte-induced corneal neovascularization: a morphologic assessment, Invest Ophthalmol Vis Sci 21:87, 1981.

53. Epstein RJ, Stulting RD: Corneal neovascularization induced by stimulated lymphocytes in inbred mice, Invest Ophthalmol Vis Sci, 28:1508, 1987.

54. Epstein RJ, Stulting RD: Lymphocyte-induced corneal neovascularization in inbred mice, Invest Ophthalmol Vis Sci 28:61, 1987.

55. Epstein RJ, Stulting RD, Hendricks RL, et al: Corneal neovascularization, pathogenesis and inhibition, Cornea 6:250, 1987.

56. Farrell RA, McCally RL, Tatham PER: Wave-length dependencies of light scattering in normal and cold swollen rabbit corneas and their structural implications, J Physiol 233:589, 1973.

57. Fatt I, Goldstick TK: Dynamics of water transport in swelling membranes, J Colloidal Sci 20:434, 1965.

58. Fischbarg J: Active and passive properties of rabbit corneal endothelium, Exp Eye Res 15:615, 1973.

59. Folkman J, Klagsbrun M: Angiogenic factors, Science 235:442, 1987.

60. Folkman J, Klagsbrun M, Sasse J, et al: A heparin-binding angiogenic protein-basic fibroblast growth factor is stored within basement membrane, Am J Pathol 130:393, 1988.

61. Folkman J, Weisz PB, Joullie MM, et al: Control of angiogenesis with synthetic heparin substitutes, Science 243:1490, 1989.

62. Foster CS, Forstot SL, Wilson LA: Mortality rate in rheumatoid arthritis patients developing necrotizing scleritis or peripheral ulcerative keratitis, Ophthalmol 91:1253, 1984.

63. Foster CS, Wilson LA, Ekins MB: Immunosuppressive therapy for progressive ocular cicatricial pemphigoid, Ophthalmol 89:340, 1982.

64. Friedenwald JS, Buscke W: Mitotic and wound healing activities of the corneal epithelium, Arch Ophthalmol 32:410, 1944.

65. Friedman MH, Green K: Swelling rate of corneal stroma, Exp Eye Res 12:239, 1971.

66. Fullard RJ, Wilson GS: Investigation of sloughed corneal epithelial cells collected by non-invasive irrigation of the corneal surface, Curr Eye Res 5:847, 1986.

67. Gachon AM, Verrelli P, Betail G, et al: Immunological and electrophoretic studies of human tear proteins, Exp Eye Res 29:539, 1979.

68. Gallar J, et al: Effects of capsaicin on corneal wound healing, Invest Ophthalmol Vis Sci 31:1968, 1990.

69. Geiger B, et al: Immunoelectron microscope studies of membrane microfilament interactions: distributions of α-actinin, tropomyosin and vinculin in intestinal brush border and chicken gizzard smooth muscle cells, J Cell Biol 91:614, 1981.

70. Geroski DH, Edelhauser HF: Quantitation of Na/K ATPase pump sites in the rabbit corneal endothelium, Invest Ophthalmol Vis Sci 25:1056, 1984.

71. Geroski DH, Kies JC, Edelhauser HF: The effects of ouabain on endothelial function in human and rabbit corneas, Curr Eye Res 3:331, 1984.

72. Geroski DH, Matsuda M, Edelhauser HF: Pump function of the human corneal endothelium; effects of age and corneal guttata, Ophthalmol 92:759, 1985.

73. Gipson IK, Kiorpes TC: Epithelial sheet movement: protein and glycoprotein synthesis, Dev Biol 92:259, 1982.

74. Gipson IK, Spurr-Michaud SJ, Tisdale AS: Anchoring fibrils form a complex network in human and rabbit corneas, Invest Ophthalmol Vis Sci 28:212, 1987.

75. Gipson IK, Spurr-Michaud SJ, Tisdale AJ: Hemidesmosomes and anchoring fibril collagen appear synchronously during development and wound healing, Dev Biol 126:253, 1988.

76. Gipson IK, et al: Hemidesmosome formation *in vitro*, J Cell Biol 97:849, 1983.

77. Gipson IK, et al: Reassembly of the anchoring structures of the corneal epithelium during wound repair in the rabbit, Invest Ophthalmol Vis Sci 30:425, 1989.

78. Glasser DB, et al: Effect of intraocular irrigating solutions on the corneal endothelium after anterior chamber irrigation, Am J Ophthalmol 99:321, 1985.

79. Goldman JN, Benedek GB: The relationship between morphology and transparency in the nonswelling corneal stroma of the shark, Invest Ophthalmol 6:574, 1967.

80. Goldman JN, Benedek GB, Dohlman CH, et al: Structural alterations affecting transparency in swollen human corneas, Invest Ophthalmol 7:501, 1968.

81. Gonnering RS, et al: The pH tolerance of the rabbit and human corneal endothelium, Invest Ophthalmol Vis Sci 18:373, 1979.

82. Goodman WM, SundarRaj N, Garone M, et al: Unique parameters in the healing of linear partial thickness penetrating corneal incisions in rabbit: immunohistochemical evaluation, Curr Eye Res 8:305, 1989.

83. Gospodarowicz D, et al: The identification and localization of fibronectin in cultured corneal endothelial cells: cell surface polarity and physiological implications, Exp Eye Res 29:485, 1979.

84. Gosset AR, and Dohlman CH. The tensile strength of corneal wounds, Arch Ophthalmol 79:595, 1968.

85. Green K, et al: Rabbit endothelial response to ophthalmic preservatives, Arch Ophthalmol 95:2218, 1977.

86. Green K, et al: Chlordexidine effects on corneal epithelium and endothelium, Arch Ophthalmol 98:1273, 1980.

87. Hamano H, Hori M, Hamano T, et al: Effect of contact lens wear on the mitosis of corneal epithelial cells and the amount of lactate in aqueous humor, Jpn J Ophthalmol 27:451, 1983.

88. Hanna C, Bicknell DS, O'Brien J: Cell turnover in the adult human eye, Arch Ophthalmol 65:695, 1961.

89. Hanna C, O'Brien JE: Cell production and migration in the epithelium layer of the cornea, Arch Ophthalmol 64:536, 1960.

90. Harris JE, Nordquist LT: Hydration of the cornea, I, The transport of water from the cornea, Am J Ophthalmol 40:100, 1955.

91. Hay ED: Development of the vertebrate cornea, Int Rev Cytol 63:263, 1980.

92. Haynes WL, Proia AD, Klintworth GK: Effect of inhibitors of arachidonic acid metabolism on corneal neovascularization in the rat, Invest Ophthalmol Vis Sci 30:1588, 1989.

93. Hazlett CD, et al: Desquamation of the corneal epithelium in the immature mouse: a scanning and transmission microscopy study, Exp Eye Res 31:21, 1980.

94. Hedbys BO: The role of polysaccharides in corneal swelling, Exp Eye Res 1:81, 1961.

95. Hedbys BO, Dohlman CH: A new method for determination of the swelling pressure of the corneal stroma in vitro, Exp Eye Res 2:122, 1963.

96. Hedbys BO, Mishima S, Maurice DM: The imbibition pressure of the corneal stroma, Exp Eye Res 2:99, 1963.

97. Hendricks RL, Barfknecht CF, Schoenwald RD, et al: The effect of flurbiprofen on herpes simplex virus type 1 stromal keratitis in mice, Invest Ophthalmol Vis Sci 31:1503, 1990.

98. Hill RM, Fatt I: How dependent is the cornea on the atmosphere? J Am Optom Assoc 35:873, 1964.

99. Hodson S, Miller F: The bicarbonate ion pump in the endothelium which regulates the hydration of the rabbit cornea, J Physiol 236:271, 1974.

100. Hodson SA, Wigham CG: Effect of glutathione on human corneal transendothelial potential difference, J Physiol 301:34, 1980.

101. Hogan MJ, Alvarado JA, Weddell E: Histology of the human eye, Philadelphia, WB Saunders. 1971.

102. Holden BA, Polse KA, Fonn D, et al: Effects of cataract surgery on corneal function, Invest Ophthalmol Vis Sci 22:343, 1982.

103. Holden BA, Sweeney DF: The oxygen tension and temperature of the superior palpebral conjunctiva, Acta Ophthalmol 63:100, 1985.

104. Holden BA, Sweeney DF, Vannas A, et al: Effects of long-term extended contact lens wear on the human cornea, Invest Ophthalmol Vis Sci 26:1489, 1985.

105. Huff J, Green K: Demonstration of active sodium transport across the isolated rabbit corneal endothelium, Curr Eye Res 1:113, 1981.

106. Hull DS, et al: Corneal endothelial bicarbonate transport and the effect of carbonic anhydrase inhibitors on endothelial permeability, fluxes and corneal thickness, Invest Ophthalmol Vis Sci 16:883, 1977.

107. Hyldahl L: Factor VIII expression in the human embryonic eye; differences between endothelial cells of different origin, Ophthalmologica 191:184, 1985.

108. Hyldahl L, Aspinall R, Watt FM: Immunolocalization of keratan sulphate in the human embryonic cornea and other foetal organs, J Cell Sci 80:181, 1986.

109. Ingber D, Folkman J: Inhibition of angiogenesis through modulation of collagen metabolism, Lab Invest 59:44, 1988.

110. Inomata H, Smelear GK, Polack FM: Corneal vascularization in experimental uveitis and graft rejection, Invest Ophthalmol Vis Sci 10:840, 1971.

111. Jentsch TJ, Keller SK, Wiederholt M: Ion transport in cultured bovine corneal endothelial cells, Curr Eye Res 4:361, 1985.

112. Johnson DH, Bourne WM, Campbell RJ: The ultrastructure of Descemet's membrane, I, Changes with age in normal corneas, Arch Ophthalmol 100:1942, 1982.

113. Joyce NC, Martin ED, Neufeld AH: Corneal endothelial wound closure in vitro; effects of EGF and/or indomethacin, Invest Ophthalmol Vis Sci 30:1548, 1989.

114. Joyce NC, Meklir B, Neufeld AH: In vitro pharmacologic separation of corneal endothelial migration and spreading responses, Invest Ophthalmol Vis Sci 31:1816, 1990.

115. Jumblatt MM, Neufeld AH: Characterization of cyclic AMP-mediated wound closure of the rabbit corneal epithelium, Curr Eye Res 1:189, 1981.

116. Junghaus BM, Collin HB: The limbal vascular response to corneal injury; an autoradiographic study, Cornea 8:141, 1989.

117. Kangas TA, Edelhauser HF, Twining SS, et al: Loss of stromal glycosaminoglycans during corneal edema, Invest Ophthalmol Vis Sci 31:1994, 1990.

118. Kaye G: Stereologic measurement of cell volume fraction of rabbit corneal stroma, Arch Ophthalmol 82:792, 1969.

119. Kenyon KR: Mesenchymal dysgenesis in Peters' anomaly, sclerocornea and congenital endothelial dystrophy, Exp Eye Res 21:125, 1975.

120. Kenyon KR: Ocular manifestations and pathology of systemic mucopolysaccharidoses, Birth Defects 12:133, 1976.

121. Kenyon KR: Recurrent corneal erosion: pathogenesis and therapy, Int Ophthalmol Clin 19(2):169, 1979.

122. Khodadoust AA, et al: Adhesion of regenerating corneal epithelium, Am J Ophthalmol 65:339, 1968.

123. Kilp H, Hersig-Salentin B, Framing D: Metabolites and enzymes in the corneal epithelium after extended contact lens wear; the effects of contact lenses on the normal physiology and anatomy of the cornea: symposium summary, Curr Eye Res 4:738, 1985.

124. Kinoshita S, Friend, J, Thoft RA: Sex chromatin of donor corneal epithelium in rabbits, Invest Ophthalmol Vis Sci 21:434, 1981.

125. Klintworth GK, Burger PC: Neovascularization of the

cornea: current concepts of its pathogenesis, Int Ophthalmol Clin 23:27, 1983.

126. Klintworth GK, Meyer R, Dennis R, et al: Macular corneal dystrophy—lack of keratan sulfate in serum and cornea, Ophthal Paed Genet 7:139, 1986.

127. Klyce SD: Electrical profiles in the corneal epithelium, J Physiol 226:407, 1977.

128. Klyce SD: Stromal lactate accumulation can account for corneal oedema osmotically following epithelial hypoxia in the rabbit, J Physiol 321:49, 1981.

129. Klyce SD, Beuerman RW, Crosson CE: Alteration of corneal epithelium in transport by sympathectomy, Invest Ophthalmol Vis Sci 26:434, 1985.

130. Klyce SD, Beuerman RW: Structure and function of the cornea, In Kaufman HE, et al: The cornea, New York, Churchill Livingstone, 1988, p 3.

131. Klyce SD, Crosson CE: Transport processes across the rabbit corneal epithelium: a review, Curr Eye Res 4:323, 1985.

132. Klyce SD, Dohlman CH, Tolpin DW: In vivo determination of corneal swelling pressure, Exp Eye Res 11:220, 1971.

133. Klyce SD, Neufeld AH, Zadunaisky JA: The activation of chloride transport by epinephrine and Db cyclic-AMP in the cornea of the rabbit, Invest Ophthalmol 12:127, 1973.

134. Koester CJ, et al: Wide-field specular microscopy; clinical and research applications, Ophthalmol 87:849, 1980.

135. Kuang K, et al: Effects of ambient bicarbonate, phosphate and carbonic anhydrase inhibitors on fluid transport across rabbit cornea endothelium, Exp Eye Res 50:487, 1990.

136. Kupfer C, Kaiser-Kupfer MI: Observations on the development of the anterior chamber angle with reference to the pathogenesis of congenital glaucomas, Am J Ophthalmol 88:424, 1979.

137. Kurpakas MA, Stock EL, Jones JRC: Expression of the 55-kD/64-kD corneal keratins in ocular surface epithelium, Invest Ophthalmol Vis Sci 31:448, 1990.

138. Kuwabara T, Perkins DG, Cogan DG: Sliding of the epithelium in experimental corneal wounds, Invest Ophthalmol 15:4, 1976.

139. Laing RH, Sandstrom MM, Leibowitz HM: *In vivo* photomicrography of the corneal epithelium, Arch Ophthalmol 93:143, 1975.

140. Lee D, Wilson G: Non-uniform swelling properties of the corneal stroma, Curr Eye Res 1:457, 1981.

141. Lemp MA: Cornea and sclera, Arch Ophthalmol 94:473, 1976.

142. Lemp MA, Holly FJ, Iwata S, et al: The precorneal tear film, I, Factors in spreading and maintaining a continuous tear film over the corneal surface, Arch Ophthalmol 83:89, 1970.

143. Lim JJ: Na^+ transport across the rabbit corneal endothelium, Curr Eye Res 1:255, 1981.

144. López Bernal D, Ubels JL: Quantitative evaluation of the corneal epithelial barrier: effect of artificial tears and preservatives, Curr Eye Res 10:645, 1991.

145. Lutty GA, Liu SH, Prendergast RA: Angiogenic lymphokines of activated T-cell origin, Invest Ophthalmol Vis Sci 24:1595, 1983.

146. MacDonald JM, Geroski DH, Edelhauser HF: Effect of inflammation on the corneal endothelial pump and barrier, Curr Eye Res 6:1125, 1987.

147. MacRae SM, et al: The effects of hard and soft contact lens wear on the corneal endothelium, Am J Ophthalmol 102:50, 1986.

148. Madigan MC, Penfold PL, Holden BA, et al: Ultrastructural features of contact lens-induced deep corneal neovascularization and associated stromal leukocytes, Cornea 9:144, 1990.

149. Malley DS, Steinert RF, Puliafito CA, et al: Immunofluorescence study of corneal wound healing after excimer laser anterior keratectomy in the monkey eye, Arch Ophthalmol 108:1316, 1990.

150. Mandell RB, Farrell R: Corneal swelling at low atmospheric oxygen pressures, Invest Ophthalmol Vis Sci 19:697, 1980.

151. Mandell RB, Fatt I: Thinning of the human cornea on awakening, Nature 208:292, 1965.

152. Matsuda M, et al: Cellular migration and morphology in corneal endothelial wound repair, Invest Ophthalmol Vis Sci 26:443, 1985.

153. Matsuda M, Suda T, Manabe R: Quantitative analysis of endothelial mosaic pattern changes in anterior keratoconus, Am J Ophthalmol 98:43, 1984.

154. Matsuda M, Suda T, Manabe R: Serial alterations in endothelial cell shape and pattern after intraocular surgery. Am J Ophthalmol 98:313, 1984.

155. Matsuda M, Ubels JL, Edelhauser HF: A larger corneal epithelial wound closes at a faster rate, Invest Ophthalmol Vis Sci 26:897, 1985.

156. Matsuda M, Ubels JL, Edelhauser HF: Kinetics of corneal wound healing, in Brightbill FS, ed: Corneal surgery, theory, technique and tissue, St Louis, CV Mosby, 1986, p 603.

157. Maurice DM: The permeability to sodium ions of the living rabbit cornea, J Physiol (Lond) 112:367, 1951.

158. Maurice DM: The location of the fluid pump in the cornea, J Physiol 221:43, 1972.

159. Maurice DM: Structures and fluids involved in the penetration of topically applied drugs, Int Ophthalmol Clin 20:7, 1980.

160. Maurice DM, Mishima S: Ocular pharmacokinetics, in Sears, ML, ed: Pharmacology of the eye, New York, Springer-Verlag, 1984.

161. Maurice DM: The structure and transparency of the cornea, J Physiol 136:263, 1957.

162. McLaughlin BJ, et al: Freeze fracture quantitative comparison of rabbit corneal epithelial and endothelial membranes, Curr Eye Res 4:951, 1985.

163. Meek KM, Glamires T, Elliot GF, et al: The organization of collagen fibrils in the corneal stroma: A synchrotron X-ray diffraction study, Curr Eye Res 6:841, 1987.

164. Meyers LA, Ubels JL, Edelhauser HF: Corneal endothelial morphology in the rat; effects of aging, diabetes and topical aldose reductase inhibitor treatment, Invest Ophthalmol Vis Sci 29:940, 1988.

165. Mishima S, Hedbys BO: The permeability of the corneal epithelium and endothelium, Exp Eye Res 6:10, 1967.

166. Mondino BJ, Laheji AK, Adamu SA: Ocular immunity to staphylococcus aureus, Invest Ophthalmol Vis Sci 28:560, 1987.

167. Murphy C, Alvarado J, Juster R, et al: Prenatal and postnatal cellularity of the human corneal endothelium; a quantitative histologic study, Invest Ophthalmol Vis Sci 25:312, 1984.

168. Muthukkaruppan VR, Auerbach R: Angiogenesis in the mouse cornea, Science 205:1416, 1979.

169. Nakazawa K, Hassell JR, Hascall VC, et al: Defective processing of keratan sulfate in macular corneal dystrophy, J Biol Chem 259:1351, 1984.

170. Newsome DA, Gross J, Hassell JR: Human corneal stroma contains three distinct collagens, Invest Ophthalmol Vis Sci 22:376, 1982.

171. Niederkorn JY, Ubelaker JE, Martin JE: Vascularization of corneas of hairless mutant mice, Invest Ophthalmol Vis Sci 31:948, 1990.

172. Nikolic L, Friend J, Taylor S, et al: Inhibition of vascularization in rabbit corneas by heparin: cortisone pellets, Invest Ophthalmol Vis Sci 27:449, 1986.

173. Nishida T, et al: Fibronectin: a new therapy for trophic corneal ulcer, Arch Ophthalmol 101:1046, 1983.

174. O'Leary DJ, Millodot M: Abnormal oxygen fragility in diabetes and contact lens wear, Acta Ophthalmol 59:827, 1981.

175. O'Neal MR, Polse KA: In vivo assessment of mechanisms controlling corneal hydration, Invest Ophthalmol Vis Sci 26:849, 1985.

176. Ohashi Y, Motokura M, Kinoshita Y, et al: Presence of epidermal growth factor in human tears, Invest Ophthalmol Vis Sci 30:1879, 1989.

177. Osgood TB, et al: Evaluation of ocular irritancy of hair care products, J Toxicol Cut and Ocular Toxicol 9:37, 1990.

178. Otori T: Electrolyte content of the rabbit cornea, Exp Eye Res 6:356, 1967.

179. Perez E, et al: Effects of chronic sympathetic stimulation on cornea wound healing, Invest Ophthalmol Vis Sci 28:221, 1987.

180. Pfister RR: The normal surface of corneal epithelium: a scanning electron microscope study, Invest Ophthalmol 12:654, 1973.

181. Pfister RR: The healing of corneal epithelial abrasions in the rabbit: a scanning electron microscope study, Invest Ophthalmol 14:648, 1975.

182. Pfister RR, Haddox JL, Paterson CA: The efficacy of sodium citrate treatment of severe alkali burns of the eye is influenced by the route of administration, Cornea 1:205, 1982.

183. Pitts DG: The human ultraviolet action spectrum, Am J Optom Arch Am Acad Optom 51:946, 1974.

184. Poggio EC, Glynn RJ, Schein OD, et al: The incidence of ulcerative keratitis among users of daily wear and extended wear contact lenses, N Engl J Med 321:779, 1989.

185. Polse KA, Mandell RB: Etiology of corneal striae accompanying hydrogel lens wear, Invest Ophthalmol 75:557, 1976.

186. Pouliquero Y, Hamada R, Giraud JP, et al: Etude analytique et statistique des lamelles, des kératocytes, des fibrilles de collagéne de la région de la cornée humaine normale (microscopie optique et électronique), Arch Ophthalmol (Paris) 32:563, 1972.

187. Quantock AJ, Meek KM, Ridgway AEA, et al: Macular corneal dystrophy: reduction in both corneal thickness and collagen interfibrillar spacing, Curr Eye Res 9:393, 1990.

188. Rae JL, Dewey J, Cooper K: Properties of single potassium-selective ionic channels from the apical membrane of the rabbit cornea endothelium, Exp Eye Res 49:591, 1989.

189. Rae JL, et al: Dye and electrical coupling between cells of the rabbit corneal epithelium, Curr Eye Res 8:859, 1989.

190. Rae JL, et al: Single potassium channels in corneal epithelium, Invest Ophthalmol Vis Sci 31:1799, 1990.

191. Rao GN, et al: Morphological appearance of the healing corneal endothelium, Arch Ophthalmol 96:2027, 1978.

192. Rao GN, et al: Morphologic variation in graft endothelium, Arch Ophthalmol 98:1403, 1980.

193. Riley MV: Glucose and oxygen utilization of the cornea, Exp Eye Res 8:193, 1969.

194. Riley MV, Meyer RF, Yates EM: Glutathione in the aqueous humor of humans and other species, Invest Ophthalmol Vis Sci 19:94, 1980.

195. Rodrigues M, Ben-Zvi A, Krachmer JH, et al: Suprabasal expression of a 64-kilodalton keratin (no. 3) in developing human corneal epithelium, Differentiation 34:60, 1987.

196. Rodrigues MM, Krachmer JH: Recent advances in corneal stromal dystrophies, Cornea 7:19, 1988.

197. Rozenman Y, Donnenfeld ED, Cohen EJ, et al: Contact lens-related deep stromal neovascularization, Am J Ophthalmol 107:27, 1989.

198. Savage CP Jr, Cohen S: Proliferation of corneal epithelium induced by epidermal growth factor, Exp Eye Res 15:361, 1973.

199. Schermer A, Galvin S, Sun T-T: Differentiation related expression of a major 64 k corneal keratin *in vivo* and in culture suggests a limbal location of corneal epithelial stem cells, J Cell Biol 103:49, 1986.

200. Schimmelpfennig B, et al: Tissue storage, in Brightbill FS, ed: Corneal surgery: theory, technique and tissue, St Louis, CV Mosby, 1986, p 60.

201. Schultz RO, Glasser DB, Matsuda M, et al: Response of the corneal endothelium to cataract surgery, Arch Ophthalmol 104:1164, 1986.

202. Schultz RO, Matsuda M, Yee RW, et al: Corneal endothelial changes in type I and type II diabetes mellitus, Am J Ophthalmol 98:401, 1984.

203. Scott JE, Haigh M: "Small"- proteoglycan: collagen interactions: keratan sulphate proteoglycan associates with rabbit corneal collagen fibrils at the "a" and "c" bands, Biosci Rep 5:765, 1985.

204. Sevel D: A reappraisal of the development of the eyelids, Eye 2:123, 1988.

205. Sharma A, Coles WH: Kinetics of corneal epithelial maintenance and graft loss. Invest Ophthalmol Vis Sci 30:1962, 1989.

206. Simonsen AH, Andreassen TT, Bendix K: The healing strength of corneal wounds in the human eye, Exp Eye Res 35:287, 1982.

207. Sliney DH: Eye protective techniques for bright light, Ophthalmol 90:937, 1983.

208. Smelser GK, Ozanics V: Importance of atmospheric oxygen for maintenance of the optical properties of the human cornea, Science 115:140, 1952.

209. Smolek MK, McCarey BE: Interlamellar adhesive strength in human eyebank corneas, Invest Ophthalmol Vis Sci 31:1087, 1990.

210. Soirbrane G, Jerdan J, Karpouzas I, et al: Binding of basic fibroblast growth factor to normal and neovascularized rabbit cornea, Invest Ophthalmol Vis Sci 31:323, 1990.

211. Soong HK: Vinculin in focal cell-to-substrate attachments of spreading corneal epithelial cells, Arch Ophthalmol 105:1129, 1987.

212. Soong HK, Cintron C: Different corneal epithelial healing mechanisms in rat and rabbit: role of actin and calmodulin, Invest Ophthalmol Vis Sci 26:838, 1985.

213. Stiemke MM, Romcen RJ, Palmer ML, et al: Sodium activities and concentrations of the corneal stroma, aqueous humor and plasma in the presence and absence of a transparent cornea, Invest Ophthalmol Vis Sci 32 (Suppl):1065, 1991.

214. Suvarnamani C, Halperin EC, Proia AD, et al: The effects of total lymphoid irradiation upon corneal vascularization in the rat following chemical cautery, Radiation Res 117:259, 1989.

215. Tervo T, Palkema A: Electron microscopic localization of adenosine triphosphatase (NaK-ATPase) activity in the rat cornea, Exp Eye Res 21:269, 1975.

216. Thoft RA, Friend J: Biochemical transformation of regenerating ocular surface epithelium, Invest Ophthalmol 16:14, 1977.

217. Thoft RA, Friend J: The X,Y,Z hypothesis of corneal epithelial maintenance, Invest Ophthalmol Vis Sci 24:142, 1983.

218. Tisdale AS, Spurr-Michaud SJ, Rodrigues M, et al: Development of the anchoring structures of the epithelium in rabbit and human fetal corneas, Invest Ophthalmol Vis Sci 29:727, 1988.

219. Tripathi RC, Raja SC, Tripathi BJ: Prospects for epidermal growth factor in the management of corneal disorders, Surv Ophthalmol 34:457, 1990.

220. Tseng SCG, et al: Expression of specific keratin markers by rabbit corneal, conjunctival and esophageal epithelium during vitamin A deficiency, J Cell Biol 99:2279, 1984.

221. Ubels JL, et al: The efficacy of retinoic acid ointment for treatment of xerophthalmia and corneal epithelial wounds, Curr Eye Res 4:1049, 1985.

222. Uusitalo H, Kootila K, Palkema A: Calcitonin gene-related peptide (CGRP) immunoreactive sensory nerves in the human and guinea pig uvea and cornea, Exp Eye Res 48:467, 1989.

223. Van Horn DL, et al: Effect of the ophthalmic preservative thimerosal on rabbit and human corneal endothelium, Invest Ophthalmol Vis Sci 16:273, 1977.

224. Van Horn DL, et al: Regenerative capacity of the corneal endothelium in the rabbit and cat, Invest Ophthalmol Vis Sci 16:597, 1977.

225. Vannas A, Holden BA, Sweeney DF, Polse KA: Surgical incision alters the swelling response of the human cornea, Invest Ophthalmol Vis Sci 26:864, 1985.

226. Verbey NLJ, van Haeringen NJ, de Jong PRVM: Modulation of immunogenic keratitis in rabbits by topical administration of inhibitors of lipoxygenase and cyclo-oxygenase, Curr Eye Res 7:361, 1988.

227. Waring GO, et al: The corneal endothelium; normal and pathologic structure and function, Ophthalmol 89:531, 1982.

228. Wechsler S: Striate corneal lines, Am J Optom Physiol Optics 51:851, 1974.

229. Weissman BA, Selzer K, Duffin RM, et al: Oxygen permeability of rabbit and human corneal stroma, Invest Ophthalmol Vis Sci 24:645, 1983.

230. Whikehart DR, Soppet DR: Activities of transport enzymes located in the plasma membranes of corneal endothelial cells, Invest Ophthalmol Vis Sci 21:819, 1981.

231. Wiederholt M, Koch M: Effect of intraocular irrigating solutions on intracellular membrane potentials and swelling rate of isolated human and rabbit cornea, Invest Ophthalmol Vis Sci 18:313, 1979.

232. Wolosin JM: Regeneration of resistance and ion transport in rabbit corneal epithelium after induced surface cell exfoliation, J Membrane Biol 104:45, 1988.

233. Yang CJ, SundarRaj N, Thonar EJ-MA, et al: Immunohistochemical evidence of heterogeneity in macular corneal dystrophy, Am J Ophthalmol 106:65, 1988.

234. Yee RW, et al: Changes in the normal corneal endothelial cellular pattern as a function of age, Curr Eye Res 4:671, 1985.

235. Yee RW, et al: Correlation of corneal endothelial pump site density, barrier function and morphology in wound repair, Invest Ophthalmol Vis Sci 26:1191, 1985.

236. Yee RW, Matsuda M, Edelhauser HF: Wide-field endothelial counting panels, Am J Ophthalmol 99:596, 1985.

237. Ytteborg J, Dohlman CH: Corneal edema and intraocular pressure, II, Clinical results, Arch Ophthalmol 74:477, 1965.

238. Zadunaisky JA: Active transport of chloride across the cornea, Nature (London) 209:1136, 1977.

239. Zantos SG, Holden BA: Transient endothelial changes soon after wearing soft contact lenses, Am J Optom Physiol Optics 54:856, 1977.

240. Ziche M, Alessandri G, Gullino PM: Gangliosides promote the angiogenic response. Lab Invest 61:629, 1989.

241. Ziche M, Jones J, Gullion DM: Role of prostaglandin E_1 and copper in angiogenesis, J Natl Cancer Inst 69:475, 1982.

242. Zieske JD, Gipson IK: Protein synthesis during corneal epithelial wound healing, Invest Ophthalmol Vis Sci 27:1, 1986.

243. Zieske JD, Bukusoglu G, Gipson IK: Enhancement of vinculin synthesis by migrating stratified squamous epithelium, J Cell Biol 109:571, 1989.

244. Zimmermann DR, Trueb B, Winterhalter KH, et al: Type VI collagen is a major component of the human cornea, FEBS Letters 197:55, 1986.

245. Zinn KM, Mockel-Pohl, S: Fine structure of the developing cornea, Int Ophthalmol Clin 15:19, 1975.

Somatic Sensations from the Eye

HAROLD BURTON, Ph.D.

A consideration of the somatic sensations from the eye and its adnexa is essential for understanding the role these sensations play in preserving vision, for making appropriate diagnoses when particular somatosensory losses or alterations indicate various pathologic conditions, and for explaining the specialized role played by the afferent endings and the central nervous system connections that are associated with some of the ocular tissues. This chapter presents the gross and microscopic neuroanatomy, physiology, and some clinicopathologic aspects of the somatic sensory structures of the eye and neighboring tissues.

Like the rest of the body, the eye is richly innervated with receptors that collectively mediate sensations of touch, light pressure, cold, warmth, and pain. However, sensations from all parts of the eye do not encompass the full range of somatosensory perceptions available from other parts of the body. For example, the somatic innervation of the cornea, iris, conjunctiva, and sclera differs from other parts of the body to such an extent that the sensations arising from these tissues are principally pain or irritation. The extent that sensations of touch, cold, or warmth can be appreciated from the cornea has been subject to some debate (see below). Limited sensations also arise from touching the lens, which has no sensory endings. In addition, innervation of other tissues surrounding or in some cases quite distant from the orbit derives from nerve branches to the eye so that pathology in the eye sometimes can be

expressed in or through these distant connections.

TRIGEMINAL NERVE: BRANCHES TO THE EYE AND SURROUNDING TISSUE

Almost all nerve terminals originating from somatosensory receptors throughout the face, including those from the eye, gather into the sensory root of the trigeminal nerve. This root arises from central processes of the semilunar or gasserian ganglion. The trigeminal root may be regarded as a compressed group of afferent dorsal roots, and the semilunar ganglion contains cell bodies from three principal peripheral divisions of the trigeminal nerve: ophthalmic, maxillary, and mandibular nerves. Respective peripheral branches for each of these nerves will be considered only as they relate to somatic sensations from the eye.

Ophthalmic nerve

This purely sensory nerve arises from the anteromedial portion of the trigeminal ganglion. At the point where it pierces and travels anteriorly in the lateral wall of the cavernous sinus, several small filaments leave the ophthalmic nerve to course with the extraocular motor nerves to provide sensory innervation for the muscles supplied by these nerves. Anteriorly, but still where the ophthalmic nerve lies next to the cavernous sinus, additional branches form a plexus of nerves known as the recurrent ophthalmic or tentorial nerves (Fig. 4-1). These supply the dura around the crista galli, cavernous

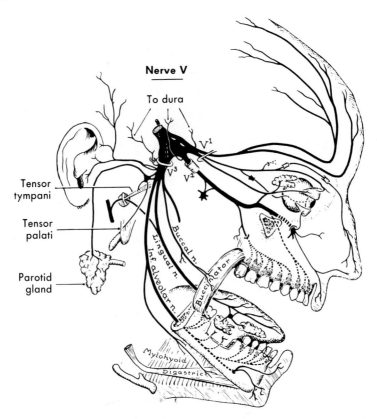

FIG. 4-1 Schematic illustration of cutaneous distribution of the trigeminal nerve. V^1, ophthalmic nerve; V^2, maxillary nerve; V^3, mandibular nerve. Note that each division supplies small twigs to dura mater close to point where main nerve exits from trigeminal ganglion. For ophthalmic nerve these twigs form into the recurrent ophthalmic or tentorial nerve shown as the branches coursing superior and posterior to the innervation for the eye (see text). (From Grant JCB: Grant's atlas of anatomy, 5th ed, Baltimore, Williams & Wilkins, 1962.)

sinus, tentorium, posterior portion of the falx, and inferior sagittal, longitudinal, transverse, and confluence of the sinuses. Some of these branches may supply pain fibers to the major cerebral arteries. Of note is that stimulation of these nerves, either directly or by mechanical disturbance of the dura or the blood vessels with which they are associated, produces pain referred to the eye and forehead.

The ophthalmic nerve divides into three major branches near the superior orbital fissure at the anterior end of the cavernous sinus: the frontal, lacrimal, and nasociliary nerves. Each of these nerves further subdivides into terminal branches that innervate the eye and surrounding tissues (Fig. 4-2).

Frontal nerve

The frontal nerve is the largest branch of the ophthalmic nerve. It enters the orbit superior to the rectus and levator palpebrae superioris muscles and runs forward obliquely just below the periosteum. Midway through the orbit it divides into a *medial supratrochlear nerve* and a larger *lateral supraorbital nerve.* These nerves exit from the orbital cavity through the orbital septum. The supratrochlear nerve supplies skin at the base of the nose, adjoining medial part of the forehead, and medial part of the upper eyelid. The supraorbital nerve, which divides into medial and lateral branches and exits via the supraorbital notch, supplies the middle two thirds of the upper eyelid and superior conjunctiva, portions of the frontal sinus, and skin on the forehead and scalp as far back as the vertex (Fig. 4-3).

Lacrimal nerve

The lacrimal nerve is the smallest branch of the ophthalmic nerve. It courses laterally within the orbital cavity above and along the upper border of the lateral rectus muscle. It divides into two terminal divisions: one supplies sensory innervation to the lacrimal gland and lateral portion

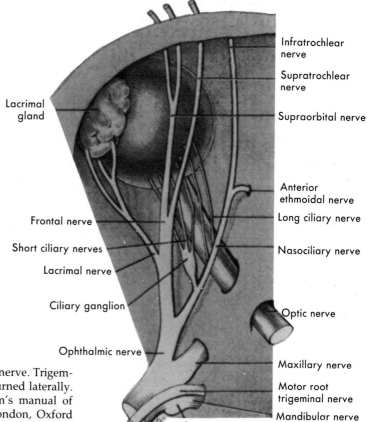

Lacrimal gland

Infratrochlear nerve

Supratrochlear nerve

Supraorbital nerve

Anterior ethmoidal nerve

Long ciliary nerve

Nasociliary nerve

Frontal nerve

Short ciliary nerves

Lacrimal nerve

Ciliary ganglion

Optic nerve

Ophthalmic nerve

Maxillary nerve

Motor root trigeminal nerve

Mandibular nerve

Trigeminal ganglion

FIG. 4-2 Branches of left ophthalmic nerve. Trigeminal nerve and ganglion have been turned laterally. (From Romanes GJ, ed: Cunningham's manual of practical anatomy, 14th ed, vol 3, London, Oxford University Press, 1979.)

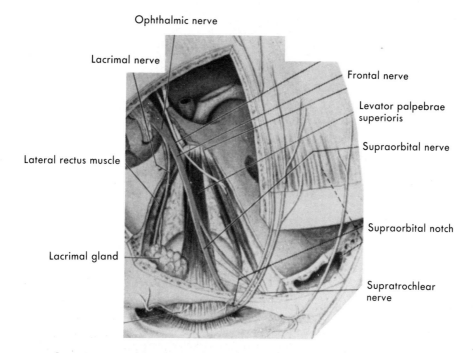

Ophthalmic nerve

Lacrimal nerve

Frontal nerve

Levator palpebrae superioris

Supraorbital nerve

Lateral rectus muscle

Supraorbital notch

Lacrimal gland

Supratrochlear nerve

FIG. 4-3 Superior view of distribution of ophthalmic nerve branches to the eye. The lacrimal and frontal nerves run through the orbit close to the periosteum. The lacrimal nerve runs along the lateral wall; frontal nerve crosses obliquely from lateral side above levator palpebrae superioris (see Fig. 4-4). Frontal nerve divides into supratrochlear and supraorbital nerves about half-way through the orbit before terminating. The lacrimal nerve receives a communication from the zygomaticotemporal nerve, a branch of the maxillary nerve. (Redrawn from Warwick R, Williams PL, Gray's anatomy, 35th ed, Philadelphia, WB Saunders, 1973.)

of the upper eyelid and conjunctiva; one (inferior) anastomoses with the zygomaticotemporal branch from the maxillary nerve to innervate skin around the temple of the forehead.

Nasociliary nerve

The nasociliary nerve, which has five divisions, conveys the principal somatosensory inputs from the eye plus sensory input from the skin and mucous membranes of the nose. It enters the orbit inferior to other branches of the ophthalmic nerve, passes through the common tendinous ring of the rectus muscles and between the two divisions of the oculomotor nerve, and courses obliquely and medially beneath the superior rectus muscle (Fig. 4-4). Before crossing to the medial side of the optic nerve, it first gives origin to the sensory root, which passes through the ciliary ganglion to contribute to the *short ciliary nerves*. When the nasociliary nerve reaches the medial side of the optic nerve, two to three slender branches arise to form the *long ciliary nerves*; these course to the eye together with the optic nerve. They penetrate the eye and pass between the sclera and choroid to supply the cornea, iris, and sensory fibers to the ciliary body, trabecular meshwork, and sclera. The third division from the nasociliary nerve is the *posterior ethmoidal nerve*; it supplies the posterior ethmoidal and sphenoidal sinuses. Near the medial border of the orbit the nasociliary nerve divides into the *infratrochlear* and *anterior ethmoidal nerves* in the vicinity of the superior oblique muscle. The infratrochlear nerve supplies skin at the medial angle of the eye and root of the nose, medial eyelid and conjunctiva, caruncle, lacrimal canaliculus, and lacrimal sac. The anterior ethmoidal nerve provides sensory input from the nasal cavity and skin on the distal part of the nose.

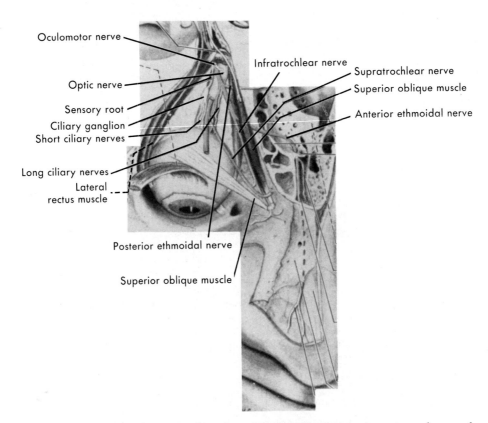

FIG. 4-4 Lateral view of the nerve branches to the eye. The intervening extraocular muscles have been removed to reveal distribution of nasociliary nerve within retrobulbar portion of the orbit. This nerve provides nearly all the somatosensory innervation of the eye (see text). Its first branch is the sensory root, which passes through the ciliary ganglion from which arise the mixed short ciliary nerves. The long ciliary, anterior ethmoidal, posterior ethmoidal (unlabeled branch between long ciliary and anterior ethmoidal n.) and infratrochlear nerves arise subsequently. (Redrawn from Warwick R, Williams PL, Gray's anatomy, 35th ed, Philadelphia, WB Saunders, 1973.)

Maxillary nerve

Only two branches of the maxillary nerve are related directly to sensory input from the eye. The *zygomatic nerve,* which enters the orbit through the inferior orbital fissure, supplies a branch, the *zygomaticotemporal nerve,* that anastomoses with the superficial extension of the lacrimal nerve along the side of the head. The *infraorbital nerve,* which also passes through the inferior orbital fissure, innervates the lower eyelid and inferior conjunctiva. It also anastomoses with the infratrochlear nerve to provide sensory input from the inferior medial corner of the eye.

Fixed peripheral boundaries for each of the trigeminal branches may, however, be less precise than previously suspected. For example, about 4% of cells of origin for corneal afferent fibers in cats reside in the maxillary division of the semilunar ganglion.[59] In monkeys Ruskell[75] has noted that one third of the innervation to the eye may come from an orbitociliary branch from the maxillary nerve. Similarly, in man observed preservation of some normal sensation in the distribution of a sectioned division of the trigeminal root could be explained as due to aberrant fibers between the trigeminal roots.[59]

Mandibular nerve

No branches from the mandibular nerve have terminations related to the eye.

INNERVATION OF THE CORNEA
Stromal plexus

In humans approximately 900 to 1200 small (0.5 to 5 μm) myelinated and unmyelinated axons from the ciliary nerves convey sensory signals from the cornea. The organization of the nerve supply to the cornea can be divided into several levels that are based on the different calibers of nerve fibers and bundles making up each plexus and on the locations of the plexus within the stroma and epithelium.[57,72,77,96] The axons first distribute radially around the periphery of the cornea in 70 to 80 bundles in humans.[57] These fibers diverge from those destined for the ciliary body, iris, and sclera just proximal to the limbus (Fig. 4-5). In humans the innervation of the epithelium comes from two sources. The central region obtains nerve terminals from a stromal plexus that traverses Bowman's membrane.[77] Nerve axons to peripheral regions of the epithelium arise more directly from the conjunctival plexus near the limbus.[57,77]

The branches enter the substantia propria (stroma) in a radial manner (Fig. 4-6) directly from the sclera, episclera, and conjunctiva. Following dichotomous branchings, these preter-

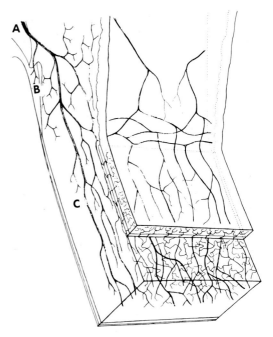

FIG. 4-5 Schematic representation of innervation of limbus and cornea. Long ciliary nerve (A) supplies limbal region, then sends branches into cornea. Nerves also supply trabecular meshwork (B) and the region of canal of Schlemm. Note paucity of nerves to deep cornea (C) and their absence in region of Descemet's membrane. (From Hogan MJ, Alvarado JA, Weddell JE: Histology of the human eye, Philadelphia, WB Saunders, 1971.)

minal fibers form a plexus with twigs, loops, or brushes whose branches mainly distribute throughout the middle one third of the substantia propria to Bowman's membrane (see Figs. 4-5 and 4-6). Once within the stroma all the myelinated axons lose their multiple myelin wrappings within ~1 mm of their entrance from the limbus; thus the entire plexus within the cornea forms from fine unmyelinated fibers. A Schwann cell covering persists in the stromal plexus, although for many axons the covering may consist only of a basal lamina.

There have been some claims that bare axon terminals exist in the stromal plexus and that these can transduce sensory signals from within the stroma.[96] Other observations have not indicated that free nerve endings occur in the stroma.[72] However, because of the general absence of any cellular covering over the axons in the stroma, it has been suggested that these axons still may be influenced physiologically by exogenous substances in the stroma.[7]

A second plexus forms in the stroma before

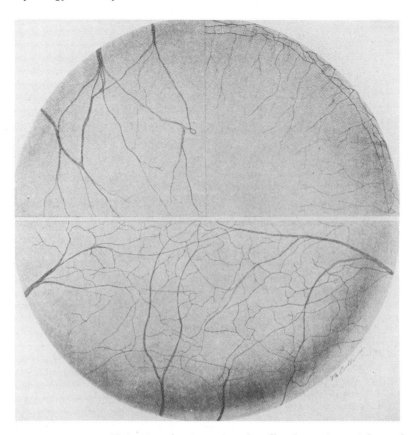

FIG. 4-6 Arrangement and behavior of various nerve bundles that enter periphery of cornea in different planes. Composite drawing based on observations from large number of methylene blue-stained rabbit corneas. Upper left quadrant shows form and behavior of nerve bundles entering the cornea from the scleral position. Upper right quadrant illustrates form and behavior of nerve bundles entering cornea from episcleral and subconjunctival positions. Lower half of drawing indicates manner in which plexiform pattern of nerve fibers arises from nerve bundles and passage of nerve bundles across center of cornea from limbus to limbus. Note that not all nerve bundles in cornea are radially disposed. (From Zander E, Weddel G: J Anat 85:68, 1951.)

individual axons enter the epithelial layer. This flattened and narrow subepithelial plexus consists of a dense mesh of smaller bundles of very thin fibers. From these filaments single or multiple leashes of axons penetrate into the basal epithelial layer completely devoid of any Schwann cell coverings (Figs. 4-7 and 4-8).

Epithelial plexus

As shown schematically in a three-dimensional reconstruction (Fig. 4-8), intraepithelial axons are distributed in two modes: "oriented and branched leashes running parallel to the base of the epithelium and unoriented terminal filaments that course anteriorly either in an oblique or vertical fashion."[72] An example of the outstanding innervation density and unorganized pattern of branches and terminals obtained

from the plexus of fibers in the epithelium is shown in Figure 4-9. In comparison with other parts of the skin, such as the finger pads, it has been estimated that corneal innervation density is 3 to 4 times greater.[72] The innervation density across the cornea is highest near the center and decreases nearly fivefold at the limbus. These relative changes in innervation density correlate remarkably well with data on the distribution of corneal sensitivity from limbus to center (Fig. 4-10 and see below).

Some sensory axons may distribute over 50 to 200 mm^2 of the corneal surface; the terminal field of an axon may lie as far as three fourths of the distance across the cornea from the axon's entry point at the limbus.[96] Recordings from single nerve fibers have confirmed this innervation pattern by finding that a fiber can be activated

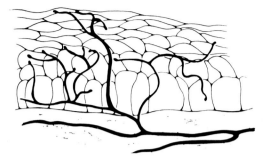

FIG. 4-7 *Camera lucida* drawing used for calculations of innervation density. Terminal arrangements shown include leashes of endings near basal epithelial cells and solitary fibers extending to middle and upper epithelial cells. (From Rozsa AJ, Beuerman RW: Pain 14:105, 1982).

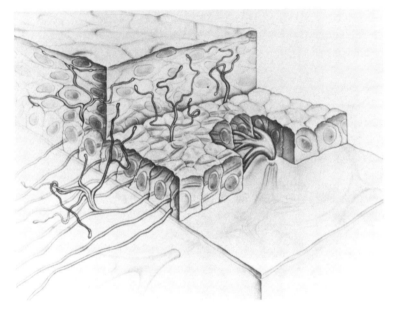

FIG. 4-8 Graphic illustration of three-dimensional organization design of innervation pattern of corneal epithelium. The construction of the figure was based on *camera lucida* drawing and photomicrographs taken at successive focal levels. Size of axon terminals relative to dimensions of epithelial cells was exaggerated for clarity. (From Rozsa AJ, Beuerman RW: Pain 14:105, 1982.)

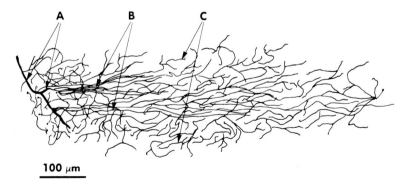

100 μm

FIG. 4-9 Reconstruction of intraepithelial arrangement of two "families" of leashes by *camera lucida* drawing: A, subepithelial plexus; B, horizontally oriented leashes; C, horizontal and vertical axon terminals and endings at wing and superficial levels of epithelium. (From Rozsa AJ, Beuerman RW: Pain 14:105, 1982.)

from receptive fields covering one fourth to one third of the corneal surface.[54] Observations involving more controlled stimulus application, however, have shown that the majority of the receptive field areas in the rabbit cornea are smaller and range from 5 to 20% (10.65 to 45.2 mm^2) of the total corneal surface.[81] These receptive fields overlap extensively (Fig. 4-11) and, in

some cases in which the fibers can be activated from the periphery of the cornea, the receptive fields include portions of adjacent conjunctiva.[1,81] According to calculations obtained from the rabbit cornea, there may be as many as 1000 branches for each corneal axon. Given this extensive distribution of axon terminals and high innervation density, it has been estimated that more than 100 terminal endings may be activated when the tip of a nylon filament aesthesiometer is applied to test the sensitivity of the cornea (discussed later). Rozsa and Beuerman[72] have calculated "that a mechanical stimulus perceived as painful by humans activates no more than 5% of the terminal endings that belong to as many as four to five different somas located in the trigeminal ganglion."

Histochemistry of epithelial axon terminals

Intense interest has been directed at histochemical characterization of the population of sensory ganglion cells associated with A delta and C fibers of the type that innervate the cornea. Two peptides, substance P and calcitonin gene-related peptide, have been particularly noted in the cornea. In addition, the cornea shows selective staining for catecholamines and acetylcholine.

Substance P (SP)

Immunohistochemical studies have demonstrated that substance P (SP) is localized in

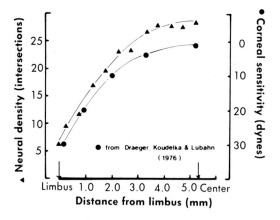

FIG. 4-10 Comparison of psychophysical corneal sensitivity threshold values and relative changes in neural density as a function of distance from center of cornea. Psychophysical data were replotted for illustration purposes. Each neural density value represents the mean of 30 corneas. Standard deviations were too small to plot. (From Rozsa AJ, Beuerman RW: Pain 14:105, 1982.)

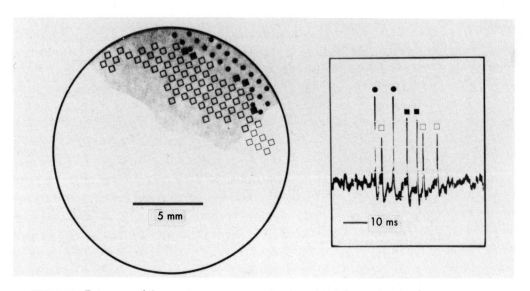

FIG. 4-11   Response of three units to punctate stimulus of 190 dynes depicting the overlap of receptive fields. *Left,* Circle represents perimeter of cornea. Symbols correspond to receptive fields where stimulation elicited action potentials indicated on the right with matching symbols. Area represented by filled circles is typical example of peripherally situated receptive field. (From Tanelian DL, Beuerman RW: Exp Neurol 84:165, 1984.)

many of the A delta and C fibers throughout the body, including the cornea, iris, and anterior sclera of humans and several other mammals.[28,37,71,82,88] In the anterior part of the eye SP-like immunoreactivity probably occurs in sensory fibers, because SP-labeled cells have been demonstrated in the gasserian ganglion and SP-like labeling of fibers in the cornea disappears after lesions to the ganglion or ophthalmic nerve but not after sympathectomy.[15,42,83] According to reports based on cryostat sections of the rabbit cornea, there are relatively few labeled fibers that arise from only 10 to 30% of the ganglion cells[15,88]; others,[76] who have used whole-mount techniques, have found a very dense plexus of SP-like immunoreactivity in the rat cornea. The significance of this discrepancy lies in trying to understand the function of this peptide in sensory endings, since a widespread distribution might indicate that release of SP from axon endings could cause dramatic changes in the tissue (see below).

The association between SP-like labeling in small-diameter fibers that possibly mediate pain has led to the suggestion that SP may be the neurotransmitter for pain.[63] However, the function of SP in the cornea is still equivocal. For example, it has been shown that the extent to which the SP content in the cornea is reduced by ganglion lesions or blocked by a SP antagonist does not correlate with a reduction in corneal sensitivity as measured by a blink reflex.[15,42] An alternative possibility is that SP may act as "a neurogenic mediator of inflammatory responses."[15] In areas of the skin with vascular beds, SP may be involved in vasodilation and plasma extravasation as a consequence of antidromic activation of sensory afferent fibers.[30,51] Inflammatory responses in the eye after an injury also may be mediated by local axon reflexes involving nociceptive sensory endings.[14,91] Bynke et al.[15] showed that an aqueous flare response in the iris after exposure to infrared could be prevented by pretreatment with an SP antagonist; a similar absence of an inflammatory response was seen in animals whose SP-like immunoreactivity had previously been eliminated through destruction of the trigeminal ganglion cells by neonatal capsaicin treatments. These results suggest that SP may contribute to local tissue reactions to painful stimuli rather than directly to the transmission of sensory signals.

The consequence of these antidromic axon reflex effects most probably is greater pain and discomfort due to inflammatory responses throughout the distribution of the branches of a nerve whose terminals have been excited by a painful stimulus in one part of the nerve's terminal field. This suggests that if some branches of the ophthalmic nerve are irritated, other branches might be antidromically activated to release SP and thereby cause local, painful inflammatory responses. For example, the intracranial tentorial branches of the ophthalmic nerve might respond to vasodilation of the blood vessels they innervate and this might lead to painful inflammations in the nasal sinuses, eye, and other areas innervated by this nerve.

Calcitonin Gene-Related Peptide (CGRP)

Another potent vasodilator found throughout the corneal nerve plexus, iris stroma, and in the vicinity of blood vessels and muscles of the ciliary body of humans and other animals is CGRP.[79,90,92] As in other parts of the body, CGRP originates in small to medium-sized sensory ganglion cells that have been associated with A delta and C fibers. The pattern of innervation of CGRP and general sensory endings in the cornea are similar,[90] as is the distribution of SP endings. These two pepitdes have also been co-localized in trigeminal ganglion cells.[49]

CGRP may, like SP, provide for a local axon reflex mechanism in sensory nerves that responds to potentially damaging stimuli. These two peptides may act in synergy to change local tissue permeability and inflammatory responses associated with noxious stimulation.

Catecholamines

A dense sympathetic innervation to the cornea has been demonstrated in several animals, including man,[26,85-87,90] Most of these inputs appear to arise from the superior cervical ganglion. The pattern of innervation is similar to that obtained from sensory fibers, including a stromal plexus, dense basal epithelial plexus, and endings throughout the thickness of the epithelium. Beta-adrenergic receptors also have been found on corneal epithelial cells.[28] These receptors have been considered as potential "first messengers" in the activation of cyclic nucleotides. It is possible that adrenergic innervation of the cornea is responsible for metabolic events within the epithelial cells that are associated with mitosis, Cl^- pump activity, and collagen production.[90] Loss of this sympathetic innervation might, therefore, be expected to lead to epithelial breakdown as in neurotropic keratitis.

Acetylcholine

According to some investigators,[55] some intra-epithelial endings resemble cholinergic endings.

This is consistent with histochemical demonstrations of acetylcholinesterase (AChE) activity in the axolemma of nerves in the stroma, epithelial cell membranes, and intraepithelial endings in the cornea of the rat.[58,85–87] These endings are not likely to come from an autonomic innervation of the cornea, because the cholinesterase reaction goes away only after ophthalmic nerve transection and not after cervical sympathectomy and ciliary ganglionectomy.[84] Corneal sensitivity also can be lowered after application of hemicholinium.[27] However, these results do not positively demonstrate that stimuli are transduced in the cornea through a cholinergic step. High levels of ACh, choline acetylase, and cholinesterase have been shown to exist in corneal epithelial cells in the absence of innervation.[28] The presence of ACh in the epithelial cells (reported to be the highest concentration of ACh in the body[57]) could be related to metabolic or neuronotropic activity in these cells. Changes in ACh content (and release from epithelial cells) could, in turn, be related to altered corneal sensitivity indirectly through effects of ACh on action potential initiation. This consequence may arise from ACh's alteration of Na^+ and Cl^- conductances in the membranes of axon terminals in the vicinity of the epithelial cells.[57]

Fine structure of epithelial axon terminals

Except for the extreme density of endings, the fine structure of the free nerve endings in the corneal epithelium is comparable to descriptions of these endings in other parts of the body.[16,45] When a collateral branch leaves the

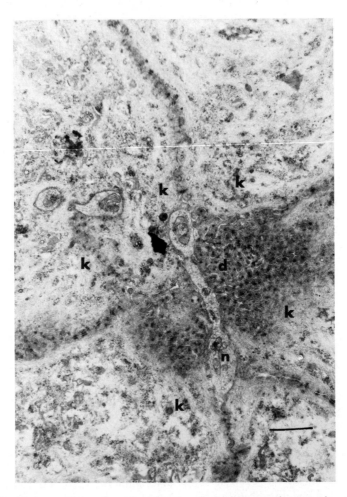

FIG. 4-12   In this tangential section of epidermis, neurite (n) passes between keratinocytes (k), and numerous desmosomes (d) are seen where the section grazes a keratinocyte surface. Bar equals 1.5 μm. (From unpublished micrographs by Dr. Adolph Cohen, Department of Ophthalmology and Visual Sciences, Washington University School of Medicine, St Louis, MO.)

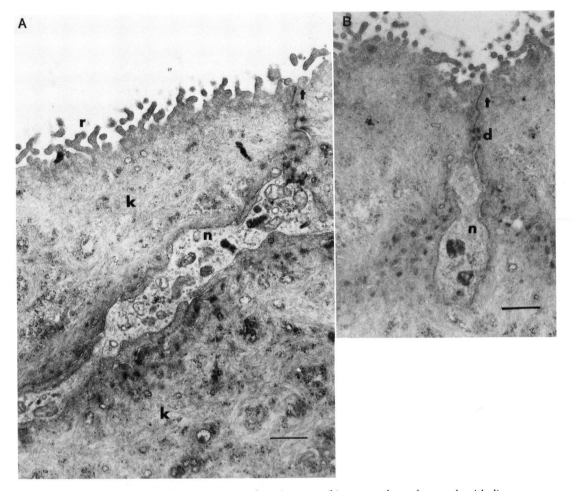

FIG. 4-13 A, Neurite (n) between two keratinocytes (k) near surface of corneal epithelium. Surface ridges (r) of outermost keratinocytes are rich in glycocalycal extensions and help anchor tear film. Tight junction (t) is evident between the two keratinocytes. Bar equals 0.75 μm. **B,** Neurite (n) near junction of two corneocytes at the epidermal surface. Note the tight junction (t) and desmosomes (d) below this level. Bar equals 0.75 μm. (From unpublished micrographs by Dr. Adolph Cohen, Department of Ophthalmology and Visual Sciences, Washington University School of Medicine, St Louis, MO.)

subepithelial plexus to penetrate the epithelium, it loses all of its remaining Schwann cell coverings. However, the sensory endings are never directly exposed to intercellular spaces, because they are always tightly surrounded by epidermal cells (Fig. 4-12). The terminal portions of individual endings are usually swollen[72] and are found throughout the epithelium. Indeed, some endings in the superficial layers extend up to the last desmosomal junction between two cells (Fig. 4-13, *A* and *B*). Some of these endings are separated from the external environment only by a complex of desmosomes and a single tight junction at the edge of the microvilli from two neighboring epithelial surface cells (Fig. 4-13,

B). The presence of tight junctions at the surface of the cornea indicates that any changes in the composition of the tear film that are to have an effect on the nerve endings might have to be conveyed to the endings through the surface epithelial cells. Because changes in the hypertonicity of the tear film are believed to be responsible for triggering normal blinking,[25] some interaction between the surface epithelial cells and the nerve terminals must be suspected.

Similarly, migration of new surface epithelial cells from more basal positions must involve construction of new tight junctions at the surface of the cornea. Significant interactions with the nerve endings also might be expected during the insertion of new epithelial cells so that the endings are always protected from direct exposure to the surface environment.

Consistent with the notion of a dynamic interaction between the nerve endings and surface epithelial cells of the cornea, there has been visualization (with fluorescent microscopy in living corneas) of remodeling of the distribution of nerve terminals. The precise alignment of terminals within a living epithelium may change over very short times. Harris and Purves[33] showed that endings within the same corneal region of adult mice shift position within 24 hours and distribute to new nearby locations after 1 week. After 1 month, the alignment of endings is completely novel. These changes occur in uninjured corneas and indicate that the endings may retract, reinsert, or shift position possibly in response to the continual turnover of epithelial cells.

The terminals usually are filled with mitochondria and various sizes of vesicles (Fig. 4-13, A and B). Some investigators[39,90] have suggested that there are two types of nerve endings in the cornea. One is associated with thicker axons, numerous mitochondria, a dense whirl of neurofilaments, many neurotubules, occasional small, round, clear vesicles, and a few small dense-core vesicles in some preparations.[90] A second type contains few neurotubules, some mitochondria, a reticular network of neurofilaments, and usually two types of vesicles consisting of a few large (100 nm), dense-cored vesicles and several small (60 nm), clear vesicles. As SP and CGRP have been localized to large dense-core vesicles in other tissues and catecholamines are found in small dense-core vesicles in the sympathetic nervous system, the two types of terminals may, respectively, reflect dual sensory and sympathetic innervation of the cornea.[90]

SENSORY INNERVATION OF OTHER OCULAR STRUCTURES

The sensory innervation of the eye excluding the cornea can be divided into three types: (1) free nerve endings as in the cornea, (2) a broad variety of endings as are generally found in other parts of the skin, and (3) endings that primarily relate to position sense.

The iris, sclera, trabecular area, ciliary body, and choroid

The iris, sclera, trabecular area, ciliary body, and choroid are supplied from the same ciliary nerves that extend to the cornea (see Fig. 4-5).[40] It is unknown whether the endings arise as collateral or separate branches of the axons destined for the cornea. The innervation in the iris is particularly dense. It arises from sensory and autonomic fibers. A fine plexus courses along the blood vessels and among the muscle fibers; many of these are probably efferent fibers. Additional unmyelinated filaments occur throughout the stroma, from which branches arise to supply the anterior epithelial cell layer. No fibers have been traced into the posterior pigmented epithelium.[36] Immunohistochemical studies have revealed that SP-positive and CGRP-positive afferent fibers distribute to all parts of the iris dilator and sphincter muscles and to all parts of the stroma.[78] As in the cornea, these peptides co-localize in many but not all endings. These peptide-labeled fibers terminate as free nerve endings throughout the iris. Additional peptide-labeled fibers distribute to the ciliary body, where the highest density occurs in the ciliary processes.

The density of nerve endings in the sclera is low; very small filaments occur interspersed throughout the lamellae. The nerve plexus in the anterior parts of the sclera forms from branches of the nasociliary nerve, whereas branches from the short ciliary nerves supply the posterior portions of the sclera near the root of the optic nerve. In the episcleral region some swollen endings have been identified as Krause end-bulbs[93]; this observation probably needs to be checked with modern fixation methods. It is more likely that all endings in the sclera are free nerve endings.

A dense and widespread plexus of nerve filaments forms in the vicinity of the scleral spur and distributes small myelinated and unmyelinated fibers to the trabecular area. The nerve filaments in the trabecular meshwork are mainly unmyelinated and distribute in a plexiform pattern. Because many of these nerve endings relate to Schlemm's canal and the ciliary body, it has been suggested that they function in regulating intraocular pressure.[92] However, observations of multiple free nerve endings enveloped by endothelial cells have also suggested possible sensory functions for many of these terminals.[37]

The ciliary body also receives a plexus of fibers from the region of the scleral spur. Most of the sensory fibers distribute in the anterior segment of the ciliary body. The morphology and function of these fibers are not known.

The eyelids and conjunctiva

The sensory nerves innervating these structures arise from the lacrimal, supraorbital, supratrochlear, infratrochlear, and infraorbital nerves (Fig. 4-14). The plexus formed by these nerves lies deep to the palpebral fibers of the orbicularis oculi muscle in a layer of loose areolar tissue. Terminal nerve fibers arise from this plexus to enter the subepithelium and penetrate the epithelium. Because of the deep position of the plexus, any attempts to anesthetize the eylids must be accomplished by injecting local anesthetics deep into the orbicularis muscle.

As in the cornea, the eyelids and conjunctiva are densely supplied with free nerve endings. However similar to the corneal free nerve endings these appear, a greater range of sensations arise from these terminals in the eyelids and conjunctiva. Thus true low-threshold temperature sensitivity exists in these tissues, which is distinct from perceptions of noxious heat or cold as are found nearly exclusively in the cornea (discussed later). These distinctions are probably due to the presence of a broader spectrum of A delta and C fibers in the palpebral area than is found in other parts of the skin. In addition, a variety of specialized nerve endings exist in the eyelids that compare to those found throughout the skin (Fig. 4-15). All of these are mechanoreceptors that can be viewed as providing a continuum of sensitivity that includes various aspects of touch. All of these specialized endings are associated with larger, myelinated nerve fibers whose diameters generally range between 5 and 15 μm. A more complete discussion of each of these receptors is available elsewhere.[21]

Innervation of extraocular muscles

A detailed discussion of the specialized afferent innervation of the extraocular muscle fibers can be found in Chapter 5.

The extraocular muscles receive a dense plexus of sensory nerve endings from branches arising near the base of the ophthalmic nerve. In the vicinity of the cavernous sinus these branches form anastomoses with the oculomotor nerve in which they travel to reach the muscles. Many of these nerve endings are found near tendinous insertions. There are few if any

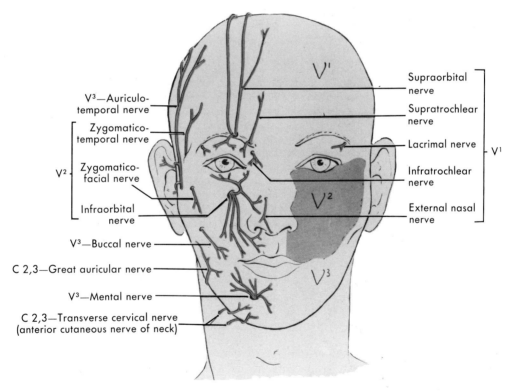

FIG. 4-14 Diagram of cutaneous nerves to face. Note that upper eyelid receives branches from four V^1 nerves (infratrochlear, supratrochlear, supraorbital, and lacrimal); lower eyelid is supplied by the superior branches of infraorbital nerve from V^2. (From Basmajians J: Grant's method of anatomy, 10th ed, Baltimore, Williams & Wilkins, copyright 1980.)

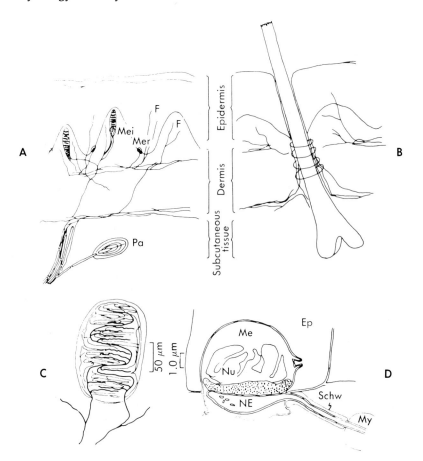

FIG. 4-15 Schematic drawings of location and morphology of some somesthetic receptor organs. **A,** Free nerve endings, F, are found within and below epidermal layer; Meissner's corpuscles, Mei, frequently are found in dermal ridges; Merkel cell-neurite complexes, Mer, generally are located in basal layer of the epidermis; pacinian corpuscles, Pa, generally occur in subcutaneous tissue, around periosteum, and in or near joints. **B,** Hair follicles have several nerve nets from different sensory units entwined around root of hair, especially above level of hair bulb. Many terminals lie parallel to root; some endings wrap around hair. **C,** Enlarged view of Meissner corpuscle shows sandwiching of sensory root terminals between connective tissue leaflets. **D,** Drawing taken from electron micrograph shows the Merkel cell, Me, and its associated nerve terminal, Ne. Merkel cell is modified epithelial cell characterized by its large, lobulated nucleus, Nu. Sensory terminal arises from myelinated fiber, My; the Schwann cell covering, Schw, extends up to region of contact between the nerve terminal and Merkel cell. (From Somjen G: Sensory coding in the mammalian nervous system, New York, Appleton-Century-Crofts, 1972.)

distinct neuromuscular spindles or tendon organs in extraocular muscles. There are, however, "grapelike" endings or a myotendinous cylinder among the extraocular muscle fibers and in the intermuscular connective tissues.[93] These major sensory organs in extraocular muscles consist of encapsulated nerve terminals situated in series with muscle fibers. There are also many free nerve endings that may be responsible for the very marked painful sensations produced when the extraocular muscles are stretched. However, pain also may arise from

the distortions produced in other ocular tissues, such as the orbital periosteum, dural sheaths, or sclera, by manipulating the muscles and their insertions.

The lens, retina, and optic nerve

Because the lens does not contain any sensory endings it lacks sensitivity to pricking or touch. However, Tower[89] demonstrated in experimental animals that pushing on the anterior curvature of the lens with a blunt glass rod provoked a small burst of nerve impulses in the long ciliary nerve. The lens appeared to be without surface sensitivity but seemed to possess what might be characterized as a position sensibility in modest proportions. The receptors responsible may be located in the ciliary body.

The retina and optic nerve, like the rest of brain tissue, lack direct sensitivity to somatosensory stimuli. However, the uvea and optic nerve dural sheaths are densely innervated with free nerve endings. Consequently, although the retina and optic nerve are insensitive to pain, moving the eye in patients with retrobulbar neuritis or photocoagulation of the posterior segment of the eye frequently produces pain because of involvement of these adjacent densely innervated tissues.

DEGENERATION AND REGENERATION OF CORNEAL NERVE FIBERS

Neurotrophic or neuroparalytic keratitis and corneal scarring are frequently present in pathologic conditions that also result in corneal anesthesia. Some of these diseases include herpetic infections of the cornea, local corneal trauma or surgery, lesions of the trigeminal ganglion, nerve, or root from infections, tumors or surgery, and various brainstem lesions of the trigeminal nuclei. The presence of corneal anesthesia in those cases in which corneal opacity impairs vision has led to the hypothesis that corneal innervation is important for maintaining epithelial function. For example, experimentally induced sensory denervation by coagulation lesions of the ophthalmic portions of the trigeminal ganglion causes increased epithelial layer permeability as a result of decreased cellular adhesion, impaired wound healing with failed reepithelization, decreased epithelial cell migration, and reduced epithelial cell mitosis.[6,52] These changes closely correlate with the degree of sensory impairment and extent of corneal denervation and thus imply maintenance of corneal function by the nerves. In contrast, in humans several reports state that corneal function persists in patients with corneal anesthesia.[22,53] However, the extent of damage to the corneal innervation may need to be assessed because some patients had neurotrophic keratitis and permanent corneal damage. There may therefore be "a limiting factor of minimal innervation necessary for maintenance of corneal function."[53,74]

Regeneration of nerve supply

Neural regeneration after corneal damage as a result of surgery, accidents, or disease is of some importance given the dual role of corneal innervation in maintaining normal sensory and epi-

thelial properties. Experimental studies[2,5,18,73] have shown that regeneration generally occurs in two phases; however, the timing and pattern of the reinnervation process vary with the type and extent of damage to the original nerve supply. During each phase the remodeling of corneal innervation is shaped by degeneration and regeneration of terminals and neurites in and bordering the wound. Generally, the extent and chronology of reinnervation are the same for those lesions (for example, local abrasions, radial or circular keratotomies, and keratectomies) that leave the main nerve supply around the limbus intact. A substantially different temporal picture characterizes reinnervation after lesions that section perilimbal nerve bundles (Fig. 4-16).

In the first phase after an epithelial wound that damages intraepithelial axons only, degeneration proceeds rapidly; by 24 hours all the original intraepithelial terminals in the wound area have degenerated and by 48 hours additional degeneration can be seen in the subepithelial plexus in and within ~0.5 mm of the wound margins. At 1 week no axonal leashes are seen within the basal epithelial regions of a wounded area.[18] During the same time that degeneration of the original innervation takes place, a hyperplasia of collateral sprouts grows from intraepithelial axons proximal to the wound from neighboring, undamaged portions of the cornea. These parallel running sprouts may travel from 2 mm beyond the original wound margins. These wound-bound neurites completely surround and, most notably, orient perpendicular to the edge of the wound[73] (Fig. 4-17). They primarily enter and ramify terminals in the basal portions of the repairing epithelium within the wound.

The second phase of remodeling begins around 7 days after injury and extends for 14 to 21 days, depending upon the extent of the original injury. During this stage, additional sprouting begins in the subepithelial plexus within the proximal stumps of the original axons that innervated the damaged areas and a second "wave" of wound-oriented neurites courses toward the wound margins. Unlike the first sprouts, the basal leashes of neurites formed from the subepithelial plexus, although still surrounding the wound, orient obliquely as is normally seen in an intact cornea (Fig. 4-18). By 2 weeks some rudimentary axonal leashes reappear in the wounded area.[18] During the same time, the "foreign" sprouts formed during the first phase of reinnervation degenerate and disappear entirely by 3 weeks (see Fig. 4-16). This second reinnervation probably reestablishes

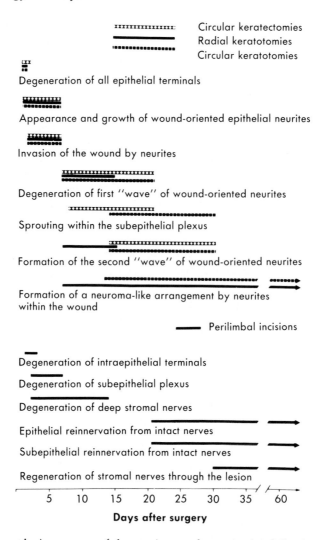

FIG. 4-16   Chronologic sequence of changes in neural organization following various lesions to nerves innervating cornea. (From Rozsa AJ, Guss RB, Beuerman RW: Invest Ophthalmol Vis Sci 24:1033, 1983.)

much of the original pattern of innervation, although neuromas may form after circular keratotomies.[73] By 4 weeks a normal innervation pattern is reestablished.

An anomalous consequence of these two phases of regeneration is that the density of innervation at the edges of the damaged area of the cornea is significantly elevated above normal levels and the intraepithelial neurite lengths are two to three times greater (Fig. 4-19). Within the wounded area, however, neural density is less than normal even after 4 weeks.[18,50] The function of the first phase of "foreign" neurites is unknown; however, a neuronotropic role in the healing process through effects on mitogenic rates of keratoblasts has been suggested.[73] The increased density of endings at the edges of a

wound do not appear to yield heightened sensitivity. The center of a wound area is devoid of sensation for more than 2 weeks and partial restoration of responses to tactile stimuli does not appear until the second phase of regeneration appears. Restitution of tactile sensitivity at 3 to 4 weeks is approximately 60% of normal, which corresponds with comparable reinnervation densities at this time.[50]

Degeneration and reinnervation also follow subsequent to perilimbal lesions that cut the main ciliary nerve bundles at the periphery of the cornea.[73,94] Unlike the observations with intracorneal lesions, collateral sprouting from intact axons is much more limited; however, the growing neurites still orient toward the wound margins. In addition, nearly all reinnervation

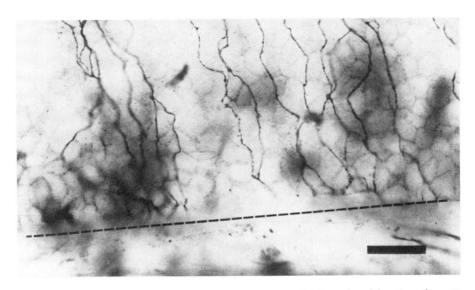

FIG. 4-17 Circular keratotomy, 24 hours. Extensive wound-oriented proliferation of neurites is seen at margin of wound *(interrupted line)*. Bar equals 25 μm. (From Rozsa AJ, Guss RB, Beuerman RW: Invest Ophthalmol Vis Sci 24:1033, 1983.)

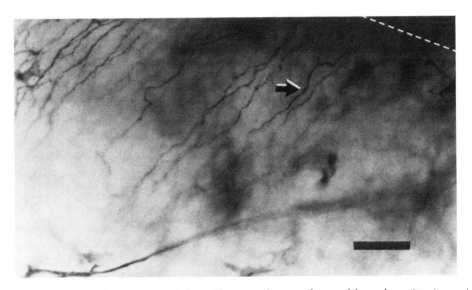

FIG. 4-18 Circular keratotomy, 14 days. The second wave of wound-bound neurites *(arrows)* appear rotated from perpendicular disposition of early wound-bound neurites. Their oblique approach to wound margin *(interrupted line)* approximates the normal orientation of basal leashes. Bar equals 25 μm. (From Rozsa AJ, Guss RB, Beuerman RW: Invest Ophthalmol Vis Sci 24:1033, 1983.)

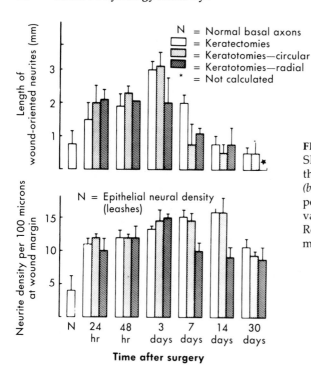

FIG. 4-19 Intraepithelial neurite lengths (mean ± SE) measured from point of penetration of basal epithelium to edge of wound *(top)*; density of neurites *(bottom)* at wound margin calculated at different time periods after surgery. Data for normal innervation values are from Rozsa and Beuerman (1982). (From Rozsa AJ, Guss RB, Beuerman RW: Invest Ophthalmol Vis Sci 24:1033, 1983.)

proceeds from regrowing stromal stumps that pass through the perilimbal scar tissue. The time course of the remodeling is much longer (greater than 60 days, Fig. 4-16), and the density of innervation is lower than normal. Stromal and epithelial plexuses and intraepithelial terminals remain distorted even after 30 months.[19] Tactile sensitivity recovers slowly and may never reach normal levels. This reduced innervation may be responsible for reports that cryosurgery of the ciliary body in patients with acute secondary glaucoma will have persisting relief from pain even after a return of some corneal sensitivity.[94]

A truly notable feature of both phases of reinnervation is the remarkably uniform orientation of the growing neurites to the denervated parts of the cornea. This feature could be a consequence of a chemotactic attraction to the wound area. One possibility might be the release of an epithelial neurotrophic factor (ENF) from corneal epithelial cells.[17] ENF leads to neurite extension from trigeminal ganglion cells grown in culture and affects protein metabolism in these cells.[18] ENF levels also rise 2 weeks following corneal injuries, which is the time when normal innervation patterns are being reestablished. Although it is tempting to speculate that ENF is responsible for regeneration, more complicated mutual interactions probably exist between corneal epithelium and its innervation. As stated by Chan and colleagues: "... the re-

generated epithelium may induce its own re-innervation, and the regenerated nerves may exert an influence on the epithelium to maintain the proper degree of innervation."[18]

SENSATIONS FROM THE CORNEA

In a clinical setting the simplest way to ascertain corneal sensitivity is to move a wisp of cotton from the limbus toward the center of the cornea while monitoring for a blink reflex or a patient's report of a sensation. A more quantitative way of measuring ocular sensations is to use an aesthesiometer (Fig. 4-20); this device employs a thin nylon monofilament for stimulus. The force necessary to bend different lengths of the filament is indirectly related to the exposed length.[4,9,20] Systematic variations in sensitivity across the anterior surface of the eye can be assessed by perpendicular applications of the aesthesiometer. For more accurate measurements of sensitivity, the aesthesiometer is held in a multidirectional micromanipulator and the probe is advanced until a 5-degree bend occurs in the filament. Corneal touch threshold is defined as the force applied by a given length of nylon monofilament that a subject feels on 50% of 4 to 8 stimulus trials. Obtaining a subjective report of a touch threshold is not always possible with all patients and is impossible in animals. Millodot[56] showed that the involuntary blink reflex was exceptionally correlated with

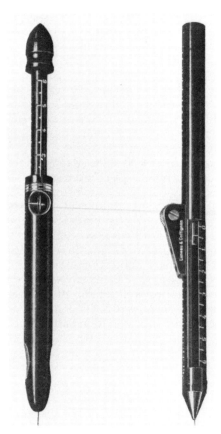

FIG. 4-20 Aesthesiometers of Boberg-Ans *(left)* and of Cochet and Bonnet *(right)*. (From Walsh FB, Hoyt WF: Clinical neuroophthalmology, 3rd ed, vol 1, Baltimore, Williams & Wilkins, 1969.)

subjective thresholds and could be used to predict the latter.

Experiments studying the distribution of touch sensitivity across the cornea and adjoining tissues[10,57,64] clearly demonstrated that the most sensitive area of the anterior portion of the eye is the center of the cornea (for example, 10 to 14mg/mm²); in decreasing order of sensitiivty are the periphery of the cornea (20 to 50 mg), the eyelids (53 to 58 mg), caruncle (63 mg), and conjunctiva (83 to 96 mg). The distribution of sensitivity across the periphery of the cornea is not uniform and the highest thresholds exist in superior regions that are generally covered by upper eyelids.

Sensations resulting from mechanical stimulation of the cornea

The question of a true sense of touch in the cornea has been the subject of lively dispute. It was maintained by earlier workers that there is no true sensation of touch or pressure from stimu-

lating the cornea. According to these observers, mechanical stimulation of the cornea results only in the sensation of pain. They claimed that failure to react to a vibratory stimulus except as a persistent pain proved the absence of touch as a mode of corneal sensation. Further proof of the absence of a pressure sense was suggested by poor stereognostic sensation in the cornea.

Quantitative studies of tactile sensibilities of the cornea showed that only one threshold could be determined for the blink reflex when the corneas of laboratory animals were stimulated.[80] Comparable force levels that caused the corneal reflex in humans also corresponded to the threshold for pain. Consequently, because of the similarities in thresholds for the corneal blink reflex in all instances, and because only a single threshold level was observed, the results were interpreted as indicating that only pain sensations could be elicited by mechanical stimulation of the cornea. In contrast, separate levels for touch and pain sensations could be determined when the skin of the eyelids was tested.

Other observations tend to suggest that a sense of touch can be appreciated from the cornea if the stimulus amplitudes are carefully controlled.[57] Recent single-fiber recordings from the long ciliary nerve have shown that some sensory units in the cornea are activated by touch.[1,32,54,81] In some cases the responses were obtained from fibers that were activated only by physiologic levels of mechanical stimuli[81]; other fibers responded to mechanical and thermal stimuli.[1] As shown in Figure 4-11, many mechanically sensitive corneal units had small receptive fields that occupied 5 to 15% of the corneal surface; others had larger receptive fields that extended over more than 20% of the cornea and sometimes included the adjacent conjunctiva. Force thresholds for mechanically sensitive cells were 170 to 350 dynes, which is also the threshold for the blink reflex in the rabbit. These sensory units did not respond to temperatures between 20° and 43°C; they were most sensitive to moving a nylon filament across the receptive field. However, repeated stimulation of the same spot within the receptive field usually resulted in decreased responses. This fatigue severely limits the ability of these endings to code mechanical stimulus properties. It also may explain previous observations of only pain sensations when a monofilament was repeatedly used against a single point on the cornea to determine psychophysical thresholds for touch, since higher force levels would be needed to overcome the refractory endings.

The presence of a response in some corneal

sensory fibers to low-threshold mechanical stimuli does not entirely define the stimulus specificity of this sensory unit, since many free nerve endings found in the cornea lie within a few microns of the surface (see previous discussion) in an uncornified epithelium. Protection of this bare epithelium is vital for the preservation of vision. Consequently, the stimulus intensity that is considered harmful to the organism must be considerably lower in the cornea; in other areas of the skin similar receptors might be activated only by frankly painful stimuli. Tanelian and Beuerman[81] have speculated that the "touch" sensitivity of the mechanical sensory units seen in the cornea might best be considered "candidates for the detection of particulate foreign bodies."

Factors affecting corneal sensitivity

A number of factors affect corneal sensitivity measurements. For example, Norn[64] has shown that sensitivity from all parts of the anterior portion of the eye declines with age. The least dramatic decrease occurs in the cornea and is greatest in the conjunctiva. Corneal sensitivity changes slowly up to 50 years but declines to less than half after 65 years of age.[57]

Changes in corneal sensitivity also appear to accompany the menstrual cycle in women who do not take contraceptive pills. Decreased sensitivity occurs during the premenstruum and continues until about the time of menstruation. Water retention and increased intraocular pressure may contribute to variations in corneal sensitivity because both of these rise during premenstruum. At other times, however, there is no difference in sensitivity between sexes.[57]

Blue-eyed individuals tend to have higher sensitivity than those with more pigmented irises. On a relative scale individuals with dark brown eyes have ~¼ the sensitivity of those with blue eyes and about ½ those with green eyes. The absence of all pigment in albinos, however, is accompanied by decreased sensitivity. No explanation currently exists for these differences.[57]

Decreased corneal sensitivity also accompanies various adverse environmental conditions (e.g., extreme cold of −14°C and UV light exposure). Similarly, most eye pathology and diabetes raises corneal touch or eye blink thresholds.[57]

Any condition that results in decreased oxygen flow to the cornea substantially reduces corneal sensitivity. Hence, extended periods of eyelid closure raises thresholds as a reduction in tear film lowers oxygen perfusion over the cornea. For example, after normal sleep, thresholds may rise >20%.[57] Similarly, comatose patients whose eyes remain closed for many hours or days will display reduced blink reflexes but not necessarily because of attendant brainstem pathology.

Contact lenses substantially reduce oxygenation of the cornea and thereby lower sensitivity. Millodot,[57] who has reviewed these changes, describes long-term and short-term declines in sensitivity in normal eyes. Several studies have shown that after long-term adaptation to hard, but not hydrophilic ("gel") contact lenses, decreased sensitivity was found from the cornea, center of the tarsus, and eyelid margin. These changes were noted after periods of adapting to contact lenses for 2 weeks to more than 1 year; in most cases greater declines in sensitivity were seen after longer periods of adaptation. However, there also may be an inverse correlation between wearing well-fitted contact lenses and changes in corneal sensitivity. Recovery to normal sensitivity has been found after the contact lens is removed in patients who have been comfortably fitted with contact lenses for a long time. The time needed to recover relates to duration of use with full corneal integrity not returning for months in people who have discontinued contact wear after several years.

The length of exposure to contact lenses within 1 day also causes short-term changes in corneal sensitivity. The decreases relate to duration of wear. Little change occurs after 1 hour, a slight reduction begins to appear at 1 to 2 hours, significant declines begin to appear after 4 hours, and potentially dangerous alterations in sensitivity are apparent after 6 to 8 hours of wear even with comfortably fitted lenses. According to Millodot,[57] "this well-documented loss of sensation with contact lens wear represents one of the most unequivocal reasons why patients should be warned against overwearing their lenses."

Progressive depression in corneal sensitivity arises with soft or extended wear lenses. These declines are less marked but still of sufficient magnitude to alter the cornea.

Sensations of temperature from the anterior eye

The presence of a sensation of temperature from the cornea has been controversial.[23,43,61] A good part of this debate has been due to problems with restricting thermal stimuli to the intended target tissue. Previous reports of thermal sensations from the cornea may have confused their results by inadvertently stimulating the large number of very sensitive temperature spots on the eyelids and conjunctiva.[3] In noncorneal skin epithelium, 0.5°C decreases in temperature elicit a sensation of cooling, comparable increases in temperature are sensed as warming, and shifts of more than 10 to 12°C above adapting skin temperatures cause pain. These separate sensations have been attributed to the unique thresholds of cold and warm thermoreceptors and polymodal heat nociceptors, respectively. All of these receptors are associated with free nerve endings. The exclusive presence of free nerve endings in the cornea has long been suggestive that similar sensations ought to arise from stimulating these endings.

Beuerman and colleagues[3,8,81] developed a device for controlling thermal stimulation of the eye; it consists of a closed chamber fitted around the cornea and a temperature-controlled microjet stream of saline solution for delivery of different temperatures. They showed that stimulation of the eyelids or conjunctiva leads to temperature sensations of cold and warm at thresholds comparable to those on other facial skin (+ or −0.5° to 1°C from an adapting temperature of 33°C). When thermal stimulation was isolated to the center of the cornea, 0.5°C shifts in either direction were not perceived. At temperatures below 30°C only aversive or nociceptive perceptions were obtained. Warming of 2.8° to 6°C above the adapting temperatures was perceived as painful; this temperature change is considerably below that established for pain sensations from activating skin polymodal nociceptors. However, the actual temperature needed to reach the nerve endings must be different in normal skin and the cornea, since free nerve endings in the former are buried and insulated in more than 50 μm of keratinized skin and are protected by less than 10 μm of a single epithelial cell process in the cornea. In control experiments these investigations showed that expected sensations of temperature were obtained when stimuli were isolated to the eyelids while the cornea was anesthetized, whereas sensations of pain and irritation were present when all stimuli to the eyelids were blocked and only the isolated cornea received thermal stimulation. These results suggest that the persistence of cold sensations shortly after local anesthetics are instilled in the eye may be due to spread of the fluid to the conjunctiva and eyelid margins, rather than to the presence of cold receptors deep in the cornea.

SOMATIC SENSATIONS FROM OTHER PARTS OF THE EYE

Few studies have specifically examined sensations evoked from other parts of the eye. In most cases stimuli that activate sensory nerve endings in the iris, sclera, trabecular area, and ciliary body elicit pain or discomfort. This is not surprising as most of these structures have only free nerve endings like those seen in the cornea. The eyelids have a broader range of sensory endings like that generally found in other parts of the body. Consequently, a true sense of touch, some stereognosis, vibratory sensations, and a full range of temperature sense (cold, warm, and noxious heat) can be elicited from the eyelids. The functions of peptide-containing sensory endings throughout the iris, including the muscles, are unknown. As in other tissues, release of SP through axon reflexes leads to vasodilation. In addition, in the iris the changes include miosis, breakdown of the blood-aqueous barrier, and increased intraocular pressure.[78] SP release triggers noncholinergic and nonadrenergic contraction of iris sphincter muscle that can be blocked by tachykinin antagonists. It has been suggested that the SP endings to the iris may monitor intraocular pressure and provide a proprioceptive feedback for the iris muscles.[78]

There is little or no proprioceptive sense of eye position despite the presence of encapsulated end organs within the extraocular muscles. The central projections of these endings (see below) correspond to those from muscle receptors in other parts of the body at the level of the brainstem where these projections are integrated with oculomotor centers within the brain.

TRIGEMINAL NUCLEI

The representation of somatic sensations from the eye in the central nervous system has been studied mainly in relation to the overall organization of the trigeminal nerve projections. A detailed consideration of these can be obtained elsewhere.[10] Presented here are only those aspects of this neuroanatomy that are of immediate relevance to ophthalmology. Specifically, the following describes the organization of ophthalmic nerve projections to the trigeminal nuclei in the pons and medulla that is relevant to understanding clinical conditions in which hyperalgesia or hypesthesia may affect the eye. The brainstem connections associated with the corneal blink reflex also will be discussed. The representation of the eye in higher levels of the somatosensory pathways, which has not received much detailed analysis, will be considered only briefly.

Trigeminal root entry

The sensory fibers from the eye gain entry through the trigeminal root at the pons and distribute projections to various divisions of the sensory nuclei of the trigeminal nerve (Fig. 4-21). Where the sensory root enters the brainstem, a segregation of the different peripheral divisions of the face exists. In experimental animals Kerr[44] established that the ophthalmic division fibers reside ventrally, mandibular division fibers are placed dorsally, and maxillary division fibers occupy an intermediate position. The segregation of these divisions in the sensory root of humans has been debated but generally agrees with findings in animals. The ophthalmic division fibers tend to occupy the rostral third of the root, and fibers from the mandibular and maxillary divisions are principally represented in the posterior two-thirds.

Principal and spinal trigeminal nuclei

Upon entering the pons, the trigeminal root fibers course dorsomedially before dividing and distributing to the trigeminal nuclei. Almost half of the sensory fibers that enter at the pons divide into a short ascending branch that reaches the *principal sensory nucleus* and a long descending branch from which collaterals distribute to the *nucleus of the spinal tract* (Figs. 4-21 and 4-22). The principal sensory nucleus is well developed in humans, receives afferent input mostly from low-threshold tactile receptors on the head, connects into the medial lemniscus together with the output from the dorsal column nuclei, and clinically appears to provide the major brainstem relay for all tactile sensations from the head, including the eye. In contrast, the spinal trigeminal nucleus resembles the spinal cord dorsal horn. It receives a broader range of afferent inputs that includes projections from pain and temperature receptors. Its central projections mostly join those from the spinothalamic tract, and, clinically, lesions to the nucleus of the spinal tract or the fiber tract that carries afferent input to it (see following discussion) produce analgesia and thermoanesthesia in the head.

Spinal trigeminal tract

The nucleus of the spinal tract receives its input through a large mass of descending sensory fibers that course along the lateral and ventral border of the nucleus in a bundle known as the *spinal trigeminal tract.* In humans this tract contains mostly thin-caliber fibers with the diameter of approximately 90% of the fibers less than 4 μm. The proportion of thin fibers increases as the tract courses caudally toward the spinal cord.[10] The spinal trigeminal tract is continuous with the dorsolateral tract of Lissauer in the spinal cord. As the spinal trigeminal tract courses caudally through the medulla, terminals are given off medially into the adjoining spinal tri-

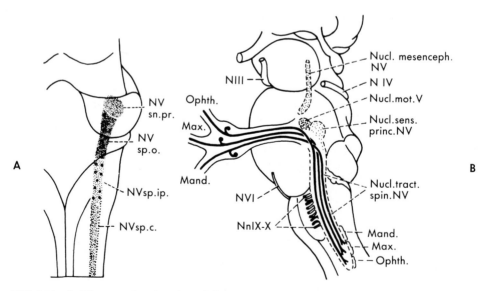

FIG. 4-21   A, Diagram showing the subdivisions of the trigeminal sensory nuclei. Upper region NV sn. pr. is main sensory nucleus in pons. Caudal to this in medulla are three subdivisions of spinal nucleus: the oralis, NS sp. o., the interpolaris, NS sp. ip., and the caudalis, NV sp. c. Latter continues caudally into dorsal horn. **B,** Diagram showing topical arrangement within spinal trigeminal tract of fibers belonging to main divisions of trigeminal nerve. Fibers terminate in nuclei according to same pattern. (From Brodal A: Neurological anatomy, 3rd ed, New York, Oxford University Press, 1981.

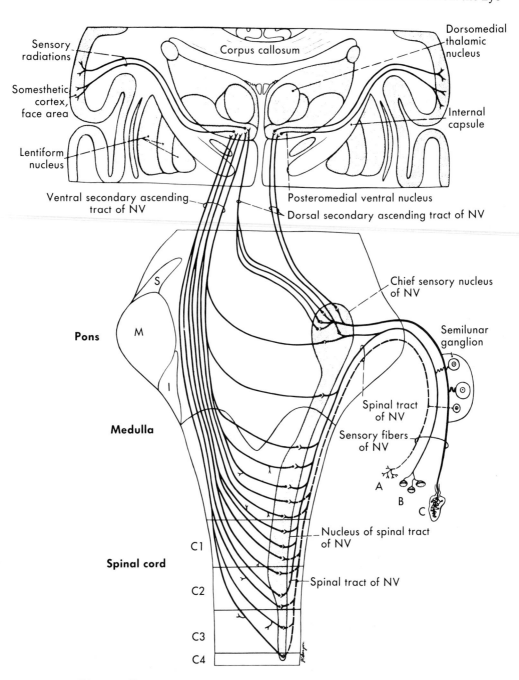

FIG. 4-22 Diagram illustrating projections to dorsal thalamus from trigeminal nuclei. Free sensory ending at A, Merkel's tactile discs at B, and Meissner's corpuscle at C are associated with fibers that function in transmission of impulses set up by pain, sustained tactile, and rapidly changing fine tactile stimuli, respectively. (From Crosby EC, Humphrey T, Lauer EW, eds: Correlative anatomy of the nervous system, New York, Macmillan, 1962, copyright © 1962 by Macmillan Publishing Company.)

geminal nucleus, which also continues into the spinal cord, where it fuses with the dorsal horn (see Figs. 4-21 and 4-22). In the medulla the spinal tract and nucleus are located laterally just underneath the surface of the brainstem in an extensive longitudinal column that reaches the second cervical segment. In the pons the spinal trigeminal nucleus is continuous with the principal sensory nucleus.

The fibers from each of the three main branches of the trigeminal root are somatotypically arranged in the spinal trigeminal tract with those from the ophthalmic divisions located most ventrally and the inputs from the mandibular division placed farthest dorsally. In humans fibers from the ophthalmic division also extend farther caudally in the tract beyond the spinomedullary junction, possibly to the upper part of spinal cord. The order of termination of the fibers in the spinal trigeminal nucleus follows the somatotopic organization in the tract such that inputs from the eye are located ventrally and laterally and those from the mouth are placed farthest medially and dorsally. A similar somatotopic, dorsoventral organization is present in the principal sensory nucleus in the pons.

Components of the spinal trigeminal nucleus

The nucleus of the spinal tract is divisible into three respective rostral to caudal portions known as the oralis, interpolaris, and caudalis nuclei (see Fig. 4-21). Each nucleus receives input from all components of the descending trigeminal tract. These nuclei have separable central connections as well, although a full discussion of these is beyond the scope of this chapter. The organization of the nucleus caudalis is of special interest because it appears to be a major terminus for specific pain and temperature afferent fibers from the head.[60,69,70] This view has received strong clinical support from findings of analgesia in the face subsequent to transection of the spinal trigeminal tract at caudal levels in the medulla for the treatment of trigeminal neuralgia.[10] These results have been interpreted as providing a selective deafferentation of projections to the nucleus caudalis. An important component of this operation is the preservation of tactile sensations from the eye, including possibly some "touch" from the cornea. (See section: Sensations resulting from mechanical stimulation of the cornea.) Consequently, patients treated with a trigeminal tractotomy will retain some corneal sensitivity and thereby be protected against the development of neuroparalytic keratitis.

Topography of projections from the eye to the nucleus caudalis

Structurally, the nucleus caudalis resembles the longitudinal layering of cells common throughout the dorsal horn of the spinal cord. The outer layer consists of a thin, one- or two-cell border known as the marginal zone. Ventral to this is a layer that contains very small cells and unmyelinated, thin-caliber fibers called the substantia gelatinosa after a similarly organized region in the spinal cord. Deep to this is a heterogeneous collection of medium to large cells that in its most ventral position is known as the magnocellular layer. Projections to the substantia gelatinosa and marginal layer have been traced from the cornea in cats and other mammals (Fig. 4-23, A and B).[66] The projections to these outer layers are much denser from those parts of the eye in which the primary sensations are pain. The deeper layers of nucleus caudalis receive far more substantial projections from those nerves supplying the eyelids, although the outer layers of the nucleus also receive some projections from these nerves (Fig. 4-23, C and D).

In contrast to the rest of the trigeminal nuclei, the somatotopic organization in the marginal zone and substantia gelatinosa of nucleus caudalis follows a medial to lateral and rostrocaudal pattern. Thus the ophthalmic representation is located farthest laterally; in this lateral part of substantia gelatinosa the inputs from more inferior and medial parts of the eye are located rostral to inputs from lateral and superior parts of the eye. This is shown diagrammatically in Figure 4-24, in which the distribution of projections to the substantia gelatinosa from the various terminal branches of the ophthalmic nerve is summarized. For example, medial and anterior receptive fields innervated by the infratrochlear nerve are represented close to the obex, whereas more lateral and posterior parts of the face that are innervated by the lacrimal nerve are located at more caudal locations.

The significance of this rostrocaudal organization of inputs to substantia gelatinosa is that it correlates better with the topographic picture of zones of analgesia and thermoanesthesia found in patients with syringomyelia or syringobulbia or in those subjected to trigeminal tractotomies.[24,31,48,95] According to the clinical observations, the peripheral distribution of the divisions of the trigeminal nerve is superimposed on an "onion peel" representation (Fig. 4-25). In this pattern the different branches of the same trigeminal division are not necessarily found in the same concentric band and all three trigeminal divisions represent anterior and posterior parts of the face.

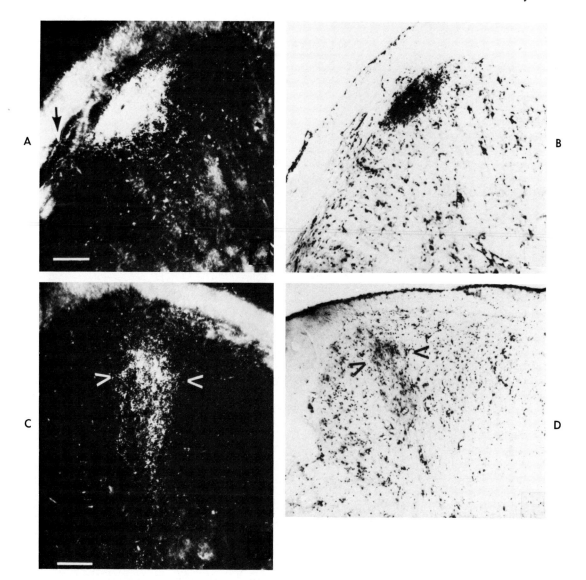

FIG. 4-23 **A** and **C**, Darkfield photomicrograph and **B** and **D**, brightfield photomicrograph showing distribution of transganglionically transported horseradish peroxidase to subnucleus caudalis from cornea (**A**, **B**) and frontal nerve (**C**, **D**). Arrow in **A** indicates labeling of sparse projection to marginal layer, which contrasts with dense corneal projections to substantia gelatinosa shown to right of arrow. Open arrowheads in **C** and **D** indicate border between substantia gelatinosa and deeper layers of trigeminal dorsal horn. Note that dense projections from frontal nerve extend into deeper laminae. Bars equal 100μm.

A number of studies have shown that mainly small-caliber sensory fibers project to substantia gelatinosa and the outer marginal layer and that they transmit nociceptive and thermal information to these layers of the spinal and trigeminal dorsal horns.[46,47,53,70,71] The topographic organization of these projections further suggests that the sensory projections to substantia gelatinosa in the trigeminal dorsal horn are a major determinant in defining the somatotopical arrangement for pain and temperature sensations from the head. "Thus, the 'onion peel organization,' which was first proposed in the clinic mainly on the basis of analgesic zones in patients, is supported by anatomic data on the topography of projections to (substantia gelatinosa)."[66]

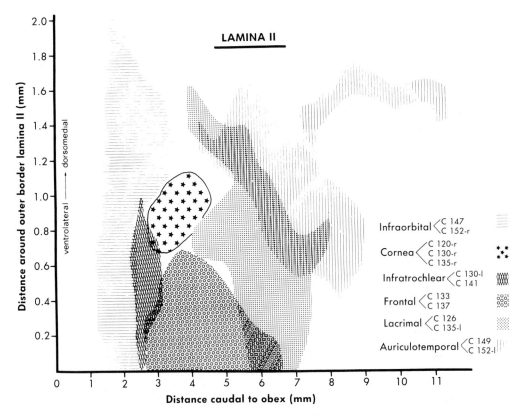

FIG. 4-24 Summary diagram showing distribution of projections to substantia gelatinosa layer (lamina *II*) of trigeminal dorsal horn from various cutaneous nerves supplying the eye and neighboring skin. Organization of projections has been reconstructed onto a two-dimensional map of lamina *II* on the basis of caudal distance from obex, which arbitrarily was set at 0 mm on abscissa, and medial to lateral position around margin of the substantia gelatinosa (ordinate). Note central location of corneal representation. (From Panneton WM, Burton H: J Comp Neurol 199:327, 1981.)

Connections responsible for the unconditioned corneal blink reflex

Various protective unconditioned blink reflexes were described in Chapter 1. These have an initial fast and a subsequent slow component.[34,35] The series of connections responsible for this reflex must lead to activation of the facial motoneurons controlling the orbicularis oculi muscle. These motoneurons are grouped together in the dorsal part of the facial nucleus as the intermediate subnucleus. On the ipsilateral side input reaching one or more subdivisions of the spinal trigeminal nucleus and principal trigeminal nucleus contact neurons that form monosynaptic connections with the ipsilateral facial nucleus.[38] This reflex arc is activated by nociceptive and tactile stimulation. This three-neuron, disynaptic reflex arc is responsible for the fast component (latency of 10 to 15 msec) of the ipsilateral blink response. The second, slower, multisyn-

aptic bilateral phase (20 to 35 msec) of the contraction of the orbicularis muscle is a result of additional connections from the ipsilateral trigeminal nuclei to various brainstem centers that subsequently project to medullary and pontine blink premotor areas with final projections to the facial nucleus. Some of the intermediate nuclei include the deep layers of the superior colliculus, portions of the red nucleus, and several pretectal nuclei.[38] These centers, in turn, receive projections from cortex and cerebellum that provide overall coordination of movement, including the eyes, and provide the anatomic substrate for linking blinking behavior with various learned responses.

The source of the fast crossed blink response is less certain because the connections are not completely understood. Some evidence suggests that the ipsilateral trigeminal nuclei send crossed fibers directly to the motor nuclei,[34] but

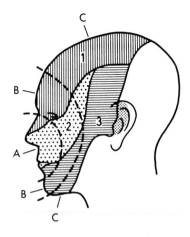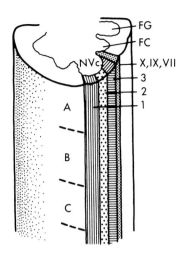

FIG. 4-25 Diagram to explain how pattern of segmental distribution in spinal trigeminal tract (and its nucleus) of fibers from the three divisions of trigeminal nerve (1, 2, and 3) can be reconciled with onion-skin pattern of anesthesia (particularly analgesia and thermoanesthesia), often seen in patients in whom parts of spinal trigeminal tract and its nucleus are damaged. Diagram to right shows segmental termination of fibers from trigeminal divisions. 1, 2, and 3 from ventral to dorsal, and termination of fibers from cranial nerves VII, IX, and X most dorsally. Within each of the cutaneous territories of trigeminal divisions (1, 2, 3), fibers from middle (anterior, perioral, and perinasal) facial regions (zone A) are assumed to terminate most rostral in nucleus of spinal tract, whereas fibers from zones B and C end at successively lower levels. FC and FG, Nuclei of cuneate and gracile fasciculi; NV c., nucleus of spinal trigeminal tract. (From Brodal A: Neurological anatomy, 3rd ed, New York, Oxford University Press, 1981.)

others suggest that the crossed connections travel primarily to the reticular formation[13,65,67] and from there reach the facial nucleus. Multisynaptic connections for the crossed response are likely, because the fast component of the contralateral blink response is slower than the ipsilateral response.

Central projections of extraocular muscle afferents

Projections from the extraocular muscles are conveyed to the trigeminal nuclear complex, especially spinal interpolaris nucleus, and the rostral and lateral third of the medial cuneate nucleus.[68] The latter subdivision of the cuneate nucleus also receives joint and muscle receptor inputs from other parts of the body in a medial-lateral somatotopy. Within this organization the cuneate eye muscle projections converge with muscle afferent projections from the neck. This anatomic convergence from muscle receptors could be critical for coordinating eye and head movements.[68] Additional projections also distribute to other trigeminal nuclei, especially nucleus caudalis. These inputs may convey pain sensibility from the many free nerve endings found in eye muscles.

The oculocardiac reflex

The oculocardiac reflex consists of bradycardia, nausea, and faintness after applying pressure on or in the orbit, stretching the extraocular muscles, or applying pressure on the orbit during enucleation operations. The bradycardia may be of such severity as to produce cardiac arrest during ocular surgery. The reflex can be eliminated entirely by retrobulbar anesthesia or premedication with intravenous atropine to block the motor aspects of the reflex.[93] The afferent pathway involves the ophthalmic division fibers to the spinal trigeminal nuclei. In most instances it probably is triggered by activity in nociceptive fibers. The reflex response may be based on the projections from the spinal trigeminal nuclei to the reticular formation in and around the vicinity of the visceral motor nuclei of the vagus nerve.[13,67] Direct input to some of these motor nuclei also may be present.

Central projections of the trigeminal nuclei

The complexity and diversity of the efferent connections from the trigeminal nuclei are too great to be considered here. However, the ascending connections to the thalamus and cortex are of some interest because these are responsible for somatic sensations from the eye. All parts of the trigeminal nuclei contribute to the trigeminothalamic projections. A large, crossed projection arises from the ventrolateral part of the principal sensory nucleus where the eye is represented. These fibers join the medial part of the medial lemniscus and distribute to the contralateral ventral posterior medial nucleus (VPM) of the thalamus (see Fig. 4-22).

Crossed and a small number of uncrossed thalamic projections come from all parts of the spinal trigeminal nucleus. However, the greatest number of these arise from the caudal half of nucleus interpolaris and nucleus caudalis.[11] Although many of these projections also terminate in the VPM,[13,29] additional connections have been traced to intralaminar nuclei and other nuclei in the thalamus.[12] Some of the projections from cell groups in the marginal layer of the nucleus caudalis are specifically associated with conveying pain from structures such as the cornea; other trigeminothalamic connections from the spinal trigeminal nuclei arise from cells excited by low-threshold tactile stimuli. Consequently, the VPM region of the thalamus in humans and primates receives inputs from all aspects of somatic sensation from the eye, including pain from the cornea.

A somatotopic organization is present in the VPM, in which the eye is represented medially and dorsal to the rest of the face. Thalamocortical projections from this region travel to several areas of the cortex that are concerned with somatic sensations. A rather extensive area of the face is located along the lateral convexity of the postcentral gyrus (see Fig. 4-22), where several different subdivisions of the primary sensory cortex have been recognized. A small representation for the eye has been located medial to zones for somatic sensations for the maxillary and mandibular division.[62] However, no detailed studies exist on the orbital projections and there are no data on the corneal representation.

REFERENCES

1. Belmonte C, and Giraldez F: Responses of cat corneal sensory receptors to mechanical and thermal stimulation, J Physiol 321:355, 1981.
2. Beuerman RW, and Kupke K: Neural regeneration following experimental wounds of the cornea in the rabbit, in Hollyfield JG, ed: The structure of the eye, New York, Elsevier Science Publishers, 1982.
3. Beuerman RW, Maurice DM, Tanelian DL: Thermal stimulation of the cornea, in Anderson DJ, Mathews B, eds: Pain in the trigeminal region, Amsterdam, Elsevier Science Publishers, 1977.
4. Beuerman RW, McCulley JP: Comparative clinical assessment of corneal sensation using a new aesthesiometer, Am J Ophthalmol 85:812, 1978.
5. Beuerman RW, Rozsa AJ: Collateral sprouts are replaced by regenerating neurites in the wounded corneal epithelium, Neurosci Lett 44:99, 1984.
6. Beuerman RW, Schimmelpfennig B: Sensory denervation of the rabbit cornea affects epithelial properties, Exp Neurol 69:196, 1980.
7. Beuerman RW, Singh T: Structure of the corneal nerves at the limbus and peripheral cornea—a transitional zone ARVO abstr, Invest Ophthalmol Vis Sci 17(Suppl):237, 1978.
8. Beuerman RW, Tanelian DL: Corneal pain evoked by thermal stimulation, Pain 7:1, 1979.
9. Boberg-Ans J: Experience in clinical examination of corneal sensitivity, Br J Ophthalmol 51:325, 1956.
10. Brodal A: Neurological anatomy in relation to clinical medicine, 3rd ed, New York, Oxford University Press, 1981.
11. Burton H, Craig AD Jr: Distribution of trigeminothalamic neurons in cat and monkey, Brain Res 161:515, 1979.
12. Burton H, Craig, AD Jr: Spinothalamic projections in cat, raccoon and monkey: a study based on anterograde transport of horseradish peroxidase, in Macchi G, Rustioni A, Spreafico R, eds: Somatosensory integration in the thalamus, Amsterdam, Elsevier Science Publishers, 1983.
13. Burton H, Craig AD Jr, Poulos DA, Molt HJ: Efferent projections from temperature sensitive recording loci within the marginal zone of the nucleus caudalis of the spinal trigeminal complex in the cat, J Comp Neurol 183:753, 1979.
14. Butler JM, Unger WG, Cole DF: Axon reflex in ocular injury: sensory mediation of the response of the rabbit eye to laser irradiation of the iris. QJ Exp Physiol 65:261, 1980.
15. Bynke G, Hakason R, Sundler F: Is substance P necessary for corneal nociception? Eur J Pharmacol 10:253, 1984.
16. Cauna N: The fine structure of the sensory receptor organs in the auricle of the rat, J Comp Neurol 136:81, 1969.
17. Chan KY, Haschke RH: Action of a trophic factor(s) from rabbit corneal epithelial culture on dissociated trigeminal neurons, J Neurosci 1:1155, 1981.
18. Chan KY, Jones RR, Bark DH, et al: Release of neuronotrophic factor from rabbit corneal epithelium during wound healing and nerve regeneration, Exp Eye Res 45:633, 1987.
19. Chan-Ling T, Tervo K, Tervo T, et al: Long-term neural regeneration in the rabbit following 180° limbal incision, Invest Ophthalmol Vis Sci 28:2083, 1987.
20. Cochet P, Bonnet R: L'esthesiometrie corneenne: realisation et interet practique, Bull Soc Ophthalmol Fr 6:541, 1961.
21. Darian-Smith I: The sense of touch: performance and peripheral neural processes, in Darian-Smith I, ed: Handbook of physiology, sect I, part 2, vol III, Sensory

processes, Bethesda, MD, American Physiological Society, 1984, pp 770-792.

22. Davies MS: Corneal anesthesia after alcohol injection of the trigeminal sensory root: examination of 100 anesthetic corneas, Br J Ophthalmol 54:577, 1970.

23. Dawson, WW: The thermal excitation of afferent neurones in the mammalian cornea and iris, in Hardy, JD, ed: Temperature: its measurement and control in science and industry, New York: 1963.

24. Déjèrine J: Semiologie des affections du systeme nerveux, Paris, Masson, 1914.

25. Dohlman CH: Corneal edema, in Smolin G, Thoft RA, eds: The cornea, scientific foundations and clinical practice, Boston, Little, Brown, 1983.

26. Ehinger G, Sjoberg N-O: Development of the ocular adrenergic nerve supply in man and guinea pig. Z Zellforsch Mikrosk Anat 118:579, 1971.

27. Fitzgerald GG, Cooper JR: Acetylcholine as a possible sensory mediator in rabbit corneal epithelium, Biochem Parmacol 20:2741, 1971.

28. Friend J: Metabolism and biochemisty, in Smolin G, Thoft RA, eds: The cornea, scientific foundations and clinical practice, Boston, Little, Brown, 1983.

29. Ganchrow D: Intratrigeminal and thalamic projections of nucleus caudalis in the squirrel monkey *(Saimiri sciureus)*: a degeneration and autoradiographic study, J Comp Neurol 178:281, 1978.

30. Gazelius B, Olgart L: Vasodilatation in the dental pulp produced by electrical stimulation of the inferior alveolar nerve in the cat, Acta Physiol Scand 109:181, 1980.

31. Gerard MW: Afferent impulses of the trigeminal nerve: the intramedullary course of the painful thermal and tactile impulses, Arch Neurol Psychiatry 9:306, 1923.

32. Giraldez F, Geijo E, Belmonte C: Response characteristics of corneal sensory fibers to mechanical and thermal stimulation, Brain Res 177:571, 1979.

33. Harris LW, Purves D: Rapid remodeling of sensory endings in the corneas of living mice, J Neurosci 9:2210, 1989.

34. Harvey JA, Land T, McMaster SE: Anatomical study of the rabbit's corneal-VIth nerve reflex: connections between cornea, trigeminal sensory complex, and the abducens and accessory abducens nuclei, Brain Res 301:307, 1984,

35. Hiraoka M, Shimamura M: Neural mechanisms of the corneal blinking reflex in cat, Brain Res 125:265, 1977.

36. Hogan MJ, Alvarado JA, Weddell JE: Histology of the human eye: an atlas and textbook, Philadelphia, WB Saunders, 1971.

37. Hokfelt T, Kellerth J, Nilsson G, et al: Substance P: localization in the central nervous system and in some primary sensory neurons, Science 190:889, 1975.

38. Holstege G, Tan J, van Ham JJ, et al: Anatomical observations on the afferent projections to the retractor bulbi motoneuronal cell group and other pathways possibly related to the blink reflex in the cat, Brain Res 374:321, 1986.

39. Hoyes AD, Barber P: Ultrastructure of the corneal nerves in the rat, Cell Tissue Res 172:133, 1976.

40. Huhtola A: Origin of myelinated nerves in the rat iris, Exp Eye Res 22:259, 1976.

41. Jessell TM, Iversen LL, Cuello AC: Capasaicin-induced depletion of substance P from primary sensory neurones, Brain Res 152:183, 1978.

42. Keen P, et al: Substance P in the mouse cornea: effects of chemical and surgical denervation, Neurosci Lett 29:231, 1982.

43. Kenshalo DR: Comparison of thermal sensitivity of the forehead, lip, conjunctiva and cornea, J Appl Physiol 15:987, 1960.

44. Kerr FWL: The divisional organization of afferent fibers of the trigeminal nerve, Brain 86:721, 1963.

45. Kruger L, Perl ER, Sedivec MJ: Fine structure of myelinated mechanical nociceptor endings in cat hairy skin, J Comp Neurol 198:137, 1981.

46. Kumazawa T, Perl ER: Primate cutaneous receptors with unmyelinated (C) fibers and their projection to the substantia gelatinosa, J Physiol (Paris) 73:287, 1977.

47. Kumazawa T, Perl ER: Excitation of marginal and substantia gelatinosa neurons in the primate spinal cord: indications of their place in dorsal horn organization, J Comp Neurol 177:417, 1978.

48. Kunc Z: Significant factors pertaining to the results of trigeminal tractotomy, in Hassler R, Walker AE, eds: Trigeminal neuralgia, Philadelphia, WB Saunders, 1970.

49. Lee Y, Takami K, Kawai Y, et al: Distribution of calcitonin gene-related peptide in the rat peripheral nervous system with reference to its coexistance with substance P, Neurosci 15:1227, 1985.

50. de Leeuw AM, Chan KY: Corneal nerve regeneration. Correlation between morphology and restoration of sensitivity, Invest Ophthalmol Vis Sci 30:1980, 1989.

51. Lembeck F, Holzer P: Substance P as neurogenic mediator of antidromic vasodilatation and neurogenic plasma extravasation, Naunyn Schmiedebergs, Arch Pharmacol 310:175, 1979.

52. Lewis, RA, Keltner JL, Cobb CA: Corneal anesthesia after percutaneous radiofrequency trigeminal rhizotomy: a retrospective study, Arch Ophthalmol 100:301, 1982.

53. Light AR, Trevino DL, Perl ER: Morphological features of functionally defined neurons in the marginal zone and substantia gelatinosa of the spinal dorsal horn, J Comp Neurol 186:151, 1979.

54. Mark D, Maurice D: Sensory recording from the isolated cornea, Invest Ophthalmol 16:541, 1977.

55. Matsuda H: Electron microscopic study of the corneal nerve with special reference to the nerve endings, Acta Soc Ophthalmol Jpn 72:880, 1968.

56. Millodot M: Objective measurement of corneal sensitivity, Act Ophthalmol (Copenh) 51:325, 1973.

57. Millodot M: A review of research on the sensitivity of the cornea, Ophthal Physiol Opt 4:305, 1984.

58. Mindal JS, Mittag TW: Choline acetyltransferase in ocular tissues of rabbits, cats, cattle, and man, Invest Ophthalmol 15:808, 1976.

59. Morgan C, Jannetta PJ, deGroat WC: Organization of corneal afferent axons in the trigeminal nerve root entry zone in the cat, Brain Res 68:411, 1987.

60. Mosso JA, Kruger L: Spinal trigeminal neurons excited by noxious and thermal stimuli, Brain Res 38:206, 1972.

61. Nafe J, Wagoner K: Insensitivity of cornea to heat and pain derived from high temperatures, Am J Psychol 49:631, 1937.

62. Nelson RJ, Sur M, Felleman DJ, et al: Representations of the body surface in postcentral parietal cortex of *Macaca fascicularis*, J Comp Neurol 192:611, 1980.

63. Nicoll RA, Schenker C, Leeman SE: Substance P as a transmitter candidate, Ann Rev Neurosci 3:227, 1980.

64. Norn MS: Conjunctival sensitivity in normal eyes, Acta Ophthalmol 51:58, 1973.

65. Ongerboer de Visser BW: The corneal reflex: electrophysiological and anatomical data in man, Prog Neurobiol 15:71, 1980.

66. Panneton WM, Burton H: Corneal and periocular representation within the trigeminal sensory complex in the cat studied with transganglionic transport of horseradish peroxidase, J Comp Neurol 199:327, 1981.

67. Panneton WM, Burton H: Projections from the paratrigeminal nucleus and the medullary spinal dorsal horns to the peribrachial area in the cat, Neuroscience 15:779, 1985.

68. Porter JD: Brainstem terminations of extraocular muscle primary afferent neurons in the monkey, J Comp Neurol 247:133, 1986.

69. Poulos DA, Burton H, Molt JT, et al: Localization of specific thermoreceptors in spinal trigeminal nucleus of the cat, Brain Res 165:144, 1979.

70. Price DD, Dubner R, Hu JW: Trigeminothalamic neurons in nucleus caudalis responsive to tactile, thermal, and nociceptive stimulation of the monkey's face, J Neurophysiol 39:936, 1976.

71. Price DD, Hayashi H, Dubner R, et al: Functional relationships between neurons of marginal and substantia gelatinosa layers of primate dorsal horn, J Neurophysiol 42:1590, 1979.

72. Rozsa AJ, Beuerman RW: Density and organization of free nerve endings in the corneal epithelium of the rabbit, Pain 14:105, 1982.

73. Rozsa AJ, Guss RB, Beuerman RW: Neural remodeling following experimental surgery of the rabbit cornea, Invest Ophthalmol Vis Sci 24:1033, 1983.

74. Ruben M, Colebrook F: Keratoplasty sensitivity, Br J Ophthalmol 63:265, 1979.

75. Ruskell GL: Ocular fibers of the maxillary nerves in monkeys, J Anat 118:195, 1974.

76. Sasaoka A, Ishiimoto I, Kuwayama Y, et al: Overall distribution of substance P nerves in the rat cornea and their three-dimensional profiles, Invest Ophthalmol Vis Sci 25:351, 1984.

77. Schimmelpfennig B: Nerve structures in human central corneal epithelium, Graefes Arch Clin Exp Ophthalmol, 218:14, 1982.

78. Seiger A, Selin UB, Kessler J, et al: Substance P-containing sensory nerves in the rat iris; normal distribution, ontogeny and innervation of intraocular iris grafts, Neuroscience 15:519, 1985.

79. Silverman JD, Kruger L: Lectin and neuropeptide labeling of separate populations of dorsal root ganglion neurons and associated "nociceptor" thin axons in rat testis and cornea whole-mount preparations, Somatosen Res 5:259, 1988.

80. Strughold H: Mechanical threshold of cornea-reflex of the usual laboratory animals, Am J Physiol 94:235, 1930.

81. Tanelian DL, Beuerman RW: Responses of rabbit corneal nociceptors to mechanical and thermal stimulation, Exp Neurol 84:165, 1984.

82. Tervo K, Tervo T, Eranko L, et al: Immunoreactivity for substance P in the gasserian ganglion, ophthalmic nerve and anterior segment of the rabbit eye, Histochem J 13:425, 1981.

83. Tervo K, Tervo T, Eranko L, et al: Effect of sensory and sympathetic denervation on substance P immunoreactivity in nerve fibers of the rabbit eye, Exp Eye Res 34:577, 1982.

84. Tervo T: Histochemical demonstration of cholinesterase activity in the cornea of the rat and the effect of various denervations on the corneal nerves, Histochemistry 47:133, 1976.

85. Tervo T, Joo F, Huikuri KT, et al: Fine structure of sensory nerves in the rat cornea: an experimental nerve degeneration study, Pain 6:57, 1979.

86. Tervo T, Palkama A: Sympathetic nerves to the rat cornea, Acta Ophthalmol 54:75, 1976.

87. Tervo, T, and Palkama A: Innervation of the rabbit cornea; a histochemical and electron-microscope study, Acta Anat (Basel) 102:164, 1978.

88. Tervo T, Tervo K, Eranko L, et al: Substance P immunoreaction and acetylcholinesterase activity in the cornea and gasserian ganglion, Ophthalmol Res 15:280, 1983.

89. Tower S: Unit for sensory reception in the cornea, J Neurophysiol, 3:486, 1940.

90. Ueda S, del Cerro M, LoCascio JA, et al: Peptidergic and catecholaminergic fibers in the human corneal epithelium, Acta Ophthalmol 67(Suppl 192):80, 1989.

91. Unger WG, Cole DF, Bass MS: Prostaglandin and neurogenically mediated ocular response to laser irradiation of the rabbit iris, Exp Eye Res 25:209, 1977.

92. Uusitalo H, Krootila K, Palkama A: Calcitonin gene-related peptide (CGRP) immunoreactive sensory nerves in the human and guinea pig uvea and cornea, Exp Eye Res 48:467, 1989.

93. Walsh FB, Hoyt WF: Sensory innervation of the eye and orbit, in Clinical neuro-ophthalmology, 3rd ed, Baltimore, Williams & Wilkins, 1969.

94. Werner RG, Pinkerton RMH, Robertson DM: Cryosurgical induced changes in corneal nerves, Can J Ophthalmol 8:548, 1973.

95. Woods AH: Segmental distribution of the spinal root and nucleus of the trigeminal nerve, J Nerv Ment Dis 40:91, 1913.

96. Zander E, Weddell G: Observations on the innervation of the cornea, J Anat 85:68, 1951.

The Extraocular Muscles

Movement of the globes is performed by an orbital plant that includes the connective and adipose tissues of the orbit as well as the extraocular muscles. These structures enable the eyes to rotate rapidly in a precise, coordinated manner. The orbital plant is activated by complex patterns of neural innervation that are generated by the cerebral cortex, cerebellum, and brainstem and transmitted via the ocular motor nerves. Proper control of eye movement facilitates the alignment of the foveas of both eyes toward targets of visual interest.

This chapter is divided into three sections. The first section explores the anatomy, physiology, and pharmacology of the extraocular muscles; the second section examines the neurophysiology of the ocular motor system; and the third section discusses the clinical assessment of binocular vision.

SECTION ONE

Anatomy, physiology, and pharmacology

RONALD M. BURDE, M.D.
STEVEN E. FELDON, M.D.

ANATOMIC RELATIONSHIPS BETWEEN THE EXTRAOCULAR MUSCLES AND THE ORBITS

Each eyeball is suspended in its bony orbital cavity by a complex matrix of fascia and muscle (Figs. 5-1 and 5-2). The two bony orbits are—roughly—quadrilateral pyramids whose medial walls are parallel to each other. The lateral walls produce approximately a 90-degree angle (Fig. 5-3). The widest part of each pyramid is about 1.5 cm posterior to the orbital margin, and the walls taper to the orbital opening, giving the cavity a somewhat pear-shaped appearance.

The complexity of the orbital musculofibrous apparatus required to support the orbital structures while allowing considerable freedom of movement has been detailed by Kornneef.[30] The extraocular muscles originate at the orbital apex and terminate on the globe in the spiral of Tillaux (Fig. 5-4). Throughout their course extraocular muscles also are attached by means of fibrous septa to the periosteal lining of the bony orbit (periorbita) (Fig. 5-5). Anteriorly, these fascial planes blend with Tenon's capsule, enclosing the sclera; posteriorly, they blend with the dura of the optic nerve sheath.

Individual muscles

The *levator palpebrae* and the *superior rectus muscle* originate at the anulus of Zinn near the orbital apex. Posteriorly, they are both anchored to the orbital roof. Fascial attachments between the superior rectus muscle and the levator palpebrae limit movement of one muscle with respect to the other.[10] As the muscles pass anteriorly through the orbit, the superior rectus loses its attachment to the orbital roof first and develops fibrous connections with the lateral rectus muscle (Figs. 5-5 and 5-6). Eventually, the levator becomes dissociated from the orbital roof

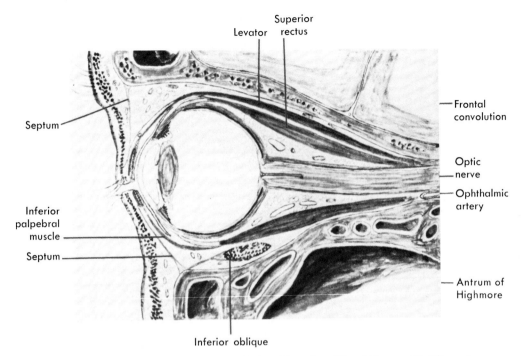

Superior
Levator   rectus

Septum

Frontal
convolution

Optic
nerve

Ophthalmic
artery

Inferior
palpebral
muscle

Septum

Antrum of
Highmore

Inferior oblique

FIG. 5-1   Vertical anteroposterior section of orbit. (From Last RL, ed: Eugene Wolff's anatomy of the eye and orbit, 6th ed, Philadelphia, WB Saunders, 1968.)

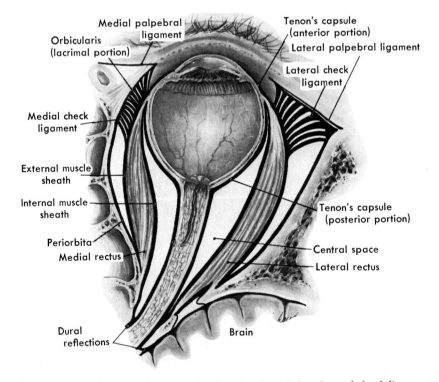

Medial palpebral
ligament

Orbicularis
(lacrimal portion)

Tenon's capsule
(anterior portion)

Lateral palpebral ligament

Lateral check
ligament

Medial check
ligament

External muscle
sheath

Internal muscle
sheath

Periorbita

Medial rectus

Tenon's capsule
(posterior portion)

Central space

Lateral rectus

Dural
reflections

Brain

FIG. 5-2   Horizontal section through orbit showing fascial sheaths and check ligaments.

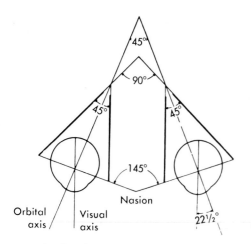

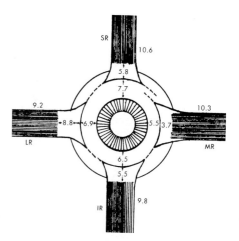

FIG. 5-3 Angles formed by walls of orbit. (From Duke-Elder S, Wybar KC: The anatomy of the visual system, in Duke-Elder S, ed: System of ophthalmology, vol 2, St Louis, CV Mosby, 1961.)

FIG. 5-4 Diagrammatic view of front of right eye, drawn to scale, showing insertions of rectus muscles. All figures are in millimeters. Spiral made by insertions of oculorotary muscle tendons is indicated by dotted line; this is called spiral of Tillaux. (From Scobee RG: The oculorotary muscles, St Louis, CV Mosby, 1952.)

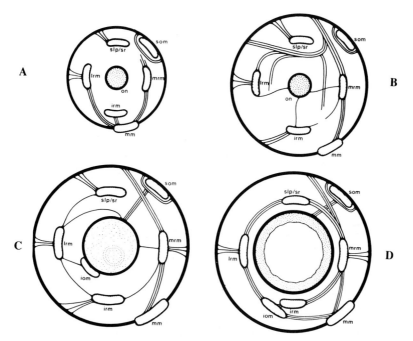

FIG. 5-5 Four highly schematic drawings illustrating directions of connective tissue septa of different eye muscles in orbit. See text for further explanation. **A,** Area near orbital apex. **B,** Area posterior from, but close to, hind surface of eye. **C,** Area lying a little anterior from hind surface of eye. **D,** Area close to eyeball equator. slp/sr, Superior levator palpebrae/superior rectus muscle complex; lrm, lateral rectus muscle; iom, inferior oblique muscle; irm, inferior rectus muscle; mm, Müller's muscle; mrm, medial rectus muscle; som, superior oblique muscle; on, optic nerve. (From Koorneef L: Spatial aspects of orbital musculo-fibrous tissue in man: a new anatomical and histological approach, Amsterdam, Swets and Zeitlinger, 1976, p 129.)

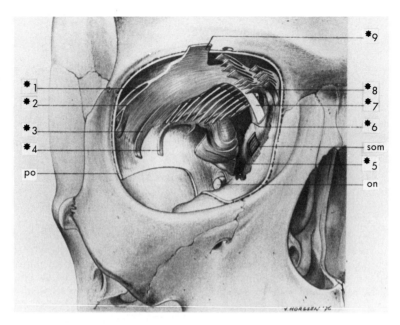

FIG. 5-6 Drawing of connective tissue of superior levator palpebrae/superior rectus muscle complex and connective tissue of superior oblique muscle. *1*, Superior part of lateral aponeurosis; *2*, middle part of aponeurosis; *3*, inferior part of aponeurosis; *4*, connections with lateral rectus muscle connective tissue; *po*, periorbit; *on*, optic nerve; *5*, contributions to superior ophthalmic vein hammock; *som*, superior oblique muscle; *6*, connections of superior oblique muscle tendon connective tissue to medial upper part and hind surface of eye; *7*, medial aponeurosis; *8*, area of superior oblique muscle trochlea; *9*, attachment to superior tarsal plate. (From Koorneef L: Spatial aspects of orbital musculo-fibrous tissue in man, Amsterdam, Swets and Zeitlinger, 1976, p 121.)

to develop its lateral aponeurosis. A small medial aponeurosis inserts into the connective tissue of the superior oblique muscle. The superior rectus inserts into the globe 7.7 mm behind the limbus.

The *lateral rectus muscle* (see Fig. 5-2) arises from an inferomedial muscle complex at the orbital apex, which also includes the inferior and medial rectus muscles. Septal connections between Müller's muscle (covering the inferior orbital fissure) and the lateral rectus muscle extend anteriorly; there are also fibrous connections between the lateral and inferior rectus muscles in the posterior orbit (Fig. 5-7). A firm attachment between the fascia of the lateral rectus muscle and the lateral orbital wall extends along the entire course of the muscle (see Fig. 5-5, *A-D*). Anteriorly, fascial bridges join the lateral rectus muscle with the inferior oblique muscle (see Fig. 5-5, *C*). Attachments also are formed with the levator palpebrae/superior rectus muscle complex (see Fig. 5-7). The lateral rectus muscle runs forward on the temporal side of the globe to insert approximately 7 mm from the limbus by means of a very long and relatively thin tendon, approximately 9 mm in length.

Throughout its course anteriorly, the *inferior rectus muscle* (see Fig. 5-1) traverses temporally within the orbit. The inferior rectus muscle has its origin within the inferomedial muscle complex at the orbital apex and, like the lateral rectus muscle, has attachments to Müller's muscle in the region of the inferior orbital fissure (see Fig. 5-5, *A*). In the midorbit, fasciae of the inferior rectus muscle then become adherent to the orbital floor (see Fig. 5-5, *B* and *C*). Septa develop to bridge the inferior and lateral rectus muscles as well as the inferior and medial rectus muscles (Fig. 5-8). At the level of the inferior oblique the inferior rectus muscle sheath inserts into the posterior border of the inferior oblique muscle sheath and contributes to the suspensory ligament of Lockwood (Figs. 5-8 and 5-9). At this point the inferior rectus and inferior oblique muscles are bound firmly together. The muscle inserts into the globe 6.5 mm from the limbus. The tendon is 5.5 mm long and about 10 mm wide.

The *medial rectus muscle* has its origin at the anulus of Zinn and hugs the medial orbital wall as it travels anteriorly (Figs. 5-2 and 5-10). Posteriorly, there are well-developed attachments

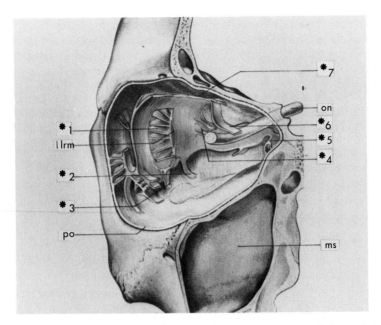

FIG. 5-7 Drawing of lateral rectus muscle connective tissue apparatus. *1*, Area of attachment to lateral orbital wall; lrm, lateral rectus muscle; *2*, connections with connective tissue of inferior rectus muscle; *3*, connections with inferior oblique muscle connective tissue septa; po, periorbit; *4*, relationships with optic nerve; *5*, connections with Müller's muscle in inferior orbital fissure; *6*, contribution to superior ophthalmic vein hammock; ms, maxillary sinus; on, optic nerve; *7*, connection to lateral aponeurosis of superior levator palpebrae/superior rectus muscle complex. (From Koorneef L: Spatial aspects of orbital musculo-fibrous tissue in man, Amsterdam, Swets and Zeitlinger, 1976, p 121.)

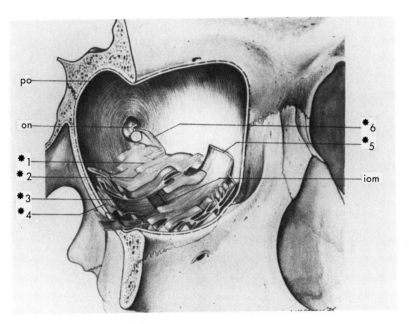

FIG. 5-8 Drawing of connective tissue of inferior rectus and inferior oblique muscle. po, Periorbit; on, optic nerve; *1*, inferior rectus muscle connective tissue; *2*, septal connections with lateral rectus muscle; *3*, connections of inferior oblique muscle connective tissue to lateral rectus muscle connective tissue; *4*, fingerlike offshoots to inferolateral orbital wall; iom, inferior oblique muscle; *5*, septal connections with medial rectus muscle connective tissue; *6*, contributions to superior ophthalmic vein hammock. (From Koorneef L: Spatial aspects of orbital musculo-fibrous tissue in man, Amsterdam, Swets and Zeitlinger, 1976, p 123.)

of the muscle to the orbital roof, floor, and underlying Müller's muscle. Connections also develop with fibrous elements of the superior and inferior rectus muscles (see Fig. 5-5, *A-D*). More anteriorly, multiple attachments develop with the medial orbital wall. These attachments join with the medial aponeurosis of the levator palpebrae/superior rectus complex (see Fig. 5-10). The muscle attaches to the globe 5.5 mm posterior to the limbus; its tendon is less than 4 mm in length.

The *inferior oblique muscle* (see Figs. 5-1 and 5-8) originates in the lateral aspect of the lacrimal fossa and passes laterally and posteriorly over a distance of 3.7 cm to insert into the globe just below the lateral rectus. The connective tissue associated with the inferior oblique muscle intermingles with that of the inferior rectus muscle to form Lockwood's ligament (see Fig. 5-9), which acts as an effective insertion of the inferior oblique muscle.[55] Fibrous connections between the inferior oblique and the lateral and

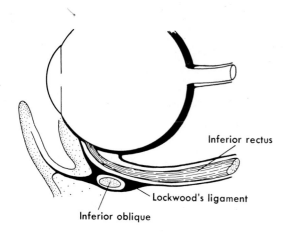

FIG. 5-9 Vertical longitudinal section through lower anterior portion of orbit showing Lockwood's ligament. (Modified from Maddox.)

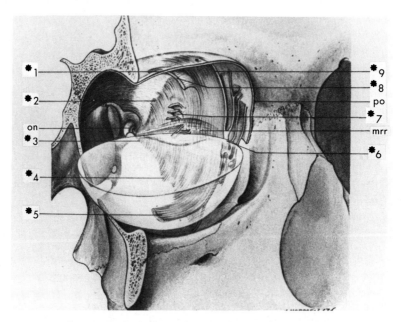

FIG. 5-10 Drawing of connective tissue system of medial rectus muscle. *1,* Superior ophthalmic vein hammock; *2,* area of attachment to orbital roof; *on,* optic nerve; *3,* connective tissue septa to Müller's muscle; *4,* area of attachment to the orbital floor; *5,* connections with the connective tissue systems of inferior oblique and inferior rectus muscles; *6,* medial conglomeration area; *mrm,* medial rectus muscle; *7,* relationships with optic nerve and hind surface of eyeball; *po,* periorbit; *8,* connection to medial aponeurosis of superior levator palpebrae muscle; *9,* connections to orbital roof. (From Koorneef L: Spatial aspects of orbital musculo-fibrous tissue in man, Amsterdam, Swets and Zeitlinger, 1976.)

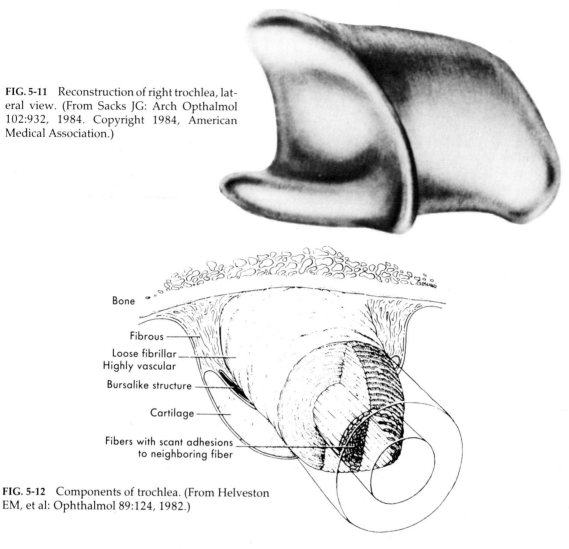

FIG. 5-11 Reconstruction of right trochlea, lateral view. (From Sacks JG: Arch Opthalmol 102:932, 1984. Copyright 1984, American Medical Association.)

Bone

Fibrous

Loose fibrillar
Highly vascular

Bursalike structure

Cartilage

Fibers with scant adhesions
to neighboring fiber

FIG. 5-12 Components of trochlea. (From Helveston EM, et al: Ophthalmol 89:124, 1982.)

medial rectus muscles also are present (see Fig. 5-5, *D*).

The *superior oblique muscle* arises from the lesser wing of the sphenoid bone above the anulus of Zinn and rises about 2 cm as it travels superomedially through its own adipose tissue compartment to reach the trochlea (see Figs. 5-5, *A-D*, and 5-6). The trochlea is a plate of cartilage forming a U-shaped pully over the trochlear fossa of the frontal bone (Fig. 5-11). At this point the muscle tendon turns sharply backward to create an angle of about 20 degrees with the muscle belly. The tendon then descends 1.4 cm over its 2.8 cm extent before inserting into the sclera just behind the equator, posterior to the center of rotation of the globe.[18] The anatomic relationship of the superior oblique tendon with its sheath facilitates muscle function (Fig. 5-12).

ACTIONS OF THE EXTRAOCULAR MUSCLES
Mechanics of ocular rotation: frames of reference

To discuss eye movements, a frame of reference that defines the *axes of rotation* is necessary.

The *center of rotation* of the globe is not fixed, being dependent upon the position of the globe in the orbit.[49,61] Nonrotational (translational) movements with rotation of the globe form a semicircular locus of points called the *space centroid* (shown for the horizontal plane in Fig. 5-13). To establish systematic reference coordinates, the globe can be considered to rotate around a fixed point that lies 13.5 mm in back of the corneal apex and 1.6 mm to the nasal side of the geometric center of the globe.

Movements of the globe are described by a coordinate system with three axes perpendicu-

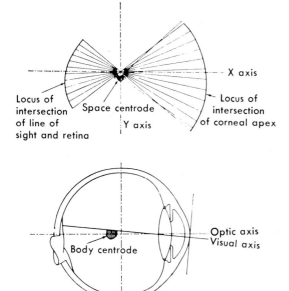

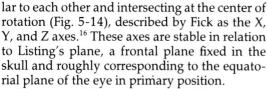

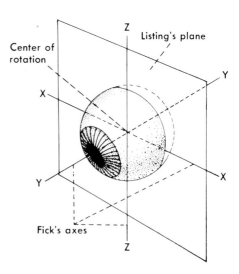

FIG. 5-13   Position of space centrode computed by Park and Park.

FIG. 5-14   Fick's axes and Listing's plane.

lar to each other and intersecting at the center of rotation (Fig. 5-14), described by Fick as the X, Y, and Z axes.[16] These axes are stable in relation to Listing's plane, a frontal plane fixed in the skull and roughly corresponding to the equatorial plane of the eye in primary position.

Rotations of either eye alone—without attention to the movements of its mate—are called ductions. Horizontal rotation (rotation around the Z axis) is termed "adduction" if the anterior pole of the eye is rotated nasally (medially, in), or "abduction" if the anterior pole of the eye is rotated temporally (laterally, out). Vertical rotation (rotation about the X axis) is called "elevation" (sursumduction, supraduction) if the anterior pole moves up, or "depression" (deorsumduction, infraduction) if the anterior pole moves down.

Primary position of gaze

The *primary position* of the eyes is that position from which all other ocular movements are initiated or that position of the eyeball in its socket against which all torsional, rotational, and translatory movements are measured. The primary position has been defined by Scobee[54] as "that position of the eyes in binocular vision when, with the head erect, the object of regard is at infinity and lies at the intersection of the sagittal plane of the head and a horizontal plane passing through the centers of rotation of the two eyeballs."

Secondary positions of gaze

Rotation solely around either the horizontal or vertical axis places the eye in a secondary position of gaze. In achieving secondary positions of gaze, there is no rotation of the globe around the Y axis. Therefore secondary positions are not associated with torsion.

Tertiary positions of gaze

The oblique positions of gaze are called *tertiary positions*. Tertiary positions are achieved by a simultaneous rotation around the horizontal and vertical axes, a movement that can be considered to occur around an oblique axis lying in Listing's plane.[39] As the eye rotates obliquely out of the primary position, the vertical axis of the globe is seen to tilt with respect to the X and Z axes of the fixed planar-coordinate system (Fig. 5-15). This tilt is termed "false torsion," because there is no real rotation around the Y axis, only an apparent movement with respect to the coordinate system. The amount of false torsion associated with any particular oblique position is constant regardless of how the eye reaches the position (Donder's law). Tertiary positions of gaze are thus positions of gaze associated with false torsion.

Torsion

True torsion (or wheel rotation) is a relative movement of the sagittal axis of the eye with respect to the sagittal plane of Fick's axis. As such,

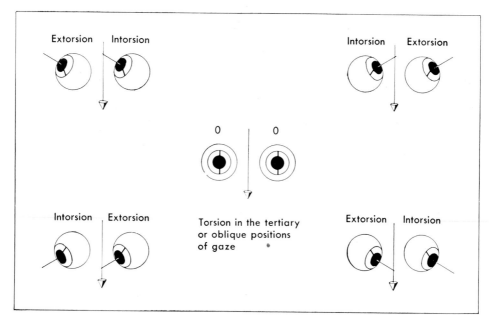

FIG. 5-15 Globe in primary and tertiary positions of gaze to demonstrate false torsion (in terms of planar coordinate system).

this is not a rotation strictly about the Y axis but rather about a point at the lateral limbus[22,23,24,26] (Fig. 5-16). Torsional movements work within a small range to keep the sensory vertical raphe of the retina perpendicular to the horizon. If the upper end of the vertical meridian of the eye tilts toward the nose, this is termed "incycloduction," and if it tilts toward the temple, "excycloduction." With a 30-degree head tilt there is a mean incycloduction of the ipsilateral eye of 7.00 ± 3.10 degrees and an excycloduction of 8.36 ± 2.50 degrees of the contralateral eye.[38]

Models of extraocular muscle functions

To discuss the independent action of any individual extraocular muscle is strictly a hypothetical convenience, because innervational and anatomic considerations necessitate the involvement of all six extraocular muscles for any rotation of the eye. The broad arclike insertions of the extraocular muscles resist movement out of their usual plane of rotation. Also, depending upon rotation, either the medial or temporal fibers of the muscle tendon can serve as the effective insertion.[23,28]

Because of the complexity of fully describing ocular rotation, models have been developed to simplify the problem and to impart a conceptual understanding of the process. The more detailed the model, the more realistic is the resulting information. Of the three models presented in the following paragraphs, the *isolated agonist model* is the simplest and has gained the greatest clin-

ical acceptance. The more complicated *paired antagonist model* described by Boeder[4] allows for the contributions of secondary muscle actions. As such, it is consistent with certain experimental data.[22,23,28] Robinson[52] has used the availability of experimental data and digital computers to formulate a *quantitative model* that calculates the relative contributions of all muscles to any given position of gaze.

Isolated agonist model

Traditionally, concepts of individual extraocular muscle function were based mostly on the writings of Duane,[11-13] who proposed that opposed vertical muscles act as synergists in certain gaze positions and that their functions vary with change in direction of gaze (for example, with increasing abduction the oblique muscles are said to cause increasing torsion and abduction). Continued development[31,32,54,60] of these concepts was based mainly on mathematic analysis of static anatomic relationships and the construction of ophthalmotropes (models of the eye in the orbit in which straps and springs represented extraocular muscles). Observations in normal human subjects were compatible with these models when movements in proximity to the primary position were studied. Therefore the models remain applicable and relevant clinically.[60] The primary and secondary actions of the individual extraocular muscles are summarized in Table 5-1.[7]

Medial rectus. The muscle plane of the me-

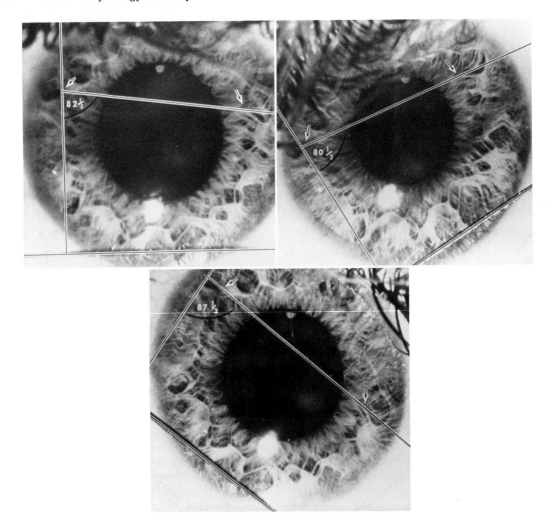

FIG. 5-16 Right eye. Lower line represents string stretched across eye. Another line is drawn perpendicular to this. Upper line connects two landmarks *(arrows)* on iris and forms angle with perpendicular line. By measuring angle, it was found that head tilt to right *(top right)* caused 2 degrees of incycloduction, and head tilt to left *(bottom)* caused 5 degrees of excycloduction. (From Linwong M, Herman SJ: Arch Ophthalmol 85:570, 1971.)

dial rectus is exactly in the horizontal plane of the globe; thus when the globe is in the primary position, contraction of the medial rectus results in internal rotation only (Fig. 5-17, *A*), that is, adduction (medial rotation). When the visual line is directed above the horizon, contraction of the medial rectus will aid in further elevation, and when the visual line is directed below the horizon, its contraction will further depress the globe (Fig. 5-18).

Lateral rectus. The plane of the lateral rectus is the same as that of the medial rectus, and when the eye is in the primary position, contraction of the lateral rectus results in abduction alone (Fig. 5-17, *B*). Like the medial rectus, when the eyeball is elevated or depressed, con-

traction of the lateral rectus will further elevate or depress the globe.

Superior rectus. The superior rectus muscle makes an angle of 23 to 25 degrees with the visual line when the eye is in primary position. Its primary action is elevation. Additional, or secondary, actions due to its angle of insertion are adduction and intorsion (Fig. 5-19). Therefore contraction of this muscle will result in a movement of the globe around several axes.

The relative strength of the individual vector forces varies according to the direction of gaze. When the visual line is directed horizontally outward to 23 degrees from the primary position, contraction of the superior rectus will produce elevation only (see Fig. 5-19, *C*). If the eye

TABLE 5-1   Actions of the Extraocular Muscles

Muscle*	Primary	Secondary	Tertiary
Medial rectus	Adduction	—	—
Lateral rectus	Abduction	—	—
Inferior rectus	Depression	Excycloduction	Adduction
Superior rectus	Elevation	Incycloduction	Adduction
Inferior oblique	Excycloduction	Elevation	Abduction
Superior oblique	Incycloduction	Depression	Abduction

From Bahill AT, et al: Invest Ophthalmol Vis Sci 14:468, 1975.
*The superior muscles are incycloductors; the inferior muscles, excycloductors. The vertical rectus muscles are adductors; the oblique muscles, abductors.

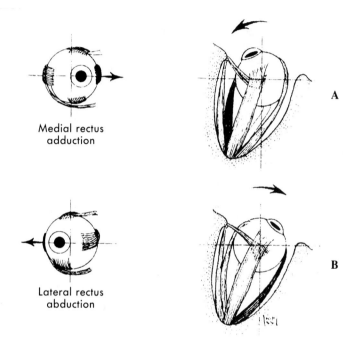

FIG. 5-17   A, Action of medial rectus muscle (adduction). **B**, Action of lateral rectus muscle (abduction). (From von Noorden GK: Atlas of strabismus, 4th ed, St Louis, CV Mosby, 1983.)

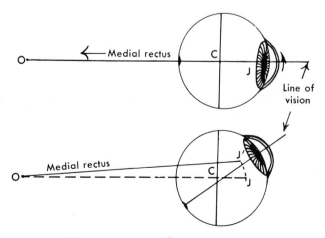

FIG. 5-18   *Top*, J, insertion of medial rectus muscle when eye is in primary position. *Bottom*, When eye turns up, J moves to J'.

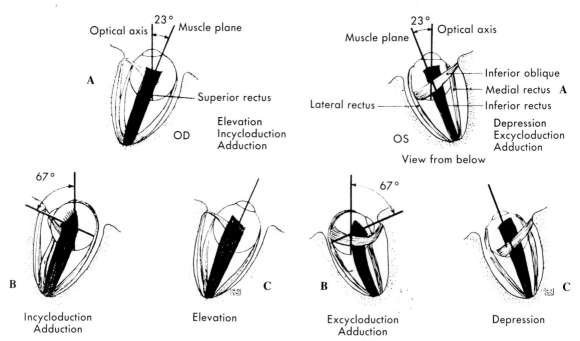

FIG. 5-19 Superior rectus. **A,** When the eye is in primary position, muscle plane of superior rectus forms angle of 23 degrees with optical axis. In this position superior rectus elevates globe. Secondary actions include incycloduction and adduction. **B,** As eye moves into adduction, superior rectus becomes less of an elevator and more of an adductor and incycloductor. In 67 degrees of adduction superior rectus would become exclusive source of incycloduction while still having adductive power. Position of 67 degrees is chosen for theoretic reasons only; eye is never adducted that far. **C,** In 23 degrees abduction superior rectus becomes a pure elevator. In this position muscle plane coincides with optical axis. (From von Noorden GK: Atlas of strabismus, 4th ed, St Louis, CV Mosby, 1983.)

FIG. 5-20 Inferior rectus. **A,** With eye in primary position inferior rectus forms angle of 23 degrees with optical axis. Thus relationship between muscle plane and optical axis is identical to that of superior rectus. In primary position inferior rectus depresses globe; secondary actions include excycloduction and adduction. **B,** As eye moves into adduction, inferior rectus becomes less of a depressor and more of an excycloductor and adductor. In 67 degrees adduction it would become exclusive source of excycloduction and would aid adduction. However, eye is never adducted that far. **C,** In 23 degrees abduction inferior rectus becomes pure depressor; in this position muscle plane coincides with optical axis. (From von Noorden GK: Atlas of strabismus, 4th ed, St Louis, CV Mosby, 1983.)

is rotated 67 degrees nasally from the primary position, so that the visual line is at a right angle to the muscle plane, contraction of the muscle will produce adduction and intorsion only (Fig. 5-19, B).[31]

Inferior rectus. The inferior rectus muscle has the same muscle plane as the superior rectus muscle (that is, it makes an angle of 23 degrees with the visual line in primary position). Accordingly, when the eye is in the primary position, contraction of the inferior rectus, like that of the superior rectus, results in a compound rotation of the globe, consisting primarily of depression and secondarily of adduction and excyclotorsion (Fig. 5-20).

Superior oblique. In primary position contraction of the superior oblique muscle produces

a compound rotation of the globe consisting of three components: the primary action, intorsion, and the secondary actions, depression and abduction. When the eye is turned 51 degrees nasally from the primary position, the visual line is parallel to the muscle pull, and contraction of the muscle will produce isolated depression of the globe. If the eye is turned temporally 39 degrees from the primary position, so that the visual line is at right angles to the muscle pull, contraction will produce nearly isolated intorsion (Fig. 5-21).

Inferior oblique. The muscle plane makes an angle of 51 degrees with the visual line when the eye is in the primary position; thus contraction of the inferior oblique will produce a compound movement of the globe consisting of

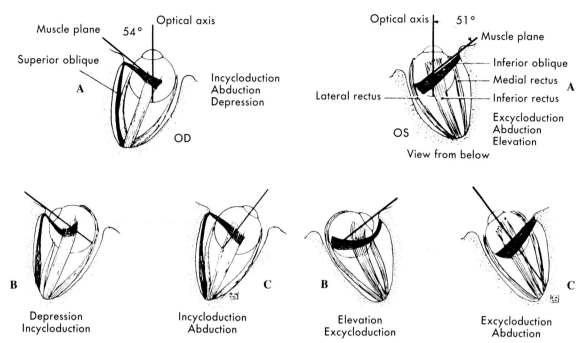

FIG. 5-21 Superior oblique. **A,** When eye is in primary position, muscle plane of superior oblique muscle forms an angle of 54 degrees with optical axis. In this position principal action of superior oblique is incycloduction; secondary actions include adduction and depression. **B,** When globe is adducted 54 degrees, optical axis coincides with muscle plane. In this position muscle still acts as an incycloductor, but its vertical action becomes more significant. **C,** When globe is abducted, superior oblique is primarily an incycloductor and secondarily an abductor. (From von Noorden GK: Atlas of strabismus, 4th ed, St Louis, CV Mosby, 1983.)

FIG. 5-22 Inferior oblique. **A,** When eye is in primary position, the muscle plane of the inferior oblique forms an angle of 51 degrees with the optical axis. In this position the principal action of the inferior oblique is one of excycloduction; secondary actions include abduction and elevation. **B,** When eye is adducted 51 degrees, optical axis approaches muscle plane. Muscle still acts as an excycloductor, but its action as an elevator becomes more significant. **C,** In abduction the inferior oblique acts primarily as an excycloductor and secondarily as an abductor. (From von Noorden GK: Atlas of strabismus, 4th ed, St Louis, CV Mosby, 1983.)

three components: the primary action, extorsion, and the secondary actions, abduction and elevation. When the eye is turned 39 degrees temporally from the primary position, the pull of the inferior oblique produces extorsion and some abduction, whereas when the eye is turned 51 degrees nasally from the primary position, the pull of the muscle produces elevation alone (Fig. 5-22).

Paired antagonist model
The simultaneous analysis of six extraocular muscle forces has been simplified by Boeder[4] into an analysis of antagonist pairs. The analysis of antagonist pairs may be reasonable because the tone of the other extraocular muscles can be assumed to be constant to prevent the eye from wobbling during movement. Boeder reasons that contraction of one member of an antagonist pair generally is associated with an extension or

lengthening of the opposite muscle in the pair. From a mechanical viewpoint, this lengthening must be regarded as a muscle action on a par with contraction. When a muscle pair functions, the eye is rotated around an axis that lies midway between the two muscles. (For more detailed discussion, see Boeder.[4]) In his analysis Boeder uses a spherical coordinate system with phi representing horizontal deviations and delta representing vertical deviations. An analysis of the action of individual antagonist pairs is shown in Fig. 5-23.

Paired vertical recti. Primary actions of the vertical recti are elevation and depression; secondary actions are adduction and torsion. Adduction increases with increasing medial movement. Note that there is relative abduction in moving from inferior or superior gaze to the primary position. Using Volkmann's figures for cross-sectional areas[17,62] and calculating torque

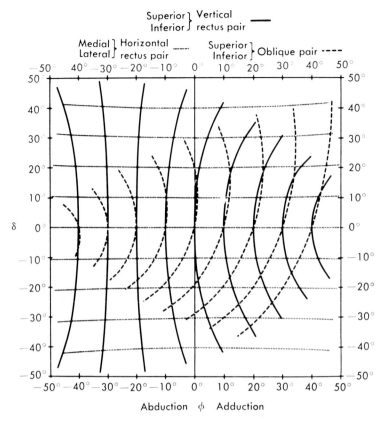

FIG. 5-23 Traces of line of fixation when three muscle pairs act individually. (From Boeder P: Am J Ophthalmol 51:469, 1961.)

(force times radius), it is theoretically possible for the vertical muscle pair, by cocontracting, to exert greater than 50% of the force required for adduction once the globe has been adducted slightly less than 30 degrees. Cocontraction is the simultaneous contraction of muscles that are normally antagonists. However, there is no physiologic evidence of increased firing of these muscles with horizontal rotation. Even at a fixed firing rate, the mechanical advantage for adduction by the vertical recti increases with increasing adduction. In abduction both muscles must lengthen (relax). When the eye is externally rotated 25 to 30 degrees, these muscles have minimal abduction function. With increasing adduction the vertical recti must take up the slack.

The superior rectus, which causes intorsion, is estimated to contribute about 30% of the force required in primary position to keep the horizontal raphe parallel to the horizon. The inferior rectus, which causes extorsion, contributes approximately 30% of the required force in primary position to keep the horizontal raphe parallel to the horizon. The torsional effect of the vertical recti is almost nil in lateral gaze and con-

tinues to increase with increasing adduction.

Paired obliques. The primary actions of the oblique muscle pair are intorsion and extorsion. The fundamental finding[23,25] on which the newer concepts of oblique muscle action are based is that the axis about which the oblique muscles rotate the eye in the orbit remains constant when the eye rotates horizontally from any position of gaze. This constancy is due to the structure of the oblique muscle tendons, which insert obliquely into the globe. The inner fibers of the fanlike tendon are elongated in adduction, whereas the outer fibers are shortened and conversely in abduction. Hence the contractile force of the muscle tends to remain concentrated at the same site on the line of insertion regardless of the horizontal rotation of the globe.[24]

The torsional movement is not a wheel movement around the visual, or Y, axis but rather is a motion relative to a fixed spot on the lateral limbus (Fig. 5-24). For a given contraction of the oblique muscles the torsional component is the same throughout the range of eye movements.

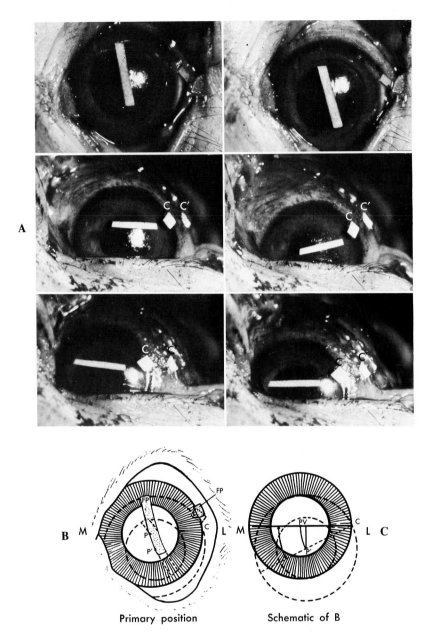

Primary position   **Schematic of B**

FIG. 5-24 Left eye of monkey. **A,** Prints taken from motion picture frames illustrating technique for demonstrating that anterior pole of rotational axis is fixed in space during horizontal eye movements. *Top left and right,* Before and after contraction of superior oblique with eye in primary position. *Center left and right,* Same situation as in top left and right except that lateral and superior walls of orbit had been removed along with lid and levator muscle. Note that marker C moved very little in relation to adnexal structures because it was placed near pole of superior oblique rotational axis. *Bottom left and right,* Before and after contraction of superior oblique with eye in adduction. Note that marker C' now moved very little because it was near pole of rotational axis. **B,** Tracing taken from successive motion picture frames (upper left and right in **A**) showing eye movement from primary position produced by superior oblique. Anterior pole of rotational axis is at C near lateral limbus. Fixation line moves from P to P', transcribing an arc. **C,** Schematic drawing of **B,** showing components of movement. M, medial; L, lateral; FP, filter paper markers; PV, outward component; P', downward component. (From Jampel RS: Arch Ophthalmol 75:535, 1966.)

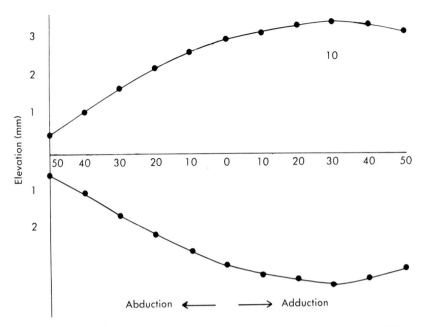

FIG. 5-25 Approximate amount of depression produced by superior oblique (SO) and elevation produced by the inferior oblique (IO) muscles in humans projected onto a frontal plane with the head in the normal erect position and eye in different positions in horizontal plane. Maximum rotation of the eye is about 17 degrees around axis of oblique muscles. Note that maximum elevation or depression occurs when eye is adducted about 30 degrees.

Because of the stability of the rotational axis in the orbit, a given contraction of one of the obliques (with relaxation of its antagonist) produces a constant rotation around its axis independent of the fixation line in the horizontal plane. The *secondary actions* of the oblique antagonist pairs are the result of horizontal and vertical displacements with increasing adduction. As shown in Fig. 5-25, the magnitude of the horizontal and vertical displacement increases as the eye adducts, until a point 90 degrees (30 degrees of adduction) from the oblique axis is reached. (The oblique axis is 60 degrees lateral to the Y axis of Fick.[25]) Further medial movement is accompanied by a decrease in magnitude of the arc movement. Whether the horizontal displacement is abduction or adduction depends on whether the fixation line is above or below the horizontal plane. From these analyses it is clear that the vector component for vertical displacement increases with increasing adduction (to 30 degrees). The vertical recti remain, in all positions of gaze, the main elevators and depressors, as shown in Boeder's calculations of percent participation of the extraocular muscles with changing position of the eye (Figs. 5-26 and 5-27).

Paired horizontal recti. The primary actions of the horizontal recti antagonist pairs are adduction and abduction; the secondary actions of the horizontal recti are minimal (see Fig. 5-23). For initial positions of elevation there is a component of excycloduction in adduction and of incycloduction in abduction; the opposite is true in depression. In addition, a change in mechanical advantage of these muscles due to upward or downward displacement of the insertions with vertical rotation can aid elevation in upgaze and depression in downgaze. Alteration of the insertion of the horizontal rectus muscles with respect to their vertical placement can be used to treat vertical deviations as well as A and V pattern syndromes.

Using the concept of muscle pairs, Boeder has calculated the changes in muscle length for each eye position. From this he has deduced each muscle's relative contribution to a given excursion (Figs. 5-25 to 5-28).

"Quantitative" model

In the interim since Boeder's model was proposed, an enormous amount of information regarding the mechanics of the extraocular muscles has become available. Furthermore, digital

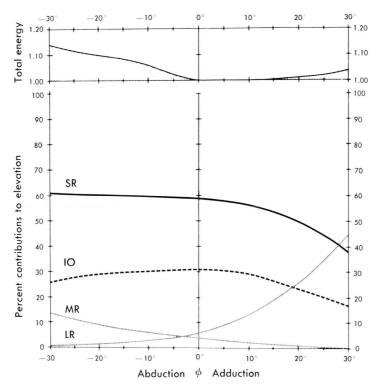

FIG. 5-26 Contributions in percent to 30-degree elevations. *Upper graph,* Relative total muscular energy spent in these elevations. (From Boeder P: Am J Ophthalmol 51:469, 1961.)

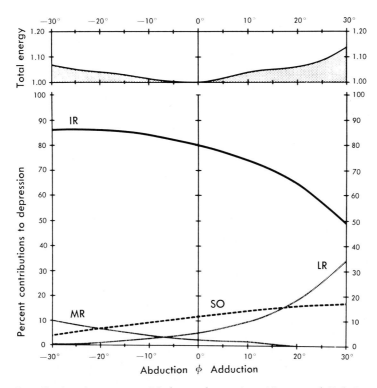

FIG. 5-27 Contributions in percent to 30-degree depressions. *Upper graph,* Relative total muscular energy spent in these elevations. (From Boeder P: Am J Ophthalmol 51:469, 1961.)

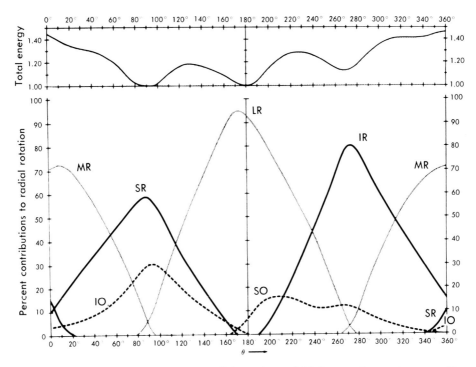

FIG. 5-28 Contributions in percent to radial rotations of 30 degrees from primary position. *Upper graph,* Relative total muscular energy spent in these rotations. (From Boeder P: Am J Ophthalmol 51:469, 1961.)

computers have allowed solutions to be found for more complex models. Robinson[52] has used data obtained in collaboration with faculty of the Smith-Kettlewell Institute of Visual Sciences in San Francisco to formulate a quantitative analysis of extraocular muscle cooperation.

The appropriate innervation to each extraocular muscle is achieved if the eye remains at rest after moving from the primary position to a new eye position represented by the horizontal angle (theta) and the vertical angle (phi); the angle of torsion (psi) is calculated by Listing's law (Fig. 5-29). Using the data of Volkmann and Helmholtz, the moments for each muscle can be determined. These moments (F_n m_n) and the passive moment (P) created by the combined nonmuscular tissues that act to return the globe to a mechanical neutral point must equal zero:

$$P + F_1 m_1 + F_2 m_2 + \ldots + F_6 m_6 = 0$$

Calculation of muscle force (F) is dependent upon its length and its innervation F (L, I). Experimental curves defining the length-tension relationships for given innervational states have been determined (Fig. 5-30). To use the experimental length-tension curves to measure innervation, a fixed muscle length must be defined at

which to measure it—primary position (L_p). The innervation (I) is defined as the isometrically developed force (in grams) of a muscle if it were set as its primary position length.

The measure of muscle length used in length-tension curves is the change in muscle length, expressed as a percent of muscle length in primary position (ΔL). The relative strengths of different muscles are expressed as a proportion of lateral rectus muscle strength (γ). Therefore the original equation defining the moments of each muscle to hold the eye in a given position can be rewritten as:

$$P + \sum_{i=1}^{i=6} \gamma_i F (\Delta L_i, I_i) m_i = 0$$

In the above equation the innervations can be determined by trial and error once the passive tissue moment (P), the unit action vector (m), and the length change (ΔL) are defined.

The unit action vector and the length change (ΔL) are determined by the path the muscle takes. Robinson shows by various examples that the shortest path is impossible, given the limitations of muscle movement within the orbit. This argument is summarized diagrammatically in Figure 5-31. Two forces that limit the muscle

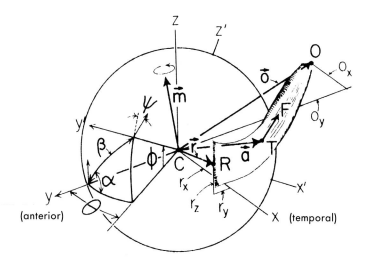

FIG. 5-29 Coordinates and muscle vectors for left eye. Primary position of gaze is along the y axis. Horizontal component of eye rotation is angle θ, vertical component is angle ϕ. Torsion of eye, ψ, is measured from local vertical meridian. Each muscle has an origin, O, and is inserted on globe at some point, R. Vector from center of globe, C, to O is origin vector $\vec{o}$ with coordinates O_x, O_y, and O_z. Vector from C to R is insertion vector r with coordinates r_x, r_y, r_z. Muscle takes same path from R to O and leaves the globe's surface at T, point where muscle force, F, acts. Vector $\vec{a}$ from C to T is moment arm of muscle. Moment exerted on eye is directed along unit moment vector $\vec{m}$, which is perpendicular to both $\vec{a}$ and $\vec{o}$. Axes x, y, and z are fixed in orbit; x', y', and z' move with eye. (From Robinson DA: Invest Ophthalmol 14:801, 1975).

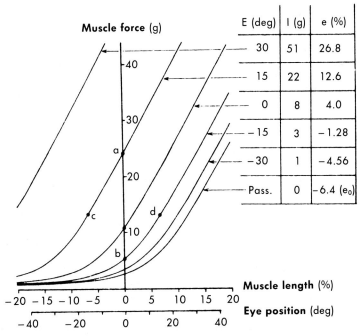

E (deg)	I (g)	e (%)
30	51	26.8
15	22	12.6
0	8	4.0
−15	3	−1.28
−30	1	−4.56
Pass.	0	−6.4 (e₀)

FIG. 5-30 Length-tension curves of detached human extraocular muscle for various innervation levels. Muscle length was measured in millimeter changes from primary position length and converted to percent change. Curves represent mean behavior of five muscles studied. E is angle, left and right of zero, of target lamps viewed by intact eye. Innervation, I, is taken as isometric developed tension at primary position length, a measure of neural activity created by the gaze angle effort E. The variable, e, is an alternate way of expressing innervation. (From Robinson DA: Invest Ophthalmol 14:801, 1975.)

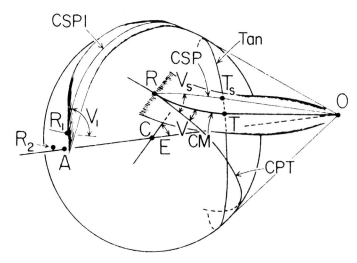

FIG. 5-31 Possible paths muscles could take from insertion to origin O. R_1 and R_2, Possible locations of LR muscle insertion near its antipodes point, A, which lead to absurd muscle locations, such as CSP_1, if muscle is allowed to take shortest path to O. R, A more general insertion location. Great circle CPT, Tract on globe's surface that tendon took in the primary position. Great circle CSP, Great circle path muscle would take if it took shortest path. CM, Nongreat circular path proposed as more realistic path than CSP. V_s, Tendon twist angle demanded by shortest path. V, Proposed, permitted, twist angle. Tan, Tangency circle of O. All muscles leave globe's surface on their way to O when they cross circle Tan (e.g., point T, T_s). E, Angle between line from C to O and perpendicular to plane of CPT. (From Robinson DA: Invest Ophthalmol 14:801, 1975.)

path are the *tendon twist angle* and *twisting force*, which are estimated in the model. The exact *muscle path* is unknown, but it is estimated using boundary conditions to avoid any sudden change in the direction of the muscle as it leaves the globe.

The *passive moment* acts to return the globe to primary position. P will be a vector perpendicular to Listing's plane, the amplitude of which increases with increasing rotation. Values for the passive moment have been determined experimentally with subjects under deep anesthesia and after death. Because the equation for the overall moment on the globe needs to be solved for each vector (X, Y, and Z), the solution is a set of three nonlinear equations. Therefore, there can be only three unknown innervations. By applying Sherrington's law of reciprocal innervation, three of the muscle moments can be calculated, thus allowing the problem to be solved. The innervational state of each muscle (I) for any given eye position can be computed (Fig. 5-32).

These data suggest that in the primary position muscle tone is about 8 g for the horizontal recti, 6 g for the vertical recti, and 4 g for the obliques. Maximum innervation 40 degrees into the field of action of the horizontal recti is 84 g,

of the vertical recti 65 g, and of the obliques 40 g. Near primary position the horizontal muscles do not participate in vertical gaze.

As is true of other models, the vertical muscles have more complicated behavior due to interference with each other when moved out of their primary muscle planes. Robinson differentiates three types of innervation: primary, without cross coupling; secondary, with increased innervation required to offset passive forces; and tertiary, with moments that act on other muscle pairs. This last innervation pattern occurs when a muscle pair is rotated out of its plane of action. Since there are six muscles operating in three axes, 18 types of interactions may occur. Even eliminating torsional and horizontal movements of the paired horizontal muscles leaves 10 interactions.

Four of the tertiary innervations are called "bridle" effects by Robinson. He likens the effect to increasing the elevation of a horse's head by pulling on the reins when the head is up or further depressing the head when the head is down. In some positions of gaze (for example, elevation and abduction) the force of the horizontal muscles may overcome as much as half the passive force (P). The horizontal muscles also develop a torsional force in some positions

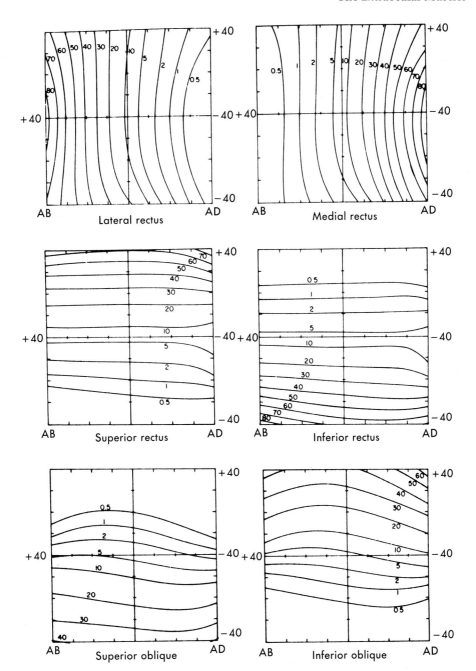

FIG. 5-32 Behavior of muscle innervation, I, for all six extraocular muscles over field of gaze out to 40 degrees horizontally and vertically. Contours are equi-innervation lines. Along them, innervation is constant and its value in grams is indicated next to each contour. (From Robinson DA: Invest Ophthalmol 14:801, 1975.)

of elevation and depression. In addition, the vertical muscles have a bridle effect on horizontal movements. The six other tertiary innervations occur due to horizontal forces that develop when both pairs of vertically acting muscles are activated. To further complicate matters, the amount of force exerted on the globe is not only a function of innervation but also of the mechanical properties of the muscle in terms of shortening per unit innervation.

The clinical value of the more complicated models of ocular rotation has not yet been established. However, in complicated extraocular muscle paralyses and in pathologic conditions of the extraocular muscles or orbit, computer models may prove to be beneficial in developing surgical strategies.

STRUCTURE OF EXTRAOCULAR MUSCLES
Review of mechanism of muscle contraction

The extraocular muscles are specialized striated muscles. As such, a review of the mechanism of muscle contraction is appropriate (see Huxley[21]). Under the microscope voluntary muscle fibers appear regularly striated at right angles to their length, whereas muscles responsible for involuntary movements, such as those of the gut, appear smooth (that is, without striation). Under the higher resolution and magnification afforded by the electron microscope, striated muscle is seen to consist of a number of individual fibers (Fig. 5-33). An individual fiber consists of parallel elements, called myofibrils, each about 1 μm in diameter. In turn, each myofibril is made of parallel thin actin (50 to 70 Å) and thick myosin (160 Å) filaments. The arrays of thick and thin filaments produce the characteristic banding pattern of striated muscle.

This pattern is constructed with a succession of dense bands, called "A bands," and light bands, called "I bands." The A bands consist of the thicker myosin filaments overlapped at each end by actin filaments. The H zone of the A band appears relatively less dense because the myosin filaments are not overlapped by the actin filaments. A dense central line in the A band, called the "M line," is caused by a slight increase in the diameter of each myosin filament. The low density of the I band is due to the fact that only thin actin filaments are present. Two sets of actin filaments are attached, one on each side, to a dense transverse structure, called the Z line, that divides the I band. The structure between two Z lines is the function unit of skeletal muscle, the *sarcomere*.

With active contraction of the muscle fiber, a distinct change is noted in the banding pattern.

First, the H zone closes as the actin filaments move over the myosin filaments, and then a new dense zone develops in the center of the A band when approaching actin filaments overlap (Fig. 5-34). The individual filaments do not change in length, but they slide past each other in a "ratchetlike" fashion.

The muscle fibers (cells) are surrounded by the surface membrane, the sarcolemma, from which invaginations in the form of tubules permeate the cell structure. Abundant sarcoplasmic reticulum may be seen surrounding individual myofibrils and associated with the surface tubules at special structures called triads[45] (Fig. 5-35). Active contraction and relaxation of the muscle units depend on the release and binding of calcium by the sarcoplasmic reticulum.

As mentioned previously, muscle contraction takes place when myosin and actin filaments are actively moved past each other. The origin of the sheer force[15] probably lies in the myosin heads that project in helical arrays from the surface of the filament. The myosin heads lie close to the thick strands in the presence of adenosine 5'-triphosphate (ATP) and in the absence of calcium. In the absence of ATP the myosin heads move out and attach to actin. Myosin can be considered to act like adenosine triphosphatase (ATPase). In relaxed muscle the relative concentration of ATP is maintained by the relaxing system composed of troponin and tropomyosin, proteins associated with the thin filaments.[6] This relaxing system is inhibited in the presence of calcium, which binds to troponin.

The proteins tropomyosin and troponin lie along the grooves of the two-stranded actin helix of the thin filaments. In resting muscle the troponin-tropomyosin strands appear to lie close to the actin helix, but in contraction, when the myosin heads are attached to actin, this complex is displaced toward the center of the groove. It is postulated that the troponin-tropomyosin combination acts to block actin and myosin interaction in the absence of calcium. When calcium is released from the sarcoplasmic reticulum, a configurational alteration occurs in the structure of troponin that causes the troponin-tropomyosin to move, unblocking the access of myosin heads to actin.

Mechanism of contraction of the extraocular muscles

The extraocular muscle fibers originally were subdivided anatomically into large- and small-diameter fibers by Kato.[27] In 1961 Hess,[19] using the electron microscope, established the presence of two distinct morphologic fiber types,

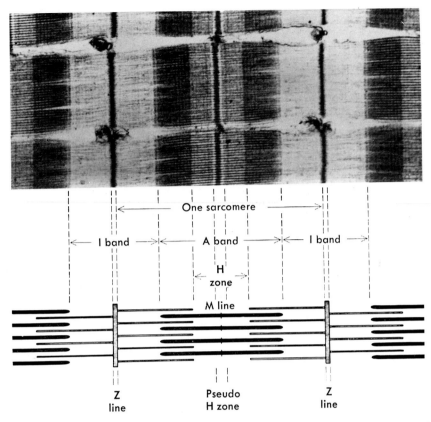

One sarcomere

I band — A band — I band

H zone

M line

Z line — Pseudo H zone — Z line

FIG. 5-33 Striated muscle from leg of frog is shown in longitudinal section in electron micrograph *(top)*: overlap of filaments that gives rise to its band pattern is illustrated schematically *(bottom)*. Part of two myofibrils (long parallel strands organized into muscle fiber) are enlarged some 23,000 diameters in micrograph. Myofibrils are separated by gap running horizontally across micrograph. Major features of sarcomere (a functional unit enclosed by two membranes, the Z lines) are labeled. I band is light because it consists of thin filaments. A band is dense (and thus dark) where it consists of overlapping thick and thin filaments; it is lighter in H zone, where it consists solely of thick filaments. M line is caused by a bulge in center of each thick filament, and pseudo H zone by bare region immediately surrounding bulge. (From The mechanism of muscular contraction by H.E. Huxley. Copyright by Scientific American, Inc. All rights reserved.)

one of which resembled the so-called slow fiber of certain vertebrates. In 1963 Hess and Pilar[20] correlated these anatomic findings of two distinct morphologic fiber types with the physiologic evidence of two forms of contractile activity in extraocular muscle: twitch or fast activity and slow or tonic activity. This finding offered a basis for the observation that eye movements can vary in a controlled fashion from very slow to extremely rapid (up to 1000 degrees of arc/sec).

The twitch fibers of extraocular muscle resemble the twitch fibers of skeletal muscle. A twitch fiber is innervated by one large motoneuron, which may have several end plates, and the fiber conducts propagated action potentials. The typical twitch fiber has a prominent sarcoplasmic reticulum and a well-developed tubule system (Fig. 5-36). The neuromuscular junction consists of a typical motor end plate or "en plaque" ending with many postjunctional folds.

The slow fiber is not found in mammalian skeletal muscle but is found in the muscles of the middle ear. The slow fiber (Fig. 5-37) is supplied along its length by small-diameter motor nerves with "en grappe" endings. These endings lie in proximity to the sarcolemma without development of a refined postjunctional apparatus.

Unfortunately, the extraocular muscle fibers

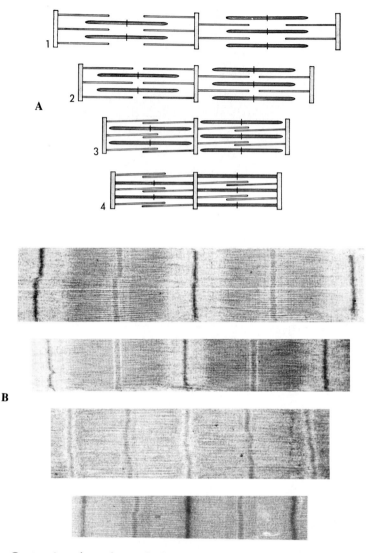

FIG. 5-34 Contraction of muscle entails change in relative position of thick and thin filaments that comprise myofibril, *A*. Effect of contraction on band pattern of muscle is indicated by four electron micrographs and accompanying schematic illustrations of muscle in longitudinal section, fixed at consecutive stages of contraction. First, H zone closes, *2;* then a new dense zone develops in center of A band, *3* and *4,* as thin filaments from each end of sarcomere overlap. (From the mechanism of muscular contraction by H.E. Huxley. Copyright 1965 by Scientific American, Inc. All rights reserved.)

cannot be so easily divided into two morphologic groups as these early studies suggested; neither can function be easily correlated with anatomy. In 1971 Peachey[50] subdivided the extraocular muscle fiber types into five groups; similar classifications have been reported by Mayr[40-42] and Alvarado and van Horn.[1] These classifications depend on variations in banding patterns, amount of sarcoplasmic reticulum, number of mitochondria, cell size, and other factors. At one end of the spectrum is the typical twitch fiber (see Fig. 5-36) and at the other the typical slow fiber (see Fig. 5-37), with atypical fibers having intermediate characteristics completing the spectrum. Working with extraocular muscle of cat, Lennerstrand[36] has correlated this ultrastructural classification with a histochemical classification, based upon staining procedures for ATPase and succinodehydrogenase (SDH) (Table 5-2).

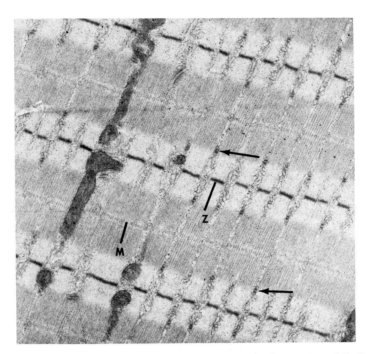

FIG. 5-35 Cat twitch muscle fiber in superior oblique muscle. Separation of fibrils by sarcoplasmic reticulum. Straight Z line, Z, regularly occurring T system *(arrows)*, and M line, *M*, are seen. Compare with Figure 5-37. (Glutaraldehyde fixation; longitudinal section; magnification × 16,000.) (From Hess A: Invest Ophthalmol 6:217, 1967.)

TABLE 5-2 Pathophysiologic and Histochemical Typing of Extraocular Muscle Fibers

EM type	1	2	3	4	5
Layer	Global	Global	Global + orbital	Global	Global + orbital
Mean diameter (μm)	30	22	12	23	12
Membranous SR + TT	Much	Much	Moderate	Poor	Poor
Mitochondria	Few/small	Moderate	Many/large	Few	Many
Proposed innervation	Single	Single	Single	Multiple	Multiple
% of global fibers	38	20	26	15	*
% of orbital fibers	—	—	60-70	*	30-40
Histochemical type	Global II	Global II	Global + orbital II	Global I	Global + orbital IIC
ATPase-9.4	+ +	+ +	+ +	0	+ +
ATPase-fix	+ +	+,+ +	+,+ +	0	+ +
ATPase-4.35	0	0	0,+	+ +	+ +
SDH	0	+	+ +	0,+	+ +
% of global fibers	36	24	17	14	9
% of orbital fibers	—	—	54		46

*Alvarado and associates (1979) report occurrence of type 4 fibers in orbital layer and type 5 fibers in global layer but not the relative proportions of each type.

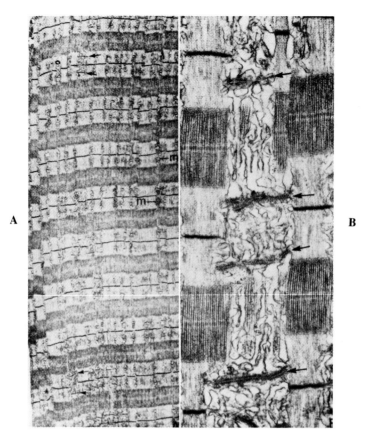

FIG. 5-36 Type I muscle fiber. **A,** Myofibrils are well aligned, clearly separated from each other by extensive transverse tubular system *(arrows)* and sarcoplasmic reticulum (SR); sarcomere has thin Z lines and prominent M line; mitochondria (M) are few and very small. (Magnification × 13,200.) **B,** Detail of sarcomere showing well-developed SR, especially along I-band region. Note complex interconnections among SR tubules, as well as triads *(arrows)* formed with transverse tubules. (Magnification × 27,000.) (From Alvarado JA, and van Horn C: Muscle cell types of the cat inferior oblique, in Lennerstrand G, Bach-y-Rita P, eds: Basic mechanisms of ocular motility and their clinical implications, Oxford, Pergamon Press, 1975, p 15.)

According to McNeer and Spencer,[44] mitochondria distribution can be affected by "overaction" and the effects of strabismus, so that function may, to some extent, dictate morphology, rather than vice versa. This view is supported by experimental studies in cats with strabismus,[36] suggesting subnormal fast fiber development.

Miller[46] has demonstrated in both monkeys and humans that the extraocular muscles undergo sequential changes with increasing age. The muscle fiber that atrophied most was predominant centrally, had fewer mitochondria, and demonstrated an M line in the center of the A band (Peachey's type 4). Miller astutely recommends that correlates from experiments involving eye movements or extraocular muscle fibers be limited to given age-groups.

As mentioned previously, the extraocular muscles are composed of two layers, an outer orbital layer (OL) and a central global layer (GL). The orbital layer consists of two fiber types, both small in diameter, one with multiple and one with focal innervation. The global layer contains three fiber types, all larger than fibers in the orbital layer, two of which are singly innervated and one of which is multiply innervated.

The works of Mayr[42] and Alvarado and van Horn[1] demonstrate that many individual muscle fibers do not extend the entire length of the muscle. In the orbital layer the fibers tend to be shorter than those in the global layer, and there

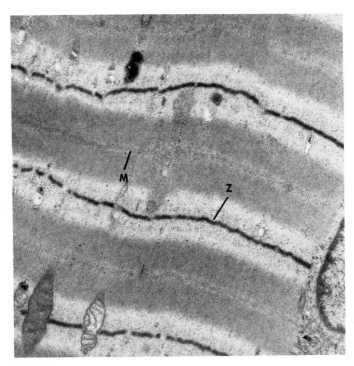

FIG. 5-37 Cat slow muscle fiber in superior oblique muscle. Poor separation of fibrils by sparse amounts of sarcoplasmic reticulum, zig-zag Z line, Z, virtual absence of T system elements (only aberrant T system elements occur), and M line, M, are illustrated. Compare with Figure 5-35 (glutaraldehyde fixation; longitudinal section; magnification × 16,000.) (From Hess A: Invest Ophthalmol 6:217, 1967.)

is usually a staggered arrangement of muscle tendon junctions. Large motor end plates are confined to a large band in the middle one third of the muscle, and myo-myous junctions are rare, existing only at either end of the muscle.

In the global layer large motor end plates are found everywhere along the muscle. Myo-myous junctions are dispersed throughout both ends of the fiber bundles, since only a few of the singly innervated fibers run the entire length of the muscle, most being approximately one third the length of the bundle. The myo-myous junctions exhibit cholinesterase activity[43,59] and are the sites of mechanical linkage between different muscle fibers.

Multi-innervated muscle fibers run the entire length of the muscle and extend about 0.5 mm farther into the distal tendon than do the focally innervated fibers. Mayr[42] has emphasized that the internal structure of the extraocular muscles (that is, the presence of serially linked muscle fibers) must have functional importance.

Miller[45] showed in 1967 that the orbital surface layer of extraocular muscle consists of two small fiber types. By histochemical means he de-termined that this surface layer corresponds with the classic red muscle, high in mitochondrial content (and oxidative enzymes). The central mass of muscle consists of three fiber types corresponding to so-called white muscle, which is relatively low in mitochondrial content and high in glycolytic enzymes. Miller's findings support the theory that there is a close correlation between histochemistry and function. Muscles that have the characteristics of red fibers are used for prolonged contractions (that is, slow movements), whereas muscles that have the characteristics of white fibers perform phasic or twitch movements. Kugelberg[33] has demonstrated that the histochemical reaction for myosin ATPase is associated with contraction speed, and mitochondrial oxidative activity with resistance to fatigue. The independent variability of both enzyme types enables a wide range of specifications with regard to speed and endurance. According to Kugelberg, careful histochemical analysis should make it possible to correlate with some accuracy the functional competence of muscle fibers and motor units.

PHYSIOLOGY OF EXTRAOCULAR MUSCLE FIBERS

Electrical and contractile properties of extraocular muscle fibers

Although Miller[46] and subsequently Peachey[50] and Alvarado and van Horn[1] identified at least five morphologic types of muscle fibers, so far only three[34,35] functional types of fiber have been identified by using sophisticated intracellular and extracellular recording methods. Lennerstrand classifies these fibers as SI (singly innervated), MINC (multiply innervated nonconducting), and MIC (multiply innervated conducting). Chiarandini and Davidowitz[8] have written an extensive review of this subject.

Twitch, single-innervated (SI) fibers

Singly innervated fibers are similar to those of other mammalian twitch fibers with resting potential of −65 to −90 mV. When depolarized to about −60 mV, they conduct an action potential of 80 mV, due principally to a rapid shift of Na^+. The resistive and capacitive characteristics of extraocular muscle fibers seem to be species specific. The end-plate activity consists of both miniature end-plate potentials (mepp) triggered by single packets of acetylcholine (ACh) occurring at random, and end-plate potentials (epp) that are evoked by a neural impulse releasing large quantities of ACh. In the cat inferior oblique, Hess and Pilar[20] demonstrated an epp rise time of 2 to 3 msec, with a half amplitude decay of 2 to 4 msec.

Singly innervated fibers respond to depolarization with a rapid contraction, having a rise time of 5 to 8 msec and a decay time of 7 msec (Fig. 5-38). These fibers have a fusion frequency to tetanic contraction of 175 to 350 pps.

Tonic, multiply innervated fibers without action potentials (MINC)

There are multiply innervated fibers without action potentials (MINC).[20] With repetitive electrical stimulation greater than 50 pps, a graded tension of a tonic or sustained nature develops (Fig. 5-39). The multiply innervated nature of these muscle fibers was confirmed by Pilar,[51] who demonstrated that the synaptic potentials are graded and have different time courses and latencies (Fig. 5-40), and by Ozawa et al.[48] using an intracellular staining technique. Although these fibers seem to have a lower resting membrane potential than do SI fibers (see Fig. 5-40), Stefani and Steinbach[58] showed this is likely to be an artifact of the measurement technique, with actual resting membrane potential similar to that of SI fibers. Compared to SI fibers, the input resistance is quite high (5 megohm vs. 1 megohm). Excitation-coupling in these fibers

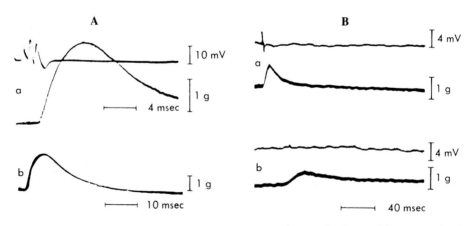

FIG. 5-38 Isometric twitches in response to nerve stimulation of inferior oblique muscle. **A,** Time courses of maximal twitch responses to cathode excitation of a nerve in which none of the three branches had been cut; initial tension 2.6 g. a, Single twitch (lower trace) and simultaneously recorded surface potential indicating both fast and slow fibers were activated (upper trace); b, total contraction time course of single twitch. **B,** Single twitch response when proximal and central branches of innervating nerve had been cut; initial tension 5.5 g. a, Single twitch of fast fibers selectively stimulated by anode block excitation (lower trace) and simultaneously recorded extracellular action potential showing only fast fiber activation (upper trace). b, Single twitch of slow fibers selectively stimulated by anode block excitation (lower trace) and simultaneously recorded extracellular action potential showing only slow fiber activation (upper trace). (From Bach-y-Rita P, Ito F: J Gen Physiol 49:1177, 1966.)

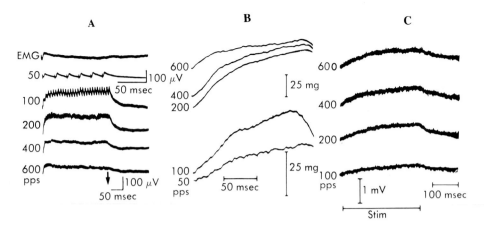

FIG. 5-39   Electrical, **A** and **C**, and mechanical, **B**, responses of MINC units to stimulation at the rates marked. In **A**, monopolar, dc-EMG is recorded from one unit. Local responses to single stimulus (top trace) summate at repetitive stimulation of 60 pps and above. Arrow in lowest trace signifies stimulus removal. **B** and **C**, From another unit. The tetanus fuses at approximately 60 pps (**B**). The electrical activity presented in **C** is recorded with a micropipette close to unit. Because of high noise level of this dc-recording, individual local responses cannot be separated. (From Lennerstrand G: Acta Physiol Scand 91:458, 1974.)

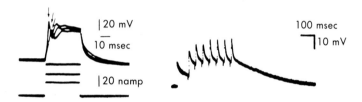

FIG. 5-40   Failure of tonic fibers to generate action potentials. *Left,* Rat inferior rectus. Fiber was identified as multiply innervated by presence of characteristic miniature small junction potentials. Intracellular application of pulses of current that depolarized the cell from a membrane potential of −70 mV up to −5 mV failed to evoke an action potential. However, a transient and fast signal appeared at the beginning of the three pulses (*arrows*). These local responses were followed by slowly rising depolarization. (Chiarandini DJ, and Stefani E, unpublished results). *Right,* Cat superior oblique. Fiber was depolarized by repetitive activation of small junction potentials. Resting potential of fiber was −65 mV. In spite of depolarization of about 35 mV, no action potentials were evoked. (Reproduced from Pilar G: The Journal of General Physiology, 1967, vol 50, p 2289, by copyright permission of the Rockefeller University Press.)

depends on Ca^{+2} release from the surface membrane rather than from the sarcoplasmic reticulum. These muscle fibers are innervated by small-diameter nerve fibers.

Multiply innervated fibers with action potentials (MIC)

Multiply innervated fibers with action potentials were first identified by Bach-y-Rita and Ito[3] (Fig. 5-38). Input resistance is about 1 megohm, similar to that of SI fibers. Although the number of multiply innervated conducting fibers in extraocular muscle is controversial, a small percentage of extraocular muscle fibers does appear to be of the MIC type.[20,51]

MIC fibers conduct action potentials at a significantly lower velocity than do singly innervated fibers (1.32 vs. 2.93 msec). In addition, the membrane potential is lower (Fig. 5-41), approximately 40 mV. These findings indicate that the fibers in the MIC units should be thinner, which is compatible with the morphologic findings. MIC units have a slower contraction time (5 to 18 msec) and lower fusion frequencies (120 to 225 pps) than do singly innervated units.

Role of different fiber types in eye movements

In the absence of eye movements the extraocular muscles have a resting tone seen as electrical

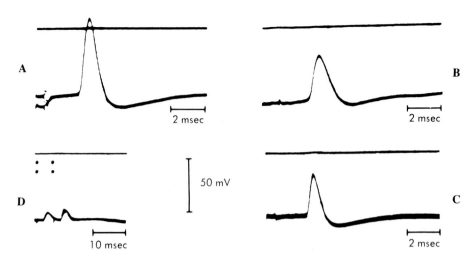

FIG. 5-41   Intracellular responses to single shocks in an SI unit, **A**, and in two different MINC units, **B** and **C**, and to double shocks in an MINC unit, **D**. Top line is reference (zero) potential. Action potentials are seen in **A**, **B**, and **C**. In the MINC unit, **D**, no action potentials were fired even at increased stimulus strength (marked by stimulus dots); two superimposed traces coincide. (From Lennerstrand G: Acta Physiol Scand 91:458, 1974.)

potentials when studied by electromyography. It has been stated that only slow fibers demonstrate spontaneous activity, and Breinin[5] inferred from this statement that the constant tonic activity characteristic of electromyography of extraocular muscle reflected potentials of the slow system only. This poses a paradox; the motor unit activity of tonic contraction as recorded by electromyography consists of propagated spikes, implying contraction of twitch fibers, and cannot arise from nonpropagated junction potentials of slow fibers. It seems apparent that the view that the fast twitch fibers are responsible for saccadic movement and that slow fibers are responsible for resting tone, vergences, and pursuit is too simplistic. Neither twitch nor slow fibers can be isolated to one function, but both probably have roles in all ocular movements. Collins and Scott,[9,57] by recording simultaneously from fibers in the different layers of human eye muscles (Fig. 5-42), have demonstrated that all fibers are active at all times and are recruited differentially during different ocular movements. At this time it still appears that multi-innervated mechanically slow units are responsible for the majority of tonic activity in all gaze positions, including the primary position. Single innervated units generate most of the initial force necessary for saccadic eye movements, but they also have a supportive role during fixation and pursuit conditions. The physiologic correlation of fiber type with move-

ment characteristics remains to be elucidated in greater detail. The two approaches that seem most promising are (1) the simultaneous recording of tension and electrical activity from precisely defined regions of muscle and (2) intracellular recording and dye marking for subsequent morphologic identification.[8]

PHARMACOLOGY OF THE EXTRAOCULAR MUSCLES

Consistent with the electrical properties of extraocular muscle, pharmacologic data also suggest the existence of a slow, tonic system and a fast, twitch system. The slow system responds with a slow chronic contraction of the extraocular muscles when subjected to acetylcholine (ACh), choline, and nicotine (Fig. 5-43). Bach-y-Rita[2] localized these tonic responses to multiply innervated fibers (types 4 and 5) occurring primarily in the orbital layer. ACh applied to fast fibers produces a characteristic twitch.[14]

Effect of neuromuscular blocking agents

The effect of neuromuscular blocking agents on the extraocular muscles is of interest since these agents are frequently used in conjunction with general anesthesia and, more recently, have become useful diagnostically and therapeutically in the care of strabismus.

Blocking agents can be classified into two groups based on whether they have a *depolarizing* or *nondepolarizing* effect on the postjunc-

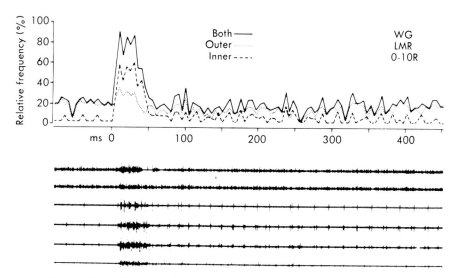

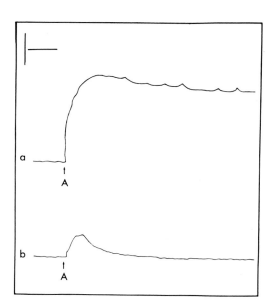

FIG. 5-42 *Bottom,* Record from six channels of the multiple electrode array. Top two channels are recordings from superficial, small, orbital fibers deeper in central part of muscle. *Top,* instantaneous frequencies of activity of both large and small fibers and total muscle activity corresponding to bottom EMG single-unit records. These represent eye movement control signal for a 10-degree "on" saccade. (From Collins CC: The human oculomotor control system, in Lennerstrand G, Bach-y-Rita P, eds: Basic mechanisms of ocular motility and their clinical implications, Oxford, Pergamon Press, 1975, p 145.)

FIG. 5-43 "Contractures" induced by 0.05 μg acetylcholine/ml bath solution. Calibration, 20 mg tension, 1 minute. *a,* From dissection comprising Felderstruktur fibers exclusively: weight of muscle piece, 1.1 mg. *b,* Same muscle as *a,* from dissection comprising Fibrillenstruktur fibers with a few Felderstruktur fibers; weight of muscle piece, 5.2 mg. (From Kern R: Invest Ophthalmol 4:901, 1965.)

tional membrane. Depolarizing agents combine with the receptors of the postjunctional membrane and cause a sustained depolarization. Thus ACh in large quantities can act as a depolarizing agent (as occasionally seen in the cholinergic crisis of the overtreated patient with myasthenia). Clinically useful depolarizing agents include succinylcholine (SCh) and decamethonium. Katz and Eakins,[28,29] studying the effects of SCh on the twitch and tonic systems of extraocular muscle, found that small dosages of SCh increased baseline muscle tension but did not depress the twitch response. Larger dosages of SCh continued to increase the baseline tension while depressing the twitch system (Fig. 5-44). The dosage of SCh required to depress the twitch response in extraocular muscle is greater than that required to depress the twitch response of skeletal muscle. Recently, the differential effect of SCh on the tonic fibers responsible for nonalignment of the eyes in strabismus has been used clinically to predict alignment of the extraocular muscles following surgery.[37,47] Intraoperatively, after repositioning of the extraocular muscles, a bolus of intravenous SCh is administered. The extraocular muscle deviation then is measured, which correlates highly with the final postoperative alignment (Fig. 5-45).

Another neuromuscular blocking agent that

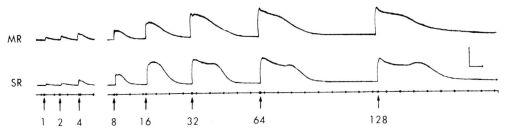

MR

SR

1 2   4   8   16   32   64   128

FIG. 5-44   Cat, 3.7 kg, pentobarbital anesthetic. Effect of increasing intravenous dosage (in μg/kg) of succinylcholine on tension of medial rectus muscle, MR, and superior rectus muscle, SR. Calibrations, 10 g tension, 1 minute. (From Eakins KE, Katz RL: Br J Pharmacol 26:205, 1966.)

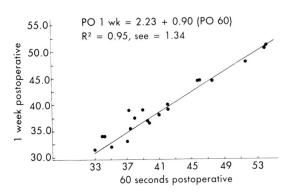

FIG. 5-45   Regression equation of interlimbal distance (ILD) in millimeters 1 week postoperatively (PO 1 wk) on the basis of the intraoperative succinylcholine-induced position 60 seconds after injection (PO 60). Data obtained from 20 congenital esotropes. (From Lingua RW: J Pediatr Ophthalmol Strabismus 20(4):146, 1983.)

has become clinically useful is botulinum toxin, which interferes with ACh release from the nerve terminal. Scott[56] has shown that small doses of botulinum toxin A, injected into extraocular muscles, alter contractility. He has used such injections as a therapeutic alternative to strabismus surgery and as a method of preventing contracture of the antagonist muscle in extraocular muscle palsies.

Nondepolarizing agents combine with postjunctional receptor sites to produce a block but do not cause depolarization. This is a competitive block, whereas depolarizing agents produce a noncompetitive block. Clinically, the most commonly used nondepolarizing agent is *d*-tubocurarine. It was widely held that mammalian extraocular muscles are more sensitive to curare than are other skeletal muscles, but this concept has been proved erroneous.[28,53] Depolarizing and nondepolarizing agents may be differentiated as follows:

Depolarizing agent	Nondepolarizing agent
Initial fasciculations	None
Tetanus is well sustained	Tetanus is poorly sustained
Posttetanic facilitation is not seen	Posttetanic facilitation is present
Cholinesterase inhibitors enhance the block	The block is antagonized by cholinesterase inhibitors

Sympathetic alpha-aminergic agents cause a modest increase in baseline muscle tension, about 10% of the effect produced by cholinergics. This response is independent of changes in intraorbital smooth muscle and cardiovascular effects. The physiologic implications of this response, which probably bears on the tonic system, are unknown.

REFERENCES

1. Alvarado J, van Horn C: Muscle cell types of the cat inferior oblique, in Lennerstrand G, Bach-y-Rita P, eds: Basic mechanisms of ocular motility and their clinical implications, Oxford, Pergamon Press, 1975, pp 5-43.
2. Bach-y-Rita P: Structural-functional correlations in eye muscle fibers: eye muscle proprioception, in Lennerstrand G, Bach-y-Rita P, eds: Basic mechanisms of ocular motility and their clinical implications, Oxford, Pergamon Press, 1975, pp 91-109.
3. Bach-y-Rita P, Ito F: In vivo studies on fast and slow muscle fibers in cat extraocular muscles, J Gen Physiol 49:1177, 1966.
4. Boeder P: The co-operation of extraocular muscles, Am J Ophthalmol 51:469, 1961.
5. Breinin GM: The structure and function of extraocular muscle—an appraisal of the duality concept, Am J Ophthalmol 72:1, 1971.
6. Bremel RD, Weber A: Cooperation within actin filament in vertebrate skeletal muscle, Nature (New Biol) 238:97, 1972.
7. Burian MB, Von Noorden GK: Binocular vision and ocular motility: theory and management of strabismus, St Louis, CV Mosby, 1974.

8. Chiarandini DJ, Davidowitz J: Structure and function of extraocular muscle fibers, Curr Top Eye Res 1:91, 1979.

9. Collins CC: The human oculomotor control system, in Lennerstrand G, Bach-y-Rita P, eds: Basic mechanisms of ocular motility and their clinical implications, Oxford, Pergamon Press, 1975, pp 145-180.

10. Crone RA: Diplopia, Amsterdam, Excerpta Medica, 1973.

11. Duane A: A new classification of the motor anomalies of the eye, Ann Ophthalmol Otolaryngol 5:969, 1896.

12. Duane A: The basic principles of diagnosis in motor anomalies of the eye, Arch Ophthalmol 48:2, 1919.

13. Duane A: Anomalies of the ocular muscles: symptoms and diagnosis of paralysis and spasms, Arch Ophthalmol 11:394, 1934.

14. Eakins KE, Katz R: The pharmacology of extraocular muscle, in Bach-y-Rita P, Collins CC, Hyde JE: The control of eye movements, New York, Academic Press, 1971, pp 237-258.

15. Editorial: Towards a unified theory of muscle contraction, Nature 238:187, 1972.

16. Fick A: Die Bewegungen des menschlichen Augapfels, Zeitschrift IV, Henle & Pfeufer, 1854, p 101.

17. Helmholtz H: Handbuch der Physiologischen Optik, 3rd ed, vol 3, Hamburg, Leopold Voss, 1910, p 47.

18. Helveston E, et al: The trochlea: a study of the anatomy and physiology, Ophthalmol 89:124, 1982.

19. Hess A: The structure of slow and fast extrafusal muscle fibers in the extraocular muscles and their nerve endings in guinea pigs, J Cell Physiol 58:63, 1961.

20. Hess A, Pilar G: Slow fibres in the extraocular muscles of the cat, J Physiol 169:780, 1963.

21. Huxley HE: The mechanism of muscular contraction, Sci Am 213(6):18, 1965.

22. Jampel RS: Extraocular muscle action from brain stimulation in the macaque, Invest Ophthalmol 1:565, 1962.

23. Jampel RS: The action of the superior oblique muscle: an experimental study in the monkey, Arch Ophthalmol 75:535, 1966.

24. Jampel RS: The fundamental principle of the action of the oblique ocular muscles, Am J Ophthalmol 69:623, 1970.

25. Jampel RS: Ocular torsion and the function of the vertical extraocular muscles, Am J Ophthalmol 79:292, 1975.

26. Jampel RS, Bloomgarden CI: Individual extraocular muscle function from faradic stimulation of the oculomotor and trochlear nerves of the macaque, Invest Ophthalmol 2:265, 1963.

27. Kato T: Über histologische Untersuchungen der Augenmuskeln von Menschen und Saugetieren, Okajimas Folia Anat Jpn 16:131, 1938.

28. Katz RL, Eakins KE: A comparison of the effects of neuromuscular blocking agents and cholinesterase inhibitors on the tibialis anterior and superior rectus muscles of the cat, J Pharmacol Exp Ther 154:304, 1966.

29. Katz RL, Eakins KE: The effects of succinylcholine, decamethonium, hexacarbacholine, gallamine, and dimethyl tubocurarine on the twitch and tonic neuromuscular systems of the cat, J Pharmacol Exp Ther 154:303, 1966.

30. Koorneef L: Spatial aspects of orbital musculofibrous tissue in man, Amsterdam, Swets & Zeitlinger, 1977.

31. Krewson WE: The action of the extraocular muscles: a method of vector-analysis with computations, Trans Am Ophthalmol Soc 48:443, 1950.

32. Krewson WE: Comparison of the oblique extraocular muscles, Arch Ophthalmol 32:204, 1964.

33. Kugelberg E: The motor unit: histochemical and functional correlations, in Lennerstrand G, and Bach-y-Rita P, eds: Basic mechanisms of ocular motility and their clinical implications, Oxford, Pergamon Press, 1975, pp 85-89.

34. Lennerstrand G: Electrical activity and isometric tension in motor units of the cat's inferior oblique muscle, Acta Physiol Scand 91:458, 1974.

35. Lennerstrand G: Motor units in eye muscles, in Lennerstrand G, Bach-y-Rita P, eds: Basic mechanisms of ocular motility and their clinical implications, Oxford, Pergamon Press, 1975, pp 119-143.

36. Lennerstrand G: Postnatal development of eye muscle function: an experimental study in cats and normal and impaired binocular vision, in Lennerstrand G, Zee DS, Keller EL, eds: Functional basis of ocular motility disorders, Oxford, Pergamon Press, 1981, pp 39-47.

37. Lingua RW, et al: Succinylcholine as a predictor in strabismus surgery, J Pediatr Ophthalmol 20(4):145, 1983.

38. Linwong M, Herman SJ: Cycloduction of the eyes with head tilt, Arch Ophthalmol 85:570, 1971.

39. Listing JB: Moleschott's Untersuch, vol 193, 1854.

40. Mayr R: Structure and distribution of fibre types in the external eye muscles of the rat, Tissue Cell 3:433, 1971.

41. Mayr R: Morphometrie von Ratten-Augenmuskelfasern, Verh Anat Ges 67:353, 1973.

42. Mayr R: Discussion remarks of R Mayr on the lecture of Doctors JA Alvarado and C van Horn on two aspects of eye muscle morphology, in Lennerstrand G, Bach-y-Rita P, eds: Basic mechanisms of ocular motility and their clinical implications, Oxford, Pergamon Press, 1975, pp 44-45.

43. Mayr R, Zenker W, Gruber H: Zwischensehnenfreie Skeletmuskelfaser-Verbindungen, Z Zellforsch 79:319, 1967.

44. McNeer KW, Spencer RF: The histopathology of human strabismic extraocular muscle, in Lennerstrand G, Zee DS, Keller EL, eds: Functional basis of ocular motility disorders, Oxford, Pergamon Press, 1981.

45. Miller JE: Cellular organization of rhesus extraocular muscle, Invest Ophthalmol 6:18, 1967.

46. Miller JE: Aging changes in extraocular muscle, in Lennerstrand G, Bach-y-Rita P, eds: Basic mechanisms of ocular motility and their clinical implications, Oxford, Pergamon Press, 1975, pp 47-61.

47. Mindel JS, et al: Succinyldicholine and the basic ocular deviation, Am J Ophthalmology 95:315, 1983.

48. Ozawa T, Cheng-Minoda K, Davidowitz J, et al: Correlation of potential and fiber type in extraocular muscle, Doc Ophthalmol 26:192, 1969.

49. Park RS, Park GE: The center of ocular rotation in the horizontal plane, Am J Physiol 104:545, 1933.

50. Peachey L: The structure of the extraocular muscle fibers of mammals, in Bach-y-Rita P, Collins CC, Hyde JE: The control of eye movements, New York, Academic Press, 1971, pp 47-66.

51. Pilar G: Further study of the electrical and mechanical

responses of slow fibers in cat extraocular muscles, J Gen Physiol 50:2289, 1967.

52. Robinson DA: A quantitative analysis of extraocular muscle cooperation and squint, Invest Ophthalmol 14:801, 1975.

53. Sanghvi IS, Smith CM: Characterization of stimulation of mammalian extraocular muscles by cholinomimetics, J Pharmacol Exp Ther 167:351, 1969.

54. Scobee RG: The oculorotary muscles, 2nd ed, St Louis, CV Mosby, 1952.

55. Scott AB: Strabismus—muscle forces and innervations, in Lennerstrand G, Bach-y-Rita P, eds: Basic mechanisms of ocular motility and their clinical implications, Oxford, Pergamon Press, 1975, pp 181-191.

56. Scott AB: Botulinum toxin injection of the eye muscles to correct strabismus, Trans Am Ophthalmol Soc 79:734, 1981.

57. Scott AB, Collins CC: Division of labor in human extraocular muscles, Arch Ophthalmol 90:319, 1973.

58. Stefani and Steinbach: Resting potential and electrical properties of frog slow muscle fibres: effect of different external solutions, Physiologie 203:383, 1969.

59. Teravainen H: Localization of acetylcholinesterase activity in myotendinous and myomyous junctions of the striated skeletal muscles of the rat, Experientia (Basel) 25:524, 1969.

60. Van der Hoeve J: Ocular movements, Trans Ophthalmol Soc UK 52:1, 1932.

61. Verrjip C: Movements of the eyes, in Behrens C, ed: The eye and its diseases, Philadelphia, WB Saunders, 1949.

62. Volkmann AW: Zur Mechanik der Augenmuskeln, Trans Leipzig Soc Sci 21:28, 1869.

63. Von Noorden GK, Maumenee AE: Atlas of strabismus, 2nd ed, St Louis, CV Mosby, 1973.

SECTION TWO

The oculomotor system

STEVEN E. FELDON, M.D.
RONALD M. BURDE, M.D.

The control and coordination of the extraocular muscles have been studied extensively using anatomic, physiologic, and bioengineering techniques. The integration of these disciplines has contributed enormously to the understanding of the oculomotor system.

AFFERENT SYSTEM

The system controlling eye position necessarily consists of an afferent limb, relaying sensory information about current eye position, as well as the efferent limb, responsible for the eye movement itself. Besides visual input, proprioceptive inputs and an internal "memory" of eye position are likely to be present. Nonvisual inputs are probably important adjuncts to guiding eye movements under all conditions and are the only means of determining eye position under conditions of darkness or low vision.

Proprioception

Controversy has surrounded the role of proprioception in the control of eye movements. There is wide species-dependent variability in the morphology of the sensory end organs. Human extraocular muscle has a generous complement of muscle spindles, similar to those of other skeletal muscle.[73] Therefore, whether or not individuals are aware of eye position in the absence of vision, proprioceptive information of considerable fidelity is definitely available to the central nervous system.

Pathways for proprioception

Proprioceptive impulses from the extraocular muscles travel via the ophthalmic branch of the trigeminal nerve to the semilunar ganglion. There is evidence that the semilunar ganglion has a somatotopic organization[128] (Fig. 5-46). The central processes of the first-order neurons

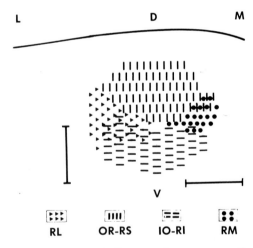

FIG. 5-46 Schematic diagram of transverse section of semilunar ganglion of the lamb showing somatotopic organization of eye muscle afferents within proprioceptive cellular pool. L, lateral; D, dorsal; M, medial; V, ventral; RL, lateral rectus; OS, superior oblique; IO, inferior oblique; RI, inferior rectus; RM, medial rectus. Calibrations: 1 mm. (From Manni E, Pettorossi VE: Arch Ital Biol 114:178, 1976.)

terminate in the ipsilateral main sensory trigeminal nucleus and in the orad portion of the ipsilateral spinal trigeminal nucleus (in the lamb), but they also may project to more caudal portions of the trigeminal nucleus. The organization of the proprioceptive fibers from the extraocular muscles within the trigeminal nucleus is also somatotopic.[129] From the trigeminal nucleus, proprioceptive impulses are relayed to the tectum and tegmentum of the mesencephalon, to the medial lemniscus, and to the ventrobasal complex of the thalamus. Within the superior colliculus, the innervation is again noted to be somatotopic.[56,130] Other pathways for proprioception may involve the lateral geniculate,[55] the visual cortex,[30,31,127] and the cerebellum.*

Physiology of proprioception

Although debated, there is likely to be little perceptual role for afferent extraocular muscle fibers.[186] There is also considerable controversy about the existence of a stretch reflex for the extraocular muscles.[70,107,148]

Proprioceptive fibers from the extraocular muscles have an important input to lobules V, VI, and VII of the cerebellar cortex, involving both the mossy and the climbing fibers.[10,65] Batini[16] showed that the feedback loop is fast enough for the cerebellum to influence the late trajectory of saccades. Proprioceptive afferents to the superior colliculus exert an inhibitory effect on visual afferents. Also, visual units are capable of modulating proprioceptive responses.[1,17,55] Proprioceptive information reaching the visual cortex may be important in binocular interaction.[25,186]

The corollary discharge

The ability of the oculomotor control system to determine eye position is essential. However, physiologic and psychophysical data suggest that proprioceptive information is likely to make only a minor contribution. Most perceptual information related to the direction of eye movements is attributed to an "efference copy" of the motor signal sent to the extraocular muscles.[186] The existence of centrally generated corollary discharges that signal changes of eye position has recently been confirmed experimentally.[76,187]

THE EFFERENT SYSTEM

The purpose of the oculomotor system is to bring the eyes into a chosen target in an efficient,

coordinated manner. The mechanisms controlling the various types of eye movements will be discussed after reviewing the direct innervation to the extraocular muscles.

Anatomy of the oculomotor nerves

The extraocular muscles are controlled by three pairs of cranial nerves: the oculomotor nerve (III), the trochlear nerve (IV), and the abducens nerve (VI). Their nuclei reside in the brainstem, sending axons via the cavernous sinus through the superior orbital fissure and into the orbit to terminate on the individual extraocular muscles.

Oculomotor nerve (cranial nerve III)

The oculomotor nerve is the most complex of the cranial nerves controlling eye movements, innervating the medial rectus, inferior rectus, inferior oblique, superior rectus, levator palpebrae superioris, and the presynaptic parasympathetic outflow to the internal muscles of the eye (the ciliary muscle and the sphincter muscle of the iris).

The oculomotor nucleus

The individual muscles each have corresponding subnuclei in the brainstem. This complex lies ventral to the central gray matter of the midbrain (Fig. 5-47). The classic description of the oculomotor nucleus of the primate was provided by Warwick,[202] using the method of retrograde chromatolysis. He proposed that the cell columns in this nucleus had both a rostrocaudal and dorsoventral arrangement (Fig. 5-48). The levator has only a single midline nucleus that supplies both sides. The medial rectus, inferior rectus, and inferior oblique are innervated ipsilaterally, whereas the superior rectus is innervated contralaterally. The visceral nuclei consist of two distinct pairs that are in continuity rostrally. The Edinger-Westphal nucleus consists of two slender columns dorsal to the rostral part of the oculomotor complex. Caudally, each of these columns divides into two smaller columns that gradually fade away. Rostrally, the two columns merge into the anterior median nucleus. Both of these subnuclei supply the presynaptic parasympathetic outflow. This anatomic organization was supported by the single unit electrophysiologic findings of Robinson.[165]

More recent studies[26] using horseradish peroxidase (HRP) and wheat germ agglutinin (WGA) as tracers have identified three separate subnuclei innervating the medial rectus muscle (Fig. 5-49). The largest, the "A" subgroup of medial rectus motoneurons, corresponds to the

_____
*References 6, 10, 16, 65, 126, 156.

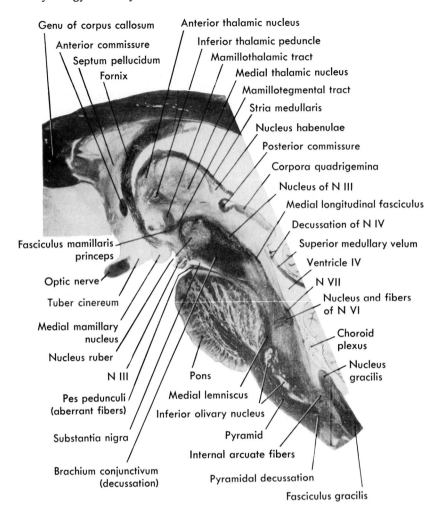

Genu of corpus callosum
Anterior commissure
Septum pellucidum
Fornix
Anterior thalamic nucleus
Inferior thalamic peduncle
Mamillothalamic tract
Medial thalamic nucleus
Mamillotegmental tract
Stria medullaris
Nucleus habenulae
Posterior commissure
Corpora quadrigemina
Nucleus of N III
Medial longitudinal fasciculus
Decussation of N IV
Superior medullary velum
Ventricle IV
N VII
Nucleus and fibers of N VI
Choroid plexus
Nucleus gracilis
Fasciculus mamillaris princeps
Optic nerve
Tuber cinereum
Medial mamillary nucleus
Nucleus ruber
N III
Pes pedunculi (aberrant fibers)
Substantia nigra
Brachium conjunctivum (decussation)
Pons
Medial lemniscus
Inferior olivary nucleus
Pyramid
Internal arcuate fibers
Pyramidal decussation
Fasciculus gracilis

FIG. 5-47 Sagittal section of brainstem through pillar of fornix and root of third nerve. (Weigert's myelin stain: photograph.) (From Strong OS, Ellwyn A: Human neuroanatomy, 3rd ed, Baltimore, Williams & Wilkins, 1953.)

localization of the medial rectus subnucleus defined by Warwick.[202] It is located in the ventral and ventrolateral part of the oculomotor nucleus (OMN). It extends from the most rostral tip of the OMN, diminishing caudally until it disappears in the caudal one third of the OMN. The cell bodies within the A subnucleus have an average diameter of 25 µm. A "B" subgroup is located in the caudal one third of the OMN dorsally. The average diameter of these cells is 30 µm. The area occupied by this medial rectus subgroup corresponds to an area considered as an inferior rectus subgroup by Warwick.[202] However, the inferior rectus subgroup is confined to the rostral two thirds of the OMN dorsally. A "C" subgroup is located at the dorsomedial border of the OMN, medial to the rostral part of subgroup B, and stretches to the rostral

tip of the OMN. The diameter of these cells is much smaller, averaging only 18 µm. The axons emanating from subgroup C terminate in the orbital layer of muscle, corresponding to the multiply innervating muscle fibers primarily mediating tonic activity.[181] As such, Buettner-Ennever and Akert[26] have speculated that medial rectus subnucleus C may be functionally related to convergence.

The course of the oculomotor nerve

The oculomotor neurons leave the nuclear complex and pass ventrally through the red nucleus, exiting the brainstem through the medial portion of each cerebral peduncle to emerge in the interpeduncular space. The nerve then passes

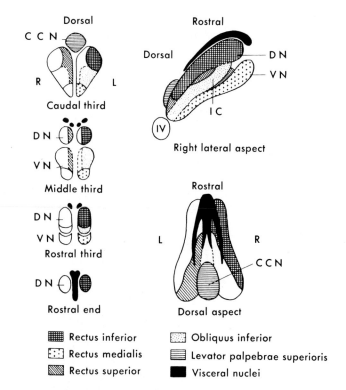

FIG. 5-48 Representation of right extraocular muscles in oculomotor nucleus of monkey. Transverse sections at levels as indicated in the complex. DN, dorsal nucleus; VN, ventral nucleus; CCN, caudal central nucleus; IC, intermediate column; IV, trochlear nucleus. (From Warwick R: J Comp Neurol 98:449, 1953.)

between the posterior cerebral and superior cerebellar arteries to travel lateral to, but parallel with, the posterior communicating artery of the circle of Willis. It pierces the dura just lateral to the posterior clinoid process. The oculomotor nerve enters the cavernous sinus, running dorsal to the fourth nerve in the lateral wall of the sinus, dividing into superior and inferior branches as it enters the orbit through the superior orbital fissure. Once in the orbit the superior and inferior divisions form multiple ramifications that then innervate the individual muscles.[172]

Trochlear nerve (cranial nerve *IV*)

The trochlear nerve arises from a pair of small compact cell groups ventral to the periaqueductal gray matter at the level of the inferior tectal plate (Fig. 5-50). The cell groups are almost continuous with the caudal part of the third nerve nucleus and indent the dorsal surface of the medial longitudinal fasciculus. The fibers course dorsolaterally and caudally to turn medially and cross completely in the superior medullary velum. The fourth cranial nerve is the only cranial nerve to exit dorsally, as well as decussate completely. It travels anteriorly and ventrally in the subarachnoid space to pierce the dura and enter the lateral wall of the cavernous sinus just caudal to the posterior clinoid process. It enters the orbit through the superior orbital fissure to innervate the superior oblique muscle as a single fascicle.[172]

Abducens nerve (cranial nerve *VI*)

The abducens nerves arise from paired groups of multipolar motoneurons situated beneath the floor of the fourth ventricle (Fig. 5-51). These nuclei lie within the loops of the internal genu of the facial nerves and produce eminences, called the facial colliculi, on the floor of the fourth ventricle. Two populations of neurons are found within the abducens nucleus. About half of the cells are motoneurons that innervate the lateral rectus muscle. These cells have smooth nuclear envelopes and well-developed granular endoplasmic reticulum.[125] Using retrograde and orthograde labeling techniques,

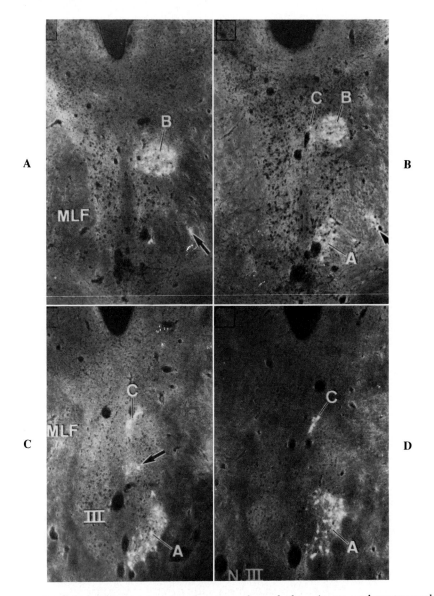

FIG. 5-49 Semi-darkfield photographs of sections through the primate oculomotor nucleus (OMN) taken in transverse plane and arranged in a caudal-to-rostral sequence, **A-D**, MR motorneurons labeled with (^{125}I) WGA (wheat germ agglutinin) lie in subgroups A, B, C. Subgroup A lies ventral and rostral, B, dorsal and caudal in OMN. Subgroup C is situated dorsomedial to the large-celled OMN. In **A** and **B** some cells of subgroup A *(arrow)* are scattered between the fascicles of the medial longitudinal fasciculus (MLF). **C,** An S-shaped continuum of labeled cells between subgroups C and A is partially visible; a group of cells associated with this is marked by an arrow. **D,** Relationship of subgroup C to subgroup A in the rostral tip of OMN. MLF, Medial longitudinal fasciculus; N III, oculomotor nerve; III, oculomotor nucleus. Calibration 1 mm. (From Buettner-Ennever JA, Akert K: J Comp Neurol 197:17, 1981.)

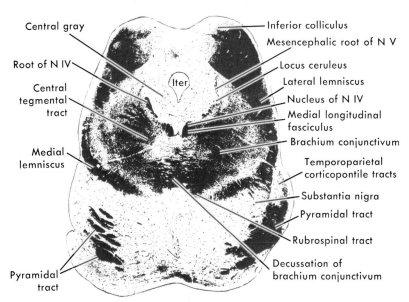

FIG. 5-50 Section of midbrain through inferior colliculi. One-month-old infant. (Weigert's myelin stain; photograph; magnification × 7). (From Strong OS, Ellwyn A: Human neuroanatomy, 3rd ed, Baltimore, Williams & Wilkins, 1953.)

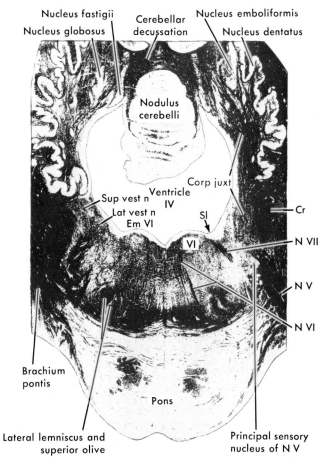

FIG. 5-51 Section through pons, pontine tegmentum, and part of cerebellum, just below entrance of trigeminal nerve. Infant, 1 month old. (Weigert's myelin stain; photograph) Cr, restiform body; Corp juxt, juxtarestiform body; Em VI, eminentia abducentis; SI, sulcus limitans; VI, nucleus of sixth nerve. (From Strong OS, Ellwyn A: Human neuroanatomy, 3rd ed, Baltimore, Williams & Wilkins, 1953.)

Graybiel and Hartwieg[74] showed another projection from the abducens nucleus to the medial rectus subnuclei of the oculomotor nerve (Fig. 5-52). Most of these interneurons are of 24 to 40 μm in diameter and are characterized by fusiform perikarya, fluted or deeply invaginated nuclear envelopes, and poorly developed, granular endoplasmic reticulum.[188] They are distributed fairly evenly throughout the nucleus.

The sixth nerve fibers course ventrally through the pons to emerge at its base at the medullopontine junction. The abducens nerve turns rostrally and laterally in the subarachnoid space, crossing over the tip of the petrous portion of the temporal bone. It is anchored there by a reflection of dura, the petrosphenoidal ligament (Gruber's ligament). The reflection of dura at the tip of the petrous pyramid resembles a canal and bears the eponym Dorello's canal. The abducens nerve pierces the dura at the level of the dorsum sellae to enter the cavernous sinus. It travels within the sinus near the carotid artery, enters the orbit through the superior orbital fissure, and supplies the lateral rectus muscle. Before entering the medial surface of the muscle, the nerve separates into multiple ramifications. It has the longest intracranial course of any nerve and is often subject to embarrassment with raised intracranial pressure. Because of its long intracranial course, an isolated lesion of the abducens nerve has no significance for anatomic localization.

Physiology of ocular motoneurons

Motor control of eye movements requires the ability to move the eyes either quickly or slowly and the ability to keep the eyes relatively stationary. The extraocular muscles demonstrate a heterogeneity that seems suited to these different tasks,[134] although Scott and Collins[48,181] have pointed out that all muscle fibers participate to various extents (Fig. 5-53). Despite the conclusion of Keller and Robinson[108] and others[66,78,165,166,176] that individual motoneurons participate in all eye movements, Henn and Cohen[77,78] found that motoneurons can be clas-

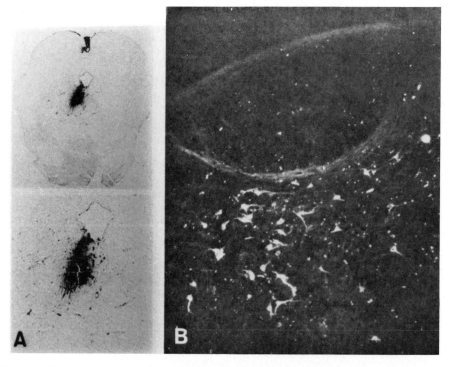

FIG. 5-52   Photomicrographs of **A,** Injection site centered in oculomotor nucleus (*above,* $\times$ 1.5; *below,* $\times$ 3). **B,** Darkfield photomicrograph of HRP-positive neurons in abducens nucleus contralateral to the site of injection ($\times$ 100). HRP, Horseradish peroxidase. (From Graybiel AM, Hartwieg EA: Brain Res 81:543, 1974.)

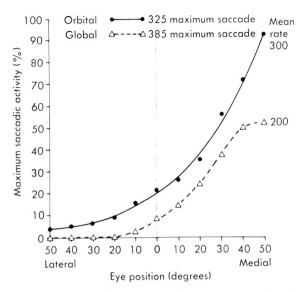

FIG. 5-53 LMR innervation—global vs. orbital fibers' fixation activity. Quantitative representation of relative contributions of large and small oculorotary muscle fibers to fixation and slow tracking movement. It can be seen that the small fibers contribute the greater activity during fixation, progressively increasing their activity across the entire gamut of eye positions. Large fibers appear to saturate at extreme gaze fixation, which suggests that they may be fatiguing. (From Collins CC: The human oculomotor control system, in Lennerstrand G, Bach-y-Rita P, eds: Basic mechanisms of ocular motility and their clinical implications, Oxford, Pergamon Press, 1975, p 145.)

sified according to their behavior during saccades and fixation. Their analysis revealed the following characteristics.

1. All motoneurons have clear on-off directions (in direction of agonist activity).
2. On-off directions for medial rectus and abducens units lie on the horizontal plane, whereas on-off directions for the other muscles are tilted 10 to 20 degrees off the vertical plane.
3. Most units are active during periods of fixation and saccades (Fig. 5-54).

These units could be subdivided into tonic units (Fig. 5-54, *A* and *B*), burst units (Fig. 5-54, *E* and *F*), and burst-tonic units (Fig. 5-54, *C* and *D*). Motoneurons form a continuous spectrum of graded response, with burst units at one end and tonic units at the other.

Tonic units are active during periods of fixation and increase their firing patterns in a steplike fashion during saccades. These units tend to have a lower threshold and a lower maximum frequency than do phasic units. The tonic units are often not totally inhibited during movement in the "off" direction. Sampling from a single medial rectus unit, Henn and Cohen[78] found a highly linear relationship between change in eye position and change in firing frequency (range ± 20 degrees, ± 200 spikes per second) (Fig. 5-55). Burst units are active over the entire range of eye movements, but they fire a train of spikes only at the onset of ocular movements in the "on" direction.[14,78] For phasic motoneurons, the relationship between change in eye position is found to be linear with the change in the phasic frequency of firing when multiplied by the duration of the burst (Fig. 5-56).

It thus appears that although specific types of eye movements are not produced by one class of motoneuron, a physiologic hierarchy exists. The more tonic motoneurons (as a broad class) are responsible for holding the eyes steady or moving them slowly, and the more phasic or burstlike motoneurons are responsible for moving the eyes rapidly. Furthermore, using antidromic stimuli,[78] it has been shown that the burstlike motoneurons have faster conduction velocities than those with more tonic activity. This suggests that the more phasic neurons have larger axons and are therefore the same neurons that singly innervate the larger eye muscle twitch fibers.

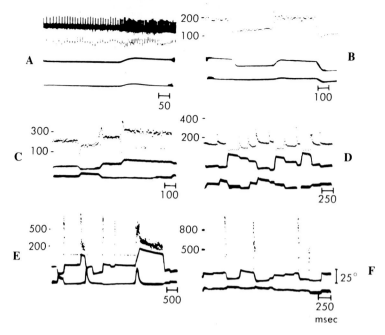

FIG. 5-54 Medial rectus units with different characteristics. **A**, Top trace is spike activity. **B** to **F**, Dot displays represent instantaneous frequency. Height of each dot is the reciprocal of the last spike interval. Numbers on the left refer to frequencies in hertz. Middle and bottom traces are the horizontal and vertical EOG respectively. Up corresponds to right or upward movements. **A** and **B** are samples of the same tonic unit; **C** and **D** are two predominantly tonic units; **E** is predominantly phasic unit; **F** is a phasic unit. Note that from **C** to **F** the phasic part of the unit activity becomes more prominent until in **F** the unit fires only during quick eye movements in the "on" direction. (From Henn V, Cohen B: Activity in eye muscle motoneurons and brainstem units during eye movements, in Lennerstrand G, Bach-y-Rita P, eds: Basic mechanisms of ocular motility and their clinical implications, Oxford, Pergamon Press, 1975, p 303.)

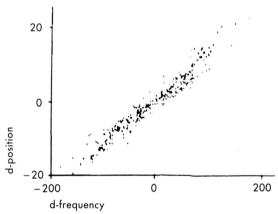

FIG. 5-55 Tonic medial rectus unit. Change in frequency of firing during periods of fixation (abscissa) is plotted against position of eyes in horizontal plane (ordinate). Linear line of regression is: $Y = -0.069 + 0.194 X$. Correlation factor is 0.954. (Reprinted with permission from Henn V, Cohen B: Activity in eye muscle motoneurons and brainstem units during eye movement, in Lennerstrand G, Bach-y-Rita P, eds: Basic mechanisms of ocular motility and their clinical implications, Oxford, Pergamon Press, copyright 1975, p 309.)

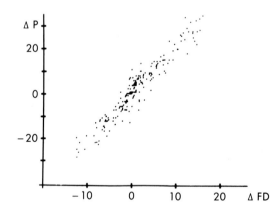

FIG. 5-56 *Abscissa*, phasic change in frequency of firing of medial rectus burst unit multiplied by duration of phasic burst. *Ordinate*, position change during that movement. Equation for linear line of regression in this case is $Y = 2.585 + 3.086X$. Correlation factor is 0.943. (Reprinted with permission from Henn V, Cohen B: Activity in eye muscle motoneurons and brainstem units during eye movements, in Lennerstrand G, Bach-y-Rita P, eds: Basic mechanisms of ocular motility and their clinical implications, Oxford, Pergamon Press, copyright 1975, p 310.)

THE CONJUGATE EYE MOVEMENT SYSTEM

The binocular coordination of the eyes that allows them to move together into a field of gaze is an important function of the oculomotor system. Such coordinated eye movements, called "versions," follow a pattern of action described by Hering.[82,83] Hering's law states that in all voluntary conjugate movements of the eyes, equal and simultaneous innervation flows from the oculomotor centers to the muscles concerned in establishing the direction of gaze. In other words, the amount of nervous energy sent to the muscles of the two eyes causes the eyes to turn equally in a particular direction. As discussed in the previous section, this equal innervation is distributed among several agonist muscles. However, in extreme positions yoked pairs of muscles are activated primarily (Table 5-3). The precision required to ensure binocularity is dependent upon complex anatomic and physiologic relationships, which only recently have been satisfactorily elucidated.

Conjugate eye movements can be rapid or slow. A summary of the various types of conjugate eye movements (and vergence movement) is shown in Table 5-4. Rapid eye move-

TABLE 5-3 Yoke Muscles of the Eyes

Right eye	Left eye
Medial rectus	Lateral rectus
Lateral rectus	Medial rectus
Superior rectus	Inferior oblique
Inferior rectus	Superior oblique
Superior oblique	Inferior rectus
Inferior oblique	Superior rectus

TABLE 5-4 Control Mechanism

	Position maintenance	Pursuit	Saccadic	Vergence	Nonoptic reflex (vestibular)
Function	Maintain eye position vis-à-vis target	Maintain object of regard near fovea; matches eye and target	Place object of interest on fovea rapidly	Align visual axes to maintain bifoveal fixation	Maintain eye position with respect to changes in head and body posture
Stimulus	Visual interest and attention(?)	Moving object near fovea	Object of interest in peripheral field	Retinal disparity	Stimulation of semicircular canals, utricle, and saccule
Latency (from stimulus to onset of eye movement)		125 milliseconds	200 milliseconds	160 milliseconds	Very short
Velocity	Both rapid (flicks, microsaccades) and slow (drifts)	To 100 degrees/sec, accurately to 30 degrees/sec	To 400 degrees/sec	Around 20 degrees/sec	To 300 degrees/sec*
Feedback Substrate	Occipitoparietal junction	Continuous Occipitoparietal junction	Sampled data Frontal lobe; occipitoparietal junction; superior colliculus(?)	Unknown	Vestibular apparatus; muscle receptors in neck → cerebellum(?)

*Slow phase only. The fast phase, although initiated in the pontine reticular formation, is discharged via the saccadic mechanism.

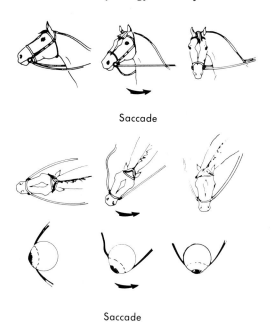

Saccade

Saccade

FIG. 5-57 On the origins of the word saccade. The horse's head (eyeball) is abruptly turned (saccade) by the jerk of the reins (extraocular muscles), one taut (agonist facilitation), the other relaxed (antagonist inhibition). Final position of head or eye may then be maintained by tonic activity of the reins of extraocular muscle. (From Troost BT, Dell'Osso LF: Fast eye movements (saccades): basic science and clinical correlations, in Thompson HS, ed: Topics in neuroophthalmology, Baltimore, Williams & Wilkins, 1979, p 247.)

ments are referred to as *saccades,* derived from the French *saquer,* which means "to pull," and is used in referring to the jerk of a horse's head when the reins are applied[196] (Fig. 5-57). Saccades occurring when an eccentric target is brought onto the fovea are called *refixation saccades* and when a command is given to move the eyes they are called *schematic saccades.* They also occur during the fast phase of jerk nystagmus. Slow eye movements are used to keep a moving target on the fovea and to generate the slow phase of nystagmus.

Anatomic substrate of horizontal eye movements

Interneurons that connect the oculomotor nuclei establish the mechanisms for coordination of eye movements at a relatively peripheral anatomic level. Highstein and Baker[84] demonstrated a monosynaptic excitatory input to the medial rectus subnucleus of the oculomotor

nerve from the contralateral abducens nucleus. This internuclear connection was found to course in the medial longitudinal fasciculus. These findings were confirmed and extended by Buettner-Ennever and Akert[26] and by Graybiel and Hartwieg.[74] Although the medial longitudinal fasciculus is a paired fiber tract that extends from the thalamus to the anterior horn cells of the spinal column, it is especially well developed between the region of the vestibular (medulla) nuclei and oculomotor (midbrain) nuclei.[123]

The supranuclear center for the control of conjugate eye movements is the paramedian pontine reticular formation (PPRF). Goebel and coworkers[68] demonstrated that lesions in this region produced paralysis of conjugate gaze, that is, paralysis of the ipsilateral lateral rectus and contralateral medial rectus muscles (Fig. 5-58). Inputs to the PPRF originate in the superior colliculi, the vestibular nuclei, the frontal eye fields, the rostral interstitial nucleus of the medial longitudinal fasciculus (riMLF), the cerebellum, and the perihypoglossal nuclei.[81] It is likely that burst signals received by the perihypoglossal nuclei are used in gaze-holding and to provide position information for use in gaze-holding directly to motoneurons.[34,35,118] In the primate there are direct pathways from the PPRF to the ipsilateral abducens motoneurons and interneurons, which in turn project to the medial rectus subnuclei of the oculomotor nerve (Fig. 5-59).[24] Additional pathways project to the riMLF and to the cerebellum.[81]

Anatomic substrate for vertical eye movements

The coordination of vertical eye movements is not as clearly elucidated as that of horizontal eye movements. The interstitial nucleus of Cajal (iC), the nucleus of Darkschewitsch (nD), the nucleus of the posterior commissure in the pretectum (npc), the posterior commissure (PC), and the rostral interstitial nucleus of the MLF (riMLF) have all been implicated (Fig. 5-60). The riMLF is the most likely premotor nucleus for vertical eye movements (both upward and downward).[2] This nucleus is situated dorsomedial to the red nucleus, lateral to the nD, and just above the iC.[27] However, the staging area for the vertical system probably resides in the medial portion of the PPRF,[1] which projects directly to the riMLF, coursing just outside the MLF.[29,30] Output from the riMLF could be segregated into a dorsal tract subserving upward movements and a ventral tract subserving downward movements.[150] In turn, these tracts would project onto

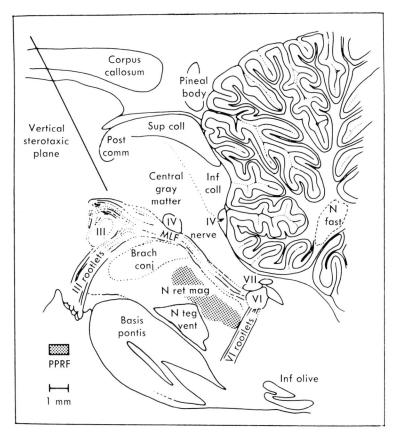

FIG. 5-58 Sagittal section of brainstem of *Macaca mulatta*, 0.75 mm from midline. Solid line shows a vertical stereotaxic plane anterior to AP-O. Dotted region shows extent of paramedian zone of pontine reticular formation. It lies in the nucleus reticularis magnocellularis, N ret mag, between level of trochlear and abducens nuclei. Destruction of this region causes paralysis of horizontal conjugate gaze. (From Goebel HH, et al: Arch Neurol 24:431, 1971.)

the trochlear nucleus[67] and the vertical subnuclei of the oculomotor nerve.[25]

Physiologic substrate coordinating horizontal and vertical eye movements

Electrical activity within cells of the PPRF and riMLF demonstrate several distinct patterns that correspond to particular types of eye movements.[43,80,105,121] Rapid eye movements are associated with neurons that discharge as a high-frequency *burst* of activity, some of which also demonstrate a level of tonic discharge. Other cells change in *tonic* firing with slow changes in eye position. There is also a group of cells that *pause* during eye movements.[110] The timing and duration of these discharge patterns relative to eye movement are used to categorize the premotor neurons (Fig. 5-61).

Medium-lead burst neurons

Neurons that discharge in a burst pattern 6 to 12 msec prior to eye movement are called medium-lead burst neurons. These cells usually are activated by eye movement to the ipsilateral side (for horizontal movements). The rate of discharge is dependent upon the size of the shift in eye position (Fig. 5-62). The cells that are activated are those whose "on" direction corresponds with the direction of the eye movement. Combinations of directionally sensitive cells thus may be used to generate any size eye movement in any direction.

Long-lead burst neurons

Long-lead burst neurons fire earlier relative to the onset of eye movement. One type of long-lead burst neuron is directionally sensitive but responds maximally prior to eye movements

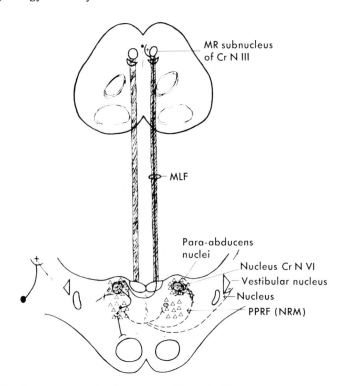

FIG. 5-59 Fiber is seen emanating from area of frontobulbar tract synapsing in the left PPRF. From the left PPRF excitatory fibers travel to left sixth cranial nerve (Cr N VI) and to the left para-abducens nucleus, wherein a synapse occurs. Excitatory fibers arise from the left para-abducens nucleus, cross the midline dorsally, and travel by way of the right MLF to the medial rectus (MR) subnucleus of the right third cranial nerve (Cr N III). Excitation of the ipsilateral sixth cranial nerve (Cr N VI) and contralateral third cranial nerve (Cr N III) MR produces a saccade to the ipsilateral side (*left*). Inhibitory fibers (*dashed lines*) also arise from the PPRF, cross the midline ventrally, and synapse in the contralateral PPRF, para-abducens nucleus, abducens nucleus, and vestibular nucleus, thus abetting the ipsilateral saccade.

that are at angles other than purely horizontal or vertical. A second class of long-lead burst neurons is not directionally sensitive but responds prior to saccades of a given magnitude. The two types of long-lead burst neurons may operate together to produce spatial encoding of saccades.[80] These neurons are likely to project directly on the medium-lead burst neurons, which in turn activate the ocular motoneurons.

Pause cells

When medium-lead burst neurons are activated, pause cells cease firing. These cells may serve as gates, providing precise timing to the medium-lead burst neurons. These cells also may participate in the integration of burst-type activity by providing input to tonically active cells.

Nuclear and supranuclear inputs to the conjugate oculomotor pathway

Activation of the oculomotor system occurs either as a response to stimulation of other brainstem mechanisms (reflexes) or as a response to volitional inputs. Calibration between eye position and these inputs also is required.

The vestibular input
Vestibular end organ

The vestibular apparatus plays a major role in coordinating the tone of body musculature, including the extraocular muscles. Maintained postural deviations are controlled by the otoliths in the utricles and saccules, whereas postural movements resulting from acceleration are controlled by impulses from the hair cells in the semicircular canals; that is, the sensory apparatus codes head position as well as angular and linear head movements. There are three semi-

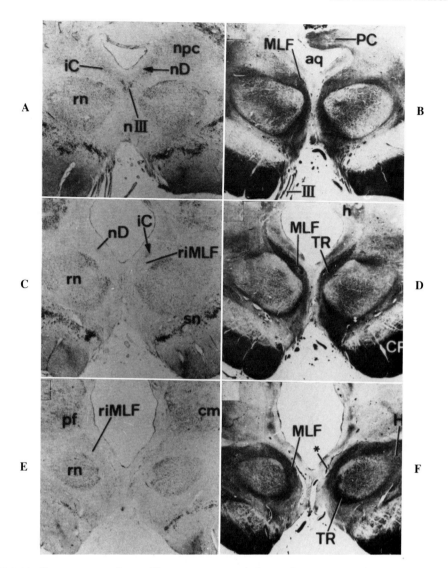

FIG. 5-60 Transverse sections of human mesencephalon to demonstrate relationship of rostral iMLF to nD, iC, and rn. Sections are stained with either cresyl violet to show cell groups (**A, C, E**) or by the Weil method for fibers (**B, D, F**). **A** and **B**, Taken caudal to rostral iMLF at the level of N III and PC. Note cell groups npc, iC, and nD. **C** and **D**, Caudal pole of rostral iMLF, anterior tip of iC dorsomedial to rostral iMLF (on the right side only), nD and TR. **E** and **F**, Taken at the level of midrostral iMLF and the rostral tip of rn (pars parvocellularis). Rostral iMLF is bordered by the posterior thalamo-subthalamic paramedian artery (*); cells are interstitial to the anterior extension of MLF. iMLF, Interstitial nucleus of the medial longitudinal fasciculus; nD, nucleus of Darkschewitsch; iC, interstitial nucleus of Cajal; rn, reticular nucleus; npc, nucleus of posterior commissure; calibration indicates mm. (From Buettner-Ennever JA, et al: Brain 105:125, 1982.)

circular canals—the horizontal, the anterior vertical, and the posterior vertical—each lying in a plane approximately 90 degrees to the others (Fig. 5-63). The anterior end of the horizontal canal is actually deviated 30 degrees superiorly to the horizontal (Fig. 5-64). The right and left horizontal canals are parallel, but the vertical canals form angles of approximately 44 degrees with the anteroposterior axis. The posterior vertical canal lies in a plane parallel to the opposite anterior vertical canal. The medial arms of the vertical canals merge to form a com-

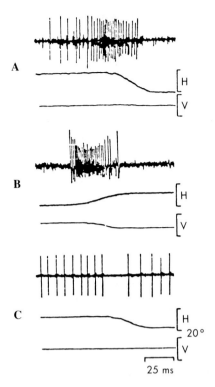

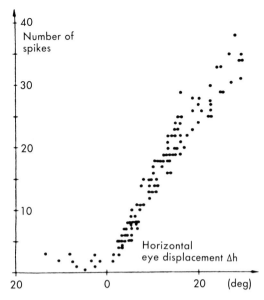

FIG. 5-61 Original records of types of neurons found in the PPRF. **A**, Long-lead burster. **B**, Medium-lead burster. **C**, Pause neuron. Top tracing in each group, spike potentials. H, horizontal eye position. V, vertical eye position. (From Henn V, et al: Hum Neurobiol 1:87, 1982.)

FIG. 5-62 Medium-lead burst neuron from the right PPRF. With most movements a burst occurs that is strongest for large movements toward the right. In the graph on the left the number of spikes was counted for individual bursts, and 100 consecutive such bursts are plotted against the horizontal position change. The greater the number of spikes *(ordinate)*, the further the eyes moved in a horizontal direction toward the ipsilateral side *(abscissa)*. (From Henn V, et al: Hum Neurobiol 1:87, 1982.)

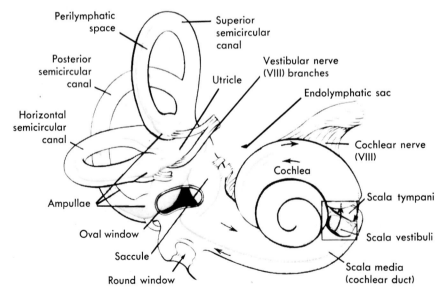

FIG. 5-63 Right auricular end organs and their nerves. Labyrinth and cochlea are viewed from horizontal aspect. Note the three ampullary nerves that conduct impulses centrally from each semicircular canal; each of these nerves is associated with specific sets of ocular muscles by means of tegmental brainstem connections between vestibular nuclei and oculomotor nuclei. Sensory input from these nerves and the nerves from the utricle and saccule plays an essential role in visuospatial perception, as well as in stabilization of ocular fixation during movements of the head. (Drawing by Ernest W. Beck; courtesy Beltone Electronics Corp., Chicago, Ill.)

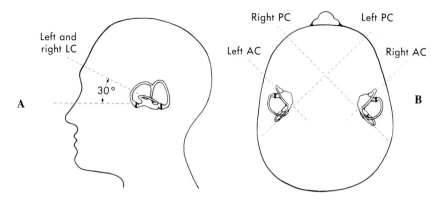

FIG. 5-64 Planes of the semicircular canals. **A**, Lateral canals. **B**, Anterior and posterior vertical canals. LC, lateral canal; AC, anterior vertical canal; PC, posterior vertical canal. Size of the canals is greatly exaggerated. (From Barber HO, Stockwell CW: Manual of electronystagmography, St Louis, CV Mosby, 1976.)

mon canal and, with the posterior end of the horizontal canal, connect with the utricle. One end of each semicircular canal has a bullous expansion, the ampulla, containing a ridge of neuroepithelium. The ridge contains ciliated somatosensory cells innervated by vestibular nerve fascicles. The cilia are embedded in a gelatinous dome-shaped structure, the cupola (Fig. 5-65). The membranous labyrinth is filled with endolymph, the formation of which is associated with a membranous structure of the auditory receiving apparatus, the cochlea. The fluid apparently flows to the membranous labyrinth through the saccule to the utricle.

The utricle is a sac connected to the semicircular canals superiorly and to the saccule inferiorly. The receptor organs in these sacs are plaques of hair cells (maculae) embedded in a gelatinous mass containing crystals of calcium carbonate (otoliths). The hair cells in the utricle are positioned parallel to the horizon, and those in the saccule are positioned perpendicular to the horizon. The entire membranous labyrinth is enveloped in the petrous portion of the temporal bone, the bony labyrinth that contains perilymph and communicates with the subarachnoid space.

Physiology of the vestibular inputs to the oculomotor system

The semicircular canals are stimulated by rotational acceleration or deceleration in their respective planes. Movement alone is insufficient if there is no change in rate. A given semicircular canal is stimulated when there is a relative flow of endolymph displacing the hair cells in the ampulla. The horizontal canal is stimulated when the relative flow of endolymph is toward the ampulla, whereas the two vertical canals are stimulated when the relative flow is away from the ampulla. For example, if a subject is stabilized in a rotating chair with his or her chin depressed 30 degrees and the chair rotated to the right, there will be a relative flow of endolymph toward the left; that is, the fluid suspended within the membranous labyrinth will have a certain inertia, resisting motion, causing a relative displacement of endolymph anteriorly in the right canal (excitatory) and posteriorly in the left horizontal canal (inhibitory) (Fig. 5-66). The opposite effect is brought on by deceleration.

Vestibular neural pathway. The cell bodies of the vestibular nerve lie in the internal auditory meatus, making up the vestibular (Scarpa's) ganglion. The ganglion contains bipolar cells whose afferent limb passes to the sensory organs of the membranous labyrinth and whose central efferents enter the upper medulla as the vestibular part of the eighth cranial nerve. After entering the brainstem, the fibers divide into two tracts: ascending and descending. The ascending tract is concerned with oculomotor control. Certain of these fibers ascend in the vestibulocerebellar fascicle to the vermis and roof nuclei of the cerebellum, but most of the fibers terminate in the vestibular nuclei. Stein and Carpenter[191] have shown that neurons from the semicircular canals synapse primarily in the rostral medial and superior vestibular nuclei, and those from the utricle and saccule go to the inferior and caudal medial vestibular nuclei (Fig. 5-67).

The "three-neuron arc" from vestibular ganglion to vestibular nuclei to oculomotor nuclei is considered the major set of projections mediating the vestibulo-ocular reflex. However, other

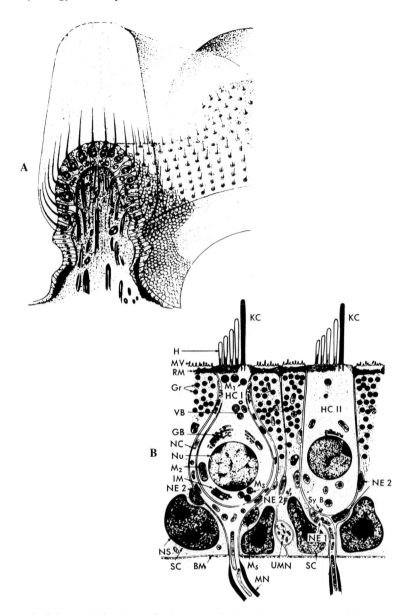

FIG. 5-65 A, Schematic drawing of crista ampullaris, the sense organ of the semicircular canal. Note ciliated vestibular sensory cells. **B,** Schematic details of two types of vestibular sensory cells. Flask-shaped type I cell, HC I, is surrounded by a nerve calyx, NC, which makes contact on its outer surface with granulated (presumably efferent) nerve endings, NE 2. Unmyelinated nerve fibers, UMN, are extensions of myelinated fibers, MN, which lose their myelin sheath as they pass through basement membrane. Type II sensory cell, HC II, is roughly cylindrical and is supplied by two types of nerve endings, NE 1 and NE 2, which can be seen at its basal end. Several groups of mitochondria, M_1, M_2, M_3, M_5, are found in sensory cells and neural elements. Two types of hair project from surfaces of sensory cells, stereocilia, H, and kinocilium, KC, single kinocilium always being the longest on each cell. Supporting cells are easily distinguished from sensory cells by virtue of their large population of rather uniformly distributed granules, Gr. (**A,** From Wersall W: Acta Otolaryngol 126(Suppl):1, 1956; **B,** From Engstrom H, Ades HW, Hawkins JE Jr: J Acoust Soc Am 34:1356, 1962.)

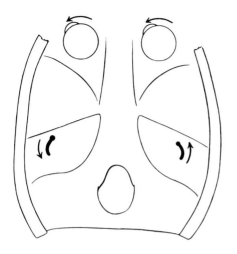

FIG. 5-66 Deviation of eyes and displacement of endolymph with rotation of head to the right. (From Cogan DG: Neurology of the ocular muscles, 2nd ed, Springfield, IL, Charles C Thomas, Publisher, 1966.)

disynaptic pathways also exist, because lesions of the medial longitudinal fasciculi do not abolish this reflex.[119] Ito et al.[99,100] have demonstrated that excitatory connections from the anterior canals and the saccule reach the oculomotor nuclei via the brachium conjunctivum (BC) rather than via the medial longitudinal fasciculus (MLF). Schematic diagrams of these connections are shown in Figure 5-68; the projections are summarized in Table 5-5. For the vertical canals the excitatory connections are crossed and the inhibitory connections are uncrossed. For the horizontal canals the lateral rectus excitatory innervation is crossed and the medial rectus excitatory innervation is uncrossed. Inhibitory pathways are opposite for each muscle group. Two types of cells are excited:

1. Tonic cells, which have continuous spontaneous activity that increases or de-

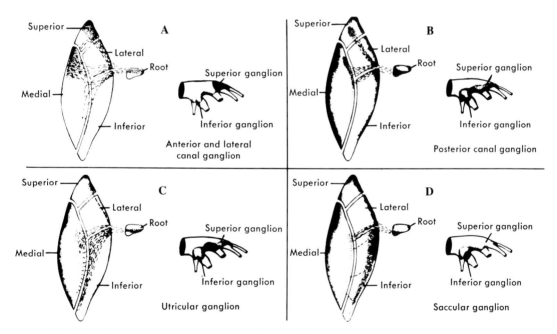

FIG. 5-67 Diagrammatic representation of central distribution of degeneration in vestibular nuclei resulting from lesions of various parts of vestibular ganglion. In **A**, lesion destroyed cells that innervate anterior and lateral canals; in **B**, posterior canal; in **C**, the utricle; in **D**, the saccule. Note that in **A** and **B** the most profuse central degeneration is present in the superior vestibular nucleus and in rostral parts of medial vestibular nucleus, whereas in **C** and **D** central degeneration is most profuse in the inferior vestibular nucleus and in caudal portions of medial vestibular nucleus. (From Stein BM, Carpenter MB: Am J Anat 120:281, 1967; modified by Cohen B, in Bach-y-Rita P, Collins CC, Hyde JE: The control of eye movements, New York, Academic Press, 1971.)

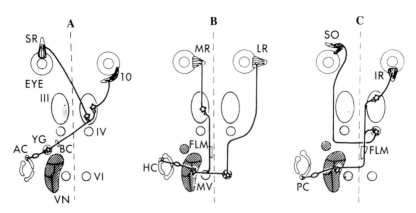

FIG. 5-68 Schematic drawing of the excitatory vestibulo-ocular reflex pathways for, **A**, the anterior canal, **B**, horizontal canal, and **C**, posterior canal. SR, Superior rectus; IO, inferior oblique; MR, medial rectus; LR, lateral rectus; SO, superior oblique; IR, inferior rectus; AC, anterior canal; HC, horizontal canal; PC, posterior canal; III, oculomotor nucleus; IV, trochlear nucleus; VI, abducens nucleus; YG, y group region; VN, vestibular nucleus; MV, medial vestibular nucleus; BC, brachium conjunctivum; FLM, medial longitudinal fasciculus. (From Ito M, Nisimaru N, Yamamoto M: Exp Brain Res 24:281, 1976.)

TABLE 5-5 Summary of Afferent Inputs to the Cerebellum: Direct Vestibulo-ocular Projections as Determined by Electrophysiologic Studies in Cat and Rabbit

Receptor	Effect	Muscle	Relay nucleus	Pathway	Motor nucleus
HC	Excitation	c-LR	MVN	MLF	c-VI
		i-MR	LVN	ATD	i-III
	Inhibition	i-LR	MVN	MLF	i-VI
		c-MR	—	Extra MLF polysyn.	c-III
AC	Excitation	i-SR	SVN	BC	c-III
		c-IO	SVN	BC	c-III
	Inhibition	i-IR	SVN	MLF	i-III
		c-SO	SVN	MLF	i-IV
PC	Excitation	c-IR	MVN	MLF	c-III
		i-SO	MVN	MLF	c-IV
	Inhibition	c-SR	SVN	MLF	i-III
		i-IO	SVN	MLF	i-III
U	Excitation	i-LR	LVN	MLF	i-VI
		c-MR	LVN	MLF	c-III
		i-SO	LVN	MLF	c-IV
S	Excitation	—	y-group	BC	—

HC, Horizontal canal; AC, anterior canal; PC, posterior canal, U, utricle; S, saccule; c, contralateral; i, ipsilateral; LR, lateral rectus; MR, medial rectus; SR, superior rectus; IO, inferior oblique; IR, inferior rectus; SO, superior oblique; MVN, medial vestibular nucleus; LVN, lateral vestibular nucleus; SVN, superior vestibular nucleus; MLF, medial longitudinal fasciculus; ATD, anterior decussation; BC, brachium conjunctivum. (Modified from Leigh RJ, Zee DS: The neurology of eye movements, Philadelphia, FA Davis, 1983.)

creases in response to ipsilateral or contralateral rotation, respectively

2. Kinetic cells, which are silent in the resting state and increase their firing only with strong ipsilateral rotation

Two types of neurons have been identified in the vestibular nuclei: type *I* cells, which increase their discharge rate for ipsilateral rotations and decrease their discharge rate for contralateral rotations; and type *II* cells, which do the opposite. Type *I* cells synapse on contralateral type *II* cells via the vestibular commissure. Leigh and Zee[114] observe: "The push-pull pairing of canals, the resting vestibular tone, and exchange of neural input through the vestibular commissure maximize vestibular sensitivity in health and provide a substrate for compensation and adaptation in disease."

Vestibulospinal inputs. The importance of tonic neck reflexes in humans is questionable. Neural pathways originate in proprioceptors in neck muscles and tendons and pass through the dorsal spinal roots of the cervical cord to enter the spinocerebellar tracts. Hikosaka and Maeda[85] reported that afferent spinal signs reach the contralateral vestibular nuclei to im-

pinge on vestibulo-ocular relay motoneurons. Effects of spinal afference under normal and pathologic conditions have been reviewed by Dichgans.[51]

Cerebellar inputs. The cerebellum is divided into the cortex and the intrinsic nuclei. The cortex is divided into a midline *vermis* and two *hemispheres*. The hemispheres, in turn, are divided into lobules of important functional significance: the *flocculonodular*, the *anterior*, and the *neocerebellum* (Fig. 5-69).

The vestibular and oculomotor connections of the cerebellum act primarily to modulate the activity of the oculomotor system and vestibulo-ocular reflexes.

Flocculonodular lobe of the cerebellum. The flocculonodular lobe is of primary importance in mediating vestibular inputs to the oculomotor system. Primary vestibular axons and secondary fibers originating in the inferior and medial vestibular nuclei ascend as mossy fibers to terminate in the flocculonodular lobe (Fig. 5-70). Indirect connections from the oculomotor and vestibular systems abound, routed via the inferior olive and the lateral reticular nucleus. Purkinje cells of the flocculonodular lobe are modulated by vestibular stimulation.[116]

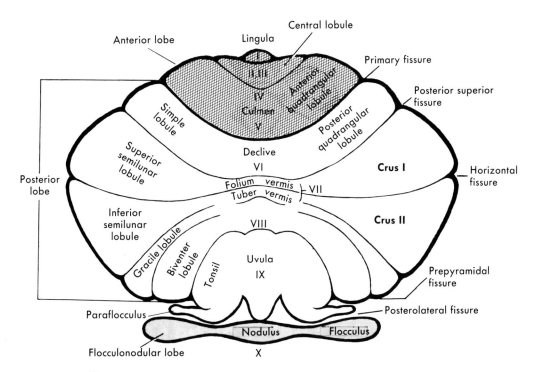

FIG. 5-69 Human neuroanatomy. Ventral surface of cerebellum after removal of lower pons and medulla. (From Strother CM, Salamon G: Topographic anatomy of the brain, in Newton TH, Potts DG, eds: Radiology of the skull and brain anatomy and pathology, vol 3, St Louis, CV Mosby, 1977.)

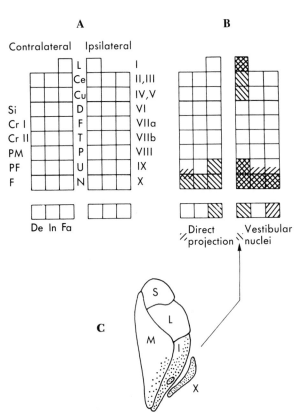

FIG. 5-70 Projection from vestibular nuclei to cerebellum. **A,** Key to highly schematic representation of cerebellar cortex and deep nuclei. The three columns represent, respectively (from inside to outside), vermal, paravermal, and lateral regions of cortex, divided horizontally as indicated; underneath them lie fastigial (Fa), interpositus (in), and dentate (De) nuclei. *L, Lingula; Ce, centralis; Cu, culmen; D, declive; F, folium; T, tuber; P, pyramis; U, uvula; N, nodulus; Si, simplex; Cr I and Cr II, crus I and crus II (ansiform lobe); PM, paramedian lobe; PF, paraflocculus; F, flocculus. On the right, corresponding roman numeral nomenclature is shown. **B,** Distribution of direct primary vestibular fibers and secondary fibers from the vestibular nucleus; the origins of the latter are shown stippled in **C.** (From Carpenter RHS: Movements of the eyes, London, Pion, Ltd, 1977.)

Efferent fibers from the flocculonodular lobe terminate directly on the vestibular complex and also project to the intrinsic nuclei. From the intrinsic nuclei, some fibers pass to the contralateral superior rectus subnuclei[37] and paramedian pontine reticular formation,[36] whereas other fibers project contralaterally to the superior vestibular nucleus and bilaterally to ventral and lateral portions of the other vestibular nuclei.

Cerebellar vermis. In contrast to the flocculonodular lobe of the cerebellum, which functions primarily to mediate the vestibular inputs to the oculomotor system, the cerebellar vermis is more directly involved in the generation of eye movements. Although the exact efferent pathways from the vermis to the brainstem centers controlling eye movement are unknown,[153] electrical stimulation produces rapid eye movements,[42,171] and lesions result in alteration of Purkinje cell activity in the vermis. Normally, Purkinje cells fire rapid eye movements, the intensity of firing being inversely proportional to the magnitude of the movement.[117,132,203] In studies by McElligott and Keller[133] Purkinje cells were found to be directionally sensitive, to fire up to 22 msec prior to the onset of eye move-

ment, and to continue discharging up to 400 msec after the eye movement (Fig. 5-71). They concluded that the extended period of activity of these neurons may relate to visual or proprioceptive inputs that compensate for inaccuracies in final eye position.

Superior colliculus. The superior colliculus consists of seven layers divided into dorsal (superficial) and ventral (deep) portions.[207] The dorsal portion is activated by visual stimuli and is retinotopically mapped. The ventral portion is associated with initiation of rapid eye movements.

Although there are no direct connections between the efferent fibers of the superior colliculus and the oculomotor nuclei, connections to the contralateral PPRF may be present.[161] Some collicular fibers terminate in the interstitial nucleus of Cajal and the nucleus of Darkschewitsch.

Stimulation of the superior colliculus in alert monkeys elicits contralateral saccades,[166,177] with the size and direction of the saccade being dependent on location (Fig. 5-72). Collicular lesions in animals and humans have only subtle effect on ocular motility. However, Schiller et al.[178] have demonstrated nearly total paralysis of

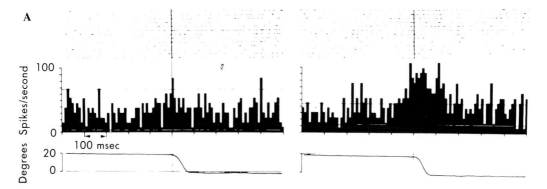

FIG. 5-71 Example of vermal Purkinje cell that showed excitatory modulation for outward (**B**) directed left saccades but not inward saccades (**A**) in the same direction. In each plate discharge rasters for individual trials, cumulative histograms, and averaged horizontal eye movements are displayed from top to bottom. In each histogram the individual discharges are summed in 10 ms bins and then are divided by the number of trials to yield average frequency. Neuronal activity was aligned in time with saccade onset (vertical line). Horizontal lines represent discharge rates, which are plus or minus two standard deviations from the mean ongoing discharge rate. On eye movement traces rightward direction of movement is shown as up, and horizontal lines show primary position. (Reprinted with permission from McElligott JG, Keller EL: Neuronal discharge in the posterior cerebellum: its relationship to saccadic eye movement generation, in Lennerstrand G, Zee DS, Keller EL, eds: Functional basis of ocular motility disorders, Oxford, Pergamon Press, copyright 1982, p 453.)

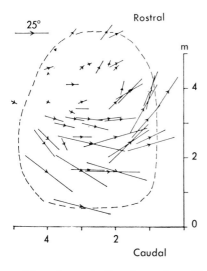

FIG. 5-72 Map of saccade direction and amplitude on dorsal view of left superior colliculus. Scale is in millimeters; m, midline. Composite of saccades *(arrows)* evoked from 50 electrode tracks in two monkeys. *Dotted line,* Reconstructed boundary of superior colliculus. (From Robinson DA: Vision Res 12:1975, 1972.)

rapid eye movements if both the frontal lobes and the superior colliculi are ablated.

Supplementary motor cortex. The supplementary motor cortex (as well as the frontal eye fields and cerebellum) is active during all types of saccadic eye movement independent of task complexity. The pathways subserving this input and its actual role are unknown.[63]

Frontal eye fields. The frontal eye fields (Brodal area 8) project to the basal ganglia, thalamus, pretectum, superior colliculus, and portions of the mesencephalic and pontine reticular formations.[112,113] The frontal eye fields receive inputs via a collosal projection from the opposite frontal eye fields, which may subserve vertical eye movements. They also receive projections from prestriate cortex (MT, V4, and intraparietal sulcus), anterior cortex (area 46, cingulate cortex) to subserve behavioral processing, and thalamus (lateral portion of medial dorsal nucleus, intralaminar nucleus, and medial pulvinar).[69]

Within the frontal eye fields Bruce and Goldberg have identified presaccadic visual cells responding to visual stimuli that become the targets of saccades, movement cells responding before and during learned saccades in the dark, and visuomovement cells responding to both conditions.[23] There are also cells that respond following saccades[21] and in relation to fixation.[21,22]

Clinical and experimental studies suggest that the frontal eye fields mediate voluntary contralateral eye movements by specifying the coordinates of a desired saccade and by influencing the saccadic initiation process.[69,75]

Thalamus and basal ganglia

The thalamus and basal ganglia participate in a pathway that is involved in the generation of voluntary saccades and in the suppression of inappropriate "reflex" saccades.[88,109] The anatomic substrate is summarized schematically in Figure 5-73. Cells within the substantia nigra appear to modulate their activity prior to memory-guided or visually-guided saccades.[87] These cells project to the intermediate layers of the superior colliculus and provide a GABA-mediated inhibitory influence.[39,64] Removal of this inhibition may directly or indirectly activate superior colliculus cells to initiate saccades. Caudate cells, with inputs primarily from the association cortex, thalamic nuclei, and frontal eye fields, are directly inhibitory to the substantia nigra.[86] Because lesions of this pathway do not result in a complete permanent paralysis of contralateral eye movements, the pathway is considered to operate in parallel with the descending motor pathway from the superior colliculus. As noted, simultaneous lesions of the ipsilateral frontal eye fields and superior colliculus result in complete abolition of rapid eye movements to the contralateral side.[178]

Posterior parietal cortex

Neurons in the posterior parietal cortex demonstrate enhanced rates of firing prior to the detection of an eccentric visual target, whether or not an eye movement is made to the target[32] (Fig. 5-74). Such firing patterns suggest that the role of this area (especially Fig 5-74,A) is to integrate sensory and motor information, perhaps mediating visual attention. Other areas may have more specialized functions. For instance, the lateral intraparietal area (LIP) is associated with the memory-linked planning of intended eye movements[4], and the medial superior temporal area (MST) is associated with smooth pursuit.[175,208]

THE SACCADIC SYSTEM
Controller signal for saccades

The neural signal that initiates saccadic eye movements consists of a *burst* of high frequency discharge to the agonist muscles with a corresponding period of inhibition to the antagonist muscles.[66,165,170] This burst of firing is coordinated by the paramedian pontine reticular formation (PPRF).[43,105] The burst or *pulse* of innervation is required to achieve the high peak velocities recorded for human eye movement (up to 1000 degrees/sec).

At the end of a saccade, a small amount of force must be applied through the extraocular muscles to hold the new eye position. The tonic firing of the extraocular muscles is referred to as the "step," in which both agonist and antago-

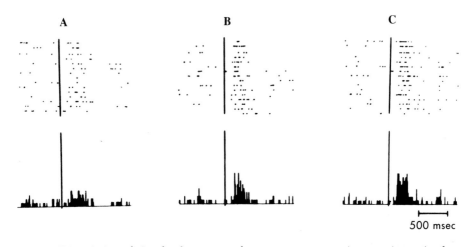

FIG. 5-73 Dissociation of visual enhancement from eye movements in posterior parietal cortex. Each diagram consists of raster *(top)* and related poststimulus histogram. Each dot in raster signifies occurrence of action potential. Each line of raster represents a 2-second epoch of cell activity. Successive trials are aligned on stimulus onset, which occurs at vertical line. Each histogram represents sum of activity in raster above. Vertical line in histogram corresponds to discharge frequency of 114 Hz; bin width is 12 msec. **A,** Response of a neuron when stimulus is irrelevant. **B,** Response of same neuron when stimulus is target for eye movement. **C,** Response of neuron when animal attends to but does not make a saccade to stimulus. (From Bushnell MC, Goldberg ME, Robinson DL: J Neurophysiol 46:755, 1981.)

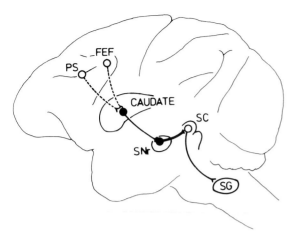

FIG. 5-74. Neural mechanism in the basal ganglia for the initiation of saccades. Excitatory and inhibitory neurons are indicated by open and filled circles, respectively. SC, superior colliculus; FEF, frontal eye field; PS, cortical area around the principal sulcus; SG, saccade generator in the brainstem reticular formation. The "axon" of substantia nigra (SNr) neuron is made thicker than others to indicate its high background activity. (From Hikosaka O: Role of basal ganglia in saccades, Rev Neurol (Paris), 1989, 145:8, 580.)

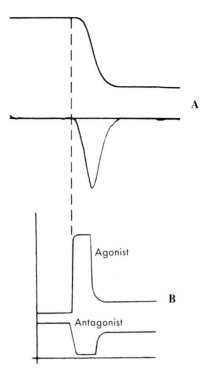

FIG. 5-75 A, Position (upper) and velocity (lower) record for saccade. B, Proposed neuronal control signal for saccade consists of pulse-step pattern of innervation to agonist muscle and pulse-step pattern of inhibition to antagonist muscle. (Reprinted by permission of the publisher from The main sequence, a tool for studying human eye movement, by Bahill AT, Clark MR, Stark L: Math Biosci 24:193, copyright 1975 by Elsevier Science Publishing Co, Inc.)

nist muscles participate. An integration of the *pulse* signal, performed by cells in the PPRF, produces a *step* appropriate to the new eye position.[105,106] Therefore the *pulse-step* of innervation (Fig. 5-75), delivered primarily via burst-tonic neurons, is the neural control signal that generates saccadic eye movements.

A hypothetical premotor organization of this signal has been proposed by Hepp and Henn.[80] They suggest that the pulse-step is initiated by an inhibition of "pause" cells that allow medium-level burst neurons to activate the oculomotor plant both directly and via burst-tonic neurons.

The main sequence of eye movements

A characteristic of saccades is that the peak velocity is proportional to the size of the eye movement, a relationship referred to as the main sequence[8] (Fig. 5-76). Because all neurons in the available pool are considered to be activated for eye movements of greater than 5 degrees, the duration of the pulse determines the magnitude of the saccade.

Ballistic nature of saccades

Instantaneous adjustment of the pulse-step of innervation to the extraocular muscles is considered impossible because there is no time for visual feedback to guide the eye to its final position. Therefore saccades are considered to be

preprogrammed or *ballistic* based on retinal error signal.[77,168] Robinson[168] has suggested that saccades are not truly ballistic, but may represent the response to an internal error signal produced by the difference between actual and desired position of the eyes in space.

Pulse-step mismatch

When the pulse and the step of innervation are perfectly matched, the saccadic trajectory is a rapid movement that terminates at the new eye position. Under both normal and pathologic conditions, pulses and steps may become mismatched, resulting in more complex saccadic trajectories.[9] The pulse may be too large for the step or vice versa. The resulting oculomotor behaviors are shown in Fig. 5-77. Lesions in patients[41,215] and in animals[144,163] suggest that the cerebellum is important in gradually adjusting the pulse-step controller signal to minimize mismatch. Recent primate studies indicate that the dorsal cerebellar vermis controls pulse size and

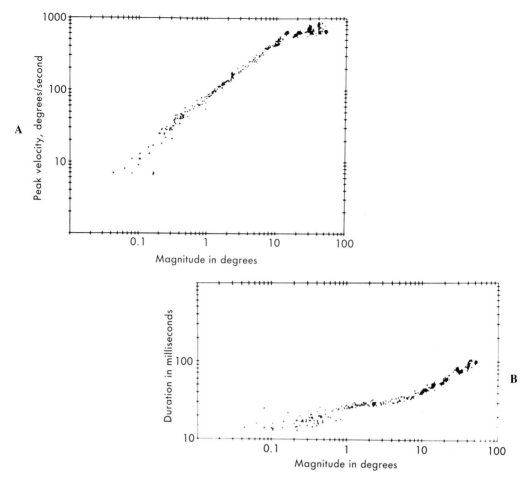

FIG. 5-76 **A**, Peak velocity vs. magnitude of human saccadic eye movements. **B**, Duration versus magnitude of human saccadic eye movements. (Reprinted by permission of the publisher from The main sequence, a tool for studying human eye movement, by Bahill AT, Clark MR, Stark L: Math Biosci 24:191, copyright 1975 by Elsevier Science Publishing Co, Inc.)

that the flocculus controls the pulse-step match.[115,144,145]

Sample data model. Saccades usually can be evoked at minimum intervals of 150 to 200 msec. This observation led to the hypothesis of intermittent rather than continuous sampling. This hypothesis, as originally proposed by Young and Stark,[211] suggests that a region of 0.3 degrees around the fovea is sampled periodically for the detection of retinal error. One reaction time later, a step change in eye position occurs. The most convincing evidence for the sampled data model is the saccadic behavior elicited under *open loop conditions.* Such conditions can be achieved by restraining the imaging eye and observing oculomotor behavior in the non-imaging eye,[210] as well as by attempting to refixate an eccentric retinal afterimage. Under all open loop conditions, attempts to fix a perifoveal target result in a series of saccadic jumps with an interval of about 200 msec (Fig. 5-78).

The smooth pursuit system

In foveating animals, smooth pursuit allows a target to be followed as it moves in space. The critical parameter for smooth pursuit to occur is probably target velocity.[157,164] Eye velocity usually matches target velocity[54] after a latency of 130 msec.[164] In bioengineering terms a perfect match is said to have *a gain of unity.* If the ratio of eye velocity to target velocity is greater than unity, the gain is increased; similarly, if the ratio of eye velocity to target velocity is less than unity, the gain is decreased. Hypotheses have emerged that include a predictive component in tracking by smooth pursuit.[57,200] Experimental

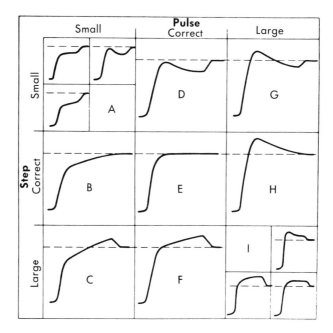

FIG. 5-77 Pulse and step components of saccadic control signal can be mismatched in a variety of ways, resulting in the 13 trajectories shown here. For example, when step is correct but pulse is too large (H), a glissadic overshoot is generated. When the pulse is too small (B), resulting saccade stops short of its final position and a glissade finishes the movement. When step component is incorrect (either too strong or too weak), saccade moves the eye to off-target position, where it remains until visual feedback instigates corrective saccade, either forward to the target (D) or backward to it (F). When both pulse and step are too large (I) or too small (A), primary saccade may be followed by rightward glissade, leftward glissade, or no glissade at all, depending on relative sizes of components. Broken line through each trajectory marks final, or target, eye position. (From Bahill AT, Stark L: Sci Am 240:115, 1979.)

support for such hypotheses has been obtained by Becker and Fuchs,[18] who demonstrated that sudden disappearance of a moving target resulted in decay of smooth pursuit to a "residual velocity" (Fig. 5-79).

The anatomic substrate of the pursuit system is poorly elucidated. The accessory optic system (for example, the nucleus of the optic tract), the cerebellar flocculus, the brainstem reticular formation, and the cerebral hemispheres all are associated with smooth pursuit. Hemispherectomy in humans interferes with smooth pursuit to the same side as the lesion.[184,195] Neurons of the middle temporal visual area,[15,98,198,199] the parietal[122] and frontal[178] cortices are modulated by smooth tracking. The descending pathway for smooth pursuit may originate in the middle temporal and middle superior temporal visual areas, projecting to the dorsolateral pontine nuclei.[197] The flocculus and possibly the mid-vermis may serve as premotor centers for smooth pursuit, which then project to the vestibular nuclei.[33,152] As the "final common path-

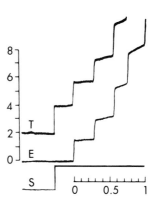

FIG. 5-78 Responses of saccadic system to conditions of variable visual feedback under open loop conditions. E, horizontal eye position; T, horizontal target position; S, initial target stimulus. (From Fuchs A: The saccadic system, in Bach-y-Rita P, Collins C, Hyde J, eds: The control of eye movements, New York, Academic Press, 1971, p 348.)

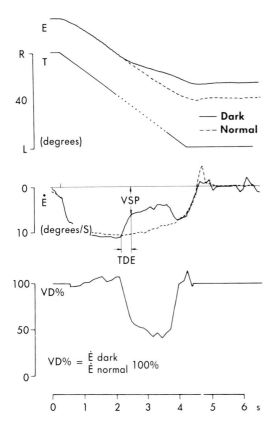

FIG. 5-79 Example of smooth pursuit response to a target movement of 10 degrees per second (deg/s). *Dashed curves,* Average (n = 20) of trials without blanking of target *(normal). Continuous curves,* Trials (n = 8) with blanking *(dark).* E, Desaccadized eye position ("smooth eye position").

way" the PPRF is likely to relay smooth pursuit signals to the ocular motor nuclei.[115] Other centers thought to mediate smooth pursuit include the superior colliculus, the thalamus, and the pulvinar.

Hoyt and Daroff[96] postulate the following ipsilateral pathway on the basis of clinical case studies:

> Occipitocollicular projections lie medial to the visual radiations (internal sagittal striatum) and pass through the retrolenticular portion of the internal capsule to the ipsilateral superior colliculus and synapse. Fibers presumably leave the superior colliculus with the mediotectospinal tract and course to the opposite side of the midbrain tegmentum in the dorsal fountain decussation of Meynert. Fibers then accompany the decussation from the mesencephalic saccadic tract and terminate in the PPRF. This requires a double decussation.

Vertical pursuit movements are probably bilaterally represented similar to the saccadic system.

The optokinetic system

The optokinetic system is closely related to the smooth pursuit system. As such, discussions of oculomotor behavior and pathways often are considered interchangeable. When a subject views a series of moving objects, such as stripes on an optokinetic drum, rotating around the patient, the eyes tend to lock onto a stripe, follow the stripe for a time (compensatory movements), and then saccade in the opposite direction (anticompensatory movement). This pattern of alternating slow and fast components is called optokinetic nystagmus (OKN). In humans this reflex is instruction and attention dependent. Looking at the stimulus results in large amplitude excursions with infrequent fast phases; staring at the stimulus results in smaller amplitude excursions with frequent fast phases; active following of the stimulus results in poor correspondence between eye position and stimulus position (Fig. 5-80).[96]

At slow target velocities there is good correspondence with slow phase eye velocity.[20] This correspondence deteriorates with increasing target velocities (Fig. 5-81). At velocities of 30 to 100 deg/sec, the eye movement progressively lags behind target movement, creating *phase lag.* At velocities greater than 100 deg/sec, optokinetic nystagmus can no longer be evoked.[91,92]

Unlike simple foveal smooth pursuit, OKN appears to have both foveal and peripheral retinal components. Patients with central scotoma are able to match higher target velocities than are normally sighted individuals,[94] and patients with small central islands of vision demonstrate reduced optokinetic responses.[93-95] Carpenter[38] concludes that selective attention is, in large part, responsible for these observations. In normal subjects instructed to "stare at the drum," the initiation of the nystagmus is a quick phase movement toward the direction from which the stimuli enter the periphery of vision. Thus the anticompensatory saccade serves an "anticipatory" function rather than a "resetting function."[11] In conditions that minimize foveal contributions the initiation of the nystagmus is a slow phase movement in the direction of target movement[93] (Fig. 5-82).

Precht[154,155] recently has reviewed the anatomic and functional organization of the optokinetic pathways. At the level of the retina, specific ganglion cells have been identified in the rabbit[146,147] and the cat.[90] These cells project pri-

Active optokinetic nystagmus

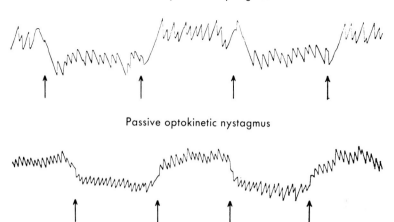

Passive optokinetic nystagmus

FIG. 5-80 Nystagmus tracings obtained with subject following stripes of drum (active opto-kinetic nystagmus) and gazing passively at drum (passive optokinetic nystagmus). *Arrows,* Reversal of drum direction. Note deviation of eye in direction of slow component of nystag-mus in case of active optokinetic nystagmus and in direction of fast component in case of passive optokinetic mystagmus. (From Hood JD, Leech J: Acta Otolaryngol 77:72, 1974.)

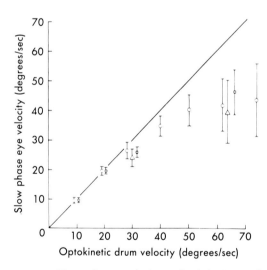

FIG. 5-81 Normal mean ± 1 standard deviation for horizontal OKN slow phase velocity at different drum velocities. Three different types of optokinetic stimuli: ramp, constant velocity, and sinusoidal. (Reprinted with permission from Baloh RW, Yee RD, Honrubia V: Clinical abnormalities of optokinetic nystagmus, in Lennerstrand G, Zee DS, Keller EL, eds: Functional basis of ocular motility disorders, Oxford, Pergamon Press, copyright 1982, p 311.)

marily to the contralateral[40] accessory optic system (AOS), nucleus of optic tract (NOT), and visual cortex via the lateral geniculate. The AOS consists primarily of the dorsal, lateral, and medial terminal nuclei. The schematic relationship between these nuclei and the NOT is shown in Fig. 5-83. In mammals lesions of NOT and the subnuclei of AOS have been associated with abolished horizontal and vertical OKN, respectively.[44-46,153,185,201] On the basis of accumulated experimental evidence, Precht has postulated three possible optokinetic pathways (Fig. 5-84): (1) a short latency pathway that takes the form of a three neuron arc (*A* in Fig. 5-83) is suggested as a pathway to rapidly increase initial eye velocity; (2) a long latency pathway (*C* in Fig. 5-84) mediated by the vestibular nucleus, probably via intermediate nuclei such as the n. reticularis tegmenti pontis (NRTP) and the n. prepositus hypoglossi, which may integrate velocity of the environment relative to the head rather than just to the retina; and (3) in primates and humans foveal OKN is likely to be mediated principally via the LGN-transcortical-floccular pathway (*B* in Fig. 5-84). Lesions of the visual cortex induced in animals with normally symmetric responses to nasotemporal and temporonasal stimulation result in marked deficits to nasotemporal stimulation,[139,206] as well as in reduced gain to temporonasal stimulation.[139] Further experiments demonstrate that both crossed and uncrossed fibers act on subcortical centers directly, as well as through the LGN-visual cortex pathway.

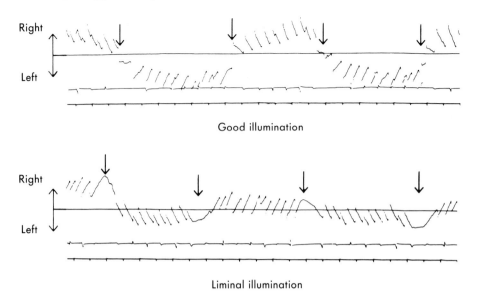

Good illumination

Liminal illumination

FIG. 5-82 Tracings of optokinetic nystagmus in good illumination and limited illumination. Under conditions of good illumination, change in direction of eyes occurs with fast phase. Under conditions of limited illumination, change in direction of eyes occurs with slow phase (i.e., develops the character of reflex, vestibular nystagmus). Drum velocity is indicated by tracing above time marker and shows each 20-degree displacement. (From Hood JD: Acta Otolaryngol 63:208, 1967.)

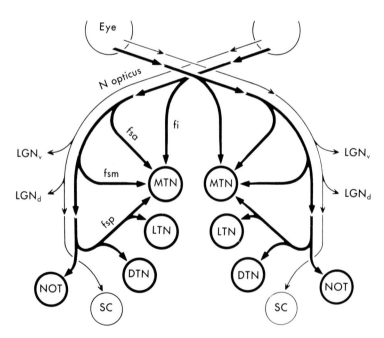

FIG. 5-83 Schematic representation of accessory optic system of optic tract. LGN$_v$, ventral lateral geniculate nucleus; LGN$_d$, dorsal lateral geniculate nucleus; MTN, medial terminal nuclei; LTN, lateral terminal nuclei; DTN, dorsal terminal nuclei; SC, superior colliculus; NOT, nucleus of optic tract; fi, fasciculus inferior; fas, fsm, fsp, fasciculus superior, pars anterior, medialis, posterior. (Reprinted with permission from Precht W: Anatomical and functional organization of optokinetic pathways, in Lennerstrand G, Zee DS, Keller EL, eds: Functional basis of ocular motility disorders, Oxford, Pergamon Press, copyright 1982.)

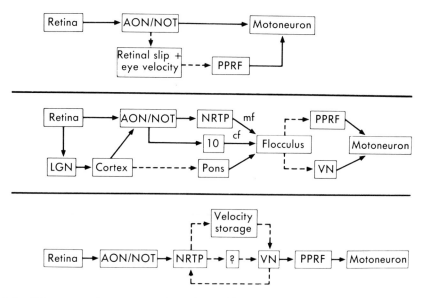

FIG. 5-84 Diagrammatic representation of possible optokinetic pathways. See text for details. AON/NOT, accessory optic nucleus/n. optic tract; PPRF, paramedian pontine reticular formation; LGN, lateral geniculate nucleus; NRTP, n. reticularis tegmentis pontis; IO, inferior olive; VN, vestibular nucleus; cf, mf, climbing and mossy fiber afferents to cerebellum. (Reprinted with permission from Precht W: Anatomical and functional organization of optokinetic pathways, in Lennerstrand G, Zee DS, Keller EL, eds: Functional basis of ocular motility disorders, Oxford, Pergamon Press, copyright 1982.)

Vestibulo-ocular reflex (VOR)

As stated by Leigh and Zee,[114] "The VOR functions to maintain steady gaze (eye position in space) during head rotation" (Fig. 5-85). A mechanical model demonstrating the response of the semicircular canal to head rotation is shown in Fig. 5-86. These mechanical displacements result in vestibular neural firing frequencies proportional to the change in angular velocity (Fig. 5-87).

Static vestibulo-ocular responses

The utricle and saccule respond to rectilinear acceleration and govern postural tone in relation to head position. These organs compensate for static head tilt by counter-rolling the eyes. The amount of static compensatory eye rolling is small. The utricular reflex of counter-rolling forms the basis of Bielschowsky's head-tilt test used in isolating paretic vertical muscles (Fig. 5-88). Rotation of the head up and down with contraversive rolling of the eyes, that is, eyes up with chin down and vice versa, is under control of the utricle and saccule (Fig. 5-89). In humans, however, only the torsional response is not dominated by vision (Fig. 5-90).

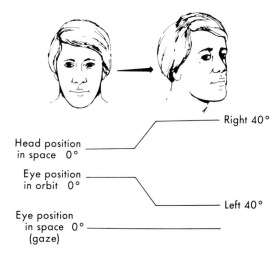

$$EYE_{space} = EYE_{orbit} + HEAD_{space}$$

FIG. 5-85 Function of vestibulo-ocular reflex. As head is rapidly turned to left, eyes move to right by a corresponding amount in the orbit. *Below,* Head position and eye position in the orbit are plotted against time. Because movements of head and eye in orbit are equal and opposite, the sum, eye position in space (gaze), remains zero (bottom equation). If gaze is held steady, then images of the seen world do not slip on the retina and vision remains clear. (From Leigh RJ, Zee DS: The neurology of eye movements, Philadelphia, FA Davis, 1983.)

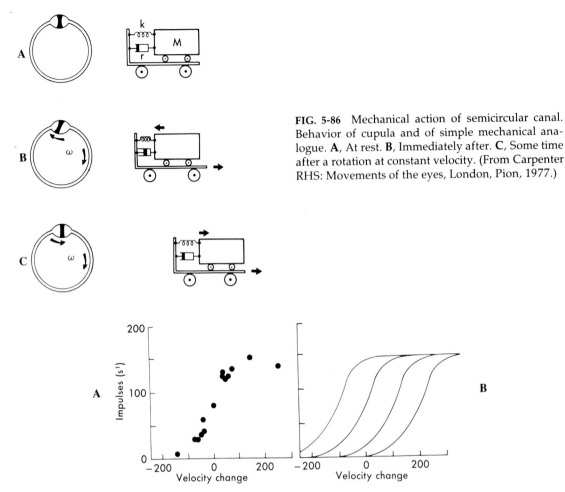

FIG. 5-86 Mechanical action of semicircular canal. Behavior of cupula and of simple mechanical analogue. **A**, At rest. **B**, Immediately after. **C**, Some time after a rotation at constant velocity. (From Carpenter RHS: Movements of the eyes, London, Pion, 1977.)

FIG. 5-87 **A**, Peak firing frequency of vestibular fibers in the ray to sudden angular velocity changes of different magnitudes. One can assume that maximum cupular deviation under these conditions is proportional to the change in velocity; thus there appears to be an S-shaped relationship between cupular deflection and firing frequency. **B**, How different units of this type, lying at different points along a scale of cupular deflection, might show the range of tonic activity that is observed. (From Carpenter RHS: Movements of the eyes, London, Pion, 1977.)

FIG. 5-88 Otostatic reflex compensating for left head tilt. *Solid line*, Normal vertical axis. *Dotted line*, Assumed vertical axis after head tilt to left shoulder. Superior oblique and superior rectus muscles are activated in eye ipsilateral to head tilt, with inferior oblique and inferior rectus activated in contralateral eye. If one were attempting to differentiate between a left superior oblique palsy and a right superior rectus palsy, both leading to a left hypertropia, the patient would be instructed to tilt head first to one side then the other, and the manifest deviation would be measured in both positions. When head is tilted to left, a larger vertical deviation would be measured if the left superior oblique were involved, because the left superior rectus would act unopposed.

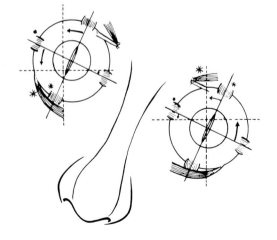

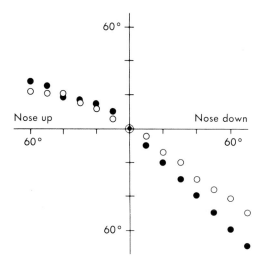

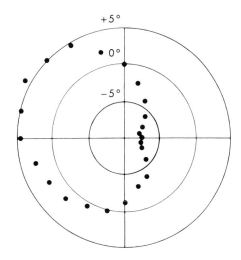

FIG. 5-89 Compensatory rotation of rabbit's eye for different degrees of tilt in sagittal plane *(filled circles)*. *Open circles,* Observations made when dorsal roots of first and second cranial nerves have been cut, that is, when influence of neck reflexes has been removed to leave response that is almost wholly vestibular in origin. (From Carpenter RHS: Movements of the eyes, London, Pion, 1977.)

FIG. 5-90 Ocular counter-rolling in humans: rotation of eye about torsional axis measured for different angles of lateral tilt of head. (From Carpenter RHS: Movements of the eyes, London, Pion, 1977.)

Dynamic vestibulo-ocular reflexes

Rotational acceleration of the head results in significant attempts by the oculomotor system to stabilize vision. The mechanical limitations of the oculomotor plant preclude compensation for large angles of head rotation. Therefore slow compensatory movements of the eyes are interrupted by fast movements in the direction of rotation. This system allows the eyes to match head *velocity* even though head *position* has been reset.[36] The transfer function, which demonstrates the amplitude and phase correspondence of the head and eyes over a range of rotation frequencies, is shown in Fig. 5-91.

Together, the slow and quick phases of eye movement constitute vestibular nystagmus. The relationships between head velocity, deviation of the cupula, and vestibular nystagmus are shown diagrammatically in Fig. 5-92.

Flourens,[61] in a series of experiments, established the following rule: each semicircular canal gives rise to nystagmus in the plane of that canal (Flourens' law). The slow phase of the induced nystagmus originates from the vestibular apparatus. The horizontal canal probably projects via at least two synapses to the contralateral parapontine reticular formation. The fast phase of nystagmus is a corrective movement, which is not generated by the vestibular system.

The deviation of the eyes corresponds to the slow phase of vestibular nystagmus and is always in the direction opposite the change in rate of motion. Thus with acceleration the eyes appear to lag, whereas with deceleration they anticipate the movement. This serves to stabilize the visual image. Simplistically, each semicircular canal can be thought of in terms of influencing yoked pairs of eye muscles, one muscle for each eye, that rotate each globe in approximately the same plane as that in which the semicircular canal is located[193] (Fig. 5-93). For the vertical canals, the anterior canal excites the ipsilateral superior rectus and contralateral inferior oblique muscles; the posterior canal excites the ipsilateral superior oblique and contralateral inferior rectus muscles; and the horizontal canal excites the ipsilateral medial rectus and contralateral lateral rectus muscles. Stimulation of one anterior canal produces upward rotation of both eyes with ipsilateral incyclotorsional and contralateral excyclotorsional movement. Stimulation of one posterior canal elicits a mixture of downward rotation with inclyclotorsion of the ipsilateral and excyclotorsion of the contralat-

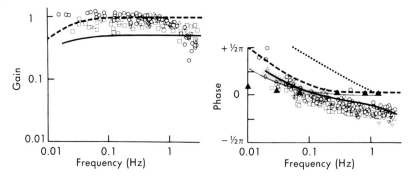

FIG. 5-91   Transfer function of vestibulo-ocular reflex in different preparations. *Thick line,* Human data; *thin line,* human data; *shading,* human data; *dashed line,* normal cat; *dotted line,* anesthetized cat; *open symbols,* decerebrate cat; *solid triangles,* normal monkey. (From Carpenter RHS: Movements of the eyes, London, Pion, 1977.)

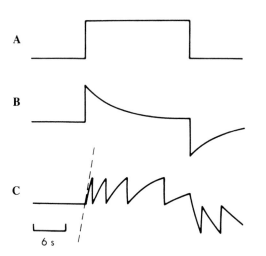

FIG. 5-92   Vestibular nystagmus during constant-velocity turn. **A,** Represents time-course of velocity of head. **B,** Resultant deviation of cupula. **C,** Very diagrammatically, ensuing vestibular nystagmus; frequency of quick phases has been drastically reduced for clarity. Velocity of slow phase is approximately proportional to cupular deviation at every point. (From Carpenter RHS: Movements of the eyes, London, Pion, 1977.)

FIG. 5-93 Relationships between semicircular canals and eye muscles. In each of the five cases, upper diagram shows a schematic frontal representation of the six canals. *Arrow,* Direction of the stimulus rotation; *thickened line,* canal that is thus stimulated; *dotted line,* canal that is inhibited. *Below,* Front view of both eyes and their muscles, active muscle shown in black and inhibited muscles in stipple. Small arrow near pupil shows resultant motion of globe. (From Carpenter RHS: Movements of the eyes, London, Pion, 1977.)

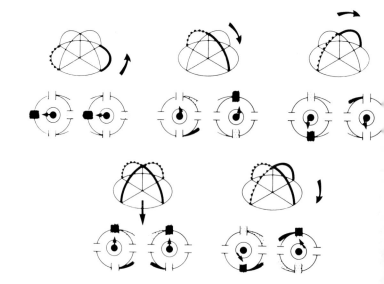

eral globe.[214] The relative degree of vertical or torsional movement depends on the position of the eye in the orbit.[44]

Semicircular canal function in humans most often is studied with caloric or rotatory stimuli. In normal individuals these stimuli do not excite individual canals. When two or more canals are simultaneously stimulated, the induced eye movements summate. Inducing caloric stimulation produces convection currents in the endolymph, causing relative displacement of the receptor cells. With this method the external auditory canal is irrigated with either warm (40° C) or cool (33° C) water. Ice water often is used clinically. A caloric stimulus in one ear simultaneously activates all the canals, but with appropriate positioning, for example, if the head is held back at 60 degrees, the horizontal canals will predominate (Fig. 5-94). If hot water is used, the relative movement will be toward the elevated ampulla and the eyes will deviate toward the contralateral side with a fast phase toward the ipsilateral side. The opposite is true for cold water stimuli; there is relative inhibition, with tonic deviation ipsilaterally with the fast phase to the contralateral side. Clinically, the mnemonic device COWS (cold, opposite, warm, same) should be remembered for the fast phase of induced nystagmus. Bilateral stimulation will induce vertical nystagmus.

Vestibular reactions are strictly reflexes and are not under voluntary control. The vestibular system is inhibited by the fixation maintenance mechanism. Optic fixation tends to inhibit vestibular nystagmus, and optokinetic stimuli can completely dominate this system. Vestibular nystagmus is exaggerated in the dark, when the eyes are closed, and by the use of high plus lenses.

Modification of the vestibulo-ocular reflex

The vestibulo-ocular reflex demonstrates a surprising capacity to adapt to alterations in environment and anatomy. This *plasticity* is due to the prominent role of the cerebellum, which acts to adjust the *gain* of the reflex. Precht[153] has summarized the likely pathways mediating the neural interactions between vestibular and oculomotor systems (Fig. 5-95).

Gonshor and Melvill Jones[71,72,135,136] demonstrated that goggles, which inverted the visual environment, worn for periods of up to 4 weeks resulted in rapid 65% attenuation of the vestibulo-ocular reflex in the horizontal direction. Complete reversal of the vestibulo-ocular reflex was achieved after 2 weeks (Fig. 5-96). In repeating these experiments in the cat, Robinson found the effect abolished by cerebellectomy.[167,168]

Eye-head coordination

The vestibulo-ocular reflex provides a primary pathway coordinating eye and head position. However, to maintain steady fixation on a visual target in the presence of head movement the VOR must be suppressed. This suppression could occur either by using the pursuit system or by generating an internal signal representing planned head movement. Robinson[169] has proposed that both systems exist as separate sys-

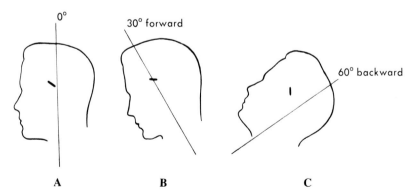

FIG. 5-94 Plane of the horizontal semicircular canal with different positions of head. In erect position of head, **A**, anterior end of horizontal canal is tilted upward approximately 30 degrees but may be made horizontal by tilting head forward 30 degrees, **B**, or be made vertical by tilting the head backward 60 degrees, **C**. (From Cogan DG: Neurology of the ocular muscles, 2nd ed, Springfield, IL, Charles C Thomas, Publisher, 1966.)

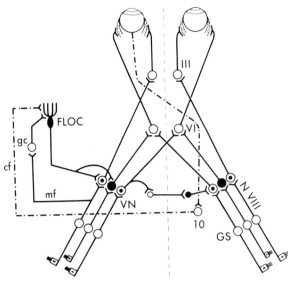

FIG. 5-95 Diagram of short latency vestibulo-ocular reflexes originating from horizontal canals and their relation to cerebellum. *Open and filled circles*, Excitatory and inhibitory neurons respectively. *Dotted circles*, Second-order excitatory vestibular neurons. *Small filled circle*, Type II inhibitory neuron mediating commissural inhibition. *Broken line*, Visual path from eye to flocculus. cf, Climbing fiber; floc, flocculus; gc, granule cell; GS, ganglion scarpae; IO, inferior olive; mf, mossy fiber; VN, vestibular nucleus; III, motoneurons of medial rectus; IV, abducens nucleus; N VIII, nerve fibers from horizontal canal. (Reprinted with permission from Lennerstrand G, Bach-y-Rita P, eds: Basic mechanisms of ocular motility and their clinical implications, Oxford, Pergamon Press, copyright 1975.)

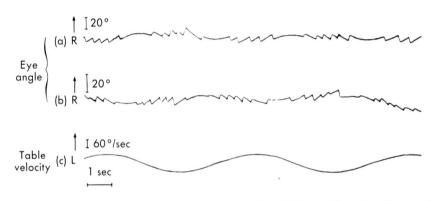

FIG. 5-96 Comparison of (*a*) control and (*b*) reversed vestibulo-ocular reflex. Reversed response was recorded in dark 14 days after donning reversing prisms. Slight phase advancement of *b* relative to true reversal was characteristic at this stimulus frequency of ⅙ Hz, and it was consistently maintained from the day 14 until removal of prisms. (Reprinted with permission from Lennerstrand G, Bach-y-Rita P, eds: Basic mechanisms of ocular motility and their clinical implications, Oxford, Pergamon Press, copyright 1975.)

tems that can be switched, depending upon whether the head movement is planned.

Eye-head coordination is also critical to the generation of large eye pursuit[47] and gaze[212,213] movements to highly eccentric visual targets. Bahill et al.[7] have shown that eye movements larger than 15 degrees seldom occur in nature. Rather, eye movements are coordinated with head movements to achieve the new gaze position (Fig. 5-97). Eye movement usually precedes head movement, although the large head mass relative to eye mass may account for these phase lags (Fig. 5-98). Zangemeister and Stark[213] have shown, however, that many types of coordinated gaze movements can occur. Studies in trained monkeys suggest that a subpopulation of burst cells, which coordinates eye-head position during change in gaze, rather than just saccades alone, exists within the pontine reticular formation[115] (Fig. 5-99). At the cortical level the frontal eye fields possess neurons that discharge in relation to head movement.[22]

Neural commands   **Eye and head movements**   **Gaze change**

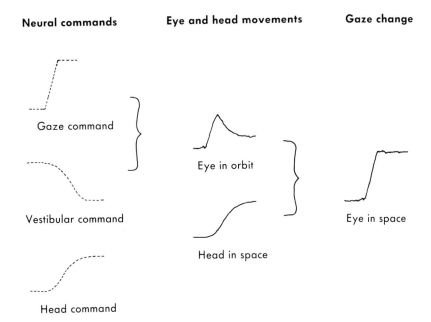

Gaze command

Vestibular command

Eye in orbit

Head in space

Eye in space

Head command

FIG. 5-97 Interaction between saccadic gaze and vestibular command signals during a combined eye-head movement to a peripheral target. Saccadic gaze and vestibular signals add centrally to produce a command for eye position in orbit. Position of eye in space (gaze) is equal to sum of positions of eye in orbit and head in space. When VOR gain is 1.0, head movement per se does not move eyes in space; thus gaze change simply reflects central saccadic gaze command. (From Leigh RJ, Zee DS: The neurology of eye movements, Philadelphia, FA Davis, 1983.)

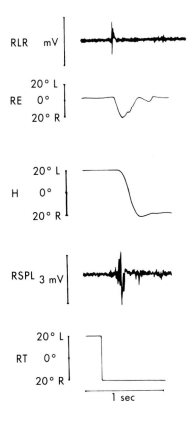

RLR mV

RE 20° L
    0°
    20° R

H 20° L
   0°
   20° R

RSPL 3 mV

RT 20° L
    0°
    20° R

1 sec

FIG. 5-98 Response to 40-degree target shift from left (L) to right (R). Random target (RT) shift. Eye movement precedes head movement (H) by 45 msec, whereas right splenius EMG (RSPL) starts about 10 msec before initial eye position changes. RE, Right eye; RLR, right lateral rectus (calibration: 1 mV). (Reprinted with permission from Zangemeister WH, Stark L: Normal and abnormal gaze types, in Lennerstrand G, Zee DS, Keller EL, eds: Functional basis of ocular motility disorders, Oxford, Pergamon Press, copyright 1982.)

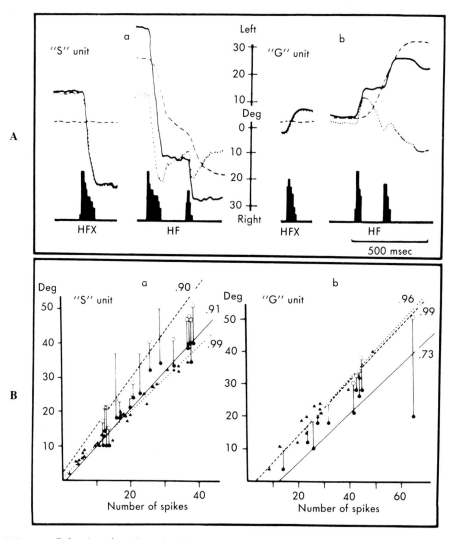

FIG. 5-99 Behavior of medium-lead burst (MLB) units. **A,** Response of two type 1 MLB units whose discharges are related to (*a*) the size of the saccadic eye movements ("S" unit) and (*b*) the total gaze shift including the head movement contribution ("G" unit). The two conditions are head fixed (HFX) and head free (HF). The three tracings are head movement (*dashed line*), horizontal eye movement (*dotted line*), and total gaze shift (*solid line*). The spike histogram shows the cumulated discharges in bins of 5 msec. **B,** Relations between movement size and number of spikes per burst for typical "G" unit and "S" unit for saccadic gaze shifts with head fixed (*triangles* and *dotted regression lines*), total gaze shifts when head was free (*open circles* and *dashed lines*), and saccade size when head was free (*solid circles* and *lines*). Vertical lines connecting data points indicate amplitude of head contribution during eye and head movement. (From Becker W, Fuchs AF: Predictive mechanisms in human smooth pursuit movement, in Roucoux A, Crommelinck M, eds: Physiologic and pathological aspects of eye movements, The Hague, Dr W Junk, 1982.)

THE NONCONJUGATE EYE MOVEMENT SYSTEM

Except under unusual pathologic conditions, nonconjugate movements, called "vergence" or "disjunctive" movements of the eyes, are slow (the exception is related to the convergence retraction nystagmus associated with periaqueductal lesions[143] rather than saccadic in nature). Maximum velocity for vergence movements is only about 21 degrees/sec.[204] Increasing the angle between the visual axes to bring the visual line to a nearer target is termed "convergence"; decreasing the angle between the visual axes to bring the visual line to a more distant target is termed "divergence." Under normal conditions the act of convergence is associated with miosis and accommodation, forming the "near triad."

Anatomic substrate of vergence eye movements

Motor substrate. The oculomotor pathways that mediate vergence eye movements, although seemingly independent,[159] are poorly characterized. Buettner-Ennever and Akert[26] found a separate medial rectus subnucleus "C" that innervates tonic muscle fibers of the orbital layer, suggesting that the version and vergence systems may remain completely isolated from the neural standpoint. However, Keller,[104] described medial rectus motoneurons that discharged to both vergence and version eye movements.

The brainstem input to medial rectus neurons mediating vergence is also unclear. Delgado-Garcia and coworkers[50] described some abducens interneurons projecting to the medial rectus subnucleus of the oculomotor complex that did not vary in frequency of discharge with vergence (Fig. 5-100). On the other hand, abducens projections to the medial rectus subnucleus "C" described by Buettner-Ennever and Akert[26] were found. Mays[131] recorded from cells in the midbrain (Fig. 5-101) that responded either tonically to a steady level of convergence or phasically to a change in level of convergence. However, he was unable to isolate vergence movement from the rest of the near triad (that is, miosis and accommodation).

Sensory substrates. At the level of the primary visual cortex, significant binocular interaction occurs within ocular dominance columns.[97] Precise alignment of receptive fields was found to increase firing rates of some cortical cells.[13] Poggio and Fischer[151] found visual cortical cells that responded selectively to the presence or absence of retinal disparity, identified as "near cells," "far cells," and "zero-disparity cells." Surgical section of the corpus collosum precludes visual stimuli presenting to temporal retinae (near to fixation point) from being processed binocularly in the visual cortex. Experiments in patients have confirmed a loss of disparity perception and a loss of convergence under such conditions.[138,204]

Higher visual cortices also may be important in the perception of disparity and the initiation of vergence eye movements. Electrical stimulation of Brodmann areas 19 and 22 in the occipital cortex of anesthetized monkeys produces different combinations of components of the near triad.[101] Light insensitive neurons within area 7 of the parietal cortex of monkeys are activated

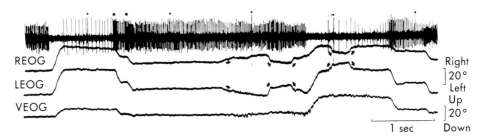

FIG. 5-100 Interneurons within the abducens nucleus modulate to conjugate but not to vergence eye movements. All conjugate eye movements are associated with changes in interneuron firing *(top track)*. No changes occur during divergence *(outward curved arrows)* or convergence *(inward curved arrows)* eye movement. Compare versional *(filled circles)* and vergence movements *(unfilled circles)* of equal magnitude. Antidromic activation by stimulating medial rectus muscle *(intervals between stars)* did not affect interneuron behavior. REOG, LEOG, VEOG: right, left, and vertical electro-oculogram. (From Delgado-Garcia J, Baker R, Highstein SM: The activity of internuclear neurons identified within the abducens nucleus of the alert cat, in Baker R, Berthoz A, eds: Control of gaze by brain stem neurons, Amsterdam, Elsevier/North-Holland Biomedical Press, 1977, p 297.)

FIG. 5-101 Instantaneous firing rate of a tonic neuron related to the convergence cycle of the eyes. Records of right horizontal (RH), left horizontal (LH), and vertical (V) eye positions are shown along with average horizontal eye position (AVE). The difference between left and right horizontal eye positions (DIFF) is a measure of convergence angle. Presentations of far target (FT, 83 cm distant) and near target (NT, 19 cm) are shown at top. Upward deflections represent rightward movements for RH, LH, and AVE, upward movement for V, and increased convergence for DIFF. (From Mays LE: Neurophysiological correlates of vergence eye movements, in Schor CM, Ciuffreda KJ, eds: Vergence eye movements: basic and clinical aspects, Stoneham, MA, Butterworth, 1983.)

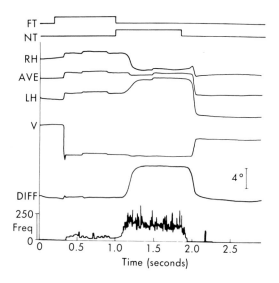

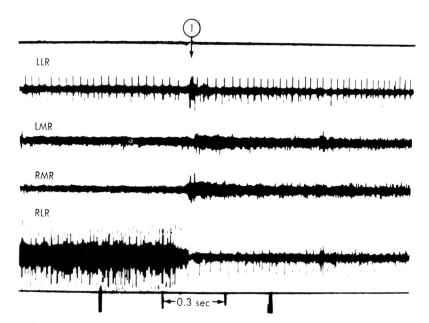

FIG. 5-102 *Arrow 1,* Uncover of exotropic right eye, followed by convergence refusion of 40Δ of intermittent exotropia. It clearly shows both reciprocity of moving eye and maintained contraction of fixing eye. Note fixation disengagement of fixing left eye in this brief but "powerful" refusion vergence. Electromyogram clearly shows all details of refusion in intermittent exotropia. (From Jampolsky A: Coordination of extraocular muscles; clinical aspects, in Lennerstrand G, Bach-y-Rita P, eds: Basic mechanisms of ocular motility and their clinical implications, Oxford, Pergamon Press, 1975, p 209.)

during visual tracking of targets moving in the sagittal plane.[140]

Physiologic substrate of vergence eye movements

Motor physiology. After a stimulus for convergence, there is a short latent period followed by a gradual increase in the activity of the medial rectus muscle, which reaches a maximum and then gradually declines. The lateral rectus shows reciprocity throughout the movement.[137] These relationships can be shown electromyographically (Fig. 5-102).

Electromyographic activity suggests two

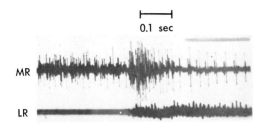

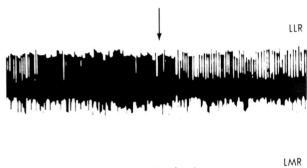

FIG. 5-103   Divergence from 20 degrees. (From Miller JE: Arch Ophthalmol 62:790, 1959.)

FIG. 5-104   Divergence from 25 degrees. (From Miller JE: Arch Ophthalmol 62:790, 1959.)

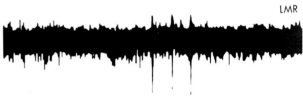

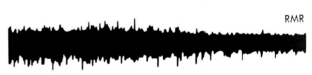

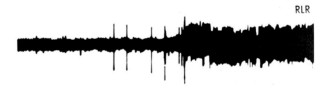

types of divergence. The first type consists of coactivity of the medial and lateral recti with a saccadic burst seen concomitantly in both muscles followed by reciprocal excitation and inhibition of agonist and antagonist (Fig. 5-103). The second type of pattern consists of an immediate saccadic burst of activity in the lateral rectus with concomitant inhibition of the medial rectus followed by irregular activity in both muscles (Fig. 5-104).

Jampolsky[102] has demonstrated a slightly different pattern for divergence associated with exophoria (Fig. 5-105). Occlusion of one eye is associated with a slow increase in activity of the lateral rectus muscle and a decrease in activity of the medial rectus muscle of the covered (deviating) eye. Interestingly, there is a concomitant and parallel decrease in activity of the medial and lateral rectus muscles of the fixating eye.

Sensory physiology. Vergence eye movements may be evoked under binocular conditions, when a visual target does not stimulate corresponding retinal points (see Section Three, Panum's area), creating diplopia. The eye movement caused by this nonalignment of the visual images between the two eyes is called "disparity vergence." Vergence eye movements also may be caused by a blurred image on the retina. This blur stimulates the accommodative mechanism, which is closely coupled to vergence by means of the near triad. This second major cause of vergence is *accommodative vergence.* Under noncontrolled situations, both stimuli to vergence are usually present simultaneously.[216]

Disparity vergence. Disparity alone is a strong and sufficient stimulus for inducing vergence eye movement.[159] Two components of disparity vergence have been identified. An initial component is elicited by retinal image disparities as large as 5 degrees.[103,205] This initial component does not require the presence of like

FIG. 5-105   *Arrow,* Covering right eye in patient with 25Δ of intermittent exotropia. Note the smooth reciprocity of the abducting right eye following the break of fusion. When this movement is free of blink artifact, as it is here, one clearly sees the usual physiologic reciprocity in the moving eye during the break from fusion. Note especially the very clear decrease in the lateral rectus of the fixing left eye *(arrow).* (From Jampolsky A: Coordination of extraocular muscles; clinical aspects, in Lennerstrand G, Bach-y-Rita P, eds: Basic mechanisms of ocular motility and their clinical implications, Oxford, Pergamon Press, 1975, p 209.)

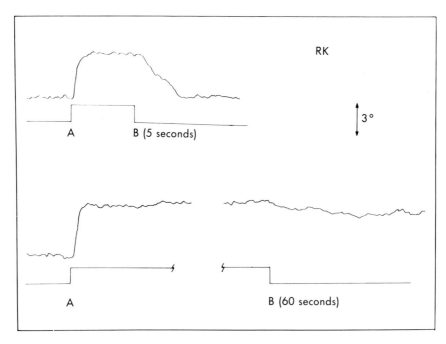

FIG. 5-106 Disparity-induced vergence showing time constants for relaxation of fusional vergence after stimulating convergence for 5 seconds *(upper trace)*. **A**, Onset of stimulation; **B**, occlusion of one eye. Incomplete relaxation of convergence after long-term stimulation of convergence demonstrates vergence adaptation *(lower trace)*. (Reprinted with permission from Lennerstrand G, Zee DS, Keller EL, eds: Functional basis of ocular motility disorders, Oxford, Pergamon Press, copyright 1982.)

stimuli. The final component, the so-called *fusional* component of disparity vergence, requires the retinal images presented to each eye to be similar and the amount of disparity to be small.[180] Fusional vergence typically has a response time of less than 1 second.[158] Vergence also may be stimulated voluntarily. Under such conditions the amplitude of the movement may be very large (up to 24 degrees) with correspondingly high peak velocities.[49,62]

Vergence movements of the fusional type are subject to long-term adaptation. After brief periods of disparity stimulation, the convergence decays with a time constant of 10 seconds,[111,120] whereas after longer periods of stimulation, the decay is greatly prolonged[79,179] (Fig. 5-106).

Accommodative vergence and its interactions with disparity vergence. As already described, the presence of a blurred image on the retina stimulates a vergence eye movement.[3,5,149,190,194] The interaction of disparity and accommodative components can be explored using a pinhole pupil that reduces blur and comparing the results to the normal accommodative mechanisms that reduce blur.[182,183] Under such conditions overaccommodation due to disparity induced

changes in the accommodative state can be identified.

COMPLEX OCULOMOTOR BEHAVIOR

In an unrestricted environment various patterns of eye movements are used to obtain and process visual information. Study of these complex oculomotor behaviors has revealed a consistency that stereotypes the eye movements associated with fixation, reading, and free visual search.

Fixation. Holding steady fixation on a visual target is not associated with lack of eye movement (Fig. 5-107). Indeed, stabilization of targets on the retina results in fading of the visual image.[209] Therefore it is not surprising that detailed oculographic recordings have demonstrated three characteristic eye movements that occur during fixation: microsaccades, drift, and high frequency tremor[209] (Fig. 5-108). Microsaccades, aside from having smaller amplitude than refixation saccades, are otherwise similar, sharing the same peak velocity-amplitude relationship.[217] These small movements, occurring 2 to 3 times per second, along with a slow drift, prevent fading of the retinal image.[174] Slow drift

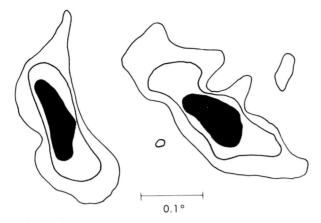

FIG. 5-107 Two typical spatial distributions of fixation dwell times. Contours define areas within which point of fixation was to be found 25%, 50%, 75%, and 100% of the time, in centrifugal order. (From Carpenter RHS: Movements of the eyes, London, Pion, 1977.)

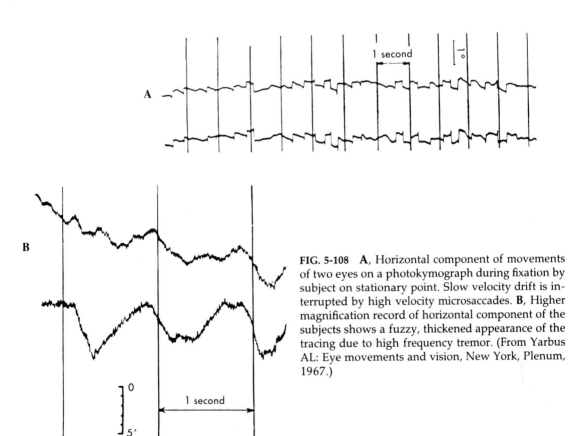

FIG. 5-108 A, Horizontal component of movements of two eyes on a photokymograph during fixation by subject on stationary point. Slow velocity drift is interrupted by high velocity microsaccades. B, Higher magnification record of horizontal component of the subjects shows a fuzzy, thickened appearance of the tracing due to high frequency tremor. (From Yarbus AL: Eye movements and vision, New York, Plenum, 1967.)

has a velocity of about 1 min/sec and amplitude about 2 to 5 min.[53] High frequency tremor (about 90 Hz)[58,59,173] is of very small amplitude (up to 40 sec of arc).[52,160,206] The exact etiology and function of tremor are unknown. The manner in which microsaccades and drifts are interposed is evidently dependent upon both attentional and perceptual factors.[12,60,192]

Reading. Eye movement recordings of reading behavior demonstrate a highly stereotyped "staircase" pattern of eye movements, consisting of alternating saccades and periods of fixation (about 100 to 500 msec each). During the pauses, semantic identification is thought to occur.[2] Each saccade moves the fovea about eight characters to the right. At the end of a line, a large saccade to the beginning of the next line occurs, and the behavior is repeated[162] (Fig. 5-109).

Free visual search. The scanpaths involved in "free" visual search are highly task dependent.[142,209] In examining complex stimuli the eye

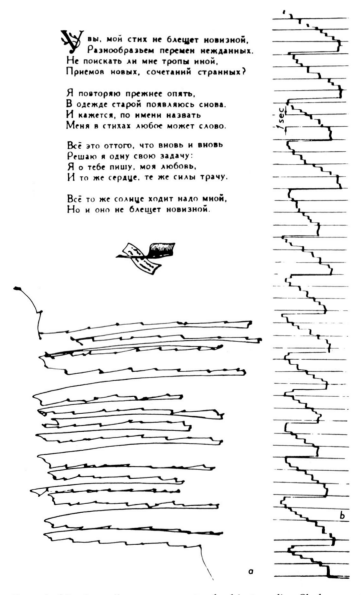

FIG. 5-109 Record of "staircase" eye movements of subject reading Shakespeare sonnet (in Russian). Record on stationary photosensitive paper (a) and on moving phototape of a photokymograph (b). (From Yarbus AL: Eye movements and vision, New York, Plenum, 1967.)

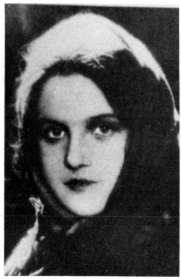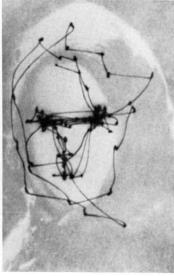

FIG. 5-110   Photograph of a girl's face. Record of eye movements during free examination of photograph with both eyes for 1 minute. Much of the image is not examined with fovea. (From Yarbus AL: Eye movements and vision, New York, Plenum, 1967.)

foveates longest on elements with relevant information, whereas many elements never are viewed foveally[209] (Fig. 5-110). One possible strategy for visual search emphasizes stereotyped oculomotor behavior.[143] Stark and Ellis[189] proposed that "habitually preferred" patterns are the initial step in visual search—"look without seeing." These authors suggested that an internal model then is formed—"see without looking." Finally, there is model verification—"look and see"—that requires foveation of salient features.

Other proposed search strategies use peripheral vision to "edit" sampling choices.[6,89,125] Nodine and colleagues[141] concluded that "survey-sampling" is responsible for identifying target areas, after which "examination-type sampling" occurs based upon cues. When close scrutiny is required in regions of "high visual noise," Mackworth[124] proposed that peripheral scanning is replaced by "tunnel vision," requiring extended periods of foveation.

REFERENCES

1. Abrahams VC: Proprioceptive influences from eye muscle receptors on cells of the superior colliculus, Prog Brain Res 50:325, 1979.
2. Abrams SG, Zuber BL: Some temporal characteristics of information processing during reading, Reading Res Q 8:40, 1972.
3. Allen MJ: The stimulus to accommodation, Am J Optom 32:422, 1955.
4. Anderson RA, Siegel RM, Essick GK, et al: Subdivision of the inferior parietal lobule and dorsal prelunate gyrus of macaque by connectional and functional criteria, Invest Ophthalmol Vis Sci 26 (Suppl):266, 1985.
5. Antes JR: The time course of picture viewing, J Exp Psychol 103:62, 1974.
6. Azzena GB, Desole C, Palmieri G: Cerebellar projections of the masticatory and extraocular muscle proprioception, Exp Neurol 27:151, 1970.
7. Bahill, AT, Adler D, Stark L: Most naturally occurring human saccades have magnitudes of 15 degrees or less, Invest Ophthalmol Vis Sci 14:468, 1975.
8. Bahill AT, Clark MR, Stark L: The main sequence, a tool for studying human eye movements, Math Biosci 24:191, 1975.
9. Bahill AT, Stark L: The trajectories of saccadic eye movements, Sci Am 240:108, 1979.
10. Baker R, Precht W, Llinas R: Mossy and climbing fiber projections of extraocular muscle afferents to the cerebellum, Brain Res 38:440, 1972.
11. Baloh RW, Yee RD, Honrubia V: Clinical abnormalities of optokinetic nystagmus, in Lennerstrand G, Zee DS, Keller EL, eds: Functional basis of ocular motility disorders, Oxford, Pergamon Press, 1982, p 311.
12. Barlow HB: Eye movements during fixation, J Physiol (Lond) 116:290, 1952.
13. Barlow HB, Blakemore C, Pettigrew JD: The neural mechanism of binocular depth discrimination, J Physiol (Lond) 193:327, 1967.
14. Barmack NH: Saccadic discharges evoked by intra-cellular stimulation of extraocular motoneurons, J Neurophysiol 37:395, 1974.
15. Bartlett JR, Doty RW Sr: Response of units in striate cortex of squirrel monkeys to visual and electrical stimuli, J Neurophysiol 37:621, 1974.

16. Batini C: Extraocular muscle input to the cerebellar cortex, Prog Brain Res SO:315, 1979.

17. Batini C, Horcholle-Bossavit G: Extraocular muscle afferents and visual input interactions in the superior colliculus of the cat, Prog Brain Res 50:335, 1979

18. Becker W, Fuchs AF: Predictive mechanisms in human smooth pursuit movement, in Roucoux A, Crommelinck M, eds.: Physiologic and pathological aspects of eye movements. The Hague: Dr W Junk, Publishers, 1982, p 33.

19. Beckstead RM: Long collateral branches of substantia nigra pars reticulata axons to thalamus, superior colliculus and reticular formation in monkey and cat; multiple retrograde neuronal labeling with fluorescent dyes, Neuroscience 10:767, 1983.

20. Bennet-Clark HC: The oculomotor response to small target replacement, Opt Acta 11:301, 1964.

21. Bizzi E: Discharge of frontal eye field neurons during saccadic and following eye movements in unanesthetized monkeys, Exp Brain Res 6:69, 1968.

22. Bizzi E, Schiller PH: Single unit activity in the frontal eye fields of unanesthetized monkeys during eye and head movement, Exp Brain Res 10:151, 1970.

23. Bruce CJ, Goldberg ME: Primate frontal eye fields, I, Single neurons discharging before saccades, J Neurophysiol 53:603, 1985.

24. Buettner-Ennever JA: Pathways from the pontine reticular formation to structures controlling horizontal and vertical eye movements in the monkey, Dev Neurosci 1:89, 1977.

25. Buettner-Ennever JA: Organization of reticular projections onto oculomotor neurons, Prog Brain Res 50:619, 1979.

26. Buettner-Ennever JA, Akert K: Medial rectus subgroups of the oculomotor nucleus and their abducens internuclear input in the monkey, J Comp Neurol 197:17, 1981.

27. Buettner-Ennever JA, Büttner U, Cohen B, et al: Vertical gaze paralysis and the rostral interstitial nucleus of the medial longitudinal fasciculus, Brain 105:125, 1982.

28. Buettner-Ennever JA, Henn V: An autoradiographic study of the pathways from the pontine reticular formation involved in horizontal eye movements, Brain Res 108:155, 1976.

29. Buettner-Ennever, JA, Lang W: Connections of a vertical eye movement are in the rostral mesencephalic tegmentum of the monkey, Soc Neurosci Abstracts 4:161, 1978.

30. Buisseret P: Does extraocular proprioception influence the development of visual processes and the oculomotor system? Prog Brain Res 50:345, 1979.

31. Buisseret P, Maffei L: Extraocular proprioceptive projections to the visual cortex, Exp Brain Res 28:421, 1977.

32. Bushnell MC, Goldberg ME, Robinson DL: Behavioral enhancement of visual responses in monkey cerebral cortex, 1, Modulation in posterior parietal cortex related to selective visual attention, J Neurophysiol 46:755, 1981.

33. Büttner, U: The role of the cerebellum in smooth pursuit eye movements and optokinetic nystagmus in primates, Rev Neurol (Paris) 145:560, 1989.

34. Cannon SC, Robinson DA: The final common integrator is in the prepositus and vestibular nuclei, in Keller EL, Zee DS, eds: Adaptive processes in visual and oculomotor systems, Adv Biosci, vol 57, Oxford, Pergamon Press, 1986, p 307.

35. Cannon SC, Robinson DA: Loss of the neural integrator of the oculomotor system from brain stem lesions in monkey, J Neurophysiol 57:1383, 1987.

36. Carpenter MB, Nova HR: Descending division of the brachium conjunctivum in the cat: a cerebello-reticular system, J Comp Neurol 114:295, 1960.

37. Carpenter MB, Stringer NL: Cerebello-oculomotor fibers in the rhesus monkey, J Comp Neurol 123:211, 1964.

38. Carpenter RHS: Movements of the eyes, London, Pion, Ltd, 1977.

39. Chevalier G, Thierry AM, Shibazaki T, et al: Evidence for a GABAergic inhibitory nigrotectal pathway in the rat, Neuroscience Lett 21:67, 1981.

40. Cochran SL, Precht W: Electrophysiological characterization of the basal optic region in the anuran, Proc Int Union Physiol Sci 14:1100, 1980.

41. Cogan DG: Neurology of the ocular muscles, Springfield, IL, Charles C Thomas, Publisher, 1956.

42. Cohen B, Goto K, Shanzer S, et al: Eye movements induced by electrical stimulation of the cerebellum in the alert cat, Exp Neurol 13:145, 1965.

43. Cohen B, Henn V: Unit activity in the pontine reticular formation associated with eye movements, Brain Res 46:403, 1972.

44. Cohen D: The vestibulo-ocular reflex arc, in Kornhuber HH, ed: Handbook of sensory physiology, vol 6, part 1: Vestibular system, Berlin, Springer-Verlag, 1974, p 477.

45. Collewijn H: Direction-selective units in the rabbit's nucleus of the optic tract, Brain Res 100:489, 1975a.

46. Collewijn H: Oculomotor areas in the rabbit's midbrain and pretectum, J Neurobiol 6:3, 1975b.

47. Collewijn H, Conijn P, Tammingar EP: Eye-head coordination in man during the pursuit of moving targets, in Lennerstrand G, Zee DS, Keller EL, eds: Functional basis of ocular motility disorders, Oxford, Pergamon Press, 1982, p 369.

48. Collins CC: The human oculomotor control system, in Lennerstrand G, Bach-y-Rita P, eds: Basic mechanisms of ocular motility and their clinical implications, Oxford, Pergamon Press, 1975, p 145.

49. Crane HD: Binocular motor adjustments for far and near vision, Opt Soc Am Annual Meeting, Oct-Nov 1978, p 1359.

50. Delgado-Garcia J, Baker R, Highstein SM: The activity of internuclear neurons identified within the abducens nucleus of the alert cat, Dev Neurosci 1:291, 1977.

51. Dichgans J: Spinal afferences to the oculomotor system: physiological and clinical aspects, in Lennerstrand G, Bach-y-Rita, P, eds: Basic mechanisms of ocular motility and their clinical implications, Oxford, Pergamon Press, 1975, p 299.

52. Ditchburn RW: Eye movements in relation to retinal action, Opt Acta 1:171, 1955.

53. Ditchburn RW: Eye movements and visual perception, Oxford, Clarendon Press, 1973.

54. Dodge R: Five types of eye movement in the horizontal

meridian plane of the field of regard, Am J Physiol 8:307, 1903.

55. Donaldson IML, Dixon RA: Excitation of units in the lateral geniculate and contiguous nuclei of the cat by stretch of extrinsic ocular muscles, Exp Brain Res 38:245, 1980.

56. Donaldson IML, Long AC: Interactions between extraocular proprioceptive and visual signals in the superior colliculus of the cat, J Physiol (Lond) 298:85, 1980.

57. Eckmiller R, Mackeben M: Pursuit eye movements and their neural control in the monkey, Pflugers Arch 377:15, 1978.

58. Fender DH, Nye PW: An investigation of the mechanisms of eye movement control, Kybernetik 1:81, 1962.

59. Findlay JM: Frequency analysis of human involuntary movement, Kybernetik 8:207, 1971.

60. Fiorentini A, Ercoles AM: Involuntary eye movements during attempted mononuclear fixation, Atti Fond Giorgio Ronchi 21:199, 1966.

61. Flourens P: Récherches experimentales sur les propriétés et les fonctions du systeme nerveux dans les animaux vertebres, 2nd ed, Paris, JB Baillière, 1842, p 516.

62. Foley JM, Richards W: Effects of voluntary eye movements and convergence on the binocular appreciation of depth, Percept Psychophys 11:423, 1972.

63. Fox PT, Fox JM, Raichle ME, et al: The role of cerebral cortex in the generation of voluntary saccades: a positron emission tomographic study, J Neurophysiol 54:348, 1985.

64. Francois C, Percheron G, Yelnik J: Localization of nigrostriatal, nigrothalamic and nigrotectal neurons in ventricular coordinates in macaques, Neuroscience 13:61, 1984.

65. Fuchs AF, Kornhuber HH: Extraocular muscle afferents to the cerebellum of the cat, J Physiol (Lond) 200:713, 1969.

66. Fuchs AF, Luschei ES: Firing patterns of abducens neurons of alert monkeys in relationship to horizontal eye movement, J Neurophysiol 33:382, 1970.

67. Fuchs AF, Luschei ES: The activity of single trochlear nerve fibers during eye movements in the alert monkey, Exp Brain Res 13:78, 1971.

68. Goebel HH, et al: Lesions of the pontine tegmentum and conjugate gaze paralysis, Arch Neurol 24:431, 1971.

69. Goldberg ME, Segraves MA: The visual and frontal cortices, in Wurtz RH, Goldberg ME, eds: The neurobiology of saccadic eye movements, Amsterdam, Elsevier Science Publishers, 1989, p 283.

70. Goldberg SJ, Lennerstrand G, Hull CD: Motor unit responses in the lateral rectus muscle of the cat: intracellular current injection of abducens nucleus neurons, Acta Physiol Scand 96:58, 1976.

71. Gonshor A, Melvill Jones G: Plasticity in the adult human vestibulo-ocular reflex arc, Proc Can Fed Biol Soc 14:11, 1971.

72. Gonshor A, Melvill Jones G: Changes of human vestibulo-ocular response induced by vision-reversal during head rotation, J Physiol (Lond) 234:102P, 1973.

73. Granit R: The probable role of muscle spindles and tendon organs in eye movement control, in Bach-y-

Rita P, Collins CC, eds: The control of eye movements, New York, Academic Press, 1971, p 3.

74. Graybiel AM, Hartwieg EA: Some afferent connections of the oculomotor complex in the cat: an experimental study with tracer techniques, Brain Res 81:543, 1974.

75. Guitton D, Buchtel HA, Douglas RM: Disturbances of voluntary saccadic eye movement mechanisms following discrete unilateral frontal lobe removals, in Lennerstrand G, Zee DS, Keller EL, eds: Functional basis of ocular motility disorders, Oxford, Pergamon Press, 1982, p 497.

76. Guthrie BL, Porter JD, Sparks DL: Corollary discharge provides accurate eye position information to the oculomotor system, Science 221:1193, 1983.

77. Henn, V, Cohen B: Quantitative analysis of activity in eye muscle motoneurons during saccadic eye movements and positions of fixation, J Neurophysiol 36:115, 1973.

78. Henn V, Cohen B: Activity in eye muscle motoneurons and brainstem units during eye movements, in Lennerstrand G, Bach-y-Rita P, eds: Basic mechanisms of ocular motility and their clinical implications, Oxford, Pergamon Press, 1975, p 303.

79. Henson DB, North R: Adaptation to prism-induced heterophoria, Am J Opt Physiol Optics 57:129, 1980.

80. Hepp K, Henn V: Physiology of horizontal gaze, in Lennerstrand G, Zee DS, Keller EL, eds: Functional basis of ocular motility disorders, Oxford, Pergamon Press, 1982, p 247.

81. Hepp K, Henn V, Vilis T, et al: Brainstem regions related to saccade generation, in Wurtz RH, Goldberg ME, eds: The neurobiology of saccadic eye movements, Amsterdam, Elsevier Science Publishers, 1989, p 105.

82. Hering E: Die Lehre über binokularen Sehen, Leipzig, Engelman, 1868.

83. Hering E: Der Raumsinn und die Bewegungen der Auges, in Ludimar H: Handbuch der Physiologie, vol 3, part 1, 1879, English translation by Radde CA, Baltimore, American Academy of Optometry, 1942.

84. Highstein SM, Baker R: Termination of internuclear neurons of the abducens nuclei on medial rectus motoneurons, Neurosci Soc Abstracts 2:278, 1976.

85. Hikosaka O, Maeda M: Cervical effects on abducens motoneurons and their interaction with vestibuloocular reflex, Exp Brain Res 18:512, 1973.

86. Hikosaka O, Wurtz RH: Visual and oculomotor functions of monkey substantia nigra pars reticulata, I, Relation of substantia nigra to superior colliculus, J Neurophysiol 49 (5):1230, 1983a.

87. Hikosaka O, Wurtz RH: Visual and oculomotor functions of monkey substantia nigra pars reticulata, III, Memory-contingent visual and saccade responses, J Neurophysiol 49 (5):1268, 1983b.

88. Hikosaka O, Wurtz RH: The basal ganglia, in Wurtz RH, Goldberg ME, eds: The neurobiology of saccadic eye movements, Amsterdam, Elsevier Science Publishers, 1989, p 257.

89. Hochberg, J: In the mind's eye, in Haber RN, ed: Contemporary theory and research in visual perception, New York, Holt, Rinehart, & Winston, 1968.

90. Hoffman KP, Schoppmann A: Retinal input to direc-

tion selective cells in the nucleus tractus opticus of the cat, Brain Res 99:359, 1975.

91. Honrubia V, Downey WL, Mitchell DP, et al: Experimental studies on optokinetic nystagmus, II, Normal humans, Acta Otolaryngol 65:441, 1968.

92. Honrubia V, Scott BJ, Ward, PH: Experimental studies on optokinetic nystagmus, 1, Normal cats, Acta Otolaryngol 64:388, 1967.

93. Hood JD: Observations upon the neurological mechanism of optokinetic nystagmus with especial reference to the contribution of peripheral vision, Acta Otolaryngol 63:208, 1967.

94. Hood, JD: Observations upon the role of the peripheral retina in the execution of eye movements, OtoRhino-Laryngology 37:65, 1975.

95. Hood JD, Leech J: The significance of peripheral vision in the perception of movement, Acta Otolaryngol 77:72, 1974.

96. Hoyt WF, Daroff RB: Supranuclear disorders of ocular control systems in man: clinical, anatomical, and physiological correlations, in Bach-y-Rita P, Collins CC, eds: The control of eye movements, New York, Academic Press, 1971, p 175.

97. Hubel DH, Wiesel TN: Receptive fields, binocular interaction and functional architecture in the cat's visual cortex, J Physiol (Lond) 160:106, 1962.

98. Hubel DH, Wiesel TN: Receptive fields and functional architecture of monkey striate cortex, J Physiol (Lond) 195:215, 1968.

99. Ito M, Nisimaru N, Yamamoto M: Pathways for the vestibulo-ocular reflex excitation arising from semicircular canals of rabbits, Exp Brain Res 24:257, 1976a.

100. Ito M, Nisimaru N, Yamamoto M: Postsynaptic inhibition of oculomotor neurons involved in vestibulo-ocular reflexes arising from semicircular canals of rabbits, Exp Brain Res 24:273, 1976b.

101. Jampel RS: Convergence, divergence, pupillary reactions and accommodations of the eyes from faradic stimulation of the macaque brain, J Comp Neurol 115:371, 1960.

102. Jampolsky A: Coordination of extraocular muscles: clinical aspects, in Lennerstrand G, Bach-y-Rita P, eds: Basic mechanisms of ocular motility and their clinical implications, Oxford, Pergamon Press, 1975, p 209.

103. Jones R, Kerr KE: Motor responses to conflicting asymmetrical vergence stimulus information, Am J Opt Arch Am Acad Opt 48:989, 1971.

104. Keller EL: Accommodative vergence in the alert monkey: motor unit analysis, Vision Res 13:1565, 1973.

105. Keller EL: Participation of medial pontine reticular formation in eye movement generation in monkey, J Neurophysiol 37:316, 1974.

106. Keller EL: The role of the brain stem reticular formation in eye movement control, in Brooks BA, Bajandas FJ, eds: Eye movements, New York, Plenum Press, 1977, p 105.

107. Keller, EL, Robinson DA: Absence of a stretch reflex in extraocular muscles of the monkey, J Neurophysiol 34:908, 1971.

108. Keller EL, Robinson DA: Abducens unit behavior in the monkey during vergence movements, Vision Res 12:369, 1972.

109. Kennard C, Lueck CJ: Oculomotor abnormalities in diseases of the basal ganglia, Rev Neurol (Paris) 145:587, 1989.

110. King WM, Precht W, Dieringer N: Connections of behaviorally identified cat omnipause neurons, Exp Brain Res 32:435, 1978.

111. Krishnan VV, Stark L: A heuristic model for the human vergence eye movement system, IEEE Trans Biomed Eng 24:44, 1977.

112. Kunzle H, Akert K: Efferent connections of cortical area 8 (frontal eye field) in *Macaca fascicularis:* a reinvestigation using the autoradiographic technique, J Comp Neurol 173:147, 1977.

113. Leichnetz GR: The prefrontal cortico-oculomotor trajectories in the monkey: a possible explanation for the effects of stimulation lesion experiments on eye movements, J Neurol Sci 49:387, 1981.

114. Leigh RJ, Zee DS: The neurology of eye movements, Philadelphia, FA Davis, 1983, p 69.

115. Lestienne F, Whittington DA, Bizzi E: Single cell recording from the pontine reticular formation in monkey: behavior of preoculomotor neurons during eye-head coordination, in Fuchs AF, Becker W, eds: Progress in oculomotor research, New York, Elsevier/North Holland, 1981, p 325.

116. Llinas R, Precht W, Clark M: Cerebellar Purkinje cell responses to physiological stimulation of the vestibular system of the frog, Exp Brain Res 13:408, 1971.

117. Llinas R, Wolfe JW: Functional linkage between the electrical activity in the vermal cerebellar cortex and saccadic eye movements, Exp Brain Res 29:1, 1977.

118. Lopez-Barneo J, Darlot C, Berthoz A, et al: Neuronal activity in prepositus nucleus correlated with eye movement in the alert cat, J Neurophysiol 47:329, 1982.

119. Lorente de No R: Vestibulo-ocular reflex arc, Arch Neurol Psychiatry 30:245, 1933.

120. Ludvigh E, McKinnon P, Zaitzeff L: Temporal course of the relaxation of binocular duction (fusion) movements, Arch Ophthalmol 71:389, 1964.

121. Luschei ES, Fuchs AF: Activity of brain stem neurons during eye movements of alert monkey, J Neurophysiol 35:445, 1972.

122. Lynch JC, McLaren JW: The contribution of parieto-occipital association cortex to the control of slow eye movements, in Lennerstrand G, Zee DS, Keller EL, eds: Functional basis of ocular motility disorders, Oxford, Pergamon Press, 1982, p 501.

123. Maciewicz RJ, Spencer RF: Oculomotor and abducens internuclear pathways in the cat, Dev Neurosci 1:99, 1977.

124. Mackworth NH: Visual noise causes tunnel vision, Psychonic Sci 3:67, 1965.

125. Mackworth N, Morandi AJ: The gaze selects informative details within pictures, Perception Psychophys 2:547, 1967.

126. Maekawa K, Kimura M: Mossy fiber projections to the cerebellar flocculus from the extraocular muscle afferents, Brain Res 191:313, 1980.

127. Maffei L, Fiorentini A: Oculomotor proprioception in the cat, Dev Neurosci 1:477, 1977.

128. Manni E, Pettorossi VE: Somatotopic organization of the eye muscle efferents in the semilunar ganglion, Arch Ital Biol 114:178, 1976.

129. Marini R, Bortolami R: Somatotopic organization of second order neurons of the eye muscle proprioception, Arch Ital Biol 117:45, 1979.

130. Marini R, Bortolami R: Somatotopic representation of eye muscle proprioception within the superior colliculus of the lamb, Exp Neurol 69:226, 1980.

131. Mays LE: Neurophysiological correlates of vergence eye movements, in Schor CM, Ciuffreda KJ, eds: Vergence eye movements: basic and clinical aspects, Woburn MA, Butterworth, 1983, pp 649-670.

132. McElligott JG: Purkinje cell activity in the vermal cerebellum of the cat during trained saccadic eye movements and fixations, Soc Neurosci Abstracts 5:104, 1979.

133. McElligott JG, Keller EL: Neuronal discharge in the posterior cerebellum: its relationship to saccadic eye movement generation, in Lennerstrand G, Zee DS, Keller EL, eds: Functional basis of ocular motility disorders, Oxford, Pergamon Press, 1982, p 453.

134. McNeer KW, Spencer RF: The histopathology of human strabismic extraocular muscle, in Lennerstrand G, Zee DS, Keller EL, eds: Functional basis of ocular motility disorders, Oxford, Pergamon Press, 1982, p 27.

135. Melvill Jones G, Gonshor A: Extreme vestibular habituation to long-term reversal of vision during natural head movements, Proceedings of Aerospace Medicine Association Annual Scientific Meeting, Bal Harbour, FL, 1972, p 22.

136. Melvill Jones G, Gonshor A: Goal-directed flexibility in the vestibulo-ocular reflex arc, in Lennerstrand G, Bach-y-Rita P, eds: Basic mechanisms of ocular motility and their clinical implications, Oxford, Pergamon Press, 1975, p 227.

137. Miller JE: The electromyography of vergence movement, Arch Ophthalmol 62:790, 1959.

138. Mitchell DE, Blakemore C: Binocular depth perception and the corpus callosum, Vision Res 10:49, 1970.

139. Montarolo PG, Precht W, Strata P: Functional organization of the mechanisms subserving the optokinetic nystagmus in the cat, Neuroscience 6:231, 1981.

140. Motter BC, Mountcastle VB: The functional properties of the light-sensitive neurons of the posterior parietal cortex studied in waking monkeys: foveal sparing and opponent vector organization, J Neurosci 1:3, 1981.

141. Nodine CF, Carmody DP, Kundel HL: Searching for Nina, in Senders JW, Fisher DF, Monty RA, eds: Eye movements and the higher psychological functions, Hillsdale, NJ, Lawrence Erlbaum Associates, 1978, p 241.

142. Norton D, Stark, L: Scanpaths in saccadic eye movements while viewing and recognizing patterns, Vision Res 11:929, 1971.

143. Ochs AL, et al.: Opposed adducting saccades in convergence-retraction nystagmus, Brain 102:497, 1979.

144. Optican LM, Robinson DA: Cerebellar-dependent adaptive control of primate saccadic system, J Neurophysiol 44:1058, 1980.

145. Optican LM, et al: Oculomotor deficit in monkeys with flocculus lesions, Soc Neurosci Abstracts 6:474, 1980.

146. Oyster CW, et al: Retinal ganglion cells projecting to the rabbit accessory optic system, J Comp Neurol 190:49, 1980.

147. Oyster CW, Takahashi E, Collewijn H: Direction-selective retinal ganglion cells and control of optokinetic nystagmus in the rabbit, Vision Res 12:183, 1972.

148. Pettorossi VE, Filippi GM: Muscle spindle autogenetic inhibition in the extraocular muscles of the lamb, Arch Ital Biol 119:179, 1981.

149. Phillips S, Stark L: Blur: a sufficient accommodative stimulus, Doc Ophthalmol 43:65, 1977.

150. Pierrot-Deseilligny C: Circuits oculomoteurs centraux, Rev Neurol (Paris) 141:349, 1985.

151. Poggio GF, Fischer B: Binocular interaction and depth sensitivity in striate and prestriate cortex of behaving rhesus monkey, J Neurophysiol 40:1392, 1977.

152. Precht W: Cerebellar influences on eye movements, in Lennerstrand G, Bach-y-Rita P, eds: Basic mechanisms of ocular motility and their clinical implications, Oxford, Pergamon Press, 1975, p 261.

153. Precht W: The functional synaptology of brainstem oculomotor pathways, Dev Neurosci 1:131, 1977.

154. Precht W: Anatomical and functional organization of optokinetic pathways, in Lennerstrand G, Zee DS, Keller EL, eds: Functional basis of ocular motility disorders, Oxford, Pergamon Press, 1982, p 291.

155. Precht W, Strata P: On the pathway mediating optokinetic responses in vestibular nuclear neurons, Neuroscience 5:777, 1980.

156. Rahn AC, Zuber BL: Cerebellar evoked potentials resulting from extraocular muscle stretch: evidence against a cerebellar origin, Exp Neurol 31:230, 1971.

157. Rashbass C: The relationship between saccadic and smooth tracking eye movements, J Physiol (Lond) 159:326, 1961a.

158. Rashbass C, Westheimer G: Disjunctive eye movements, J Physiol (Lond) 159:339, 1961b.

159. Rashbass C, Westheimer G: Independence of conjugate and disjunctive eye movements, J Physiol (Lond) 159:361, 1961c.

160. Ratliff FA, Riggs LA: Involuntary motions of the eye during monocular fixation, J Exp Psychol 40:687, 1950.

161. Raybourn MS, Keller EL: Colliculoreticular organization in primate oculomotor system, J Neurophysiol 40:861, 1977.

162. Rayner K: Eye movements in reading and information processing, Psych Bull 85:618, 1978.

163. Ritchie L: Effects of cerebellar lesions on saccadic eye movements, J Neurophysiol 39:1246, 1976.

164. Robinson DA: The mechanics of human smooth pursuit eye movement, J Physiol (Lond) 180:569, 1965.

165. Robinson DA: Oculomotor unit behavior in the monkey, J Neurophysiol 33:393, 1970.

166. Robinson DA: Eye movements evoked by collicular stimulation in the alert monkey, Vision Res 12:1795, 1972.

167. Robinson DA: The effect of cerebellectomy on the cat's vestibulo-ocular integrator, Brain Res 71:195, 1974.

168. Robinson DA: Oculomotor control signals, in Lennerstrand G, Bach-y-Rita P, eds: Basic mechanisms of ocular motility and their clinical implications, Oxford, Pergamon Press, 1975, p 337.

169. Robinson DA: A model of cancellation of the vestibulo-ocular reflex, in Lennerstrand G, Zee DS, Keller EL, eds: Functional basis of ocular motility disorders, Oxford, Pergamon Press, 1982, p 5.

170. Robinson DA, Keller EL: The behavior of eye movement motoneurons in the alert monkey, Bibl Ophthalmol 82:7, 1972.

171. Ron S, Robinson DA: Eye movements evoked by cerebellar stimulation in the alert monkey, J Neurophysiol 36:1004, 1973.

172. Sacks JG: The shape of the trochlea, Arch Ophthalmol 102(69):933, 1984.

173. St Cyr GJ: Signal and noise in the human oculomotor system, Vision Res 13:1979, 1973.

174. St Cyr GJ, Fender DH: The interplay of drifts and flicks in binocular fixation, Vision Res 9:245, 1969.

175. Sakata H, Shibutani H, Kawano K: Functional properties of visual tracking neurons in posterior parietal association cortex of the monkey, J Neurophysiol 49:1364, 1983.

176. Schiller PH: The discharge characteristics of single units in the oculomotor and abducens nuclei of the unanesthetized monkey, Exp Brain Res 10:347, 1970.

177. Schiller PH, Stryker M: Single-unit recording and stimulation in superior colliculus of the alert rhesus monkey, J Neurophysiol 35:915, 1972.

178. Schiller PH, True SD, Conway JL: Effects of frontal eye field and superior colliculus ablations on eye movements, Science 206:590, 1979.

179. Schor CM: The influence of rapid prism adaptation upon fixation disparity, Vision Res 19:757, 1979.

180. Schor CM: Vergence eye movements: basic aspects, in Lennerstrand G, Zee DS, Keller EL, eds: Functional basis of ocular motility disorders, Oxford, Pergamon Press, 1982, p 83.

181. Scott AB, Collins, C: Division of labor in human extraocular muscle, Arch Opththalmol 90:319, 1973.

182. Semmlow JL: A theory for control of the oculomotor near triad, in Lennerstrand G, Zee DS, Keller EL, eds: Functional basis of ocular motility disorders, Oxford, Pergamon Press, 1982, p 97.

183. Semmlow JL, Hung G: Accommodative and fusional components of fixation disparity, Invest Ophthalmol Vis Sci 18:1082, 1979.

184. Sharpe JA, Lo AW, Rabinovitch HE: Control of the saccadic and smooth pursuit systems after cerebral hemidecortication, Brain 102:387, 1979.

185. Simpson JI, Soodak RE, Hess R: The accessory optic system and its relation to the vestibulocerebellum, Prog Brain Res 50:715, 1979.

186. Skavenski AA: Inflow as a source of extraretinal eye position information, Vision Res 12:221, 1972.

187. Sparks DL, Mays LE, Porter JD: Eye movements induced by pontine stimulation: interaction with visually triggered saccades, J Neurophysiol 58:300, 1987.

188. Spencer RF, Sterling P: An electron microscopic study of motoneurones and interneurones in the cat abducens nucleus identified by retrograde intraaxonal transport of horseradish peroxidase, J Comp Neurol 176:65, 1977.

189. Stark L, Ellis SR: Scanpaths revisited: cognitive models direct active looking, in Fisher DF, Monty RA, Senders JW, eds: Eye movements: cognition and visual perception, Hillsdale, NJ, Lawrence Erlbaum Associates, 1981, p 193.

190. Stark L, Takahashi Y: Absence of odd-error signal mechanism in human accommodation, IEEE Trans Biomed Eng 12:138, 1965.

191. Stein BM, Carpenter MB: Central projections of portions of the vestibular ganglia innervating specific parts of the labyrinth in the rhesus monkey, Am J Anat 120:281, 1967.

192. Steinman RM, et al: Voluntary control of microsaccades during maintained monocular fixation, Science 155:1577, 1967.

193. Szentagothai J: Pathways and synaptic articulation patterns connecting vestibular receptors and oculomotor nuclei, in Bender MD, ed: The oculomotor system, New York, Harper & Row, 1964, pp 203-223.

194. Troelsta A, et al: Accommodative tracking: a trial-and-error function, Vision Res 4:85, 1964.

195. Troost BT, Dell'Osso LF: Fast eye movements (saccades): basic science and clinical correlations, in Thompson HS, et al, eds: Topics in neuro-ophthalmology, Baltimore, Williams & Wilkins, 1979, p 246.

196. Troost BT et al: Hemispheric control of eye movements, 11, Quantitative analysis of smooth pursuit in a hemispherectomy patient, Arch Neurol 27:449, 1972.

197. Tusa RJ, Ungerleider LG: Fiber pathways of cortical areas mediating smooth pursuit eye movements in monkeys, Ann Neurol 23:174, 1988.

198. Van Essen DC: Visual areas of the mammalian cerebral cortex, Annu Rev Neurosci 2:227, 1979.

199. Van Essen DC, Maunsell JHR, Bixby JL: The middle temporal visual area in the macaque: myeloarchitecture, connections, functional properties and topographic organization, J Comp Neurol 199:293, 1981.

200. Vossius G, Warner J: The functional control of the eye-tracking system and its digital stimulation, Congress of the International Federation of Automatic Control, Warsaw.

201. Walley RE: Receptive fields in the accessory optic system of the rabbit, Exp Neurol 17:27, 1967.

202. Warwick R: Representation of the extra-ocular muscles in the oculomotor nuclei of the monkey, J Comp Neurol 98:449, 1953.

203. Waterhouse BD, McElligott JG: Simple spike activity in Purkinje cells in the posterior vermis of awake cats during spontaneous saccadic eye movements, Brain Res Bull 5:159, 1980.

204. Westheimer G, Mitchell AM: Eye movement responses to convergence stimuli, Arch Ophthalmol 55:848, 1956.

205. Westheimer G, Mitchell DE: The sensory stimulus for disjunctive eye movements, Vision Res 9:749, 1969.

206. Wood CC, Spear PD, Braun JJ: Direction-specific deficits in horizontal optokinetic nystagmus following removal of visual cortex in the cat, Brain Res 80:231, 1973.

207. Wurtz, RH, Albano JE: Visual-motor function of the primate superior colliculus, Annu Rev Neurosci 3:189, 1980.

208. Wurtz RH, Newsome WT: Divergent signals encoded by neurons in extrastriate areas MT and MST during smooth pursuit eye movements, Soc Neurosci Abstr 11:1246, 1985.

209. Yarbus AL: Eye movements and vision, New York, Plenum Press, 1967.

210. Young LR: The sampled data model and foveal dead zone for saccades, in Zuber BL, ed: Models of oculomotor behavior and control, Boca Raton, FL: CRC Press, 1981, p 43.

211. Young LR, Stark L: Variable feedback experiments testing a sampled data model for tracking movements, IEEE Trans Human Factors Electron 4:38, 1963.

212. Zangemeister WH, Stark L: Active head rotations and eye-head coordination, in Cohen B, ed: Vestibular and oculomotor physiology, International Meeting of the Barany' Society, Ann NY Acad Sci 374:540, 1981.

213. Zangemeister WH, Stark L: Normal and abnormal gaze types and active head movements, in Lennerstrand G, Zee DS, Keller EL, eds: Functional basis of ocular motility disorders, Oxford, Pergamon Press, 1982, p 407.

214. Zee, DS: The organization of the brainstem ocular motor subnuclei, Ann Neurol 4:384, 1978.

215. Zee DS: Ocular motor abnormalities related to lesions in the vestibulocerebellum in primate, in Lennerstrand G, Zee DS, Keller EL, eds: Functional basis of ocular motility disorders, Oxford, Pergamon Press, 1982, p 423.

216. Zuber BL: Control of vergence eye movements, in Bach-y-Rita P, Collins CC, eds: The control of eye movements, New York, Academic Press, 1971, p 447.

217. Zuber BL, Stark L, Cook G: Microsaccades and the velocity-amplitude relationship for saccadic eye movements, Science 150:1459, 1965.

SECTION THREE

Clinical assessment of binocular vision

A. FRANCES WALONKER, C.O.
STEVEN E. FELDON, M.D.

The two eyes are capable of both conjugate and disconjugate movements. Binocular conjugate movements occur when both eyes turn equally and simultaneously in the same direction. These coordinated eye movements are called "versions." The stimulus for a rapid versional movement can be either an eccentric object of regard, which results in a step-change in eye position, called a "saccade," or a smoothly moving target that the eyes follow in a "pursuit" movement. Binocular disconjugate movements occur when the eyes turn simultaneously, but in opposite directions. These movements are called "vergences." The stimulus for a vergence movement can be either a double image (disparity vergence) or a blurred image (accommodative vergence). Maintenance of a single or a clear image requires continued vergence control.

FUSION

The process of coordinating eye movements to produce a single binocular image is called "fusion." For fusion to occur, it is necessary to have (1) overlapping visual fields, (2) corresponding retinal elements, and (3) normally functioning extraocular muscles capable of maintaining alignment of the visual axes.

Corresponding points: the cyclopean eye

All object points that simultaneously stimulate the *two foveas* appear in one and the same subjective visual direction. This direction is attributed to both the right and the left foveas and is called the "principal subjective visual direction" (Fig. 5-111). For any given nonfoveal retinal point in one eye, there will be a nonfoveal point in the fellow eye, which, when stimulated, will give rise to the same visual direction. Retinal elements of the two eyes that share this common subjective visual direction are called "corresponding points" (Fig. 5-112). All other retinal points are noncorresponding or disparate with respect to the other eye. The stimulus to sensory fusion or binocular single vision is the excitation of corresponding retinal points.

All common subjective visual directions can be represented in a drawing as an intersection of the principal visual axes (that is, the line from the fovea to the fixation point) (Fig. 5-113). In binocular vision a single visual direction is needed in which the frame of reference is related to the head rather than to the eyes. When both eyes are used, we imagine that the world is viewed from an imaginary *cyclopean eye* centered at the area of the root of the nose (Fig. 5-114).

Horopter

For any given distance there is a series of corresponding points for which there is no disparity between the two eyes. These points form a curved line called the "horopter" (Fig. 5-115). Formally stated, the horopter is the locus of all points in external space that stimulate corresponding points.

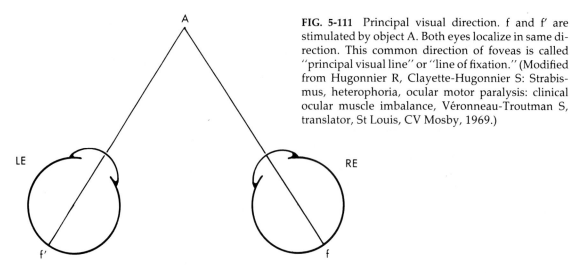

FIG. 5-111 Principal visual direction. f and f' are stimulated by object A. Both eyes localize in same direction. This common direction of foveas is called "principal visual line" or "line of fixation." (Modified from Hugonnier R, Clayette-Hugonnier S: Strabismus, heterophoria, ocular motor paralysis: clinical ocular muscle imbalance, Véronneau-Troutman S, translator, St Louis, CV Mosby, 1969.)

FIG. 5-112 Corresponding points. Points f and f' and a and b are corresponding points; each pair of corresponding points has a common visual direction. (Modified from Hugonnier R, Clayette-Hugonnier S: Strabismus, heterophoria, ocular motor paralysis: clinical ocular muscle imbalance, Véronneau-Troutman S, translator, St Louis, CV Mosby, 1969.)

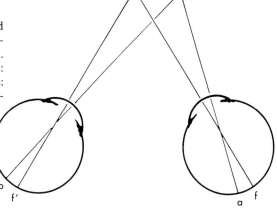

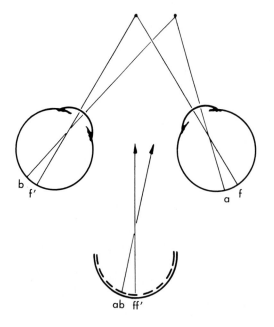

FIG. 5-113 Egocentric visual direction, or the cyclopean eye. The cyclopean eye is formed by the superimposition of the retina of the right eye and that of the left eye in such a way that the fixing fovea and the retinal point corresponding to it in the opposite eye meet. Points f and f' are superimposed at a single point; a and b, another pair of corresponding points, also meet at the same distance in the cyclopean eye as they do on each eye (abff' = fa = f'b). (From Hugonnier R, Clayette-Hugonnier S: Strabismus, heterophoria, ocular motor paralysis: clinical ocular muscle imbalance, Véronneau S, translator, St Louis, CV Mosby, 1969.)

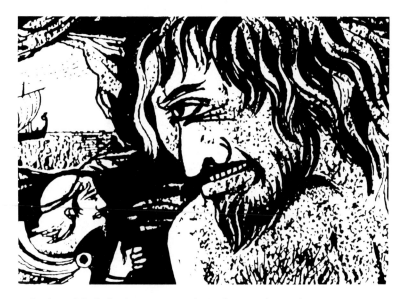

FIG. 5-114   Cyclops. Mythologic creature with single eye at base of nose, suggesting term "cyclopean eye" to represent egocentric visual direction. (From Clarke HW, ed: Twentieth century interpretations of the Odyssey, Englewood Cliffs, NJ, Prentice-Hall, 1983. Jacket illustration by E. Blakney.)

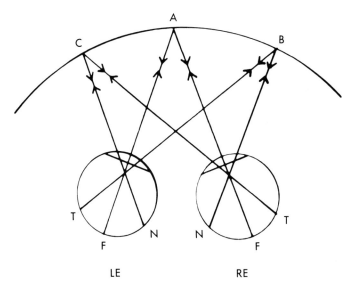

FIG. 5-115   Horopter: the curved line joining C, A, and B. Image from object A falls on fovea of each eye and is seen straight ahead. Image from object B falls on nasal retina of right eye and temporal retina of left eye, which are corresponding points. Images from the object C fall on temporal retina of right eye and nasal retina of left eye, which also are corresponding points. F-LE F-RE; T-LE N-RE; and N-LE T-RE are pairs of corresponding points.

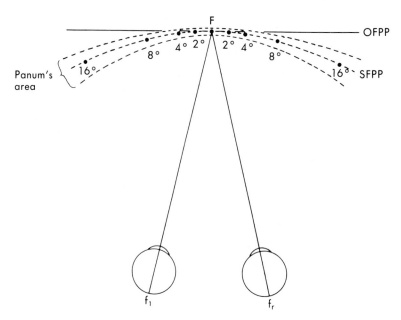

FIG. 5-116   Panum's fusional space or area. F, fixation point; OFPP, objective frontoparallel plane; SFPP, subjective frontoparallel plane—the horopter. (From Burian HK, von Noorden GK: Binocular vision and ocular motility: theory and management of strabismus, 3rd ed, St Louis, CV Mosby, 1985.)

Panum's area

Although points on the horopter are seen singly without disparity, there is a region of single vision surrounding the horopter that does have disparity. This area, where disparate or noncorresponding points transmit the impression of single vision, is called "Panum's area" (Panum's fusional space) (Fig. 5-116). The horizontal extent of this area is small at the center (6 to 10 minutes of arc near the fovea) and increases toward the periphery (30 to 40 minutes of arc at 12 degrees from the fovea).

Stereopsis

A solid object placed in the midline creates slightly different images when viewed with both eyes.[3] This phenomenon is called binocular parallax (Fig. 5-117). It is binocular parallax that provides the retinal disparity essential for stereopsis. The perception of depth is dependent on the fusion of disparate retinal elements within Panum's space.

The *presence of fusion* may be estimated by the Worth Dot Test[8] (Fig. 5-118). The test consists of four lights in a diamond formation, two green, one red, and one white. The test can be performed for both distance (visual angle of 1.25 degrees) and for near at 33 cm (visual angle

of 6 degrees). The patient wears glasses with a red filter before one eye and a green filter before the fellow eye. When fusion is present, four appropriately colored lights are seen, the white light being either green or red depending on ocular dominance (Fig. 5-119).

The *range of fusion* may be measured on a projection perimeter. Both eyes are open, and a moderately sized target is moved into the area of comfortable single vision. The patient follows the target out of this area and reports when diplopia occurs. This area of single vision is then plotted on an appropriate chart (Fig. 5-120).

The *degree of stereopsis* is estimated by measuring the disparity necessary to produce the impression of depth. The Titmus Stereo test is used for near (Fig. 5-121) and the American Optical vectograph slide is used for distance (Fig. 5-122). Polarized viewers are used with these two tests, and the disparity is graded from 800 to 40 seconds of arc at near and from 240 to 60 seconds of arc for distance. The Random Dot Test and TNO test (Fig. 5-123) are similar but use random-dot stereograms to eliminate monocular clues.

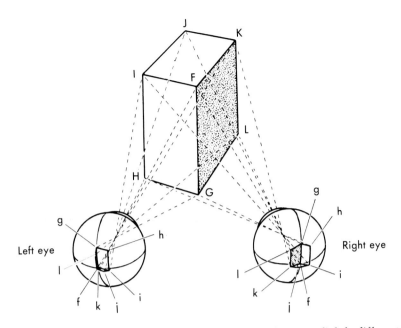

FIG. 5-117 Stereopsis. Solid object placed in midline of head creates slightly different or disparate retinal images, the fusion of which results in a three-dimensional sensation. (From Burian HK, von Noorden, GK: Binocular vision and ocular motility: theory and management of strabismus, 3rd ed, St Louis, CV Mosby, 1985.)

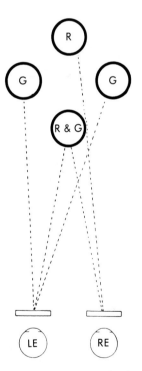

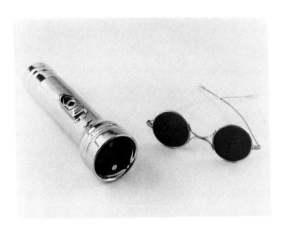

FIG. 5-118 Hand-held Worth light with red and green goggles. (From Stein HA, Slatt BJ: The ophthalmic assistant: fundamentals and clinical practice, 4th ed, St Louis, CV Mosby, 1983.)

FIG. 5-119 A fusion response with Worth lights. The red glass is in front of the right eye and the green glass is in front of the left eye. The bottom light will be either red (R) or green (G), depending on ocular dominance. (From Gonzales C: Strabismus and ocular motility, Baltimore, Williams & Wilkins, 1983.)

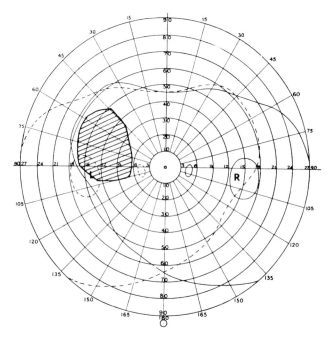

FIG. 5-120 Abnormal field of binocular single vision represented by shaded area. This area is obtained by having the patient follow a test object and indicate when the test object appears to double. Shaded area represents fusion present 20 to 60 degrees to the left and superiorly. (From Lyle and Jackson's Practical orthoptics in the treatment of squint, revised by Lyle TK, 4th ed, London, HK Lewis, 1953.)

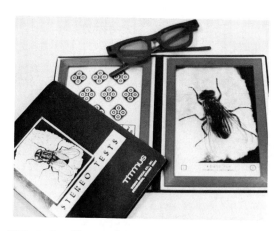

FIG. 5-121 Titmus Stereopsis Test with polaroid glasses. (From Gonzales C: Strabismus and ocular motility, Baltimore, Williams & Wilkins, 1983.)

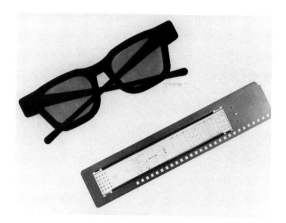

FIG. 5-122 American Optical Vectographic Project-O-Chart. (From Gonzales C: Strabismus and ocular motility, Baltimore, Williams & Wilkins, 1983.)

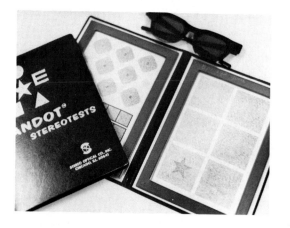

FIG. 5-123 TNO test for stereopsis with red and green goggles. (From Gonzales C: Strabismus and ocular motility, Baltimore, Williams & Wilkins, 1983.)

DIPLOPIA

The concept and evaluation of fusion have been described in the previous paragraphs. In particular, Panum's area has been defined as an area where stimulation of noncorresponding points is fused. Stimulation of noncorresponding points that fall outside the fusional area produces diplopia. This diplopia occurs under both physiologic and nonphysiologic conditions.

Physiologic diplopia

Physiologic diplopia occurs only in the presence of binocular vision. The fovea projects images straight ahead; the nasal retina projects images temporally (that is, it interprets images as having come from a temporal direction), and the temporal retina projects images nasally (that is, it interprets images as having come from a nasal direction) (Fig. 5-124). In Fig. 5-125, if the eyes are looking at F (the fixation point), it will be seen singly because corresponding points are stimulated. Another point in space, *A*, situated beyond or distant to the fixation point and lying outside Panum's fusional area, will stimulate noncorresponding retinal points nasal to the two foveas, and the images will be projected temporally. This phenomenon results in diplo-

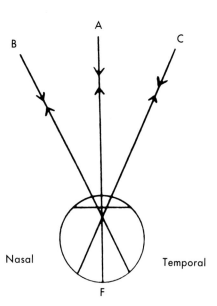

FIG. 5-124 A, Fixation object; B, object in the nasal field; C, object in the temporal field. Image from object A falling on fovea is interpreted as coming from straight ahead. Image from object B in nasal field falls on temporal retina and is projected nasally. Image from object C in temporal field falls on nasal retina and is projected temporally.

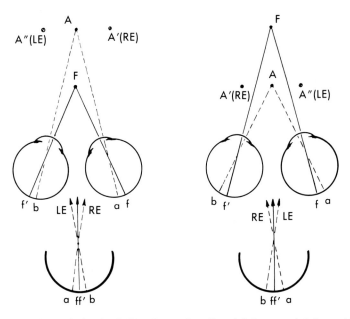

FIG. 5-125 Physiologic diplopia. F, Fixation point; f' and f, foveas of right and left eye. A, Object point stimulating noncorresponding points b and a. There are both binocular and cyclopean representations of physiologic diplopia. *Left*, Object, point A, stimulates noncorresponding points b and a, which fall nasally to foveas, f and f'. These are then projected temporally, resulting in homonymous or uncrossed diplopia. *Right*, Object, point A, stimulates noncorresponding points b and a, which fall temporally to foveas, f and f'. These are then projected nasally, resulting in heteronymous or crossed diplopia. (From Hugonnier R, and Clayette-Hugonnier S: Strabismus, heterophoria, ocular motor paralysis: clinical ocular muscle imbalance, Véronneau-Troutman S, translator, St Louis, CV Mosby, 1969.)

pia, termed "homonymous" or "uncrossed" diplopia. Similarly, if the eyes are looking at F, and another point in space, A, is situated nearer than the fixation point but outside Panum's space, noncorresponding retinal points temporal to the two foveas will be stimulated and the images will be projected nasally. This phenomenon results in "heteronymous" or "crossed" diplopia.

Nonphysiologic diplopia

Conditions that preclude fusion and cause disruption of binocular coordination are called "heterotropias." In the presence of a heterotropia images from an object fall on noncorresponding retinal areas outside the horopter and Panum's fusional space and are seen as double. Heterotropia can be either *concomitant* or *incomitant*. In a concomitant heterotropia the measured deviation is the same regardless of (1) the eye chosen for fixation and (2) the direction of gaze. In an incomitant heterotropia, the measured deviation varies with (1) the eye chosen for fixation and (2) the direction of gaze.

There are three types of binocular diplopia: horizontal, vertical, and torsional. For instance, in a right *esotropia* (right eye turned in) an object in space is imaged on the fovea of the left eye and on a nasal retinal point of the right eye (that is, noncorresponding points). The left eye projects its image straight ahead; the right eye projects its image temporally, resulting in *uncrossed* or *homonymous diplopia* (Fig. 5-126). In a right *exotropia* (right eye turned out) an object in space is imaged on the fovea of the left eye and on a temporal retinal point of the right eye. Again, the left eye projects its image straight ahead, but the right eye projects its image nasally. This results in *crossed or heteronymous diplopia* (Fig. 5-127). The same logic applies to vertical deviations. Objects in space that are imaged on the upper retina are projected inferiorly and vice versa. For example, in a right hypertropia the left eye projects its image straight ahead and the right eye projects its image inferiorly (Fig. 5-128). Torsional diplopia results when the involved eye is rotated along the line of the visual axis. In a superior oblique palsy, for instance,

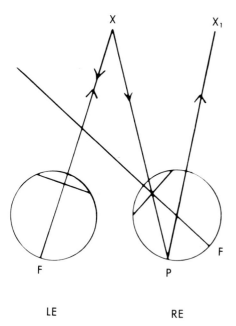

FIG. 5-126 Right esotropia, with homonymous or uncrossed diplopia. F, fovea; X, object point; X_1, projected image; P, peripheral retinal point (noncorresponding). Image of X falling on fovea of left eye is projected straight ahead. Image of X falling on nasal retina of right eye is projected temporally, resulting in a diplopic mental image, X_1, of object X.

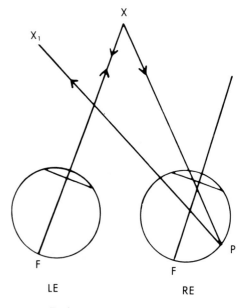

FIG. 5-127 Right exotropia, with heteronymous or crossed diplopia. F, fovea; X, object point; X_1, projected image; P, peripheral retinal point (noncorresponding). Image of X falling on fovea of left eye is projected straight ahead. Image of X falling on temporal retina of right eye is projected nasally, resulting in a diplopic mental image, X_1, of object X.

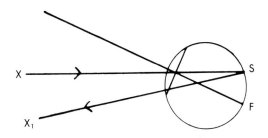

FIG. 5-128   Hypertropia. F, fovea; X, object point; X_1, projected image; S, peripheral retinal point (noncorresponding). Image of X falling on S (superior retina) is projected inferiorly, below the straight ahead foveal projection of the other eye (not shown).

there is an outward rotation or *extorsion* of the eye. Therefore the resultant image is projected as an intorsion. The amount of perceived intorsion increases as the eye is brought into the field of action of the defective superior oblique.

Sensory evaluation of diplopia

In the sensory evaluation of heterotropia the subjective separation between a single object point imaged on the fovea of one eye and the extrafoveal retinal point of the fellow eye is determined. The test often is performed with a red filter placed before one eye (usually the right eye). The filter is used for several reasons: (1) to dissociate the eyes in a manner that prevents fusion of the two images, (2) to allow the patient to separately identify each light, and (3) to determine the relative position of the two lights (for example, the red light is higher and to the left of the white light). The presence of cyclotorsion can be assessed by using a linearly extended light to estimate the relative tilt of the two images. The patient is instructed to follow the light into the various positions of gaze to determine where the greatest separation of the images occurs. If the deviation is incomitant, the largest degree of separation corresponds to the action of the defective muscle; the more peripheral image (for example, the lower image in downgaze) is projected from the eye with the defective muscle. Most patients will try to avoid diplopia by moving their eyes into an area of minimal separation, adopting a compensatory head position.

Torsional diplopia is evaluated by using a bar light and a red filter and noting the greatest deviation from the true vertical. Again, if the deviation is incomitant, the direction of the greatest tilt of the image is the direction of the rotation of the paretic muscle, with the more peripheral and torted image being projected from the affected eye. Torsional diplopia may be quantitated by using the double Maddox rod test. A flashlight is observed through two Maddox rods, one white and one red, placed in a trial frame parallel to each other. The rods produce two lines of light that can be rotated until the imaged lines appear parallel to the patient. The angle of deviation then can be determined from the scale on the trial frame. Bagolini lenses, Burian's cyclophorometer, and Franceshetti's cyclophorometer are other examples of tests that quantitate the degree of torsion.

Motor evaluation of deviation

To measure the deviation in different positions and to estimate the presence of concomitance or incomitance, the *prism cover test* is used.

The patient fixes on a target either at near or distance and an opaque occluder is placed before one eye. The appropriate prism (either base up, base down, base in, or base out) is placed before the fellow eye. The occluder then is moved to cover the eye with the prism. As the occluder is moved, the previously occluded eye will shift its position to bring the fovea into line with the target. This shift is eliminated when the appropriate prismatic correction is placed before the fellow eye. The test is repeated with the patient looking up, down, right, and left.

When an incomitant deviation is present, the primary and secondary deviations must be measured. If the uninvolved eye is used for fixation, the measured deviation is termed the "primary deviation." If the involved eye is used for fixation, the deviation is termed the "secondary deviation." The secondary deviation is always greater than the primary one in the acute stages of the palsy. For example, in a right lateral rectus palsy there is a moderate amount of esotropia in the primary position with the left eye fixating the target (Fig. 5-129, *A*). With the right eye fixating the target, additional innervation will be required to bring the right lateral rectus muscle into the primary position of gaze. The yoked left medial rectus muscle (contralateral synergist) also will receive this increased level of innervation. The result is an overaction of the left medial rectus muscle, which increases the amount of esotropia compared to the amount when the nonparetic eye is fixating. The measured secondary deviation continues to increase as the affected eye is moved further into the action of the paretic muscle (Fig. 5-129, *B*).

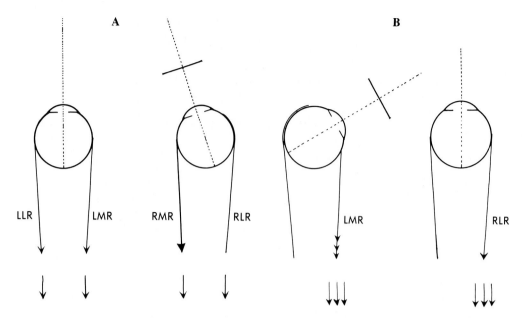

FIG. 5-129 Primary and secondary deviation for a right lateral rectus (RLR) palsy. **A,** Fixing with the uninvolved eye, demonstrating moderate esotropia (primary deviation). **B,** Fixing with the involved eye. (From Hugonnier R, Clayette-Hugonnier S: Strabismus, heterophoria, ocular motor paralysis: clinical ocular muscle imbalance, Véronneau-Troutman, translator, St Louis, CV Mosby, 1969.)

Comparative innervational outputs in incomitant deviations: Hering's law. Incomitance is based on Hering's law of equal innervation[4]: "one and the same impulse of will directs both eyes simultaneously as one can direct a pair of horses with single reins." In the acute stage of the paresis there will be an obvious difference between the primary and secondary deviations, but over a period of time overaction of the ipsilateral antagonist and underaction of the contralateral antagonist may occur.

Development of a secondary underaction was termed by Chavasse[6] "secondary inhibitional palsy of the contralateral antagonist." With improvement in the function of the paretic muscle and the development of an underaction of the contralateral antagonist, the manifest deviation may appear to be almost concomitant. This change in the deviation is termed the "spread of concomitance," and it may be impossible to determine with any assurance which muscle was paretic primarily.

The measurements of the comparative innervational outputs to each of the extraocular muscles can be done in various ways.

Passpointing. If a subject viewing a target with the paretic eye is asked to use the hand to quickly point at the target, the subject will tend to point beyond its actual location in space. Extraocular muscle innervation may be an impor-

tant cue for egocentric localization. If so, the disproportionate innervation caused by paresis of an extraocular muscle may explain this phenomenon.[3]

Projection tests. Projection tests, such as the ones designed by Hess[5] in 1916, depend on dissociating the two eyes. The patient, wearing goggles that have a red lens before one eye and a green lens before the other eye, is seated in front of a screen (Fig. 5-130). A red flashlight held by the examiner is used to control fixation, and a green flashlight is held by the patient. The red light is projected onto the screen, and the patient is asked to superimpose the green light on the red light. The red filter is always before the eye that is fixating. A measure of the innervational effort required by this eye to maintain fixation in different positions of gaze is obtained by marking the position at which the patient directs the green light onto a chart (Fig. 5-131). The fellow eye is tested by reversing the glasses and repeating the procedure. By comparing the two plotted charts, the examiner can estimate the primary and secondary deviations, even when there has been some spread of concomitance.

Head tilting test

If a normal individual tilts his or her head to one side, two physiologic eye movements occur that

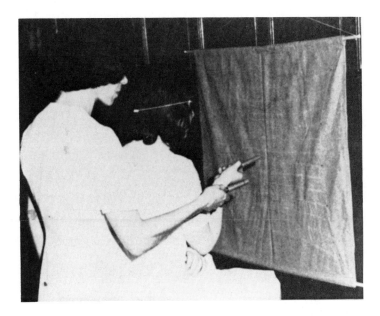

FIG. 5-130 Hess Screen. The patient sits 50 cm from chart wearing red and green goggles. Red projection light is held by examiner, and green projection light is held by patient. (From Crone RA: Diplopia, Amsterdam, Excerpta Medica, 1973.)

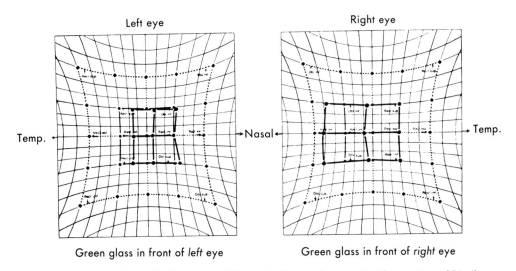

FIG. 5-131 Hess Chart. Darker *dots* and *lines,* Positions where patient has projected his/her green light onto screen. *Left,* Right eye fixing (green before left). There is an inability to superimpose lights in the action of left lateral rectus. *Right,* Left eye fixing (green before right). There is an overshoot when attempt is made to superimpose lights in the action of right medial rectus. Smaller plotted field, Primary deviation, fixation with the uninvolved eye. Larger plotted field, Secondary deviation, fixation with the involved eye. Therefore this chart depicts results for a left lateral rectus palsy (small grid fixing right, large grid fixing left). (From Lyle and Jackson's Practical orthoptics in the treatment of squint, revised by Lyle TK, 4th ed, London, HK Lewis, 1953.)

form the *compensatory fixation reflex.* There is incyclotorsion of the lower eye (to the side of the head tilt) and excyclotorsion of the higher eye (Fig. 5-132), associated with a small amount of elevation of the lower eye and depression of the higher eye (Fig. 5-133). In principle these eye movements allow each eye to maintain a constant vertical meridian relative to the horizon.

Based on the compensatory fixation reflex (Fig. 5-134), Bielschowsky[2] described how it was possible to differentiate between a superior oblique palsy in one eye and a superior rectus palsy in the fellow eye. This original test evolved into the more popular Three-Step Test of Parks[7] to diagnose the presence of an isolated cyclovertical muscle paresis. This test asks three questions.

1. Is there a right hypertropia or a left hypertropia?
2. Does the deviation increase on right or left gaze?
3. Does the deviation increase on right or left head tilt?

For example, if a patient has a right hypertropia, one of the four vertical muscles can be paretic: the agonist muscles that cause supraduction of the left eye (that is, left superior rectus/left inferior oblique) or the agonist muscles that cause infraduction of the right eye (that is, right inferior rectus/right superior oblique). If the deviation increases on right gaze, then those vertically acting muscles that are most functional when the right eye is abducted and the left eye is adducted must be implicated. This would limit the alternatives to either the right inferior rectus or the left inferior oblique. If the deviation increases on head tilting to the left shoulder, then the vertically acting muscles responsible for producing extorsion of the right eye or for producing intorsion of the left eye must be implicated. Because the left inferior oblique does *not* produce intorsion and the right inferior

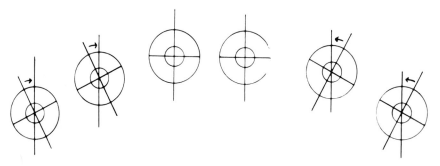

FIG. 5-132 Head tilting to right produces intorsion of right eye and extorsion of left eye, while tilting to left produces intorsion of left eye and extorsion of right eye.

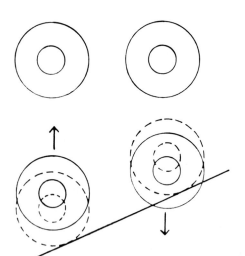

FIG. 5-133 Head tilting to right produces slight elevation of right eye and slight depression of left eye.

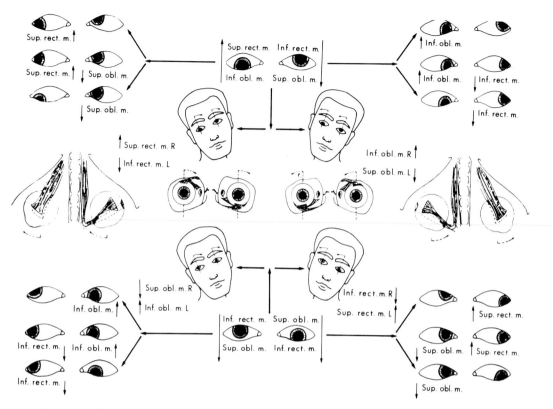

FIG. 5-134 Hagerdoorn's diagram for differential diagnosis of muscle paralysis (see text). (From Crone RA: Diplopia, Amsterdam, Excerpta Medica, 1973.)

rectus *does* produce extorsion, the paretic right inferior rectus muscle has been identifed. The increased hyperdeviation on head tilt is due to the participation of the right inferior oblique in the attempt to extort the right eye. The maneuver may be quantitated by incorporating the prism cover test.

Sensory adaptation to diplopia

Abnormal retinal correspondence. If the onset of the heterotropia occurs before the optomotor reflexes are fixed (that is, plasticity is still present), there is an associated loss of normal retinal correspondence. An adaptive process occurs that attempts to fuse misaligned images. This fusion is termed "abnormal retinal correspondence" (ARC). Under binocular conditions the visual axis and the anatomic axis (the line through the nodal point of the eye) of the deviating eye fail to correspond (Fig. 5-135). All points of the deviating eye assume a changed directional value. The fovea of the fixing eye and the eccentric area of the deviating eye assume

the same visual direction, that is, become corresponding retinal points. This eccentric area of fixation is sometimes called the pseudofovea.

Bagolini striate lenses[1] can be used to evaluate the abnormal retinal correspondence associated with heterotropia. If ARC is present, the response to the test would simulate fusion despite the presence of the heterotropia (Fig. 5-136). To establish how deeply seated this adapation has become, a linear afterimage flash can be given to each fovea in turn, one flash being horizontal and the other being vertical. If the foveas are no longer corresponding points, the resultant afterimage of the crossed lines would not bisect (Fig. 5-137).

If abnormal retinal correspondence has become well established, it is possible, under certain circumstances, to experience *triplopia* or *paradoxical diplopia.* In such instances the capacity for normal retinal correspondence never becomes totally inoperative. When the angle of deviation is changed, both the true fovea and the pseudofovea of the deviating eye are stim-

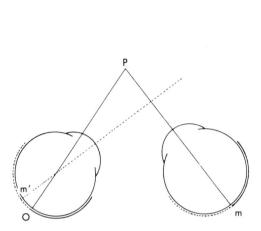

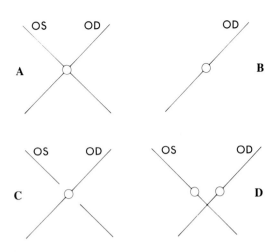

FIG. 5-135 Abnormal retinal correspondence (ARC). Object point, P, projects to O, a nonfoveal point that corresponds to foveal point m in the other eye. m' (macula), the true fovea, projects temporally. (From Hugonnier R, Clayette-Hugonnier S: Strabismus, heterophoria, ocular motor paralysis: clinical ocular muscle imbalance, Véronneau-Troutman S, translator, St Louis, CV Mosby, 1969.)

FIG. 5-136 Images seen in the Bagolini Striate Lens Test. A, Fusion. In fusion, lines formed by striations are seen bisecting light source with no areas of suppression. B, Suppression. No line formed by striations are seen by left eye. C, Abnormal retinal correspondence. Striations are seen to bisect light source with small area of suppression present around center belonging to eye fixing para-foveally. D, Diplopia. Two light sources with line going through each light, representing uncrossed diplopia. (From Gonzales C: Strabismus and ocular motility, Baltimore, Williams & Wilkins, 1983.)

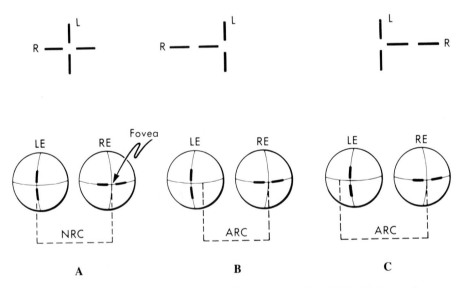

FIG. 5-137 After-Image Test. A, Normal localization (cross) in NRC. Flash has been presented vertically to right eye and horizontally to left eye. B, Abnormal retinal correspondence in esotropia. Flash has been presented vertically to right eye, in which fovea is now a noncorresponding point, and horizontally to left eye, the normally fixing eye. C, Abnormal retinal correspondence in exotropia. Flash has been presented vertically to right eye, in which fovea is now a noncorresponding point, and horizontally to left eye, the normally fixing eye. (From Burian HK, von Noorden GK: Binocular vision and ocular motility: theory and management, 3rd ed, St Louis, CV Mosby, 1985.)

ulated, producing monocular diplopia in the deviating eye in addition to the single image from the nondeviating eye—hence the term "triplopia." Paradoxical diplopia occurs postoperatively when the objective angle of deviation is changed mechanically and the subjective angle does not adapt to the new objective angle. For example, if surgery for the correction of a 30-diopter esotropia has been performed and a residual esotropia of 10 diopters remains, there is paradoxical or crossed diplopia in the presence of esotropia. The diplopia is subjectively neutralized by a 20-diopter base-in prism, but the objective angle of deviation is neutralized by a 10-diopter base-out prism.

Suppression

An alternate means of coping with diplopia in the presence of a heterotropia is by *suppression* or by mentally ignoring the image on one retina. When suppression occurs in incomitant deviations, it is governed by the direction of gaze, being present when diplopia is present and absent when fusion recurs. This type of supression is called "facultative suppression." When one eye is used exclusively for fixation, the suppression can become fixed and obligatory, leading to amblyopia.

Although most of the adaptations to diplopia relate to concomitant deviations occurring at an early age, adults with acquired (usually incomitant) deviations also may develop a form of conscious or unconscious suppression of the false image. The false image is identifiable because it does not correspond with the subjective localization of the object in space.

REFERENCES

1. Bagolini A: Technica per l'esame della visione binoculare senza introduzione di elementi dissocianti: "test del vetro striato," Boll Ocul 37:195, 1958.
2. Bielschowsky A: Lectures on motor anomalies, Hanover, NH, Dartmouth College Publications, 1943.
3. Burian HM, von Noorden GK: Binocular vision and ocular motility: theory and management of strabismus, St Louis, CV Mosby, 1974, p 27.
4. Hering E: Theory of binocular vision, translated by Bridgeman B, Stark L, New York, Plenum Press, 1977.
5. Hess WR: Ein einfaches messendes Verfahren zur Motilitatsprufung der Augen, Z Augenheilkd 35:210, 1916.
6. Lyle TK, ed: Worth and Chavasse's squint: the binocular reflexes and the treatment of strabismus, 8th ed, Philadelphia, Blakiston, 1950.
7. Parks MM: Isolated cyclovertical muscle palsy, Arch Ophthalmol 60:1027, 1958.
8. Worth C: Squint, its causes, pathology and treatment, London, John Bale, 1903, p 103.

GENERAL REFERENCES

1. Burian HM, von Noorden GK: Binocular vision and ocular motility: theory and management of strabismus, St Louis, CV Mosby, 1974.
2. Crone RA: Diplopia, Amsterdam, Excerpta Medica BV, 1973.
3. Hugonnier R, Clayette-Hugonnier S: Strabismus, heterophoria, ocular motor paralysis: clinical ocular muscle imbalance, translated by Veronneau-Troutman S, St Louis, CV Mosby, 1969.
4. Lang J: Strabismus, translated by Cibis GW, Slack Inc, 1984.
5. Solomons H: Binocular vision: a programmed text, London, William Heineman Medical Books.

Ocular Circulation

ALBERT ALM, M.D.

During the last few years, two interesting developments in circulatory research have added to our understanding of blood flow through the normal and diseased eye. One is based on research into the important role of the vascular endothelium in regulation of vascular tone; the other has enabled new possibilities for clinical studies of ocular blood flow. These two new approaches are included in this revision, although their application to ocular research is still in its initial stage. Thus the vascular endothelium has been the subject of intensive research during the last decade, but only a few studies on ocular vessels have been reported so far. Recent improvements in instruments for angiography, laser Doppler velocimetry, and blue field entoptoscopy have encouraged clinical research, but much remains unknown about the pathophysiology of ocular blood flow. These approaches are, however, particularly relevant for vascular diseases, and in the next few years we can expect useful information on blood flow through the diseased eye from these two lines of research.

ANATOMY

Two separate vascular systems are involved in the nutrition of the eye: the retinal vessels and the uveal, or ciliary, blood vessels. The uveal blood vessels include the vascular beds of the iris, the ciliary body, and the choroid. The main function of the choroid is to serve the retina. In some lower mammals, e.g., rabbits and guinea pigs, the retina is almost completely dependent on the choroid, since retinal vessels are found only within a small area of the retina or are totally lacking. In many higher mammals, including humans and other primates, the retina depends upon both the retinal vessels and the choroid.

In humans the ocular vessels are derived from the ophthalmic artery, which is a branch of the internal carotid.[109] The ophthalmic artery branches into the central retinal artery, two or three posterior ciliary arteries, and several anterior ciliary arteries.[86] Figure 6-1 shows schematically the blood vessels of the human eye. The central retinal artery enters the optic nerve about 10 mm behind the eyeball and appears at the optic disc, where it branches into four major vessels each supplying one quadrant of the retina (Fig. 6-2). Small arterioles and veins interdigitate in a characteristic way (Fig. 6-3). A capillary-free zone surrounds the arterioles.[119] This is probably due to high local oxygen tension, which causes vascular remodeling during maturation.[90]

The retinal vessels are distributed within the inner two thirds of the retina, whereas the outer layers, including the photoreceptors, are avascular and nourished from the choroid (Fig. 6-4). An avascular zone, which enables light to reach the central photoreceptors without encountering a single blood vessel, is seen centrally in the fovea (Fig. 6-5). Arteries and veins are located within the nerve fiber layer. The capillaries are arranged in a laminated fashion with two layers of flat capillary networks in a large part of the

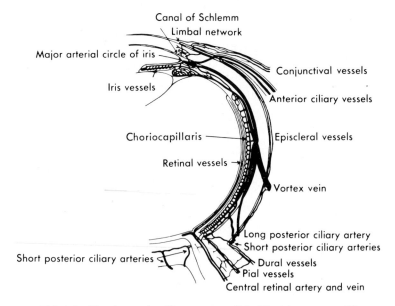

FIG. 6-1 Blood vessels of human eye. (Modified from Leber.[109])

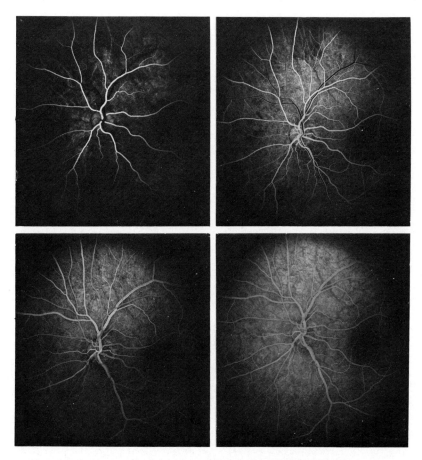

FIG. 6-2 Fluorescein angiogram from normal eye. In arterial phase *(top left)* choroidal filling is still incomplete. In early venous phase *(top right)* laminar streaming is prominent in the veins, the choriocapillaris is not filled completely, and some large choroidal arteries can still be seen. Later retinal veins and choroid show a more homogenous fluorescence. Fading of fluorescence is observed first in the arteries *(bottom right).*

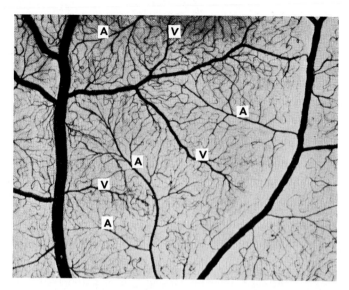

FIG. 6-3 Field from equatorial zone in retina. *Left,* vein; *right,* artery. Note interdigitation of venae efferentes (V) with arteriae afferentes (A). Note also capillary-free zone around artery. (From Michaelson J, Campbell ACP: Trans Ophthalmol Soc UK 60:71, 1940.)

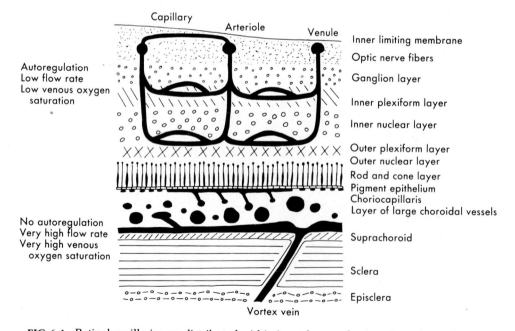

FIG. 6-4 Retinal capillaries are distributed within inner layers of retina. Outer layer, 130 μm thick, has no blood vessels. It is nourished mainly from choroidal capillaries.

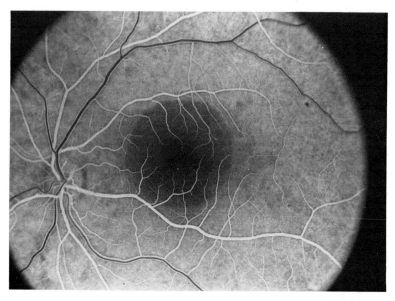

FIG. 6-5   Fluorescein angiogram showing the fovea with its capillary-free area in the center of the figure.

retina.[119,193] In the central part of the retina these capillary networks are dense and may become three- or four-layered, whereas in the periphery the networks are less dense and reduced to one layer. The extreme periphery is avascular. A separate superficial layer of capillaries, the radial peripapillary capillaries, extends from the optic disc, with its main extensions in the upper and lower temporal directions. A cilio-retinal artery is sometimes seen. It is a direct branch from the ciliary arteries, emerging from the rim of the optic cup and supplying a small area of the retina.

The retro-ocular part of the optic nerve is furnished by branches from the central retinal artery and from pial vessels, whereas the intra-ocular part of the nerve receives no branches from the central retinal artery with the exception of the most superficial layers of the optic disc. The remaining part of the optic nerve head and the lamina cribrosa receive their main supply by direct branches from choroidal arteries and short posterior ciliary arteries.[89] The peripapillary choriocapillaris does not contribute to the vascular supply of the optic nerve head (Fig. 6-6).

The posterior ciliary arteries branch behind the globe into 10 to 20 short posterior ciliary arteries and, as a rule, two long posterior ciliary arteries. The short posterior ciliary arteries pierce the sclera at the posterior pole and form the choriocapillaris, a dense, one-layered network adjacent to Bruch's membrane and the retinal pigment epithelium. In the posterior pole the choriocapillaris is arranged in a lobular fashion with alternating feeding arterioles and draining venules,[87,199] and the transition from arteriole to choriocapillaris is unusually abrupt (Fig. 6-7). In the equatorial area and at the periphery the lobular arrangement becomes gradually replaced by more spindle- or ladder-shaped patterns.[199] Interarterial and intervenous shunts between medium-sized vessels have been observed in the human choroid.[199] Some of the short posterior ciliary arteries may form either a partial or complete intrascleral vascular ring around the optic nerve, the circle of Zinn-Haller. The long posterior ciliary arteries furnish a sector each in the nasal and temporal periphery of the choroid, respectively.[87]

The anterior ciliary arteries are the major source of blood supply to the anterior uvea.[197] They travel with the rectus muscles, pierce the sclera anteriorly to form an intramuscular circle, and, with the long posterior ciliary arteries, form the major iridial circle of the iris, which is the main supply of the iris and ciliary body (Fig. 6-8). They also send some recurrent branches to the peripheral choroid.[71]

The vascular supply of the ciliary processes is complex and large species variations have been observed.[123] In the human eye the vascular anatomy of the ciliary processes has been described as divided into three territories (Figs. 6-8 and 6-9).[71] The first territory consists of anterior arterioles with a capillary network situated mainly at the broadened base of the anterior edge of the

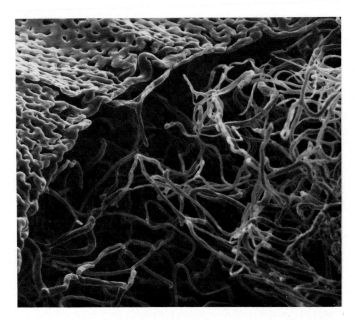

FIG. 6-6   Retinal view at edge of juxtapapillary choroid. *Above,* choriocapillaris does not send branches to prelaminar portion of optic nerve. *Below,* choriocapillaris, larger choroidal vessels penetrate prelaminar portion of optic nerve and anastomose with outermost retinal capillaries seen in right side of micrograph (retina is artifactually detached). (From Risco JM, Grimson BS, Johnson PT: Arch Ophthalmol 99:864, 1981. Copyright 1981, American Medical Association.)

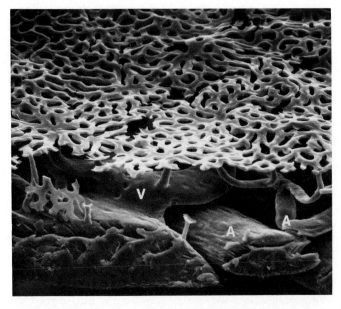

FIG. 6-7   Scanning electron micrograph of cast of cat choroid. Choroidal arteries (A) and veins (V) are seen beneath choriocapillaris. Note abrupt transition from arterioles to choriocapillaris. (From Risco JM, Nopanitaya W: Invest Opthalmol Vis Sci 19:5, 1980.)

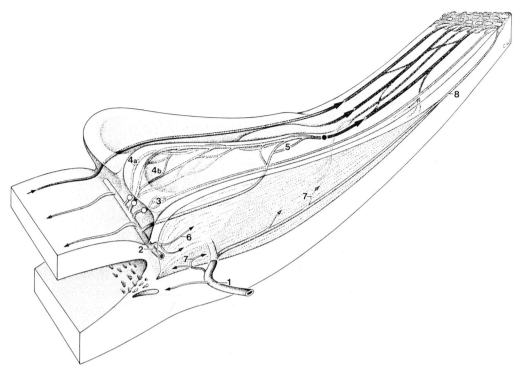

FIG. 6-8 Schematic drawing of the vascular architecture in the human ciliary body, sagittal section. 1, perforating branches of the anterior ciliary arteries; 2, major arterial circle of iris; 3, first vascular territory; 4, second vascular territory; 4a, marginal route, 4b, capillary network in the center of this territory; 5, third vascular territory; 6 and 7, arterioles to the ciliary muscle; 8, recurrent choroidal arteries. *Light circles,* terminal arterioles; *dark circle,* efferent venous segment. (Modified from Funk R, Rohen JW: Exp Eye Res 51:651, 1990.)

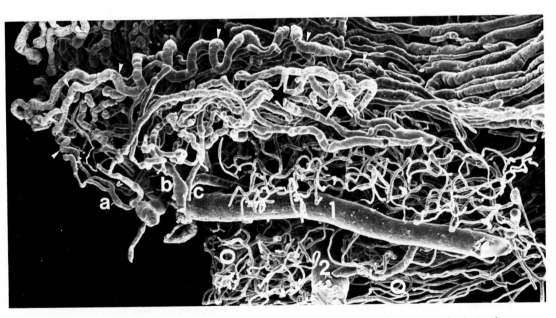

FIG. 6-9 Scanning electron micrograph of a vascular resin cast of the ciliary body in the human eye; lateral aspect. 1, branch of the long posterior ciliary artery bending into the major arterial circle of the iris; 2, further branch of the major arterial circle of the iris; a, anterior arterioles of the major processes *(arrows)*; b, arteriole for the central portion of the major process; c, arteriole for the minor processes *(asterisk); circles,* ciliary muscle capillaries. Note the marginal venule *(arrowheads).* (From Funk R, Rohen JW: Exp Eye Res 51:651, 1990.)

major ciliary process. The capillaries drain into venules located deep in the ciliary processes with little connection to the other vascular territories or to the marginal ciliary vein. These vessels form a transition zone between the fenestrated capillaries of the ciliary processes and the nonfenestrated capillaries of the iris. The second territory is also derived from the anterior portion of the major ciliary processes, but these vessels drain into a broad marginal vein at the inner edge of the ciliary process. The third and final territory provides blood to the posterior portion of the major ciliary processes and the minor ciliary processes. If exposed to epinephrine, the terminal arterioles of the two first vascular territories show marked focal constrictions.[71] This may well be to protect the blood-aqueous barrier; a sympathetic tone prevents breakdown of the blood-aqueous barrier when arterial blood pressure is suddenly raised.[31]

Retinal venous blood is drained by a central retinal vein that leaves the eye through the optic nerve and drains into the cavernous sinus. Choroidal blood leaves the eye via the vortex veins, as a rule one vein in each quadrant of the posterior pole of the eye. Blood from the anterior uvea is drained mainly through the vortex veins, although there are minor anastomotic communications with anterior episcleral vessels. Aqueous humor is drained into these episcleral vessels from the collector channels leaving the canal of Schlemm. These episcleral veins, containing aqueous humor, were described by Ascher.[16]

Experimental occlusion of the retinal arteries in pigs has demonstrated that these vessels are end arteries without any anastomoses.[49] Occlusion of retinal vessels therefore destroys the inner retinal layers.[170] Irreparable damage occurs if ocular ischemia exceeds 1 hour.[70] Occlusion of choroidal arterioles destroys the outer layers of the retina.[44] Interarterial shunts between medium-sized choroidal arteries[199] may reduce the damage caused by occlusion of a single large or medium-sized choroidal artery, but the anatomic continuity of the choriocapillaris will not prevent choroidal ischemia. The reason is that occlusion of a terminal choroidal arteriole cannot be compensated by flow through adjacent venules, since there will be no adequate pressure gradient promoting blood flow. The situation is very different in the anterior segment of the eye, where the anastomotic circles supplied by the anterior and long posterior ciliary arteries permit rather extensive muscle surgery without anterior segment ischemia.

FINE STRUCTURE AND BLOOD-OCULAR BARRIERS

The fine structure of the various vascular beds of the eye differs markedly with corresponding differences in permeability. All vascular beds are highly permeable to lipid-soluble substances, such as oxygen and carbon dioxide, which pass readily through the endothelial cells. Water also diffuses rapidly through the vessel wall, most likely both between and through the endothelial cells. For water-soluble substances the permeability of the vessel wall is determined by the structure of the capillary endothelium. Capillaries may be classified as continuous, fenestrated, or discontinuous. Continuous capillaries are the most impermeable type and they can be found, for example, in mesentery, skeletal muscle, and brain. Adjacent endothelial cells are connected by more or less continuous networks of membranous ridges, tight junctions (zonula occludentes) (Fig. 6-10). The wall of fenestrated capillaries is thin, with fenestrations covered by a thin, porous membrane. They are generally found in tissues where there are large fluid movements between the intravascular and extravascular compartments, such as the kidney, the intestinal mucosa, and exocrine and endocrine glands.[116] Liver, spleen, and bone marrow contain discontinuous capillaries that permit blood cells to pass easily through the capillary walls. Continuous and fenestrated capillaries are represented in the eye but no discontinuous capillaries are found.

Functional studies have demonstrated that even the continuous capillaries behave as porous membranes and that there are two populations of pores. The smaller pores, with a diameter of about 9 nm, are practically impermeable to albumin and large proteins.[135] They correspond to small interruptions in the junctional bindings between the cells.[39] Large pores are much less frequent and have an estimated diameter of 24 to 70 nm.[79] They may be due to occasional wide slits between endothelial cells.

Continuous capillaries in various tissues show a wide range of permeability due to a difference in continuity and complexity of the junctions corresponding to a difference in number and sizes of the small pores. Thus the small pores of cerebral vessels have been estimated to have a diameter as small as 0.8 nm,[59] and the endothelial permeability of the brain is less than 1% of that in skeletal muscle and less than 0.1% of that in the mesentery.[45] The tight junctions between the endothelial cells in the cerebral capillaries are the anatomic counterparts of the

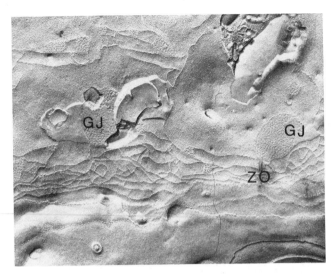

FIG. 6-10 Freeze-fracture view of membrane cleavage face at junctional complexes of frog pigment epithelial cells. Apex of cells lies toward top of figure. GJ, gap junction; ZO, zonula occludentes. (From Hudspeth AJ, Yee AG: Invest Ophthalmol 12:354, 1973.)

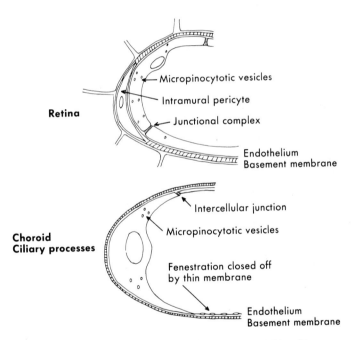

FIG. 6-11 Schematic representation of capillary wall in retina and in ciliary process and choroid.

blood-brain barrier. The retina, being part of the brain, has a similar arrangement, the blood-retinal barrier, with tight junctions between the endothelial cells of the retinal capillaries[46] (Fig. 6-11) and between the cells of the retinal pigment epithelium (see Fig. 6-10).[97] A defect in the blood-retinal barrier exists at the level of the optic disc, where water-soluble substances may enter the optic nerve head by diffusion from the extravascular space of the choroid.[78]

In the anterior segment of the eye there is a corresponding blood-aqueous barrier that has tight junctions between the endothelial cells of the iris capillaries[196] and between the nonpigmented cells of the ciliary epithelium.[169,171] Also within the eye there is a considerable variation in degree of "leakiness" of tight junctions. Thus the permeability of the retinal capillaries is similar to that of cerebral vessels with no, or only minimal, leakage of fluorescein,[78] or even sodium ions,[191] whereas the junctional complexes of the primate iris vessels have a complexity intermediate between cerebral vessels and those of striated muscle.[67] Species differences exist; the iris vessels of the cat seem to be more permeable than those of primates.[18]

Since the blood-ocular barriers are largely impermeable even to small water-soluble substances, such as glucose and amino acids, important metabolic substrates have to be transported through these barriers by means of carrier-mediated transport systems. Such transport systems can be found both in the blood-aqueous[144] and the blood-retinal barriers.[13,120,190]

Recent studies have demonstrated that rapid, modest, and reversible increments in permeability can occur even in cerebral vessels through a variety of stimuli, including such drugs as histamine, serotonin, and bradykinin.[45] This is assumed to take place through contractions of the endothelial cells in the cerebral venules causing widening of intercellular clefts. A receptor-mediated increase in vascular permeability has been observed in the rat iris, where isoproterenol increases permeability to carbon particles[185] through development of clefts between the endothelial cells of the venules.[184] Thus, we may expect some normal variation in the permeability of the blood-aqueous and blood-retinal barriers.

Several ocular diseases and surgical trauma alter the permeability of the blood-ocular barriers. Thus the integrity of these barriers is of primary concern for the clinician. Ocular fluorophotometry permits clinical assessment of the permeability of the blood-retinal and blood-aqueous barriers, and this technique has been used to demonstrate increased permeability of the blood-retinal barrier in diabetes[106] and arterial hypertension,[107] and of the blood-aqueous barrier after surgery.[164]

The retinal capillaries have a diameter of 5 to 6 μm.[109] The continuous layer of endothelial cells is surrounded by a thick basement membrane within which there is a discontinuous layer of intramural pericytes. Junctions between endothelial cells and pericytes occur through fenestrations in the basement membrane.[41] The function of the pericytes is not known, but they are reduced in number in diabetic retinopathy.[48]

In the ciliary processes and the choroid the capillaries are quite different from those of the retina and the iris (see Fig. 6-11) in that these tissues contain fenestrated capillaries.[19,95] In the choriocapillaris the fenestrations are more numerous and larger in the submacular area compared to the periphery.[183] Such fenestrae result in high permeability to low molecular weight substances, and in both the ciliary processes and the choroid the permeability even to substances as large as myoglobin (molecular weight 17,000) is high. The still larger albumin and gamma globulin molecules (molecular weight 67,900 and 156,000 respectively) also pass at high rates when compared with the conditions in many other tissues.[27] For the choriocapillaris, this high permeability is probably necessary to maintain a high concentration of glucose at the retinal pigment epithelium and to permit passage of proteins involved in the supply of vitamin A to the retina.[36]

The uveal capillaries are wider than those of the retina. The branches of the choriocapillaris have been considered to be unusually wide. It was surprising therefore that only about 5% of intraarterially injected microspheres with a diameter of 8 to 10 μm could pass through the rabbit choroid, whereas about 50% of these spheres passed through the vascular beds of the anterior uvea.[14] Casts from the rabbit choroid indicate that the spheres are caught in narrow or flat parts of the capillaries.[34]

TECHNIQUES FOR MEASURING OCULAR BLOOD FLOW

Much of our information on blood flow through the normal eye has been obtained with techniques that can only be used in animal experiments. A few techniques that have proved particularly useful will be presented here along with some recent clinical techniques. For more details I refer readers who have a particular interest in clinical techniques to a recent review on laser Doppler velocimetry and the blue field entoptic technique.[147]

Techniques used in animal experiments

For animal experiments four basic techniques have proved very valuable. Direct cannulation of uveal veins has made it possible to obtain quantitative data for uveal blood flow in rabbits[24] and cats.[23] Rabbits must be pretreated with indomethacin to prevent release of prostaglandins and uveal vasodilation.[127] In cats there is a large intrascleral venous plexus that permits sampling of venous blood from either the anterior uvea or the choroid. This plexus has been used to determine arteriovenous differences for oxygen[7] and glucose.[188] Retinal arteriovenous differences can be studied in pigs, in which the retinal veins form a ring-shaped plexus around the optic nerve.[191]

Labeled microspheres permit determination of blood flow through all the different tissues of the undisturbed eye.[9,131] The precision of the technique depends on the number of spheres trapped in the tissue sample, but blood flow through small pieces of tissue, such as the iris or the retina, can still be determined with adequate precision if enough experiments are made.[94] For measurements in very small pieces of tissue, such as the optic nerve head, precision is improved by using nonlabeled spheres and counting them in tissue sections in a microscope.[75]

Continuous recording of the oxygen tension in the vitreous body close to the retina can give information on changes in retinal blood flow.[8] Studies of the oxygen profile within the retina with microelectrodes have the advantage of supplying information on the relative importance of the choroidal and the retinal circulation in providing oxygen to the retina.[3] Glucose consumption in vivo can be studied by determining the tissue uptake of labeled 2-deoxy-D-glucose. Although it is not a direct measure of blood flow, this technique may indicate inadequate blood supply as well as increased metabolic demands and has proved very useful for studying the effects of increased intraocular pressure and lighting conditions on the retina and the optic nerve head.[33,175]

Clinical methods

Fluorescein angiography has provided a great deal of clinical information on retinal circulation (see Fig. 6-2). Angiograms normally provide only qualitative information, but various attempts have been made to obtain quantitative or semiquantitative information from fluorescein angiograms based on the assumption that there is a constant relationship between fluorescence and fluorescein concentration. Thus densitometric measurements of the film can be used to calculate the mean transit time of the retinal circulation from fluorescein angiograms.[91] Mean transit time is defined as the ratio of blood volume to blood flow. The calculation is based on mathematics derived for a bolus injection,[149] and it requires that the complete concentration-time curve can be reconstructed. The technique involved in such measurements is simple, but it has not achieved widespread use. The major problem is the badly defined and prolonged bolus reaching the eye after an injection into the antecubital vein. Together with the rapid recirculation of dye, this makes extrapolation of the downslope of the venous curve difficult. The injection technique is important. Injecting a small volume with a rapid saline flush improves the dye-dilution curve in the eye.[63] and an even better bolus can be achieved by injecting into a catheter with its tip in the superior vena cava.[148] An interesting approach to obtaining a perfect bolus is the introduction of fluorescein into liposomes that can be released by a laser in the retinal arteries (Fig. 6-12).[102,201] The lack of choroidal background gives a beautiful demonstration of single retinal capillaries even outside the macula, and combined with high-speed angiography and image analysis this technique should provide good opportunities for measuring various aspects of local retinal blood flow.

For studies on the choroidal circulation indocyanin green (ICG) is a more suitable dye.[38] ICG has two significant advantages for choroidal angiography: The fluorescence is not blocked by the pigment epithelium as it fluoresces at near infrared; further it is almost completely bound to proteins, which means that it does not easily pass the walls of the choriocapillaris. Single choroidal vessels can be observed even late in the angiogram (Fig. 6-13). Despite these obvious advantages, the technique has not become a routine clinical tool. Apart from the requirement of a special camera, the difficulty in interpretation of these angiograms has been an obstacle. An obvious use for ICG is to examine subretinal neovascular membranes, where it seems to be a valuable complement to, but not a substitute for, fluorescein angiography.[85] Recent attempts with image analysis techniques[103] have demonstrated that the choroidal filling pattern is fairly constant for the same individual (Fig. 6-14), and interpretation of ICG-angiograms based on image analysis may well be a viable approach to clinical studies on choroidal blood flow.

Laser Doppler velocimetry has become a routine technique for measurements of blood flow through many tissues. The first measurement of blood flow velocity in any tissue was made in the rabbit retina,[158] and the first measurement in the human eye was presented only 2 years later.[186] That it is still not widely used for studies of retinal circulation illustrates the difficulty of making measurements in the eye. The instrument is complicated and its use requires great expertise. Present instruments permit absolute measurements of flow velocity in large retinal vessels by bidirectional laser Doppler velocimetry.[150] The laser Doppler signal can also be used to estimate blood volume, which has enabled semiquantitative measurements of blood flow in the optic nerve head.[157] An alternative method is to combine laser Doppler velocimetry with disc reflectometry.[166] A noninvasive tech-

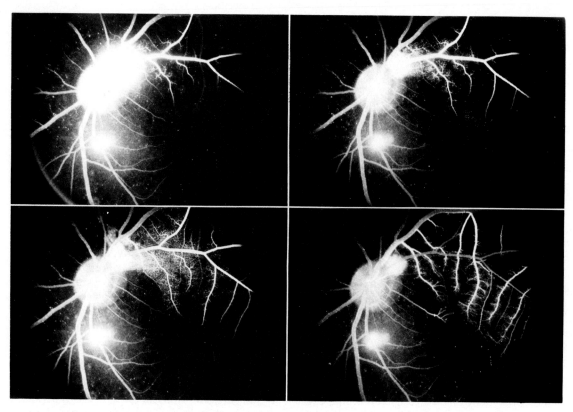

FIG. 6-12 Fluorescein angiogram with targeted dye delivery in a monkey retina. Fluorescein is encapsulated in lipid vesicles and injected intravenously. Fluorescein is then released in the retinal artery by heating the artery with an argon laser. (Courtesy R. Zeimer, Ph.D.)

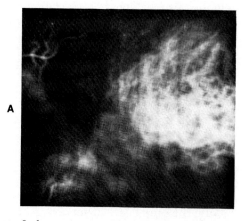

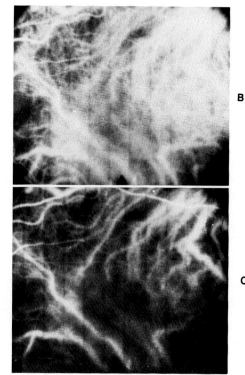

FIG. 6-13 Indocyanin green choroidal angiogram. **A**, choroidal arterial phase; **B**, choroidal capillary phase; **C**, choroidal venous phase. (From Niederberger H, Bischoff P: Journal of Ophthalmic Photography 9:90, 1986.)

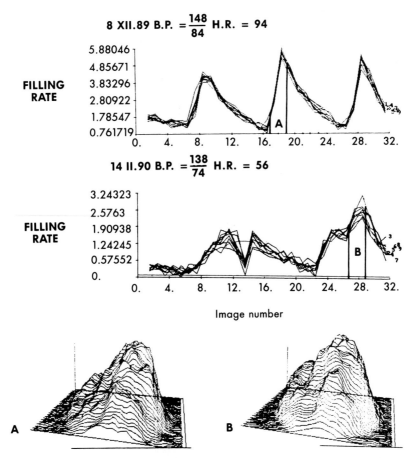

8 XII.89 B.P. = $\frac{148}{84}$ H.R. = 94

FILLING RATE

14 II.90 B.P. = $\frac{138}{74}$ H.R. = 56

FILLING RATE

Image number

A   B

FIG. 6-14 Computer-based reconstruction of choroidal filling in the normal human eye with indocyanin green (ICG). The angiogram is recorded with a CCD camera and images are stored at a rate of 15 frames/sec. The frames are aligned and divided into a grid pattern with 150 sectors, each sector corresponding to a fundus area of about 0.25 sq mm (roughly corresponding to the size of a choroidal lobule). The change in average grey level for each area is recorded as a function of time, and the first derivative of that function is the instantaneous filling rate of that particular sector of the choroid. The two top curves represent the filling rates of 9 clustered choroidal sectors on two different occasions in the same individual. Cyclic variation in filling rates corresponds to heart rate. The two three-dimensional surfaces at the bottom of the graph represent the filling rates during systole (A and B) in all 150 choroidal sectors included in the angiogram, where the x- and y-axis correspond to fundus location and the z-axis to filling rate. Note the similarity of the two filling patterns despite marked difference in heart rate (H.R.). For details see Klein et al.[103] (Courtesy R.W. Flower.)

nique to determine oxygen saturation in retinal vessels[47] is another interesting clinical technique, which, combined with laser Doppler velocimetry, permits calculations of oxygen delivery from retinal circulation.[167]

The observation of the retinal shadow produced by leukocytes[172] flowing through the paramacular retinal capillaries, the blue field entoptic phenomenon, is another noninvasive technique for studies of retinal blood flow. Leukocyte velocity is estimated by matching the speed of the perceived leukocytes to the speed of computer-simulated particles on a video screen.[155] The method is subjective and is based on the assumption that the macular capillaries have a fixed diameter and that the number of capillaries open to flow is constant. If these requirements are met, leukocyte velocity is proportional to blood flow through the macular area.

RATE OF BLOOD FLOW AND OXYGEN SUPPLY

With the previously described techniques the following information on normal blood flow through the eye has been obtained. Blood flow

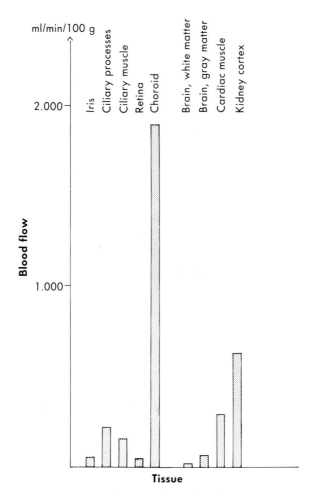

FIG. 6-15   Blood flow through tissues of monkey eye. Flow through other tissues is included for comparison. (Values for blood flow through ocular tissues from Alm et al, 1973.[12] Values for extraocular tissues are taken from Folkow and Neil, 1971.[64])

through the undisturbed eye of anesthetized monkeys, with some other tissues included for comparison, is presented in Figure 6-15. Reported blood flow values for the human retina, 35 and 80 μl/min,[57,154] are in the same range as flow values obtained in monkeys. The mean retinal circulation time in humans has been reported to be 4 to 5 seconds.[52,91]

In monkeys there are marked regional differences in blood flow through the retina and choroid; blood flow near the fovea and around the optic nerve head is much higher than blood flow in the peripheral parts (Fig. 6-16).[11] As shown in Figure 6-15, blood flow through the choroid is extremely high, and if the combined retinal and choroidal blood flow per 100 g retina is calculated, the resulting figure is about 10 times that of gray matter of the brain. A corresponding difference in metabolic requirements does not exist. Consequently, oxygen extraction from

each milliliter of uveal blood is very low. Thus the arteriovenous difference for choroidal blood in cats is about 3%, and the difference for mixed blood from the choroid and anterior uvea is 4 to 5%.[7] Similar figures have been obtained for mixed uveal blood in dogs and pigs.[43,189] In contrast, the oxygen content of retinal venous blood in humans is about 38% lower than that in arterial blood.[92] A similar figure was obtained in a study with direct measurements of the oxygen content of venous blood from pigs.[189]

Despite the low oxygen extraction from choroidal blood, the choroid is of great importance for the supply of nutrients to the retina. This is evident for primates in which the avascular fovea is nourished mainly by the choroid, but also in lower mammals, where a major part of the nutrients consumed by the retina is derived from the choroidal blood vessels. Thus in anesthetized cats about 80% of the oxygen con-

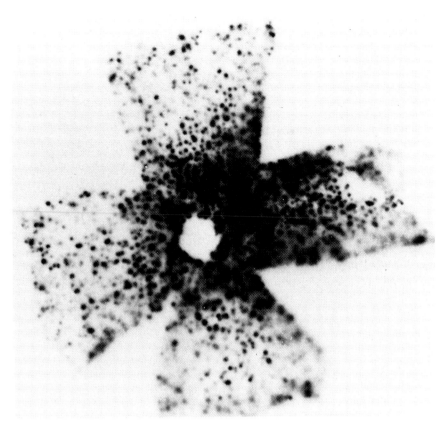

FIG 6-16 Autoradiograph of flat mount of monkey choroid after injection of labeled micro-spheres into left heart ventricle. Flow is proportional to number of microspheres per unit area. High flow in central choroid corresponds to fovea and region around optic nerve. Four incisions were made from periphery into choroid. Optic nerve gave central hole. (Technique reported in Alm and Bill.[10]) (From Alm A: Microcirculation of the eye, in Mortillaro NA, ed: The physiology and pharmacology of the microcirculation, vol 1, New York, Academic Press, 1983, pp 299-359.)

sumed by the retina is delivered by the choroid.[9] The corresponding figure for the monkey is about 65%.[11] In pigs the total consumption in vivo of oxygen and glucose is 330 and 150 nmol/min, respectively.[189] About 60% of the oxygen and 75% of the glucose were delivered by the choroidal vessels. The dependence of the retina on both retinal and choroidal blood flow is illustrated by the retinal tissue oxygen tension profile (Fig. 6-17).[3]

Undoubtedly, the high rate of blood flow through the uvea is very important. Not only does it give a high oxygen tension in the uvea, which inhances the diffusion of oxygen into the retina, but it also helps to protect the eye from thermal damage even under extreme conditions, e.g., an Arctic snow storm, a Finnish sauna bath, or observation of very bright objects. A high rate of choroidal blood flow seems to prevent damaging increments in tissue tem-perature when light is focused on the fovea.[34,136]

In many tissues only some of the capillaries are open at a given time, the number depending mainly on the metabolic needs of the tissue. The precapillary sphincter or arteriolar smooth muscle regulates opening and closing of the capillaries. Recent studies with laser Doppler flowmetry[157] have demonstrated that there are rhythmic changes in both vascular volume and red cell velocity in the optic nerve head, retina, and choroid, with the most pronounced but slow changes in the optic nerve head. These fluctuations were out of phase by almost 180 degrees, resulting in much smaller fluctuations in flow. Whether these fluctuations are due to variation in the number of open capillaries or changes in volume of the small venules is not clear. In a study with direct observation of the retinal and choroidal vasculature no precapillary sphincters were found; the blood flow ap-

FIG. 6-17 Oxygen tension profile through the cat retina. Oxygen tension was determined with a microelectrode. In this example oxygen tension at the internal limiting membrane (left on the graph) is 33 mm Hg. It stays at that level for the first 20% of retinal depth and then falls to a minimum of about 5 mm Hg at a depth most likely corresponding to the inner nuclear layer. It then increases toward the choroid with a maximum of almost 85 mm Hg close to the choriocapillaris, clearly demonstrating the dual supply of oxygen to the retina. (Courtesy V.A. Alder, S. Cringle, and D.-Y. Yu).

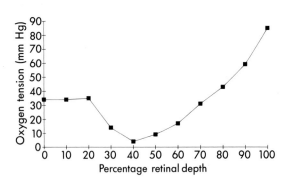

peared to be uninterrupted in all capillaries observed.[68,69] In the retina of young cats there are some spontaneous contractions and dilations in the small arterioles and precapillary sphincters, but there is much less vasomotion in the retinal vessels of adult cats.[111]

CONTROL OF CIRCULATION
The vascular endothelium

Vascular pressure, the tone in vasoactive nerves, exogenous and endogenous vasoactive substances, and metabolic activity influence blood flow, either by acting directly on the vascular smooth muscles or by influencing the vascular endothelial cells to release vasodilators or vasoconstrictors. The key role of the vascular endothelium in regulation of blood flow has become increasingly clear over the last decade. It is involved in regulation of vascular tone, platelet activity,[122] and vascular permeability.[98] The importance of the vascular endothelium as a selective barrier for exchange between blood and tissue has long been recognized. In the brain and retina part of the role of the vascular endothelium in regulation of vascular tone is due to its barrier function. The blood-brain and blood-retinal barriers prevent circulating nonlipid-soluble vasoactive substances from reaching the vascular smooth muscles. The vascular endothelial cells also inactivate such vasoactive substances as norepinephrine, serotonin, bradykinin, and adenosine, and they convert the inactive precursor angiotensin I to angiotensin II. Recently, it has become known that the vascular endothelium also takes an active part in regulation of vascular tone by releasing potent vasoactive agents. Endothelial cells synthesize prostacyclin (PGI$_2$) from arachidonic acid. It is a vasodilator but also a potent inhibitor of platelet aggregation.[122] The vasodilatory effect of acetylcholine depends on an intact vascular endothelium.[73] Stimulation of endothelial muscarinic receptors releases an endothelium-derived relaxing factor (EDRF), which stimulates the guanylate cyclase of the vascular smooth muscles, causing an increase in cGMP and relaxation.[72] EDRF has been identified as nitric oxide (NO),[121] and is synthesized from the amino acid L-arginine.[134]

The endothelium also releases a vasoconstrictive peptide, endothelin (ET).[198] ET is a 21-amino-acid peptide, closely related to the snake venom sarafotoxin.[104] Endothelin occurs in at least three different forms[99] but only one, ET-1, is produced by the vascular endothelium.

There is no known role for PGI$_2$ or ET in regulation of normal blood flow, but inhibition of the synthesis of EDRF increases blood pressure[145] and reduces resting blood flow,[195] suggesting that EDRF may be engaged in sustaining a constant vasodilation. Experimental atherosclerosis significantly impairs acetylcholine-induced relaxation in the rabbit aorta,[100] and one may speculate that vasoconstriction is an important consequence of a diseased endothelium.

The role of these endothelial autacoids in the regulation of ocular blood flow is unclear. EDRF has been demonstrated in retinal arteries in vitro.[125] ET binding sites and mRNA have been found in the vessels of the rat iris,[113] and ET receptors in pericytes of retinal capillaries.[110] However, these receptors might not mediate vasoconstriction. At least in cats and rabbits the major effect of intracameral injections of ET is a release of prostaglandins, which induces miosis in cats and increased intraocular pressure in rabbits.[77]

Perfusion pressure

The pressure head promoting blood flow through a tissue, the perfusion pressure, is the difference between the pressure in the arteries entering the tissue (Pa) and the veins leaving it (Pv). With the viscosity assumed to be constant, the relationship between blood flow (BF), perfusion pressure, and vascular resistance (R) is expressed by:

$$BF = \frac{Pa - Pv}{R}$$

The pressure in the ocular arteries just outside the eye (Pa) cannot be determined accurately with available clinical methods. Ophthalmodynamometry is based on the appearance of pulsations and cessation of blood flow through the central retinal artery at increased eye pressures. The high eye pressures that are used reduce blood flow through the ophthalmic artery, which results in a corresponding reduction in the pressure fall between the internal carotid and the peripheral ocular arteries. Consequently, the pressures measured are closer to those existing in the internal carotid artery than to those in the arteries of the undisturbed eye. A reasonable figure for the normal pressure in the ocular arteries can be calculated. At a blood pressure measured in the brachial artery of 140/80 mm Hg the mean arterial blood pressure at the level of the heart is 100 mm Hg (the diastolic pressure plus one third of the pulse pressure). Sitting or standing, with the eyes positioned at least 25 cm above the heart, the pressure in the internal carotid at the level of the ophthalmic artery is about 80 mm Hg. The difference corresponds to a blood column with a height of 25 cm. A further reduction in blood pressure takes place along the ophthalmic artery. In rabbits this pressure drop has been estimated to be 14 mm Hg.[25] In monkeys the difference between mean arterial blood pressure and the mean pressure in the anterior ciliary artery at the point where it enters the eye is 20 to 25 mm Hg.[114] Thus a reasonable estimate of the pressure in the arteries entering the eye is 60 to 70 mm Hg in the upright position. Lying down will increase this pressure, roughly corresponding to the change in height of the eyes over the heart.

A good estimate of the pressure in the veins leaving the eye (Pv) can be made by measuring the intraocular pressure, since these two pressures are almost equal at normal and high intraocular pressure.[26,114] Thus with an intraocular pressure of 15 mm Hg the normal perfusion pressure for ocular blood flow is only about 50 mm Hg, and it may even be considerably lower in healthy individuals without any obvious disturbance of normal eye function.

The spontaneous pulsations of the central retinal vein at the optic disc are a consequence of the fact that the pressure within the vein is practically equal to the intraocular pressure, and at the peak pulse pressure the vein and other parts of the ocular vascular bed expand slightly.

This leads to small changes in blood volume within the eye, and as a consequence the intraocular pressure also varies with the pulse. The variation in intraocular pressure is about 1 to 2 mm Hg, which corresponds to volume changes of 1 to 4 μl.

Outside the eye the pressure in the ocular veins is lower than the intraocular pressure. In the normal human eye the mean pressure in the episcleral veins is 7 to 8 mm Hg.[200] In anesthetized monkeys the episcleral venous pressure at a spontaneous IOP of about 14 mm Hg was 10 to 11 mm Hg, and increasing IOP above 35 mm Hg had very little effect on pressure in the episcleral veins.[115] The pressure in the vortex veins just outside the eye may be expected to be similar to that in the episcleral veins. This means that there may be a pressure drop of 5 to 10 mm Hg in the ocular veins as they pass through the sclera, resulting in partial collapse of the veins.[21] Small increments in the extraocular venous pressure tend to reverse this collapse and reduce the pressure drop without affecting the intraocular venous pressure. At larger increments of the pressure in the extraocular veins part of the pressure will be transmitted into the intraocular veins, causing venous congestion (Fig. 6–18). Congested ocular veins with capillary leakage and hemorrhages are seen when the intracranial pressure or the pressure within the sheath of the optic nerve is increased.[88] Another example may be the engorgement of retinal veins seen in early diabetic retinopathy, which indicates that the transmural pressure in the capillaries is increased.

As explained previously, the transmural pressure (the pressure inside the vessel minus the pressure outside the vessel) in the intraocular veins and the venous parts of the capillaries is very small. In a recent study on rabbits the pressure in the choroidal veins was about 2 mm Hg above the IOP.[114] Thus even a small increase in intravascular pressure may raise the transmural pressure to several times its normal value. This raises the possibility that the development of microaneurysms in diabetic retinopathy may be due in part to venous stasis. Clinical reports have suggested that in cases with impaired blood flow to one eye, diabetic retinopathy in that eye is less pronounced than in the other eye.[74] In this situation it seems likely that a reduction of the transmural pressure in the veins and capillaries contributes to protection of the walls of the vessels.

The ocular perfusion pressure (Pa − Pv) can be reduced by either a reduction in arterial pressure or an increase in intraocular pressure. From the equation above it follows that this will result

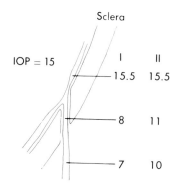

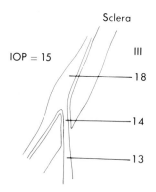

FIG. 6-18 At intraocular pressure of 15 mm Hg vortex vein is partially collapsed at place where it enters sclera. I, Venous pressure at this point is practically equal to intraocular pressure. II, Small rise in extraocular venous pressure does not change uveal venous pressure unless there is a change in intraocular pressure. III, Large rise in pressure in extraocular part of vortex vein raises pressure in choroid and produces intraocular venous congestion.

in a reduction in ocular blood flow (BF) unless the vascular resistance (R) is reduced to the same extent as the perfusion pressure. In most tissues, e.g., the brain and the kidney, such a reduction in vascular resistance takes place when the perfusion pressure is reduced. This autoregulation of blood flow tends to ensure constant levels of flow despite moderate variations in perfusion pressure. Such autoregulation has been demonstrated in the vascular beds of the anterior uvea in cats[9] and monkeys[11] and in the retina in rabbits,[29] cats,[8,9] pigs,[62] and monkeys.[11] Some species variation exists; blood flow through the anterior uvea in rabbits is not autoregulated.[29] In most of these studies the ocular perfusion pressure was reduced by increments in the intraocular pressure; but as expected, at least in cats, reductions in blood pressure have the same effect on retinal oxygen tension as increments in intraocular pressure.[8]

In the human eye there is no information on the effect of increased IOP on uveal blood flow, but blood flow through the retina is autoregulated.[151,159] In these studies the upper limit for autoregulation of retinal blood flow was about 30 mm Hg. The remaining ocular perfusion pressure was probably no more than 30 mm Hg, which is about the same as the upper limit for autoregulation in experimental animals.

Autoregulation also means that blood flow should remain normal if blood pressure is increased. However, a sufficiently large increment in blood pressure will overcome autoregulation and increase blood flow (see also Fig. 6-22). Such a mechanism has been observed in the human eye, where an increase in blood pressure of about 40% increases retinal blood flow.[161]

Considering the deleterious effect of glaucoma on the optic disc, the effect of increased IOP on blood flow through the optic nerve head is of special interest. However, the optic nerve head does not seem to differ from the retina in this respect. At least in healthy eyes blood flow through the prelaminar part of the optic nerve is autoregulated both in monkey[75,175] and human eyes.[152]

For the choroid the situation is quite different. Moderate increments in intraocular pressure cause concomitant reductions in choroidal blood flow in both cats and monkeys.[9,11] Figure 6-19 summarizes the effects of reductions in ocular perfusion pressure on blood flow through the various vascular beds of the primate eye.

The lack of autoregulation of choroidal blood flow is of interest, since most vascular beds are autoregulated. The mechanism behind autoregulation is twofold,[64] with one myogenic and one metabolic component that, as a rule, operate together. The stimuli for the myogenic mechanism are variations in the transmural pressure difference. When this pressure difference is decreased, as with increased intraocular pressure, the activity of pacemaker cells in the arteriolar wall is reduced, resulting in reduced arteriolar tone and consequently lowered vascular resistance. The lack of response of choroidal blood vessels to increments in intraocular pressure suggests that no such pacemaker cells operate in the choroidal arterioles. The stimulus for the metabolic mechanism is local accumulation of vasodilatory metabolites, such as carbon dioxide, and hypoxia. The choroidal vessels respond to carbon dioxide and thus could be expected to show some "metabolic autoregulation." Normally, however, the choroidal arteriovenous difference for carbon dioxide is very small.[7] Even marked reductions in choroidal blood flow will cause only a minor increase in tissue carbon dioxide tension and consequently no measurable

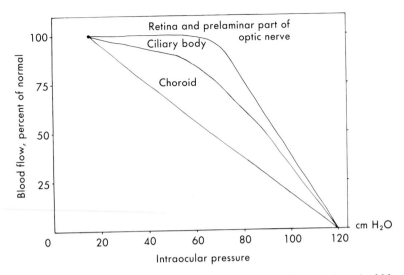

FIG. 6-19 When intraocular pressure is increased, there is no decrease in retinal blood flow and optic nerve head blood flows up to a certain level. Change in flow in ciliary body is also small. In the choroid even moderate increments in eye pressure reduce blood flow. At high intraocular pressure further increments in pressure reduce flow in all intraocular tissues.

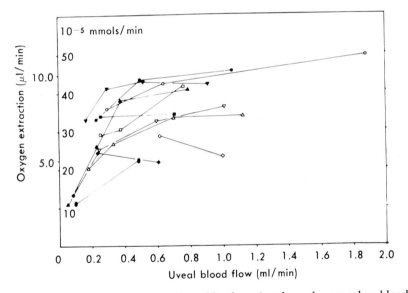

FIG. 6-20 Changes in oxygen extraction from blood passing through uvea when blood flow is reduced by increase in intraocular pressure. (From Alm A, Bill A: Acta Physiol Scand 80:19, 1970.)

effect on choroidal vascular resistance. At very low levels of choroidal blood flow, however, further reductions may be expected to cause a significant accumulation of vasodilatory metabolites and thus some autoregulatory response.

As a result of the autoregulation of retinal blood flow, the oxygen tension in the inner parts of the retina is maintained at a constant level even during large variations in intraocular pressure or blood pressure.[8] The reduction in choroidal blood flow that follows moderate increments in intraocular pressure does not seem to reduce the supply of nutrients to the retina, since the extraction of oxygen and glucose from each milliliter of blood is increased. Thus the net extraction is maintained at the same level despite large variations in blood flow[7,189] (Fig. 6-20).

The autoregulation of blood flow through the optic nerve head is of interest as these very small vessels originate from offshoots from choroidal and ciliary arteries that apparently do not alter resistance in response to increased intraocular pressure. It is possible that changes in optic nerve head vascular resistance are mediated by the vascular endothelium, which can induce vasodilation in response to changes in blood flow.[133,143]

NERVOUS CONTROL OF BLOOD FLOW

Histologic studies and stimulation experiments have revealed a rich and powerful supply of different autonomic vasoactive nerves to the various vascular beds of the uvea but not to the retina (Fig. 6-21). Thus sympathetic nerves, derived from the superior cervical sympathetic ganglion, innervate the central retinal artery up to the lamina cribrosa but not beyond, whereas all uveal vascular beds are innervated.[53,108] Many sympathetic nerves contain neuropeptide Y (NPY). In several species, including primates, NPY immunoreactive nerves have been observed close to uveal blood vessels. Their distribution resembles that of the adrenergic innervation.[180] Ocular parasympathetic nerves with effects on ocular blood flow include the oculomotor and the facial nerves. The facial nerve innervates mainly choroidal vessels.[163] The transmitter is probably vasoactive intestinal peptide (VIP) and vascular nerves with VIP-like immunoreactivity have also been found in the human eye.[182] Sensory nerves of trigeminal origin containing the peptides substance P (SP) and calcitonin gene-related peptide (CGRP) are also associated with uveal blood vessels, mainly in the ciliary body and, to some extent, in the choroid.[179,181]

Sympathetic stimulation reduces blood flow through all parts of the uvea in rabbits, cats, and monkeys, whereas retinal blood flow is unaffected.[5,10,22] Only alpha receptors seem to be present in the uvea.[10,22] At least in rabbits not all of the vasoconstriction is adrenergic; part of it remains after alpha-adrenergic blockade. It is reasonable to assume that the nonadrenergic component is due to NPY as is the case in other vascular beds.[76] One important physiologic role of the sympathetic nerves in ocular blood flow control—possibly the only one—is to help maintain the blood flow at a suitable level during sudden increments in blood pressure[31] (Fig. 6-22). Such increments, occurring in everyday life in acute stress situations and during work are the result of a general increase in sympathetic activity. They tend to cause overperfusion of the eye, resulting in breakdown of the blood-aqueous and blood-retinal barriers. However, with simultaneous activity in the sympathetic nerves to the eye, these effects are prevented. Thus sympathetic activity assists autoregulatory mechanisms in maintaining the intraocular blood flow and volume constant.

The role of the parasympathetic nerves in the eye is much less clear than that of the sympathetic nerves. Oculomotor nerve stimulation has marked, complex effects on blood flow through the anterior uvea but no marked effect on choroidal or retinal blood flow.[35,178] Thus blood flow through the iris is reduced in rabbits, cats, and monkeys, whereas blood flow through the ciliary body is reduced in rabbits but increased in cats and monkeys. The latter effect may be caused by vasodilatory metabolites accumulated during contraction of the ciliary muscle. The vasoconstriction in the iris is a combined aminergic and cholinergic effect. The nature of the aminergic transmitter and its physiologic role are not known. The cholinergic component is muscarinic, and it results in a cholinergic vasoconstrictor tone in conscious rabbits. It is interesting to note that this tone is almost eliminated by anesthesia with pentobarbital. As stated above, the vasodilating effect of acetylcholine is due to a receptor-mediated release of EDRF. Vasoactive cholinergic nerves in lower

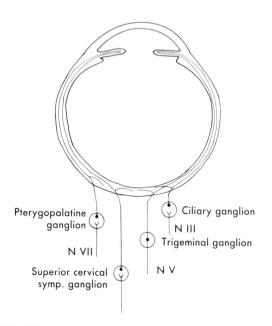

FIG. 6-21 Schematic representation of innervation of ocular blood vessels.

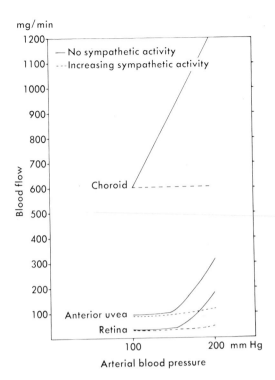

FIG. 6-22 Studies on the effect of sympathetic stimulation at different arterial blood pressures indicate that with increasing pressure due to sympathetic activation the blood flow in the different parts of the eye changes very little.[31] If acute blood pressure increments are not paralleled by increasing sympathetic tone to the eye, the blood flow in the choroid increases in proportion to the blood pressure. In the anterior uvea and the retina autoregulatory mechanisms prevent overperfusion at moderate pressure increments. However, they fail at very high pressures, and as a result the tissues are overperfused and there is small-vessel extravasation of plasma, resulting in a tendency toward breakdown of blood-aqueous and blood-retinal barriers.

species are mainly vasoconstrictive, but in mammals most vascular beds lack cholinergic vasoactive innervation. The coronary vessels form an exception with dual cholinergic regulation of vascular tone: vasoconstrictive cholinergic nerves and vasodilatory endothelial receptors.[101] The iridial vessels are another example. A cholinergic vasoconstrictor tone is also present in primates,[178] but topical application of neostigmine causes a marked vasodilation in the anterior uvea of monkeys.[12] This discrepancy may be due to the different vasoactive effects of acetylcholine when acting directly on vascular smooth muscle and when acting on vascular endothelial cells. The normal cholinergic tone in the anterior uvea releases acetylcholine, which acts mainly on the vascular smooth muscles, causing them to contract. Neostigimine treatment, on the other hand, probably results in large amounts of acetylcholine and a direct cholinergic effect on the vascular endothelium. The endothelial cells will then respond by releasing EDRF.

Intracranial stimulation of the facial nerve in rabbits, cats, and monkeys causes a moderate vasodilation in the anterior uvea and a marked vasodilation in the choroid.[129] The effect cannot be blocked by atropine and can be simulated by vasoactive intestinal peptide.[128] The physiologic role of these potent, vasodilatory, "peptidergic" nerves may well be the reflexive increase in choroidal blood flow induced by light.[137]

A peculiar type of neural influence on the blood vessels is seen in rabbits. Stroking the iris in this animal gives rise to a local dilation of the arteriole that spreads all over the iris. The vascular permeability is increased, and there is prolonged miosis and a rise in intraocular pressure.[165] A substance with vasodilating and smooth muscle-contracting properties is released when stroking the iris.[15] This substance, irin, seems to be a single prostaglandin or a mixture of several.[51] It is interesting to note that aspirin, which inhibits the synthesis of prostaglandins, modifies the effects of paracentesis in the rabbit eye.[124] Mechanical or electrical stimulation of the sensory nerve to the eye produces a reaction similar to that of stroking the iris, but, surprisingly, nerve stimulation seems to cause little release of prostaglandins.[51] The effect of sensory nerve stimulation seems to be mediated by SP and CGRP.[37,132] Prostaglandins and SP have similar effects on the anterior segment of the rabbit eye, and there seems to be some interaction between them. Thus the miosis caused by prostaglandin application depends on an intact trigeminal innervation. Indomethacin pretreatment, which inhibits prostaglandin synthesis, reduces the effects of intracamerally injected SP.[118]

Although vascular nerves with SP and CGRP immunoreactivity have been observed in the human eye, mainly in the ciliary body,[179,181] their effect on blood flow is not known. There are large species differences in the ocular effects of these transmitters. In rabbits[117] but not in cats[132] intracameral injections of SP cause a marked vasodilation in the ciliary body, while in cats a similar effect can be achieved with CGRP.[132] In rabbits SP causes an accumulation of inositoltriphosphate (IP$_3$) and contraction of the iris sphincter, but the human iris sphincter does not contract as a response to SP, and there is an accumulation of cyclic AMP instead of IP_3.[1]

EFFECT OF DRUGS ON BLOOD FLOW THROUGH THE EYE

Intravenous and close-arterial injections of vasoactive drugs usually have different effects on choroidal blood flow.[42] Intravenous injections will have an effect on most vascular beds of the body, which in turn influences the arterial blood pressure and thus the ocular perfusion pressure. As discussed previously, choroidal blood flow lacks autoregulation; thus effects of systemically administered vasoactive drugs on choroidal blood flow may be secondary to changes in blood pressure. Although the other vascular beds of the eye are autoregulated, this might not be true in a diseased eye. Thus systemic administration of vasodilators can at most be expected to have no effect on ocular blood flow. They might even reduce it if given in sufficient doses to affect blood pressure. Therefore, in general, there is no therapeutic benefit to be expected from systemic administration of vasodilators. Topical application as eye drops will circumvent this problem, but in phakic eyes therapeutic concentrations can be expected to be reached mainly in the anterior uvea. Retro-ocular or close-arterial injections may give therapeutic concentrations in the posterior pole of the eye without systemic effects. However, they may still have no effect on retinal blood flow, since the blood-retinal barrier will prevent most drugs from reaching the smooth muscles of the retinal vessels. Thus at present there seems to be no indication for the use of vasodilators in ocular therapy. However, there are other reasons to investigate the pharmacology of ocular blood vessels. Some drugs that we use for other purposes, e.g., in the treatment of glaucoma, have known effects on vascular smooth muscles in other tissues. In addition, vascular pharmacology gives information on normal regulation of blood flow, in that vasoactive drugs often engage regulatory mechanisms involved in vascular tone.

Vasoconstrictors

Topical administration of epinephrine reduces blood flow through the anterior uvea in monkeys,[6] and vasoconstriction in the uvea is provoked by arterial injections of dihydroergotamine.[20] Studies of the effects of various drugs on the oxygen tension of the vitreous body close to the retina indicate that none of the vasoconstricting drugs norepinephrine, angiotensin, or dihydroergotamine has any effect on retinal vascular resistance.[4] Angiotensin does not contract retinal vessels in vitro,[130] but in the case of epinephrine the blood-retinal barrier may be decisive for the lack of effect. Norepinephrine applied outside the blood-retinal barrier in vitro constricts retinal arteries,[96] and retinal vessels bind adrenergic agonists, indicating the presence of both alpha$_1$ and alpha$_2$ receptors.[65]

Vasodilators

Acetylcholine,[22,126] papaverine, aminophylline,[20] theophylline,[126] and amyl nitrite,[20,126] but not nicotinic acid,[20,126] dilate uveal blood vessels, and topical administration of pilocarpine or neostigmine increases blood flow through the anterior uvea in monkeys.[12] The oxygen tension in the vitreous body close to the retina in cats is unaffected by arterial administrations of the vasodilators isoproterenol, histamine, nicotinic acid, and xanthinol nicotinate, but is markedly increased by papaverine.[4] The vasodilating effect of papaverine may well be due to its high lipid solubility, which enables it to pass the blood-retinal barrier easily. Papaverine inhibits adenosine uptake. Adenosine, a natural vasodilator involved in hypoxic vasodilation, is released during hypoxia in the brain.[195] Papaverine potentiates cerebral hypoxic vasodilation, while caffeine, an adenosine-antagonist, reduces it.[139] The adenosine-receptor antagonist theophylline increases cellular ischemic damage in the brain.[162] A similar role for adenosine in the retina and optic nerve seems possible. Intravitreal injections of adenosine cause retinal vasodilation and hemorrhages.[40]

Cholinergic receptors and the ability to synthesize acetylcholine have been demonstrated in retinal vessel preparations.[61] The presence of an endothelium-dependent relaxation of retinal arteries in vitro[125] suggests an endothelial origin for these receptors. Endothelial receptors may also explain the binding sites for beta$_1$- and beta$_2$-agonists in retinal vessels,[60] as beta-adrenergic agonists have no effect on retinal vessels either in vitro[96] or after intravitreal[40] or intra-arterial injections.[4]

METABOLIC CONTROL OF OCULAR BLOOD FLOW

In the brain high tissue concentrations of oxygen produce vasoconstriction and low concentrations produce vasodilation. High concentrations of carbon dioxide lead to vasodilation and low concentrations lead to vasoconstriction. In the uvea of adult cats and rabbits the effect of moderate oxygen excess or lack seems to be too small to be detected.[23] However, the effect of oxygen tension on some of the vascular beds of the uvea may be concealed in studies on total uveal blood flow. Photographic studies of the iris vessels of the albino rabbit indicate that they respond with contraction and dilation at increased and reduced levels of oxygen tension respectively.[177] Excessive carbon dioxide gives marked vasodilation in all parts of the uvea.[9]

Arterial oxygen tension has a significant effect on retinal vascular tone and blood flow in the human eye. Breathing pure oxygen constricts retinal vessels[66] and reduces blood flow by 60%.[153] The vasoconstriction is not sufficiently marked to prevent a rise in retinal oxygen tension.[2,8] Hyperoxia reduces and hypoxia increases leukocyte velocity in the macular capillaries.[55]

In immature eyes a high oxygen concentration in the inhaled gas has dramatic effects on both humans and experimental animals[17]: vasoconstriction, inhibition of vascular development, and, after some time, obliteration of the vessels (Fig. 6-23). After withdrawal of the extra oxygen, there may be vasoproliferation, retinal edema, and hemorrhage. These changes constitute retinopathy of prematurity, which may lead to traction detachment of the retina and blindness.

Inhalation of 7% carbon dioxide in 21% oxygen gives a moderate dilation of visible retinal vessels.[66] There is, however, a marked dilation of the small resistance vessels, and at an arterial carbon dioxide tension of 80 mm Hg retinal blood flow is increased by 300 to 400% in cats.[9] With combinations of carbon dioxide and oxygen, the oxygen tension in the inner parts of the retina can be increased by more than 300%.[8]

Breathing pure oxygen increases the oxygen tension of choroidal venous blood, and consequently the amount of oxygen delivered by the choroid to the retina. However, this is not enough to supply the whole retina in case of a retinal arterial occlusion.[141] Adding 4 to 6% carbon dioxide to the oxygen will increase choroidal blood flow and oxygen supply to the retina and may help relieve vascular spasm. The clinical value of inhaling such a mixture of oxygen and carbon dioxide is doubtful. It had no effect in fully developed retinal venous occlusions, whereas some improvement was reported for selected cases of preocclusion of retinal veins.[168] Thus presently there are not enough clinical data to support the value of oxygen, with or without added carbon dioxide, in the treatment of retinal vascular occlusions.

Illumination of the retina influences retinal metabolism and blood flow. The photoreceptors

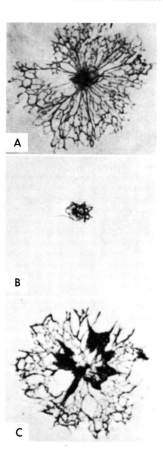

FIG. 6-23   **A**, Normal mouse retina at 1 day old. **B**, Total vaso-obliteration after 5 days in 98% to 100% oxygen. **C**, Five days after return to air. New vessels have grown into retina and into vitreous (dense central vessel). (India ink injection.) (From Ashton N: Br J Ophthalmol 52:505, 1968.)

consume more oxygen in the dark,[112,202] and preretinal oxygen tension is 26% lower in dark-adapted rabbits compared to light-adapted ones.[187] The rabbit retina is avascular and increased oxygen consumption in the photoreceptor layer will affect the oxygen tension also in the inner layers of the retina. The situation is different in a vascularized retina. Studies of glucose consumption in the monkey retina during different lighting conditions show that glucose uptake in the photoreceptor layer is higher in darkness than during constant daylight illumination, but that there is no significant difference in glucose uptake in the inner retinal layers[33] (Fig. 6-24, *bottom*). Flickering light at 4 to 8 Hz, on the other hand, increased glucose uptake in the ganglion cell layer (Fig. 6-24, *top*). A corresponding brief increase in retinal blood flow ve-

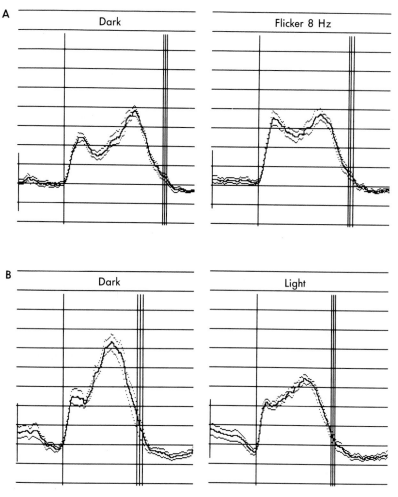

FIG. 6-24 Optical density profiles from autoradiograms of the central retina at a position 1 to 4 mm temporal to the optic disc at different lighting conditions after an intravenous injection of labeled 2-deoxy-D-glucose. High density indicates high glucose uptake. Vitreous to the left, triple vertical lines indicate position of retinal pigment epithelium. **A**, Flickering light increases glucose uptake in ganglion cell layer compared to glucose uptake in the dark. **B**, The glucose uptake in the photoreceptor layer is lower during constant illumination than in darkness. Technique reported in Bill and Sperber.[33] (Courtesy A. Bill and G. Sperber.)

locity has been observed in the human retina when light was turned on after a period of darkness.[156]

FORMATION AND DRAINAGE OF TISSUE FLUID IN THE EYE

Fluid movement through small pores from one compartment to another depends on the hydrostatic and colloid osmotic pressures in the two compartments and the permeability of the barrier or wall between them. The flow of fluid across the capillary wall through small ion-permeable pores is expressed by a modified concept of Starling's hypothesis:

$$F = C \times [(P_{hc} - P_{ht}) + (P_{collt} - P_{collc})]$$

where

C = constant
P_{hc} = mean hydrostatic pressure in capillary
P_{collc} = mean colloid osmotic pressure in capillary
P_{ht} = hydrostatic pressure in tissue fluid
P_{collt} = colloid osmotic pressure in tissue fluid

The hydrostatic pressure in most tissues of the

eye corresponds to the intraocular pressure, but in the suprachoroidal space it is a few mm Hg less.[54] Outside the eye, in the orbit, the hydrostatic pressure is close to zero. The blood-aqueous and blood-retinal barriers prevent passage of large molecules such as proteins into the aqueous humor, vitreous body, and extracellular spaces of the iris and the retina. This results in a colloid osmotic pressure in these compartments that is close to zero. In the extracellular spaces of the ciliary processes and the choroid the situation is quite different. The permeability of the capillaries even to proteins leads to a protein content in these compartments between 60 and 70% of that in plasma.[27,28] The normal colloid osmotic pressure in plasma is about 25 mm Hg. Thus the colloid osmotic pressure in the stroma of the ciliary processes and the choroid is about 16 mm Hg. This means that there is a colloid osmotic pressure gradient tending to absorb fluid into the vessels, which corresponds to about 25 mm Hg across the capillary walls of the iris and the retina and about 9 mm Hg across the capillary walls of the ciliary processes and the choroid. The hydrostatic pressure in the capillaries is obviously higher than that in the veins and higher than the intraocular pressure. This results in a hydrostatic pressure gradient over the capillary walls in the eye, tending to move fluid into the extravascular compartments by ultrafiltration. In the choriocapillaris of the rabbit the average pressure has recently been determined to be about 10 mm Hg above the IOP.[114] Thus in the choroid the colloid osmotic and the average hydrostatic pressure gradients are very similar and there will be very little net flow of fluid over the capillary wall. The pressures in the capillaries of the iris and retina have never been determined and we do not know whether there is a net inflow or outflow through these capillaries. It has been demonstrated, however, that the net inflow or outflow through the iris capillaries is negligible compared to the rate of formation and outflow of aqueous humor.[30] Ultrafiltration must take place through the capillary walls of the ciliary processes to provide fluid for the aqueous humor formation. It is not clear if the rate of aqueous formation adjusts itself to the net ultrafiltration from the blood vessels or if the latter is adjusted to the rate of secretion. A hybrid model, in which the extravascular albumin concentration plays a central role, is a likely possibility.[27]

The pores that are permeable to proteins are fewer than the small pores. Flow through large pores depends mainly on hydrostatic pressure differences.[27]

The high protein concentration of the tissue fluid in the choroid and the absence of protein in the tissue fluid in the retina have an interesting consequence. The colloid osmotic pressure of the choroidal tissue fluid will tend to cause water movement through the pigment epithelium from the retina into the choroid. This may be one of several important mechanisms for the attachment of the rest of the retina to the pigment epithelium.

Lymph vessel-like structures have been observed in the monkey choroid,[105] but they are probably not necessary for the removal of extravascular proteins. The sclera is permeable even to large molecules and proteins that have passed out of the vascular beds of the ciliary processes, and the choroid can leave the eye mainly by direct flow or diffusion through the sclera.[27] The fact that the sclera is permeable even to proteins means that the colloid osmotic pressure has no effect on transscleral flow. There is an adequate hydrostatic pressure gradient promoting flow through the sclera. This pressure gradient is of the same order as the intraocular pressure, since the pressure in the orbit is about zero and the pressure in the suprachoroidal space is almost as high as the intraocular pressure. There is a pressure gradient, albeit small, between the anterior chamber and the suprachoroidal space. Part of the aqueous humor is drained by this pressure gradient into the suprachoroidal space through the tissue spaces of the ciliary muscle. In monkeys such flow is quite pronounced;[30] in adult humans it seems to be less than 15% of the total drainage.[32]

OCULAR BLOOD FLOW IN OCULAR DISEASE

Blood flow through the retina and the optic nerve head can now be determined noninvasively with quantitative or semi-quantitative methods. So far most clinical studies have addressed the correlation between blood flow and other signs of ocular disease. Long-term studies will be needed to determine to what extent a disturbed blood flow is a cause or a consequence of the disease and to what degree medical or surgical therapy improves blood flow.

Neurogenic optic atrophy

In neurogenic optic atrophy there is a loss of the number of optic disc capillaries proportionate to the loss of tissue.[142] The remaining capillaries are smaller than normal, and clinical studies with laser Doppler velocimetry and optic disc reflectometry indicate that the loss of blood flow may exceed the tissue loss.[166] A study with combined retinal vessel oximetry and laser Doppler velocimetry showed that in neurogenic optic disc atrophy there is also a reduction of retinal metabolism and an overall decrease in retinal oxygen delivery of about 40%.[167]

Glaucoma

Migraine or an increased vasospastic reaction to cold is more common among patients with low-tension glaucoma than in the average population of the same age.[50,138] A marked rise in eye pressure, as often seen in angle-closure glaucoma, can be expected to cause partial ischemia in the optic nerve head, as well as in the retina, and may damage both of these tissues. The situation in chronic open-angle glaucoma may be very different. Both experimental and clinical studies support the assumption that optic nerve head blood flow is as efficiently autoregulated as retinal blood flow. However, these studies have been performed on healthy eyes and most likely under constant illumination. The metabolic demands on the retina under anesthesia and constant illumination are rather low, and under other conditions the eye may be more vulnerable to an increased IOP.[33] It is also possible that the autoregulation is deficient in the average elderly glaucoma patient. In one group of glaucoma patients studied with the blue field entoptoscope the upper limit for normal leukocyte velocity was an IOP of about 25 mm Hg compared to about 30 mm Hg in normal eyes.[84] Retinal blood flow may also be affected in glaucoma. A positive correlation between macular leukocyte velocity and visual function has also been reported.[176] Indirect studies of the optic nerve indicate that autoregulation in the optic disc vessels may also be disturbed.[140,160] It is worth noting that if autoregulation is deficient, reducing IOP and thus increasing ocular perfusion should be a rational therapeutic approach.

Diabetes mellitus

In diabetic retinopathy one may expect changes in retinal blood flow that differ in magnitude depending on the stage of the disease. In diabetic dogs without retinopathy, retinal blood flow was significantly reduced.[174] A similar reduction of retinal blood flow was not seen in patients,[83] but there are many indications that a disturbed retinal blood flow exists in diabetes. Reduced retinal vasoconstriction in response to breathing oxygen is an early sign in diabetes,[93] and the normal reduction of retinal blood flow observed during hyperoxia is progressively impaired in diabetic patients with retinopathy.[82] Arterial flow pulsatility is reduced in mild retinopathy,

but increases with progression and becomes above normal in severe retinopathy.[58] Furthermore, there is a progressive reduction in macular leukocyte velocity in eyes with nonproliferative diabetic retinopathy.[146] The autoregulatory response of retinal blood flow to an increased IOP is also progressively impaired in diabetics.[173] The effects of photocoagulation on the retinal vessels provide other indications of reduced blood flow in eyes with severe retinopathy. After photocoagulation, arterial pulsatility and venous diameters are reduced,[56] and the response to hyperoxia is improved.[80] Improved facilities for determinations of retinal blood flow may well become a valuable tool in gauging the effect of surgical or medical treatment of diabetic retinopathy.[81]

REFERENCES

1. Abdel-Latif AA, Akhtar RA, Yousufzai SYK, et al: Substance P and IP₃, cAMP and contraction in iris sphincter of different mammalian species, Proc Int Soc Eye Res 6:227, 1990.
2. Alder VA, Cringle SJ: The effect of the retinal circulation on vitreal oxygen tension, Curr Eye Res 4:121, 1985.
3. Alder VA, Cringle SJ, Constable IJ: The retinal oxygen profile in cats, Invest Ophthalmol Vis Sci 24:30, 1983.
4. Alm A: Effects of norepinephrine, angiotensin, dihydroergotamine, papaverine, isoproterenol, nicotinic acid and xanthinol nicotinate on retinal oxygen tension in cats, Acta Ophthalmol 50:707, 1972.
5. Alm A: The effect of sympathetic stimulation on blood flow through the uvea, retina, and optic nerve in monkeys, Exp Eye Res 25:19, 1977.
6. Alm A: The effect of topical l-epinephrine on regional ocular blood flow in monkeys, Invest Ophthalmol Vis Sci 19:487, 1980.
7. Alm A, Bill A: Blood flow and oxygen extraction in the cat uvea at normal and high intraocular pressures, Acta Physiol Scand 80:19, 1970.
8. Alm A, Bill A: The oxygen supply to the retina, I, Effects of changes in intraocular and arterial blood pressures and in arterial Po₂ and Pco₂ on the oxygen tension in the vitreous body of the cat, Acta Physiol Scand 84:261, 1972a.
9. Alm A, Bill A: The oxygen supply to the retina, II, Effects of high intraocular pressure and of increased arterial carbon dioxide tension on uveal and retinal blood flow in cats: a study with labelled microspheres including flow determinations in brain and some other tissues, Acta Physiol Scand 84:306, 1972b.
10. Alm A, Bill A: The effect of stimulation of the sympathetic chain on retinal oxygen tension and uveal, retinal and cerebral blood flow in cats, Acta Physiol Scand 88:84, 1973.
11. Alm A, Bill A: Ocular and optic nerve blood flow at normal and increased intraocular pressures in monkeys (Macaca irus): a study with radioactively labelled microspheres including flow determinations in brain

and some other tissues, Exp Eye Res 15:15, 1973.

12. Alm A, Bill A, Young FA: The effects of pilocarpine and neostigmine on the blood flow through the anterior uvea in monkeys: a study with radioactively labelled microspheres, Exp Eye Res 15:31, 1973.

13. Alm A, Törnquist P, Mäpea O: The uptake index method applied to studies on the blood-retinal barrier, II, Transport of several hexoses by a common carrier, Acta Physiol Scand 113:81, 1981.

14. Alm A, Törnquist P, Stjernschantz J: Radioactively labeled microspheres in regional ocular blood flow determinations, Bibl Anat 16:24, 1977.

15. Ambache N, Kavanagh L, Whiting J: Effect of mechanical stimulation on rabbit eyes: release of active substance in anterior chamber perfusate, J Physiol 176:378, 1965.

16. Ascher KW: The aqueous veins, Springfield IL: Charles C Thomas, Publisher, 1961.

17. Ashton N: Lecture, Glasgow, Scotland, 1968, William Mackenzie Centenary Symposium.

18. Bellhorn RW: Permeability of blood-ocular barriers of neonatal and adult cats to fluorescein-labeled dextrans of selected molecular sizes, Invest Ophthalmol Vis Sci 21:282, 1981.

19. Bernstein MH, Hollenberg MJ: Fine structure of the choriocapillaris and retinal capillaries, Invest Ophthalmol 4:1016, 1965.

20. Bill A: Aspects of physiological and pharamacological regulation of uveal blood flow, Acta Soc Med Ups 67:122, 1962.

21. Bill A: Aspects of regulation of the uveal venous pressure in rabbits, Exp Eye Res 1:193, 1962.

22. Bill A: Autonomic nervous control of uveal blood flow, Acta Physiol Scand 56:70, 1962.

23. Bill A: A method for quantitative determination of blood flow through the cat uvea, Arch Ophthalmol 67:156, 1962.

24. Bill A: Quantitative determination of uveal blood flow in rabbits, Acta Physiol Scand 55:101, 1962.

25. Bill A: Blood pressure in the ciliary arteries of rabbits, Exp Eye Res 2:20, 1963.

26. Bill A: The uveal venous pressure, Arch Ophthalmol 69:780, 1963.

27. Bill A: Capillary permeability to and extravascular dynamics of myoglobin, albumin and gammaglobulin in the uvea, Acta Physiol Scand 73:204, 1968.

28. Bill A: A method to determine osmotically effective albumin and gammaglobulin concentrations in tissue fluids, its application to the uvea and a note on the effects of capillary "leaks" on tissue fluid dynamics, Acta Physiol Scand 73:511, 1968.

29. Bill A: Effects of acetazolamide and carotid occlusion on the ocular blood flow in unanesthetized rabbits, Invest Ophthalmol 13:954, 1974.

30. Bill A: Blood circulation and fluid dynamics in the eye, Physiol Rev 55:383, 1975.

31. Bill A, Linder M, Linder J: The protective role of ocular sympathetic vasomotor nerves in acute arterial hypertension, in Proceedings of the Ninth European Conference on Microcirculation, Antwerp, Belgium, 1976, Bibl Anat 16:30, 1977.

32. Bill A, Phillips CI: Uveoscleral drainage of aqueous humor in human eyes, Exp Eye Res 12:275, 1971.

33. Bill A, Sperber GO: Aspects of oxygen and glucose consumption in the retina; effects of high intraocular pressure and light, Graefe's Arch Clin Exp Ophthalmol 228:124, 1990.

34. Bill A, Sperber G, Ujiie K: Physiology of the choroidal vascular bed, Int Ophthalmol 6:101, 1983.

35. Bill A, Stjernschantz J, Alm A: Effects of hexamethonium, biperiden and phentolamine on the vasoconstrictive effects of oculomotor nerve stimulation in rabbits, Exp Eye Res 23:614, 1976.

36. Bill A, Törnquist P, Alm A: The permeability of the intraocular blood vessels, Trans Ophthalmol Soc UK 100:332, 1980.

37. Bill A, et al: Substance P-release on trigeminal nerve stimulation: effects on pupil, eye pressure and capillary permeability, Acta Physiol Scand 106:371, 1979.

38. Bishoff PM, Flower RW: Ten years experience with choroidal angiography using indocyanine green dye: a new routine examination or an epilogue? Doc Ophthalmol 60:235, 1985.

39. Bundgaard M: The three-dimensional organization of tight junctions in a capillary endothelium revealed by serial-section electron microscopy, J Ultrastruct Res 88:1, 1984.

40. Campochiaro PA, Sen A: Adenosine and its agonists cause retinal vasodilation and hemorrhage; implications for ischemic retinopathies, Arch Ophthalmol 107:412, 1989.

41. Carlson ES: Fenestrated subendothelial basement membranes in human retinal capillaries, Invest Ophthalmol Vis Sci 30:1923, 1989.

42. Chandra SR, Friedman E: Choroidal blood flow, II, The effects of autonomic agents, Arch Ophthalmol 87:67, 1972.

43. Cohan BE, Cohan S: Flow and oxygen saturation in the anterior ciliary vein of the dog eye, Am J Physiol 205:60, 1963.

44. Collier RH: Experimental embolic ischemia of the choroid, Arch Ophthalmol 77:683, 1967.

45. Crone C: The Malpighi lecture; from "Porositates carnis" to cellular microcirculation, Int J Microcirc Clin Exp 6:101, 1987.

46. Cunha-Vaz JG, Shakib M, Ashton N: Studies on the permeability of the blood-retinal barrier, Br J Ophthalmol 50:441, 1966.

47. Delori FC: Noninvasive technique for oximetry of blood in retinal vessels, Appl Optics 27:1113, 1988.

48. de Oliveira F: Pericytes in diabetic retinopathy, Br J Ophthalmol 50:134, 1966.

49. Dollery CT, et al: Focal retinal ischaemia, I, Ophthalmoscopic and circulatory changes in focal retinal ischaemia, Br J Ophthalmol 50:283, 1966.

50. Drance SM, Douglas GR, Wijsman, et al: Response of blood flow to warm and cold in normal and low-tension glaucoma patients, Am J Ophthalmol 105:35, 1988.

51. Eakins KE: Prostaglandin and nonprostaglandin mediated breakdown of the blood-aqueous barrier, Exp Eye Res 25 (Suppl.):483, 1977.

52. Eberli B, Riva CE, Feke GT: Mean circulation time of fluorescein in retinal vascular segments, Arch Ophthalmol 97:145, 1979.

53. Ehinger B: Adrenergic nerves to the eye and to related

structures in man and the cynomolgus monkey, Invest Ophthalmol 5:42, 1966.

54. Emi K, Pederson JE, Toris CB: Hydrostatic pressure of the suprachoroidal space, Invest Ophthalmol Vis Sci 30:233, 1989.

55. Fallon TJ, Maxwell CD, Kohner EM: Retinal vascular autoregulation in conditions of hyperoxia and hypoxia using the blue field entoptic phenomenon, Ophthalmol 92:701, 1985.

56. Feke GT, Green GJ, Goger DG, et al: Laser Doppler measurements of the effect of panretinal photocoagulation on retinal blood flow, Ophthalmol 89:757, 1982.

57. Feke GT, Tagawa H, Deupree DM, et al: Blood flow in the normal human retina, Invest Ophthalmol Vis Sci 30:58, 1989.

58. Feke GT, Tagawa H, Yoshida A, et al: Retinal circulatory changes related to retinopathy progression in insulin-dependent diabetes mellitus, Ophthalmol 92:1517, 1985.

59. Fenstermacher JD, Johnson JA: Filtration and reflection coefficients of the rabbit blood-brain barrier, Am J Physiol 211:341, 1966.

60. Ferrari-Dileo G: Beta$_1$ and beta$_2$ adrenergic binding sites in bovine retina and retinal blood vessels, Invest Ophthalmol Vis Sci 29:695, 1988.

61. Ferrari-Dileo G, Davis EB, Anderson DR: Biochemical evidence for cholinergic activity in retinal blood vessels, Invest Ophthalmol Vis Sci 30:473, 1989.

62. ffytche TJ, et al: Effects of changes in intraocular pressure on the retinal micro-vasculature, Br J Ophthalmol 58:514, 1974.

63. Flower RW: Injections technique for indocyanine green and sodium fluorescein dye angiography of the eye, Invest Ophthalmol Vis Sci 12:881, 1973.

64. Folkow B, Neil E, eds: Circulation, New York: Oxford University Press, 1971.

65. Forster BA, Ferrari-Dileo G, Anderson DR: Adrenergic alpha$_1$ and alpha$_2$ binding sites are present in bovine retinal blood vessels, Invest Ophthalmol Vis Sci 28:1741, 1987.

66. Frayser R, Hickam JB: Retinal vascular response to breathing increased carbon dioxide and oxygen concentrations, Invest Ophthalmol 3:427, 1964.

67. Freddo TF, Raviola G: Freeze-fracture analysis of the inter-endothelial junctions in the blood vessels of the iris in *Macaca mulatta*, Invest Ophthalmol Vis Sci 23:154, 1982.

68. Friedman E, Oak SM: Choroidal microcirculation in vivo, Bibl Anat 7:129, 1965.

69. Friedman E, Smith TR, Kuwabara T: Retinal microcirculation in vivo, Invest Ophthalmol 3:217, 1964.

70. Fujino T, Hamasaki DI: Effect of intraocular pressure on the electroretinogram, Arch Ophthalmol 78:757, 1967.

71. Funk R, Rohen JW: Scanning electron microscopic study on the vasculature of the human anterior eye segment, especially with respect to the ciliary processes, Exp Eye Res 51:651, 1990.

72. Furchgott RF: Role of endothelium in responses of vascular smooth muscle, Circ Res 53:557, 1983.

73. Furchgott RF, Zawadzki JV: The obligatory role of the endothelium in the relaxation of arterial smooth muscle by acetylcholine, Nature 398:373, 1980.

74. Gay AJ, Rosenbaum AL: Retinal artery pressure in asymmetric diabetic retinopathy, Arch Ophthalmol 75:758, 1966.

75. Geijer C, Bill A: Effects of raised intraocular pressure on retinal, prelaminar and retrolaminar optic nerve blood flow in monkeys, Invest Ophthalmol Vis Sci 18:1030, 1979.

76. Granstam E, Nilsson SFE: Non-adrenergic sympathetic vasoconstriction in the eye and some other facial tissues in the rabbit, Eur J Pharmacol 175:175, 1990.

77. Granstam E, Wang L, Bill A: Effects of endothelin on pupil size and intraocular pressure in the rabbit and the cat, Acta Physiol Scand 140:5AC4, 1990.

78. Grayson MC, Laties AM: Ocular localization of sodium fluorescein, Arch Ophthalmol 85:600, 1971.

79. Grotte G: Passage of dextran molecules across the blood-lymph barrier, Acta Chir Scand (Suppl)211:1, 1965.

80. Grunwald JE, Brucker AJ, Petrig BL, et al: Retinal blood flow regulation and the clinical response to panretinal photocoagulation in panretinal diabetic retinopathy, Ophthalmol 96:1518, 1989.

81. Grunwald JE, Brucker AJ, Schwartz SS, et al: Diabetic glycemic control and retinal blood flow, Diabetes 39:602, 1990.

82. Grunwald JE, Riva CE, Brucker AJ, et al: Altered retinal vascular response to 100% oxygen breathing in diabetes mellitus, Ophthalmol 91:1447, 1984.

83. Grunwald JE, Riva CE, Sinclair SH, et al: Laser Doppler velocimetry study of retinal circulation in diabetes mellitus, Arch Ophthalmol 104:991, 1986.

84. Grunwald JE, Riva CE, Stone RA, et al: Retinal autoregulation in open-angle glaucoma, Ophthalmol 91:1690, 1984.

85. Hasegawa Y, Hayashi K, Tokoro T, et al: Klinische Anwendung von Indozyanin-grün-Angiographie zur Diagnose choroidaler neovaskulärer Erkrankungen, Fortsch Ophthalmol 85:410, 1988.

86. Hayreh SS: The ophthalmic artery, III, Branches, Br J Ophthalmol 46:212, 1962.

87. Hayreh SS: Segmental nature of the choroidal vasculature, Br J Ophthalmol 59:631, 1975.

88. Hayreh SS: Optic disc edema in raised intracranial pressure, V, Pathogenesis, Arch Ophthalmol 95:1553, 1977.

89. Hayreh SS: Pathogenesis of optic nerve damage and visual field defects, in Heilman LK, Richardson KT, eds: Glaucoma, Stuttgart, West Germany, Georg Thieme Verlag KG, 1978.

90. Henkind P, de Oliveira F: Development of the retinal vessels in the rat, Invest Ophthalmol 6:520, 1967.

91. Hickam JB, Frayser R: A photographic method for measuring the mean retinal circulation time using fluorescein, Invest Ophthalmol 4:876, 1965.

92. Hickam JB, Frayser R, Ross J: A study of retinal venous blood oxygen saturation in human subjects by photographic means, Circulation 27:375, 1963.

93. Hickam JB, Sieker HO: Retinal vascular reactivity in patients with diabetes mellitus and atherosclerosis, Circulation 22:243, 1960.

94. Hillerdal M, Sperber GO, Bill A: The microsphere method for measuring low blood flows: theory and

computer simulations applied to findings in the rat cochlea, Acta Physiol Scand 130:229, 1987.

95. Holmberg Å: The ultrastructure of the capillaries in the ciliary body, Arch Ophthalmol 62:949, 1979.

96. Hoste AM, Boels PJ, Brutsaert DL, et al: Effect of alpha-1 and beta agonists on contraction of bovine retinal resistance arteries in vitro, Invest Ophthalmol Vis Sci 30:44, 1989.

97. Hudspeth AJ, Yee AG: The intercellular junctional complexes of retinal pigment epithelia, Invest Ophthalmol 12:354, 1973.

98. Huxley VH: Physiological regulation of capillary permeability, J Reconstr Microsurg 4:34, 1988.

99. Inoue A, Yanagisawa M, Kimura S, et al: The human endothelin family: three structurally and pharmacologically distinct isopeptides predicted by three separate genes, Proc Natl Acad Sci USA 86:2863, 1989.

100. Jayakody L, Senaratne M, Thomson A, et al: Endothelium-dependent relaxation in experimental atherosclerosis in the rabbit, Circ Res 60:251, 1987.

101. Kalsner S: Cholinergic constriction in the general circulation and its role in coronary artery spasm, Circ Res 65:237, 1989.

102. Khoobehi B, Peyman GA, Niesman MR, et al: Measurement of retinal blood velocity and flow rate in primates using a liposome-dye system, Ophthalmol 96:905, 1989.

103. Klein GJ, Baumgartner RH, Flower RW: An image processing approach to characterizing choroidal blood flow, Invest Ophthalmol Vis Sci 31:629, 1990.

104. Kloog Y, Ambar I, Sokolovsky M, et al: Sarafotoxin, a novel vasoconstrictor peptide: phosphoinositide hydrolysis in rat heart and brain, Science 242:268, 1988.

105. Krebs W, Krebs IP: Ultrastructural evidence for lymphatic capillaries in the primate choroid, Arch Ophthalmol 106:1615, 1988.

106. Krogsaa B, Lund-Andersen H, Mehlsen J, et al: Blood-retinal barrier permeability versus diabetes duration and retinal morphology in insulin dependent diabetic patients, Acta Ophthalmol 65:686, 1987.

107. Krogsaa B, et al: The blood-retinal barrier permeability in essential hypertension, Acta Ophthalmol 61:541, 1983.

108. Laties AM: Central retinal artery innervation, Arch Ophthalmol 77:405, 1967.

109. Leber T: Circulations and Ernährungsverhältnisse des Auges. In Graefe A, Saemisch T, eds: Handbuch der gesamten Augenheilkunde, Leipzig, Germany, Springer-Verlag, 1903.

110. Lee T-S, Hu K-Q, Chao T, et al: Characterization of endothelin receptors and effects of endothelin on diacylglycerol and protein kinase C in retinal capillary pericytes, Diabetes 38:1643, 1989.

111. Lemmingson W: Über das Vorkommen von Vasomotion im Retinalkreislauf, Graefes Arch Clin Exp Ophthalmol 176:368, 1968.

112. Linsenmeier RA: Effects of light and darkness on oxygen distribution and consumption in cat retina, J Gen Physiol 88:521, 1986.

113. MacCumber MW, Ross CA, Glaser BM, et al: Endothelin: visualization of mRNAs by in situ hybridization provides evidence for local action, Proc Natl Acad Sci 86:7285, 1989.

114. Mäepea O: Pressure in the anterior ciliary artery, choroidal veins and choriocapillaries, Exp Eye Res (In press).

115. Mäepea O, Bill A: The pressure in the episcleral veins, Schlemm's canal and the trabecular meshwork in monkeys: effects of changes in intraocular pressure, Exp Eye Res 49:645, 1989.

116. Majno G: Ultrastructure of the vascular membrane, in Handbook of physiology, sect 2: Circulation, vol 3, Baltimore, Williams & Wilkins, 1965, p 2293.

117. Mandahl A: Effects of substance P on regional ocular blood flow, intraocular pressure and blood-aqueous barrier in rabbits, Acta Ophthalmol 67:378, 1989.

118. Mandahl A, Bill A: Ocular responses to antidromic trigeminal stimulation, intracameral prostaglandin E1 and E2, capsaicin and substance P, Acta Physiol Scand 112:331, 1981.

119. Michaelson IC: Retinal circulation in man and animals, Springfield, IL: Charles C Thomas, Publisher, 1954.

120. Miller S, Steinberg RH: Transport of taurine, L-methionine and 3-0-methyl-D-glucose across frog retinal pigment eipthelium, Exp Eye Res 23:177, 1976.

121. Moncada S, Radomski MW, Palmer RMJ: Endothelium-derived relaxing factor; identification as nitric oxide and role in the control of vascular tone and platelet function, Biochem Pharmacol 37:2495, 1988.

122. Moncada S, Vane JR: Pharmacology and endogenous roles of prostaglandins endoperoxides, thromboxane A_2 and prostacyclin, Pharmacol Rev 30:293, 1979.

123. Morrison JC, DeFrank MP, Van Buskirk EM: Comparative microvascular anatomy of mammalian ciliary processes, Invest Ophthalmol Vis Sci 28:1325, 1987.

124. Neufeld AH, Jampol LM, Sears JL: Aspirin prevents the disruption of the blood-aqueous barrier in the rabbit eye, Nature 238:58, 1972.

125. Nielsen PJ, Benedito S, Prieto D, et al: Endothelium dependent relaxation of isolated bovine retinal small arteries in vitro, Invest Ophthalmol Vis Sci (Suppl) 31:170, 1990.

126. Niesel P: Messungen von experimentell erzeugten Aenderungen der Aderhautdurchblutung be Kaninchen, Basel, Switzerland, S Karger AG, 1962.

127. Nilsson S, Bill A: Role of uveal prostaglandins in the response to facial nerve stimulation, Acta Physiol Scand Suppl 508:59, 1982.

128. Nilsson SFE, Bill A: Vasoactive intestinal peptide (VIP): effects on the eye and on regional blood flow, Acta Physiol Scand 121:385, 1984.

129. Nilsson SFE, Linder J, Bill A: Characteristics of uveal vasodilation produced by facial nerve stimulation in monkeys, cats and rabbits, Exp Eye Res 40:841, 1985.

130. Nyborg NCB, Nielsen PJ, Prieto D, et al: Angiotensin II does not contract bovine retinal resistance arteries in vitro, Exp Eye Res 50:469, 1990.

131. O'Day DM, Fish MB, Aronson SB, et al: Ocular blood flow measurements by nuclide labelled microspheres, Arch Ophthalmol 86:205, 1971.

132. Oksala O: Effects of calcitonin gene-related peptide and substance P on regional blood blow in the cat eye, Exp Eye Res 47:283, 1988.

133. Olesen S-P, Clapham DE, Davies PF: Haemodynamic shear stress activates a K^+ current in vascular endothelial cells, Nature 331:168, 1988.

134. Palmer RMJ, Ashton DS, Moncada S: Vascular endothelial cells synthesize nitric oxide from L-arginine, Nature 333:664, 1988.

135. Pappenheimer JR: Passage of molecules through capillary walls, Physiol Rev 33:387, 1953.

136. Parver LM, Auker C, Carpenter DO: Choroidal blood flow as a heat dissipating mechanism in the macula, Am J Ophthalmol 89:641, 1980.

137. Parver LM, Auker CR, Carpenter DO: Choroidal blood flow, III, Reflexive control in human eyes, Arch Ophthalmol 101:1604, 1983.

138. Phelps CD, Corbett J: Migraine and low-tension glaucoma, Invest Ophthalmol Vis Sci 26:1105, 1985.

139. Phillips JW, Preston G, Delong RE: Effects of anoxia on cerebral blood flow in the rat brain: evidence for a role of adenosine in autoregulation, J Cerebr Blood Flow Metab 4:586, 1984.

140. Pillunat LE, Stodtmeister R, Wilmanns I, Christ T: Autoregulation of ocular blood flow during changes in intraocular pressure, Preliminary results, Graefe's Arch Clin Exp Ophthalmol 223:219, 1985.

141. Pournaras CJ, Riva CE, Tsacopoulos M, et al: Diffusion of O_2 in the retina of anesthetized miniature pigs in normoxia and hyperoxia, Exp Eye Res 49:347, 1989.

142. Quigley HA, Hohman RM, Addicks EM: Quantitative study of optic nerve head capillaries in experimental optic disk pallor, Am J Ophthalmol 93:689, 1982.

143. Ralevic V, Milner P, Hudlicka O, et al: Substance P is released from the endothelium of normal and capsaicin-treated rat hind-limb vasculature, in vivo, by increased flow, Circ Res 66:1178, 1990.

144. Reddy VN: Dynamics of transport systems in the eye: Friedenwald Lecture, Invest Ophthalmol Vis Sci 18:1000, 1979.

145. Rees DD, Palmer RMJ, Moncada S: Role of endothelium-derived nitric oxide in the regulation of blood pressure, Proc Natl Acad Sci USA 86:3375, 1989.

146. Rimmer T, Fallon TJ, Kohner EM: Long-term follow-up of retinal blood flow in diabetes using the blue light entoptic phenomenon, Br J Ophthalmol 73:1, 1989.

147. Riva CE: Retinal blood flow: Laser Doppler velocimetry and blue field simulation technique, in Masters BR, ed: Noninvasive diagnostic techniques in ophthalmology, New York, Springer Verlag, 1990, pp 390-409.

148. Riva CE, Ben-Sira I: Injection method for ocular hemodynamic studies in man, Invest Ophthalmol Vis Sci 13:77, 1974.

149. Riva CE, Feke GT, Ben-Sira I: Fluorescein dye-dilution technique and retinal circulation, Am J Physiol 234:H315, 1978.

150. Riva CE, Feke GT, Eberli B, et al: Bidirectional LDV system for absolute measurements of retinal blood speed, Appl Opt 18:2302, 1979.

151. Riva CE, Grunwald JE, Petrig BL: Autoregulation of human retinal blood flow; an investigation with laser Doppler velocimetry, Invest Ophthalmol Vis Sci 27:1706, 1986.

152. Riva CE, Grunwald JE, Sinclair SH: Laser Doppler measurement of relative blood velocity in the human optic nerve head, Invest Ophthalmol Vis Sci 22:241, 1982.

153. Riva CE, Grunwald JE, Sinclair SH: Laser Doppler velocimetry study of the effect of pure oxygen breathing on retinal blood flow, Invest Ophthalmol Vis Sci 24:47, 1983.

154. Riva CE, Grunwald JE, Sinclair SH, et al: Blood velocity and volumetric flow rate in human retinal vessels, Invest Ophthalmol Vis Sci 26:1124, 1985.

155. Riva CE, Petrig B: Blue field entoptic phenomenon and blood velocity in the retinal capillaries, J Opt Soc Am 70:1234, 1980.

156. Riva CE, Petrig BL, Grunwald JE: Near infrared retinal laser Doppler velocimetry, Lasers Ophthalmol 1:211, 1987.

157. Riva CE, Pournaras CJ, Poitry-Yamate CL, et al: Rhythmic changes in velocity, volume, and flow of blood in the optic nerve head tissue, Microvasc Res 40:36, 1990.

158. Riva C, Ross B, Benedek GB: Laser Doppler measurements of blood flow in capillary tubes and retinal arteries, Invest Ophthalmol Vis Sci 11:936, 1972.

159. Riva E, Sinclair SH, Grunwald JE: Autoregulation of retinal circulation in response to decrease of perfusion pressure, Invest Ophthalmol Vis Sci 21:34, 1981.

160. Robert Y, Steiner D, Hendrickson P: Papillary circulation dynamics in glaucoma, Graefe's Arch Clin Exp Ophthalmol 227:436, 1989.

161. Robinson F, Riva CE, Grunwald JE, et al: Retinal blood flow autoregulation in response to an acute increase in blood pressure, Invest Ophthalmol Vis Sci 27:722, 1986.

162. Rudolphi KA, Keil M, Hinze H-J: Effect of theophylline on ischemically induced damage in mongolian gerbils: a behavioral and histopathological study, J Cerebr Blood Flow Metab 7:74, 1987.

163. Ruskell GL: Facial parasympathetic innervation of the choroidal blood vessels in monkeys, Exp Eye Res 12:166, 1971.

164. Sanders DR, et al: Quantitative assessment of postsurgical breakdown of the blood-aqueous barrier, Arch Ophthalmol 101:131, 1983.

165. Sears M: Miosis and intraocular pressure changes during manometry, Arch Ophthalmol 63:707, 1960.

166. Sebag J, Delori FC, Feke GT, et al: Anterior optic nerve blood flow decrease in clinical neurogenic optic atrophy, Ophthalmol 93:858, 1986.

167. Sebag J, Delori F, Feke GT, et al: Effects of optic atrophy on retinal blood flow and oxygen saturation in humans, Arch Ophthalmol 107:222, 1989.

168. Sedney SC: Photocoagulation in retinal vein occlusion, The Hague: W Junk, Publisher, 1976, pp 100-111.

169. Shabo AL, Maxell DS: The blood-aqueous barrier to tracer protein: a light and electron microscopic study of the primate ciliary process, Microvasc Res 4:142, 1972.

170. Shakib M, Ashton N: Ultrastructural changes in focal retinal ischemia, Br J Ophthalmol 50:325, 1966.

171. Shiose Y: Electron microscopic studies on blood-retinal and blood-aqueous barrier, Jpn J Ophthalmol 14:73, 1971.

172. Sinclair SH, Azar-Cavanagh M, Soper KA, et al: Investigation of the source of the blue field entoptic phenomenon, Invest Ophthalmol Vis Sci 30:668, 1989.

173. Sinclair SH, Grunwald JE, Riva CE, et al: Retinal vascular autoregulation in diabetes mellitus, Ophthalmology 89:748, 1982.

174. Small KW, Stefánsson E, Hatchell DL: Retinal blood flow in normal and diabetic dogs, Invest Ophthalmol Vis Sci 28:672, 1987.

175. Sperber GO, Bill A: Blood flow and glucose consumption in the optic nerve, retina and brain; effects of high intraocular pressure, Exp Eye Res 41:639, 1985.

176. Sponsel WE, DePaul KL, Kaufman PL: Correlation of visual function and retinal leukocyte velocity in glaucoma, Am J Ophthalmol 109:49, 1990.

177. Stefansson E, et al: Iris arteriolar diameters in hypoxia and hyperoxia: a photographic study in albino guinea pigs, Invest Ophthalmol Vis Sci 24:741, 1983.

178. Stjernschantz J, Bill A: Effect of intracranial stimulation of the oculomotor nerve on ocular blood flow in the monkey, cat and rabbit, Invest Ophthalmol Vis Sci 18:90, 1979.

179. Stone RA, Kuwayama Y: Substance P-like immunoreactive nerves in the human eye, Arch Ophthalmol 103:1207, 1985.

180. Stone RA, Laties AM, Emson PC: Neuropeptide Y and the ocular innervation of rat, guinea pig, cat and monkey. Neuroscience 17:1207, 1986.

181. Stone RA, McGlinn AM: Calcitonin gene-related peptide immunoreactive nerves in human and rhesus monkey eyes, Invest Ophthalmol Vis Sci 29:305, 1988.

182. Stone RA, Tervo T, Tervo K, et al: Vasoactive intestinal polypeptide-like immunoreactive nerves to the human eye, Acta Ophthalmol 64:12, 1986.

183. Sugita S, Hamasaki M, Higashi R: Regional difference in fenestration of choroidal capillaries in Japanese monkey eye, Jpn J Ophthalmol 26:47, 1982.

184. Szalay J: Effect of beta adrenergic agents on blood vessels of the rat iris, II, Morphological modifications of the vessel wall, Exp Eye Res 31:299, 1980.

185. Szalay J, Fliegenspan J, Zaager A, et al: Effect of beta adrenergic agents on blood vessels of the rat iris, I, Permeability to carbon particles, Exp Eye Res 31:289, 1980.

186. Tanaka T, Riva C, Ben-Sira I: Blood velocity measurements in human retinal vessels, Science 186:830, 1974.

187. Tillis TN, Murray DL, Schmidt GJ, et al: Preretinal oxygen changes in the rabbit under conditions of light and darkness, Invest Ophthalmol Vis Sci 29:988, 1988.

188. Törnquist P: Capillary permeability in cat choroid studied with the single injection technique, Acta Physiol Scand 106:425, 1979.

189. Törnquist P, Alm A: Retinal and choroidal contribution to retinal metabolism in vivo: a study in pigs, Acta Physiol Scand 106:351, 1979.

190. Törnquist P, Alm A: Carrier-mediated transport of amino acids through the blood-retinal and blood-brain barriers; a study with the uptake index method, Graefe's Arch Clin Exp Ophthalmol 224:21, 1986.

191. Törnquist P, Alm A, Bill A: Studies on ocular blood flow and retinal capillary permeability to sodium in pigs, Acta Physiol Scand 106:343, 1979.

192. Reference deleted in proofs.

193. Toussaint D, Kuwabara T, Cogan DG: Retinal vascular patterns, Arch Ophthalmol 65:575, 1961.

194. Vallance P, Collier J, Moncada S: Effects of endothelium-derived nitric oxide on peripheral arterial tone in man, Lancet 2:989, 1989.

195. Van Wylen DGL, Park TS, Rubio R, et al: Increases in cerebral interstitial fluid adenosine concentration during hypoxia, local potassium infusion, and ischemia, J Cerebr Blood Flow Metab 6:522, 1986.

196. Vegge T: A study of the ultrastructure of the small iris, Z Zellforsch Mikosk Anat 123:195, 1972.

197. Wilcox LM, Keough EM, Connolly RJ, et al: The contribution of blood flow by the anterior ciliary arteries to the anterior segment of the primate eye, Exp Eye Res 30:167, 1980.

198. Yanagisawa Y, Kirihara H, Kimura S, et al: A novel vasoconstrictor peptide produced by vascular endothelial cells, Nature 332:311, 1988.

199. Yoneya S, Tso MOM: Angioarchitecture of the human choroid, Arch Ophthalmol 105:681, 1987.

200. Zeimer RC, et al: A practical venomanometer: measurement of episcleral venous pressure and assessment of the normal range, Arch Ophthalmol 101:447, 1983.

201. Zeimer RC, Khoobehi B, Niesman MR, et al: A potential method for local drug and dye delivery in the ocular vasculature, Invest Ophthalmol Vis Sci 29:1179, 1988.

202. Zuckerman R, Weiter JJ: Oxygen transport in the bullfrog retina, Exp Eye Res 30:117, 1980.

CHAPTER
7

The Ciliary Epithelia and Aqueous Humor

JOSEPH CAPRIOLI, M.D.

The secretion of aqueous humor generates the intraocular pressure required for an optically efficient globe. The flow of aqueous provides nutrition for the avascular ocular tissues that it bathes: the posterior cornea, trabecular meshwork, crystalline lens, and anterior vitreous. The volume of aqueous in the anterior chamber turns over approximately once every 100 minutes. This constant flow of aqueous replenishes nutrients that have been taken up by avascular ocular tissues and carries away their metabolic wastes.

The aberrations of aqueous humor dynamics that produce abnormally high intraocular pressures have been studied at length in animals and humans. The elucidation of the biochemistry of the aqueous and the precise mechanisms of its production have lagged behind the study of its flow dynamics. Modern research techniques hold the promise of providing an understanding of the molecular physiology of the ciliary epithelia and of the biochemical functions of the aqueous.

Morphological and physiological approaches have been used to study the mechanisms of aqueous humor formation.[49,56,210,211] The wide-spread use of drugs that suppress aqueous formation to treat glaucoma (beta blockers, alpha$_2$-agonists, and carbonic anhydrase inhibitors) have provided additional impetus to investigate the mechanisms of aqueous humor production.

The ciliary processes secrete aqueous humor by active secretion of solutes into the posterior chamber by the nonpigmented epithelium (NPE). The exact nature by which the pigmented epithelium (PE) contributes to this process is yet unknown but undoubtedly helps provide substrates for the NPE. The tight junctions between the nonpigmented epithelial cells and the nonleaky endothelial cells of the iris capillaries exclude large molecules from the aqueous, and together they form the anterior blood-ocular barrier. This "blood-aqueous barrier" maintains the clarity of the aqueous required for the optical integrity of the eye. In this chapter we shall explore what is known about how the ciliary epithelia produce aqueous humor, the composition of the aqueous, and the functions of this unique fluid.

THE CILIARY EPITHELIA
Gross structure

The ciliary body, iris, and choroid comprise the vascular uveal coat of the eye. The ciliary body forms a ring along the inner wall of the globe and extends from the iris anteriorly to the ora serrata posteriorly. The largest mass of the ciliary body is smooth muscle that is arranged in three bundles: longitudinal, radial, and circular (Figs. 7-1 and 7-3). The ciliary body is anatomically divided into two segments: the anterior

ACKNOWLEDGMENT

Dr. Marvin Sears has sparked and kindled my interest in aqueous humor, glaucoma, and the pursuit of truth. I am indebted to him for his encouragement and guidance, and greatly value his enduring friendship.

Joseph Caprioli, M.D.

228

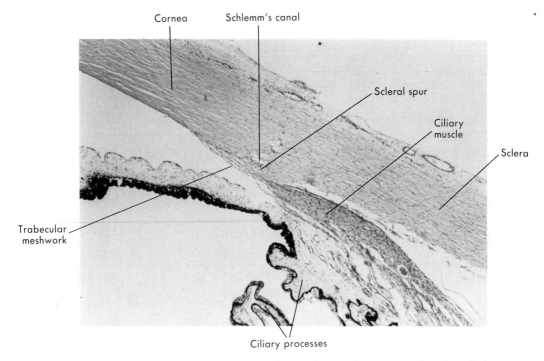

Cornea

Schlemm's canal

Scleral spur

Ciliary muscle

Sclera

Trabecular meshwork

Ciliary processes

FIG. 7-1 Low-power light photomicrograph of ciliary body in human eye, showing relationships of ciliary muscle, ciliary processes, iris, scleral spur, trabecular meshwork, and Schlemm's canal.

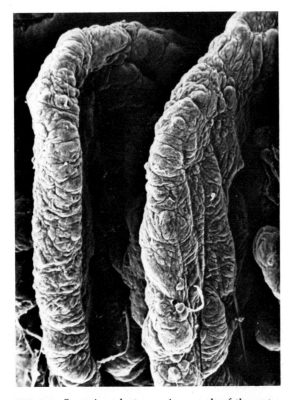

FIG. 7-2 Scanning electron micrograph of the anterior tips *(above)* of human ciliary processes. Notice the highly convoluted ridgelike structure. (Magnification × 1200.) (Courtesy Drs. N. Mori and M. Sears.)

pars plicata and the smooth posterior pars plana. The ciliary processes, approximately 70 in the human, project inward from the pars plicata region as radial ridges (Fig. 7-2). Each process is about 1 mm high, 2 mm long antero-posteriorly, and 0.5 mm wide.[102] The processes are highly involuted and have an overall surface area in rabbits of approximately 5.7 cm^2.[49] The ciliary body is firmly attached to the sclera at the scleral spur, which is located approximately 1.5 mm posterior to the corneolimbal junction. The supraciliary space is a potential space between the ciliary body and the sclera. A collection of fluid or blood in the supraciliary space will rotate the ciliary body away from the sclera, while the apex of the ciliary body remains hinged anteriorly at the scleral spur.

Blood supply

The ciliary body is well vascularized and has a high rate of blood flow.[5,41] Arterial supply is by the anterior ciliary and long posterior ciliary arteries, which anastomose to form the major arterial circle of the iris. The major arterial circle is located at the base of the iris in the ciliary body (Fig. 7-3). Woodlief suggested that direct anastomoses may be lacking between the anterior and long posterior ciliary arteries.[212] Each of the ciliary processes receives at least one, and usually several, small arterial branches from the

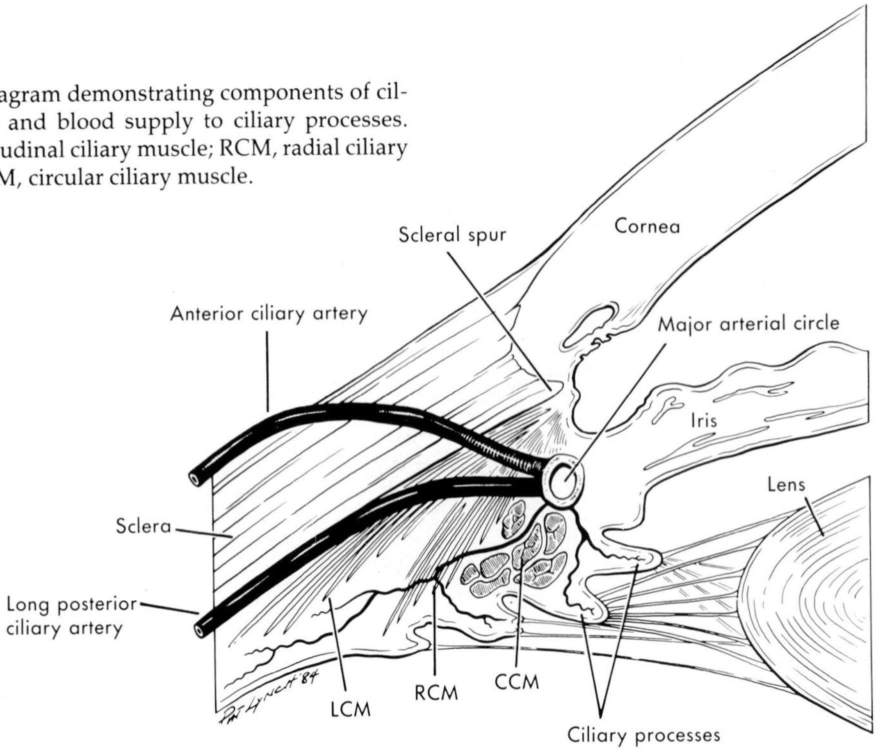

FIG. 7-3   Diagram demonstrating components of ciliary muscle and blood supply to ciliary processes. LCM, longitudinal ciliary muscle; RCM, radial ciliary muscle; CCM, circular ciliary muscle.

major arterial circle that supply a rich capillary network within the ciliary process stroma. The arterial supply in humans may be regulated by a sphincter mechanism located near the branching point of the arterioles from the major arterial circle.[212] Venules drain the ciliary processes into pars plana veins that empty posteriorly into the vortex system.

Nerve supply

The ciliary body is innervated by a plexus of myelinated and unmyelinated nerves that branch from the long posterior ciliary and short ciliary nerves that accompany the vessels of the same name. Parasympathetic fibers originate in the Edinger-Westphal nucleus of the third cranial nerve, travel with the inferior division of this nerve in the orbit, and synapse in the ciliary ganglion, within the short ciliary nerves, and in the ciliary body.[36] Postsynaptic fibers form extensive plexuses within the ciliary muscle and subserve accommodation. Sympathetic fibers synapse in the superior cervical ganglion and are distributed to the muscles and blood vessels of the ciliary body. Numerous unmyelinated nerve fibers surround the stromal vessels of the ciliary processes; these are likely noradrenergic and subserve vasomotion.[179] Sensory fibers arise

from the ophthalmic division of the trigeminal nerve and enter the ciliary body, but their distribution and function have not been well studied in the human.

Ultrastructure

The ciliary processes consist of a central core of highly vascularized connective tissue stroma and a specialized double layer of epithelium that covers the stromal core (Fig. 7-4). The capillaries of the stroma have large fenestrations of approximately 300 to 1000 Å and are somewhat less numerous than those of the choriocapillaris.[198] The inner epithelial layer (NPE) is in direct contact with the aqueous humor, and the outer pigmented epithelium (PE) lies between the NPE and the stroma. Bruch's membrane continues anteriorly beneath the retinal pigment epithelium and constitutes the basement membrane of the PE. The PE cells are cuboidal and contain numerous melanosomes but are relatively poor in intracellular organelles compared to the NPE. The internal limiting membrane of the ciliary body forms the basement membrane of the NPE. The NPE cells are columnar and contain numerous mitochrondria and rough and smooth endoplasmic reticulum characteristic of a highly metabolically active

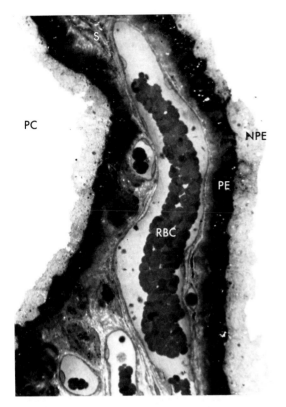

FIG. 7-4 Cross-section of human ciliary process. NPE, nonpigmented epithelium; PC, posterior chamber; PE, pigmented epithelium; RBC, red blood cells; S, stroma. (Magnification × 500.) (Courtesy Drs. N. Mori and M. Sears.)

cell. The cell membrane of the NPE cells has numerous basal infoldings and multiple convoluted lateral interdigitations (Fig. 7-5. See also Fig. 7-8).

Various types of intercellular junctions join the NPE and PE cells; desmosomes, gap junctions, puncta adherentia, and tight junctions are all present.[161] Tight junctions are always present near the apexes of the NPE cells. Many gap junctions are found between the lateral surfaces of the PE cells and less frequently between the lateral surfaces of the NPE cells. Gap functions and puncta adherentia are located between the PE and NPE cells. Desmosomes are found most frequently between the lateral surfaces of the NPE cells (Fig. 7-5. See also Fig. 7-8).

As a consequence of the invagination of the optic vesicle, the pigmented and nonpigmented ciliary epithelia lie apex to apex. Between the apexes are well developed ciliary channels that have been demonstrated with electron micros-

copy.[88] The physiology of these channels and how they may be related to fluid transport are unknown.

Blood-aqueous barrier

Physiologists have long conceptualized the presence of blood-brain and blood-ocular barriers. The classic experiments of Ehrlich, published in 1885[74] and elaborated by Goldmann,[95] demonstrated that trypan blue injected intravascularly in experimental animals stained all tissues except the central nervous system and stained the central nervous system only when injected in the subarachnoid space. Ocular physiologists noted a similar exclusion phenomenon in the eye; many substances present in the plasma were preferentially excluded from the aqueous humor. For example, the normal protein concentration in the aqueous is a tiny fraction of that in the plasma. "Ray" or "flare" evident on slit-lamp examination is caused by light scattered by increased levels of protein in the anterior chamber (Rayleigh scattering). In humans normal plasma protein levels are approximately 6 g/100 ml, compared with less than 20 mg/100 ml in the aqueous.[126,127] Bill[25,26] showed that albumin and other proteins pass through the ciliary vessel walls at a much faster rate than they enter the aqueous humor and concluded that a barrier to these substances existed at a site other than the vessel walls. Horseradish peroxidase has been used as a tracer to study the permeability characteristics of the ciliary processes.[160,186,191,201,202] This substance easily exits the vessels of the ciliary processes through endothelial fenestrations, but is blocked by the tight junctions at the apical segments of the NPE cells. Regional differences of permeability in the ciliary body have been noted. For instance, the epithelia of the anterior portions of the ciliary processes of the rabbit (the iridial processes) are less permeable than the epithelia of the pars plana.[202]

The tight junctions between the NPE cells together with the nonfenestrated iris vessels comprise the morphologic contributions to the blood-aqueous barrier. The junctions between the ciliary epithelial cells have been described by freeze-fracture techniques.[161] These consist of a network of anastomosing strands that firmly unite adjacent cells. The tight junctions, once thought to be somewhat "leaky" compared with other epithelia because of high hydraulic conductivity and low transport-potential measurements,[49,155] have subsequently been shown in edge-damage-free specimens in rabbits[35] to have lower values for hydraulic con-

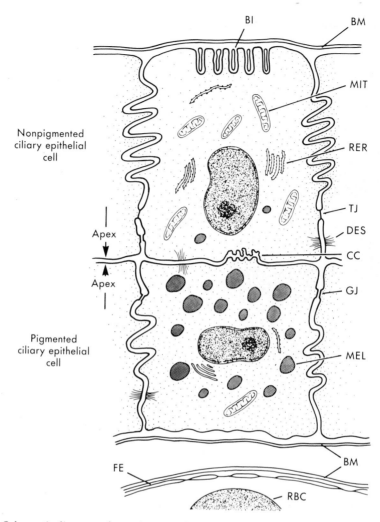

FIG. 7-5 Schematic diagram of nonpigmented and pigmented epithelial cells. Note apices of cells facing each other. BI, basal infoldings; BM, basement membrane; CC, ciliary channels; DES, desmosomes; FE, fenestrated capillary endothelium; GJ, gap junction; MEL, melanosome; MIT, microchondrion; RBC, red blood cell; RER, rough endoplasmic reticulum; TJ, tight junction.

ductivity than previously thought: 210 μm/sec compared with >4000 μm/sec. Electrical potential and fluid secretion measurements also suggest that the ciliary epithelia form a "tight" rather than "leaky" barrier and that fluid secretion is a result of an active process rather than ultrafiltration.[37] Destabilization of the blood-aqueous barrier with leakage of plasma proteins into the anterior chamber has important clinical consequences. Breakdown of the blood-aqueous barrier occurs after paracentesis of the anterior chamber in rabbits and primates.[3,11,16,133,152,153,190] Fragmentation of the tight junctions, particularly in the anterior pars plicata region of the ciliary body, occurs after paracentesis, with subsequent leakage of plasma protein into the aqueous.[16,152] This inflow of plasmalike, or "plasmoid," aqueous (also called "secondary" aqueous) is responsible, at least in part, for the increased intraocular pressure that is found after paracentesis in rabbits.[3]

A variety of noxious stimuli can break the blood-aqueous barrier. Ambache isolated a substance from the irides of various species that was released into the aqueous after trauma.[6,8] Later, this substance (which Ambache called irin) was found to contain both E and F prostaglandins.[7,10] Prostaglandins have been implicated in the irritative response after mechanical trauma to the eye, and cause miosis, vasodilation, release of protein into the aqueous, and increased intraocular pressure. This response can be blocked by pretreatment with inhibitors of prostaglandin synthesis such as aspirin or indomethacin.[23,24,70,149] Prostaglandins applied topically to the eye in sufficiently high concentrations cause breakdown of the tight junctions of the NPE and increase the protein content of the aqueous humor; the highest levels of protein are found in the posterior chamber.[97,150] Damage to the blood-aqueous barrier has been induced by intracarotid infusion of hyperosmotic agents; this causes separation of the ciliary epithelial layers, opening of the blood-aqueous barrier, and severe, permanent damage to the PE cells.[92,159] Disruption of the blood-aqueous barrier has been reported in the contralateral eyes of patients who have had cataract extraction and lens implantation surgery[146] and in the eyes of patients after argon laser trabeculoplasty.[124] Severe damage to the blood-aqueous barrier occurs with cyclodestructive procedures used to treat advanced glaucoma and is evidenced by the prolonged or chronic presence of aqueous flare.

In vitro preparations of the ciliary epithelia

Friedenwald used suspensions of bovine ciliary epithelia as early as 1943 to study the regional distribution of cytochrome oxidase.[87] DeRoetth, Ballantine, and others used similar preparations to study respiration, glycolysis, and oxidative phosphorylation.[12,13,59] Shimizu and coworkers studied oxidative metabolism of ciliary epithelia separated on a concentration gradient of colloidal silica.[188] Whole-mounted iris-ciliary body preparations were used to show that ascorbate and certain amino acids are transported against a concentration gradient. Ion transport and electrophysiological studies have been performed in an iris-ciliary body isolated in specialized transport (Ussing-type) chambers.[35,200] The latter preparation has been used to show that the ciliary epithelia constitute a moderately tight barrier to the movement of substances from the plasma rather than a leaky one.[35,37]

Cell cultures of ciliary epithelium have been used to study transepithelial transport. Separate cultures of PE and NPE (usually virally transformed or supplemented with hormonal growth factors) can be maintained.[44,45,111,173] Epithelial tissues reconstituted in cell culture can provide an accessible system for studying cell layers with normally complicated geometric relationships as a simplified monolayer in vitro. Isolated, mechanically stripped, pigmented and nonpigmented ciliary epithelium from the shark have provided convenient flat sheets of tissue to model epithelial transport.[209]

A completely new sort of bilayered ciliary epithelial preparation has recently been developed.[182] The bilayered rabbit ciliary epithelium is floated free after in vitro perfusion and mounted in an Ussing-type chamber for studies of its bioelectrical and vectorial transporting properties. This preparation holds particular promise for further study of the complex mechanisms involved in aqueous humor formation.

AQUEOUS HUMOR FORMATION

There are three mechanisms by which materials may cross an epithelial barrier: diffusion, ultrafiltration, and active transport. Diffusion of solutes across cell membranes occurs down a concentration gradient; lipid-soluble substances that easily penetrate cell membranes readily move across epithelia in this fashion. Ultrafiltration is a bulk flow of material across epithelia and is increased by augmenting its hydrostatic driving force. Active transport requires cellular energy (usually in the form of adenosine triphosphate) to secrete solute against a concentration gradient. Although all three processes may contribute to the formation of aqueous humor, the greatest contribution is from active transport of solute. The active solute pump sets up a concentration gradient that forces an osmotic flow of water into the posterior chamber.

Active secretion

Aqueous humor formation was once considered a simple process of diffusion or ultrafiltration of fluid from the plasma across the ciliary epithelia. The concentrations of solutes in the aqueous humor in comparison with their plasma concentrations are inconsistent with this view.[55,85,165] It is now well accepted that active transport of certain solutes by the ciliary epithelia is the most important process in the formation of aqueous humor. The rate of aqueous formation is a function of the rate of active solute transport by the ciliary epithelia.[53] The membrane-bound enzyme complex sodium-potassium adenosine triphosphatase (Na^+/K^+ ATPase) is an energy-dependent active transport system present in the NPE and is found in highest concentrations along the lateral cellular interdigitations.[48,110,187] Aqueous formation is substantially decreased after poisoning Na^+/K^+ ATPase with ouabain.[34,53,93,205] It is likely that Na^+ is the actively transported ion, though the relative rates of Cl^-

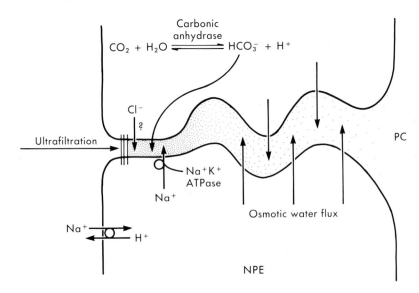

FIG. 7-6 Hypothetical diagram of aqueous production with standing gradient osmotic flow model. N_a^+/K^+ ATPase is located in highest concentration along lateral cellular interdigitations. Role of transport of Cl^- is still in question. NPE, nonpigmented epithelium; PC, posterior chamber.

and HCO_3^- transport remain unclear. Measurements of the electric potential across the ciliary epithelia indicate that the aqueous is positive with respect to the stroma; ouabain reduces this potential.[47,144] These data are consistent with the hypothesis that Na^+ is the primary mover. Active transport of Cl^- may also occur, although the magnitude of this transport is probably small compared with that of Na^+.[50] Interspecies differences in the aqueous-plasma ratios of Cl^- (e.g., high in humans, low in rabbits) might be explained by the relative proportions of Cl^- actively transported.[121] Transepithelial electrical measurements in the isolated rabbit iris-ciliary body indicate that Na^+/K^+ ATPase and HCO_3 are required for active ion transport.[128] The relationship between these experimental observations about ciliary metabolism and the actual site(s) of ion and fluid transport is complex because of the unique anatomic relationship between the ciliary epithelial layers.

Histochemical studies have demonstrated a number of active enzyme systems in the NPE layer. These include nucleotide phosphatases (especially ATPase), adenylate cyclase, and carbonic anhydrase.[22,110,145,187,199] There is greater development of intracellular organelles and a higher metabolic rate in the NPE compared with the PE.[38,185] The NPE probably plays the dominant role in aqueous humor formation, but the exact nature of its interaction with the PE remains unclear.

Fluid formation by transporting epithelia is described best by the standing gradient osmotic flow model proposed by Diamond and Bossert.[62,63] A steady-state, standing osmotic gradient is maintained in the lateral intercellular channel. Solute is at its highest concentration in the proximal channel near the tight junction (Fig. 7-6). The hypertonic fluid in the proximal region of the channel favors an osmotic flux of water into the channel. The solute concentration decreases from the proximal to the distal end of the channel as water enters; slightly hypertonic fluid flows into the posterior chamber as nascent aqueous. The successful explanation of aqueous production by this model requires the restriction of fluid and solute entry into the intercellular channels by the tight junctions of the NPE.

Ultrafiltration

Ultrafiltration of fluid from the plasma into the posterior chamber has been held by some to be responsible for as much as 70% of aqueous humor formation.[98,99,210] The following experimental observations indicate that ultrafiltration does not contribute significantly to aqueous humor formation. First, ouabain decreases aqueous formation by some 70% by inhibiting Na^+/K^+ ATPase[53]; this could not occur if the largest proportion of aqueous humor formation was ultrafiltrative. Second, Bill[27] pointed out that the hydrostatic and oncotic forces across the ciliary epithelia would, if anything, favor re-

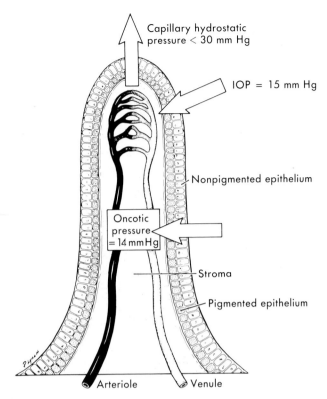

Capillary hydrostatic
pressure < 30 mm Hg

IOP = 15 mm Hg

Nonpigmented epithelium

Oncotic pressure = 14 mm Hg

Stroma

Pigmented epithelium

Arteriole   Venule

FIG. 7-7   Schematic diagram of hydrostatic forces involved in argument against ultrafiltration as important process in production of aqueous humor. (See text for discussion.)

absorption of aqueous humor into the ciliary process (Fig. 7-7). The ciliary process stroma has an oncotic pressure of approximately 14 mm Hg because of its protein content. If one assumes an intraocular pressure of 15 mm Hg, a capillary hydrostatic pressure in excess of 29 mm Hg would be required to drive an ultrafiltrate. Values for capillary hydrostatic pressure in the ciliary processes have been estimated by Bill[28] to be 27 to 28 mm Hg and by Cole[53] to be 25 to 33 mm Hg. Green and Pederson have calculated that a capillary pressure greater than 50 mm Hg would be necessary to promote ultrafiltration.[98] The values of capillary hydrostatic pressure in the ciliary processes and a consideration of the hydrostatic and oncotic forces involved do not favor ultrafiltration as an important mechanism of aqueous humor formation.

Carbonic anhydrase inhibition

Acetazolamide is a potent inhibitor of carbonic anhydrase, which catalyzes the reaction $H_2O + CO_2 \rightleftharpoons HCO_3^- + H^+$. Systemic treatment with acetazolamide and other carbonic anhydrase in-

hibitors decreases intraocular pressure by reducing aqueous humor formation.[17,19] It has been postulated that acetazolamide causes constriction of afferent ciliary arteries, thereby decreasing ultrafiltration and aqueous humor formation.[136] This is not a likely explanation of its mechanism of action based on the foregoing consideration of ultrafiltration. There is substantial evidence that acetazolamide directly affects the transport mechanisms of the ciliary epithelia.[53] Inhibition of carbonic anhydrase lowers the aqueous Cl^- concentration in primates and the HCO_3^- concentration in rabbits.[19,179] Acetazolamide decreases the rate of Na^+ and HCO_3^- transport into the posterior chamber by equimolar amounts, suggesting a linkage of the accession of these two solutes into the posterior chamber of dogs and monkeys.[137] Knowledge of the mechanism by which carbonic anhydrase activity is coupled to Na^+ and HCO_3^- movement into the posterior chamber is still sought. Several hypotheses could explain the decrease of active transport of sodium by the NPE: (1) inhibition of carbonic anhydrase

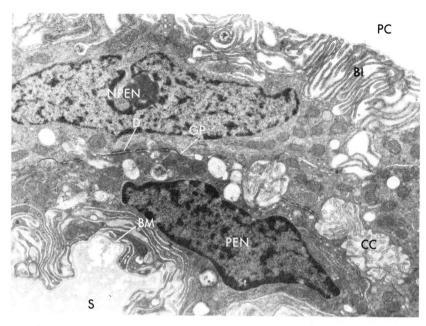

FIG. 7-8 Electron micrograph of pigmented and nonpigmented ciliary epithelia of the albino rabbit. Notice the convoluted ciliary channels between the pigmented and nonpigmented cells. BI, basal infoldings; BM, basement membrane; CC, ciliary channels; D, desmosome; GP, gap junction; NPEN, nonpigmented epithelium nucleus; PC, posterior chamber; PEN, pigmented epithelium nucleus; S, stroma. (Magnification × 14,400.) (Courtesy Drs. N. Mori and M. Sears.)

causes a decrease in HCO_3^- available for movement with Na^+ to the aqueous side to maintain electroneutrality; (2) a change in intracellular pH may inhibit Na^+/K^+ ATPase; and (3) decreased availability of H^+ produced by the reaction catalyzed by carbonic anhydrase decreases H^+/Na^+ exchange and reduces the availability of intracellular sodium for transport into the intercellular channel.

Control of aqueous formation

The homeostatic regulators of intraocular pressure remain largely unidentified. Clinical observations and experimental data suggest that neural or humoral pathways influence the steady-state level of intraocular pressure by altering the rate of aqueous production.[42,135,181] The enzyme-receptor complex adenylate cyclase, which is responsible for the formation of cyclic AMP, may play a role in the regulation of aqueous production.[15,39,42,100,176]

The rate of aqueous flow is lower in humans during sleep than during waking hours, with an average relative reduction during sleep of 45%.[167] This magnitude of flow reduction during sleep is similar to the suppression that can be achieved with carbonic anhydrase inhibitors or beta-blockers. Subsequent measurements of diurnal fluctuations of aqueous flare in rabbits have confirmed these findings.[143] The well-known diurnal fluctuation of intraocular pressure in humans can be reproduced in rabbits entrained to 12-hour-light–12-hour-dark cycles. The circadian rhythm of measured aqueous flow explains the magnitude of circadian intraocular pressure fluctuation.[192] The neural and humoral controls that underlie this diurnal rhythm of aqueous flow are not yet understood.

COMPOSITION OF NORMAL AQUEOUS HUMOR

Information about how aqueous humor is produced was first obtained by measuring the relative concentrations of substances in the aqueous and plasma.[56,204] Kinsey and Reddy[121] analyzed the composition of aqueous in the anterior and posterior chambers separately and made mathematical deductions about aqueous formation. The composition of aqueous depends on the nature of the freshly secreted fluid, the subsequent passive and active solute exchanges across the tissues it bathes, and the rate of its exit from the eye. The metabolic requirements of avascular tissues such as the cornea, lens, trabecular meshwork, and perhaps the anterior vitreous are met by the continuous flow of aqueous through the posterior and anterior chambers.

Exchange of substances between aqueous and surrounding tissues

The vitreous humor is a gel that consists of a network of collagen fibers bound by hyaluronic acid. Approximately 98% of this gel is water; diffusion of low-molecular-weight solutes such as inorganic ions, glucose, and amino acids is unimpeded through the vitreous.[157] The diffusion of solutes from the posterior aqueous into the vitreous contributes significantly to the concentration gradients of low-molecular-weight substances in the vitreous.[36]

Solute exchange between aqueous and cornea promotes normal corneal metabolism. Oxygen is supplied largely by the atmosphere. Although the limbal vasculature can supply some of the nutritional needs of the peripheral cornea,[141] the central cornea must derive its nutrition from the aqueous.[142] The flux of glucose into and lactic acid out of the cornea has been measured[142] and contributes to the lower concentration of lactic acid found in the anterior aqueous compared to the posterior aqueous.[121] Amino acids supplied to the cornea by aqueous probably enter by diffusion.[170] The corneal endothelium functions as a fluid pump to keep the cornea in a clear, deturgesced state. Approximately 10 μl/hr of fluid is pumped back into the anterior aqueous[82] by the corneal endothelium. This does not contribute significantly to the normal flow of aqueous humor, which occurs at the rate of approximately 150 μl/hr.

Removal of the crystalline lens causes an increase in the glucose content of the anterior chamber aqueous and a decrease in its lactic acid content in rabbits.[28,170] The lens takes up amino acids from the aqueous under normal conditions and may release accumulated amino acids into the aqueous when aqueous amino acid concentrations are low.[32,112,122] Active transport of potassium occurs across the anterior surface of the lens.[29] The lens thus alters the aqueous by using glucose, amino acids, and other solutes, releases metabolic products such as lactic acid, and may act as a homeostatic reservoir for amino acids.

Relatively little is known about transport processes across the iris. The anterior border of the iris does not consist of a continuous cell layer, and therefore the extracellular space of iris tissue is in continuity with the aqueous humor.

The nonfenestrated endothelial cells of iris vessels are joined by tight junctions and contribute to the blood-aqueous barrier. Although diffusional exchange across the iris vessels is likely, no data indicate that there is active transport of any material across these vessels.[29,30]

Osmolarity

The aqueous humor is slightly hyperosmotic to plasma in a number of mammalian species.[20,52,116,132,172] A recent study of pooled aqueous humor samples from the eyes of rhesus monkey showed no significant difference in osmolarity between the aqueous and plasma.[91] This result in pooled samples does not reflect the osmolarity of the aqueous near the surface of the ciliary epithelia, where local solute concentrations may be much higher. No significant differences in osmolarity between samples of anterior and posterior chamber aqueous have been found.[117]

Electrolytes

The concentrations of electrolytes in anterior and posterior aqueous and in plasma are shown in Table 7-1. Most studies have shown the Na^+ concentration in plasma and aqueous to be similar, although there have been a few reports of a slight excess of Na^+ in the aqueous.[51,91] Despite equimolar concentrations of Na^+ in aqueous and plasma, a slightly higher effective osmotic pressure caused by Na^+ occurs in the aqueous humor when the Gibbs-Donnan effect is taken into account. (For a discussion of the Gibbs-Donnan equilibrium with respect to the aqueous see Kinsey[117] and Sears.[179]) When evaluating the concentrations of electrolytes as they may reflect aqueous humor formation, it is not the concentration of anterior or even posterior aqueous that is crucial; it is the concentration adjacent to NPE cells, particularly in the intercellular channels, that is important. Actual measurements of concentration gradients in this microenvironment await the development of more advanced techniques.

Significant species differences exist regarding the concentration of the predominant anions in the aqueous. In humans there is an apparent excess of Cl^- and deficit of HCO_3^- in relation to their plasma concentrations. In rabbits the reverse situation holds.[118] Active Cl^- transport across the isolated ciliary body of the cat has been reported.[103,104] However, the role of active Cl^- transport in the formation of aqueous humor remains speculative. The apparent interspecies differences in the aqueous/plasma distribution of Cl^- may depend on the relative pro-

TABLE 7-1 Concentrations of Inorganic Substances in the Aqueous Humor

Substance	Concentration			Species	Investigator
	Anterior aqueous	Posterior aqueous	Plasma		
Bicarbonate (μmol/ml)	27.7	34.1	24.0	Rabbit	Kinsey,[117] 1953
	33.6		27.4	Rabbit	Davson,[57] 1962
	20.2		27.5	Human	DeBernadinis et al.,[58] 1965
	22.5		18.8	Monkey	Gaasterland et al.,[91] 1979
Chloride (μmol/ml)	131.6		124.0	Human	Remkey,[168] 1956, 1957
	105.7		106.2	Rabbit	Cole,[46] 1959
	131.0		107.0	Human	DeBernadinis et al.,[58] 1965
	105.1	100.0	111.8	Rabbit	Kinsey and Reddy,[121] 1964
	124.8		107.3	Human	Gaasterland et al.,[91] 1979
Calcium (μmol/ml)	1.7		2.6	Rabbit	Davson,[57] 1962
	2.5	2.5	4.9	Monkey	Bito,[29] 1970
Hydrogen ion (pH)	7.60	7.57	7.40	Rabbit	Kinsey and Reddy,[121] 1964
	7.49			Monkey	Gaasterland et al.,[91] 1979
Magnesium (μmol/ml)	0.8	·	1.0	Rabbit	Davson,[57] 1962
	1.2	1.3	1.2	Monkey	Bito,[29] 1970
	0.8		0.7	Monkey	Gaasterland et al.,[91] 1979
Oxygen (mm Hg)	55		100-500	Rabbit	Heald and Langham,[101] 1956
	53		*	Human	Kleifeld and Neumann,[122] 1959
	30		77	Rabbit	Wegener and Moller,[208] 1971
	32		*	Rabbit	Stefansson et al.,[194] 1983
Phosphate (μmol/ml)	0.62		1.11	Human	Walker,[207] 1933
	0.86	0.57	1.11	Rabbit	Constant and Falch,[54] 1963
	0.89	0.52	1.49	Rabbit	Kinsey and Reddy,[121] 1964
	0.14		0.68	Monkey	Gaasterland et al.,[91] 1979
Potassium (μmol/ml)	5.1	5.6	5.6	Rabbit	Reddy and Kinsey,[162] 1960
	5.2		5.5	Rabbit	Davson,[57] 1962
	3.6	4.1	4.2	Monkey	Bito,[29,31] 1970
	3.9		4.0	Monkey	Gaasterland et al.,[91] 1979
Sodium (μmol/ml)	146	144		Rabbit	Kinsey and Reddy,[121] 1964
	143		146	Rabbit	Kinsey and Reddy,[121] 1964
	145	150	144	Sheep	Cole,[51] 1970
	153	153	152	Dog	Maren,[137,138] 1976, 1977
	152		148	Monkey	Gaasterland et al.,[91] 1979

*Breathing room air.

portions of Na^+ and Cl^- actively transported into the posterior chamber.[119]

Glucose and lactate

The aqueous concentration of glucose is approximately 80% of that in plasma (Table 7-2). Glucose probably enters the aqueous by simple diffusion. Transport of glucose across the ciliary body in the streptozotocin-diabetic rat is increased, probably a result of an increase in the permeability of the ciliary epithelia in this disease.[67] Glucose diffuses into the cornea, where its concentration in corneal endothelium and the extracellular stromal space is approximately half that of the aqueous.[166] Lactic acid is found

in the anterior chamber in much higher levels than in plasma. Lactate enters the posterior chamber readily across the ciliary epithelia, but does not accumulate in the posterior chamber appreciably above the plasma level. Tracer studies indicate that the metabolism of glucose by the ciliary epithelia and retina, in addition to the lens and cornea, contributes significantly to the lactate content of the aqueous.[169]

Oxygen

Estimates of oxygen tension in aqueous humor range between 13 and 80 mm Hg depending on the method used.[101,112,123] Continuous measurements of oxygen tension in the mid-anterior

TABLE 7-2 Concentrations of Organic Substances in Aqueous Humor

Substance	Concentrations			Species	Investigator
	Anterior aqueous	Posterior aqueous	Plasma		
Ascorbate (μmol/ml)	0.96	1.30	0.02	Rabbit	Kinsey,[117] 1953
	1.06		0.04	Human	DeBernadinis et al.,[58] 1965
	1.18		0.02	Monkey	Gaasterland et al.,[91] 1979
Citrate (μmol/ml)	0.38-0.46			Rabbit	Granwall,[96] 1937
	0.12			Human	Granwall,[96] 1937
Creatinine (μmol/ml)	0.18		0.18	Horse	Duke-Elder,[68] 1927
	0.11			Rabbit	Furuichi,[90] 1961
	0.04		0.03	Monkey	Gaasterland et al.,[91] 1979
Glucose (μmol/ml)	4.9		5.3	Rabbit	Reddy and Kinsey,[162] 1960
	2.8		5.9	Human	DeBernadinis et al.,[58] 1965
	6.9		7.2	Rabbit	Reim et al.,[166] 1967
	3.0		4.1	Monkey	Gaasterland et al.,[91] 1979
Hyaluronate (μg/ml)	4.0			Ox	Duke-Elder and Goldsmith,[69] 1951
	4.4			Cattle	Laurent,[129] 1981
	1.1			Human	Laurent,[129] 1981
Lactate (μmol/ml)	12.1	11.2	8.2	Rabbit	Kinsey,[117] 1953
	9.3	9.9	10.3	Rabbit	Reddy and Kinsey,[162] 1960
	4.5		1.9	Human	DeBernadinis et al.,[58] 1965
	9.9	9.0	5.6	Rabbit	Riley,[169] 1972
	4.3		3.0	Monkey	Gaasterland et al.,[91] 1979
Protein (mg/100 ml)	13.5			Human	Krause and Raunio,[126] 1969
	100.3			Rat	Stjernschantz et al.,[196] 1973
	33.3			Monkey	Gaasterland et al.,[91] 1979
	25.9			Rabbit	Dernouchamps,[60] 1982
	23.7			Human	Dernouchamps,[60] 1982
Urea (μmol/ml)	6.3	5.8	7.3	Rabbit	Kinsey,[117] 1953
	7.0		9.1	Rabbit	Davson,[57] 1962
	6.1		7.3	Monkey	Gaasterland et al.,[91] 1979

chamber with a polarographic method yield values of 30 to 40 mm Hg.[193,194] Polymethylmethacrylate corneal contact lenses produce outer corneal hypoxia by restricting access of atmospheric oxygen to the cornea. Under these circumstances an increase in the flux of oxygen from the anterior chamber increases and the partial pressure of oxygen in the aqueous humor decreases.[193] Topical epinephrine causes a significant decrease in aqueous humor oxygen tension,[194] probably the result of vasoconstriction in the anterior uvea.[4,41]

Ascorbate

The high ascorbate content of the aqueous humor of many species has been an enigma for years.[14,86] Linner[134] suggested that the amount of ascorbate secreted into the aqueous may depend directly on the quantity reaching the site of se-cretion. He used this compound to estimate changes in the rate of plasma flow through the ciliary processes, similar to the way in which p-aminohippuric acid was used in studies of renal blood flow. Kinsey[115] demonstrated that ascorbate in the aqueous increases to a certain limiting level (approximately 50 mg/100 ml) with increasing concentration in the blood. With higher blood levels, no further increase occurs in the aqueous concentration of ascorbate, even though the concentration in the blood is more than twice that of the aqueous. Furthermore, the isolated ciliary body can accumulate ascorbate against a concentration gradient.[18,43] The transepithelial transport of ascorbate appears to require energy and a Na^+ gradient. These observations show that ascorbate is secreted actively by a specific, saturable transport mechanism.

The functions of ascorbate in the eye remain

speculative. Sears's experiments[178] suggested a relationship between ascorbate and the storage of catecholamines in the iris. The lens epithelium actively takes up ascorbate, though the reason for this is unknown.[66] Ascorbate in the aqueous may serve as an antioxidant, regulate the sol-gel balance of mucopolysaccharides in the trabecular meshwork,[133] or serve to partially absorb ultraviolet radiation.[171] Diurnal mammals have high aqueous ascorbate levels, whereas nocturnal mammals do not; the diurnal species of spiny mice has an aqueous ascorbate concentration 35 times higher than its closely related nocturnal species.[125] It has therefore been suggested that ascorbate may help protect the eye from harmful effects of ultraviolet light.

Amino acids

The concentrations of amino acids in the aqueous humor in rabbits, monkeys, and humans are summarized in Table 7-3. In the rabbit the concentration of most amino acids in the aqueous is higher than that in plasma,[163] consistent with active secretion into the aqueous. However, certain species (e.g., dogs) have lower concentrations of amino acids in the aqueous than in plasma.[33] The relative deficiency of amino acids in the aqueous of some species may be caused by a sink effect of the vitreous, while active transport of amino acid across the ciliary epithelia probably occurs in all mammalian species.[65,164,206] Kinsey and Reddy[120] postulated at least three transport systems for amino acids: one each for the basic, acidic, and neutral groups. It was later discovered that the kidney has at least four genetically determined mechanisms for amino acid transport: a neutral system, a basic system, an acidic system, and an amino-glycine system.[183] A statistical study of the covariation of the concentration of amino acids and related compounds in human aqueous suggested the existence of six transport systems in the ciliary epithelia: three independent mechanisms for neutral amino acids and independent

TABLE 7-3   Concentrations of Amino Acids in Aqueous Humor and Aqueous/Plasma Ratio in Rabbits, Monkeys, and Humans

Amino acid (µmol/kg H₂O)	Rabbit* Aqueous	Rabbit* Aqueous/plasma	Monkey† Aqueous	Monkey† Aqueous/plasma	Human‡§ Aqueous	Human‡§ Aqueous/plasma
Alanine	480	1.59	208.5	0.76	306	0.94
Arginine	272	2.83	51.0	0.49	105	1.50
Aspartate	55	1.90	Trace	—	—	—
Citrulline	—	—	4.0	0.12	—	—
Cysteine	—	—	217.0	1.01	—	—
Glutamate	295	1.66	13.0	0.18	9	0.19
Glycine	614	0.52	44.5	0.12	24	0.11
Histidine	210	1.81	40.5	0.45	67	0.85
Isoleucine	116	1.04	47.5	0.82	65	1.30
Leucine	174	1.07	110.5	1.16	139	1.42
Lysine	423	2.00	85.0	0.53	159	0.64
Methionine	23	1.64	46.5	1.42	44	2.54
Methylhistidine	—	—	8.5	0.27	—	—
Ornithine	—	—	9.0	0.25	—	—
Phenylalanine	97	1.00	73.0	1.45	93	2.01
Proline	267	0.83	27.0	0.16	44	0.19
Serine	585	1.39	718.0	1.38	—	—
Taurine	—	—	11.5	0.09	66	1.02
Threonine	138	0.84	61.5	0.83	128	1.17
Tryptophan	24	1.85	11.5	0.62	—	—
Tyrosine	101	1.74	65.0	1.26	91	1.84
Valine	230	1.18	167.0	1.02	285	1.35

*From Reddy DVN, Rosenberg C, Kinsey VE: Exp Eye Res 1:175, 1961.[163]
†From Gaasterland DR, et al: Invest Ophthalmol Vis Sci 18:1139, 1979.[91]
‡From Ehlers N, Schonheyder F: Acta Ophthalmol [Suppl.]123:179, 1974.[73]
§Aqueous samples were taken just prior to cataract extraction in 30 patients.

mechanisms for basic amino acids, acidic amino acids, and urea.[72] Although it may be concluded that amino acids enter the posterior chamber across the ciliary epithelia by an active process, the specific transport systems have not been defined.

Proteins

The blood-aqueous barrier normally limits the protein of aqueous humor to less than 1% of its plasma concentration. The aqueous protein composition differs from that of plasma: lower-molecular-weight proteins such as albumin and the beta-globulins are more prominent in the electrophoretic pattern of normal aqueous. The heavy-molecular-weight proteins such as beta-lipoproteins and heavy immunoglobulins are present only in trace quantities. The albumin/globulin ratio of the aqueous is many times higher than that of the plasma because of the exclusion of heavy globulin.[196] Dernouchamps[60] found that aqueous/plasma ratios for various proteins were inversely proportional to the molecular weight of the proteins; this relationship did not hold in cases in which the aqueous protein level was higher than 1 g/100 ml because of inflammation. Based on these protein studies, it was calculated that the blood-aqueous barrier behaves as a semiporous membrane with a pore radius of about 104 Å. In patients with uveitis and aqueous humor protein levels greater than 1 g/100 ml there has been total breakdown of the selectivity of the blood-aqueous barrier, and the aqueous humor protein fractions become qualitatively similar to those of plasma.[127] Recently, diffusion of proteins from the ciliary process stroma through the iris stroma and into the aqueous humor has been proposed to account for the major fraction of protein in normal rabbit aqueous.[84]

Immunoglobulin levels in the aqueous of normal and diseased eyes have been measured.[81,94,184] Immunoglobulin (Ig) G normally is found in the aqueous humor in a concentration of approximately 3 mg/100 ml.[81] IgD, IgA, and IgM are not normally present in detectable amounts because of their larger size. In patients with uveitis levels of IgG tend to increase, and IgM and IgA become detectable.[94] Complement can be found in minute quantities in normal human aqueous, which contains functional C2, C6, and C7 fractions.[147]

Primary (normal) aqueous humor contains only traces of the components of the coagulation and fibrinolytic systems, with the exception of plasminogen and plasminogen proactivator, that are contained in primary aqueous in signif-

icant amounts. Only traces of the inhibitors of plasminogen activation are found in normal aqueous.[154] The presence of plasminogen and plasminogen proactivator and the paucity of their inhibitors may help keep the aqueous outflow pathways free of fibrin. Secondary (diseased) aqueous contains considerable amounts of all the major components of coagulation and fibrinolysis. Recent evidence suggests that human aqueous humor promotes coagulation by shortening the prothrombin and partial thromboplastin times, and may act as a procoagulant rather than a thromboplastin-like substance.[105,112] The unique properties of the aqueous are responsible for the difference in evolution of intracameral clots compared to intravascular clots; true histologic organization of the intracameral clot does not take place during the first 7 days after clot formation.[40] Secondary aqueous humor stimulates the proliferation of cultured corneal endothelial cells and may play a role in cellular regeneration after ocular injury.[130]

The alpha and gamma lens crystallines are present in small amounts in the aqueous humor of eyes with clear lenses. The concentration of these lens crystallines increases in eyes with cataract, which indicates that these proteins may leak through the intact lens capsule.[89,174]

Lipids

Lipids were first detected in the aqueous humor in 1832 by Berzelius,[21] who found traces of fat in bovine aqueous. Modern studies have demonstrated less than 1 mg/100 ml of lipoprotein in aqueous.[195] Lysophosphatidylcholine, sphingomyelin, and phosphatidylcholine were reported in the aqueous by Varma and Reddy.[203] A significant blood-aqueous barrier apparently exists for the phospholipids; their concentrations range from 1/30 to 1/2 of the corresponding plasma concentrations.[114]

Other substances

Other substances, such as hyaluronic acid,[129] sialic acid,[76] trivalent chromium ions,[77] vitamin B_{12},[2] endogenous corticosteroids,[151] and monoamine metabolites,[9] have been found in the normal aqueous humor of various species. The significance of their presence, if any, is unknown.

ALTERATIONS OF AQUEOUS HUMOR IN DISEASE
Intraocular malignancy

The aqueous protein profile of patients may be altered by intraocular malignancies. Retinoblastoma causes an increased globulin content of aqueous and a decreased albumin/globulin ratio, whereas nonmalignant inflammatory conditions are generally associated with a rise of the albumin fraction and an increase in the albumin/globulin ratio.[64] Lactic dehydrogenase (LDH) has been found in small quantities in the normal human aqueous. Isoenzymes 3, 4, and 5 predominate.[107] The aqueous/plasma ratio of LDH was reported to be greater than 1.50 in patients with retinoblastoma and less than 0.60 in a variety of other ocular conditions, including rubeosis iridis, persistent hyperplastic primary vitreous, retrolental fibroplasia, and malignant melanoma.[197] The source of aqueous LDH in patients with intraocular malignancy probably is the release and diffusion of cytosol enzymes into the surrounding medium by dying cells. Areas of necrosis are typically found in retinoblastomas, allowing more free enzyme to reach the aqueous.[78] The isoenzyme pattern of LDH in the aqueous and serum of patients with retinoblastoma does not help to identify the lesion, because this pattern is similar to normal aqueous.[1] Although aqueous LDH activity of eyes with other intraocular tumors (for example, melanoma) is not elevated compared with controls,[158] LDH release into the aqueous is not specific to retinoblastoma. Increased aqueous LDH levels have been measured in Coats' disease.[108] Recent reports indicate that aqueous and serum levels of enolase may be of value in the diagnosis of retinoblastoma and ocular malignant melanoma.[189]

Uveitis

Complement components found in increased amounts in the aqueous humor of inflamed eyes are increased in proportion to aqueous IgG levels. Immune complexes, which have been detected in the aqueous of patients with Fuchs's heterochromic iridocyclitis, other forms of endogenous uveitis, and sympathetic ophthalmia, were not found in the aqueous of a control group of 20 patients with senile cataract.[61] Aqueous immune complexes also have been demonstrated in experimental immunogenic uveitis.[106] Patients with active forms of toxoplasmosis and toxocariasis have specific antibodies against *Toxoplasma gondii* and *Toxocara canis* in their aqueous.[79,113,156] Serum and aqueous sialic acid levels are elevated in patients in the active and remission stages of Behçet's disease.[213] Raised levels of interleukin-6 were found in patients with Fuchs's heterochromic cyclitis and suggests that this substance may play a role as an inflammatory mediator in uveitis.[148]

Retinal disease

Tapetoretinal degenerations can cause specific abnormalities in the concentration of certain amino acids of the aqueous,[71] though the analysis of amino acid profiles of the aqueous has not generally been found to be of any diagnostic significance in chronic ocular diseases.[175] Glaucoma associated with rhegmatogenous retinal detachment was described by Schwartz in 1973.[177] The aqueous of such patients was subsequently found to contain outer segments of photoreceptor cells, and their presence in the trabecular meshwork has been thought to cause elevated intraocular pressure.[139,140]

Glaucoma

Heavy-molecular-weight soluble proteins have been detected in the aqueous of patients with phacolytic glaucoma. These proteins have a molecular weight greater than 150×10^6 daltons and have been postulated to increase IOP by obstructing aqueous outflow.[75,83] A 140,000 to 160,000 dalton protein has recently been reported in the aqueous of patients with primary open-angle glaucoma but not in the aqueous of control cataract patients.[131] If its presence is substantiated, any relationship of this protein to abnormalities of the aqueous outflow pathway will require investigation. The chemotactic activity of aqueous humor in glaucoma patients has been implicated in the failure of glaucoma filtering surgery from fibrosis.[109]

REFERENCES

1. Abramson DH, et al: Lactate dehydrogenase levels and isoenzyme patterns, Arch Ophthalmol 97:870, 1979.
2. Ainley RG, et al: Aqueous humor vitamin B_{12} and intramuscular cobalamins, Br J Ophthalmol 53:854, 1969.
3. Al-Ghadyan A, Mead A, Sears ML: Increased pressure after paracentesis of the rabbit eye is completely accounted for by prostaglandin synthesis and release plus pupillary block, Invest Ophthalmol Vis Sci 18:361, 1979.
4. Alm A: The effect of topical l-epinephrine on regional ocular blood flow in monkeys, Invest Ophthalmol Vis Sci 19:487, 1980.
5. Alm A, Bill A: Ocular and optic nerve blood flow at normal and increased intraocular pressure in monkeys (*Macaca iris*): a study with radioactively labelled microspheres including flow determination in brain and some other tissues, Exp Eye Res 15:15, 1973.
6. Ambache N: Properties of irin, a physiological constituent of the rabbit iris, J Physiol (Lond) 135:114, 1957.
7. Ambache N, Brummer HC: A simple chemical procedure for distinguishing E from F prostaglandins with application to tissue extracts, Br J Pharmacol 33:162, 1968.
8. Ambache N, Kavanagh L, Whiting JMC: Effect of me-

chanical stimulation on rabbit eyes: release of active substance in anterior chamber perfusates, J Physiol (Lond) 176:378, 1965.

9. Andersson H: Monoamine metabolites in aqueous humor, J Pharm Pharmacol 24:998, 1972.

10. Anggard E, Samuelsson B: Smooth muscle stimulating lipids in sheep iris: the identification of prostaglandin F_2, Biochem Pharmacol 13:281, 1964.

11. Bairati A, Orzalesi N: The ultrastructure of the epithelium of the ciliary body: a study of the junctional complexes and of the changes associated with the production of plasmoid aqueous humor, Z Zellforsch Milrosk Anat 69:635, 1966.

12. Ballintine EJ, Peters L: Effects of intracarotid injection of a basic dye on the ciliary body, Am J Ophthalmol 38:153, 1954.

13. Ballintine EJ, Waitzman M: Oxidative phosphorylation by ciliary processes, Am J Ophthalmol 42:349, 1956.

14. Barany EH, Langham M: On the origin of the ascorbic acid in the aqueous humor of guinea pigs and rabbits, Acta Physiol Scand 34:99, 1955.

15. Bausher LP, Gregory DS, Sears ML: Alpha 2-adrenergic and VIP receptors in rabbit ciliary processes interact, Curr Eye Res 8:47, 1989.

16. Bartels SP, et al: Sites of breakdown of the blood-aqueous barrier after paracentesis of the rhesus monkey eye, Invest Ophthalmol Vis Sci 18:1050, 1979.

17. Becker B: Carbonic anhydrase and the formation of aqueous humor, Am J Ophthalmol 47:342, 1959.

18. Becker B: Ascorbate transfer in guinea pig eyes, Invest Ophthalmol 6:410, 1967.

19. Becker B, Constant MA: Experimental tonography: the effect of carbonic anhydrase inhibitor acetazolamide on aqueous flow, Arch Ophthalmol 54:321, 1955.

20. Benham GH, Duke-Elder WS, Hodgson TH: The osmotic pressure of the aqueous humor in the normal and glaucomatous eye, J Physiol (Lond) 92:355, 1938.

21. Berzelius JJ: Lehrbuch der Chemie, Reutlingen 4:442, 1832.

22. Bhattacherjee P: Distribution of carbonic anhydrase in the rabbit eye as demonstrated histochemically, Exp Eye Res 12:356, 1971.

23. Bhattacherjee P: Autoradiographic localization of intravitreally or intracamerally injected [^{3}H]prostaglandins, Exp Eye Res 18:181, 1974.

24. Bhattacherjee P, Hammond BR: Inhibition of increased permeability of the blood-aqueous barrier by non-steroidal anti-inflammatory compounds as demonstrated by fluorescein angiography, Exp Eye Res 21:499, 1975.

25. Bill A: The albumin exchange in the rabbit eye, Acta Physiol Scand 60:18, 1964.

26. Bill A: Capillary permeability to and extravascular dynamics of myoglobin, albumin, and gammaglobulin in the uvea, Acta Physiol Scand 73:204, 1968.

27. Bill A: The role of ciliary blood flow and ultrafiltration in aqueous humor formation, Exp Eye Res 16:287, 1973.

28. Bill A: Blood circulation and fluid dynamics in the eye, Physiol Res 55:383, 1975.

29. Bito L: Intraocular fluid dynamics, I, Steady state concentration gradients of magnesium, potassium and calcium in relation to the sites and mechanisms of ocular cation transport processes, Exp Eye Res 10:102, 1970.

30. Bito LZ: The physiology and pathophysiology of intraocular fluids, Exp Eye Res 25(Suppl):273, 1977.

31. Bito LZ, Davson H: Steady state concentrations of potassium in the ocular fluids, Exp Eye Res 3:283, 1964.

32. Bito LZ, Slavador EV, Petrinonvic L: Intraocular fluid dynamics, IV, Intraocular sites of solute utilization transport as revealed by studies on aphakic eyes, Exp Eye Res 26:47, 1978.

33. Bito LZ, et al: The relationship between the concentrations of amino acids in the ocular fluids and blood plasma of dogs, Exp Eye Res 4:374, 1965.

34. Bonting SL, Becker B: Studies on Na^+-K^+ activated adenosine triphosphatase, Invest Ophthalmol 3:523, 1964.

35. Brodwall J, Fischbarg J: The hydraulic conductivity of rabbit ciliary epithelium in vitro, Exp Eye Res 34:121, 1982.

36. Bryson JM, Wolter JR, O'Keefe NT: Ganglion cells in the human ciliary body, Arch Ophthalmol 75:57, 1966.

37. Burstein NL, Fischbarg J, Liebovitch L, et al: Electrical potential, resistance, and fluid secretion across isolated ciliary body, Exp Eye Res 39:771, 1984.

38. Cameron E, Cole DF: Succinic dehydrogenase in the rabbit ciliary epithelium, Exp Eye Res 2:25, 1963.

39. Caprioli J, Sears ML: The adenylate cyclase receptor complex and aqueous humor formation, Yale J Biol Med 57:283, 1984.

40. Caprioli J, Sears ML: The histopathology of blackball hyphema: a report of two cases, Ophthalmol Surg 15:491, 1984.

41. Caprioli J, Sears ML, Mead A: Ocular blood flow in phakic and aphakic monkey eyes, Exp Eye Res 39:1, 1984.

42. Caprioli J, et al: Stimulation of ciliary adenylate cyclase by forskolin lowers intraocular pressure by reducing net aqueous humor inflow, Invest Ophthalmol Vis Sci 25:268, 1984.

43. Chu TC, Candia OA: Active transport of ascorbate across the isolated rabbit ciliary epithelium, Invest Ophthalmol Vis Sci 29:594, 1988.

44. Coco-Prados M, Kondo K: Separation of bovine pigmented ciliary epithelial cells by density gradient and further characterization in culture, Exp Eye Res 40:731, 1985.

45. Coco-Prados M, Wax MB: Transformation of human ciliary epithelial cells by simian virus 40: induction of cell proliferation and retention of beta 2-adrenergic receptors, Proc Natl Acad Sci 83:8754, 1986.

46. Cole DF: Some effects of decreased plasma sodium concentration on the composition and tension of the aqueous humour, Br J Ophthalmol 43:268, 1959.

47. Cole DF: Electrochemical changes associated with the formation of the aqueous humor, Br J Ophthalmol 45:202, 1961.

48. Cole DF: Location of ouabain-sensitive adenosine triphosphatase in ciliary epithelium, Exp Eye Res 3:72, 1964.

49. Cole DF: Aqueous humor formation, Doc Ophthalmol 21:116, 1966.

50. Cole DF: Evidence for active transport of chloride in ciliary epithelium of the rabbit, Exp Eye Res 8:5, 1969.

51. Cole DF: Aqueous and ciliary body, in Graymore CM,

ed: Biochemistry of the eye, London, Academic Press, 1970.

52. Cole DF: Electrolyte composition of anterior and posterior aqueous humor in the sheep, Ophthalmol Res 4:1, 1972/1973.

53. Cole DF: Secretion of the aqueous humor, Exp Eye Res 25(Suppl):161, 1977.

54. Constant MA, Falch J: Phosphate and protein concentrations of intraocular fluids, I, Effect of carbonic anhydrase inhibition in young and old rabbits, Invest Ophthalmol 2:332, 1963.

55. Davson H: A comparative study of the aqueous humor and cerebrospinal fluid in the rabbit, J Physiol 129:111, 1955.

56. Davson H: Physiology of the ocular and cerebrospinal fluids, Edinburgh, Churchill Livingstone, 1956.

57. Davson H: The eye, New York, Academic Press, 1962.

58. DeBarnadinis E, et al: The chemical composition of the human aqueous humor in normal and pathological conditions, Exp Eye Res 4:179, 1965.

59. deRoetth A: Glycolytic activity of ciliary processes, Arch Ophthalmol 51:599, 1954.

60. Dernouchamps JP: The proteins of the aqueous humor, Doc Ophthalmol 53:193, 1982.

61. Dernouchamps JP, et al: Immune complexes in the aqueous humor and serum, Am J Ophthalmol 84:24, 1977.

62. Diamond JR, Bossert WH: Standing-gradient osmotic flow: a mechanism for coupling of water and solute transport in epithelia, J Gen Physiol 50:2061, 1967.

63. Diamond JR, Bossert WH: Functional consequences of ultrastructural geometry in "backwards" fluid transporting epithelia, J Cell Biol 37:694, 1968.

64. Dias PLR: Post-inflammatory and malignant protein patterns in aqueous humor, Br J Ophthalmol 63:161, 1979.

65. Dickinson JC, Durham SG, Hamilton PB: Ion exchange chromatography of free amino acids in aqueous fluids and lens of the human eye, Invest Ophthalmol 7:551, 1981.

66. DiMatteo J: Active transport of ascorbic acid into lens epithelium of the rat, Exp Eye Res 49:873, 1989.

67. DiMatteo J, et al: Glucose transport across ocular barriers of the streptozotocin-diabetic rat, Diabetes 30:903, 1981.

68. Duke-Elder WS: Monograph, Br J Ophthalmol 3(Suppl):1, 1927.

69. Duke-Elder WS: The circulation of the intraocular fluids, in Goldsmith AJB, ed: Recent Adv Ophthalmol, p 338, 1951.

70. Eakins KE: Prostaglandin and non-prostaglandin mediated breakdown of the blood-aqueous barrier, Exp Eye Res 25(Suppl):483, 1977.

71. Ehlers N: Aqueous humor and plasma amino acids in tapetoretinal degenerations, Acta Ophthalmol 59:576, 1981.

72. Ehlers N, Kristensen K, Schonheyder F: Amino acid transport in human ciliary epithelium, Acta Ophthalmol 56:777, 1978.

73. Ehlers N, Schonheyder F: Concentration of amino acids in aqueous humor and plasma in congenital cataract or dislocation of the lens, Acta Ophthalmol 123(Suppl):179, 1974.

74. Ehrlich P: Eine Farbenanalytische Studie, Das Sauer-

stoff-Bedurfnis des Organismus, Berlin, 1885.

75. Epstein DL, Jedziniak JA, Grant WM: Identification of heavy molecular-weight soluble protein in aqueous humor in human phacolytic glaucoma, Invest Ophthalmol Vis Sci 17:398, 1978.

76. Falbe-Hansen L, Degn JK: Sialic acid in the aqueous humor and the vitreous of normal human eyes and of eyes with malignant melanoma of the choroid, Acta Ophthalmol 47:972, 1969.

77. Farkas TG, Pluscec J: The occurrence of trivalent chromium in the aqueous and lens of rats, Invest Ophthalmol 5:398, 1966.

78. Felberg NT, McFall R, Shields JA: Aqueous humor enzyme patterns in retinoblastoma, Invest Ophthalmol Vis Sci 16:1039, 1977.

79. Felberg HT, Shields JA, Federman JL: Antibody Toxocara canis in the aqueous humor, Arch Ophthalmol 99:1563, 1981.

80. Feller D, Weinreb R: Breakdown and reestablishment of blood-aqueous barrier with laser trabeculoplasty, Arch Ophthalmol 102:537, 1984.

81. Fielder AR, Rahi AHS: Symposium on immunology: immunoglobulins of normal aqueous humor, Trans Ophthalmol Soc UK 99:120, 1979.

82. Fischbarg J, Lim JJ: Role of cations, anions and carbonic anhydrase in the transport across rabbit corneal endothelium, J Physiol (Lond) 241:647, 1974.

83. Francois J, et al: Further perfusion studies on the outflow of aqueous humor in human eyes, Arch Ophthalmol 53:683, 1958.

84. Freddo TF, Bartels SP, Barsotti MF, et al: The source of proteins in the aqueous humor of the normal rabbit, Invest Ophthalmol Vis Sci 31:125, 1990.

85. Friedenwald JS: Formation of the intraocular fluid, Am J Ophthalmol 32:9, 1949.

86. Friedenwald JS, Buschke W, Michel HO: The role of ascorbic acid (vitamin C) in the secretion of the intraocular fluid, Arch Ophthalmol 29:535, 1943.

87. Friedenwald JS, Herrmann H, Moses R: The distribution of certain oxidative enzymes in the ciliary body, Johns Hopkins Bulletin 73:421, 1943.

88. Fujita H, Kondo K, Sears M: A new function of the non-pigmented epithelium of ciliary processes in the formation of the aqueous humor, Klin Monatsbl Augenheilkd 185:28, 1984.

89. Fujiwara H: Lens crystallin reactive protein in the aqueous humor of cataract patients, Jpn J Ophthalmol 33:418, 1989.

90. Furuichi C: The influence of various experimental injuries on creatine, creatinine metabolism of aqueous fluid of the rabbit's eye, Acta Soc Ophthalmol 65:561, 1961.

91. Gaaserland DF, et al: Rhesus monkey aqueous humor composition and a primate ocular perfusate, Invest Ophthalmol Vis Sci 18:1139, 1979.

92. Gaasterland DF, et al: Long-term ocular effects of osmotic modification of the blood brain barrier in monkeys, 1, Clinical examination, aqueous ascorbate and protein, Invest Ophthalmol Vis Sci 24:153, 1983.

93. Garg LC, Oppelt WW: The effect of ouabain and acetazolamide on transport of sodium and chloride from plasma to aqueous humor, J Pharm Exp Ther 175:237, 1970.

94. Ghose T, et al: Immunoglobulins in aqueous humor

and iris from patients with endogenous uveitis and patients with cataract, Br J Ophthalmol 57:897, 1973.

95. Goldmann EE: Vitalfarbung am Zentralnervensystem, Abhandl König Preuss Akad Wis 1:1, 1913.

96. Granwall H: Citric acid studies referring to the eye, Acta Ophthalmol (Suppl):14, 1937.

97. Green K: Permeability properties of the ciliary epithelium in response to prostaglandins, Invest Ophthalmol Vis Sci 12:752, 1973.

98. Green K, Pederson JE: Contribution of secretion and filtration to aqueous humor formation, Am J Physiol 222:1218, 1972.

99. Green K, Pederson JE: Aqueous humor formation, Exp Eye Res 16:273, 1973.

100. Gregory D, et al: Intraocular pressure and aqueous flow are decreased by cholera toxin, Invest Ophthalmol Vis Sci 20:371, 1981.

101. Heald K, Langham ME: Permeability of the cornea and the blood-aqueous barrier to oxygen, Br J Ophthalmol 40:705, 1956.

102. Hogan MJ, Alvarado JA, Weddell JE: Histology of the human eye, Philadelphia, WB Saunders, 1971.

103. Holland MG, Gipson CC: Chloride ion transport in the isolated ciliary body, Invest Ophthalmol 9:20, 1970.

104. Holland MG, Stockwell M: Sodium ion transport of the ciliary body in vitro, Invest Ophthalmol 6:401, 1967.

105. Hollinshead MB, Spillert CR, Lazara EJ: Procoagulant effect of aqueous humor on in vitro clotting of blood and plasma, Curr Eye Res 8:819, 1988.

106. Holmes EL, Char DH, Christensen M: Aqueous immune complexes in immunogenic uveitis, Invest Ophthalmol Vis Sci 23:715, 1982.

107. Jacq C, et al: Lactic dehydrogenase isoenzymes in the ocular tissues and liquids, Ophthalmol 184:174, 1982.

108. Jakobiec FA, Abramson D, Scher R: Increased aqueous lactate dehydrogenase in Coats' disease, Am J Ophthalmol 85:686, 1978.

109. Joseph JP, Grierson I, Hitchings RA: Chemotactic activity of aqueous humor; a case of failure of trabeculectomies? Arch Ophthalmol 107:69, 1989.

110. Kaye GL, Pappas GD: Studies on the ciliary epithelium and zonule, III, The fine structure of the rabbit ciliary epithelium in relation to the localization of ATPase activity, J Microsc 4:497, 1965.

111. Keam HL: Efflux of amino acids from the lens, Invest Ophthalmol 9:692, 1970.

112. Khodadoust AA, Stark WJ, Bill WR: Coagulation properties of intraocular humors and cerebrospinal fluid, Invest Ophthalmol Vis Sci 24:1616, 1983.

113. Kijlstra A, Luyendijk L, Baarsma GS, et al: Aqueous humor analysis as a diagnostic tool in toxoplasma uveitis, Int Ophthalmol 13:383, 1989.

114. Kim JO, Cotlier E: Phospholipid distributions and fatty acid composition of lysophosphatidylcholine and phosphatidylcholine in rabbit aqueous humor, lens and vitreous, Exp Eye Res 22:569, 1976.

115. Kinsey VE: Transfer of ascorbic acid and related compounds across the blood-aqueous barrier, Am J Ophthalmol 30:1262, 1947.

116. Kinsey VE: The chemical composition and the osmotic pressure of the aqueous humor and plasma of the rabbit, J Gen Physiol 34:389, 1950.

117. Kinsey VE: Comparative chemistry of aqueous humor in posterior and anterior chambers of rabbit eye: its physiologic significance, Arch Ophthalmol 40:401, 1953.

118. Kinsey VE: Further study of the distribution of chloride between plasma and intraocular fluids of the rabbit eye, Invest Ophthalmol 6:395, 1967.

119. Kinsey VE: Ion movement in ciliary processes, vol 3, Membranes and ion transport, New York, John Wiley, 1971.

120. Kinsey VE, Reddy DVN: Transport of amino acids into the posterior chamber of the rabbit eye, Invest Ophthalmol 1:355, 1962.

121. Kinsey VE, Reddy DVN: Chemistry and dynamics of aqueous humor, in Prince JH, ed: The rabbit in eye research, Springfield, IL, Charles C Thomas, Publisher, 1964.

122. Kleifeld O, Neumann HC: Der Sauerstoffgehalt des menschlichen Kammerwassers, Klin Monatsbl Augenheilkd 135:224, 1959.

123. Kleinstein RN, et al: In vivo aqueous humor oxygen tension—as estimated from measurements on bare stroma, Invest Ophthalmol Vis Sci 21:415, 1981.

124. Kondo K, Coca-Prados M, Sears ML: Human ciliary epithelia in monolayer culture, Exp Eye Res 38:423, 1984.

125. Koskela TK, Reiss GR, Brubaker RF, et al: Is the high concentration of ascorbic acid in the eye an adaptation to intense solar irradiation? Invest Ophthalmol Vis Sci 31:2265, 1989.

126. Krause U, Raunio V: Proteins of the normal human aqueous humor, Ophthalmologica 159:179, 1969.

127. Krause U, Raunio V: The proteins of the pathologic human aqueous humor, Ophthalmologica 160:280, 1970.

128. Krupin T, Reinach PS, Candia OA, et al: Transepithelial electrical measurements on the isolated rabbit iris-ciliary body, Exp Eye Res 38:115, 1984.

129. Laurent VBG: Hyaluronate in aqueous humor, Exp Eye Res 33:147, 1981.

130. Ledbetter SR, Hatchell DL, O'Brien WJ: Secondary aqueous humor stimulates the proliferation of cultured bovine corneal endothelial cells, Invest Ophthalmol Vis Sci 24:557, 1983.

131. Lee IS, Yu YS, Kim DM, et al: Detection of specific proteins in the aqueous humor in primary open-angle glaucoma, Korean J Ophthalmol 4:1, 1990.

132. Levene AZ: Osmolarity in the normal state and following acetazolamide, Arch Ophthalmol 59:597, 1958.

133. Lieb WA, Stark N: Interrelationship of ascorbic acid and facility of outflow: steroid hormones is possible regulating mechanism of intraocular pressure, in Patterson G, Miller SJH, Paterson GD, eds: Drug mechanisms in glaucoma, Edinburgh, Churchill Livingstone, 1966.

134. Linner E: Ascorbic acid as a test substance for measuring relative changes in the rate of plasma flow through the ciliary processes, Acta Physiol Scand 26:1, 1952.

135. Macri FJ, Cevario SJ: Ciliary ganglion stimulation, I, Effects on aqueous humor inflow and outflow, Invest Ophthalmol 14:28, 1975.

136. Macri FJ, Cevario SJ: A possible vascular mechanism for the inhibition of aqueous humor formation by ouabain and acetazolamide, Exp Eye Res 20:563, 1975.

137. Maren TH: The rates of movement of Na^+, Cl^-, and

HCO$_3^-$ from plasma to posterior chamber: effect of acetazolamide and relation to the treatment of glaucoma, Invest Ophthalmol 15:356, 1976.

138. Maren TH: Ion secretion into the posterior aqueous humor of dogs and monkeys, Exp Eye Res 25 (Suppl):245, 1977.

139. Matsuo N, Takabatake M, Ueno H, et al: Photoreceptor outer segments in the aqueous humor in rhegmatogenous retinal detachment, Am J Ophthalmol 101:673, 1986.

140. Matsushita M, Matsuo T, Matsuo N: Retinal detachment with oral dialysis: differences in clinical features between cases with and without photoreceptor outer segments in aqueous humor, Jpn J Ophthalmol 34:338, 1990.

141. Maurice DM: The cornea and sclera, in Davson H, ed: The eye, New York, Academic Press, 1969.

142. Maurice DM, Riley MV: The cornea, in Graymore CN, ed: Biochemistry of the eye, New York, Academic Press, 1970.

143. McLaren JW, Trocme SD, Relf S, et al: Rate of flow of aqueous humor determined from measurements of aqueous flare, Invest Ophthalmol Vis Sci 31:339, 1990.

144. Miller JE: Inter-relations of the blood-aqueous potential and acetazolamide in the rabbit, Invest Ophthalmol 1:363, 1962.

145. Mishima H, et al: Ultracytochemistry of cholera toxin binding sites on ciliary processes, Cell Tissue Res 223:241, 1982.

146. Miyake K, Asakura M, Maekubo K: Consensual reactions of human blood-aqueous barrier to implant operations, Arch Ophthalmol 102:558, 1984.

147. Mondino BJ, Rao H: Complement levels in normal and inflamed aqueous humor, Invest Ophthalmol Vis Sci 24:38, 1983.

148. Murray PI, Hoekzema R, van Haren MA, et al: Aqueous humor interleuken-6 levels in uveitis, Invest Ophthalmol Vis Sci 31:917, 1990.

149. Neufeld AH, Jampol LM, Sears ML: Aspirin prevents the disruption of the blood-aqueous barrier in the rabbit eye, Nature 238:158, 1972.

150. Neufeld A, Sears M: The site of action of prostaglandin E$_2$ on the disruption of the blood-aqueous barrier in the rabbit eye, Exp Eye Res 17:445, 1973.

151. Obenberger J, Starka L, Hampl R: Quantitative determination of endogenous corticosteroids in the rabbit plasma and aqueous humor, Albrecht v Graefes Arch Klin Exp Ophthalmol 183:203, 1971.

152. Ohnishi Y, Tanaka M: Effects of pilocarpine and paracentesis on occluding junctions between the nonpigmented ciliary epithelial cells, Exp Eye Res 32:635, 1981.

153. Okisaka S: Effects of paracentesis on the blood-aqueous barrier: a light and electron microscopic study on cynomolgus monkey, Invest Ophthalmol 15:824, 1976.

154. Pandolfi M, Neilsson IM, Martinson G: Coagulation and fibrinolytic components in primary and plasmoid aqueous humor of rabbits, Acta Ophthalmol 42:820, 1964.

155. Pederson JE, Green K: Aqueous humor dynamics: experimental studies, Exp Eye Res 15:277, 1973.

156. Pederson O, Lorentzen-Styr AM: Antibodies against Toxoplasma gondii in the aqueous humor of patients with active retinochoroiditis, Acta Ophthalmol (Copenh) 59:719, 1981.

157. Pine A: The vitreous body, in Davson H, ed: The eye, New York, Academic Press, 1969.

158. Porter R, Skillen AW: Lactic dehydrogenase activity in the aqueous humor of eyes containing malignant melanomas, Br J Ophthalmol 56:709, 1972.

159. Rapoport S: Osmotic opening of blood-brain and blood-ocular barriers, Exp Eye Res 25(Suppl):449, 1977.

160. Raviola G: Effects of paracentesis on the blood-aqueous barrier: an electron microscope study on Macaca mulatta using horseradish peroxidase as a tracer, Invest Ophthalmol 13:828, 1974.

161. Raviola G: The structural basis of the blood-ocular barriers, Exp Eye Res 25(Suppl.):27, 1977.

162. Reddy DVN, Kinsey VE: Composition of the vitreous humor in relation to that of plasma and aqueous humors, Arch Ophthalmol 63:715, 1960.

163. Reddy DVN, Rosenberg C, Kinsey VE: Steady state distribution of free amino acids in the aqueous humors, vitreous body and plasma of the rabbit, Exp Eye Res 1:175, 1961.

164. Reddy DVN, Thompson MR, Chakrapani B: Amino acid transport across blood-aqueous barrier of mammalian species, Exp Eye Res 25:555, 1977.

165. Reddy H: Die Cl Verteilung des Kammerwasser-Serum beim Menschen, Doc Ophthalmol 11:176, 1957.

166. Reim M, et al: Steady state levels of glucose in the different layers of the cornea, aqueous humor, blood, and tears in vivo, Ophthalmologica 154:39, 1967.

167. Reiss GR, Lee DA, Topper JE, et al: Aqueous humor flow during sleep, Invest Ophthalmol Vis Sci 25:776, 1984.

168. Remky H: Die Chlorverteilung Kammerwasser/Serum beim Menschen und ihre Bedeutung fur den Wasseraushalt des Auges, Albrecht v Graefes Arch Ophthalmol 157:506, 1956.

169. Riley MV: Intraocular dynamics of lactic acid in the rabbit, Invest Ophthalmol 11:600, 1972.

170. Riley MW: A study of the transfer of amino acids across the endothelium of the rabbit cornea, Exp Eye Res 24:35, 1977.

171. Ringvold A: Aqueous humor and ultraviolet radiation, Acta Ophthalmol (Copenh) 58:69, 1979.

172. Roepke RR, Hetherington WA: Osmotic regulation between aqueous humor and blood plasma, Am J Physiol 130:340, 1940.

173. Runyan TE, et al: Human ciliary body epithelium in culture, Invest Ophthalmol Vis Sci 24:687, 1983.

174. Sandberg HO, Class O: The alpha and gamma crystallin content in aqueous humor of eyes with clear lens and with cataracts, Exp Eye Res 28:601, 1979.

175. Schonheyder F, Ehlers N, Hust B: Remarks on the aqueous humor/plasma ratios for amino acids and related compounds in patients with various chronic ocular disorders, Acta Ophthalmol (Copenh) 53:627, 1975.

176. Seamon KB, Daly JW: Forskolin: a unique diterpene activator of cyclic AMP generating systems, J Cyclic Nucleotide Protein Phosphor Res 7:201, 1981.

177. Schwartz A: Chronic open-angle glaucoma secondary to rhegmatogenous retinal detachment, Am J Ophthalmol 75:205, 1973.

178. Sears ML: Adrenergic supersensitivity of the scorbutic iris, Trans Am Ophthalmol Soc 71:536, 1973.

179. Sears ML: The aqueous, in Moses RA, ed: Adler's physiology of the eye, 7th ed, St Louis, CV Mosby, 1981.

180. Sears ML, Mead A: A major pathway for the regulation of intraocular pressure, Int Ophthalmol 6:201, 1983.

181. Sears ML, et al: A mechanism for the control of aqueous humor formation, in Drance SM, Neufeld A, eds: Applied pharmacology in the medical treatment of glaucoma, New York, Grune & Stratton, 1984.

182. Sears M, Yamada E, Cummins D, et al: The isolated ciliary epithelial bilayer is useful for in vitro studies of aqueous humor formation, Suppl Invest Ophthalmol Vis Sci 32: 978, 1991.

183. Segal S, Thier SO: Renal handling of amino acids, in Orloff J, Berliner RW, eds: Handbook of physiology, renal physiology, Washington, DC, American Physiological Society, 1973.

184. Sen DK, Saren GS, Saha K: Immunoglobulins in human aqueous humor, Br J Ophthalmol 61:216, 1977.

185. Shantaveerappa TR, Boume GH: Histochemical studies on the distribution of oxidative and dephosphorylating enzymes of the rabbit eye, Acta Anat (Basel) 57:192, 1964.

186. Shiose Y: Electron microscopic studies on blood-retinal and blood-aqueous barriers, Jpn J Ophthalmol 14:73, 1970.

187. Shiose Y, Sears ML: Fine structural localization of nucleotide activity in the ciliary epithelium of albino rabbits, Invest Ophthalmol 5:152, 1966.

188. Shimizu H, Riley MV, Cole DF: The isolation of whole cells from the ciliary epithelium, Exp Eye Res 6:141, 1967.

189. Shine BSF, Hungerford J, Vaghela B, et al: Electrophoretic assessment of aqueous and serum neurone-specific enolase in retinoblastoma and ocular malignant melanoma, Br J Ophthalmol 74:427, 1990.

190. Smelser GK, Pei YF: Cytological basis of protein leakage into the eye following paracentesis: an electronic microscopic study, Invest Ophthalmol 4:249, 1965.

191. Smith RS: Ultrastructural studies of the blood-aqueous barrier. 1. Transport of an electron dense tracer in the iris and ciliary body of the mouse, Am J Ophthalmol 71:1066, 1971.

192. Smith SD, Gregory DS: A circadian rhythm of aqueous flow underlies the circadian rhythm of IOP in NZW rabbits, Invest Ophthalmol Vis Sci 30:775, 1989.

193. Stefansson E, Wolbarsht ML, Landers MB: The corneal contact lens and aqueous humor hypoxia in cats, Invest Ophthalmol Vis Sci 24:1052, 1983.

194. Stefansson E, et al: Effect of epinephrine on PO_2 in anterior chamber, Arch Ophthalmol 101:636, 1983.

195. Stephanik J, Averswald W, Doleschel W: On the problem of permeation of proteins and lipoproteins into the aqueous humor, Electrophoretic and sedimentation-flotation analysis studies on the aqueous humor of the cow, Albrecht v Graefes Arch Ophthalmol 161:282, 1959.

196. Stjernschantz J, Uusitalo R, Palkama A: The aqueous proteins of the rat in the normal eye and after aqueous withdrawal, Exp Eye Res 16:215, 1973.

197. Swartz M, Herbst R, Goldberg M: Aqueous humor lactic acid dehydrogenase in retinoblastoma, Am J Ophthalmol 4:612, 1974.

198. Taniguchi Y: Fine structure of blood vessels in the ciliary body, Jpn J Ophthalmol 6:93, 1962.

199. Tsukahara S, Maezawa N: Cytochemical localization of adenyl cyclase in the rabbit ciliary body, Exp Eye Res 26:99, 1978.

200. Ussing H, Zerahn K: Active transport of sodium as the source of electric current in the short-circuited isolated frog skin, Acta Physiol Scand 23:110, 1951.

201. Uusitalo R, Palkama A: Some observations on the mechanism regulating the blood-aqueous barrier in the rabbit eye, Scand J Clin Lab Invest (Suppl.) 116:21, 1971.

202. Uusitalo R, Palkama A, Stjernschantz J: An electron microscopic study of the blood-aqueous barrier in the ciliary body and iris of the rabbit, Exp Eye Res 17:49, 1973.

203. Varma SD, Reddy DVN: Phospholipid composition of aqueous humor plasma and lens in normal and alloxan diabetic rabbits, Exp Eye Res 13:120, 1972.

204. Vegge T: An epithelial blood-aqueous barrier to horseradish peroxidase in the ciliary processes of the vervet monkey (Cercopithecus ethiops), Z Zellforsch Mikrosk Anat 114:309, 1971.

205. Waitzman MB, Jackson RT: Effects of topically administered ouabain on aqueous humor dynamics, Exp Eye Res 4:135, 1965.

206. Walinder P: The accumulation of alpha aminoisobutyric acid by rabbit ciliary body-iris preparations, Invest Ophthalmol 7:67, 1968.

207. Walker AM: Comparison of the chemical composition of aqueous humor, cerebrospinal fluid, lymph, and blood from frogs, higher animals and man, J Biol Chem 101:269, 1933.

208. Wegener JK, Moller PM: Oxygen tension in the anterior chamber of the rabbit eye, Acta Ophthalmol (Copenh) 49:577, 1971.

209. Wiederholt M, Zadunaisky JA: Effects of ouabain and furosemide on transepithelial electrical parameters of the isolated shark ciliary epithelium, Invest Ophthalmol Vis Sci 28:1353, 1987.

210. Weinbaum S, et al: The rise of secretion and pressure dependent flow in aqueous humor formation, Exp Eye Res 13:266, 1972.

211. Weingeist TA: The structure of the developing and adult ciliary complex of the rabbit eye: a gross, light and electron microscopic study, Doc Ophthalmol 28:205, 1970.

212. Woodlief NF: Initial observations on the ocular microcirculation in man, I, The anterior segment and extraocular muscles, Arch Ophthalmol 98:1268, 1980.

213. Yagci A, Karcioglu ZA, Akkin C, et al: Serum and aqueous humor sialic acid levels in Behçet's disease, Ophthalmol 97:1153, 1990.

Intraocular Pressure

WILLIAM M. HART, Jr., M.D., Ph.D.

The vertebrate eye is a fluid-filled spheroid having a flexible and partially elastic wall. Maintenance of a stable shape is necessary for the important optical properties of the eye. The tissue pressure of the intraocular contents is called the intraocular pressure, commonly abbreviated IOP or P_i. The intraocular pressure is maintained within a fairly narrow range by a complex and dynamic equilibrium in which a nearly constant rate of aqueous humor production is matched by a nearly constant rate of aqueous humor escape from the eye through drainage pathways. Small variations in either the rate of production or in the rate of outflow from the eye can result in large changes in IOP. Thus any variation in a host of parameters affecting aqueous humor production or filtration (including body position, blood pressure, external forces applied to the surface of the globe, and central venous pressure) may result in dramatic changes in intraocular pressure. However, in the healthy eye a remarkably stable homeostasis is maintained.

INTRAOCULAR PRESSURE: A DYNAMIC EQUILIBRIUM

The aqueous humor is produced by the ciliary body epithelia (see Chapter 7) through a complex, energy-dependent active transport process. It then moves by bulk flow through the interstices of the posterior chamber, across the anterior surface of the lens, past the gentle resistance in the narrow space where the posterior aspect of the iris rests against the anterior surface of the lens, to then pass through the pupillary aperture and into the anterior chamber. The vast majority of aqueous flow then exits the eye in the anterior chamber angle by passing through the trabecular meshwork into Schlemm's canal, from where it then passes through a series of collector channels into the network of episcleral veins.

The flow of aqueous humor meets variable resistances during its passage through the posterior and anterior chambers and through the trabecular meshwork. At constant rates of aqueous humor production, intraocular pressure will rise until the resistance to outflow is exceeded. When outflow is exactly equal to the rate of aqueous humor production, intraocular pressure stabilizes at a level determined by these variables. Thus the intraocular pressure at any given moment is the result of a dynamic equilibrium exactly matching aqueous production and the rate of aqueous outflow.

The intraocular flow of aqueous and anatomy of the outflow system

Aqueous flow from the ciliary processes into the posterior chamber is principally the result of metabolic pump activity in the ciliary epithelia. The pump operates at a constant rate that is not sensitive to intraocular pressure,[8] but that can be slowed by pharmacologic agents such as carbonic anhydrase inhibitors and beta-adrenergic blocking agents. The pump operates across a semipermeable membrane that blocks the flow of all macromolecules, resulting in a blood-aqueous barrier that is closely analogous to the blood-brain barrier. The absence of large molecules such as protein from the aqueous humor is in part responsible for the high optical quality of the aqueous, which in the normal state has no significantly detectable scattering of light. The chemical composition of the aqueous is a further result of diffusional interchange of low-molecular-weight solutes with the anterior portions of the vitreous body, the lens, the iris, and the cornea. The metabolic needs of the lens epithelium, principally oxygen and glucose, are provided by the aqueous humor as it flows across the surface of the lens capsule. There is a small resistance to aqueous flow between the iris and the lens caused by a variable area of close approximation between the posterior surface of the iris and the anterior lens capsule. At the steady state of dynamic equilibrium in the normal eye, in which aqueous humor is constantly moving by bulk flow from the posterior chamber through the pupillary aperture, there is a small but significant difference in pressure between posterior and anterior chamber pressures. In some eyes this small difference in pressure is reflected in a

bowing forward of the mid peripheral portions of the iris, sometimes referred to physiologic iris bombé (Fig. 8-1). Aqueous entering the anterior chamber through the pupillary aperture then flows in a radially symmetrical fashion toward the periphery of the anterior chamber, where it exits the eye through the trabecular meshwork.

The trabecular meshwork lies in the periphery of the anterior chamber angle. It has a triangular shape in cross section with its base located posteriorly at the scleral spur and its anterior tip located at Schwalbe's line, which is a raised ridge marking the terminus of Descemet's membrane (Fig. 8-2). The trabecular mesh proper consists of a series of parallel layers of connective tissue that are thin and flat and stacked on top of one another. Each lamina is perforated by a series of pores of variable size, resulting in a criss-cross series of overlapping trabeculae of connective tissue. Each trabeculum in turn is covered by a monocellular layer of endothelium. The triangular cross-sectional shape of the trabecular tissue results from a smaller number of the parallel laminae reaching the anterior end of the trabecular layer. There

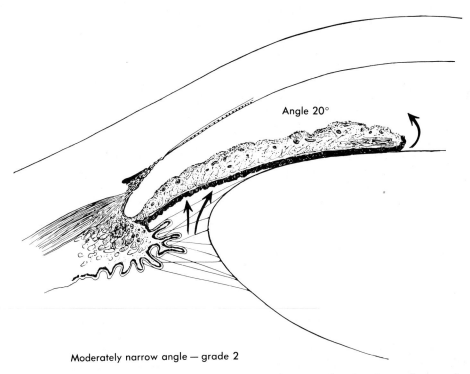

Moderately narrow angle — grade 2

FIG. 8-1 Aqueous flow from the ciliary body through the posterior chamber and across the anterior lens surface to the pupil. Slightly greater pressure in posterior chamber than in anterior chamber causes the iris to bow anteriorly, so-called physiologic iris bombé.[20] (From Kolker AE, Hetherington J Jr: Becker-Shaffer's diagnosis and therapy of the glaucomas, 4th ed, St Louis, CV Mosby, 1976.)

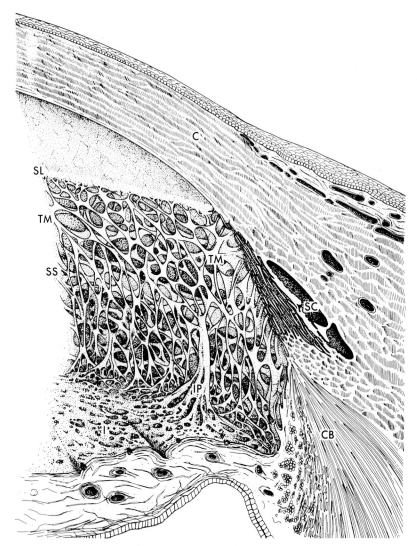

FIG. 8-2 Anatomic features of anterior chamber angle and trabecular meshwork. In cross-section the meshwork has a triangular shape. Parallel, perforated laminae of trabecular tissue are greatest in number posteriorly (base of triangle), and fuse with one another to become smaller in number anteriorly (apex of triangle). Aqueous flows through perforations in laminar sheets to enter Schlemm's canal. C, cornea; CB, ciliary body; I, iris; IP, iris process; SC, Schemm's canal; SL, Schwalbe's line; SS, scleral spur; TM, trabecular meshwork. (From Tripathi RC, Tripathi BJ: Functional anatomy of the anterior chamber angle, in Duane TD, Jaeger EA, eds: Biomedical foundations of ophthalmology, vol 1, New York, Harper & Row.)

are approximately three to five such layers present at the anterior apex of the triangle and as many as 15 to 20 layers located posteriorly at the scleral spur. This results from a progressive anatomic fusion of adjacent layers when proceeding from posterior toward anterior.

The innermost layers of the trabecular laminae that border the anterior chamber are referred to as the uveal meshwork, whereas the deeper layers constitute the corneoscleral meshwork. The corneoscleral portion of the trabecular meshwork is in turn separated from the endothelium lining Schlemm's canal by a thin strip called the juxtacanalicular tissue. Whereas the trabeculae of the meshwork tend to be radially oriented in the uveal meshwork, successive layers in the corneoscleral meshwork tend to be progressively oriented in a circumferential pat-

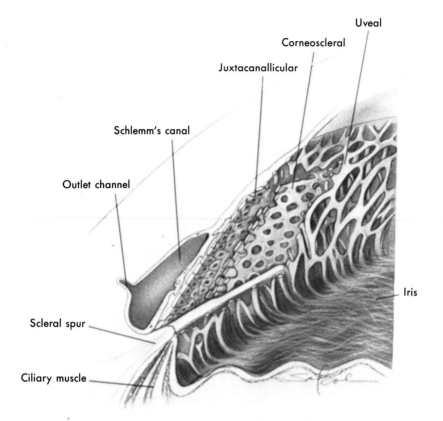

Uveal

Corneoscleral

Juxtacanallicular

Schlemm's canal

Outlet channel

Iris

Scleral spur

Ciliary muscle

FIG. 8-3 Cutaway diagram of layers of trabecular meshwork in aqueous outflow system. (Modified from Shields MB: Textbook of glaucoma, Baltimore, Williams & Wilkins, 1987.)

tern (Fig. 8-3). The monocellular layer of endothelium covering the trabecular beams contains a series of gap junctions that tightly bind adjacent endothelial cells to one another (Fig. 8-4). The trabecular beams in turn contain a complex mixture of connective tissues including collagen types I and III at the central core surrounded by cortical zones containing types III, IV, and V intermixed with heparin sulfate, proteoglycan, fibronectin, and laminin.[11,29]

The juxtacanalicular tissue of the trabecular meshwork that separates the corneoscleral portions of the meshwork from Schlemm's canal is comprised of a connective tissue ground substance containing glycosaminoglycans and glycoproteins. The principal resistance to aqueous flow through the eye is encountered in the trabecular meshwork. Resistance to flow rises gradually through the progressively smaller pores of the trabecular mesh, and it is thought that the juxtacanalicular tissue is the locus of the highest resistance to aqueous outflow in the normal eye. The juxtacanalicular tissue has a ground substance of glycosaminoglycans and

glycoproteins and is covered on the side facing Schlemm's canal by a monocellular layer of endothelial cells, sometimes referred to as juxtacanalicular cells.[17,30] The aqueous enters the endothelial cells through small (1.5 μm) passages.[16,18] These cells then give rise to giant vacuoles, projecting into the lumen of the canal,[2,10,18] that are thought by some to serve as a pathway for aqueous flow.[35] Once within the canal of Schlemm, aqueous flow through connector channels into the episcleral veins is determined principally by the resistance provided by the level of episcleral venous pressure. The collector channels that exit from Schlemm's canal consist of a series of approximately 20 to 30 radially oriented endothelial lined conduits. Occasionally, examination of the perilimbal tissue under high magnification with a slit-lamp biomicroscope will reveal the presence of visible laminar flow of aqueous into a vein (called an aqueous vein), in which one can see adjacent layers of smooth-flowing blood and clear aqueous fluid.

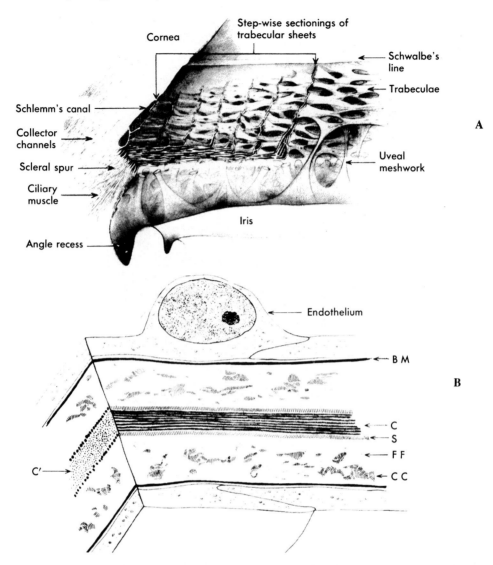

FIG. 8-4 Diagram of trabecular structures. **A**, Note large trabecular openings in uveal (inner) portions of meshwork and progressive decrease in size of openings as Schlemm's canal is approached. **B**, Cross-sectional diagram of corneoscleral trabecular lamina. C, central collagenous tissue; S, sheath of thick fibers; FF and CC, ground substance containing irregular clumps of material and fine fibrils; BM, basement membrane; C', collagen fibers cut in cross-section with lamina sectioned in meridional plane of eye. (From Garron LK, Feeney ML: Arch Ophthalmol 62:966, 1959.)

Escape of aqueous from the eye

There are two measurable pathways by which aqueous leaves the eye. One of these is pressure dependent and the other is relatively constant and pressure independent.

The principal outflow pathway for aqueous is the pressure-dependent flow through the trabecular meshwork. As outlined above, the aqueous must percolate through a progressively smaller series of channels, through the pores of the trabecular meshwork, across the juxtacanalicular tissue into Schlemm's canal, and from

there into the collector channels and the aqueous veins. Flow through this system is pressure dependent and hydrodynamic. The rate of flow is determined by the hydrostatic pressure head and the resistance to flow.

Resistance to aqueous flow is frequently referred to as the coefficient of facility of aqueous outflow, or simply facility. Whereas resistance to flow is analogous to the electrical measure of resistance to the flow of electrons, facility of aqueous flow is likewise analogous to the electrical measure of conductance. The relationship

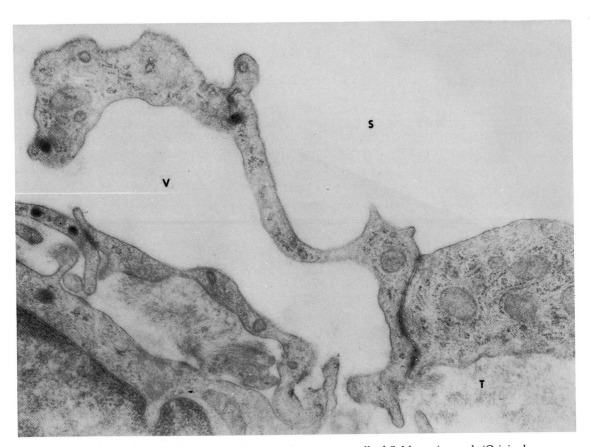

FIG. 8-5 Juxtacanalicular endothelial cells along inner wall of Schlemm's canal. (Original magnification × 32,500.) S, Schlemm's canal; V, vacuole forming passage through endothelial cell; T, trabecular space. (From Kayes J: Invest Ophthalmol 6:381, 1967.)

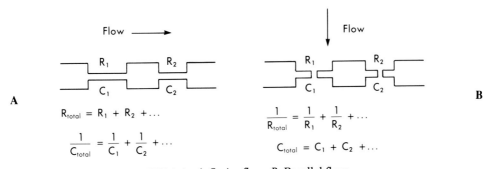

FIG. 8-6 *A,* Series flow. *B,* Parallel flow.

$$\text{Facility} = \frac{1}{\text{Resistance}} \text{ or } C = \frac{1}{R}$$

between aqueous flow, hydrostatic pressure head, and facility may be written:

$$F = \Delta PC$$

where C is facility, expressed in units of μl/min/mm Hg. For the sake of convenience, units of facility are used to express the passive resistance of the trabecular meshwork to the passage of aqueous. For flow through a series of passages (Fig. 8-6, *A*), total resistance is the sum of individual resistances in series, whereas if expressed as facility, the reciprocal of facility is

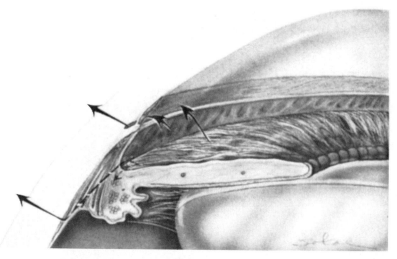

FIG. 8-7 Two principal pathways of aqueous flow: trabeculocanalicular and uveoscleral. (From Kass MA, Hoskins HD: Becker-Schaffer's diagnosis and therapy of the glaucomas, 6th ed, St Louis, CV Mosby, 1989.)

equal to the sum of reciprocals of individual facilities. For flow through a series of parallel passages, on the other hand (Fig. 8-6, *B*), the situation is reversed. Total facility is then the sum of individual facilities, whereas the reciprocal of the total resistance equals the sum of the reciprocals of individual resistances. This simple additivity of facilities in parallel flow systems like that of the trabecular meshwork makes the use of facility more convenient than the same calculations for resistances.

The second principal outflow passage for aqueous is referred to as uveoscleral outflow. It has been experimentally demonstrated that aqueous at normal levels of intraocular pressure slowly weeps through the face of the ciliary body in the region just posterior to the scleral spur in the apex of the anterior chamber just posterior to the scleral spur in the apex of the anterior chamber angle between the root of the iris and the scleral spur[6] (Fig. 8-7). Aqueous moves by bulk flow through this tissue to be subsequently absorbed into blood vessels or to leak through the scleral wall into the surrounding periocular orbital tissues. The measured rate of this flow appears to be quite constant and independent of intraocular pressure. Uveoscleral flow (commonly designated by the constant U) behaves much like a constant rate pump, although there is no evidence of a metabolically dependent process. It is thought that the constancy of uveoscleral flow may be related to an effect of IOP on uveoscleral flow, in which compression of uveal tissue against the sclera by elevated levels of intraocular pressure produces a

valve effect, preventing the elevated pressure from resulting in increasing rates of uveoscleral flow.

Aqueous flow formulas

Aqueous flow from the ciliary processes into the posterior chamber is the result of two separate processes: ultrafiltration and metabolic pumping. Ultrafiltration is the result of a hydrodynamic pressure head, $P_{blood} - P_i$ through a parallel series of microscopic passages having a total facility of C_{in}. Thus ultrafiltration flow can be expressed by the formula:

$$F_{in} = (P_{blood} - P_i)C_{in}$$

(C_{in} should not be confused with C_{trab}, the outflow facility. Hence some authors have refered to C_{in} as "pseudofacility.")[3]

Aqueous flow from the metabolic pump is not pressure sensitive, but can be represented by the constant S, expressed in units of $\mu l/min$.

Just as there are two principal pathways for flow into the eye, ultrafiltration and metabolic pumping, there are two principal pathways for flow out of the eye: trabecular flow and uveoscleral flow. The hydrodynamic pressure head for trabecular flow is the difference between the intraocular pressure (IOP or P_i) and the opposite end of the flow circuit, which is the episcleral venous pressure or P_e. The rate of flow through the trabecular system can be expressed by

$$F_{trab} = (P_i - P_e)C_{trab}$$

where C_{trab} is the outflow facility across the trabecular meshwork. A reduction in C_{trab} (in-

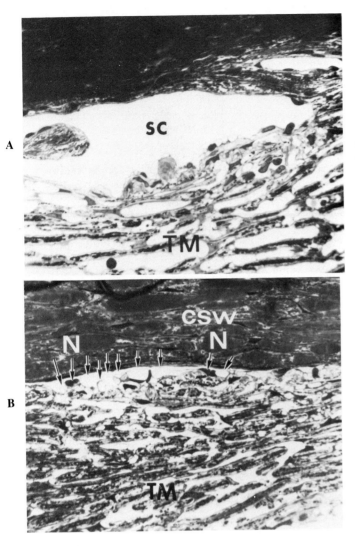

A

B

FIG. 8-8 Effect of IOP on spacing of trabecular laminae. Enucleated human eyes fixed at varying levels of IOP. **A,** Fixed at 5 mm Hg. Schlemm's canal, SC, is wide, and laminae of trabecular meshwork, TM, are spread out. **B,** Fixed at 50 mm Hg. Nuclei, N, and vacuoles *(arrows)* of inner wall endothelium contact external (corneal) wall of canal, CSW. Canal is flattened, and laminae of meshwork are compressed. (Magnification × 550.) (From Johnstone MA, Grant WM: Am J Ophthalmol 75:365, 1973.)

creased resistance to trabecular flow) is the proximate cause of elevated IOP in primary open-angle glaucoma.

This expression for trabecular flow is not entirely accurate, since it is known that the facility of trabecular outflow decreases at increasingly higher levels of intraocular pressure due to collapse of the trabecular laminae against one another[7] (Fig. 8-8). Brubaker has accordingly modified the trabecular outflow equation to yield

$$R_{trab} = R_o + R_oQ(P_i - P_e)$$

where R_o is the resistance when the outflow pressure head $(P_i - P_e)$ is zero and Q is the obstruction coefficient in units of $(mm\ Hg)^{-1}$. The mechanism of increased resistance to outflow as IOP rises is thought to be the result of collapse of Schlemm's canal. Apposition of inner and outer walls results in increased resistance to flow into and through the canal.[19,27]

Since facility (conductance) is the inverse of resistance, we have

$$C_{trab} = \frac{1}{R_{trab}} = \frac{1}{R_o + R_oQ(P_i - P_e)}$$

Uveoscleral outflow mimics the behavior of a constant rate pump and is expressed by the constant U. Unlike trabecular flow (F_{trab}), U is a constant that is unaffected by small variations in intraocular pressure. (U will diminish with large elevations in IOP.)

In experimental preparations direct measurement of C_{trab} is complicated by numerous artifacts. It has been found, for instance, that retrodisplacement of the lens will put traction on the zonular ligament, tensing the trabecular meshwork. Thus deepening of the anterior chamber during experimental perfusion of the eye will artificially widen the trabecular spaces and increase the value of C_{trab}.[25,36] Trabecular facility is also prone to artifactual elevation during prolonged ocular perfusion with saline, a phenomenon referred to as "washout." This is thought to be the result of elution of material from the trabecular surfaces,[13,32] and can be minimized by using perfusates most closely matched to the chemical composition of aqueous.

In the normal physiologic state of dynamic equilibrium, in which IOP is relatively constant over any given time period, the total flow of aqueous into the eye will be exactly equal to the rate of flow of aqueous out of the eye. By convention, inflow variables are assigned a positive sign while outflow variables are assigned a negative sign. Thus at the steady state the two inflows, ultrafiltration plus metabolic pumping when added to the two outflows, trabecular outflow plus uveoscleral outflow, will yield a value of 0 when intraocular pressure is steady. This is expressed as

total flow in + total flow out = 0.

Substituting the above-defined symbols into this expression, we have

$$F_{in} + S - F_{trab} - U = 0.$$

Expanding this expression somewhat further, but without including Brubaker's correction, we have

$$(P_{blood} - P_i)C_{in} + S - (P_i - P_e)C_{trab} - U = 0$$

Thus expressed, this equation summarizes all of the principally important variables determining intraocular pressure.

If we incorporate Brubaker's correction into this equation, we then have

$$(P_{blood} - P_i)C_{in} +$$
$$S - \frac{(P_i - P_e)}{R_o + R_oQ(P_i - P_e)} - U = 0$$

As shown in Figure 8-9, steady-state IOP (as predicted from the above equations) is directly

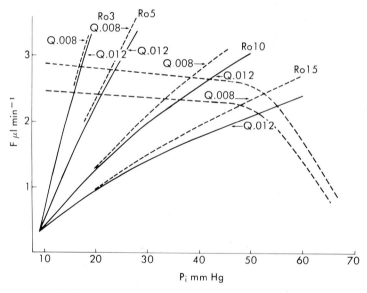

FIG. 8-9 Dynamic equilibrium (steady state), when rate of aqueous production equals total rate of outflow. Rising curves are sum of trabecular and uveoscleral flows (at various levels of outflow facility and assuming uveoscleral flow = constant 0.3 μl/min), and include Brubaker's correction (see text, Q = obstruction coefficient, the increase of trabecular resistance/mm Hg).The dashed curves falling down to the right represent estimated rates of aqueous inflow. Rate of aqueous formation falls gradually as P_i increases, until ciliary artery blood pressure is reached, above which aqueous formation rate drops sharply. Intersections of inflow and outflow curves give P_i for each R_0, where R_0 is the trabecular resistance (1/C) at P_i = 0.

and nearly linearly related to the rate of aqueous flow. Changes to this closed system by, for instance, artificially elevating the intraocular pressure through some means or pharmacologic reduction in the rate of aqueous production, will result in predictable changes in pressure and flow. In reality, however, the eye is more complex than can be expressed by this simple series of equations.[24] Experimental observations of behavior in such biological systems are always superior to the predictions of simplifying models.

Effect of episcleral venous pressure on intraocular pressure

Increases in episcleral venous pressure can be expected to result linearly in identical increases in intraocular pressure.[21] Any sudden increase in episcleral venous pressure, such as that produced by the Valsalva maneuver, will result in an immediate rise in intraocular pressure. The initial rapid increase in intraocular pressure is not solely the result of a decreased pressure head for aqueous outflow but is also initially related to engorgement of the intraocular vascular bed, principally the choroidal vessels. Since the scleral coat of the eye has a limited degree of elasticity (see discussion below of "ocular rigidity"), a small increase in intraocular volume will result in a rather substantial increase in intraocular pressure. Thus, following a sudden increase in episcleral venous pressure, a new steady state will not be reestablished until the resulting vascular engorgement has been diminished by continued pumping of aqueous into the eye. The time course of this replacement is not known accurately but is thought to be in the range of 15 to 30 minutes.

Elevation of episcleral venous pressure P_e to a new value P_e' will result in a decreased outflow of aqueous through the trabecular meshwork until the intraocular pressure has risen to a new value, reestablishing the flow at a new steady state. However, since ultrafiltration at the ciliary body is also determined by a hydrostatic pressure head, the new higher level of intraocular pressure will also decrease aqueous inflow a small amount.

To determine how a rise in episcleral venous pressure will result in a predictable increase in intraocular pressure, the new steady-state equation can be expressed as follows:

$$(P_{blood} - P_i')C_{in} + S - (P_i' - P_e')C_{trab} - U = 0$$

The normal steady state relationship prior to elevation of episcleral venous pressure was

$$(P_{blood} - P_i)C_{in} + S - (P_i - P_e)C_{trab} - U = 0$$

If we subtract these two equations from one another, we obtain the following expression:

$$(P_i' - P_i)(C_{in} + C_{trab}) - (P_e' - P_e)C_{trab} = 0$$

Since inflow facility C_{in} and trabecular outflow facility C_{trab} are in parallel, we can write

$$C_{in} + C_{trab} = C_{total}$$

We may further substitute

$$\Delta P_i = P_i' - P_i$$

and

$$\Delta P_e = P_e' - P_e$$

Following substitution and rearrangement we have

$$\frac{\Delta P_i}{\Delta P_e} = \frac{C_{trab}}{C_{total}}$$

This relationship has allowed investigators to estimate what proportion of facility is due to C_{trab} and which is C_{in}. Approximately 90% of total facility is trabecular, with less than 10% of the total being attributable to inflow facility. A normal value for total facility is approximately 0.3 $\mu l/min/mm$ Hg, where trabecular facility is approximately 0.28 and inflow ("pseudo") facility is approximately 0.02 $\mu l/min/mm$ Hg.

Throughout the above discussion we have assumed that P_{blood}, C_{in}, C_{trab}, S and U are all constants within the ranges of intraocular pressure investigated. This is at best a simplifying assumption. It is probable that all components of the above flow equations change with significant alterations in intraocular pressure.

Measurement of intraocular pressure

Tonometers are devices for the estimation of intraocular pressure, a measure referred to as tonometry. Tonometers are of two principal varieties: applanation and indentation types. In applanation tonometry the force necessary to flatten a measured area of the cornea is determined. Since pressure is defined as the force per unit area, this technique provides a nearly direct method of intraocular pressure estimation (Fig. 8-10).

There are four factors that may diminish the accuracy of applanation tonometric estimates of intraocular pressure:

1. When applanating the cornea, a small volume of aqueous beneath the cornea must be displaced. This displacement results in a small but measurable increase in IOP.
2. The precorneal tear film forms a meniscus in the angle between the surface of the ap-

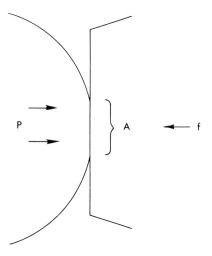

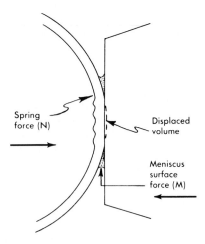

FIG. 8-10   Principle of applanation tonometry based on definition of pressure. Pressure = force per unit area.

FIG. 8-11   Potential sources of error in corneal applanation tonometry. By design, an area of applanation has been chosen such that N and M will be approximately equal, thus canceling one another.

planating instrument and the cornea, and may be mistaken for a part of the corneal contact area.

3. The surface tension of the tear meniscus adds a small force (M) to the applied force of the applanating instrument.

4. The cornea resists the flattening of its surface. A spring force (N) is needed to flatten the cornea to the desired degree, thereby increasing the measured force applied to achieve a given area of applanation (Fig. 8-11).

The Goldmann tonometer

The Goldmann applanation tonometer (Fig. 8-12) has become the global clinical standard for estimation of IOP. The design of this instrument minimizes the potential error factors (outlined above) by keeping the contact area small, so that only a small portion of aqueous is displaced by the applanating instrument, and only a small volume of corneal tissue is depressed beneath the applanating surface. The tear meniscus is stained with fluorescein dye, and when viewed in blue light the fluorescence of the dye-stained meniscus is easily distinguishable from the flattened area of cornea beneath the instrument's contact surface.

The tonometer displays the force in grams necessary to achieve the applanation criterion, a flattened circular area of cornea having a diameter of 3.06 mm. This area was chosen in part as one at which the surface tension of the tear meniscus and the force N resisting tissue compres-

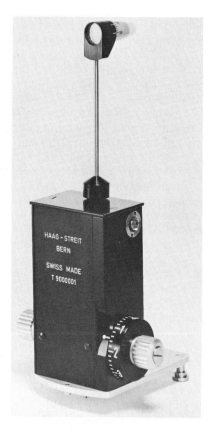

FIG. 8-12   The Goldmann applanation tonometer. During use, instrument is mounted on clinical slit lamp biomicroscope, and force against prism head of instrument (the small, truncated cone at the top) is adjusted to flatten corneal surface to a standard diameter. Circular knob at bottom adjusts force, and is calibrated in grams.

sion approximately cancel one another. The force in grams against the applanating tonometer head, when multiplied by 10, is the estimate of intraocular pressure in millimeters of mercury. The examiner uses a slit-lamp biomicroscope to view the surface of the applanated cornea through the center of the prism, which is illuminated with a blue light. The tear meniscus surrounding the circular area of applanation is seen as a yellow-green circle that is split in half by a prismatic doubling device in the tonometer head. The rotating knob of the tonometer is manipulated by the examiner to vary the force against the prism to reach the standard end point at which the inner borders of the two semicircular halves of the tear meniscus just barely touch one another (Fig. 8-13).

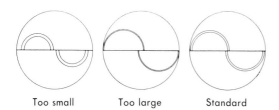

Too small   Too large   Standard

FIG. 8-13 Tonometer head contains doubling prism that splits the circle of tear meniscus into two overlapping semicircles, seen as yellow green arcs against a blue background. (From Moses RA: Am J Ophthalmol 46:865, 1958. Published with permission from The American Journal of Ophthalmology. Copyright by The Ophthalmic Publishing Company.)

Non-contact ("air puff") tonometry

The American Optical non-contact tonometer applanates the surface of the cornea by directing a calibrated jet of pressurized air against the surface. Surface flattening is sensed photoelectrically and intraocular pressure is calculated from the known force and diameter of the jet at the exact moment of applanation.

The Mackay-Marg tonometer

The Mackay-Marg tonometer contains a spring-mounted plunger having a diameter of 1.5 mm that protrudes by a distance of 10 microns through the center of a metallic, flat footplate. As the surface of the tonometer is lowered onto the surface of the cornea, the plunger initially counteracts the intraocular pressure and corneal bending force (Fig. 8-14). As the tonometer head moves farther in toward the surface of the eye, the footplate surrounding the plunger makes contact with the surface of the cornea, at which time the force on the central plunger is momentarily decreased, producing a notch in the timed record of force. The distance between the baseline and the lowest level of the notch is then taken as an estimate of the intraocular pressure. This type of tonometer is somewhat more difficult to calibrate than the Goldmann variety and is principally used in clinical situations where applanation tonometery via the Goldmann instrument is not practical, such as in patients that have recently undergone corneal surgery.

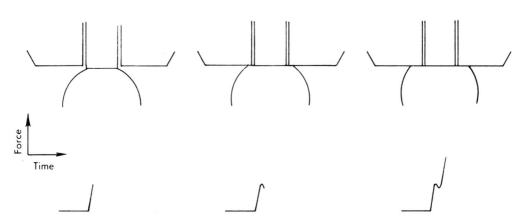

FIG. 8-14 Operating principle of Mackay-Marg Tonometer. *Left,* As central plunger first contacts corneal surface it supports both IOP and spring force of cornea. *Center,* As cornea is applanated further, footplate begins to support pressure and force on central plunger drops momentarily. *Right,* As tonometer is advanced further, displaced aqueous raises IOP. *Upper diagrams,* exaggerated representations of probe and corneal surface. *Lower diagrams,* time record of central plunger movement.

Indentation (Schiøtz) tonometry

The principle of indentation tonometry involves the measurement of the extent of indentation of the cornea by a smoothly polished metallic probe contained within a cylindrical footplate and carrying a known weight. The Schiøtz tonometer is the classical prototype of this kind of tonometer. It has a freely sliding plunger that passes through the center of a small concave footplate. The plunger can carry weights of 5.5, 7.5, or 10.0 grams (Fig. 8-15). A drop of topical anesthetic is applied to the cornea and with the patient supine the tip of the instrument is allowed to rest on the surface of the eye. The weighted plunger then forms an indentation below the level of the footplate and the depth of this indentation is then registered on a scale. One scale reading unit of the instrument corresponds to an indentation of $\frac{1}{20}$ of a millimeter.

Since indentation tonometry results in a significant increase in intraocular pressure with indentation of the cornea (P_i is raised to P_t, which can be as much as 10 mm Hg greater than P_i), a great deal of empirical testing was required to

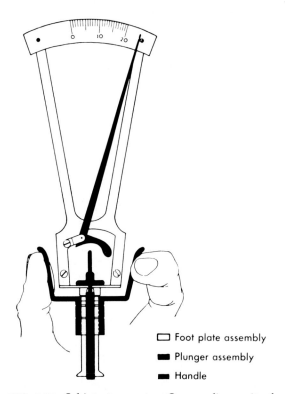

Foot plate assembly
Plunger assembly
Handle

FIG. 8-15 Schiøtz tonometer. One reading unit of scale at top corresponds to 0.05 mm of corneal indentation. (From Kronfeld PC, in Berens C, ed: The eye and its diseases, 2nd ed, Philadelphia, WB Saunders, 1949.)

produce accurate calibration charts for this instrument.[12,23] When properly used, Schiøtz tonometry produces accurate and reproducible clinical estimates of intraocular pressure. It is, however, rather less convenient than Goldmann applanation tonometry and aside from its use in tonographic measurements (see below) it has been largely discarded from routine clinical use save for those areas of the world where slit-lamp instrumentation is not readily available. In such areas its portability, ease of use, and low expense make it a practical alternative.

The original experimental work used to establish empirically the accuracy and reproducibility of Schiøtz tonometry determined that when the volume of the eye was changed linearly, the pressure of the eye changed exponentially. By convention the intraocular pressure just prior to application of the Schiøtz tonometer is symbolized as P_i, while the pressure estimate obtained immediately after application of the tonometer head is symbolized by P_t. The subsequently calculated value for IOP just prior to application of the tonometer is P_o. Thus we have

$$\log P_t - \log P_o = EV_c$$

where V_c is the volume displaced by the plunger and

$$\log P_{t1} - \log P_{t2} = E(V_{c2} - V_{c1})$$

where

$$
\begin{aligned}
P_t &= \text{tonometric pressure} \\
P_{t1}, P_{t2} &= \text{tonometric pressures with differing} \\
&\quad \text{plunger loads} \\
P_o &= \text{IOP prior to tonometry} \\
E &= \text{coefficient of ocular rigidity, and} \\
V_{c1}, V_{c2} &= \text{volumes of corneal indentation corresponding to pressures of } P_{t1}, P_{t2}
\end{aligned}
$$

The term "ocular rigidity" used in the above relationship actually refers to the elasticity (ability to deform under stress and then reform after removal of stress) of the ocular wall, hence the symbol "E". In the absence of a positive intraocular pressure to maintain tension on the ocular wall, it is of course not rigid at all. It was empirically determined that although ocular rigidity varied from one eye to another, its average value in the human was .0215. (Note that E is a dimensionless coefficient.) Similarly, values for P_t and V_c corresponding to tonometer scale readings for each of the three separate plunger weights were obtained experimentally. The results of these numerous experiments are summarized in the Friedenwald nomogram (Fig. 8-16). If for a given eye one plots the tonometer scale readings obtained with each of the differ-

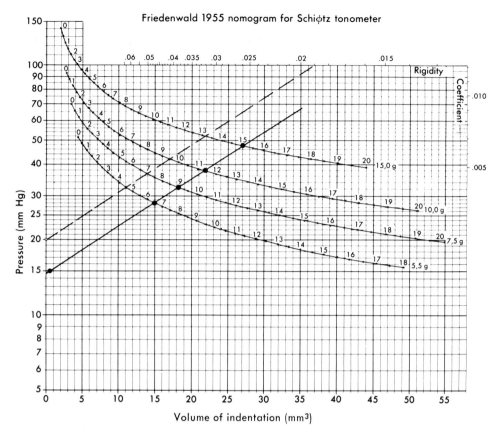

FIG. 8-16 Friedenwald nomogram for Schiøtz tonometer. Tonometric distortion (corneal indentation by plunger) considered equivalent to injection of additional intraocular volume into eye. Pressure rises exponentially with increasing injected volume. Tonometric measurements with differing plunger weights will yield a set of points along a straight line, having a slope equal to ocular rigidity (solid line). Points indicated on line are values obtained by Goldmann applanation tonometry during corneal indentation by Schiøtz instrument with four different plunger loads.

ing plunger weights and joins them by a straight line, one obtains an estimate of P_o, a derivation of the intraocular pressure present in the eye just prior to application of the indentation tonometer. The nomogram is further constructed so that the slope of the line connecting the points of two or more tonometer readings can be read from the scale where the line intersects the upper or right-hand edge of the nomogram. The slope corresponds to E, the estimate of ocular rigidity.

TONOGRAPHY

If a Schiøtz tonometer is rested on the cornea for a period of time, the plunger will slowly increase the degree of corneal indentation. The elevated intraocular pressure caused by the corneal indentation (an increase in IOP to the level of P_t)

causes an increased aqueous outflow, resulting in a gradual volume loss from the eye. This loss is made up of two parts, that which is due to the deepening of the corneal indentation and that which is due to the loss of intraocular volume.[14]

Following application of the tonometer to the eye, an immediate increase in the rate of aqueous escape through the trabecular meshwork occurs. As the volume of the eye slowly decreases, the tonometer scale reading will diminish from P_{t1} to P_{t2} (Fig. 8-17). The volume loss from the eye can be expressed as

$$\Delta V_{sclera} = \frac{1}{E} (\log P_{t1} - \log P_{t2})$$

The total volume loss during the time period (t) that the tonometer is left on the surface of the globe is

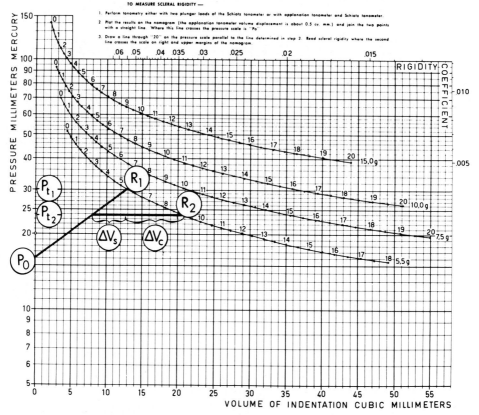

FRIEDENWALD 1955 NOMOGRAM FOR SCHIOTZ TONOMETER

FIG. 8-17 Tonography with the Schiøtz instrument. (In practice the head of the Schiøtz tonometer is modified to incorporate an electromagnetic sensor that replaces the scale of the hand-held instrument.) R_1, tonometric reading immediately after application of instrument with 5.5 gram load; R_2, tonometric reading after 4 minute tonographic interval; ΔV_c, change in corneal indentation during tonographic interval, while tonometric pressure fell from P_{t1} to P_{t2}; ΔV_s, loss of ocular volume with drop in P_t from P_{t1} to P_{t2}; P_o, estimate of P_i, assuming ocular rigidity = 0.019.

$$\frac{\Delta V_{total}}{t} = \frac{(\Delta V_c + \Delta V_s)}{t}$$

A source of error in this estimate is caused by a transient increase in episcleral venous pressure following application of the tonometer head (ΔP_e).[22] Correcting for this error, the average intraocular pressure during the tonographic time period is approximated by

$$\frac{(P_{t1} + P_{t2})}{2} - (P_o + \Delta P_e)$$

The combined expression is thus

$$C_{total} = \frac{V_{c2} - V_{c1} + \frac{1}{E}(\log P_{t1} - P_{t2})}{t(P_{tav} - P_o - \Delta P_e)}$$

where P_{tav} is the average tonometric pressure.

During clinical tonography it is ordinarily assumed that ocular rigidity (E) is 0.0215, and ΔP_e has a value of 1.25 mm Hg. The usual tonographic time period by convention is 4 minutes. Referring to the nomogram in Figure 8-17, recognize that V_{c1}, V_{c2}, P_{t1}, P_{t2} and P_o are read directly from the nomogram or taken from accompanying tables, and the only measured quantities necessary to determine C_{total} are the tonometer scale readings at the beginning and end of the tonographic time period and the time elapsed between the two readings. Although clinical estimation of outflow facility is not routinely used in the clinical management of glaucoma patients, tonographic studies in the past have provided a firm foundation for our understanding of the pathophysiology of the glaucomas. This technique furthermore remains one of the most readily available means of estimating total outflow facility in the human eye.

Distribution of IOP in the population

The IOP, like many other biological variables, has been found not to fit a normal distribution curve, but rather tails off somewhat gradually toward higher pressures.[9] In the jargon of the statistician, the curve is said to be skewed to the right (Fig. 8-18). This finding was most dramatically illustrated in a study of approximately 10,000 normal individuals undergoing Schiøtz tonometry; a mean pressure of 15.8 mm Hg ± 1 standard deviation of 2.6 mm Hg was found. The skewness to the right in the IOP distribution means that one cannot conveniently define a statistical criterion for abnormal elevation of IOP. In fact, one finds a disproportionately large number of people in the general population who have higher intraocular pressures than would be predicted by a normal distribution. It has been empirically found that if one selects for study a group of individuals whose intraocular pressures exceed the population mean by 2 standard deviations, subsequent study of these individuals (who have statistically defined "ocular hypertension") will find them to be at very low risk for disease. For follow-up periods of 5 years 90% or more of such individuals will show no evidence of damage to visual function. Thus there can be no useful statistical definition of glaucomatous or abnormally elevated intraocular pressure. Unfortunately, the level of IOP capable of resulting in disease can be defined only empirically by the observation of visual damage. This of course means that for some individuals statistically normal or even "low" pressures may be found associated with damage to visual function.

Variations in IOP

Despite the relative constancy of IOP, there are factors that contribute to both long- and short-term variations in IOP. Long-term variations are associated with age, blood pressure, and calendar seasons. Typical contributors to short-term variations include body posture, exercise, eye movements, and drug effects.

Long-term variations

Several population studies have reported an association between age and increasing IOP.[4,9,33] Most of this long-term variation is thought to be the result of a co-correlation between age, systemic blood pressure, and body weight.[9,33] This finding, however, has not been universal and a number of studies have found no significant correlation between IOP and age.

There is also a reported correlation between calendar season and IOP.[4] A small variation is found with higher intraocular pressures being present during the winter months. The mechanism for the observation is not known, although some have speculated that changes in diurnal light exposure or atmospheric temperature or pressure may be the controlling factors. Also, there may be a correlation between season, diet, body weight, and blood pressure that could account for the small increases in IOP found during the winter months.

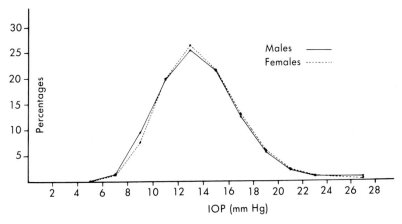

FIG. 8-18 Population distribution of IOP for 12,803 individuals, expressed as percentages for males and females. Note skewness to the right. Values obtained with A-O Non-contact tonometer. (From Carel RS, et al: Ophthalmol 91:311, 1984.)

Short-term fluctuations

There is a well-established diurnal variation in IOP, and this variation tends to be accentuated in patients with open-angle glaucoma.[15] The diurnal variation is fairly reproducible, with maximum pressure levels being reached during the early morning hours, often prior to awakening, and with minimum pressure levels being recorded late at night or in the early morning just after retiring. Most of the variation in IOP that occurs during the diurnal cycle is attributable to changes in the rate of aqueous humor production.[8,31] The rate of aqueous formation varies synchronously with endogenous levels of circulating cortisol and catecholamines. There is a 3 to 4 hour shift in cycle peaks, with IOP reaching a maximum approximately 3 to 4 hours after peak of plasma cortisol. In eyes with primary open-angle glaucoma the pattern of diurnal fluctuation is exaggerated (Fig. 8-20).

Changes in central venous pressure produce changes in episcleral venous pressure and are immediately reflected in rapid changes in IOP.[34] Change in body position from erect to supine can result in an immediate increase of IOP of up to 16 mm Hg. In patients with impaired outflow facility the elevation in IOP is even greater. Complete inversion of body position from erect to upside down can result in a doubling of measured IOP from the mid teens into the low 30s. While such variations in IOP are dramatic, they clearly are not damaging to vision in the normal population. However, in patients with glaucoma for whom the swings are even greater in magnitude, prolonged assumption of such postures may be harmful to vision.

Similar to postural changes, changes in eye movement, especially against mechanical resistance, can result in short-term swings in IOP.[26] This phenomenon is clinically very important in patients with restrictive ocular motor disease such as the ophthalmopathy of Graves' disease. Inflammatory scarring of extraocular muscles with an attendant restriction of the muscles' range of motion can result in substantial pressures being brought to bear on the globe during attempts to move the eye against the resistance of the fibrotic muscle. Since the inferior rectus is the most commonly affected muscle in Graves' disease, moving the eye into the primary gaze position may result in significant traction on the eye against the resistance of a fibrotic inferior rectus muscle. Since applanation tonometry with a Goldmann tonometer at the slit-lamp requires the patient to hold the eye in the primary gaze position, an artifactual increase in IOP at the moment of applanation is commonly observed. In such patients, if applanation pressures are remeasured with the eye held in a slightly downgaze pattern and compared with the results of the primary and upgaze positions, a transient and significant variation in IOP can be demonstrated, with increasing pressures present at ever-increasing levels of gaze. Even

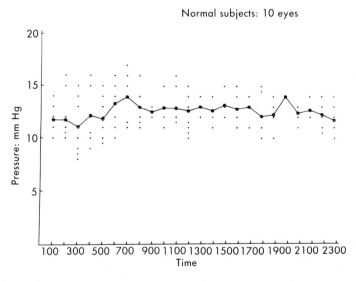

Normal subjects: 10 eyes

FIG. 8-19 Diurnal variation in IOP of normal eyes. Pressure is lowest during sleep, but peaks in the early morning hours just before or at the time of arising. Pressures remain higher during the day, but variations are relatively small. (From Henkind P, Leitman M, Weitzman E: Invest Ophthalmol 12:705, 1973.)

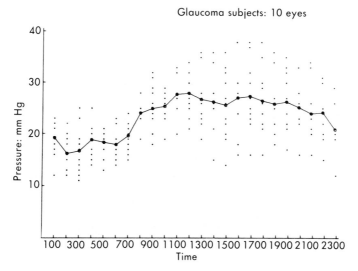

Glaucoma subjects: 10 eyes

FIG. 8-20 Diurnal variation in IOP of eyes with glaucoma; has appearance of exaggerated version of pattern seen in normals with broad swings in pressure. (From Henkind P, Leitman M, Weitzman E: Invest Ophthalmol 12:705, 1973.)

voluntary widening of the palpebral fissure in normal eyes can produce measurable, though transient, increases in IOP.[28]

Strenuous exercise can result in short-term but measurable reductions in IOP. It is thought that these variations are related to the metabolic acidosis of exercise and changes in extracellular fluid volume and osmolarity. The results are at best transient, however. Although exercise has beneficial consequences for general levels of fitness, it has not been established that exercise is in any way beneficial in the therapy of glaucoma.

Pharmacology of the IOP

Miotic drugs (those that cause the pupil to constrict) generally result in a lowered IOP. In addition to producing contraction of the iris sphincter muscle, these drugs also stimulate contraction of the ciliary muscle. The trabecular meshwork, being attached to the scleral spur, is in effect a tendon of origin for the ciliary muscle, traction on which will result in a significant change in the geometry of the trabecular meshwork (Fig. 8-21). Miotic drugs reduce uveoscleral outflow facility and produce a simultaneous increase in trabecular outflow facility. Since trabecular facility is approximately an order of magnitude greater than uveoscleral facility, the net effect is a marked elevation in outflow facility with a concomitant decrease in IOP. This effect is particularly magnified in eyes that

have abnormally high IOP (abnormally low outflow facility.)

The miotic drugs are in the parasympathomimetic group, including direct parasympathetic agonist drugs such as pilocarpine and carbachol and indirect agonists such as the cholinesterase inhibitors (eserine or phospholine iodide).

Conversely, mydriatic agents commonly produce increases in IOP. This is particularly true for eyes that have anatomically shallow anterior chambers and narrow anterior chamber angles. Additionally, some eyes have a so-called "plateau iris" configuration, where the most peripheral portion of the iris stroma is positioned very close to the uveoscleral meshwork while the rest of the anterior chamber has a more normal depth. Mydriasis (pupillary dilation) allows the most peripheral portions of the anterior iris stroma to move forward toward the inner aspect of the uveoscleral meshwork, commonly resulting in diminished trabecular outflow facility. In susceptible eyes this may result in acute and complete obstruction to trabecular outflow, producing an acute, rapid increase of IOP to very high levels, a disease known as acute angle-closure glaucoma.

Sympathetic agonists and antagonists that have minimal effects on pupillary size can nonetheless have substantial effects on IOP. For instance, epinephrine hydrochloride is a valuable drug for treating primary open-angle glaucoma.

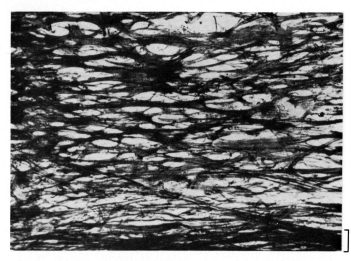

]Scleral
spur

FIG. 8-21   Tangential section through trabecular meshwork in eye fixed after application of pilocarpine. Anterior meshwork at top; posterior meshwork (and scleral spur) at bottom. Interlamellar spaces of meshwork are widened.

Tonographic studes have shown that the long-term administration of epinephrine hydrochloride results in a reduction of aqueous humor production of 30% or more.[20] The exact mechanism for this effect is not known, but it has been suggested that it is the result of chronic vasoconstriction within the ciliary body, reducing blood flow to the ciliary epithelia.[1]

Paradoxically, adrenergic beta blocking agents similarly result in a reduction in aqueous humor production, again without having significant effect on pupillary size. Fluorometric studies have demonstrated a 16 to 47% decrease in the rate of aqueous humor formation following administration of this class of drug. Clinically, the most commonly used topical beta blocking agent is timolol maleate.

Carbonic anhydrase is an enzyme involved in the membrane transport of bicarbonate and water across the ciliary epithelia. Inhibitors of this enzyme result in a decreased rate of aqueous humor formation. Acetazolamide has been in use for approximately four decades as a systemic agent for lowering IOP. In oral doses of approximately 1 gram per day or less it results in a substantial reduction in IOP, the effect being greatest in individuals with pathologically elevated IOP.

Substances that rapidly and significantly elevate blood osmolarity will result in a fluid shift out of the eye toward the blood stream, accompanied by a rapid and dramatic drop in IOP. Again this effect is likely to be most pronounced in eyes with pathologically elevated pressures. Oral ingestion of hypertonic solutions of glyc-erin or intravenous infusion of concentrated solutions of urea or mannitol are very useful in the management of acute and markedly elevated IOPs. Oral glycerin is the drug of choice when its use has not been precluded by nausea and vomiting. Rapid reduction in IOP by these hyperosmotic agents is frequently effective in interrupting an attack of acute angle-closure glaucoma, allowing a brief period for clinical stabilization prior to surgical intervention.

Conversely, ingestion of large quantities of hypotonic solution (water drinking) can result in significant and measurable increases in IOP. This effect is magnified in patients with abnormally low outflow facilities. In such patients drinking of one quart of water may result in a rise in IOP of 8 mm Hg or greater. This simple test has been proposed as a quick and inexpensive means for detecting patients with significantly reduced outflow facilities.

Corticosteroid drugs can have a significant long-term effect of raising IOP.[5] There appears to be an inherited susceptibility to this effect, which is present in a small portion of the normal population. Topical or oral administration of any corticosteroid in such individuals can produce a pressure rise in otherwise normal eyes. This effect ordinarily requires several weeks of constant exposure and is more likely to result from topical than systemic administration.

REFERENCES

1. Alm A: The effect of topical l-epinephrine on regional ocular blood flow in monkeys, Invest Ophthalmol Vis Sci 19:487, 1980.

2. Anderson DR: Scanning electron microscopy of primate trabecular meshwork, Am J Ophthalmol 71:90, 1971.

3. Barany EH: Mathematical formulation of intraocular pressure as dependent on secretion, ultrafiltration, bulk outflow, and osmotic reabsorption of fluid, Invest Ophthalmol 2:584, 1963.

4. Bengtsson B: Some factors affecting the distribution of intraocular pressures in a population, Acta Ophthalmol (Copenh) 50:23, 1972.

5. Bernstein HN, Schwartz B: Effects of long-term systemic steroids on ocular pressure and tonographic values, Arch Ophthalmol 68:742, 1962.

6. Bill A: Conventional and uveoscleral drainage of aqueous humor in the cynomolgus monkey *(Macaca irus)* at normal and high intraocular pressure, Exp Eye Res 5:45, 1966.

7. Brubaker RF: The effect of intraocular pressure on conventional outflow resistance in the enucleated human eye, Invest Ophthalmol 14:286, 1975.

8. Brubaker RF: The physiology of aqueous humor formation, in Drance S, Neufeld A, ed: Applied pharmacology in the medical treatment of glaucoma, Orlando, Grune & Stratton, 1984.

9. Carel RS, et al: Association between ocular pressure and certain health parameters, Ophthalmol 91:311, 1984.

10. Feeney L, Wissig S: Outflow studies using an electron dense tracer, Trans Am Acad Ophthalmol Otolaryngol 70:791, 1966.

11. Fine BS: Structure of the trabecular meshwork and the canal of Schlemm, Trans Am Acad Ophthalmol Otolaryngol 70:777, 1966.

12. Friedenwald JS: Tonometer calibration: an attempt to remove discrepancies found in the 1954 calibration scale for Schiøtz tonometers, Trans Am Acad Ophthalmol Otolaryngol 61:108, 1957.

13. Gaasterland DE, et al: Rhesus monkey aqueous humor composition and a primate ocular perfusate, Invest Ophthalmol Vis Sci 18:1139, 1979.

14. Grant WM: Tonographic method for measuring the facility and rate of aqueous flow in human eyes, Arch Ophthalmol 44:204, 1950.

15. Henkind P, Leitman M, Weitzman E: The diurnal curve in man: new observations, Invest Ophthalmol 12:705, 1973.

16. Holmberg AS: Our present knowledge of the structure of the trabecular meshwork, in Leydhecker W, ed: Glaucoma, Twentieth International Congress of Ophthalmology, Tutzing Symposium, Basel, Switzerland, S. Karger, 1966.

17. Inomata H, Bill A, Smelser GK: Aqueous humor pathways through the trabecular meshwork and into Schlemm's canal in the cynomolgus monkey *(Macaca irus)*, Am J Ophthalmol 73:760, 1972.

18. Johnstone MA: Morphology of the aqueous outflow system, in Drance SM, Neufeld AH, eds: Glaucoma: applied pharmacology of medical treatment, New York, Grune & Stratton, 1984.

19. Johnstone MA, Grant WM: Pressure-dependent changes in structures of the aqueous outflow system of human and monkey eyes, Am J Ophthalmol 75:365, 1973.

20. Kolker AE, Hetherington J Jr: Becker-Shaffer's diagnosis and therapy of the glaucomas, St Louis, CV Mosby, 1983.

21. Krakau CET, Widakowich J, Wilke K: Measurements of the episcleral venous pressure by means of an air jet. Acta Ophthalmol (Copenh) 51:185, 1973.

22. Linner E: Episcleral venous pressure during tonography, XVII, Concilium Ophthalmol Acta 3:1532, 1954.

23. Moses RA: Theory of the Schiøtz tonometer and its empirical calibration, Trans Am Ophthalmol Soc 69:494, 1971.

24. Moses RA: The effect of intraocular pressure on resistance to outflow: a review, Surv Ophthalmol 22:88, 1977.

25. Moses RA, Etheridge EL, Grodzki WJ Jr: The effect of lens depression on the components of outflow resistance, Invest Ophthalmol Vis Sci 22:37, 1982.

26. Moses RA, Lurie P, Wette R: Horizontal gaze position effect on intraocular pressure, Invest Ophthalmol Vis Sci 22:551, 1982.

27. Moses RA, et al: Schlemm's canal: the effect of intraocular pressure, Invest Ophthalmol Vis Sci 20:61, 1981.

28. Moses RA, et al: Proptosis and increase of intraocular pressure in voluntary lid fissure widening, Invest Ophthalmol Vis Sci 25:989, 1984.

29. Murphy CG, Yun AH, Newsome DA, et al: Localization of extracellular proteins of the human trabecular meshwork by indirect immunofluorescence, Am J Ophthalmol 104:33, 1987.

30. Raviola G, Raviola E: Paracellular route of aqueous in the trabecular meshwork and canal of Schlemm, Invest Ophthalmol Vis Sci 21:52, 1981.

31. Reiss GR, et al: Aqueous humor flow during sleep, Invest Ophthalmol Vis Sci 25:776, 1984.

32. Ruben JB, Moses RA, Grodzki WJ Jr: Perfusion outflow in the rabbit eye: stabilization by EACA, Invest Ophthalmol Vis Sci 26:153, 1985.

33. Shiose Y: The aging effect on intraocular pressure in an apparently normal population, Arch Ophthalmol 102:883, 1984.

34. Tarkkanen A, Leikola J: Postural variations of the intraocular pressure as measured with the Mackay-Marg tonometer, Acta Ophthalmol (Copenh) 45:569, 1967.

35. Tripathi RC: Mechanism of the aqueous outflow across the trabecular wall of Schlemm's canal, Exp Eye Res 11:116, 1971.

36. Van Buskirk EM, Grant WM: Lens depression and aqueous outflow in enucleated primate eyes, Am J Ophthalmol 76:632, 1973.

CHAPTER
9

The Vitreous

J. SEBAG, M.D., F.A.C.S., F.C.Ophth.

GENERAL BACKGROUND

The vitreous is located between the lens and the retina and fills the center of the eye. Its approximate volume of 4 ml constitutes about 80% of the globe, making it the largest structure within the eye. Nevertheless, our understanding of vitreous composition, morphology, and function, and its role in disease is less than perhaps of any other part of the eye. Until relatively recently, few of the modern techniques of scientific investigation have been employed to study the vitreous. In a certain sense the advent of surgical techniques for vitreous removal has lessened academic interest in furthering our understanding of this structure. To counteract this trend this chapter will pressent current information on the molecular composition and organization of the vitreous as well as the physiology and pathology of this structure during development and aging. The various functions of the vitreous will be considered and the role of the vitreous in the pathogenesis of ocular disorders will be analyzed in terms of alterations in normal structure and physiology. It is anticipated that this approach will provide a useful reference for clinicians desiring more information on the basic science of the vitreous and for scientists needing a better understanding of clinical issues of concern to vitreoretinal physicians and surgeons.

Large portions of this chapter have been published previously in Sebag J: *The Vitreous—Structure, Function and Pathobiology*, New York, Springer-Verlag, 1989, and are reproduced here with permission of the publisher.

Historical perspective
Vitreous structure

During the eighteenth and nineteenth centuries no less than four different theories of vitreous structure prevailed. Demours[149] formulated the *"Alveolar Theory."* After freezing and slowly thawing the vitreous, he described a multitude of membranes oriented in all possible directions, enclosing compartments or alveoli containing the fluid portion of the vitreous. The studies of Von Haller[597] and later Virchow[593] supported this concept.

In 1780 Zinn[644] proposed that the vitreous is arranged in a concentric lamellar configuration similar to the layers of an onion. The dissections and histologic preparations of Von Pappenheim[599] and Brucke[84] provided evidence for the *"Lamellar Theory."* Stilling[537] and Iwanoff[293] modified this theory by stating that only the peripheral third of the vitreous has a lamellar structure.

The *"Radial Sector Theory"* was first proposed by Hannover.[254] Studying coronal sections at the equator, he described a multitude of sectors approximately radially oriented about the central antero-posterior core that contains Cloquet's canal. Hannover likened this structure to the appearance of a *"cut orange."* For many years a controversy existed between proponents of the "Lamellar Theory" and supporters of the "Radial Sector Theory." Smith[520] and Gerlach[222] attempted to unify the two theories by stating that the peripheral vitreous has concentric lamellae, while the central vitreous is organized in "radial sector" structures.

Bowman[77] introduced the *"Fibrillar Theory."* Employing microscopy, he described fine fibrils that form bundles with "nuclear" granules. Blix[70] proposed that these nuclear granules were actually the intersection sites of fibers coursing in all directions. Retzius[462] described fibrous structures arising in the peripheral anterior vitreous that assume an undulating pattern similar to a "horse's tail" in the central vitreous but maintain a concentric configuration at the periphery. Virchow[592] attempted to unify the "Alveolar" and "Fibrillar" theories by stating that compartments or alveoli are separated by fibrils. The elegant studies of Szent-Gyorgi[558] supported the descriptions of Retzius and introduced the concept that vitreous structure changes with age. He claimed that between the ages of 40 and 60 years the central vitreous undergoes dissolution and loss of structure, while in the periphery fibers fuse to form "membranes."

The work of Baurmann,[51] Stroemberg,[543] and Redslob[454] showed that many of the early studies were flawed by artefacts due to the use of tissue fixatives. Thus it was anticipated that the use of slit-lamp biomicroscopy in the study of vitreous structure would eliminate this problem, since investigations could be performed without introducing artefacts. Yet the use of in vivo slit-lamp biomicroscopy spawned an equally varied set of descriptions. Gullstrand[247] saw membranes composed of a network of weblike structures. Keoppe[338] described vertical and horizontal fibers arranged in regularly intercrossing systems. Baurmann[52] saw a grill-like pattern of darker and lighter bands resembling several layers of chain-link fences. Even the use of postmortem dark-field microscopy resulted in various interpretations, ranging from Goedbloed's[233] description of fibrillar structures to Friedenwald and Stiehler's[212] description of concentric sheets and Eisner's[160] observation of "membranelles."

In Eisner's meticulous studies dissections of human vitreous were observed to contain membranous structures that coursed from the region about the lens in a circumferential pattern, parallel with the vitreous cortex, to insert at the posterior pole. Eisner[160] has described these "membranelles" as funnels that are packed into one another and diverge outward and anteriorly from the prepapillary vitreous. He named these membranelles "tractae" according to their location (Fig. 9-1). The outermost (peripheral) vitreous tract is the "tractus preretinalis," which separates the vitreous cortex from the inner vitreous. Further inward are the "tractus medianus," which extends to the ligamentum me-

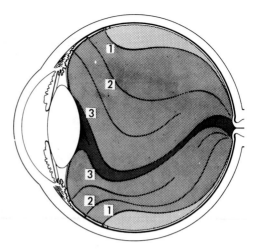

FIG. 9-1 Schematic diagram of Eisner's interpretation of vitreous structure (according to slit-lamp examinations of eyes obtained at autopsy). The vitreous body is divided into three zones: externally, as far as the retina extends, there is a relatively thick vitreous cortex (whitish gray here). It has holes at characteristic locations: in front of papilla, in region of fovea centralis, in front of vessels, and in front of anomalies of ora serrata region (enclosed ora bays, meridional folds, zonular traction tufts). Intermediate zone (light gray here) contains vitreal tracts; membranelles that form funnels packed into one another and diverge from region of papilla anteriorly. Central channel is space (dark gray here) delimited by hyaloid tract. It is closed off anteriorly by retrolental section of anterior vitreous membrane. It contains no typical tracts but only irregularly arranged vitreous fibers, part of which are residua of Cloquet's canal. The outermost vitreous tract, the preretinal tract, 1, separates intermediary substance from vitreous cortex. The innermost tract, the hyaloid tract, 3, inserts at edge of lens. Between them extends median tract, 2, to median ligament of pars plana, and coronary tract to coronary ligament.[160] (Modified from Eisner G: Biomicroscopy of the peripheral fundus, Berlin, Springer-Verlag, 1973.)

dianum of the pars plana, and the "tractus coronarius," which extends to the ligamentum coronarium of the pars plana. The innermost tract is the "tractus hyaloideus," which arises peripheral to the edge of the lens and courses posteriorly along Cloquet's canal (Fig. 9-1).

Worst[630] has also studied preparations of dissected human vitreous and has described that the "tracts" of Eisner constitute the walls of "cisterns" within the vitreous. In Worst's studies these cisterns are visualized by filling with white India ink (Fig. 9-2). Worst has named these cisterns the "hyaloid cistern" (Cloquet's canal), whose walls are the "tractus hyal-

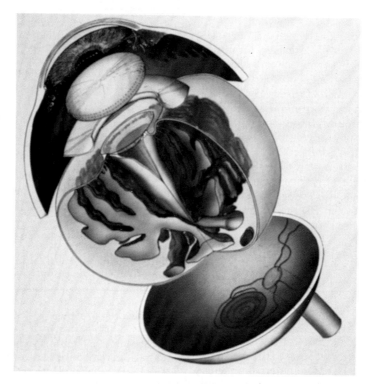

FIG. 9-2 Schematic diagram of Worst's interpretation of vitreous structure. "Cisterns" are visualized using white India ink to fill areas of the vitreous that take up this opaque dye. There are retrociliary, equatorial, and perimacular cisternal rings and a bursa premacularis. (Reprinted with permission from Jongbloed WL, Worst JGF: The cisternal anatomy of the vitreous body, Doc Ophthalmol 67:183, 1987.)

oideus," the "coronary cistern," whose walls are the "tractus coronarius," the "accessory," "equatorial," and "petalliform" cisterns. Worst has also studied the premacular vitreous in great detail and has proposed the existence of a "bursa premacularis," which he described as a pear-shaped space that is connected to the cisternal system in front of the ciliary body, the "cisterna petalliformis." Whether this observation represents a true anatomic bursa or the result of the physiologic properties and organization of the molecular components in that region will be discussed below.

Vitreous biochemistry

Before the turn of the twentieth century it was already suspected that the vitreous is, to some extent, collagenous. Morner[403] found a protein residue that was retained by a filter after passage of fresh vitreous and termed it "residual protein." Both he and Young[639] considered the residue, also named "vitrosin," to be collagenous, since it dissolved when boiled and gelled on cooling. Much later Pirie et al.[436] documented the presence of collagen by chemical analy-

sis. Soon thereafter Matoltsky et al.[383] and Schwarz[494] described the ultrastructure of the vitreous as a random network of thin, uniform filaments. Using phase-contrast microscopy, Bembridge et al.[57] demonstrated the existence of fibrous filaments in the vitreous of several species including man. Both electron microscopy and x-ray diffraction studies confirmed the collagenous nature of the filaments.

Young and Williams[640] determined that "vitrosin" contained 18% glycine, 8.4% proline, 15.4% hydroxyproline, and small amounts of cysteine. Swann and Sotman,[555] among others, later ascertained the more specific chemical characteristics of vitreous collagen.

Balazs[30] and later Schwarz[495] described how collagen fibrils are organized within the vitreous, particularly in relation to other molecular components of the vitreous. Bettelheim and Balazs[64] then studied the scattering of laser beams in untreated, intact bovine vitreous and demonstrated an optical anisotropy. This was interpreted to result from variations in the density and orientation of the collagen fibril network.

It is only relatively recently that the presence of hyaluronic acid in the vitreous was recognized. Although hyaluronic acid is found throughout the body, it was from the bovine vitreous that Meyer and Palmer[397] first isolated this macromolecule. Consequently, hyaluronic acid's name is derived from the fact that it was first discovered in the clear, colorless vitreous ("hyalos," meaning glass) and that it contains uronic acid. Subsequent studies by Meyer,[396] Balazs,[30] Comper and Laurent,[125] and others characterized this macromolecule and its configuration within the vitreous.

STRUCTURE
Vitreous biochemistry
Collagen

Collagen is the major structural protein of the vitreous. Throughout the body collagen is composed of three individual polypeptides, known as alpha chains, organized in a triple helix configuration forming fibrils. Gross[244] initially claimed that the collagen fibrils of the vitreous were morphologically distinct from collagen in other connective tissues. Yet Swann[548] demonstrated that the amino acid composition of the insoluble residue of vitreous is similar to that of cartilage collagen, and he later determined that the composition is most similar to cartilage collagen composed of alpha 1 type II chains.[551] Comparisons of the arthritogenic and immunologic properties of collagens from bovine articular cartilage (type II) and vitreous showed that the two were indistinguishable by these assays.[544] However, subsequent studies[555] demonstrated that although vitreous collagen contained an alpha (II) chain similar to cartilage, there was a lower alanine content. Furthermore, these studies found that vitreous collagen had additional peptides that were present as uncleaved extension peptides containing an amino acid composition that was different from the alpha chain component. The investigators concluded, however, that the overall similarities of amino acid composition and the types of cyanogen bromide cleavage peptides indicate that the fibers of the central and posterior peripheral regions of the vitreous are composed of a collagen that should be classified as type II. Linsenmeyer et al.[365] measured in vivo synthesis of types I and II collagen in chick embryo vitreous by radioimmunoprecipitation after tritiated proline labeling and found that over 90% of the labeled material in the vitreous was type II collagen. Snowden[526] provided further physicochemical evidence in support of the similarities between vitreous and cartilage collagens.

There are, however, distinct differences in the chemical compositions of vitreous and cartilage collagens that are only partly due to the presence of terminal peptide constituents in vitreous collagen.[555] Swann[548] has demonstrated that the carbohydrate content of pepsin-solubilized vitreous alpha chains is significantly greater than cartilage alpha chains, indicating that the carbohydrate side chains of vitreous collagen are largely composed of disaccharide units similar to those found in basement membrane collagen. Swann proposed that these distinct chemical features are related to the special structure of the mature vitreous fibers in vivo. Liang and Chakrabarti[359] have shown that there are differences between bovine cartilage and vitreous with respect to collagen fibril growth, melting temperature, and fluorescence with a hydrophobic fluorescent probe (TNS). These investigators and others[596] proposed that vitreous collagen should be considered a "special" type II collagen. Schmut et al.[488] employed differential salt precipitation of pepsin-solubilized collagen from bovine vitreous and found that type II collagen is a major component of native vitreous fibers. Polyacrylamide gel electrophoresis showed a major alpha-1 chain and at least three minor alpha-chain components of slower electrophoretic mobility.

Gloor[230] has pointed out that the collagen content of the vitreous is highest where the vitreous is a gel (vitreous cortex and vitreous base). Recently, Ayad and Weiss[23] studied bovine vitreous collagen to determine whether the gel-like structure of vitreous could be explained on the basis of chemical composition. Their findings demonstrated that type II is the major vitreous collagen but that 1 alpha, 2 alpha, and 3 alpha collagens as well as C-PS disulfide-bonded collagen were present in concentrations similar to those in cartilage. In contrast to cartilage, however, the vitreous type II collagen was significantly more hydroxylated in the lysine and proline residues. The 1 alpha, 2 alpha, and 3 alpha collagens were interpreted by Van der Rest[589] to represent type IX collagen, although Eyre et al.[170] felt that these were actually evidence of type V collagen presence in the vitreous. Furthermore, with respect to the disulfide-bonded collagen, vitreous had three times more C-PS1 and C-PS2 collagens than cartilage, although the molar ratio of C-PS1:C-PS2 in both was 1:1, suggesting that in both tissues these collagens are components of a larger molecule. Subsequent studies[589] demonstrated that these disulfide-linked triple-helix fragments were actually derivatives of type IX collagen. In this regard vitreous is once again similar to cartilage insofar as both contain type IX collagen,[170] although the two tissues differ in terms of the sizes of type IX collagen chains.[631]

Hong and Davison[274] have identified a procollagen in the soluble fraction of rabbit vitreous that was identified as type II by segment-long-spacing banding patterns. Detection of a propeptide extension only at the N-terminus prompted these investigators to conclude that this was a novel type II procollagen.

Thus it appears that although vitreous collagen should be considered as a type II collagen, there are unique features that distinguish it from other collagens in the same class. These distinctive characteristics are possibly related to the unique physiologic roles of the vitreous, in particular mechanical functions.

Hyaluronic acid

Hyaluronic acid (HA) is one of many known glycosaminoglycans (GAGs). GAGs are polysaccharides composed of repeating disaccharide units, each consisting of hexosamine (usually N-acetyl glucosamine or N-acetyl galactosamine) glycosidically linked to either uronic (glucoronic or iduronic) acid or galactose. The nature of the predominant repeating unit is characteristic for each GAG and the relative amount, molecular size, and type of GAG are said to be tissue-specific.[576] A sulfated group is attached to oxygen or nitrogen in all GAGs except HA. GAGs do not normally occur in vivo as free polymers, but are covalently linked to a protein core, the ensemble called a proteoglycan. Balazs et al.[46] documented the presence of sulfated galactosamine-containing GAGs in bovine vitreous (less than 5% of total vitreous GAGs). Breen et al.[79] and Allen et al.[7] identified these as chondroitin-4-sulfate and under-sulfated heparan sulfate. Studies in the rabbit[314] found a total vitreous GAG content of 58 ng with 13% chondroitin sulfate and 0.5% heparan sulfate.

Hyaluronic acid (HA) is the major GAG present in the vitreous. In the human HA first appears after birth and is believed to be synthesized primarily by hyalocytes. Although the synthesis of HA seems to stabilize at a constant level in the adult (see Fig. 9-15), there does not appear to be any extracellular degradation.[285,556] Thus HA levels remain constant due to escape of HA molecules from the vitreous via the anterior segment of the eye[38] and because of re-uptake by hyalocytes. Laurent and Fraser[355] showed that the escape of hyaluronic acid from the vitreous to the anterior segment is strongly molecular-weight-dependent, indicating a diffusion-controlled process. In contrast, disappearance of HA from the anterior chamber is independent of molecular weight, suggesting that this is controlled by bulk flow.

Meyer and Palmer[397] first isolated HA from bovine vitreous. Meyer[396] and Balazs[30] later identified HA as a long, unbranched polymer of repeating disaccharide (glucuronic acid beta 1-3 N-acetylglucosamine) linked by beta 1-4 bonds. Swann[548] has reviewed the subject and defined the following criteria for the recognition of HA: characteristic electrophoretic mobility, typical infrared spectrum, absence of sulfate, susceptibility to cleavage by specific enzymes, presence of equimolar amounts of glucuronic acid and N-acetyl glucosamine, and high intrinsic viscosity after treatment with proteolytic enzymes. With these criteria, HA has the same primary chemical structure in all connective tissues and in this respect is unique among the macromolecules of connective tissues.[548] However, the values ascribed to the molecular weight of vitreous HA in different studies range widely depending upon analytic methodologies,[549] species variations, and age-related differences. Balazs[38] has stated that, in general, the sodium salt of HA has a molecular weight of 3 to 4.5×10^6 in all normal human and animal tissues investigated and in all parts of the vitreous.[429] Laurent and Granath[356] used gel chromatography and found the average molecular weight of rabbit vitreous to be 2 to 3×10^6 and of bovine vitreous to be 0.5 to 0.8×10^6. In these studies there were age-related differences in the bovine vitreous, where HA molecular weight varied from 3×10^6 in the newborn calf to 0.5×10^6 in old cattle. Furthermore, there may be several species of HA within the vitreous that have polysaccharide chains of different lengths.[354] Topographic studies[60] have identified five HA fractions in the cortical vitreous (intrinsic viscosities 420 to 1800 ml/gm) and seven HA fractions in the central vitreous (intrinsic viscosities 510 to 3320 ml/gm).

The volume of the unhydrated HA molecule is about 0.66 cc/gm, whereas the hydrated specific volume is 2000 to 3000 cc/gm.[38] Thus the degree of hydration (and any pathologic condition that alters hydration) can have a significant influence on the size and configuration of the molecular network in the vitreous. Because the solution domains are so large, the long unbranched HA chains form widely open coils, which at concentrations greater than 1 mg/cc become highly entangled.[125] The large domain of HA spreads the anionic charge of the molecule over a wide space. Due to its entanglement and immobilization in tissue, HA acts much like an ion-exchange resin in that an electrostatic interaction occurs between the small charges of mobile ions in the tissue and the electrostatic envelope of the stationary polyelectrolyte. This electrostatic interaction forms the basis for various properties of HA, including its influence upon osmotic pressure, ion transport and distribution, and electric potentials within the vitreous.[25]

Based on X-ray diffractograms, Atkins and Sheehan[19] described HA as a linear helix. Further studies[18] demonstrated a left-handed, threefold helix with a rise per disaccharide on the helix axis of 0.98 nm. As described in a detailed review by Chakrabarti and Park,[109] this periodicity can vary depending on whether the helix is in a "compressed" or "extended" configuration. The existence of the molecule in either of these two states can greatly influence an HA molecule's interactions with neighboring molecules. A compressed HA chain has extensive "interdigitations," since it interacts with its nearest antiparallel as well as parallel neighbors (totaling 8 molecules), whereas extended forms only interact with 3 antiparallel neighbors.[109] It is known that changes in the microenvironment and in the types of surrounding counterions can cause changes in the conformation of the HA polyanion.[125] For example, a decrease in ionic strength can cause the anionic charges on the polysaccharide backbone to repel one another and result in an extended configuration of the macromolecule. Thus changes in the ionic milieu surrounding vitreous HA may be converted to mechanical energy on extension or contraction of the HA macromolecule and, in turn, swelling or shrinkage of the vitreous. This can be important in certain pathologic conditions, such as diabetes mellitus. Early studies by Christiansson[116] showed that alloxan-induced experimental diabetes in rabbits resulted in an increase in glucosamine content and viscosity of vitreous and a decrease in vitreous volume. Recent studies[632] showed a slight increase in the tonicity of human diabetic vitreous (324 ± 23 mOsm vs. 316 ± 21 mOsm in controls). In diabetes mellitus there can be significant fluctuations in the systemic concentrations of a variety of molecules, which can alter the ionic milieu of the vitreous. Such shifts could induce structural (on a molecular level) and volumetric changes in the diabetic vitreous. Furthermore, shifts in systemic metabolism and in turn osmolarity and hydration of the vitreous could result in periodic swelling and contraction of the entire vitreous, with resultant traction upon structures attached to the vitreous cortex such as new blood vessels.

These events could influence the course of diabetic retinopathy by contributing to the proliferation of neovascular fronds[634] and perhaps even by inducing rupture of the new vessels and causing vitreous hemorrhage. Indeed, Tasman[565] has found that in 53 cases of vitreous hemorrhage due to proliferative diabetic retinopathy, 62.3% of bleeding episodes occurred between midnight and 6 A.M., while the remaining parts of the day had only an 11 to 13% incidence. Although the author speculated that this could be due to nocturnal hypoglycemia, other metabolic or hormonal fluctuations could be influencing the vitreous in the ways described above and lead to vitreous hemorrhage.

Another important property of HA is that of steric exclusion, a phenomenon first described by Ogston and Phelps.[415] HA, with its flexible linear chains and random coil conformation, occupies a large volume and resists the penetration of this volume by other molecules to a degree dependent upon their size and shape.[109] The excluded volume effect can influence equilibria between different conformational states of macromolecules and alter the compactness or extension of these molecules. Although there is evidence to suggest that steric exclusion by collagen is more important than HA,[125] the relative contribution by these two components to this activity in the vitreous is not known. Steric exclusion occurs on a molecular level and is an entropic phenomenon in that it does not directly produce heat effects between interactive components. Comper and Laurent[125] extensively reviewed the influence that steric exclusion can have upon chemical phenomena within the vitreous. Among the most important are effects upon osmotic pressure and enzyme activity.

Vitreous osmotic pressure was long ago determined by freezing point depression as $-0.55°$ to $-0.518°C$.[403] Steric exclusion causes an excess of osmotic pressure when such compounds as albumin and hyaluronic acid are mixed, since the resultant osmotic pressure is greater than the sum of the two components. This could be important in diabetes mellitus where vascular incompetence can increase vitreous levels of serum proteins such as albumin. Thus osmotic effects can induce contraction and expansion of the vitreous, which can in turn play an important role in neovascularization and vitreous hemorrhage. Enzyme reactions can be affected, since steric exclusion will alter the Michaelis-Menten constant as well as the inhibitor constant. An increase in the chemical activity of a compound due to steric exclusion can cause its precipitation if the solubility limit is reached. This could be important in the formation of pathologic vitreous opacities in such conditions as asteroid hyalosis and amyloidosis.

Collagen-HA interaction

The vitreous is composed of interpenetrating networks of HA molecules and collagen fibrils. The collagen fibrils provide a solid structure to the vitreous, which is "inflated" by the hydrophilic contribution of hyaluronic acid (HA). Comper and Laurent[125] found that if collagen is removed from the vitreous, the remaining HA forms a viscous solution; if HA is removed, the gel shrinks. There is substantial evidence to support the concept that there exists some sort of interaction between HA and collagen, and that the structure and function of these macromolecules is influenced by this interaction.

Studies have shown that throughout the body there is a striking correlation between the distribution of different types of interstitial collagen and the association of different GAGs, suggesting a specific interaction between these components.[310] In all extracellular matrices collagen-proteoglycan interaction determines the morphology of the matrix. The nature of this interaction is a function of collagen type and proteoglycan concentration. Type I collagen is associated with small amounts of proteoglycan and has a weak interaction with this proteoglycan, thus appearing as compact fibrils. The appearance is different in extracellular matrices with predominantly type II collagen, which is rich in proteoglycans and has strong collagen-proteoglycan interaction. Thus in such extracellular matrices the type II collagen fibrils are widely separated and the spaces between are filled with proteoglycan. It has been hypothesized that in cartilage the hydroxylysine amino acids of collagen mediate polysaccharide binding to the collagen chain via O-glycosidic linkages. Thus the number of hydroxylysine residues per alpha chain should be proportional to the amount of polysaccharide bound. This was substantiated by the finding that type II collagen, which in cartilage is found in a matrix with significant amounts of proteoglycan, contains 4 to 9 times more hydroxylysine than collagen types I and III.[310] Furthermore, these polar amino acids are present in clusters along the collagen molecule, explaining why proteoglycans attach to collagen with a periodic pattern (see Fig. 9-3). Studies by Hong and Davison[274] have identified a type II procollagen in the soluble fraction of rabbit vitreous and raised the question of a possible role for this molecule in mediating collagen-HA interaction.

Physiologic observations also suggest the existence of an important interaction between HA and collagen. Jackson[296] was the first to propose that proteoglycans had a "stabilizing effect" upon collagen. Gelman and Blackwell[220] and Gelman et al.[221] have shown that several glycosaminoglycans, including HA, stabilized the helical structure of collagen so that the melting temperature of collagen was increased from 38° to 46°C. Snowden[526] demonstrated that the shrinkage temperature of tendon collagen is linearly dependent upon the concentration of chondroitin sulfate in the surrounding fluid. Hyaluronidase decreased the thermal stability of cartilage collagen and the addition of chondroitin-6-sulfate to hyaluronidase-treated collagen in turn increased the thermal stability. The temperature-dependent denaturation of collagen was found to be very different for vitreous collagen as compared to cartilage. This confirmed the findings of Snowden and Swann,[528] who noted different shrinkage behaviors in vitreous and articular cartilage collagens. Snowden[526] concluded that a concentration-dependent stabilization of collagen by GAG would explain the difference in the shape of the denaturation-temperature profile for the two tissues, and that this stabilization was greater for cartilage than vitreous.

Measurements of the dynamic viscoelasticity of bovine vitreous showed that the shapes of the master relaxation curves of the vitreous are quite similar to those of lightly cross-linked polymer systems.[574] Notably, the behavior of these relaxation curves is different from that of solutions of hyaluronic acid and collagen. This suggests that the physicochemical properties of the vitreous in vivo are not simply the result of a combination of these two molecular elements, but that HA and collagen form a lightly cross-linked polymer system. Furthermore, these investigations suggest that the molecular weight at the cross-linking points is about 10^6. This corresponds closely to the molecular weight of hyaluronic acid and according to these investigators suggests that this molecule might serve as the cross-linking element in this polymer system.

HA-collagen interaction in the vitreous may be mediated by a third molecule. Swann et al.[554] have demonstrated large amounts of noncollagenous protein associated with collagen in the insoluble residue fraction of vitreous. In cartilage "link glycoproteins" have been identified that interact with proteoglycans[105] and HA.[256,260] Supramolecular complexes of these glycoproteins are believed to occupy the interfibrillar spaces. Asakura[17] has studied bovine vitreous by ruthenium red staining and demonstrated the presence of amorphous structures on collagen fibrils at 55 to 60 nm intervals along the fibrils that are believed to be HA (Fig. 9-3). There are filaments connecting the collagen fibrils and these amorphous masses. These filaments may represent "link" structures of either a glycoprotein or proteoglycans nature. HA is known to interact with link proteins[414] as well as an HA-binding glycoprotein, hyaluronectin.[148] Thus HA could bind to vitreous collagen fibrils via such linkage molecules.

Many investigators believe that HA-collagen interaction occurs on a physiocochemical rather than chemical level. Mathews[382] observed reversible formation of complexes of an electrostatic nature between solubilized collagen and various GAGs. Both the sulfate and carboxyl groups of a GAG could be the binding sites for cations.[109] Podrazky et al.[438] demonstrated that the sulfate group of a GAG was largely responsible for interactions with the guanidino groups of arginine and epsilon-amino groups of lysine in collagen. Comper and Laurent[125] proposed that electrostatic binding occurs in the vitreous between negatively charged polysaccharides and positively charged proteins. These authors extensively reviewed the existing data characterizing the electrostatic properties of GAG and the factors influencing their electrostatic interactions with different ions.

The phenomenon of steric exclusion within the vitreous probably also influences the interactions of HA and collagen. This is particularly important with respect to the effect that steric exclusion can have on the conformation and solubility of macromolecules such as collagen.[125] Studies by Meyer et al.[395] and Wiederhielm and Black[614] suggest that in this regard collagen is more important than HA.

It may well be that there are several types of collagen-HA interactions that are at play in different circumstances. Further investigation must be undertaken to identify the nature of HA-collagen interaction(s) in the vitreous. This question is important not only with respect to the normal physiology of vitreous and its structure but in understanding the mechanisms of vitreous liquefaction and posterior vitreous detachment.

Amino acids and proteins

Free amino acids are present in the vitreous but at levels about one-fifth that of plasma.[451] Within the vitreous there exists a concentration gradient with anterior vitreous amino acid concentrations being greater than posterior levels.[451] There are two possible explanations for this finding: either the retinal pigment epithelium is able to transport free amino acids out of the posterior vitreous across the retina, or the amino acids in the posterior vitreous are utilized by the neural retina[453] and cells of the posterior vitreous cortex (hyalocytes). This latter consideration has led Reddy[453] to propose that the vitreous can act as a metabolic repository for retinal protein metabolism. Such metabolism has been cited as the reason that vitreous levels of glutaminic acid are similar to plasma, a phenomenon attributed to the release of this substance by retinal metabolism.[436]

Early studies by Laurent et al.[357] and Cooper

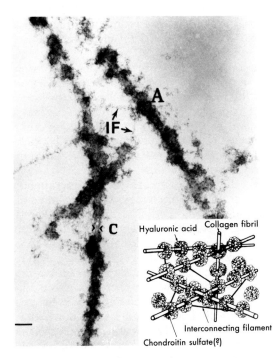

FIG. 9-3 Ultrastructure of hyaluronic acid/collagen interaction in the vitreous. Specimen was fixed in glutaraldehyde/paraformaldehyde and stained with ruthenium red. Collagen fibrils (C) are coated with amorphous material (A) believed to be hyaluronic acid. The amorphous material may connect to the collagen fibril via another glycosaminoglycans, possibly chondroitin sulfate (see inset). Interconnecting filaments (IF) appear to bridge between collagen fibrils, inserting or attaching at sites of hyaluronic acid adhesion to the collagen fibrils (Bar = 0.1 μm). (Courtesy Dr. Akiko Asakura.) (Reprinted with permission from Asakura A: Histochemistry of hyaluronic acid of the bovine vitreous body as studied by electon microscopy, Acta Soc Ophthalmol Jpn 89:179, 1985.)

et al.[128] demonstrated the existence of nine vitreous-specific proteins in the cow and six in the human vitreous. Swann and Caulfield[550] compared rabbit, sheep, and bovine vitreous and found marked differences in the amounts and types of proteins in the different species. Ishizaki[290] studied 68 fetal and adult human vitreous specimens by single radial immunodiffusion. He found relatively high concentrations of prealbumin as compared to plasma levels and noted that total protein concentrations in the fetus were greater than in the adult, especially in the case of albumin. Transferrin concentration was higher in the vitreous than aqueous, while alpha-acid glycoprotein was present in low concentrations in the vitreous. There were no topographical differences within the vitreous for any of the proteins studied.

Electrofocusing techniques have been employed by Chen and Chen,[113] who found that the soluble proteins of vitreous resemble the serum proteins of PI <6.0. The response to hyperoxygenation in dogs, aging in dogs and cows, and maturation from fetal to adult stages in the cow led these investigators to conclude that the soluble proteins of the vitreous derive from plasma and are constantly renewed. Beebe et al.[55] recently investigated vitreous protein concentrations in the developing chicken embryo and neonate. They found that the major portion of vitreous proteins in the embryo entered the vitreous by diffusion from the plasma. Vitreous levels were about 13% of plasma concentrations during days 6 to 15 of embryonic development. Following hatching, vitreous protein levels fell to 4% of plasma concentration. This was presumed to be due either to postnatal regulation of vascular permeability or dilution effects.

Swann[548] found that the protein concentration in human eyes ranged from 200 to 1400 μg/ ml (n = 21) with a tendency to higher values with increasing age. Studies of 920 human eyes[39,41] found the following age-related protein concentrations: ages 10 to 50 = 400 to 600 μg/ ml; ages 50 to 80 = 700 to 800 μg/ml; greater than 80 years of age = about 1000 μg/ml. These age-related findings may be due to increased leakage of plasma proteins from the intravascular compartment into the vitreous that results from increasing vascular incompetence with aging of the retinal and ciliary body vasculature.

Glycoproteins

Glycoproteins are macromolecules of the "ground substance" existing as heteropolysaccharides rather than homogeneous, repeating disaccharide units. They are mostly proteinaceous and contain only a minor carbohydrate

component (5 to 10% by weight). According to Balazs,[38] the most important difference between vitreous and serum proteins is the high content of glycoproteins in the vitreous, since these constitute 20% of the total non-collagenous protein content of the vitreous. There are two types of vitreous glycoproteins: those found associated with collagen fibrils and those that freely diffuse in the interfibrillar space.[31] For example, 0.3% of sialic acid in the vitreous is associated with collagen fibrils while the remainder is present as soluble vitreous glycoprotein.[45] Although some of the soluble glycoproteins enter the vitreous from serum, many are believed to be specific to the vitreous.[63] Sialic acid-containing glycoproteins constitute a much larger fraction of the soluble proteins of the vitreous than serum and aqueous.[298] The concentration of sialic acid in the vitreous is highest in the cortical layer anterior to the retina and lowest in the anterior vitreous adjacent to the lens and ciliary body.[45] This suggests that hyalocytes synthesize sialic acid-containing glycoproteins.[298] Other studies[249] in the rabbit have led to the consideration that the inner layer of the ciliary epithelium is responsible for vitreous glycoprotein synthesis. This was based upon immunohistochemical localization of a disulfide-bonded 550-KDa cartilage matrix glycoprotein with 116-KDa subunits in the ciliary epithelium.

Rhodes et al.[465] studied the incorporation of tritiated fucose into rabbit vitreous and surrounding tissues. They concluded that there is continuous renewal of the glycoproteins in and around the vitreous and suggest that this process could serve as an index of metabolic activity in normal and pathologic states. In subsequent studies Rhodes[463] showed that the binding of a horseradish peroxidase-conjugated lectin specific for fucose had the same distribution pattern as that seen in the labeled-fucose study. Using this lectin in humans, Rhodes found heavy staining at the vitreous base, zonules, and vitreous cortex (anterior and posterior). He concluded that fucosyl glycoproteins were present at these sites. Hageman and Johnson[250,251] documented the morphologic distribution of vitreous glycoproteins in several species, including human, and characterized these glycoproteins on the basis of differential staining to various FITC-conjugated lectins. There is currently no clear understanding as to the exact role of these macromolecules.

Low-molecular-weight substances

Table 9-1 lists the vitreous concentrations of low-molecular-weight substances and other molecules in bovine, rabbit, and human eyes.

TABLE 9-1 Chemical Composition of the Vitreous

Constituent	Cattle	Rabbits	Humans
Inorganic Constituents (mmol/kg H$_2$O)			
Sodium	130.5	133.9 to 152.2	137.0
Potassium	7.7	5.1 to 10.2	3.8
Calcium	3.9	1.5	—
Magnesium	0.8	—	—
Chloride	115.6	104.3	112.8
Phosphate	0.92 to 0.42	0.40	—
Sulfate	1.2	—	—
Bicarbonate	19.6 to 32.4 mEq/kg H$_2$O	19.6 to 32.4 mEq/kg H$_2$O	19.6 to 32.4 mEq/kg H$_2$O
Water and Organic Constituents (mg/100 ml H$_2$O)			
Water	99,000	99,000	99,000
Total nitrogen	22	13	23.5
Nonprotein nitrogen	10.4	18 to 25	
Amino acid nitrogen	3.0		
Peptide nitrogen	1.2		
Urea	14.2		
Uric acid	2.8		
Creatine	1.6		
Creatinine	1		
Total protein nitrogen	11.5		
Proteins	40 to 70		40
Lipids	0.6		
Glucose	55 to 62	55 to 80	30 to 70
Lactic acid	14.8	65	70
Pyruvic acid	1.2	5 to 6	7.3
Citrate	13.7	1.8	1.9
Ascorbate		8 to 15	

From Nordmann J: Biologie du corps vitre, Chapter III, Chimie, in Brini A, et al, eds: Biologie et chirurgie du corps vitré, Paris, Masson, 1968.

Since the vitreous is predominantly composed of water, it is of interest to consider the osmolarity of the vitreous and the various molecules and ions that influence this property. Molecules in this category are too small to be restricted by the usual blood-ocular barriers. Thus one would expect similar levels in the vitreous, cerebrospinal fluid, and aqueous. However, this is not the case. Human vitreous osmolality has been measured postmortem[545] and ranged from 288 to 323 mOsm/kg, which was slightly higher than serum (275 to 295 mOsm/kg) and cerebrospinal fluid (269 to 304 mOsm/kg). The possible underlying causes will be considered individually for each substance discussed below.

Sodium. Reddy and Kinsey[450] found that plasma sodium concentration is greater than aqueous, which is in turn greater than vitreous. The highest vitreous concentration of sodium is found anteriorly, with distinct topographical variations, suggesting that there is no "mixing"

between the different parts of the vitreous.[328] More recent studies in humans[557] found a closer correlation between vitreous and plasma levels of sodium immediately after death. With increasing postmortem time, however, vitreous sodium levels decreased.

Potassium. The concentration gradient between vitreous and plasma potassium is half the gradient between vitreous and aqueous, suggesting that there exists active transport of potassium from the ciliary body into the posterior chamber and anterior vitreous.[450] The lens may also contribute to the high vitreous levels of potassium by active accumulation in the anterior vitreous cortex in conjunction with passive diffusion from the posterior surface of the lens.[68] Vitreous potassium levels have been used in forensic medicine to determine the time elapsed since death.[186,535]

Chloride. Vitreous concentrations of chloride are greater than in the posterior chamber, anterior chamber, or plasma, since much exchange occurs across the retina.[450] In comparison to sodium, chloride exchange is more rapid.[328]

Calcium. Vitreous levels are equal to aqueous and plasma. It is important to include this substance, as well as magnesium, at physiologic concentrations when perfusing the vitreous cavity during vitrectomy surgery so as to maintain the integrity of intercellular tight junctions in surrounding tissues.[159]

Phosphate. Posterior vitreous concentration of phosphate is lower than anterior vitreous, which is in turn lower than aqueous concentration, suggesting that this substance is pumped from the posterior chamber into the anterior vitreous.[431] However, the overall level of vitreous phosphates is very low, primarily due to utilization by the retina.[139] Experimental induction of retinal degeneration is associated with an increase in vitreous levels of phosphate.[151]

Bicarbonate. Posterior vitreous concentration is lower than anterior vitreous, which is in turn lower than aqueous concentration,[143] suggesting an origin from the ciliary body. Disruption of retinal metabolism increases vitreous bicarbonate content.[20] Conversely, the lack of bicarbonate in infusion solutions used during vitrectomy surgery has adverse effects upon retinal electrophysiology.[273]

Miscellaneous compounds

Ascorbic acid. High-performance liquid chromatography measurements of vitreous ascorbic acid concentration recently showed values of about 0.43 mmol/kg,[391] confirming earlier findings.[211,450] The vitreous to plasma ratio for ascorbic acid is 9:1. Vitreous levels this much higher than plasma concentrations are believed to be due to active transport by the ciliary body epithelium.[211,327] Certain species, such as rats, are able to synthesize ascorbic acid in the liver, and circulating ascorbic acid enters the vitreous by passive diffusion.[152] However, in man, as in lower primates and guinea pigs, the liver is unable to synthesize ascorbic acid[92] and intraocular levels are dependent upon dietary ingestion and active transport by the ciliary epithelium.[152]

The purpose of having high concentrations of ascorbic acid in the vitreous may relate to the abilities of this compound to absorb ultraviolet light[467] and serve as a free-radical scavenger.[26] This would protect the retina and lens from the untoward effects of metabolic and light-induced singlet oxygen generation.[582] A recent study[421] showed that dietary supplementation with ascorbic acid reduced the irreversible type I form of light damage in dark-reared rats and shifted light damage to the type II form typical of cyclic-light-reared animals. Ascorbic acid may also protect against oxidative damage due to inflammation.[619] Studies[391] in a rabbit model found that endotoxin-induced ocular inflammation was associated with an increase in the concentration of ascorbic acid in the vitreous that was not derived from aqueous. This may be due to an increase in ascorbic acid synthesis in response to inflammatory mediators such as histamine.[111] Vitreous levels of serum-derived cerruloplasmin and transferrin also increase following experimental inflammation,[392] presumably to provide additional anti-oxidant protection.

Lactic acid. There is a high concentration of lactic acid in the posterior vitreous, presumably due to the high level of aerobic glucose metabolism by the neural retina.

Lipids. Swann et al.[554] found that the residual fraction of vitreous contained a significant quantity of lipids. Palmitic and stearic acids accounted for 6.9% W/W of the total residual fraction. Kim and Cotlier[326] demonstrated that the major fatty acid in the rabbit vitreous is palmitic acid. In their studies the distribution of phospholipids in the vitreous was similar to that in the lens and aqueous. In all these tissues phospholipid concentrations were lower than serum levels. These investigators concluded that there exists a blood-vitreous barrier restricting phospholipid transport into the eye. Reddy et al.[452] found evidence to suggest active lipid metabolism in the vitreous of dogs and humans. They also found that 55% of the acyl groups were unsaturated fatty acids. The major components were oleate (18:1) and arachidonate (20:4), with moderate amounts of linoleate (18:2) and docosahexaenoate (22:6). The major saturated fatty acids were palmitate (16:0) and stearate (18:0). Interestingly, these investigators found no significant changes in human vitreous lipid composition between the ages of 37 and 82 years.

Trace metals. Traces of strontium, barium, aluminum, molybdenum, manganese, iron, nickel, copper, zinc, and lead have been found in the vitreous.[230]

Species variations

The vitreous of all species is composed of essentially the same extracellular matrix elements organized to fill the center of the eye with a clear viscous substance surrounded by a dense cortex that is attached to the basal laminae of surrounding cells. There are, however, species variations in the relative concentrations of the major structural components of the vitreous, i.e., hyaluronic acid (HA) and collagen. These differences account for variations in the rheologic (gel-liquid) state of the vitreous in different species. These chemical and rheologic differences are summarized in Table 9-2 and discussed individually below. It should be emphasized that in more advanced species there are also age-related differences. Consequently, the selection of an appropriate animal with which to model human disease for scientific investigation must take into consideration these species variations and age-related differences.

Glycosaminoglycans. Hyaluronic acid (HA) is present in the vitreous of all species studied except for fish. In these organisms the posterior and peripheral vitreous adjacent to the retina is in a gel state. The anterior and central vitreous is liquid. Since there is no anterior vitreous cortex, this liquid vitreous is continuous with the posterior and anterior chambers, thereby surrounding the lens. In place of HA, the fish vitreous contains icthyosan: a nonsulfated polysaccharide of large molecular size (2 to 4×10^6) that consists of a Na-hyaluronate and a chon-droitin chain held together by noncovalent bonds.[15] The posterior and peripheral gel vitreous consist of icthyosan V whose molar ratio of NaHA:chondroitin = 1:1, whereas the liquid vitreous consists of icthyosan A, with a molar ratio of NaHA:chondroitin = 2:1.

HA concentration in the human vitreous is about the same as in the rhesus monkey (about 192 $\mu g/ml$),[425] which is less than the concentrations determined by high-performance liquid chromatography in the owl monkey (291.8 $\pm$ 18.8 ng/ml) and bovine (469.9 $\pm$ 44.0 ng/ml) vitreous.[224] The molecular weight of HA in the rhesus monkey is $2.9 \pm 0.06 \times 10^6$, which is significantly less than in the human (4.6×10^6; $p < 0.001$).[150]

Collagen. Snowden and Swann[528] demonstrated that collagen fibrils in the rabbit vitreous measure 7 nm in diamter, while bovine and canine vitreous collagen fibrils are between 10 and 13 nm in diameter. Human vitreous collagen fibrils are 10 to 25 nm in diameter.[272,541]

Thermal stability of collagen was determined by viscosity measurements and showed that all species gave identical viscosity-temperature curves. Burke[87] studied rabbit vitreous collagen peptides obtained by pepsin extraction and

TABLE 9-2 Species Variation in Vitreous Rheology and Biochemistry

| Adult | Rheology | | Range of HA* concentration $\mu g/mL$ | Protein concen ($\mu g/mL$)† | | Collagen† (% of total protein) |
	Gel (% of total)	Liquid (% of total)		Insoluble	Soluble	
Human	80-40	20-60	100-400	—	280-1360	—
Rhesus monkey	60	40	100	—	113-139‡	—
Owl monkey	2	98	300-600 (liquid)	—	66-77‡	—
Cow	100	0	800-900 (gel)	91	684	90
Sheep	100	0	100-1070	81	384	69
Dog	100	0	40-60	113	144	88
Cat	100	0	20-50	—	—	—
Rabbit	100	0	20-40	198	385	40
Guinea pig	100	0	10-20	—	—	—
Chicken, turkey	37	63	15-30	—	—	—
Owl	40	60	20-40	—	—	—
Carp	40	60§	600-700‖	—	—	—
Tuna	40	60§	200-700‖	—	—	—
Shark	40	60§	200-300‖	—	—	—

*From Balazs EA: Functional anatomy of the vitreus, in Duane TD, Jaeger EA, eds: Biomedical foundation of ophthalmology, vol 1, Philadelphia, Harper & Row, 1984, Ch 17, p 14.
†From Swann DA: Chemistry and biology of the vitreous body, Int Rev Exp Pathol 22:1, 1980.
‡From Denlinger J, et al: Age-related changes in the vitreous and lens of Rhesus monkeys, Exp Eye Res 31:67, 1980.
§Including the viscoelastic liquid of the anterior chamber.
‖Ichthyosan, glucosamine- and galactosamine-containing glycosaminoglycan.

TABLE 9-3   Comparison of Chemical Values in Bovine and Porcine Serum and Vitreous

	Bovine (N = 120)		Porcine (N = 120)	
	Serum	Vitreous	Serum	Vitreous
Urea nitrogen (mg/dL)	12.6 ± 0.2*	10.3 ± 6.4	14.0 ± 9.2	12.3 ± 7.0
Creatinine (mg/dL)	1.3 ± 0.7	0.6 ± 0.3	2.1 ± 0.8	0.5 ± 0.2
Sodium (mEq/L)	145 ± 9	137 ± 9	151.6 ± 8	148 ± 9
Potassium (mEq/L)	6.3 ± 2.2	4.6 ± 1.6	7.5 ± 2.0	5.0 ± 1.6
Calcium (mg/dL)	9.9 ± 1.9	5.4 ± 2.5	11.2 ± 1.5	5.7 ± 2.2
Magnesium (mg/dL)	2.2 ± 0.7	2.3 ± 0.3	2.6 ± 0.6	2.6 ± 0.8
Chloride (mEq/L)	103 ± 14	120 ± 13.4	103 ± 8	118 ± 7
Phosphorus (mg/dL)	6.7 ± 2.6	1.0 ± 0.7	7.5 ± 2.0	0.7 ± 0.4

Adapted from McLaughlin PS, McLaughlin BG: Chemical analysis of bovine and porcine vitreous humors—correlation of normal values with serum chemical values and changes with time and temperature, Am J Vet Res 48:467, 1987, with permission of American Veterinary Research Association.
*All values are means ± SD.

found that when similar techniques are employed, the chemical and physical properties of rabbit vitreous collagen resemble those of bovine vitreous collagen.

In the pig both collagen and HA are found in half the concentration as in man. Weber et al.[608] believed that this difference explains the different mechanical properties between pig and human vitreous. They found that the spring constant in humans was 60% greater than in pigs, while the friction constant was 25% greater.

In the baby owl monkey the vitreous is a gel with a collagen-like network of fibrils that have a diameter of 11.3 nm.[283] In the adult owl monkey, however, all collagen disappears and the vitreous is a viscous fluid that contains mostly high-molecular-weight HA.[108]

Protein. Monkey vitreous contains lower levels of soluble proteins than human. However, rhesus monkey concentrations (126 ± 13 μg/ml) were greater than owl monkey (71 ± 5 μg/ml).[150] Other studies[548,549] showed that rabbit vitreous contains a large amount of noncollagenous protein (60% of total protein), whereas bovine and canine vitreous have relatively small amounts (10% and 12% of total protein, respectively). Snowden and Swann[528] suggested that the smaller collagen fibril diameter in the rabbit vitreous may be the result of an abundance of noncollagenous protein in the insoluble fraction.

Glycoproteins. Rhodes[464] found that rabbit eyes had heavier staining for fucosyl glycoproteins in the vitreous base and vitreous cortices (anterior and posterior) than rodent eyes.

Lipids. Rabbits contain a much higher vitreous concentration of lipids (56 μg/ml) than sheep (14 μg/ml), young bovine vitreous (8 μg/ml), human and adult bovine (2 μg/ml), and canine vitreous (1 μg/ml).

Miscellaneous. Table 9-3 contains the findings of chemical analyses in the serum and vitreous of cattle and swine, determined by McLaughlin and McLaughlin.[393]

Vitreous morphology
Organization and distribution of molecular components

Collagen and hyaluronic acid are the major structural components of the vitreous. In man collagen is organized as thin fibrils 10 to 25 nm in diameter with cross-striations. Snowden and Swann[528] identified a major period in the cross-striations of 62 nm (unfixed, dried bovine vitreous), while others[206,272,541] describe a banding pattern with a periodicity of 12 to 25 nm. Vitreous collagen fibrils appear to be continuous and unbroken from the anterior peripheral vitreous to the posterior vitreous. If retinal Müller cells are primarily responsible for vitreous collagen synthesis, assembly of procollagen molecules into newly synthesized collagen can be achieved by adding to existing fibrils at their most posterior end, nearest the Müller cell. Alternatively, if fibroblasts are responsible for vitreous collagen synthesis and assembly into fibrils, the orientation of these fibrils could be the consequence of high fibroblast concentrations at the vitreous base and posterior vitreous. The continuity of these fibrils and their course through the vitreous could result from fibroblasts moving through the vitreous, which while migrating to these locations in the anterior and posterior vitreous assemble collagen fibrils in their wake.[67,635]

The distance between collagen fibrils in the rabbit vitreous has been studied by freeze-cleavage replica techniques.[430] The interfibril distance was found to be 1.2 to 3.5 μm, which approximated estimates for the bovine vitreous[30] and measurements in the albino rat.[255] Vitreous collagen fibrils are unbranched[29,35] and in the normal state are not cross-linked.[34] This is supported by studies of the mechanical properties of vitreous[608] that demonstrate a softening of the spring constant with increased elongation, suggesting that vitreous collagen is organized in a network in which fibrils can slip alongside each other.

There is heterogeneity in the distribution of collagen throughout the vitreous. Chemical[29,43] and light-scattering studies[64] have shown that the highest density of collagen fibrils is present in the vitreous base, followed by the posterior vitreous cortex anterior to the retina and then the anterior vitreous cortex behind the posterior chamber and lens. The lowest density is found in the central vitreous and adjacent to the anterior cortical gel.

Hyaluronic acid (HA) molecules have a different distribution than collagen. They are most abundant in the posterior cortical gel with a gradient of decreasing concentration as one moves centrally and anteriorly.[26,29,43,62,429] Balazs[38] has hypothesized that this is due to the fact that vitreous HA is synthesized by hyalocytes in the posterior vitreous cortex and cannot traverse the internal limiting lamina of the retina. HA leaves the vitreous to enter the posterior chamber via the annulus of anterior vitreous cortex that is not adjacent to a basal lamina. Bound water (nonfreezable) has a similar distribution within the vitreous to that of HA,[6] presumably due to binding by HA. Schwarz[495] has shown that after staining with ruthenium red, aggregates of precipitated HA molecules can be seen on electron microscopy as 8 nm granules situated in the interfibrillar space. Balazs[37] describes that HA molecules fill the spaces between the collagen fibrils and provide a "stabilizing effect" on the collagen network. In this regard there are two important functions provided by this molecular arrangement. First, the large domains of the HA molecules spread apart the collagen fibrils and minimize light scattering by these structures, thereby contributing to the transparency of the vitreous. Second, the viscoelastic properties and mechanical functions of the vitreous are the result of the presence of *both* HA and collagen and are very likely related to their association on a molecular level. Adjacent collagen fibrils would tend to cross-link and alter these properties. Consequently, the presence of HA molecules to spread apart the collagen fibrils "stabilizes" the viscoelasticity of the vitreous. Streeten[541] has claimed that large polymeric aggregates of HA "coat" the collagen fibrils (see Fig. 9-3) and that remnants can often be seen after routine staining for transmission electron microscopy. As described above, there may be physicochemical binding sites for HA along the collagen fibrils that could explain the finding of an intimate association between collagen fibrils and HA. Alterations in the interaction between these structural components with, for example, aging could influence the physical properties of the vitreous.

The topographical heterogeneity in the distribution and density of both collagen and HA molecules creates a heterogeneous bimolecular network. This inhomogeneity renders an optical anisotropy to the vitreous, which has been measured using laser light-scatting techniques.[64] The phenomenon of light scattering in the human vitreous has also been measured in vivo[643] and has been proposed as a noninvasive means to measure the viscoelastic properties of the vitreous.

Vitreous body

The vitreous of an emmetropic human eye is approximately 16.5 mm in axial length with a depression anteriorly just behind the lens (patellar fossa). Various structures and regions within the vitreous are named after the anatomists and histologists who first described them (Fig. 9-4). The hyaloideocapsular ligament (of Weiger) is the annular region 1 to 2 mm in width and 8 to 9 mm in diameter where the vitreous is attached to the posterior aspect of the lens. "Erggelet's"[169] or "Berger's"[93] space is at the center of the hyaloideocapsular ligament. Arising from this space and coursing posteriorly through the central vitreous is Cloquet's canal (Figs. 9-4 and 9-7,G), which is the former site of the hyaloid artery in the primary vitreous. The former lumen of the artery is an area devoid of vitreous collagen fibrils, surrounded by multi-fenestrated sheaths that were previously the basal laminae of the hyaloid artery wall.[72,253,294,295] Posteriorly, Cloquet's canal opens into a funnel-shaped region anterior to the optic disc known as the area of Martegiani.

In the laboratory, investigations of vitreous structure have long been hampered by the absence of easily recognized landmarks within the vitreous body. Consequently, removal of the

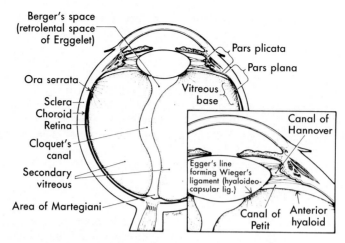

FIG. 9-4 Schematic diagram of vitreous anatomy according to classical anatomic/histologic studies. (Reprinted with permission from Schepens CL, Neetens A: Vitreous and vitreoretinal interface, New York, Springer-Verlag, 1987, p 20.)

vitreous from the eye results in a loss of orientation. The transparency of the vitreous renders observation in conventional diffuse light unrewarding. Attempts to study vitreous structure with opaque dyes do visualize the areas filled by dye but obscure the appearance of adjacent structures. The use of histologic contrast-enhancing techniques usually involves tissue-fixation, which often includes dehydration of the tissue. Since the vitreous is 98% water, dehydration induces profound alteration of the internal morphology. Consequently, any investigation of vitreous structure must overcome these difficulties.

Dissection of the outer layers of the eye (sclera, choroid, and retina) can be performed and the "naked" vitreous body can be maintained intact and attached to the anterior segment of the eye (Fig. 9-5,A). This enables study of internal vitreous morphology without a loss of intraocular orientation. However, depending upon the age of the individual and consequently the degree of vitreous liquefaction (see Fig. 9-18), the dissected vitreous will remain solid and intact (young individuals, Fig. 9-5,A) or will be flaccid and collapse. The latter is most often the case in specimens from older adults (see Fig. 9-20) and consequently vitreous turgescence must be maintained so as to avoid distortion of intravitreal structure. Immersion of a dissected vitreous specimen that is still attached to the anterior segment into a physiologic solution maintains vitreous turgescence and avoids structural distortion (Fig. 9-5,B).

The limitations induced by the transparency of the vitreous were overcome by Eisner,[160] who employed dark-field slit illumination of the vitreous body to achieve visualization of intravitreal morphology. Illumination with a slit-lamp beam directed into the vitreous from the side and visualization of the illuminated portion from above produces an optical horizontal section of the vitreous (Fig. 9-6). The thickness of this cross-section can be adjusted, as can the vertical position (level) of the cross-section. This enables visualization of any portion of the vitreous that is of interest. The illumination/observation angle of 90 degrees that is achieved using this technique maximizes the Tyndall effect and thus overcomes the limitations induced by vitreous transparency. Furthermore, the avoidance of any tissue fixation eliminates the introduction of many of the artefacts that flawed earlier investigations.

Recent studies[497,502,504,505] have utilized these techniques to study human vitreous structure. Within the adult human vitreous there are fine, parallel fibers coursing in an antero-posterior direction as shown in Figs. 9-7,B, 9-7,C, 9-8, and 9-11,A.[502,504,505] The fibers arise from the vitreous base (Figs. 9-7,H and 9-8), where they insert anterior and posterior to the ora serrata (Fig. 9-7,H). As the peripheral fibers course posteriorly they are circumferential with the vitreous cortex, while central fibers "undulate" in a configuration parallel with Cloquet's canal.[462] The fibers are continuous and do not branch. Posteriorly, these fibers insert into the vitreous cortex (Fig. 9-7,E and F).

Ultrastructural studies[505] have demonstrated that collagen fibrils are the only microscopic structures that could correspond to these fibers.

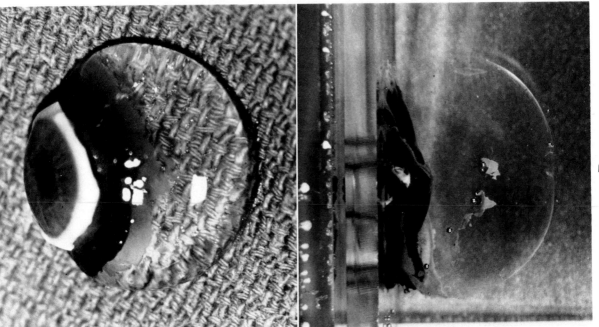

B

FIG. 9-5 Human vitreous dissection. **A,** Vitreous of a 9-month-old child. The sclera, choroid, and retina were dissected off the vitreous, which remains attached to the anterior segment. A band of gray tissue can be seen posterior to the ora serrata. This is peripheral retina that was firmly adherent to the posterior vitreous base and could not be dissected. The vitreous is solid and although situated on a surgical towel exposed to room air maintains its shape because at this age the vitreous is almost entirely gel. **B,** Human vitreous dissected of the sclera, choroid, and retina and still attached to the anterior segment. The specimen is mounted on a lucite frame using sutures through the limbus and is then immersed in a lucite chamber containing an isotonic, physiologic solution that maintains the turgescence of the vitreous and avoids collapse and artifactual distortion of vitreous structure. (Reprinted with permission from Sebag J, Balazs EA: Survey of Ophthalmology 28 (Suppl):493, 1984.)

FIG. 9-6 Schematic diagram of dark-field illumination system for the study of vitreous structure. The dissected specimen is mounted and immersed in a lucite chamber containing a physiologic solution (Fig. 9-5,*B*). A slit lamp beam is shone in from the side through the intact vitreous. The beam enters and exits laterally, avoiding any scattering of light by the structures of the anterior segment. The position of the beam can be raised or lowered and the thickness of the illuminated portion can be modified. Observation from above, perpendicular to the plane of illumination, achieves a 90-degree illumination/observation angle and thus maximizes the Tyndall effect.

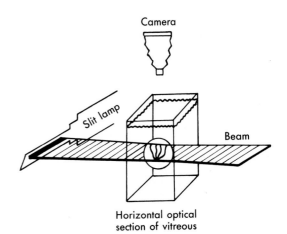

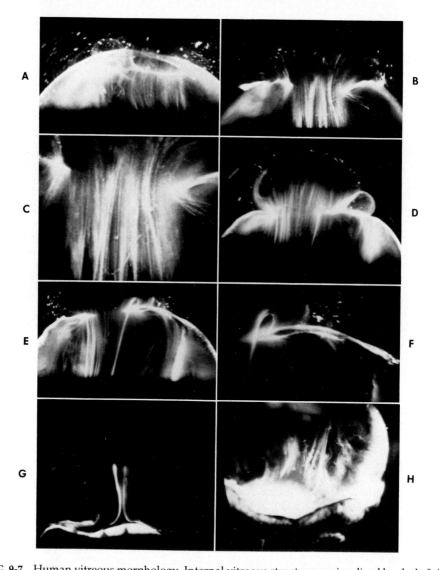

FIG. 9-7 Human vitreous morphology. Internal vitreous structure as visualized by dark-field slit illumination (Fig. 9-6). All photographs are oriented with the anterior segment below and the posterior pole above. Photographs are designated **A** to **H** sequentially beginning in the upper left-hand corner and moving left to right. (Figures **A, E** and **F** are reprinted with permission from Sebag J, Balazs EA: Survey of Ophthalmology 28 (Suppl):493, 1984. Figures **B** and **C** are reprinted with permission from Sebag J, Balazs EA: Morphology and ultrastructure of human vitreous fibers, Invest Ophthalmol Vis Sci 30:1867, 1989. All remaining figures are reprinted with permission from Sebag J: The vitreous—structure, function and pathobiology, New York, Springer-Verlag, 1989, p 41.) **A,** Posterior vitreous in the left eye of a 52-year-old male. The vitreous is enclosed by the vitreous cortex. There is a hole in the prepapillary (small, to the left) vitreous cortex. Vitreous fibers are oriented toward the premacular region. **B,** Posterior vitreous in a 57-year-old male. A large bundle of prominent fibers is seen coursing antero-posteriorly and entering the retrohyaloid space via the premacular vitreous cortex. **C,** Same as **B** at higher magnification. **D,** Posterior vitreous in the right eye of a 53-year-old female. There is posterior extrusion of vitreous out the prepapillary hole (to the right) and premacular (large extrusion to the left) vitreous cortex. Fibers course antero-posteriorly out into the retrohyaloid space. **E,** Horizontal optical section of the same specimen as **D** at a different level. A large fiber courses posteriorly from the central vitreous and inserts into the viterous cortex at the rim of the premacular hole in the vitreous cortex. **F,** Same view as **E** at higher magnification. The large fiber has a curvilinear appearance because of traction by the vitreous extruding into the retrohyaloid space (**D**). However, because of its attachment to the posterior vitreous cortex the fiber arcs back to its point of insertion. **G,** Anterior and central vitreous in a 33-year-old woman. The posterior aspect of the lens is seen below: Cloquet's canal is seen forming the retrolental space of Berger. **H,** Anterior and peripheral vitreous in a 57-year-old male. The specimen is tilted forward to enable visualization of the posterior aspect of the lens and the peripheral anterior vitreous. Behind and to the right of the lens there are fibers coursing antero-posteriorly that insert into the vitreous base. These fibers "splay out" to insert anterior and posterior to the ora serrata.

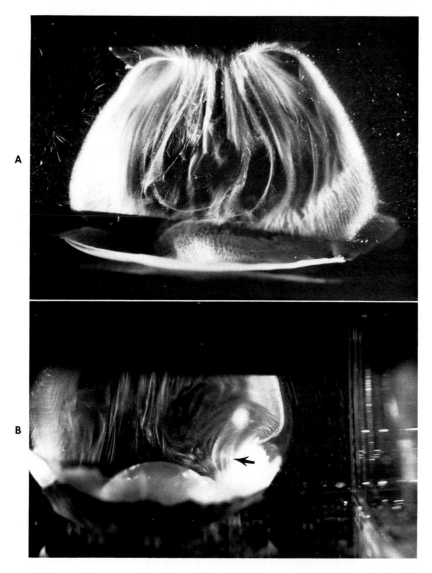

FIG. 9-8 Vitreous base morphology. **A,** Vitreous structure in a 58-year-old female. Fibers course antero-posteriorly in the central and peripheral vitreous. Posteriorly, fibers orient to the premacular region. Anteriorly, the fibers "splay out" to insert into the vitreous base. (Reprinted with permission from Sebag J, Balazs EA: Survey of Ophthalmology 28 (Suppl):493, 1984.) **B,** Central, anterior, and peripheral vitreous structure in a 76-year-old male. The posterior aspect of the lens is seen below. Fibers course antero-posteriorly in the central vitreous and insert at the vitreous base. The "anterior loop" configuration at the vitreous base is seen on the right side of the specimen *(arrow)*. (Reprinted with permission from Sebag J: The vitreous—structure, function and pathobiology, New York, Springer-Verlag, 1989, p 42.)

These studies also detected the presence of bundles of packed, parallel collagen fibrils (Fig. 9-9,*A*). It has been hypothesized that the visible vitreous fibers form when HA molecules no longer separate the microscopic collagen fibrils, resulting in the aggregation of collagen fibrils into bundles from which HA molecules are excluded. Eventually the aggregates of collagen fibrils attain sufficiently large proportions so as to be visualized in vitro (Figs. 9-7, 9-8 and 9-11,*A*) and clinically. The areas adjacent to these large fibers have a low density of randomly oriented collagen fibrils in association with HA molecules and therefore do not scatter light as intensely as the larger bundles of aggregated collagen fibrils. These adjacent "channels" (Fig. 9-9,*B*) probably

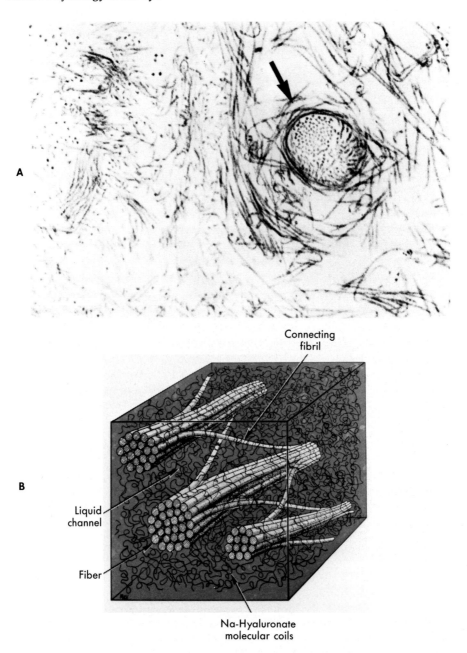

FIG. 9-9 Ultrastructure of human vitreous. **A**, Specimens were centrifuged to concentrate structural elements, but contained no membranes or membranous structures. Only collagen fibrils were detected. There were also bundles of parallel collagen fibrils such as the one shown here in cross-section (*arrow*). (Reprinted with permission from Sebag J, Balazs EA: Morphology and ultrastructure of human vitreous fibers, Invest Ophthalmol Vis Sci 30:1867, 1989.) **B**, Schematic diagram of vitreous ultrastructure, depicting the dissociation of HA molecules and collagen fibrils. The fibrils aggregate into bundles of packed parallel units. The HA molecules fill the spaces between the packed collagen fibrils and form "channels" of liquid vitreous. (Reprinted with permission from Sebag J, Balazs EA: Morphology and ultrastructure of human vitreous fibers, Invest Ophthalmol Vis Sci 30:1867, 1989.)

offer relatively little resistance to bulk flow through the vitreous and are the areas visualized in studies[308,309] using India ink to fill the channels. There are changes that occur in these fibrous structures throughout life.[497] These changes are probably the result of age-related biochemical alterations in the composition and organization of the molecular components that simultaneously result in vitreous liquefaction and fiber formation. A recent report[333] described the presence of a "posterior vitreous pocket" that the authors interpreted to represent an anatomic entity. However, over 95% of the eyes examined in this study were from individuals aged 65 years or older. Thus, these findings probably represent the result of age-related vitreous liquefaction in the precortical posterior vitreous.[500a]

Vitreous base

The vitreous base is a three-dimensional zone. It extends 1.5 to 2 mm anterior to the ora serrata, 1 to 3 mm posterior to the ora serrata[270] and several millimeters into the vitreous body itself.[456] The posterior extent of the posterior border of the vitreous base varies with age.[568] Vitreous fibers enter the vitreous base by splaying out (Fig. 9-8,A) to insert anterior and posterior to the ora serrata (Figs. 9-7 and 9-8). The most anterior fibers form the "anterior loop" of the vitreous base (Fig. 9-8,B), a structure that is important in the pathogenesis of anterior proliferative vitreoretinopathy. In the posterior portion of the vitreous base vitreous fibers are closer together than elsewhere. Gartner[218] has found that in humans the diameters of collagen fibrils in the vitreous base range from 10.8 to 12.4 nm, with a major period of cross-striations of 50 to 54 nm. Hogan[270] demonstrated that just posterior to the ora serrata heavy bundles of vitreous fibrils attach to the basal laminae of retinal glial cells. Studies by Gloor and Daicker[232] showed that cords of vitreous collagen insert into gaps between the neuroglia of the peripheral retina. They likened this structure to "Velcro" and proposed that this would explain the strong vitreoretinal adhesion at this site. In the anterior vitreous base fibrils interdigitate with a reticular complex of fibrillar basement membrane material between the crevices of the nonpigmented ciliary epithelium.[217] The vitreous base also contains intact cells that are fibroblast-like anterior to the ora serrata and macrophage-like posteriorly.[217] Damaged cells in different stages of involution and fragments of basal laminae, presumed to be remnants of the embryonic hyaloid vascular system, are also present in the vitreous base.[217]

Vitreous cortex

The vitreous cortex is defined as the peripheral "shell" of the vitreous that courses forward and inward from the anterior vitreous base to form the anterior vitreous cortex, and posteriorly from the posterior border of the vitreous base to form the posterior vitreous cortex.

The anterior vitreous cortex, clinically referred to as the "anterior hyaloid face," begins about 1.5 mm anterior to the ora serrata. Fine and Tousimis[181] described that in this region the collagen fibrils are parallel to the surface of the cortex. Studies by Faulborn and Bowald[175] described dense packing of collagen fibrils in the anterior cortex with looser collagen fibril packing in the subjacent vitreous, giving the impression of lamellae. Rhodes[464] studied mouse vitreous and found that the anterior vitreous cortex varied in thickness from 800 to 2000 nm. He also found that there are connections between the loose fibrils in the anterior vitreous and the anterior vitreous cortex. Rhodes also claimed that there are multiple interconnections between the anterior vitreous cortex and a branching fibrillar network in the posterior chamber.

The posterior vitreous cortex is 100 to 110 μm thick[30,541] and consists of densely packed collagen fibrils[571] (Fig. 9-10). There is no vitreous cortex over the optic disc (Figs. 9-7,A and 9-11) and the cortex is thin over the macula due to rarefaction of the collagen fibrils.[541] The prepapillary hole in the vitreous cortex can sometimes be visualized clinically when the posterior vitreous is detached from the retina (Fig. 9-11,B). If peripapillary glial tissue is torn away during posterior vitreous detachment and remains attached to the vitreous cortex about the prepapillary hole, it is referred to as Vogt's or Weiss's ring. Vitreous can extrude through the prepapillary hole in the vitreous cortex (Fig. 9-7,A) but does so to a much lesser extent than through the premacular vitreous cortex (Figs. 9-7B,D and 9-11,A). Jaffe[303] has described how vitreous can extrude into the retrohyaloid space created following posterior vitreous detachment and has proposed that persistent attachment to the macula can produce traction and certain forms of maculopathy.[302] Although there are no direct connections between the posterior vitreous cortex and the retina, the posterior vitreous cortex is adherent to the internal limiting lamina of the retina, which is actually the basal lamina of retinal Müller cells. The exact nature of this adhesion between the posterior vitreous cortex and the internal limiting lamina is not known, but probably results from extracellular matrix molecules.[500b]

Hyalocytes. Reeser and Aaberg[456] consider

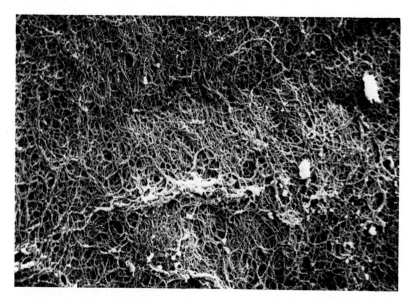

FIG. 9-10   Ultrastructure of human vitreous cortex. Scanning electron microscopy demonstrates the dense packing of collagen fibrils in the vitreous cortex. To some extent this arrangement is exaggerated by the dehydration that occurs during specimen preparation for scanning electron microscopy (magnification = 3750 ×).

the vitreous cortex to be the "metabolic center" of the vitreous because of the presence of hyalocytes (Figs. 9-11,*A*, 9-12 and 9-13). These cells were first described in 1840 by Hannover.[254] Doncan[156] first suggested that these cells were responsible for the synthesis of the vitreous. Schwalbe[491] placed these cells into the group of "Wanderzellen" (wandering cells, i.e., leukocytes or macrophages) on the basis of their morphology, distribution, and behavior. He later named them "subhyaloidale zellen".[492] Balazs[28] modified this term and named the cells "hyalocytes." These mononuclear cells are embedded in the vitreous cortex (Figs. 9-11,*A* and 9-13,*A*), widely spread apart in a single layer situated 20 to 50 μm from the internal limiting lamina of the retina posteriorly and the basal lamina of the ciliary epithelium at the pars plana and vitreous base. Quantitative studies of cell density in the bovine[47] and rabbit vitreous[228] fround the highest density of hyalocytes in the region of the vitreous base, followed by the posterior pole, with the lowest density at the equator. Hyalocytes are oval- or spindle-shaped, 10 to 15 μm in diameter, and contain a lobulated nucleus, a well-developed Golgi complex, smooth and rough endoplasmic reticula, many large PAS-positive lysosomal granules and phagosomes.[71,541] Hogan et al.[272] indicated that the posterior hyalocytes are flattened and spindle-shaped, whereas anterior hyalocytes are larger, rounder,

and at times star-shaped. Saga et al.[477] indicated that different ultrastructural features can be present in different individual cells of the hyalocyte population in an eye. Whether this relates to different origins for the different cells or different states of cell metabolism or activity is not clear.

Balazs[26] pointed out that hyalocytes are located in the region of highest hyaluronic acid concentration and suggested that these cells are responsible for vitreous hyaluronic acid synthesis.[28] In support of this hypothesis is the finding that the enzymes needed for hyaluronic acid synthesis are present within hyalocytes.[298] Osterlin[423] demonstrated that labeled intermediates destined to become incorporated into hyaluronic acid are taken up and internalized by hyalocytes. Several studies in vivo[423,424] and in vitro[46,61,284] have shown that hyalocytes synthesize large amounts of hyaluronic acid. Bleckmann[69] found that in contrast to in vivo metabolism, hyaluronic acid synthesis by hyalocytes grown in vitro is reduced in favor of sulfated polysaccharide synthesis. He suggested that when these cultured cells are reimplanted into the vitreous there must be a retransformation of hyalocyte GAG synthesis to the normal state, since vitreous clarity is maintained in these types of experimental conditions.[207]

Swann[548] claims that there is as yet no evidence that hyalocytes are responsible for the

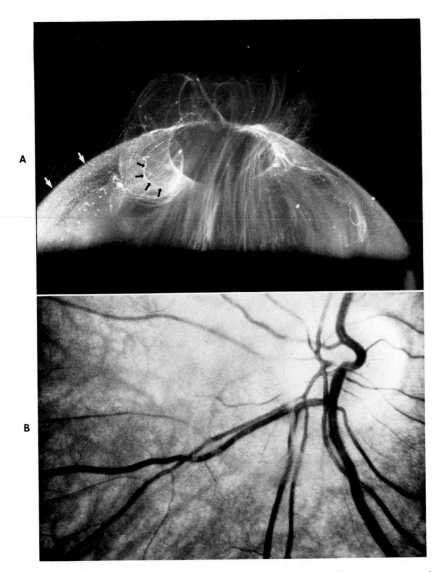

FIG. 9-11 **A**, Posterior vitreous in the left eye of a 59-year-old man. The vitreous cortex is the outer "shell" of the vitreous and contains multiple, small, highly refractile points that scatter light intensely (small white arrows, see Figs. 9-12 and 9-13). There are two locations in the posterior vitreous cortex through which vitreous extrudes into the retrohyaloid space. The prepapillary hole is to the left (black arrow), and has a small amount of extruding vitreous. Larger amounts of vitreous extrude via the premacular vitreous cortex and fibers course from the central vitreous into the retrohyaloid space. (Reprinted with permission from Sebag J, Balazs EA: Human vitreous fibres and vitreoretinal disease, Trans Ophthalmol Soc UK 104:123, 1985.) **B**, Fundus photograph (left eye). The posterior vitreous is detached and the prepapillary hole in the posterior vitreous cortex can be seen anterior to the optic disc (slightly below and to the left in this photograph).

synthesis of vitreous hyaluronic acid. There is, however, evidence to suggest that hyalocytes maintain ongoing synthesis and metabolism of glycoproteins within the vitreous. Rhodes et al.[465] have used autoradiography to demonstrate the active incorporation of fucose into rabbit vit-

reous glycoproteins. Recent studies[298] have demonstrated the presence of sialyl and galactosyl transferase activity in calf vitreous hyalocytes, suggesting that these cells are responsible for vitreous glycoprotein synthesis.

Hyalocyte capacity to synthesize collagen

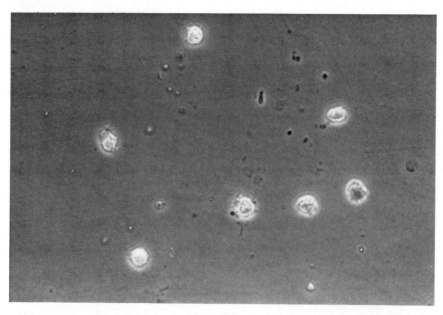

FIG. 9-12 Phase contrast microscopy of flat mount preparation of hyalocytes in the vitreous cortex from an 11-year-old girl obtained at autopsy. (Courtesy the New England Eye Bank, Boston, MA). No stains or dyes were used in this preparation. Round mononuclear cells are distributed in a single layer within the vitreous cortex. (Magnification × 290.)

was first demonstrated by Newsome et al.[411] Recent studies by Ayad and Weiss[23] showed the presence of C-PS1 and C-PS2 collagens adjacent to hyalocytes. These investigators concluded that in similar fashion to chondrocyte metabolism, hyalocytes synthesize these collagens. Hoffman et al.[269] also proposed that the distribution of high-molecular-weight substances in the vitreous, including enzymes, suggests synthesis by hyalocytes.

The phagocytic capacity of hyalocytes has been described in vivo[567] and demonstrated in vitro.[47,208,560] This activity is consistent with the presence of pinocytic vesicles and phagosomes[71,210] and the presence of surface receptors that bind IgG and complement.[238] Balazs[37] has proposed that in their resting state, hyalocytes synthesize matrix glycosaminoglycans and glycoproteins and that the cells internalize and reutilize these macromolecules via pinocytosis. They become phagocytic cells in response to inducting stimuli and inflammation. Interestingly, hyaluronic acid may have a regulatory effect upon hyalocyte phagocytic activity.[197,506] Saga et al.[477] have identified that different cells in the hyalocyte population can have different morphologic appearances, depending upon their activity at any given time.

Fibroblasts. There is a second population of cells in the vitreous cortex, which in some cases may be mistaken for hyalocytes. Several investigations[37,48,217] have determined that fibroblasts are present in the vitreous cortex. These cells constitute less than 10% of the total vitreous cell population and are localized within the vitreous base, adjacent to the optic disc and ciliary processes. It may be that these cells are involved in vitreous collagen synthesis, especially in pathologic situations. The argument for a role in normal vitreous collagen synthesis is mostly by analogy to studies of fibrillogenesis in tendon where investigations[67,635] have found that secreted collagen molecules are assembled into fibrils within invaginations of secreting fibroblasts. The locations of fibroblasts in the anterior peripheral vitreous (vitreous base and near the ciliary processes) and posterior vitreous may explain how vitreous fibers appear to be continuous structures spanning the distance between these locations.

Balazs et al.[48] have found that near the pars plana vitreous fibroblasts decrease in number with age. Gartner[218] has suggested that changes in these cells are responsible for aging changes in the collagen network of the vitreous base.

Basal laminae and vitreoretinal interface

The vitreous is situated adjacent to the retina posteriorly and behind the ciliary body and lens anteriorly. At all these sites the interface with

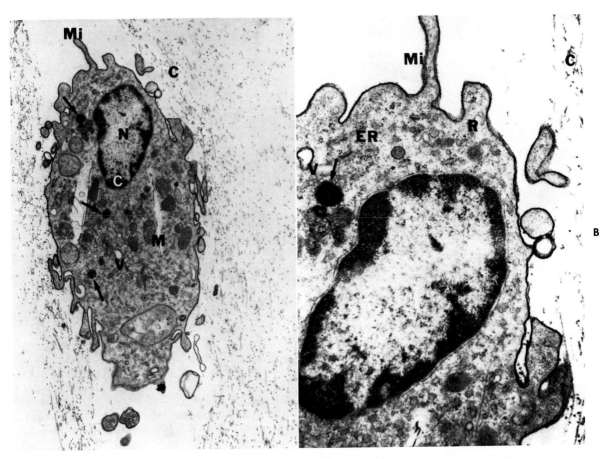

FIG. 9-13 Ultrastructure of human hyalocytes. **A,** A mononuclear cell is seen embedded within the dense collagen fibril (C) network of the vitreous cortex. There is a lobulated nucleus (N) with dense marginal chromatin (white C). In the cytoplasm there are mitochondria (M), dense granules (*arrows*), vacuoles (V), and microvilli (Mi). (Magnification × 11,670.) **B,** Higher magnification view (× 33,000) demonstrates dense granules (*arrows*), rough endoplasmic reticulum (ER), vacuoles (V), ribosomes (R), surface microvilli (Mi) and adjacent cortical collagen fibrils (C). (Photographs courtesy J.L. Craft and D.M. Albert, Harvard Medical School, Boston, MA.)

adjacent tissues consists of a complex formed by the vitreous cortex and the basal laminae of the adjacent cells. These basal laminae are firmly attached to their cells,[47,122,500b] and vitreous cortex collagen fibrils are reported to insert into the basal laminae.[181,214] The only region not adjacent to a basal lamina is the annulus of anterior vitreous cortex that is directly exposed to the zonules and the aqueous humor of the posterior chamber. Balazs[37] has pointed out the structural similarities between this zone and the surface of articular cartilage in joints that are exposed to synovial fluid. The significance of such an arrangement in the vitreous is not known, although it probably accounts for the ability of aqueous to enter the vitreous and the propensity

of various substances (red blood cells, hyaluronic acid, growth factors) to exit the vitreous anteriorly.

The basal laminae about the vitreous are composed of type IV collagen closely associated with glycoproteins.[324] Laminin has been found in the internal limiting lamina of the monkey retina but not of the rabbit.[235] At the ciliary body the basal lamina of the pars plicata is a meshwork of lamina densa that is 0.05 to 0.1 μm thick and is organized in a reticular, multilayered structure that is 2 to 6 μm thick and fills the spaces between the crevices of the ciliary epithelium. At the pars plana the basal lamina has a true lamina densa with insertions of vitreous collagen fibrils. The basal lamina posterior to the ora serrata is actually the basement membrane of retinal Müller cells, known as the internal limiting lamina (ILL) of the retina. Immediately adjacent to the Müller cell is a lamina rara 0.03 to 0.06 μm thick that demonstrates no species variations nor changes with topography or age. The lamina densa is thinnest at the fovea (0.01 to 0.02 μm) and disc (0.07 to 0.1 μm). It is thicker elsewhere in the posterior pole (0.5 to 3.2 μm) than at the equator or vitreous base.[8,189,583,633] The anterior surface of the ILL (vitreous side) is always smooth, while the posterior aspect is irregular, filling the spaces created by the irregular surface of the subjacent retinal glial cells.[8,474] This feature is most marked at the posterior pole, while in the periphery both the anterior and posterior aspects of the ILL are smooth. The significance, if any, of this topographic variation is not known.

At the rim of the optic nerve head the retinal ILL ceases, although the basement membrane continues as the "inner limiting membrane of Elschnig."[259] This membrane is 50 nm thick and is believed to be the basal lamina of the astroglia in the optic nerve head.[259] At the most central portion of the optic disc the membrane thins to 20 nm, follows the irregularities of the underlying cells of the optic nerve head, and is composed only of glycosaminoglycans and no collagen.[259] This structure is known as the "central meniscus of Kuhnt." Balazs[37] has stated that the Müller cell basal lamina prevents the passage of cells as well as molecules larger than 15 to 20 nm and proposed that the complex of the posterior vitreous cortex and ILL could act as a "molecular sieve." Consequently, the thinness and chemical composition of the central meniscus of Kuhnt and the membrane of Elschnig may account for, among other effects, the frequency with which abnormal cell proliferation arises from or near the optic nerve head.

Zimmerman and Straatsma[643] showed the existence of fine, fibrillar attachments between the posterior vitreous cortex and the ILL and claimed that this results in an extremely intimate union between normal vitreous and retina. The composition of these fibrillar structures is not known. The vitreous is known to be most firmly attached at the vitreous base, the disc and macula, and over retinal blood vessels. The posterior aspect (retinal side) of the ILL demonstrates irregular thickening the farther posteriorly one goes from the ora serrata.[189] So-called "attachment plaques" between the Müller cells and the ILL have been described in the basal and equatorial regions of the fundus but not in the posterior pole, except for the fovea.[189] It has been hypothesized that these develop in response to vitreous traction upon the retina. The thick ILL in the posterior pole dampens the effects of this traction except at the fovea, where the ILL is thin.[189] The thinness of the ILL and the purported presence of attachment plaques at the central macula could explain the predisposition of this region to changes induced by traction.[498,503]

There is an unusual vitreoretinal interface overlying retinal blood vessels. Kuwabara and Cogan[342] described "spider-like bodies" in the peripheral retina that coiled about blood vessels and connected with the ILL. Pedler[433] found that the ILL was thin over blood vessels and hypothesized that this was due to the absence of Müller cell inner processes. Wolter[625] noted the existence of pores in the ILL along blood vessels and found that vitreous strands inserted where the pores were located. Mutlu and Leopold[408] indicated that these strands extend through the ILL to branch and surround vessels in what they termed "vitreoretinovascular bands." Such structures would explain the strong adhesion between the vitreous and retinal blood vessels. This may provide a shock-absorbing function, dampening arterial pulsations during the cardiac cycle. However, pathologically, this structural arrangement could also account for the proliferative and hemorrhagic events associated with vitreous traction upon retinal blood vessels.

Zonules

Although it is arguable whether zonules are actually part of the vitreous, these structures have in the past been referred to as the "tertiary vitreous." Zonule fibers resemble vitreous collagen fibrils in that they have a diameter of 8 to 12 nm.[216,446] They differ from vitreous collagen fibrils in that they are tightly packed, resist collagenase,[446] and are solubilized by alpha-chymotrypsin.[50,561] Furthermore, zonules have an amino acid composition that more closely resembles elastin than collagen.[548,561] Streeten et al.[542] have used immunohistochemical techniques to show that zonules have structural similarity and perhaps identity with microfibrils of elastic tissue.

Zonules course through the posterior chamber from the crevices between the ciliary processes to insert onto the equatorial lens capsule in two bundles: the orbiculo-anterocapsular and orbiculo-posterocapsular fibers. Between them is the canal of Hannover and between the orbiculoposterocapsular bundle and the anterior vitreous cortex is the space (or canal) of Petit (see

Fig. 9-4). Kaczurowski[311] has described "vitreo-zonules," which he claims arise from the region of the ciliary body and enter the anterior vitreous cortex, where they terminate in non-branched fibrils. Whether these are actually the orbiculo-posterocapsular zonule fibers is not clear.

The two well-defined canals of the posterior chamber have recently gained importance as anatomic structures to be recognized clinically. This is due to an increase in the number of cases of rhegmatogenous retinal detachment treated by pneumatic retinopexy.[264,580] This procedure involves the injection of a gas into the vitreous by passing a needle through the pars plana. On occasion this gas is inadvertently injected into the posterior chamber and assumes the appearance of a "sausage" or "doughnut." This appearance probably results from the bubble being situated in one of the two perilenticular circumferential canals in the posterior chamber as a result of the needle entry being too far anterior or escape of the bubble anteriorly into the posterior chamber via a rent in the anterior vitreous cortex. In this location the bubble will move in a rotational direction with tilting of the head. Injection into the vitreous base, however, will be loculated and there will be no movement of the bubble with head tilting, even though the bubble may have a "sausage" or "doughnut" appearance.

VITREOUS DEVELOPMENT
Embryology

Vitreous embryogenesis can be considered from three interrelated, yet separable perspectives (Table 9-4). The first is the classical perspective of anatomists and histologists who described vitreous embryogenesis in terms of *structural* events. A second perspective concerns *cellular* development of the vitreous, in particular the origin and development of the resident cells of the adult vitreous (hyalocytes and fibroblasts). A third perspective considers vitreous embryogenesis from the standpoint of the major *molecular* constituents (collagen and hyaluronic acid) and their influence upon vitreous and ocular development. The following considers vitreous embryogenesis from each of these three perspectives.

Structural development

Primary vitreous. The first evidence of vitreous formation is present during the third to fourth week of gestation (4 to 5 mm stage), when the neural ectoderm becomes separated from the surface ectoderm.[376] The space that results is bridged by PAS-positive and Alcian blue-positive material. The PAS-positive structures are fibrillar processes that are in contact with the basal laminae of the two ectodermal tissues. These fibrils are believed to be collagenous in nature, consistent with their PAS-positivity. Posteriorly, they are continuous with the foot-plates of developing Müller cells.[530] The Alcian blue-positive material is most likely interfibrillar glycoprotein or glycosaminoglycans.[38]

At the 10 mm stage the optic vesicle becomes concave and mesodermal cells enter the vitreous space via the fetal fissure. These cells develop into the hyaloid artery with branches throughout the vitreous, known as the vasa hyaloidea propria. This posterior vascular network forms anastomoses with the tunica vasculosa lentis surrounding the lens. The fine structure of the hyaloid artery is characteristic of an arteriole with typical endothelial cell tight junctions,[36,295] while the vasa hyaloidea propria has the characteristic A-1-2 structure of capillaries.[295] In the hyaloid artery the medial layer contains smooth muscle cells surrounded by a multilayered basal lamina.[48] There are no fenestrations and pericytes are found in the walls of these blood vessels.[295] In the adventitia surrounding these vessels there are mononuclear phagocytes and fibroblasts. The fibroblasts are reported to synthesize collagen similar to that found in the adult vitreous.[36] This cellular vitreous has been termed by many the "primary vitreous" and conceptually can be thought of as an extension of the hyaloid artery adventitia.[48]

Closure of the optic fissure begins during the fifth week of gestation (8 to 10 mm stage). Fusion of the anterior portion of the optic fissure closes the optic cup by the 10 to 12 mm stage. Abnormal closure of the optic fissure results in the various colobomata seen later in life. At the point of final closure of the optic fissure, the eye becomes a closed system and pressure is exerted by the burgeoning structures within the optic cup. Vitreous development may contribute to this pressure rise and may thereby play a significant role in determining the ultimate size of the developing eye. Growth of the eye must occur to exact specifications, since the various ocular tissues must bear precise geometric relations to one another if effective optic and photoreceptive functions are to be possible. As summarized by Curtin,[137] there is strong support for the concept that the retina organizes ocular growth. Although growth factors probably play a mediating role, there is evidence to suggest that the retina induces various effects on growth of the

TABLE 9-4   Human Vitreous Embryogenesis

| Embryologic stage | | | | | |
Chronologic (wks)	Size (mm)	Structural development	Cellular development	Molecular development	Comment
3-4	4-5	Neural and surface ectoderms separate			
	10	Optic vesicle becomes concave	Mesodermal cells enter via fetal fissure		Progenitors of vasa hyaloidea propia
5	10-12	Optic fissure fuses, closing optic cup	Fibroblasts appear anterior to optic disc		
6	13	Lens capsule separates neural and sensory ectoderms			End of contribution by surface ectoderm
6		Secondary vitreous formation begins		Collagen synthesis begins posteriorly	Pushes primary vitreous anteriorly
7				Collagen (type II) differentiation begins	
7-9				Glycosaminoglycans synthesis begins	Synthesized by primary vitreous cells?
9	40	Hyaloid vascular systems attain maximum prominence			
10				Ascorbic acid = 0.3 mg/100mL	
	48	Marginal bundle of Druault identified			"Anterior loop" in adult
	65	Demarcation line between primary and secondary vitreous			Shaped like a "funnel" containing tunica vasculosa lentis, vasa hyaloidea propia and hyaloid artery

*Reprinted with permission from Sebag J: The vitreous—structure, function and pathobiology, New York, Springer-Verlag, 1989, pp 8-9.

TABLE 9-4 Human Vitreous Embryogenesis—cont'd

| Embryologic stage | | | | | |
Chronologic (wks)	Size (mm)	Structural development	Cellular development	Molecular development	Comment
12	70	Secondary vitreous prominent	Mononuclear cells migrate posteriorly		Progenitors of hyalocytes
	70-100	Zonule formation			
13-16				Decrease in GAG synthesis	Atrophy of adventitia of primary vitreous?
20			Hyalocytes developed and reside in posterior vitreous cortex		
20-36				Second wave of GAG synthesis	Hyalocyte-derived?
24				Ascorbic acid concen = 2 mg/ 100 mL	
28-32	240	Hyaloid artery blood flow ceases			

eye by influencing the development of the vitreous.

Following closure of the embryonic optic fissure at the 10 to 12 mm stage (end of fifth week), the vitreous becomes a closed compartment and the walls of the eye are brought under tension from within. Coulombre[131] demonstrated that at this point any increase in the size of the eye is dependent upon an increase in the size of the vitreous body. His studies of experimental models showed that when a drainage tube was inserted into the vitreous cavity intravitreal pressure dropped and the forces that normally act upon the developing eye wall were eliminated. As a consequence, the eye failed to increase in size. Subsequent studies[132] demonstrated that under these experimental conditions the retinal pigment epithelium (RPE) also did not continue to grow and the area occupied by the RPE was appropriate for the size of the eye. These investigators concluded that the growth of the eye and the RPE are dependent upon growth of the vitreous and the forces generated within the eye by the burgeoning vitreous. More recent studies[14] confirmed these findings by showing that vitrectomized rabbit eyes experienced less ocular growth than controls.

An alternative hypothesis for the control of eye growth was proposed by Porte et al.[439] who suggested that the volume of the embryonic eye is controlled by intraocular pressure that is influenced by fluid transport at the ciliary epithelium. More recent studies by Beebe et al.[55] seem to support this hypothesis.

The antero-posterior continuity between the neural and surface ectoderms persists until the sixth week of gestation (13 mm stage) when the bridging PAS-positive fibrils are interrupted anteriorly by the capsule of the developing lens, ending the contribution of the surface ectoderm to vitreous formation.

Secondary vitreous. Development of the so-called "secondary vitreous" spans the 13 to 70 mm stages. This acellular structure begins to appear at the end of the sixth week between the retina and the posterior blood vessels of the vasa hyaloidea propria. The secondary vitreous is in essence an extracellular matrix consisting primarily of type II collagen.[365,380,521] At this stage there are, as yet, no appreciable amounts of hyaluronic acid.[38] The secondary vitreous encroaches upon the vascular primary vitreous, pushing it forward and centrally. By the third month of gestation (65 mm stage) the junction of the primary and secondary vitreous is seen anteriorly as a demarcation line that extends laterally from the anterior portion of the central hyaloid artery over the posterior aspect of the lens.[36,376] The demarcation line between the primary and secondary vitreous extends posteriorly along the walls of the central hyaloid artery, the entirety forming a funnel-shaped structure. This central vitreous junction between the primary and secondary vitreous ultimately becomes the walls of Cloquet's canal. When all blood vessels have regressed, the anterior interface between the primary and secondary vitreous becomes the annular anterior vitreous cortex about the lens. Experiments in developing sheep have suggested that the retina is responsible for formation of the secondary vitreous. In these studies,[162] photocoagulation of the retina subsequently resulted in disturbed formation of the vitreous overlying the photocoagulated regions. These studies, however, did not address which cells synthesize the molecular elements needed for secondary vitreous formation and did not control for the differential effects upon various tissues in the path of incident laser energy.

At the 48 mm stage the marginal bundle of Druault can be identified at the edge of the optic cup anteriorly as a bundle of thicker fibrils of collagen that extend from the rim of the cup to the equator of the globe and also loop anteriorly to the mesoderm of the iris. Later in development this bundle atrophies anteriorly but persists around the ora serrata to form that part of the vitreous base known to vitreous surgeons as the "anterior loop" (see Fig. 9-8,B). The vitreous base also contains cell breakdown products and

fragments of basal lamina resulting from the transformation of the cellular primary vitreous to the acellular secondary vitreous.[217] This fact may be important in understanding the pathogenesis of peripheral anterior vitritis[500] commonly known as peripheral uveitis or pars planitis.

The hyaloid vascular system attains its maximum prominence during the ninth week of gestation (40 mm stage). Atrophy of the vessels begins posteriorly with drop-out of the vasa hyaloidea propria, followed by the tunica vasculosa lentis. At the 240 mm stage (seventh month) blood flow in the hyaloid artery ceases.[294] Regression of the vessel itself begins with glycogen and lipid deposition in the endothelial cells and pericytes of the hyaloid vessels.[294] Endothelial cell processes then fill the lumen and macrophages form a plug that occludes the vessel. The cells in the vessel wall then undergo necrosis and are phagocytized by mononuclear phagocytes.[36] Gloor[227] claims that macrophages are not involved in vessel regression within the embryonic vitreous but that autolytic vacuoles form in the cells of the vessel walls, perhaps in response to hyperoxia.[230]

The sequence of cell disappearance from the primary vitreous begins with endothelial and smooth muscle cells of the vessel walls, followed by adventitial fibroblasts and lastly by phagocytes.[48] Toole and Trelstad[578] point out that the vitreous differs from other connective tissues in that after regression of the hyaloid artery system and atrophy of the cellular primary vitreous there is no replacement by a second generation of cells, such as occurs in remodeling of the cornea and other connective tissues. Teleologically, this seems necessary to minimize light scattering and achieve media transparency.

It is not known what stimulates regression of the hyaloid vascular system, but studies have identified a protein native to the vitreous that inhibits angiogenesis in various experimental models.[300,369,447] Activation of this protein and its effect upon the primary vitreous may be responsible for the regression of the embryonic hyaloid vascular system as well as the inhibition of pathologic neovascularization in the adult.

The structural remnants of the transition from the primary to secondary vitreous were first described by the early anatomists and many structures bear their names (see Fig. 9-4). Anteriorly, the demarcation line between the primary and secondary vitreous is known as the capsula peri-lenticularis. The space formed by the "splaying out" of Cloquet's canal behind the lens is the previous site of anastomosis between the hyaloid artery and the tunica vasculosa lentis (see Fig. 9-7,G). It is known as Berger's space according to Busacca[93] or the retrolental space of Erggelet, according to Erggelet.[169] A variety of anomalies are due to improper transition from the primary to the secondary vitreous stages.

Anomalies of hyaloid vessel regression. Regression of the hyaloid artery and embryonic vascular system of the vitreous (vasa hyaloidea propria) and lens (tunica vasculosa lentis) usually occurs completely and without complications. Persistence of the hyaloid vascular system occurs in 3% of full-term infants but in 95% of premature infants,[307] and can be associated with prepapillary hemorrhage.[146] Anomalies involving inadequate regression of the embryonic hyaloid vascular system occur in more than 90% of infants born earlier than 36 weeks of gestation and in over 95% of infants weighing less than 5 pounds at birth.[460]

Mittendorf's dot is a remnant of the anterior fetal vascular system located at the site of anastomosis between the hyaloid artery and the tunica vasculosa lentis. It is usually found inferonasal to the posterior pole of the lens and is not associated with any known dysfunction.

Bergmeister's papilla is the occluded remnant of the posterior portion of the hyaloid artery with associated glial tissue. It appears as a gray, linear structure anterior to the optic disc and adjacent retina and does not cause any known functional disorders. Exaggerated forms can present as prepapillary veils.

Vitreous cysts are generally benign lesions that are found in eyes with abnormal regression of the anterior[367] or posterior[534] hyaloid vascular system; otherwise normal eyes[86,179]; and eyes with coexisting ocular disease such as retinitis pigmentosa[434] and uveitis.[81] Some vitreous cysts contain remnants of the hyaloid vascular system,[205] supporting the concept that the cysts result from abnormal regression of these embryonic vessels.[157] However, one histologic analysis of aspirated material from a vitreous cyst purported to reveal that the cells originated from the retinal pigment epithelium.[420] These cysts are generally not symptomatic and thus do not require surgical intervention. However, argon laser photocoagulation has been employed and a recent report[475] described the use of Nd:YAG laser therapy to rupture a free-floating posterior vitreous cyst.

Persistent hyperplastic primary vitreous (PHPV) was first described by Reese[455] as a congenital malformation of the anterior portion of the primary vitreous appearing as a plaque of retrolental fibrovascular connective tissue. This tissue is adherent to the posterior lens capsule and extends laterally to attach to the ciliary processes, which are elongated and displaced centrally. Although 90% of cases are unilateral, many of the fellow eyes in these cases have a Mittendorf dot or other anomaly of anterior vitreous development.[22] A persistent hyaloid artery, often still perfused with blood, arises from the posterior aspect of the retrolental plaque in the affected eye. In severe forms there is microphthalmos with anterior displacement of the lens-iris diaphragm, shallowing of the anterior chamber, and secondary glaucoma. PHPV is believed to arise from abnormal regression and hyperplasia of the primary vitreous.[455] Experimental data[74] suggest that the abnormality begins at the 17 mm stage of embryonic development (Table 9-4). Manschot[377] has claimed that there are associated neuroglial extensions from the retinal surface believed to be derived from Müller cells. Wolter and Flaherty[626] claimed that the hyperplastic features result from generalized hyperplasia of retinal astrocytes and a separate component of astroglial hyperplasia arising from the optic nerve head. The fibrous component of the PHPV membrane is presumably synthesized by these astrocytic and glial cells. A recent case report[3] with clinicopathologic correlation found that collagen fibrils in this fibrous tissue had diameters of 40 to 50 nm with a cross-striation periodicity of 65 nm. The investigators concluded that the collagen fibrils differed from those of the primary vitreous and suggested that they arose either from a different population of cells or were the result of abnormal metabolism by the same cells that normally synthesize vitreous collagen.

The retina is usually not involved in anterior PHPV. Indeed, Spitznas et al.[531] have suggested that the anterior form is due to a primary defect in lens development and that vitreous changes are all secondary. There are rare instances of posterior PHPV[377,444] where opaque connective tissue arises from Bergmeister's papilla and the persistent hyaloid vessels. These can cause congenital falciform folds of the retina and, if severe, can cause tentlike retinal folds leading on rare occasions to tractional and rhegmatogenous retinal detachment. Font et al.[187] have demonstrated the presence of adipose tissue, smooth muscle, and cartilage within the retrolental plaque and suggest that PHPV arises from metaplasia of the mesenchymal elements found in the primary vitreous.

Zonules. Previously referred to as the "tertiary vitreous," the zonules are in fact neither structurally nor biochemically part of the vitreous. The lens zonule of Zinn develops between the 70 and 100 mm stages. Investigations[229] with labeled amino acids (proline, glycine, methionine, and cysteine) suggest that zonules are synthesized by the ciliary epithelium. The developing zonular fibers course between the marginal bundle of Druault to span the space between the pars plana region and the equator of the lens in two distinct bundles of fibers: the orbiculo-anterocapsular and orbiculo-posterocapsular fibers. Formation of these two bundles of fibers defines a space between them known as the "canal of Hannover" (see Fig. 9-4). Between the orbiculo-posterocapsular fibers and the compacted primary vitreous (destined to be the anterior vitreous cortex) is the "space (or canal) of Petit" (see Fig. 9-4).

Cellular development

Several early investigators reported the appearance of cells in the embryonic vitreous of mammals. Virchow[593] believed that these cells were derived from mesoderm. Henle[262] proposed an ectodermal origin, while von Szilly[559] suggested that vitreous cells are derived from both germ layers. Various reports in the early literature[560,575] proposed that vitreous cells derived from blood, fibroblasts, retinal cells, connective tissue cells, and vasoformative cells.

The vitreous cells of greatest interest are the hyalocytes, for their metabolism may be important in the maintenance or dissolution of vitreoretinal adhesion and vitreous macromolecular composition, as well as fibroblasts, for they may play a role in various pathologic processes.

Hyalocytes. Hyalocytes are believed to be remnants of the cellular primary vitreous.[71,210] In the chick hyalocytes first appear on day 6 and migrate from the adventitia of the hyaloid artery to the preretinal vitreous cortex, where they are found on day 11.[48] It is at this time that PAS-positive granules are first seen within the cells and that the major site of vitreous glycosaminoglycans synthesis shifts from its previous origin in the retina to production by hyalocytes.[522] Balazs et al.[48] have shown that in the chick the number of hyalocytes increases between days 12 and 21 and that this is followed by the synthesis of macromolecules containing hyaluronic acid and hexosamine. After birth there is no new migration of cells to the vitreous cortex and, under normal circumstances, existing cells do not divide.[47] This means that with increasing globe size and vitreous cortex surface area there is a decrease in hyalocyte density. Balazs et al.[48] have studied the embryonic development of

cells within the vitreous of the hamster, mouse, rabbit, cat, cow, and man. In these studies hyalocytes first appeared as monocytes derived either from mesenchymal cells originating from the rim of the optic cup and the embryonic fissure or from blood elements in the vasa hyaloidea propia. The relative contribution of these two sources is not clear, and it may be that in early development the mesenchymal sources predominate, whereas later blood-derived monocytes are the major source. Balazs et al.[48] observed these monocytes undergo slow migration through the vitreous beginning at 26 days in the rabbit, 7½ weeks in the cat, 3½ months in the cow and 12 weeks (70 mm stage) in the human. The migrating cells come to rest in the cortical layer of the vitreous and are recognized as fully developed hyalocytes at the fifth month of gestation in man, 7½ months of gestation in the cow, and the first few postpartum days in the mouse, rabbit, and cat.

Gloor[227,231] takes issue with this hypothesis and states that hyalocytes are derived from blood monocytes that traverse the retinal blood vessel walls,[271] reside in the vitreous cortex where their half-life is less than one week, and are continually replaced throughout adult life by new blood-derived monocytes. Gloor furthermore contends that it is difficult to conceive how such cells could be responsible for the synthesis of the vitreous macromolecules that comprise vitreous structure. However, more recent studies[238] of human hyalocytes have found positive intracellular staining for nonspecific esterase and surface receptors for IgG and complement. The controversies pertaining to these questions await analysis using modern techniques of molecular biology for their resolution.

Fibroblasts. When the embryonic optic fissure closes and only a small opening is present at the optic disc to allow the mesenchymal cells and developing hyaloid artery to enter the vitreous, fibroblasts are found in the region anterior to the disc. These cells do not migrate and do not have the same cytoplasmic granules as hyalocytes.[48] Their physiologic role, if any, is not known, although the capacity of fibroblasts to synthesize collagen may be important. The role of these cells in pathologic cell proliferation and membrane formation within the vitreous and at the vitreoretinal interface may be considerable.

Molecular development

Collagen. Mann[376] described three potential sources for the embryonic synthesis of vitreous collagen: surface ectoderm, neural ectoderm, and mesoderm. Balazs[38] claimed that most of the gel-forming collagen fibrils synthesized during prenatal vitreous development are produced by the fibroblasts in the perivascular adventitia of the hyaloid artery system. Newsome et al.[411] showed that in the chick the neural retina is the chief source of the vitreous collagen during early development and that vitreous cells assume the responsibility for this synthesis during later development. Linsenmayer and Little[366] showed that the neural retina of the 6- to 7-day-old chick embryo synthesizes type II collagen. However, Burke and Kower[89] found that adult rabbit retinal astroglia synthesize type I collagen in vitro but no type II. Even when these cells were injected into the vitreous cavity they only synthesized type I collagen. Although this may be due to species differences, there is evidence to suggest that different collagen types are synthesized at different times during development. Akiya et al.[5] studied human embryos and found that the differentiation of vitreous collagen as type II begins at about 7 weeks of gestation. Their results suggest that during earlier embryonic development the human vitreous may contain only type I collagen. Interestingly, Balazs[38]

claims that there is no evidence that the vitreous collagen fibril network is actively synthesized in the normal adult vitreous, since following vitrectomy there is no regeneration of collagen fibrils. Thus the capacity of the retina to synthesize vitreous collagen during early development may be either lost or inhibited in later life.

Hyaluronic acid. In the embryos of many species vitreous polysaccharides consist primarily of galactosaminoglycans.[40,171] Hyaluronic acid (HA) synthesis does not begin until later in development. In the chick, Smith and Newsome[522] showed that chondroitin sulfates are the major early constituents. Recent histochemical studies suggest that there are two waves of polysaccharide synthesis in vitreous embryogenesis. During the seventh to ninth weeks of gestation in humans, Akiya et al.[3] found a material with strong positive staining to Alcian blue. This material was found to contain a mixture of hyaluronic acid and chondroitin sulfate or dermatan sulfate. By the twelfth to thirteenth weeks of gestation there was a marked decrease in this material. Saga[478] indicated that this Alcian blue-positive material was

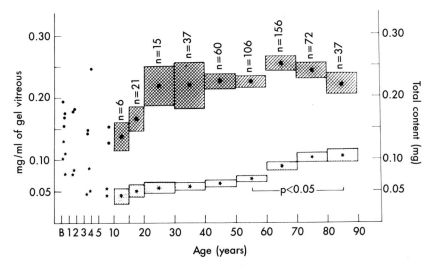

FIG. 9-14 Age-related changes in human vitreous collagen. Collagen content (mg; right ordinate) is indicated by solid dots (means) and darkly hatched boxes (height = standard error). Collagen concentration (mg/ml; left ordinate) is indicated by asterisks (means) and lightly hatched boxes (height = standard error). Vitreous collagen concentration decreases during the first decade of life, because there is no net synthesis of collagen during this period of active growth of the eye. There are no significant changes in collagen content following the age of 20, consistent with the long life span of this molecule. However, collagen concentration in the gel vitreous increases after the age of 40 to 50. This is due to the decrease in gel vitreous that occurs during this time (Fig. 9-18), concentrating the remaining collagen in an ever-decreasing volume of gel vitreous. The increase in gel vitreous collagen concentration between the ages of 50 to 60 and 80 to 90 is statistically significant ($p < 0.05$). (Reprinted with permision from Balazs EA, Denlinger JL: Aging changes in the vitreous, in Aging and human visual function, New York, Alan R Liss, 1982, pp 45–57.)

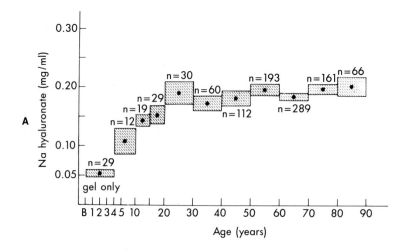

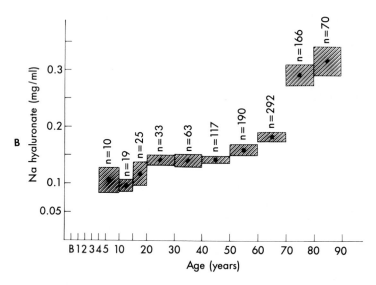

FIG. 9-15 Age-related changes in human vitreous hyaluronic acid (HA) concention. The dots represent the means of the samples. The vertical height of the boxes represents the standard error of the means. The horizontal width of the boxes represents the age ranges in the sample group. Between the ages of 5 and 10 the HA concentration is about the same (0.1 mg/ml) in both gel and liquid vitreous. (Reprinted with permission from Balazs EA, Denlinger JL: Aging changes in the vitreous, in Aging and human visual function, New York, Alan R Liss, 1982, pp 45–57.) **A**, HA concentration in the gel vitreous. There is a fourfold increase in the concentration of HA during the first two decades of life. Considering that this is also a period of active growth of the eye and substantial increase in vitreous volume, there must be prolific synthesis of HA to increase concentrations so dramatically. After the age of 20, HA concentrations in the gel vitreous are stable. Since this is a period of decreasing amounts of gel vitreous (Fig. 9-18), there must be a net decrease in the HA content of the gel to result in the absence of substantial changes in concentration. **B**, HA concentration in the liquid vitreous. There are no data for the first four years, since there is no liquid vitreous during this time. From the ages of 5 to 50 or 60 there is a 50% increase in the concentration of HA in the liquid vitreous. After this time, there is a substantial increase in liquid vitreous HA concentration. The magnitude of this accumulation of HA in the liquid component of the vitreous is even greater when one considers that this occurs during the time when the volume of liquid vitreous is increasing twofold (Fig. 9-18).

again found in 20- to 36-week-old fetuses. Bremer[80] has studied vitreous development in the mouse and has identified four stages on the basis of glycosaminoglycans (GAG) synthesis:

During the *first stage* (prenatal days 10 to 12) there is a high concentration of acid GAG in the entire vitreous. These are probably sulfated GAG, most likely chrondroitin A or C.[609] The *second stage* (prenatal days 13 to 16) features a marked decrease in the concentration of acid GAG in the posterior part of the vitreous and a concomitant slight increase in PAS positivity, probably relating to collagen synthesis. The acid GAG, which remain at the equatorial vitreous, are nonsulfated and probably represent hyaluronic acid. The decrease in acid GAG synthesis is believed to correspond to the same phenomenon of decreased GAG synthesis during the thirteenth to sixteenth week of human gestation,[3,478] since it occurs at similar developmental periods. The *third stage* of mouse vitreous embryogenesis begins at the seventeenth day of the prenatal period and extends to the first postpartum day. During this period a new surge of acid GAG synthesis occurs in the posterior vitreous. Sulfated GAGs (chondroitin A or C) reappear posteriorly while nonsulfated GAGs (HA) persist at the equator. It is during this stage that the hyaloid vessels begin to disappear. During the *fourth stage* (first two postnatal weeks) the nonsulfated GAGs disappear from the equatorial vitreous and are replaced by fibers composed of sulfated GAGs.

The cells responsible for GAG synthesis during development may also differ at different stages. Smith and Newsome[522] demonstrated that chondroitin sulfates are synthesized by the neural retina during early development but by days 10 to 11 there was a shift to production by cells in the vitreous, perhaps hyalocytes. Indeed GAG synthesis is believed to be one of the major functions of adult hyalocytes. In humans, however, this synthesis begins after birth and maximum levels of vitreous HA concentration are not achieved until adulthood.[38] A recent histochemical study[24] found that in the developing human, Müller cells produce hyaluronic acid transiently from 12 weeks gestation to the neonatal stage.

It would appear from these recent studies that the classical descriptions of vitreous morphogenesis do not adequately describe the underlying biochemical events occurring within the vitreous. Although the concept of a primary vascular and secondary avascular vitreous may have been useful to date, the future will probably see more precise subdivisions of vitreous embryogenesis based upon further understanding of more fundamental molecular events.

Other molecular components. *Glycoproteins* are found in high concentrations during early embryonic stages. Concentrations decrease toward the end of the prenatal period and level off at adult levels after birth.[43,45,171] Falbe-Hansen et al.[171] furthermore found an acidic glycoprotein that was present until the time when the primary vitreous was being replaced by the secondary vitreous. The existence of a gradient of glycoprotein concentration, with highest levels in the preretinal vitreous cortex and lowest levels anteriorly, suggests that these molecules originate either from hyalocytes or the neural retina. However, recent studies[249] suggest that in the rabbit vitreous glycoproteins are synthesized by the ciliary epithelium.

Ascorbic acid levels in the bovine embryonic vitreous are less than in the adult. A study[509] in humans found that ascorbic acid concentration increased gradually from 0.32 mg/100 ml at 10 weeks of gestation to 2 mg/100 ml at 24 weeks.

Calcium levels in the bovine vitreous are higher during embryogenesis and decrease to adult levels after birth.

Noncollagenous proteins in chick vitreous were found to be derived from the blood up to day 15, and then decline to levels of about 4% of plasma protein concentration at hatching.[55]

Development to the adult
Structural development

During childhood the vitreous undergoes significant growth. A study[348] of 926 children showed that, on average, the length of the newborn vitreous is 10.5 mm in the male and 10.2 mm in the female. By the age of 13 years the axial length of the vitreous increases to 16.1 mm (male) and 15.6 mm (female). Fledelius[184,185] used ultrasound to measure ocular dimensions in adolescent humans and found that in the absence of changes in refractive status growth from ages 10 to 18 resulted in a mean vitreous elongation of 0.35 mm. The emmetropic male adult vitreous is approximately 16.5 mm in length.[372]

Immediate postnatal development was recently studied[573] in the rhesus monkey. Axial length was found to increase most rapidly during the first 5 to 7 months, increase at a slower pace during the next 6 months, and continue to increase slowly until 4 years of age. This pattern is reported by Tigges et al.[573] to correspond closely to axial elongation in humans. Derangements in ocular growth that result in ametropia are associated with abnormal vitreous dimensions. In children born prematurely (birth weight less than 2000 gm), eye and vitreous axial lengths at age 10 are less than normal.[184] This deficiency is also present at age 18,[185] suggesting that prematurity does not simply induce a temporary delay of eye growth but a permanent deficit.

Myopia. In axial myopia progressive elongation of the globe can occur between the ages of 10 and 18 years. In cases where this introduces an additional 2.5 diopters or more of myopia, the vitreous undergoes a mean elongation of 1.44 mm.[185] Studies[381] in experimental models of this phenomenon have found that lid-suturing in the tree shrew induces 0.32 ± 0.17 mm axial elongation of the globe, attributed primarily to a 0.35 ± 0.19 mm elongation of the vitreous chamber. There are various hypotheses on the etiology of myopia,[638] but it is primarily the developmental theories that emphasize a causative role for the vitreous. During normal development, invagination of the optic vesicle, fusion of the optic fissure, and closure of the optic cup result in a closed system. At this point expansion of the developing eye is dependent upon the increase in intraocular pressure provided either by fluid transport at the ciliary epithelium[55] or by the developing vitreous.[131,132] Ultrasound studies[185] in humans would seem to support the concept that there is a primary role for vitreous development in inducing expansion of the globe. The application of the vitreous growth concept to the phenomenon of axial myopia is in essence the "ectodermal-mesodermal growth disparity theory of Vogt." This theory has been revised by Curtin,[137] who stated that excess formation of vitreous by the retina expands the sclera in a generalized fashion or focally (in the presence of a localized scleral abnormality or weakness), producing a posterior staphyloma. Other lines of investigation have formulated the concept that the vitreous mediates retinal control over growth of the eye. There have been several studies[237,598,610] of experimental models that used visual deprivation to induce axial myopia. The results of these investigations suggested that derangements in visual imagery influence retinal structure and metabolism, thereby altering vitreous development and affecting the ultimate size of the globe. Studies by Enoch and Birch[167] have demonstrated that alterations in visual input can affect photoreceptor anatomy. Other studies[602] demonstrated that local retinal factors mediate differential axial elongation. Furthermore, studies[291,361,539] have shown that on a biochemical level, form-deprivation myopia induces marked reductions in retinal dopamine and its metabolites. Stone et al.[539] also reported elevation in vasoactive intestinal polypeptide. Such altered neurochemical activity could influence retinal metabolism and the synthesis of vitreous constituents such as collagen,[365,412] thereby altering growth of the vitreous and in turn the eye. Interestingly, ganglion cell activity does not influence this phenomenon[616] and it is plausible that some other element(s) of the neural retina, possibly Müller cells, underlie these findings. The importance of vitreous growth in mediating growth changes in the eye assumes a greater degree of credibility when one considers that retinal Müller cells contribute to the formation of the secondary vitreous (see below) and induction of the internal growth forces of the eye. Indeed, collagen structure and synthesis may be important mediating factors in controlling vitreous volume and eye growth during embryogenesis particularly during "secondary vitreous" formation. Studies on experimental myopia have shown that axial elongation in experimental models results primarily from vitreous elongation.[381,387] Other studies in experimental models[381] have found that drugs such as beta amino proprionitrile and D-pennicillamine, which influence collagen synthesis and structure, result in a further increase in vitreous chamber size and axial myopia. The exact mechanisms of this phenomenon remain unclear. In addition to the role of collagen metabolism during embryogenesis and development, one must consider the possible role of hyaluronic acid metabolism during postnatal development.

Balazs[29,30] has demonstrated that vitreous volume can be influenced by changes in hyaluronic acid (HA) volume. Cationic dyes, detergents, ionizing radiation, and hyaluronidase all decrease the volume of the HA molecule (albeit by different mechanisms) and in turn reduce the volume of the vitreous gel.[38] The volume of the vitreous can be increased by chemically causing an expansion of the HA molecule, since this large non-cross-linked polyanion presses apart the network of collagen fibrils in the vitreous. The hydrophilic properties of HA attract and trap water, further expanding the collagen and HA networks within the vitreous. Thus the synthesis, molecular configuration, and hydration of HA molecules during postnatal development could also influence vitreous volume and secondarily affect growth of the eye to its ideal size. Interestingly, experimental surgical aphakia in monkeys[573] results in shortening of the axial length, regardless of whether eyes were optically corrected or not. It may be that in these circumstances the molecular alterations, especially in hyaluronic acid,[428,429] and structural effects[188] of cataract extraction upon the vitreous override the visual imagery effects and limit vitreous expansion and thus axial elongation.

Whether cause or effect, there are prominent changes within the vitreous in axial myopia and consequently a predisposition to vitreoretinal abnormalities. Rieger[466] and more recently Brandt and Leedhoff[78] found advanced vitreous "degeneration" in highly myopic children. Biomicroscopic observations by Hruby,[277] Pischel,[437] and Busacca et al.[95] established that the characteristic vitreous changes seen in old age appear much earlier in the myopic eye, especially in the high myope. Sanna and Nervi[480] claimed that myopic patients between the ages of 20 and 50 were more likely to have vitreous liquefaction and posterior vitreous detachment (PVD) than emmetropes or hyperopes of similar ages. This was confirmed in a study of 250 eyes from individuals ages 10 to 60, where Singh et al.[515] demonstrated a progressive increase in the incidence of liquefaction and PVD when comparing hyperopes, emmetropes, myopes of less than -6 diopters, and myopes of more than -6 diopters. A recent clinical study[412] found that of 172 eyes with a PVD, 26% had myopia in excess of -3 diopters. The mean age at PVD in these myopes was 56 years, as compared to 61 years in nonmyopes ($p < 0.01$). This degree of myopia, however, cannot be considered advanced, and the results of this study may not be statistically significant when performing a comparison of the control population with the appropriate test group, i.e., high myopes.

Morphologically, the vitreous of an axial myope is said to be liquefied and to contain filaments with localized nodules and thickenings.[137] Biochemical studies in the human[62] found that vitreous collagen content and concentration are lower in the central portions of myopic eyes as compared to nonmyopes. Hexosamine concentration, an index of hyaluronic acid, was also lower in the central and cortical vitreous of myopes as compared to nonmyopes. Although these investigators suggested that the findings were due to "dilution" in the enlarged cavity of the myopic vitreous, it is not clear whether these changes are part of the cause or an effect of myopia.

Further support for these concepts derives from the fact that myopia is seen in disorders such as Marfan's syndrome, Ehlers-Danlos syndrome, Stickler syndrome, Wagner's disease, and Laurence-Moon-Bardet-Biedl syndrome.[500] As pointed out by Maumenee,[385] all these conditions manifest a vitreous "degeneration" and all have varying degrees of myopia. It is perhaps more appropriate therefore to consider that the vitreous changes in such generalized connective tissue disorders (including myopia) are due to "dysgenesis" rather than "degeneration" and that the myopia may result in part from a widespread developmental abnormality of all connective tissues, including the vitreous.

Molecular development

There is ongoing synthesis of both collagen and hyaluronic acid (HA) during development to the adult (Figs. 9-14 and 9-15). Since the synthesis of collagen only keeps pace with increasing vitreous volume, the overall concentration of collagen within the vitreous is unchanged during this period of life (see Fig. 9-14). There is, however, net synthesis of HA during this time[43,426] (Fig. 9-15,A). Studies in bovine eyes[43] showed that vitreous HA concentration increases from 67.7 μg/ml at 1 to 2 months of age to 245 μg/ml at 1 to 3 years of age. In humans the concentration of HA in the gel vitreous increases from about 0.05 mg/ml during the first 4 years of life to just under 0.2 mg/ml in the third decade[39,41] (see Fig. 9-15,A). The significant increase in HA concentration during this time results from the fact that although the eye is growing in size, HA is being synthesized at a greater rate than globe enlargement. Indeed this synthesis may contribute to growth of the eye. During adulthood there is a continuous turnover of HA that is strongly dependent upon molecular weight, suggesting that the process is governed by diffusion.[230] Laurent and Tengblad[358] used radioassay techniques to determine that the turnover rate of HA was 0.45 μg per day.

HA molecules come to be situated between the collagen fibrils in an as yet unknown manner. This results in a "spreading apart" of the collagen fibrils, decreasing their light-scattering effect and increasing the optical transparency of the vitreous. Total collagen content in the gel vitreous decreases during the first few years of life and then remains at about 0.05 mg until the third decade[39,41] (see Fig. 9-14). Since collagen concentration does not increase appreciably while the size of the vitreous increases, the network density of collagen fibrils effectively decreases. This could potentially weaken the collagen network and destabilize the gel. However, the dramatic increase in HA concentration is believed to "stabilize" the thinning collagen network.[40]

In addition to developmental changes in the synthesis and concentration of collagen there are changes in the molecular configuration of vitreous collagen during development to the adult. Snowden et al.[527] found that dihydroxylysinonorleucine is the major reduced crosslink of fetal bovine vitreous collagen. Yet fetal vitreous collagen has half the amount of this crosslink as fetal articular and tendon collagens. In the adult, however, vitreous collagen has more than three times the content of dihydroxylysinonorleucine as articular collagen, and only trace amounts are present in tendon collagen. The 3-hydroxypyridinium content of adult vitreous collagen is about half that of articular cartilage collagen, indicating a more complete disappearance of the reducible 5-ketoimine crosslink from adult cartilage than from adult vitreous. The investigators suggest that this is due either to incomplete vitreous maturation to hydroxypyridinium residues or more active collagen synthesis in adult vitreous than adult articular cartilage, providing a higher proportion of younger collagen containing immature crosslinks. The physiologic significance of this phenomenon is not known. Such abnormal vitreous collagen crosslinks have, however, been detected in certain pathologic conditions, the most important of which is diabetic retinopathy.[508]

Morphologic changes

The molecular events described above probably underlie the morphologic changes observed during development to the adult. In the human embryo there is a dense, highly light-scattering appearance (Fig. 9-16) that becomes less dense and more transparent during childhood (Fig. 9-17). The occurrence of these morphologic changes during the period of active HA synthesis (see Fig. 9-15) suggests that newly synthesized HA molecules separate collagen fibrils, decreasing light scattering and achieving optical transparency. The HA-collagen interaction maintains gel stability even though the collagen network is thinned to enhance transparency. The physicochemical nature of this important interaction remains to be determined.

During development in the adult there are further changes in vitreous morphology. In childhood there is a homogeneous appearance to the vitreous (Fig. 9-17). There are no discernible structures other than the vitreous cortex and Cloquet's canal. In the adult there are macroscopic fibers coursing antero-posteriorly with insertions at the vitreous base and the posterior vitreous cortex[504,505] (Figs. 9-7,H, 9-8, and 9-11,A). Ultrastructural studies have shown that

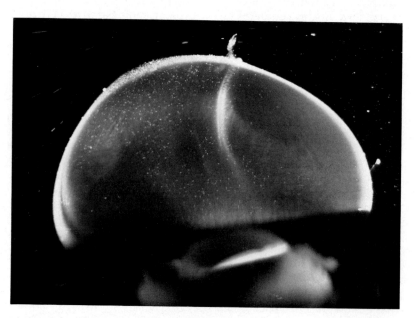

FIG. 9-16   Vitreous structure in a human embryo at 33 weeks of gestation. The posterior aspect of the lens is seen below. The vitreous is enclosed by the dense, highly light-scattering cortex. Parapapillary glial tissue was torn away during dissection and hangs from the prepapillary vitreous cortex seen above. Within the vitreous, Cloquet's canal arcs from the prepapillary vitreous cortex toward the lens. Since its course undulates through the vitreous, not all of Cloquet's canal can be visualized in a single horizontal section. (Reprinted with permission from Sebag J: Age-related changes in human vitreous structure, Graef Arch Clin Exp Ophthalmol 225:89, 1987.)

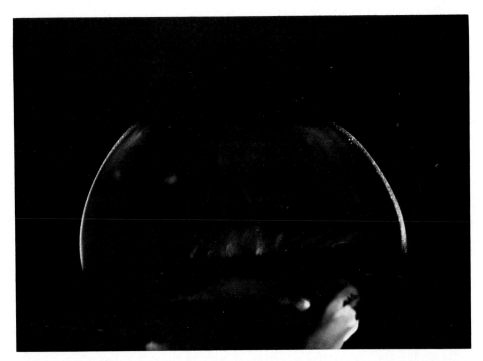

FIG. 9-17   Human vitreous structure during childhood. This view of the central vitreous from an 11-year-old child demonstrates a dense vitreous cortex with hyalocytes. The posterior aspect of the lens is seen below, though dimly illuminated. No fibers are present in the vitreous.

these fibers consist of parallel collagen fibrils packed into bundles[505] (Fig. 9-9,A). This metamorphosis probably results from changes in the association between the existing collagen network, which is purportedly not actively synthesized in the adult, and newly synthesized HA. An alteration in HA-collagen interaction is hypothesized to cause dissociation of these two components of the vitreous, resulting in aggregates of collagen fibrils packed into bundles and pooling of HA molecules in areas adjacent to the fibers.[497,498,504,505] The consequent formation of "liquid" vitreous, which becomes advanced during aging, is an important component in the pathogenesis of posterior vitreous detachment.

PHYSIOLOGY AND FUNCTIONS OF THE VITREOUS
Physiology and metabolism

The vitreous plays an important role in various physiologic processes within the eye. Oxygenation of interocular tissues is an important aspect of ocular physiology, especially crucial in retinal metabolism, which could be influenced by vitreous. Oxygen tension was recently measured in the human vitreous for the first time.[479] The lowest oxygen tension was found in the central vitreous (15.9 ± 2.8 mm Hg), followed by the peripheral anterior vitreous (16.7 ± 3.7 mm Hg), and the highest levels were in the posterior vitreous (19.9 ± 4.8 mm Hg). Interestingly, vitreous oxygen tension adjacent to detached retina showed a marked increase in man (30.0 ± 4.8 mm Hg) but not in the rabbit. It has been hypothesized that one mechanism by which vitrectomy improves the course of diabetic retinopathy is by permitting increased posterior oxygen transfer from the ciliary body via the vitreous to the inner retina.[533]

Walker and Patrick[601] suggested that the vitreous serves as a metabolic repository for the retina, hyalocytes, and neighboring tissues. These investigators were referring to the presence in the vitreous of galactose, glucose, mannose, fructose, and the hyaluronic acid (HA) precursors glucuronic acid and glucosamine. Indeed, studies[611] of experimental ischemia in the rabbit demonstrated that after 1 hour of pressure ischemia to the eye, retinal glycogen was reduced to 35% and vitreous glucose was reduced to 60% of normal levels. There was also an increase in vitreous concentration of lactic acid. Subsequent studies[606] confirmed these findings and found that vitreous glycogen was also depleted although less so than in the retina. Thus the vitreous can serve as a metabolic repository for short-term nutrients needed by the retina in emergency situations. Studies by Reddy[453] suggest that the vitreous may also serve as a repository for amino acids destined for utilization by the retina. Newman[410] has demonstrated that Müller cell membrane permeability to potassium is largely concentrated at the foot plates that insert onto the vitreous cortex-internal limiting lamina complex. It has been suggested by Newman that this specialization is intended to transfer potassium to and from the large reservoir in the vitreous. As pointed out by Gardner-Medwin[213] alterations in such activity could have a significant influence upon neuronal behavior in the retina. Studies in vivo have detected the release of glycine into the vitreous following photic stimulation in pigmented rats[129] but not albino rats.[130] Whether re-uptake occurs at a later time is not known.

The vitreous may also serve as a depository for metabolic wastes, such as lactic acid. Since high levels of this compound could be deleterious, vitreous ascorbic acid may play a protective role as a scavenger for free radicals resulting from retinal and lens metabolism as well as free radicals generated by photochemical reactions.[421,582] Comper and Laurent[125] pointed out that one consequence of the immobilization of charged polysaccharides in the vitreous is that a Donnan-type distribution is introduced between the vitreous and adjacent non-polyion-containing compartments or those with low polyion concentrations. Although the physiologic significance of this is not known, Comper and Laurent[125] suggest that this may have a protective function against the untoward effects of highly reactive, potentially destructive hydrated electrons such as those produced by ionizing radiation and water. In this regard vitreous HA may furnish an "anionic shield" for the retina and lens. Dysfunction in this protective mechanism could alter the metabolism of these adjacent tissues. Clinical evidence in support of this concept is found in the fact that there are many conditions where vitreous abnormalities are associated with lens opacification. The concept that lens transparency is somewhat dependent upon vitreous metabolism is also supported by experimental studies.[117,288,632] In experiments on lens regeneration[246] the vitreous was found to play an important role in providing a preferential pathway for the movement of growth factors from the neural retina to the dorsal iris. Movement of prostaglandins and other similar inflammatory agents in the reverse direction (from the iris to the macula) may contribute to the development of aphakic/pseudophakic cystoid macular edema. The channels adjacent to vitreous fibers may be the pathway these molecules travel. The orientation of these fibers and adjacent channels to the macula could facilitate this phenomenon.

Vitreous plays an important role in the movement of solutes and solvents within the eye. Early studies[330] showed that water movement within the vitreous is very active, with 50% of labeled water turning over every 10 to 15 minutes. Subsequent studies[53] have confirmed this finding. Several mechanisms can influence transvitreal movement of molecules. These include diffusion, hydrostatic pressure, osmotic pressure, convection, and active transport by surrounding tissues. Intrinsic properties of vitreous and its molecular components very likely have a major influence upon the first few of these processes. However, the active transport of substances from the vitreous is very much dependent upon the tissues surrounding the vitreous, and the relative importance of vitreous composition and structure upon active transport in different species and at different ages is not known. Studies[399] have found that in man the sensory retina is responsbile for 43% of the active transport of sodium fluorescein from the vitreous, while in the cynomologus monkey it contributes 25%, and in the rabbit only 7%. These studies also determined that the retinal pigment epithelium-choroid complex is responsible for about a third of the active transport in man and the cynomologus monkey and over half of the active transport of sodium fluorescein from the rabbit vitreous. Whether species variations in vitreous biochemistry account for these differences is not known. These findings nevertheless underscore the importance of considering species and age-related differences when selecting animals with which to model human physiology and disease.

Mosely[405] has developed a mathematical model for the diffusion of tracers from the vitreous to surrounding tissues and removal from the posterior segment by the choriocapillaris. He found good agreement between the predictions of this model and experimental results for xenon diffusion in the rabbit vitreous. Maurice[386] and Kinsey et al.[329] showed that diffusion is the main process influencing transvitreal movement of molecules the size of glucose (posterior diffusion) and lactic acid (anterior diffusion). Fatt and Hedbys[174] postulated the existence of appreciable transvitreal bulk flow. Although this appeared to contradict earlier findings, Fatt[172] pointed out that while both diffusion and bulk flow occur in the vitreous, the former is eight times greater than the latter for a small ion. This appears to be true of any low-molecular-weight substance, since the velocity of posteriorly directed bulk flow is too small to influence transport. Thus low-molecular-weight substances diffuse in response to a concentration gradient (in either direction), while high-molecular-weight substances and colloidal particles travel as a front with convective flow, since the diffusion constant is very low.

Hyaluronic acid (HA) represents the major resistance to the transvitreal flow of water.[204,350,416] Preston et al.[441] showed that a 1% HA solution increases resistance to the flow of water through a 0.1 mm diameter capillary tube more than a hundredfold. The resistance to bulk flow resulting from collagen is variable and dependent upon the density of the collagen fibril network. Measurements of hydraulic flow conductivity of the entire rabbit[83] and bovine[173] vitreous showed values on the order of 10^{-9} cm^4/sec/dyne. These values are substantially higher than more dense connective tissue matrices, such as skin, cartilage, and cornea (10^{-14} to 10^{-11} cm^4/sec/dyne), and probably result from the influence of HA. Indeed, Fessler[178] and Disalvo and Schubert[153] showed that the resistance to compression of collagen gels is increased by the presence of proteoglycans and interpreted this as being due to the very high resistance to solvent flow by the highly entangled polysaccharides. Studies by Foulds et al.[204] have shown that the diffusion of tritiated water from the rabbit vitreous through the vitreous cortex, and its recovery from the vortex veins is enhanced following treatment with hyaluronidase. These investigators concluded that hyaluronic acid serves as a barrier to the diffusion of water, particularly across the vitreous cortex. Even within the vitreous, HA influences water movement. Ali and Bettelheim[6] have shown that as much as 20% of the water present in bovine vitreous is nonfreezable (i.e., bound mostly to HA). As these investigators point out, this is remarkably high, since the lens, which has a 35% macromolecular content, has a nonfreezable water content of 25 to 60%.[65] Vitreous macromolecular content is only 1 to 2%, and yet the nonfreezable water content is 20%. This is due to the hydrophilic characteristics of HA. Thompson et al.[572] found that in the rabbit vitreous the transvitreal diffusion of molecules such as tritiated water, inulin, dextran (20K and 70K), and myosin decreased proportionally with increasing molecular weight of the tracer. This is probably due not only to HA, but to the collagen network as well.

Laurent et al.[350] showed that HA decreases the transvitreal transport of macromolecules and that this effect increases with increasing macromolecule size and increasing concentration of HA. These investigators claimed that this was due more to a "molecular sieve" effect than frictional resistance. This was supported by studies[351,413,442] showing that rotational movement of albumin in polysaccharide solutions is only slightly suppressed while translational movement is markedly retarded. Thus large macromolecules act as if enclosed in holes within a network where the frictional interaction is small but the large molecules cannot escape because of steric restriction. Linear polymers, however, move through polysaccharide networks more easily,[353] presumably because they move end-on through the network in a wormlike fashion. The diffusion of random-coil molecules also appears to increase in the presence of a polysaccharide matrix.[334,443] Whether these phenomena occur in the double network of HA and collagen within the vitreous is not presently known. However, studies in the intact rabbit and bovine vitreous enabled Fatt[173] to calculate that the diameter of the "pores" available for flow of water and particles through the vitreous is 400 nm. Balazs[38] has indicated that once inside the vitreous the diffusion of a large molecule is higher than would be expected, due to the "excluded volume" effect. Since the volume of solvent in the vitreous is decreased by the volume of the double network of collagen and HA, the effective concentration of the solute is higher, resulting in a faster rate of diffusion. This effect is, of course, proportional to the network densities and may vary considerably in different physiologic and pathologic states.

Such physiologic properties within the vitreous could be important with regard to the supply of nutrients and removal of waste products to and from surrounding tissues. Drug delivery to both the anterior and posterior segments of the eye could be altered by changes in vitreous composition or structure. Indeed, in an experimental model,[155] amphotericin B clearance was substantially more rapid from vitrectomized eyes than controls. A less drastic, although clearly more common, effect is that induced by aging. Vitreous fluorophotometry studies[322] have detected higher mid and anterior vitreous levels in humans aged 55 to 65 than controls aged 20 to 40 years. Although the investigators concluded that this is due to a decreased resistance in the more liquefied vitreous of the older subjects, there may also be a contribution from age-related vascular incompetence or other interactions between the vitreous components and fluorescein.[337] Furthermore, the presence of posterior vitreous detachment can also influence vitreous fluorophotometry measurements,[440] a variable that was not considered in Kayazawa's studies.

Transvitreous diffusion and bulk flow may also be involved in maintaining retinal attachment. Studies[432] in an animal model of rhegmatogenous retinal detachment demonstrated that in control eyes there is flow from the posterior vitreous of 0.19 ± 0.1 μl/min and from the anterior vitreous of 0.38 ± 0.06 μl/min. These investigators concluded that there exists a low level, constant flow of fluid through the vitreous and across the intact retina, which may help maintain retinal apposition to the retinal pigment epithelium. Clinical observations by Foulds[202] support this concept. Alterations in this activity may contribute to the development of retinal detachment.

Optical roles of the vitreous
Media transparency

The index of refraction of vitreous is 1.3349, nearly the same as of aqueous. Vitreous transmits 90% of light between 300 and 1400 nm and none above or below this range,[73] although in the infrared range transmission begins to drop off at 800 nm.[615] Since the lens absorbs ultraviolet wavelengths, vitreous transmission in this range becomes important in aphakic eyes or eyes with intraocular lenses that do not have UV filters. Swann[548] has stated that the primary function of the vitreous is to allow the unhindered transmission of light to the retina. He has pointed out that in contrast to the cornea, vitreous transparency is achieved by the existence of an extremely low concentration of macromolecular solutes. Swann concluded that the features of the vitreous that distinguish it from other extracellular matrices are related to the structure of collagen and that these are responsible for the maintenance of optical transparency. The unique amino acid composition, high content of galactosyl-glucose side chains and the existence of additional terminal peptides are thought to be important in the organization of vitreous collagen as fibers of small diameter, minimizing the scattering of light. Balazs[38] points out that the presence of large hyaluronic acid (HA) molecules serves to keep the collagen fibrils widely dispersed, further minimizing

light scattering by these structural proteins.

To ensure optical clarity the vitreous must also serve as a barrier to the influx of cells and macromolecules. Laurent and Pietruszkiewicz[354] and Ogston and Phelps[415] suggested that HA may act as a physicochemical barrier to the entry of macromolecules into the vitreous. The in vivo studies of Hultsch[281] showed that the inflammatory response elicited by intravitreal endotoxin depended upon the vitreous concentrations of HA. Protein exudation was highest when the concentration of HA was lowest. This was not due to endotoxin-induced depolymerization of HA nor to changes in the outflow of HA from the vitreous. Hultsch concluded that the diffusion barrier, which prevented the influx of macromolecules, was at least in part dependent upon the "molecular sieve" effect of HA described by Balazs.[33]

Breakdown in the aforementioned function(s) of the vitreous may result in various vitreous opacities and cell invasion of different types.

Vitreous opacities. *Synchisis scintillans.* This term is used to describe vitreous opacification related to any pathologic process that results in chronic vitreous hemorrhage. When frank hemorrhage dissipates, synchisis scintillans can appear as flat, refractile bodies that are golden brown in color and are freely mobile. They are associated with liquid vitreous, so that they settle to the most dependent portion of the vitreous when eye movement stops. The vitreous about these opacities is degenerated and liquefied such that collagen is displaced peripherally.[530] Chemical studies[10] have demonstrated the presence of cholesterol crystals in these opacities and the condition is sometimes referred to as a "cholesterolosis bulbi." Free hemoglobin sperules in the vitreous have also been reported.[245]

Asteroid hyalosis. Benson[58] was the first to identify asteroid hyalosis as being different from synchisis scintillans. Asteroid hyalosis is a generally benign condition characterized by small white or yellow-white spherical or disc-shaped opacities throughout the vitreous. The prevalence of this condition in the general population is about 0.042 to 0.5%, affecting all races, but with a male to female ratio of 2:1. When advanced, asteroid hyalosis can reduce visual acuity and obscure an adequate view of the posterior pole. Curiously, asteroid hyalosis is unilateral in over 75% of cases. In contrast to synchisis scintillans, asteroid bodies are intimately associated with the vitreous gel and more with typical vitreous displacement during eye movement. This fact may link the process more closely to collagen than HA and led Rodman et al.[470] to suggest that there was a relationship with vitreous fibril degeneration. However, posterior vitreous detachment, either complete or partial, occurs less frequently in asteroid hyalosis than in age-matched controls,[605] partly contradicting this hypothesis.

Voerhoeff[594] first described the histopathologic features of asteroid hyalosis and suggested that the opacities were calcium soaps. Subsequent histologic studies[470] demonstrated a crystalline appearance to asteroid bodies with a positive staining pattern to fat and acid mucopolysaccharide stains that was unaffected by hyaluronidase pretreatment. Electron diffraction studies[378] showed the presence of calcium oxalate monohydrate and calcium hydroxyphosphate. Miller et al.[398] demonstrated that asteroid bodies had a lamellar arrangement with a periodicity of 4.6 nm, and suggested that they are phospholipid crystals in an intermediate state between true crystals and a true liquid. Streeten[541] performed ultrastructural studies and found intertwined ribbons of multilaminar membranes with a 6 nm periodicity that she interpreted as characteristic of complex lipids, especially phospholipids, lying in a homogeneous background matrix. In these investigations energy dispersive x-ray analysis showed calcium and phosphorous to be the main elements in these structures. Electron-diffraction structural analysis demonstrated calcium hydroxyapatite and possibly other forms of calcium-phosphate crystals.

The etiology of asteroid hyalosis is not clearly understood. Voerhoeff[594] suggested that the condition resulted from "vascular sclerosis." There have been reports[49,121,501,523] suggesting an association between asteroid hyalosis and diabetes mellitus. Others[258,323,371] dispute such an association. Yu and Blumenthal[641] proposed that in aging collagen calcium binds to the free polar groups on vitreous fibers forming "nucleation" sites. They also suggested that sulfated glycosaminoglycans may be important as chelators in the binding of calcium to these sites. Studies in a rabbit experimental model[345] showed that asteroid formation is preceded by depolymerization of hyaluronic acid. Streeten[541] was impressed by the unilaterality of the condition and the presence of large quantities of complex lipids and calcium. She suggested that asteroid hyalosis is a local phenomenon involving diffusion of substances from tissues outside the vitreous.

Amyloidosis. Vitreous opacities secondary to systemic amyloidosis were first reported by Kantarjian and DeJong.[318] Amyloidosis can result in the deposition of opacities in the vitreous of one or both eyes. Bilateral involvement can be an early manifestation of the dominant form of familial amyloidosis,[135,320] although rare cases of vitreous involvement in nonfamilial forms have been reported.[82,493] The opacities first appear in the vitreous adjacent to retinal blood vessels and later appear anteriorly.[629] Initially, the opacities are granular with wispy fringes and later take on a "glass wool" appearance.[530] When the opacities form strands, they appear to attach to the retina and the posterior aspect of the lens by thick footplates.[541] Following posterior vitreous detachment, the posterior vitreous cortex is observed to have thick, linear opacities that follow the course of the retinal vessels. The opacities seem to aggregate by "seeding" on vitreous fibrils and along the posterior vitreous cortex.[541]

When visually significant, the opacified vitreous can be safely removed surgically. Specimens that have been studied histopathologically contained starlike structures with dense, fibrillar centers. The amyloid fibrils are 5 to 10 nm in diameter and are distinguished from the 10 to 15 nm vitreous fibrils by stains for amyloid and by the fact that the vitreous fibrils are very straight and long.[541] Electron microscopic studies[268] have confirmed the presence of amyloid, and immunocytochemical studies[154] have identified the major amyloid constituent as a protein resembling prealbumin. More recent investigations[236] used two-dimension gel electrophoresis and immuno-electron microscopy to study human vitreous samples from patients with amyloidosis. Specimens from both familial and nonfamilial amyloidosis were found to contain material with the molecular weight and isofocusing coordinates of prealbumin monomer. Streeten[541] has considered that hyalocytes could perform the role of macrophage-processing of the amyloid protein before its polymerization. This may further explain why the opacities initially appear at the posterior vitreous cortex where hyalocytes reside (Figs. 9-11,A, 9-12, and 9-13).

Cell invasion. To minimize light scattering and maintain vitreous clarity, certain functions of the vitreous involve the inhibition of cell migration and proliferation. HA has been shown to inhibit lymphocyte stimulation,[139,282] macrophage phagocytosis,[196,197,506] and macrophage prostaglandin synthesis.[506] Streeten[541] points out that true cellular membranes with collagen-secreting fibroblastic cells usually grow along the posterior surface of the posterior vitreous cortex and not within the vitreous. Unless there is penetrating trauma to the vitreous, at which time cells are implanted centrally, or unless the vitreous cortex is markedly disrupted, cells seldom grow within the vitreous itself.

Penetrating trauma. Constable and Swann[126] found that even minimal penetration of the vitreous is associated with substantial internal change. Aspiration of fluid vitreous from the owl monkey and immediate reinjection was followed by a rapid influx of serum proteins, prolonged increases in vascular permeability, and profound degradation of hyaluronic acid. These alterations were exaggerated if the eye wall was "injured" by cryopexy or diathermy. The same experimental conditions in the rabbit resulted in a cellular infiltrate not seen in the monkey.[126] This suggests that there are intrinsic differences between the owl monkey and rabbit vitreous that are associated with cell invasion in the rabbit but not the monkey. One possible explanation is that the high concentration of hyaluronic acid in the owl monkey vitreous inhibits cell migration and proliferation. Another possibility is that the solid gel state of the rabbit vitreous provides a better substrate for cell migration and proliferation than the liquid owl monkey vitreous.

Faulborn and Topping[177] found that intravitreal cell proliferation was already in progress 2 to 4 days after penetrating trauma and was well-established by 1 week. Winthrop et al.[620] found that in the presence of a retinal detachment, penetrating trauma resulted in periretinal proliferation by 1 to 2 weeks and resulted in a cyclitic membrane at 6 weeks following trauma. A number of authors[126,201,579] have emphasized the importance of the vitreous as a "scaffold" for cell migration and proliferation, particularly as it relates to fibroblast activity and the formation of scar tissue within the eye. Ussman et al.[584] showed that after penetrating injury, vitreous collagen fibrils are intertwined and have focal condensations. These investigators proposed that such alterations could provide the scaffold along which cells migrate into the vitreous. Studies of an experimental model in the rhesus monkey[120] showed that fibroblast proliferation within the vitreous arises from the choroid at the wound and nonpigmented and pigmented ciliary epithelium of the ciliary body. Exactly how the inhibition of cell migration and proliferation normally exerted by the vitreous is overcome in these clinical and experimental settings is currently not known. It is also not known whether the types or extent of vitreous alterations differ for different types of foreign material that enter the vitreous during penetrating trauma.

Ultrastructural studies[571] of vitreous in experimental models of penetrating trauma have found that normal collagen is replaced by a newly formed collagen. Pilkerton et al.[435] determined that only a small amount of new collagen is synthesized during the first 2 weeks following penetrating trauma. However, by 4 weeks there is a marked increase in new collagen formation that is accelerated by the presence of blood. Raymond et al.[448] have identified the newly formed collagen as type I collagen and suggest that it is synthesized by fibroblasts originating from the sclera and uvea at the site of penetration. The synthesis of collagen forms membranes and bands within the vitreous. The association of these bands with cells in the vitreous that have contractile properties can result in substantial traction upon the retina. Ussman et al.[585] found that there were increasing amounts of intracellular actin filaments in 12- to 21-day-old vitreous membranes. These authors suggested that the reason the process of wound healing in the posterior segment of the eye differs from elsewhere in the body is that the specialized anatomy of the vitreoretinal interface and at the vitreous base accounts for the development of traction retinal detachment.

Neovascularization and hemorrhage. Vitreous can inhibit some of the pathologic processes that result in neovascularization and vitreous hemorrhage. Raymond and Jacobson[447] partially purified a protein of MW = 6200, which inhibited retina-derived growth factor-induced thymidine incorporation and proliferation by vascular endothelial cells in vitro. Jacobson et al.[300] found this activity in hyalocyte-conditioned culture medium and hypothesized that hyalocyte synthesis of this "anti-angiogenic" factor may trigger the regression of the hyaloid artery system during development and inhibit neovascularization in the adult. This activity has been demonstrated in normal and pathologic vitreous as well.[299] Taylor and Weiss[566] attribute this "anti-angiogenic" activity to a glycoprotein of Mr 5,700, which they have isolated from bovine vitreous. This substance was also found to inhibit collagenase activity. Interestingly, Lutty et al.[369] found that the vitreous inhibitor of capillary endothelium is a stimulant of pericyte proliferation. Pericytes are known to inhibit retinal capillary endothelial cells in vitro[422] and in vivo.[312] Thus vitreous stimulation of pericyte activity may be a further anti-angiogenic effect. A breakdown or deficiency of these vitreous anti-neovascular activities may contribute to pathologic angiogenesis, by the lack of inhibition on capillary endothelial cells, and the lack of pericyte stimulation. Lutty et al.[369,370] also showed that the vitreous antineovascular activity was dose-dependent and effective on capillary endothelial cells, aortic endothelium, aortic smooth muscle cells, and corneal endothelium. Thus this antiproliferative activity could act upon the many different types of cells that border the vitreous, inhibiting cell invasion of the vitreous and maintaining optical transparency.

The properties of the vitreous that maintain media clarity are often overwhelmed by vitreous hemorrhage. Bleeding within the eye can be curtailed to some extent by vitreous, as evidenced by the capacity of vitreous to shorten the partial thromboplastin time[325] and the ability of vitreous collagen to cause platelet aggregation.[552] Anecdotal reports by ocular surgeons employing synthetic hyaluronic acid solutions ("viscosurgery") have demonstrated hemostatic properties clinically.

Blood in the vitreous results in several important changes that cannot always be readily observed clinically because the view of the posterior segment of the eye is obscured. Recent studies[368] showed that ultrasonography can be used to monitor blood-induced changes in the echographic characteristics of the vitreous. Forrester et al.[200] noted that vitreous liquefaction begins during the first week of vitreous hemorrhage. This was confirmed by studies in the rabbit,[321] where vitreous viscosity was decreased following hemorrhage. Further destablization of the vitreous can result from abnormal collagen metabolism. After injecting blood into the rabbit vitreous, Swann[547] found a different type of collagen fibril, by ultrastructural criteria. In a rabbit model of penetrating trauma with intravitreal hemorrhage Raymond et al.[448] identified this fibril as type I collagen.

Forrester and Grierson[199] studied the histopathology of the cellular response to blood in the vitreous and likened it to a "low-turnover granuloma." The polymorphonuclear leukocyte response was minimal but there were substantial numbers of mononuclear cells, which by 6 weeks began to form multinucleated giant cells. Interestingly, these investigators interpreted the presence of giant cells as evidence that the macrophages suffered from impaired phagocytic capacity. This is consistent with in vitro studies[197,506] demonstrating a dose-dependent inhibition of macrophage phagocytosis by hyaluronic acid. LaNauze et al.[346] also found that the inflammatory reaction to blood in the vitreous was diminished even though chemotactic activity was still in effect.

Some of the mononuclear cells involved in the chronic inflammatory reaction to blood in the vitreous may be hyalocytes. Burke et al.[90] showed that hemoglobin stimulates hyalocyte DNA synthesis. A shift in the activity of this population of cells from their normal functions in vitreous metabolism to a phagocytic action could result in further destabilization of the vitreous and liquefaction. Burke[88] also found that the invasion of mononuclear cells in the third week following vitreous hemorrhage resulted in excess vitreous levels of superoxide anion. She proposed that this may contribute to vitreous liquefaction and toxicity to adjacent tissues by free radical action. McCord's[388] finding that enzymatically generated superoxide anion can depolymerize hyaluronic acid in bovine synovial fluid supports this hypothesis. In the vitreous experimental singlet oxygen generation has been shown to induce liquefaction.[582] Furthermore, Katami et al.[319] found that following the injection of autologous erythrocytes into the rabbit vitreous there was a shift of glycosaminoglycan content. Normally in this model 91% of the total glycosaminoglycans is hyaluronic acid. Following erythrocyte injection, only 26% was hyaluronic acid, while 59% was chondroitin sulfate. Such a departure from normal vitreous macromolecular composition could further contribute to structural destabilization and liquefaction.

Regnault[458] studied an experimental model of vitreous hemorrhage and noted that after 3 days there were pyknotic changes in rod nuclei and edema of the inner nuclear, ganglion cell, and nerve fiber layers of the retina. Such changes could be due to the effects of free radicals within the vitreous. Van Bockxmeer et al.[588] found that the iron-binding proteins (transferrin and lactoferrin) of the rhesus monkey had the capacity to bind an amount of hemoglobin iron equivalent to that found in more than ½ million red blood cells. They concluded that in this way the vitreous serves a protective role in avoiding or minimizing retinal iron toxicity. Studies by McGahan and Fleisher[392] found that during endotoxin-induced ocular inflammation in rabbits there is an influx of serum-derived transferrin into the vitreous. Thus, in cases of vitreous hemorrhage the presence of endogenous as well as exogenous transferrin in the vitreous could protect against the potentially harmful effects of iron released from red blood cells.

Premacular ("epiretinal") membranes. Premacular membrane formation, often referred to as "epiretinal," is another pathologic condition in which there is a breakdown or deficiency in the properties of the vitreous that attempt to maintain media clarity by inhibiting cell migration and proliferation. Iwanoff[292] was the first to describe the existence of a membrane on the anterior surface of the retina. This condition often arises from cell proliferation at or near the optic disc that extends into the macula. Vision is affected due to disruption of macular anatomy. However, this does not occur in all cases, since evidence of abnormal cell proliferation at the optic disc has been found in about one half of "normal" human autopsy eyes.[193,474] The high prevalence of cell proliferation at this site may be due to differences between the basal laminae interfacing with the vitreous at the disc, compared with elsewhere in the posterior pole. The membrane of Elschnig and meniscus of Kuhnt, which replace the thicker internal limiting lamina (ILL) of the retina at the optic nerve head, are likely to have diminished barrier properties compared with a true basal lamina such as the ILL. Consequently, this anatomy may predispose the area about the optic disc to cell proliferation. Furthermore, the absence of a posterior vitreous cortex in the prepapillary region (see Fig. 9-11) would also diminish the inhibitory effects of the vitreous cortex on cell migration and proliferation. Other areas that are predisposed to cell proliferation due to thinness of the ILL are the fovea along major blood vessels and at retinal tufts.[240] There are also acquired sites of discontinuity in the ILL such as retinal tags, retinal pits, avulsed retinal vessels, and lattice degeneration.[240]

Clinically, the prevalence of "epiretinal" membranes is 3.5%,[473] and the condition is unilateral in 80% of cases.[621] These membranes are usually only recognized clinically at the posterior pole when the macula has an irregular surface and there are traction lines in the inner retina. With increasing severity, the retinal vessels become dilated and tortuous.[621] Small white spots can be seen as well as yellow exudates, blot hemorrhages, and microaneurysms.[622] Gass[219] has classified these membranes according to the severity of retinal distortion, concurrent biomicroscopic changes, and associated ocular disorders. In its mildest form a premacular membrane appears as so-called "cellophane maculopathy," which can advance to a wrinkled appearance in the macula when the membrane contracts, causing the underlying retina to develop small irregular folds. Further contraction causes "macular pucker" and vision is greatly disturbed due to opacification of the membrane and marked distortion of the retina. Vision can also be reduced due to macular edema sometimes exacerbated by incomplete

posterior vitreous detachment (PVD) and vitreous traction upon the macula. In a study[265] of 250 cases with premacular membranes there was a significantly higher prevalence of poor vision, cystoid macular pathology, or angiographic macular edema in cases with a partial PVD. When there was no PVD or complete PVD, there were very few cases of such maculopathy. A subsequent study[11] demonstrated that in 324 patients with premacular membranes, 303 (84.9%) had partial or complete PVD. Angiographic cystoid macular edema (CME) was present in 77 (20.6%) eyes. Of these eyes 20 (26%) had partial PVD with attachment to the macula, while only 23 of the 296 eyes without CME (7.8%) has such vitreomacular adhesion (p < 0.001). In certain cases progression from partial to complete PVD can dissect the membrane off the macula and symptoms resolve.[394]

Histopathologic studies of premacular membranes show fibrocellular sheets with varying degrees of cellularity.[119] Identifying the exact cell types in these membranes is difficult, because astrocytes, hyalocytes, fibrocytes, macrophages, and retinal pigment epithelial cells can all transform into cells with similar appearances on light and electron microscopy.[315] Many of these cell types also have the ability to develop the myofibroblast characteristics intrinsic to the pathophysiology of this disorder.[603] Immuno-staining studies[532] have shown that most cells in premacular membranes stain positively for glial fibrillary acidic protein, consistent with the presence of fibrous astrocytes. In a recent study[374] fibrous astrocytes were more commonly found in women (84% of cases), while retinal pigment epithelial cells were more common in men. The results of this study also suggested that myofibroblastic features may be characteristic of more rapidly proliferating membranes, while the presence of retinal pigment epithelial (RPE) cells is typical of more chronic, indolent membranes. Vinores et al.[591] used electron-immunocytochemical techniques to identify that RPE and retinal glial cells are most prominent in these membranes, but that macrophages also have a role.

The pathogenesis of premacular membrane formation is poorly understood. Posterior vitreous detachment (PVD) is said to be present in 80 to 95% of cases.[11,473,513,621,623] In a prospective study[623] of 34 eyes with acute PVD 9% had evidence of premacular membranes at presentation. Follow-up 18 months later found that such membranes had formed in 41%, suggesting that once the vitreous detaches from the retina there is a loss of some inhibitory effect(s). Gass[219] points out that premacular membranes are often likely to develop following transient vitreomacular traction during PVD. There are two sequences of events that could possibly explain this observation: (1) During PVD with transient vitreoretinal traction dehiscences could arise at the optic nerve head and along retinal blood vessels (where vitreoretinal adhesion is strong) that would allow migration and proliferation of fibrous astrocytes onto the anterior aspect of the ILL. (2) In cases of premacular membranes it is possible that during PVD vitreoretinal separation does not occur cleanly between the vitreous cortex and the ILL of the retina but splits the vitreous cortex ("vitreoschisis"), leaving cortical remnants and hyalocytes adherent to the ILL.[35] In an autopsy series of normal human eyes with spontaneous PVD 26 of 59 (44%) had cortical vitreous remnants at the fovea.[332] On scanning electron microscopy the adherent vitreous cortex appeared either disc-shaped, ringlike, or cystic. It is likely that these vitreous cortex remnants also contained hyalocytes, although in this study the use of scanning electron microscopy made it impossible to analyze this feature. Proliferation, fibrous metaplasia, and contraction of hyalocytes can result in premacular membranes that are confined to the central macula[219] and are hypocellular on histopathology.[119] In these cases surgical membrane peeling procedures are technically easier and far less traumatic to the underlying retina. Membranes that arise following true PVD and proliferation of fibrous astrocytes from the retina are more difficult to dissect, because their origin from the retina maintains firm connections between the membrane and the retina. Thus there are probably subcategories of premacular membranes whose etiologies and responses to surgical intervention are very different. Preoperative identification of the more favorable cases would enable better case selection.

Proliferative vitreoretinopathy (PVR). Proliferative vitreoretinopathy (PVR) following retinal detachment is a major cause of failed detachment surgery.[461] Clinically, an increase in the number and size of pigmented cells in the vitreous of patients with retinal detachment pre- or postoperatively heralds the development of massive PVR.[343,496] Early in the course of PVR, membranes are very cellular, while later there is an increase in extracellular collagen.[127] Experimental and clinical evidence suggest that this collagen is predominantly type I. Burke and Kower[89] showed that the injection of rabbit retina astroglia into the rabbit vitreous results in

the synthesis of type I collagen by these cells. Sheiffarth et al.[483] found type II collagen in pathologic vitreous membranes in only 6 of 19 patients with PVR, while 12 of 13 patients with proliferative diabetic retinopathy had type II collagen. It is therefore likely that the collagen in PVR membranes is newly synthesized by cells that do not normally synthesize vitreous collagen. The finding of type II collagen in almost one third of the PVR cases in Scheiffarth's series probably results from the fact that PVR membranes are intimately associated with the posterior vitreous cortex in some cases.[127,485]

The cells of PVR membranes are fibroblast-like but have several progenitors, particularly astrocytes[56,119,344] and retinal pigment epithelial (RPE) cells.[343,406,604] Recent immunohistochemical studies[305] have demonstrated that glial and RPE cells predominate in PVR membranes and that a small but significant macrophage population is also present. Blood-derived monocytes could be the source of these macrophages, but hyalocytes are another type of mononuclear cell that might also be involved in membrane formation at the vitreoretinal interface.

The prominence of RPE cells in PVR probably relates to the access of RPE cells to the vitreous afforded by the retinal break and the dispersion of viable RPE cells into the vitreous during cryopexy treatment of retinal tears. Clinically, a patient with a localized superior rhegmatogenous retinal detachment treated by techniques employing significant amounts of cryopexy, occasionally develops an inferior retinal detachment postoperatively due to inferior PVR. Singh et al.[516] have shown that RPE cells dispersed into the vitreous come to lie in the most dependent portion of the vitreous, where they form membranes. In a recent study[612] mononuclear phagocytes were identified by mouse antihuman macrophage antibody in a human vitreous specimen removed at surgery for PVR. Due to the unknown specificity of this antibody, it is not presently possible to state whether the stained cells were blood-derived monocytes, undifferentiated RPE cells, or hyalocytes. However, Hui et al.[280] have produced membrane formation and tractional retinal detachment that simulated PVR by injecting activated peritoneal macrophages into the rabbit vitreous. In clinical cases both RPE cells and macrophages could be involved because blood-derived monocytes can become macrophages and release chemoattractants that stimulate the migration of RPE cells,[91] further increasing the population of RPE cells within the vitreous.

Since one of the functions of vitreous is to inhibit cell invasion of the vitreous cavity, it is not clear how the vitreous is altered to permit cell migration and proliferation in PVR. In an experimental model of PVR, Kain[313] has shown that hyaluronidase-induced degradation of the vitreous is an essential prerequisite for PVR. Such alterations in vitreous physiology and molecular structure could readily exist in eyes with postoperative inflammation, intravitreal blood, or injected exogenous agents (e.g., air, gas). Furthermore, vitreous alterations in this setting could facilitate cell migration and proliferation. Such phenomena have been demonstrated in studies of the influence of different extracellular matrices upon the growth of retina-derived cells.[618] Campochiaro et al.[104] studied the influence of human vitreous aspirates upon the migration of retinal pigment epithelial cells in vivo. Vitreous from cases of PVR had much greater stimulatory activity than vitreous from patients with premacular membranes and uncomplicated retinal detachment. There are probably extrinsic as well as intrinsic factors involved in this process.

Extrinsic factors derive from migratory and proliferative stimuli not normally present in the vitreous. For example, the presence of macrophages within the vitreous in PVR could stimulate RPE cell migration[91] via chemoattractants such as platelet-derived growth factor[103,511] and fibronectin.[581] Not surprisingly, macrophages are not a prominent cell type in premacular membranes, explaining why this condition does not feature aggressive cell proliferation.

Intrinsic factors relate to alterations within the vitreous that increase inherent stimulatory activity and decrease inhibitory activity. Cell stimulatory properties have been found in normal vitreous. Wiedemann et al.[613] studied the in vivo mitogenic activity of vitreous upon several cell types in different species. They found that vitreous stimulated the proliferation of porcine retinal pigment epithelial cells, bovine and lapine dermal fibroblasts, but not the proliferation of bovine aortic endothelial and smooth muscle cells. On the basis of the experimental data these investigators concluded that this mitogenic activity was not derived from leakage of circulating growth factor(s) into the vitreous. Vidaurri-Leal et al.[590] also found that in vivo exposure of RPE cells to vitreous resulted in changes in cell morphology, whereby the RPE cells became fibrocyte-like and induced an increase in migratory activity. In addition to RPE cell dispersion into the vitreous following retinal detachment surgery, the vitreous or components of the vitreous (such as liquid vitreous) may come in contact with RPE cells in situ by entering the subretinal space via retinal tears, especially large ones. Indeed, a recent study[642] found that subretinal injection of explants of autologous vitreous in the rabbit induced retinal pigment epithelial and retinal glial cell proliferation in the subretinal space. Thus it is plausible that one element in the pathogenesis of PVR involves a vitreous-induced increase in mitogenic activity and cell migration.

PVR may also result from a decrease in the properties of the vitreous that normally inhibit cell migration and proliferation. There may be individual variations in the levels of these inhibitory properties with predisposition for the development of PVR in those individuals with low levels. It is known that the presence of blood within the vitreous alters normal vitreous metabolism and potentiates cell migration and proliferation. Kirchoff et al.[331] found that human vitreous stimulates the migration, but not proliferation, of human RPE cells when cultured without serum. The addition of serum albumin, however, stimulated RPE cell proliferation. Thus retinal tears and detachment can expose the RPE to vitreous and result in cell migration. The disruption of the blood-vitreous barrier following retinal detachment and retinal detachment surgery may have potentiating effects inducing cell proliferation. Campochiaro et al.[102] showed that in an experimental model without intravitreal blood the use of cryotherapy induced breakdown of the blood-ocular barrier and resulted in cell proliferation and the development of traction retinal detachment. Vitrectomy surgery could also result in a reduction of the antiproliferative, inhibitory properties of the vitreous. Hsu et al.[278] found that in a rabbit model, vitrectomy aggravated intraocular fibroblast proliferation and traction retinal detachment. Thus, although vitrectomy is indispensable in the management of PVR, it should be reserved for cases of established PVR. In the absence of appropriate indications vitrectomy should probably not be performed as prophylaxis against PVR.

The consequence of traction by PVR membranes is not simply wrinkling of the retina, as is the case for premacular "epiretinal" membranes, but actual retinal detachment. This may relate to the contractility of the cells in PVR[243,546] and their linking to one another by gap junctions, resulting in compact sheets.[243] Experimental studies[267] have demonstrated that some cells contain microfilaments composed of actinomyosin. Other studies[375] have identified myofibroblasts with prominent intracellular contractile myofilaments. Studies[166] of human vitrectomy specimens have demonstrated the presence of myofibroblasts associated with extracellular collagen fibrils of about 20 nm diameter. These fibrils are entwined with normal vitreous collagen and are thus able to transmit any contractile forces from the cells to the surrounding vitreous and in turn to the retina wherever the vitreous is still attached. Recent studies[449] have demonstrated that human RPE cell contraction of collagen gels is inhibited by colchicine and stimulated by transforming growth factor beta. Glial cell membranes have also been shown to exert such traction upon the retina,[279] possibly via vitreous collagen mediation.[145] Future investigations employing the vitreous as a model for cell proliferation and migration[198] may further elucidate the exact mechanisms by which this debilitating condition arises. However, while investigations with animal models have elucidated the pathogenesis of PVR considerably, one must exercise caution in drawing conclusions from some of the data. This is because species variations in vitreous composition and metabolism could influence the results of such experimentation. Reeser and Van Horn[457] showed that a technique for experimentally producing PVR worked well in rabbits but not in cats. These investigators questioned whether there were intrinsic differences in the vitreous of these species that allowed PVR to develop in the rabbit but not in the cat. It is interesting that the same was true of experimental models of penetrating trauma wherein intravitreal cell proliferation occurred in the rabbit but not in the owl monkey.[126] The structure and composition of the rabbit vitreous could thus potentiate the biologic phenomena involved in cell migration and proliferation. The appropriateness of the rabbit as a model for human intravitreal cell proliferation is thus in question.

Accommodation

Accommodation is the process by which the dioptric power of the eye is increased for seeing at near by changing the curvature of the lens. Helmholz[261] explained this phenomenon as the result of zonule relaxation, which allows lens capsule elasticity to induce "rounding-up" of the lens. The concept of a role for the vitreous in accommodation dates back to 1851, when Cramer (as cited by Fincham[180]) proposed that the vitreous pushes against the lens to alter its shape. Tscherning (as cited by Fincham[180]) and Von Pflug[600] demonstrated that the conoidal shape of the anterior lens surface could be altered by the forces of vitreous pressure. However, theories based on these findings largely ignored the influence of zonule relaxation and lens capsule elasticity. Kaczurowski[311] described the presence of "vitreozonules," which he proposed mediated an effect of vitreous on the lens during accommodation.

Coleman[123] attempted to integrate the concepts of an active role of vitreous pressure and the relaxed zonule hypotheses into a unified model for accommodation. His hypothesis is based upon the existence of a gradient of fluid or hydraulic pressure between the vitreous body, lens, and anterior chamber. Contraction of the ciliary muscle causes a decrease in the diameter of the circular component of this muscle and moves the vitreous base-zonule-lens diaphragm forward as the ora serrata and choroid move forward.[12,389,587] The anterior vitreous presses on the posterior lens, causing it to protrude forward into a more steeply curved lens-zonule diaphragm. The smaller diameter of the ciliary muscle ring sphincter opening would therefore result in an increase in axial lens distance and a decrease in the equatorial lens diameter. Ultrasound measurements of lens displacement during accommodation demonstrated that there was indeed a forward translational movement of the lens with forward movement of the anterior pole of the lens and axial elongation of the lens.[123] In support of these concepts are the studies of Koretz and Handelman,[340] who developed a mathematical model of the lens in which the various forces during accommodation are expressed in the form of equations. Solution of these equations indicated that the lens capsule acts as a force distributor, evenly spreading tension applied by the zonules over the surface of the lens. The authors concluded that the vitreous provides an essential "support" function during accommodation.

However, Fisher[183] described the case of a 32-year-old man who underwent unilateral vitrectomy for chronic vitreous hemorrhage and who had a "normal" fellow eye. In this patient there was no significant difference between the two eyes in terms of the range of accommodation and the movement of the anterior pole of the lens. Fisher concluded that the vitreous is not essential for either human accommodation or anterior displacement of the lens. He claimed that the differences in the degree of displacement of the anterior and posterior poles of the lens during accommodation result solely from inherent topographic differences in the elastic properties of the intact lens.[182] However, recent ultrasound studies[54] detected that the axial length of the vitreous decreased by 0.12 mm as the dioptric response to accommodative demand increased from 0.2 to 7 diopters. This decrease in vitreous axial length was felt to be due to posterior displacement of the posterior lens and capsule into the anterior vitreous. It would seem, therefore, that there may be a passive role for vitreous in accommodation insofar as the ability to compress the vitreous by 0.12 mm, as demonstrated by Beachamp and Mitchell,[54] could be influenced by the physicochemical properties of the vitreous. It may well be that presbyopia is in some way related not only to changes in the zonular apparatus and lens capsule elasticity but also the age-related changes in the physicochemical and structural properties of the vitreous. Further investigation will, it is hoped, resolve this controversy and elucidate whether aging changes in the vitreous play a role in the pathogenesis of presbyopia, the most common ocular affliction known to man.

Mechanical role of the vitreous

Balazs[38] has stated that optical clarity between the lens and retina would be best served by a waterlike fluid similar to aqueous humor. Thus the existence of structural elements within the vitreous suggests that there are other functions in addition to transparency of the ocular media. In a most simplistic perspective the turgescence of the vitreous prevents the globe from collapsing in the event of ocular perforation. The vitreous is probably also very important in protecting the internal structures of the eye during eye movement and physical activity.

Throughout the body there are two general types of connective tissue matrices. Cartilage, bone, tendon, and subcutaneous tissues provide mechanical support and therefore have significant structural rigidity and just enough elasticity to be able to withstand heavy mechanical stresses of low frequency. Vitreous, synovial fluid, and fasciae separate tissues and protect against friction and vibration. Thus these tissues are built less rigidly and, since they protect against high frequency stresses, they are viscoelastic.[38] In human, simian, bovine, and ovine vitreous the concentration of hyaluronic acid (HA) is high enough (greater than 100 μg/ml) to respond to mechanical stresses with a frequency above 0.4 cycles/sec as an elastic body rather than a viscous solution.[32,33,225] The HA component of the vitreous will further respond more as an elastic body as the frequency of stress increases.[42,225] This is not true of collagen, however, since under high-frequency stress, collagen (with more than 30% water) acts as a

viscous solution[115] and demonstrates very little elasticity.[562,636]

Bettleheim and Wang[66] performed compression measurement of bovine vitreous to determine the dynamic viscoelastic properties. The elastic and viscous components of the dynamic modules were similar to HA but not exactly the same as in a pure HA solution. The temperature-dependence was found to be similar to collagen gels. These investigators concluded that vitreous is a unique viscoelastic entity that cannot be described by the behavior of HA or collagen alone. Tokita et al.[574] came to essentially the same conclusion and suggested that the dynamic viscoelasticity of vitreous is not simply the result of a combination of HA and collagen but that the vitreous behaves like a lightly cross-linked gel of the HA and collagen networks. Weber et al.[608] compared the mechanical properties of pig and human vitreous. They found a 60% greater spring constant in the human vitreous and attributed this to the two-fold higher concentration of HA and collagen in the human vitreous as compared to the pig. These physical characteristics would therefore seem to be well-suited to a shock absorption function for the vitreous. Considering the rapidity of eye movements and the potential hazards to the retina and lens of eye movement and strenuous physical activity, the viscoelastic properties of the vitreous seem ideal protectors of these fragile tissues.

Zimmerman[644] has stated that the viscoelastic behavior of human vitreous has a topographic gradient that he interprets to be the result of the topographic variation in HA and collagen distribution. Both Balazs[38] and Swann[548] view the role of HA as a "stabilizer" of the collagen fibril network. Balazs[29,33] has shown that removal of HA by washing, electrophoresis, ionizing radiation ($<$ 10,000 rads), free radicals, and hyaluronidases results in a gel that is mechanically weaker but not destoyed. The efficiency of the stabilizing effect of HA increases with increasing molecular size and concentration of HA. Swann[548] states that the presence of HA in the vitreous probably stabilizes the distribution of structural proteins and contributes to homeostasis by decreasing the susceptibility of these proteins to disruption by mechanical insults. Balazs[38] further suggests that the role of HA as a stabilizer of the collagen fibril network may become important only when the local density of the collagen fibrils is so low that the distance between them becomes too large to maintain a stable network.

Such properties of the vitreous are likely to be

important as protection against blunt trauma. Little is known about the effects of blunt trauma on the vitreous, although these can be theoretically predicted on the basis of the known physical properties of vitreous viscoelasticity. Delori et al.[147] studied globe deformation and its relation to contusion injuries. Studies[13] of pressure transmission between the anterior chamber and the vitreous demonstrated that the lens-iris-zonule complex behaves like a diaphragm in that pressure is transmitted posteriorly in a linear fashion. However, traumatic disruption of this diaphragm would influence the distribution of shock waves incurred during anterior segment blunt trauma. Topographical variations in vitreous composition and structure would also alter transmission of shock waves posteriorly. Shock waves that are transmitted to the vitreous would theoretically undergo a "dissipation" interaction with the vitreous that has a friction constant that has been measured.[608] Which molecular component most influences this dissipating phenomenon is not known, although one might predict that the viscoelasticity of hyaluronic acid would be important in this regard.

Clinically, many cases of severe blunt trauma to the globe exhibit retinal edema and occasionally hemorrhages.[158] Although somewhat attenuated by the "shock-absorption" properties of the vitreous, the concussive forces of blunt trauma to the eye are largely transmitted to the retina via the vitreous. Whether passage of such shock waves through the vitreous alters the molecular structure and physiology of the vitreous itself is not known. Severe blunt trauma is at times associated with retinal dialysis (peripheral tear at the ora serrata) due to traction at the firmly attached vitreous base during "contre-coup" vitreous displacement. The dialysis can be either at the anterior or posterior borders of the vitreous base.[134] Other common types of retinal tears that result from blunt trauma and lead to retinal detachment are horseshoe-shaped tears at the posterior border of the vitreous base, the posterior end of a meridional fold, or at the equator. There can also be avulsion of the vitreous base or retinal detachment due to a macular hole. It has also been described that large retinal holes can be caused by postcompression, possibly ischemic, tissue necrosis.

The vitreous also plays an important mechanical role in the prevention and treatment of retinal detachment. Foulds[203] has divided retinal detachments into two categories: simple and complex. "Simple" retinal detachments have an intact, albeit detached, posterior vitreous cortex. Consequently, in a "simple" retinal detachment

volume-reducing operations (scleral buckling) or procedures utilizing internal tamponade of retinal breaks (pneumatic retinopexy) are successful because they utilize the intact vitreous cortex to close the retinal break and prevent fluid within the vitreous from entering the subretinal space. Indeed, such action by the vitreous cortex may explain why the overwhelming majority of retinal breaks do not result in retinal detachments. Additionally, the properties of the vitreous that inhibit cell migration and proliferation would ensure proper healing without complications such as proliferative vitreoretinopathy. In "complex" retinal detachments there are significant derangements in the structure and physiology of the vitreous such that the vitreous cortex is unable to adequately tamponade retinal breaks.[418] This disturbance of normal vitreous structure causes detachment of the retina to persist. In cases where postoperative complications develop, such as proliferative vitreoretinopathy, there is probably also a deficiency in the normal inhibitory activity of the vitreous, allowing pathologic cell migration and proliferation.

AGING OF THE VITREOUS
Substantial rheologic, biochemical, and structural alterations occur in the vitreous during aging.

Rheology
Rheology is a term that refers to the gel-liquid state of the vitreous. Using slit-lamp biomicroscopy in a clinical setting, Busacca[94] and Goldmann[234] observed that after the ages of 45 to 50 there is a decrease in the gel volume and an increase in the liquid volume of human vitreous. Eisner[161] qualitatively confirmed these findings in his postmortem studies of dissected human vitreous and observed that liquefaction begins in the central vitreous. In a large autopsy study of formalin-fixed human eyes, O'Malley[419] provided quantitative confirmation of these observations. He found that more than half of the vitreous was liquefied in 25% of individuals aged 40 to 49 and that this increased to 62% of individuals aged 80 to 89. Oksala[417] used ultrasonography in vivo to detect echoes from gel-liquid interfaces in 444 normal human eyes. He observed evidence of vitreous "degeneration" in 5% of individuals aged 21 to 40, in 19% of those aged 41 to 50, in 63% aged 51 to 60 and in greater than 80% of individuals over the age of 60. The vitreous was acoustically homogeneous in all individuals younger than 20 and in 10% of those older than 60.

Zimmerman[644] has evaluated the rheologic state of human vitreous by studying vitreous motion in vivo. Using head movement to displace the vitreous, he found that vitreous motion is overdamped with a settling time of 2 seconds and an overshoot of 25 to 50%. Buschbaum et al.[96] have derived a mathematical model for vitreous motion whose predictions fit well with Zimmerman's findings.

Vitreous liquefaction actually begins much earlier than the ages at which clinical examination or ultrasonography detect changes. Balazs and Flood[39,41] found evidence of liquid vitreous after the age of 4 and observed that by the time the human eye reaches its adult size (ages 14 to 18) approximately 20% of the total vitreous volume consists of liquid vitreous (Fig. 9-18). In these postmortem studies of fresh, unfixed human eyes it was observed that after the age of 40 there is a steady increase in liquid vitreous, which occurs simultaneously with a decrease in gel volume. By the ages of 80 to 90 years more than half the vitreous is liquid. The central vitreous is the region noted to undergo liquefaction first, as determined clinically and in postmortem studies.[161] The finding[497,504,505] that the central vitreous is where fibers are first observed is consistent with the concept that dissolution of the HA-collagen complex results in the simultaneous formation of liquid vitreous and aggregation of collagen fibrils into bundles of parallel fibrils seen as large fibers[504,505] (see Figs. 9-7, 9-8, and 9-11,A). In the posterior vitreous such age-related changes often form large pockets of liquid vitreous.[333]

Vitreous liquefaction does not occur in most mammals[150] and only a few, if any, fibers develop.[163,164] However, studies on rhesus monkeys[150] have demonstrated that in this species there exists an age-related process of liquefaction similar to that in man. Interestingly, there were no differences in protein or HA concentration between the ages of 6 and 21 (human age equivalent of 68 years), and no change in the size of the HA molecule. In the owl monkey there is a gel to liquid transformation that occurs by the age of 2 (human age 8 to 10 years). In the baby owl monkey the vitreous has a gel structure and contains a network of collagen fibrils.[283] In the adult there is disappearance of collagen and a simultaneous transformation from a gel state to a viscous fluid that contains mostly high-molecular-weight HA.[108]

The mechanism of vitreous liquefaction is poorly understood. Gel vitreous can be liquefied in vitro by removing collagen via filtration[403] and centrifugation[212] or by enzymatic destruc-

tion of the collagen network.[436] While it is unlikely that such phenomena are at play in vivo, the importance of collagen in the maintenance of the gel state of the vitreous can be deduced from the aforementioned biochemical findings in the owl monkey.[108] This was also recently demonstrated in studies employing NMR spectroscopy.[1] In these experiments performed with bovine vitreous collagenase injection induced a decrease in macroscopic viscosity and a shortening of longitudinal and transverse relaxation times on NMR spectroscopy. The drop in viscosity was proportional to the shortening of relaxation times for collagenase-treated eyes, more so than hyaluronidase-treated eyes. This suggests that the transition from gel to liquid vitreous is in some way related to the disappearance or displacement of collagen from the collagen-HA double network, resulting in a drop in viscosity and liquefaction as detected by NMR spectroscopy. This is consistent with the structural changes noted during development and

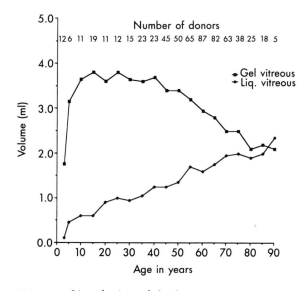

FIG. 9-18 Liquefaction of the human vitreous. The volumes of gel and liquid vitreous in 610 fresh, unfixed human eyes were measured postmortem. The results are plotted versus the age of the donor. Liquid vitreous appears by the age of 5 and increases throughout life until it constitutes more than 50% of the volume of the vitreous during the tenth decade. Gel vitreous volume increases during the first decade while the eye is growing in size. The volume of gel vitreous then remains stable until about the age of 40, when it begins to decrease in parallel with the increase in liquid vitreous. (Recreated with permission from Balazs EA, Denlinger JL: Aging changes in the vitreous, in Aging and human visual function, New York, Alan R Liss, 1982, pp 45–57.)

aging. Kammei and Totani[314] have suggested that liquefaction may be the result of changes in the minor glycosaminoglycans of the vitreous. In their studies on the rabbit vitreous liquefaction was associated with the disappearance of lower-charged chondroitin sulfate and the appearance of a higher-charged chondroitin sulfate. Heparan sulfate was also noted to disappear. However, these findings may be due to the means by which vitreous liquefaction was achieved (naphthalene), which is clearly not a physiologic process.

As mentioned earlier, age-related rheologic changes in the vitreous may result from an alteration in HA-collagen interaction. Chakrabarti and Park[109] claimed that the interaction between collagen and HA is dependent upon the conformational state of each macromolecule and that a change in the conformation of HA molecules could result in vitreous liquefaction and aggregation or cross-linking of collagen molecules. Armand and Chakrabarti[16] have detected differences in the structure of the HA molecules present in gel vitreous and those in liquid vitreous, suggesting that such conformational changes occurred during liquefaction. Whether these changes are cause or effect is not known. However, Andley and Chapman[9] have demonstrated that singlet oxygen can induce conformational changes in the tertiary structure of HA molecules. Ueno et al.[582] have suggested that free radicals generated by metabolic and photosensitized reactions could alter HA and collagen structure and trigger a dissociation of collagen and HA molecules, ultimately leading to liquefaction. This is plausible, since the cumulative effects of a lifetime of daily exposure to light may influence the structure and interaction of collagen and HA molecules by the proposed free radical mechanism(s). The importance of vitreous liquefaction in the pathogenesis of posterior vitreous detachment is discussed below.

Biochemistry

Total vitreous collagen content does not change after the ages of 20 to 30[39,41] (see Fig. 9-14). However, in studies of a large series of normal human eyes obtained at autopsy Flood and Balazs[41] found that the collagen concentration in the gel vitreous at the ages of 70 to 90 (approximately 0.1 mg/ml) was greater than at the ages of 15 to 20 (approximately 0.05 mg/ml; $p < 0.05$) (see Fig. 9-14). Since the total collagen content does not change, this finding is most likely due to the decrease in the volume of gel vitreous that occurs with aging, and a consequent increase in the concentration of the col-

lagen remaining in the gel. The collagen fibrils in this gel become packed into bundles of parallel fibrils[504,505] (Fig. 9-9,A), perhaps with cross-links between them.

Aging of collagen throughout the body is associated with increased cross-linking as manifested by decreased solubility,[489] increased collagen "stiffness",[339] and increased resistance to enzymatic degradation.[252] There is also an increase in a reducible lysine-carbohydrate condensation product with increasing age.[469] Although similar investigations have not been performed on vitreous collagen, studies by Snowden et al.[527] demonstrated that with aging there is a decrease in the quantity of bovine vitreous collagen solubilized by heat alone. This could result from an increase in collagen cross-linking, or, as suggested by the authors, from changes in the surrounding glycoproteins and proteoglycans. Abnormal collagen cross-links have been identified in human diabetic vitreous,[508] and the findings were consistent with "precocious senescence" of vitreous collagen that has been described for other organs and tissue in diabetes.[85,400,471,490]

Vitreous hyaluronic acid (HA) concentration increases until about the age of 20, when adult levels are attained[39,41] (see Fig. 9-15). Hyaluronic acid concentration does not change in either the liquid or gel vitreous from the ages of 20 to 70[33,39,41,62] (see Fig. 9-15). This necessarily means that there is an increase in the HA content of liquid vitreous and a concomitant decrease in the HA content of gel vitreous, since the amount of liquid vitreous increases and the amount of gel vitreous decreases with age (see Fig. 9-18). This is consistent with the concept that vitreous liquefaction is associated with a "redistribution" of HA molecules from the gel to the liquid vitreous.

Liquefaction has also been related to physicochemical changes in vitreous HA molecules. Studying postmorten samples of human vitreous, Armand and Chakrabarti[16] found subtle but definite differences in the chromatographic elution profiles and optical properties of HA molecules isolated from liquid as compared to gel vitreous. These investigators suggested that the conformational differences between HA molecules in gel and liquid vitreous are likely to be at least partly responsible for the gel-liquid transformation observed during aging.

Vitreous soluble protein concentrations also increase from 0.5 to 0.6 mg/ml at ages 13 to 50, to 0.7 to 0.9 mg/ml at ages 50 to 80, and 1.0 mg/ml above the age of 80.[33,39,41,62] This increase may result from an age-related breakdown in the blood-ocular barriers of the retinal vasculature, retinal pigment epithelium, and ciliary body epithelium.

Morphology

Aging is associated with substantial structural changes within the central vitreous. During perinatal development there is a transition from a dense, highly light-scattering structure to a transparent, homogeneous body. As described above, the redistribution of HA and collagen during maturation to the adult results in the aggregation of collagen fibrils into packed bundles of parallel fibrils that appear as fibers. During the latter decades of life the fine parallel fibers in the central vitreous become thickened and tortuous (Fig. 9-19,A). Immediately adjacent to these coarse structures are areas with little or no light-scattering properties that are filled with "liquid" vitreous. When advanced, this vitreous degeneration forms large pools of liquid vitreous identified clinically as "lacunae" (Fig. 9-20). When the posterior vitreous detaches from the retina, there is an overall reduction in the size of the vitreous due to the collapse (syn-

eresis) of the vitreous that occurs when liquid vitreous enters the retrohyaloid space anterior to the retina (Fig. 9-20,B). This displacement of liquid vitreous occurs via the prepapillary "hole" and the premacular vitreous cortex (see Fig. 9-11) and is an important event in the pathogenesis of posterior vitreous detachment.

Basal laminae and vitreous base

The basal laminae surrounding the vitreous thicken with age,[216,459] a phenomenon that occurs in basal laminae throughout the body.[106,223] Hogan et al.[272] claimed that the thickening of the internal limiting lamina of the retina occurs after it is initially laid down, probably as a result of synthesis by the subjacent Müller cells. This phenomenon may play a role in weakening vitreoretinal adhesion, thus contributing to the development of posterior vitreous detachment.

Teng and Chi[568] found that the vitreous base posterior to the ora serrata varies in width depending upon the age of the individual. More than half of eyes from people older than 70 had a posterior vitreous base wider than 1.0 mm.

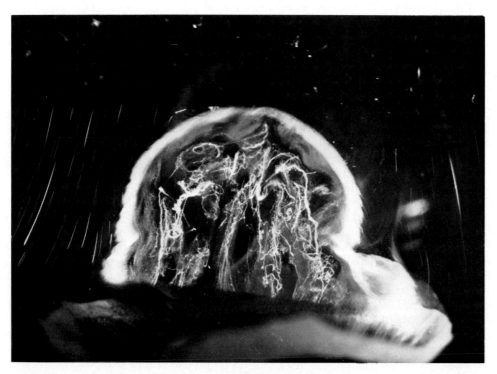

FIG. 9-19 Fibrous structure of human vitreous during old age. The vitreous of an 88-year-old woman demonstrates substantial degeneration in the fibrous structure. Fibers are thickened and tortuous. The entire inner vitreous appears to have undergone dissolution with empty spaces adjacent to the thickened fibers. (Reprinted with permission from Sebag J: Age-related changes in human vitreous structure, Graef Arch Clin Exp Ophthalmol 225:89, 1987.)

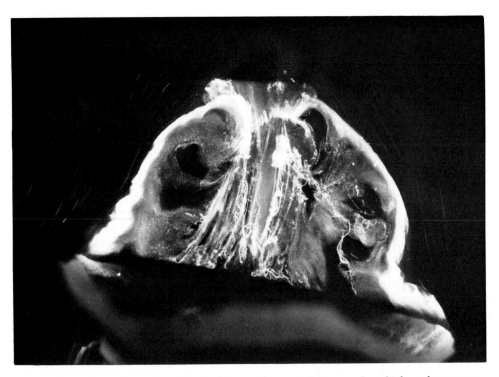

FIG. 9-20   Human vitreous lacunae in old age. The central vitreous has thickened, tortuous fibers. The peripheral vitreous has pockets devoid of any structure. These contain liquid vitreous and correspond to lacunae as seen clinically on biomicroscopy. (Reprinted with permission from Sebag J, Balazs EA: Human vitreous fibres and vitreoretinal disease, Trans Ophthalmol Soc UK 104:123, 1985.)

The width increased with increasing age to nearly 3.0 mm, bringing the posterior border of the vitreous base closer to the equator. This widening of the vitreous base was also found to be most prominent in the temporal portion of the globe. The posterior migration of the vitreous base probably plays an important role in the pathogenesis of peripheral retinal breaks and rhegmatogenous retinal detachment, since this is the area of strongest vitreoretinal adhesion. Gartner[218] found no differences in the thickness of collagen fibrils in the vitreous base when comparing five eyes from humans aged 9 months, 29, 39, 61, and 71 years. He did, however, note that there was "lateral aggregation" of the collagen fibrils in the eyes from older individuals. Such aggregation at the vitreous base is similar to aging changes within the vitreous where collagen fibril aggregation results in bundles of parallel collagen fibrils. These aging changes at the vitreous base could also contribute to increased traction on the peripheral retina and play a role in the development of retinal tears and detachment.

Peripheral traction, retinal tears, and detachment. Schepens[485] first described the clinical appearance of peripheral vitreoretinal traction as "white-without-pressure" when a geographic area of whiteness is present in the equatorial and peripheral retina. When this appearance is present only during scleral depression, it is termed "white-with-pressure." Subsequent reports[577] considered that these findings predisposed to peripheral retinal tears. Daicker[138] proposed that this appearance results from collagenous formations in the peripheral retina, while Gartner[214] suggested that they were due to irregularities of the internal limiting lamina. Green[240] described that the appearance of these lesions results from incident light (from the ophthalmoscope) that is tangential to dense bundles of vitreous collagen. All of these interpretations would be consistent with the concept that these areas are at greater risk of developing retinal tears as a result of an abnormal vitreoretinal interface in these locations. However, Byer[99] does not believe that this ophthalmoscopic appearance has any diagnostic or prognostic significance. Watzke[607] studied the clinicopathologic correlation of a case with this finding and indicated that the lesion was due to remnants of the vitreous cortex that remained attached to the retina following posterior vitreous detachment (PVD). Since the vitreous base is the site of strongest vitreoretinal adhesion, it is here, usually at the posterior border, that vitreoretinal traction causes peripheral retinal tears.

Green[240] has recently reviewed all clinical and postmortem studies on the prevalence of peripheral retinal tears. Clinical studies found that the prevalence ranged from 0.59 to 7.2%, while autopsy studies showed a prevalence from 3.3 to 8.8%. Other studies have focused upon the relationship between PVD and peripheral retinal tears. Autopsy studies[188] found that retinal breaks are present in 14.3% of all eyes with PVD. Clinical studies[304,363,412,564] found retinal tears in 8 to 15% of eyes with acute PVD. Lindner[363] and Jaffe[304] found that these retinal tears occurred in the superior fundus in over 94% of cases. In the presence of high myopia (greater than −6 diopters) PVD is associated with peripheral retinal breaks in 11.1%.[286] In high myopes who underwent uncomplicated cataract extraction (presumably by intracapsular techniques) the prevalence of retinal breaks following PVD was as high as 16.2%.[287] It is surprising that the prevalence of retinal tears in high myopes is not greater than reported, particularly in those patients who underwent cataract extraction. Further studies may be needed to confirm these observations. If, however, this finding is correct, it may point out that peripheral retinal traction and retinal tears result from changes within the vitreous that occur in the presence of irregularities at the vitreoretinal interface. Thus, although there may be a higher incidence of liquefaction and PVD in myopia, the vitreoretinal interface may not be similarly abnormal, and consequently peripheral retinal traction does not result in a significantly higher incidence of retinal tears than that observed in these patients. However, once a retinal tear develops in a myopic eye it may be more likely to produce a retinal detachment because of the biochemical and rheologic abnormalities in the myopic vitreous that cause advanced liquefaction.

Various conditions of the peripheral retina are associated with increased vitreoretinal traction. In *lattice degeneration* there are discrete oval areas of retinal thinning associated with localized vitreous liquefaction, separation of the overlying vitreous, and increased vitreoretinal adhesion at the margins of the degenerated areas.[484] Retinal breaks are found at these margins and posterior to the areas of lattice degeneration. However, retinal tears resulting from

vitreous traction are relatively infrequent as compared to atrophic retinal holes. Clinical studies[98] found retinal tears in only 1% of eyes with lattice degeneration, while 16.3%[98] and 18.2%[476] of lattice lesions had atrophic retinal holes. The risk of retinal tears is greater when the area of lattice degeneration is located juxtabasal or extrabasal relative to the vitreous base.[190,514] The retinal tears are believed to result from aggregated vitreous fibrils inducing traction upon the retina.[540] Obliterative fibrosis of the blood vessels in areas of lattice degeneration is present in only 11.9% of lesions[98] and is seen as a "lattice-wicker" of white lines, for which the condition is named. The presence of this vascular anomaly has led to the hypothesis that retinal circulatory abnormalities are the primary cause of this condition.[481] According to this theory, the vitreous changes are secondary and only important in the subsequent development of retinal tears as a local phenomenon. Overall liquefaction of the vitreous[195] and PVD[194] may not be important contributing factors in this local traction,[195] but may be important in the subsequent development of retinal detachment.[100] Nevertheless, clinical retinal detachments only developed in 3 of 276 (1.1%) patients in Byer's original study population and he has recently stated that prophylactic treatment of lattice degeneration is not indicated in phakic eyes where there is no history of retinal detachment in the fellow eye.[101]

The incidence of retinal detachment varies between 9 per 100,000 per year[409] and 24.4 per 100,000 per year.[75] In a study of the natural history of retinal detachment Davis[141] found that 31 out of 166 (18%) eyes with retinal tears progressed to develop retinal detachments. This author identified aphakia, the presence of subclinical retinal detachment, and symptomatic horseshoe-shaped retinal tears as important risk factors. In a study of 100 patients with bilateral surgical aphakia (presumably intracapsular) and rhegmatogenous retinal detachment in one eye Hovland[276] found that 26% eventually developed peripheral tears and retinal detachments in the fellow eye. In this study the absence of PVD in the fellow eye at the time of retinal detachment in the first eye was the poorest prognostic sign for the fellow eye. Indeed, Bradford et al.[77a] found that in those rhegmatogenous retinal detachments that developed within 6 months after cataract surgery, about half were due to moderately sized, posteriorly located horseshoe tears. As this is not the typical profile of an "aphakic" retinal detachment Wilkinson hypothesized that these retinal tears occurred at the time of PVD and were due to anomalous vitreoretinal adhesions. Since this appearance is no different from phakic rhegmatogenous retinal detachments, cataract surgery was probably not an important factor in these cases, although it may have precipitated the PVD as a result of biochemical changes within the vitreous.[427,428]

The relationship of a retinal tear to the vitreous base is an important prognostic feature that determines the risk of a peripheral retinal tear resulting in a retinal detachment.[514] Juxtabasal tears are the most dangerous due to the degree of peripheral vitreous traction associated with these retinal tears. Thus there are certain types of peripheral retinal tears and clinical circumstances that are predisposed to develop retinal detachments. Eyes with retinal breaks that occur at the time of symptomatic PVD are generally considered good candidates for prophylactic treatment.[97] Some authors[124] consider that prophylactic treatment of retinal tears that have persistent vitreous traction significantly reduces the risk of retinal detachment. How to best evaluate the presence or absence of vitreous attachment and how to quantitate the degree of vitreous traction is presently not known.

Vitreous liquefaction and PVD seem to be important factors in the development of peripheral traction and retinal tears. O'Malley[419] found that in 23 eyes with peripheral breaks, all had more syneresis than age-matched controls and 21 of 23 (91%) had extensive PVD. Indeed, Machemer and Norton[373] found that in order to create and maintain experimental retinal detachment in the monkey it was necessary to use hyaluronidase to degrade vitreous hyaluronic acid and alter the gel state of the vitreous. The presence of liquid vitreous and a detached posterior vitreous cortex places the eye at risk of developing a peripheral retinal tear.

Lindner[364] was among the first to point out the importance of eye movements in the pathogenesis of retinal tears and detachment. Rosengren and Osterlin[472] provided experimental evidence in support of this concept. Following PVD, the retrohyaloid space is occupied by liquid vitreous. During eye movements, liquid vitreous, which is lighter than gel, is set in motion before gel vitreous. Because all eye movements are rotational, the liquid vitreous acts as a wedge in the retrohyaloid space, further separating detached vitreous cortex from retina. Where the vitreous is firmly attached to the retina (at the vitreous base as well as at pathologic sites) traction will be exerted by the force of the liquid vitreous moving in the retrohyaloid space and

pressing against the vitreous cortex. Furthermore, when an ocular saccade stops, it is usually sudden. This causes the heavier gel vitreous to continue moving due to inertia. It is believed that substantial traction is thus placed upon sites of firm vitreoretinal adhesion, resulting in peripheral tears of the retina.[486]

Detachment of the entire vitreous base can occur following blunt trauma and results in detachment of both the ciliary epithelium anterior to the ora serrata and the retina posterior to the ora serrata.[158] Spontaneous detachment of the vitreous base can occur in high myopia, Marfan's syndrome, and Ehlers-Danlos syndrome.[577]

In penetrating trauma involving the vitreous, fibers composed of collagen fibrils are often incarcerated in the wound and radiate to the vitreous base. In animal model studies[120] fibroblasts grew into the vitreous from the stroma of the ciliary body and formed membranes along the course of the vitreous fibers. These cellular membranes probably contribute to the development of PVD at 1 to 2 weeks after injury and retinal detachment at 7 to 11 weeks. Cleary and Ryan[120] believed that blood was an important factor in stimulating the cell proliferation and traction at the vitreous base that caused the retinal detachments. This is supported by the finding that blood in the vitreous has chemotactic properties.[346]

In senile retinoschisis there is a split in the outer nuclear layer of the neural retina. Studies[76] have shown that in 85% of cases of senile retinoschisis there is PVD but that the vitreous cortex remains attached to the inner layer of the schisis cavity, a variant of "vitreoschisis."[35] Schepens[486] states that liquefaction and PVD are frequent findings in senile retinoschisis and that a prominent fibrous structure in the gel adjacent to the schisis cavity may be responsible for peripheral retinal traction, thus contributing to schisis formation.

Posterior vitreous detachment

The most common age-related event in the vitreous is posterior vitreous detachment (PVD). True PVD can be defined as a separation between the posterior vitreous cortex and the internal limiting lamina (ILL) of the retina, as demonstrated by histopathologic study.[188,270] PVD can be localized, partial, or total (up to the posterior border of the vitreous base). PVD should be distinguished from other forms of vitreoretinal separation that clinically may be mistaken for PVD. One of these forms involves separation of the ILL and some of the inner retina along with the detached posterior vitreous cortex. Separation of the ILL from the neural retinal can follow severe tractional events in the young, where the posterior vitreous cortex-ILL adhesion is strong.[33,500b] Juvenile sex-linked retinoschisis is a bilateral condition that features splitting of the retina at the level of the nerve fiber layer in the macula and sometimes the inferotemporal quadrant. In 50% of cases there is no peripheral schisis cavity.[219] The macular schisis cavity does not progress if the overlying vitreous is detached and is progressive in areas of persistent vitreous attachment.[577] This suggests that vitreous traction may contribute to the pathogenesis of this disorder. Schepens[486] has described the presence of a membrane between the retina and posterior vitreous. Whether this is composed of the vitreous cortex, the internal limiting lamina of the retina, or parts of both is not known. Yanoff et al.[637] have studied the histopathology of this condition and have postulated that the causative defect may lie in the Müller cell. This is consistent with Schepens's hypothesis that a localized failure of development of the secondary vitreous enables the schisis cavity to form, since Müller cells are at least partly responsible for vitreous formation.

Kloti[335] has shown that experimental embolization of the central retinal artery can cause total PVD. However, in some of these experiments occlusion of the central retinal artery was not complete. In these eyes Kloti found a distinct membranous layer adherent to the detached posterior vitreous, which he identified as the ILL of the retina. He concluded that partial embolization in these eyes resulted in Müller cell ischemia and dysfunction that was not sufficiently severe to cause dissolution of the ILL/cortical vitreous adhesion. However, the central portion of the Müller cell was damaged and the inner segments were torn away with the ILL that was attached to the posterior vitreous cortex. In experiments with completely occluded central retinal arteries Kloti found that Müller cell infarction caused dissolution of the ILL-cortical vitreous adhesion, resulting in true PVD. This suggests that Mueller cell metabolism is at least partly responsible for vitreoretinal adhesion at the ILL/vitreous cortex interface. This adhesion is strong at the macula and can result in traction upon the retina.

Another form of vitreoretinal separation that can mimic true PVD features forward displacement of the anterior portion of the posterior vitreous cortex, leaving part of the posterior layer of the vitreous cortex still attached to the retina. Balazs[35] has coined the term "vitreoschisis" to denote prominent liquefaction with cavitation in the posterior vitreous but persistent attachment of the outermost layers of the posterior vitreous cortex to the ILL. Clinically, this is often mistaken as true PVD and occurs in cases of advanced liquefaction without PVD, such as advanced axial myopia. The skilled examiner can distinguish this from PVD, since true PVD displays a characteristic ascension/descension movement of the posterior vitreous cortex on vertical saccades. However, in the absence of an actual split in the vitreous cortex this does not constitute vitreoschisis. True vitreoschisis may or may not have a large lacuna in the posterior vitreous, since splitting of the vitreous cortex can occur in the absence of advanced liquefaction. Green[241] has recently reported that splitting of the posterior cortical vitreous may be present in eyes with proliferative diabetic retinopathy and vitreous hemorrhage. It is possible that in these cases vitreoschisis cavities in the posterior vitreous cortex result from dissection of blood as suggested by Green. However, a split in the vitreous cortex can also *cause* bleeding, since neovascular complexes grow into the vitreous cortex.[176] The inner wall of the vitreoschisis cavity may be clinically and echographically confused with a PVD if the posterior layer of the split vitreous cortex remains attached to the ILL. Kishi et al.[332] have reported that PVD was associated with vitreous cortex remnants at the fovea in 26 of 59 (44%) human eyes studied at autopsy with scanning electron microscopy. The presence of sheets of cortical vitreous remnants at the macula following PVD could be important in the pathogenesis of premacular membranes, particularly if there are hyalocytes in the vitreous cortex remnants.

Lindner[363] and Jaffe[304] have described that in some cases of PVD there is herniation of vitreous through the vitreous cortex of the posterior pole (Fig. 9-21). Gartner[215] has drawn an analogy between this phenomenon and the herniation of the nucleus pulposus in the intervertebral discs (of the spine). In a study of 20 emmetropic patients between the ages of 21 and 54 with nucleus pulposus herniation of the intervertebral disc Gartner found evidence of presenile vitreous degeneration in 8 (40%). He proposed that a generalized connective tissue disorder resulted in disc herniation and presenile vitreous degeneration in these cases. When a PVD involves herniation of the vitreous into the retrovitreal space via the premacular and prepapillary vitreous cortex, there can be persistent attachment to the macula and traction. Other important examples of generalized con-

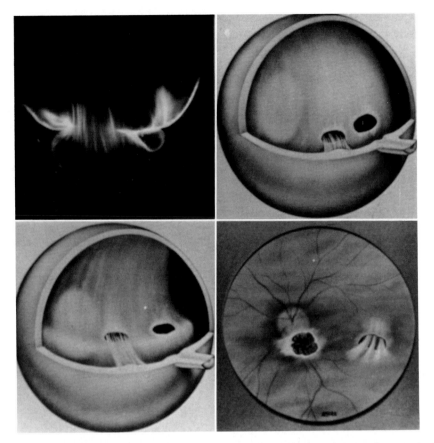

FIG. 9-21 Vitreomacular traction. Vitreous can remain attached to the macula even in the presence of posterior vitreous detachment. In such cases vitreous can extrude through the premacular vitreous cortex and fibers can insert into the macula. The diagrams in the upper right, lower left, and lower right are an artist's rendition of this phenomenon. The upper left-hand corner photograph demonstrates actual vitreous extrusion into the retrohyaloid space in a postmortem human specimen (Fig. 9-7,D). (Upper right and lower left photographs reprinted with permission from Jaffe NS: The vitreous in clinical ophthalmology, St Louis, CV Mosby, 1969. Lower right photograph reprinted with permission from Jaffe NS: Vitreous traction at the posterior pole of the fundus due to alterations in the posterior vitreous, Trans Am Acad Ophthalmol Otolaryngol 71:642, 1967.)

nective tissue disorders with vitreous degeneration can be found in patients with joint disease. Maumenee[385] has identified several different disorders with single gene autosomal dominant inheritance where dysplastic connective tissue primarily involves joint cartilage. In these conditions there is associated vitreous liquefaction, collagen condensation, and vitreous syneresis (collapse). Since type II collagen is common to both cartilage and vitreous, Maumenee[385] suggested that the various arthro-ophthalmopathies result from different mutations, perhaps of the same or neighboring genes, on the chromosome involved with type II collagen metabolism. In these disorders the fundamental prob-

lem in the posterior segment of the eye is that the vitreous is liquefied and unstable, tending to syneresis at an early age. However, there is no dehiscence at the vitreoretinal interface in concert with the changes inside the vitreous. Recall that the internal limiting lamina of the retina is composed of type IV collagen and the vitreoretinal interface may therefore not be affected in such cases. Thus, in these cases abnormal type II collagen metabolism causes destabilization of the vitreous and results in traction on the retina that can lead to large posterior tears and retinal detachments that are difficult to repair. The most common disorders of connective tissue metabolism with prominent vitreous changes are Marfan's syndrome,[486] Ehlers-Danlos syndrome,[486] Stickler syndrome,[530,536] and other variants.[336]

Epidemiology of PVD

In clinical studies the incidence of apparent PVD has been reported to be 53% in people older than 50 and 65% over the age of 65.[363,437] Autopsy studies revealed an incidence of 27 to 51% in the seventh decade and 63% in the eighth decade.[188,195] It is not certain, however, that these figures are not overestimates due to the methods employed in these postmortem studies. PVD is more common in myopes, occurring 10 years earlier than in emmetropes and hyperopes.[304,363] This likely results from effects of myopia upon the structure of the vitreous. Cataract extraction in myopes introduces additional effects.[188,427,428] In one study[287] PVD was present in all but one of 103 myopic (greater than −6 diopters) eyes that had undergone cataract extraction (presumably intracapsular).

Several studies[195,412] have found a higher incidence of PVD in women than men, a finding that may be due to hormonal changes following menopause. This hypothesis is supported by findings that glycosaminoglycans (GAG) synthesis can be influenced by a variety of hormones.[524,525] There is also evidence that sex hormones in particular can affect GAG metabolism. In studies[360] on the bovine abdominal aorta, GAG content was highest when blood concentrations of estrogen were maximal during the sexual cycle. Sirek et al.[517] showed that pituitary ablation in dogs decreased hyaluronic acid (HA) content in the aortic arch and thoracic aorta, while subsequent estrogen administration raised HA concentration to twice the normal levels. In the rabbit vitreous Larsen[347] found variations in the concentration of HA following hormonal treatment. It is interesting to note that Larsson and Osterlin[349] found that vitreous HA concentration in men (120.89 ± 75.44 μg/ml) was significantly greater than in women (79.53 ± 48.17 μg/ml; p < 0.01). This may be related to low estrogen levels in postmenopausal women and may thus explain why PVD is more common in women than men. Furthermore, all these lines of evidence support the concept that insufficient or abnormal HA destabilizes the gel state of the vitreous, contributing to liquefaction and PVD.

Pathogenesis of PVD

True PVD results from rheologic changes within the vitreous that lead to synchisis (liquefaction), in conjunction with weakening of the vitreous cortex-ILL adhesion. Spencer[530] has stated that aging as well as numerous pathologic processes cause a depolymerization of hyaluronic acid and dissolution of the collagen network. The combination of these two molecular phenomena results in synchisis. Once "liquid" vitreous forms and the collagen network is destabilized, owing to a loss of the stabilizing effect of hyaluronic acid (HA) molecules upon the collagen network, collapse (syneresis) of the vitreous body can occur. Two possible mechanisms for syneresis have been proposed: Shortening and condensation of vitreous fibrils could contract the vitreous body and pull the posterior vitreous forward.[341] More likely, however, is the hypothesis that dissolution of the posterior vitreous cortex-ILL adhesion at the posterior pole allows liquid vitreous to enter the retrocortical space via the prepapillary hole and premacular vitreous cortex.[160,363,497,498] With rotational eye movements, the liquid vitreous can dissect a plane between the vitreous cortex and the ILL, leading to true PVD. This volume displacement from the central vitreous to the preretinal space causes the observed collapse of the vitreous body (syneresis).

The latter mechanism is supported by the observations of Foos,[188] Foos and Gloor,[192] and Foos and Wheeler[195] that PVD begins at the macula. Vitreoretinal dehiscence at the macula may result from a predisposition or an increased stimulus for vitreous degeneration in the premacular region. It is here that studies[333] have identified a large pocket of liquid vitreous related to aging. Foos and Wheeler[195] proposed that preferential liquefaction in the posterior pole results from light toxicity to the premacular vitreous, since this is where the eye focuses incident light. There can also be a contribution of toxicity caused by metabolic waste products resulting from the high density of metabolically active neurons in the macula. Both light irradiation and metabolic processes can generate free radicals, which could alter HA or collagen structure and disrupt the collagen-HA association, causing liquefaction.[582]

O'Malley[419] suggested that PVD was strongly correlated with synchisis, since both are correlated with age, although PVD had a later onset than synchisis. Foos and Wheeler[195] studied 4492 autopsy eyes and found a statistically significant correlation between the degree of synchisis and the incidence of PVD. Larsson and Osterlin[349] studied 61 human eyes postmortem and correlated the degree of vitreous liquefaction with the extent of PVD. In eyes with no PVD about 10% of the vitreous was liquid; with partial PVD 23% of the vitreous was liquefied. These studies also showed that the concentration of hyaluronic acid (HA) in eyes with no PVD (131.88 ± 70.72 µg/ml) was significantly higher than those with total PVD (82 ± 66.5 µg/ml; p < 0.04). It is not clear whether this was an effect of PVD or part of the cause. Balazs[30] has induced synchisis experimentally by precipitating HA, binding HA molecules with metallic ions, or depolymerizing HA with free radicals and hyaluronidase. The same effects occur with almost all forms of high-energy radiation.[63] Other studies[62,426] have demonstrated that lacunae (pockets of liquid vitreous) contain no collagen. Morphologic studies[497] have documented that in old age there is aggregation of collagen fibrils into bundles and fibers, and segregation of hyaluronic acid into lacunae (see Figs. 9-19 and 9-20), which ultimately form large pockets of liquid vitreous.[333]

The concept that arises from all these observations and findings is that PVD results from concurrent changes within the vitreous and at the vitreoretinal interface. Whether due to age-related changes in collagen structure, HA configuration or concentration, light-induced or metabolically derived free radicals, hormonal effects, or combinations of all these factors, there is a disruption of the normal collagen-HA association, transforming the gel vitreous to liquid. Dissolution of the ILL-vitreous cortex adhesion at the posterior pole allows this liquid vitreous to dissect a retrohyaloid plane, resulting in collapse of the vitreous body. Further studies on the nature of HA-collagen interactions and the forces underlying posterior vitreous cortex-ILL adhesion should help to further identify the changes that result in PVD. Elucidating these mechanisms may enable the development of techniques by which liquefaction and PVD could be induced or prevented, depending upon the clinical circumstances.

Sequelae of PVD

In youth the vitreous is normally quite clear and has little or no effect upon glare sensitivity.[624] In old age the aggregation of vitreous collagen fibrils into thick, irregular, visible fibers (see Fig. 9-19) can induce glare sensitivity, which may be subjectively bothersome. Furthermore, the high incidence of posterior vitreous detachment in old age may also induce glare due to scattering of light by the dense collagen fibril network in the posterior vitreous cortex. One group of individuals in whom discomfort glare is a common complaint are patients who have undergone scleral buckle surgery for rhegmatogenous retinal detachment. The complaint of glare appears to be due to postoperative vitreous turbidity and not a change in the threshold sensitivity of retinal receptors.[144] Since vitreous biochemical and structural changes predispose these patients to rhegmatogenous retinal detachment, prominent vitreous fibers are probably already present preoperatively. Scleral buckle surgery adds to the preexisting vitreous turbidity by breaking down the normal vitreous barriers and mechanisms that maintain vitreous clarity. This involves inducing temporary dysfunction of the blood-ocular barriers and causing a resultant influx of serum proteins and other macromolecules as well as creating an inflammatory response and resultant influx of cellular elements.

"Floaters" are probably the most common complaint of patients with PVD. These usually result from entopic phenomena caused by condensed vitreous fibers, glial tissue of epipapillary origin that adheres to the posterior vitreous cortex, intravitreal blood, or both.[118,404,530] Floaters move with vitreous displacement during eye movement and scatter incident light, casting a shadow on the retina that is perceived as a gray, "hairlike" structure.[643] In an autopsy series of 320 cases with complete PVD, 57% had glial tissue on the posterior vitreous cortex.[193] Vogt's or Weiss's ring are the terms applied when peripapillary tissue is torn away during PVD and forms a ring around the prepapillary hole in the posterior vitreous cortex (see Fig. 9-11,B). Murakami et al.[407] studied 148 cases of floaters and detected glial tissue on the posterior vitreous cortex in 83%. They claimed that patients complaining of multiple small floaters usually have minimal vitreous hemorrhage, frequently associated with retinal tears. Lindner[363] found that minimal vitreous hemorrhage occurred in 13 to 19% of cases with PVD.

Light flashes are sometimes a complaint resulting from PVD.[404] These are generally thought to result from vitreoretinal traction and are considered by most to signify a higher risk of retinal tears. Voerhoeff[595] suggested that the light flashes are actually due to the detached vitreous cortex impacting upon the retina during eye movement. Wise[621] has noted that light flashes occurred in 50% of cases at the time of PVD and were generally vertical and temporally located.

It is of interest to consider the physiologic effects of PVD. Transvitreal flow from the posterior pole to the anterior segment may be altered by PVD, as suggested by studies of vitreous fluorophotometry.[440] How this influences lens metabolism and cataractogenesis, particularly posterior subcapsular cataracts, is open to conjecture. Flow in an antero-posterior direction may also be affected. As described above, the posterior flow of aqueous is believed to play a role in retinal adhesion. Alterations in posterior flow could be induced by vitreous liquefaction and PVD and could thus contribute to a decrease in retinal adhesion, perhaps predisposing to retinal detachment. Derangements in posterior flow of aqueous could also be involved in chronic open-angle glaucoma, especially in aphakes.[510] Abnormal transvitreal flow of aqueous has been proposed as part of the pathophysiology in malignant glaucoma.[110,168,510]

Hyalocyte metabolism may also be affected after true PVD, since these cells would be situated farther from their source of oxygen and nutrients.[479] A consequent alteration in hyaluronic (HA) acid metabolism by hyalocytes might explain Larsson and Osterlin's[349] finding of a significant reduction in HA concentration in eyes with PVD. The progression from partial PVD to total PVD is a rapid event, which probably results from the entry of liquid vitreous into the retrohyaloid space and the inertial forces generated during eye movement.[486]

Once PVD occurs there are differences in the characteristics of the detached vitreous that influence, for example, vitreous movement following displacement by ocular excursions. Differences in the "stiffness" of the detached vitreous have been identified using ultrasonic Doppler techniques.[627] These probably relate to the biochemical composition and organization of the vitreous and are likely to change with time, depending upon the effects of vitreous detachment on retinal and vitreous metabolisms.

During posterior vitreous detachment (PVD), traction on retinal blood vessels can cause retinal and vitreous hemorrhage. Retinal hemorrhages resulting from PVD are most often located along the vitreous base,[118,412] although peripapillary[118] and macular[482] hemorrhages have also been reported. These locations correspond to those areas known to have strong vitreoretinal adhesions. The anatomic causes of increased vitreoretinal adhesion over retinal blood vessels have been described above. Histopathologic studies in humans[529] have shown the presence of paravascular retinal rarefaction, which was hypothesized to be associated with abnormal vitreous attachments. Foos[191] noted a thinning of the internal limiting lamina of the retina over blood vessels and hypothesized that this results in breaks through which vitreous fibers attach or glial cells migrate to form small epiretinal membranes, resulting in abnormal

vitreoretinal adhesions. Furthermore, the absence of the stabilizing influence of Müller cell processes in these regions may make the retinal blood vessels more susceptible to the effects of vitreous traction.

The effects of mechanical traction upon tissue orientation during growth and repair have long been recognized as important in the phenomenon of bone remodeling. Among vitreoretinal pathobiologists, there has been conjecture as to whether the vitreous can have similar effects upon adjacent tissues to which it is attached. Recent studies[634] found that placing traction upon the chick chorioallantoic membrane caused an increase in the growth of mesodermal vessels and an orientation along the lines of the tractional forces. Considering the evidence that in proliferative diabetic retinopathy new blood vessels grow onto and into the vitreous cortex,[140,176,275] traction by the vitreous might induce further proliferation of these new blood vessels as well as vitreous hemorrhage. Indeed, Wong et al.[628] found "abortive neovascular outgrowths" in more than a third of cases undergoing vitrectomy for vitreous hemorrhage secondary to proliferative diabetic retinopathy. These investigators noted the absence of cortical vitreous in these locations and suggested that the benign nature of these new vessels was due to the absence of a scaffold for vessel growth and the lack of vitreous traction, which could induce hemorrhage. Furthermore, Sebag et al.[506b] studied the relationship of PVD to panretinal laser photocoagulation (PRP) and found a significantly higher incidence of PVD in treated patients as compared to controls. These investigators suggested that part of the therapeutic effect of PRP may thus be the induction of PVD, which would render any subsequent neovascularization "abortive."

Lindner[363] found that vitreous hemorrhage was present in 13 to 19% of cases with PVD. Jaffe[304] noted that in the presence of vitreous hemorrhage, PVD was associated with retinal breaks in 69% of cases. Other clinical studies[317,564] have found that two thirds of cases with PVD and retinal tears had vitreous hemorrhage. Spencer and Foos[529] claimed that the strong vitreoretinal adhesion over blood vessels accounted for the presence of paravascular retinal tears in 11% of 252 eyes studied at autopsy. In eyes with PVD 29% had full-thickness paravascular tears and 46% had full or partial thickness tears. These partial-thickness tears, referred to as "retinal pits," consist of discrete areas in the paravascular retina where the inner retinal layers are avulsed as a result of traction during PVD.[240] Spencer and Foos[529] found retinal pits in association with both retinal arteries and veins. It is also quite common for large horseshoe- or arrowhead-shaped tears of the retina to have bridging blood vessels across the anterior and posterior edges of the tear.[486]

Several authors[112,468,569] have described a syndrome of recurrent vitreous hemorrhage that is due to avulsion of retinal vessels with persistent attachment of the intact vessel to an operculum overlying a retinal break. Theodossiadis et al.[570] proposed that the recurrent bleeding was related to the mobility and size of the vessel overlying the retinal break. These authors also described six different patterns of avulsed vessels.[569] Lincoff et al.[362] treated nine cases of avulsed vessels and noted that six were associated with retinal veins and three with arteries. There were retinal breaks in six cases and retinal detachments in five of these cases. There have, however, been case reports of retinal vessel avulsion without associated full-thickness retinal tears.[263,569,586]

Vitreomacular traction. Traction on the central retina could play a role in several vitreomacular disorders. Vitreous traction at the macula has been implicated as contributing to the development of aphakic cystoid macular edema.[289,484,487,498,503] The high prevalence of an attached posterior vitreous in youth is believed to contribute to the high incidence of cystoid macular edema in peripheral anterior vitritis.[266] Jaffe[303] and Maumenee[384] have reported a vitreomacular traction syndrome in phakic patients that results in macular edema, which does not have a petalloid pattern on fluorescein angiography. Jaffe[303] described some cases with PVD in which there is persistent attachment of vitreous to the macula with visible vitreous strands that traverse the retrohyaloid space and insert into the macula (see Fig. 9-21). He further indicated that in many cases symptoms disappear and vision returns when the posterior vitreous completely detaches. Smiddy et al.[519] found that all patients with this vitreomacular traction syndrome had incomplete PVD with persistent attachment to the macula. The most common form was vitreous attachment to the disc and to the macula in an area 1 to 2 disc diameters in size surrounding the fovea. These findings confirm the original observations and concepts of Schepens, Jaffe and others, depicted in Figure 9-21. Furthermore, Smiddy et al.[519] found cystic changes in the macula of 12 of 16 cases, supporting the aforementioned hypothesis that vitreous traction can cause or at least contribute to the formation of cystoid macular edema. These authors also reported favorable results following vitrectomy for macular traction. Other cases of vitreous-induced macular dysfunction result from contraction of the premacular cortical vitreous causing a cellophane-like appearance of the internal limiting lamina, tortuosity of blood vessels, and thickening of the retina, although no fluorescein leakage is present.

Macular holes. There has recently been considerable discussion as to the role of vitreous traction in macular hole formation, the nature of such traction, and whether prophylactic or therapeutic surgery is indicated. It is important to realize that although clinically many cases may appear the same, there can be several different forms of macular hole, each with a different pathogenesis. Consequently, no single therapeutic approach will be effective in all cases.

In the formation of spontaneous macular holes, sometimes called senile or idiopathic, there can be different forms of vitreous traction at the posterior pole: localized antero-posterior traction at the fovea with or without posterior vitreous detachment (PVD) and tangential traction due either to contraction of the posterior vitreous cortex or a premacular membrane. In approximately 25% of cases there is an operculum lying immediately in front of the macular hole and no PVD.[219] In these cases vitreous traction is localized at the fovea due either to "tangential" contraction of the prefoveal vitreous cortex[306] or sagittal traction transmitted to this site by intravitreal fibers.[498,504] In the latter case vitreous fibers are often seen attached to an operculum after the macular hole is formed.[21,379]

Gass believes that "tangential" prefoveal vitreous traction is the primary cause of spontaneous macular holes.[219,306] Initially, this traction causes a retinal detachment localized to the fovea with radiating retinal folds (Gass's stage 1). At this stage there is greater visibility of xanthophyll pigment accounting for the central yellow spot or ring. Several weeks later a single or several minute holes develop near the center of the fovea (Gass's stage 2). These holes continue to enlarge in a "can-opener" fashion over the ensuing weeks and months until an operculated full-thickness hole develops (Gass's stage 3). If a PVD occurs, this operculum can be found attached to the posterior vitreous cortex in the mid-vitreous (Gass's stage 4). In 10% of cases a PVD occurs before stage 2 develops and patients will experience a spontaneous improvement in symptoms, similar to what has been observed in certain cases of macular epiretinal membranes.

Morgan and Schatz,[402] however, believe that

PVD can actually contribute to the pathogenesis of macular holes. They propose that deficient choroidal blood flow and ischemia to the retinal pigment epithelium and fovea are the first steps in spontaneous macular hole formation. Cystic changes subsequently develop in response to this ischemia (step 2). The development of atrophic changes in the fovea (step 3) then results in "involutional macular thinning." In step 4 PVD is believed to pull upon this susceptible, thinned fovea, causing a macular hole. To support this hypothesis the authors cite the finding that in their study 10 of 12 eyes (83%) with involutional macular thinning that developed PVD experienced a full-thickness macular hole. This was also noted by McDonnel et al.[390] who found that 11 of 22 eyes (50%) with macular cysts developed a macular hole following PVD. The results reported by Frangieh et al.[209] support the concept of a role for PVD in the development of macular holes. In their series of 35 cases with lamellar or full-thickness holes partial or complete PVD was present in all 35 of the eyes. Vitreous fibers were found inserting to the macula or onto a detached operculum in 8 out of 35 eyes (22.8%). Margherio and Schepens[379] found evidence of vitreous traction in 36 out of 56 eyes (64.2%) with macular holes.

It is likely that macular holes represent the end stage manifestation of more than one pathophysiologic sequence. The group of macular hole disorders can be divided (Table 9-5) on the basis of the presence or absence of an operculum, a PVD[2] and a premacular membrane.[248,518] In this context a PVD is strictly defined as clean separation between the posterior vitreous cortex and the internal limiting lamina (ILL) of the retina. A premacular membrane (PMM) can be retinal glial cell migration and proliferation, or the posterior portion of the vitreous cortex with hyalocytes left attached to the macula at the time of vitreous collapse during PVD ("vitreoschisis"). When the vitreous is attached but undergoing syneresis, localized antero-posterior traction can be exerted at the central macula by large fibers located in the central liquefied vitreous.[500] Thus even in the absence of PVD an operculated hole can result from sagittal intravitreal fibers that exert isolated antero-posterior traction localized to the central macula (type "O" macular hole—Table 9-1). Previous studies[219] have shown that in approximately 25% of cases of macular hole there is an operculum lying immediately in front of the macular hole and no PVD. Other studies found vitreous fibers inserting to the macula,[306,519] or onto a detached operculum.[21,379]

Contraction of the vitreous cortex, as Gass described, could induce tractional forces on the central macula that are either inward ("centripetal," i.e., toward the fovea) and forward (into the vitreous) or outward ("centrifugal," i.e., away from the fovea) and forward. The former would elevate the central macula and tear an operculum whose center would be the fovea. Thus, during PVD centripetal (toward the fovea) traction on the perifoveal retina can create an operculated macular hole by what Gass[219,306] described as a "can-opener" process (type "OP" macular hole—Table 9-5). Furthermore, this could occur in the presence of a premacular membrane (type "OM" macular hole, Table 9-5) or be due to centripetal (toward the fovea) contraction of an attached posterior vitreous cortex. Such mechanisms are most likely at work in those cases of operculated macular holes described by Akiba et al.[2] to have an attached vitreous. Indeed these authors found that in 73% of cases with established macular hole and 94% of so-called "early" macular holes there was no biomicroscopic evidence of PVD. In the presence of established PVD, a premacular membrane with centripetal contractile forces could also produce an operculated macular hole, although in the absence of forward (into the vitreous) movement of the membrane a true operculum may not be observed (type "OPM" macular hole—Table 9-5).

Centrifugal (outward) forces would elevate the central macula, pulling the retina away from the center of the macula and thereby open a rent in the foveola that widens with further elevation of the central macula. This can occur following pseudo-PVD with vitreoschisis or can result from incomplete (extramacular) PVD with persistent attachment at the macula (type "P" macular hole—Table 9-5). It is also conceivable that a premacular membrane that grows following true PVD can induce such centrifugal forces and create a non-operculated macular hole (type "M" macular hole—Table 9-5). Since retinal tissue is not torn away from this site (as in operculated holes), surgery to relieve this "centrifugal" outward traction could allow the macula to reattach and the central hole to decrease in size, although it is not likely to disappear completely on a microscopic level. The same can occur following spontaneous completion of incomplete PVD, relieving traction on the macula and allowing reattachment and reapposition of the perifoveal retina.

It should be emphasized that this classification system is based primarily upon theoretical considerations of pathogenesis. Since clinical examination cannot presently accurately ascertain the presence or absence of PVD and the di-

TABLE 9-5 Types of Macular Holes and Their Possible Mechanism of Formation

Type	Operculated	PVD	PMM	Mechanism/contents
O	+	−	−	Intravitreal fibers with traction on central macula cause operculated hole, without PVD.
OM	+	−	+	Premacular membrane or attached vitreous cortex with tangential traction forces directed inward toward the fovea ("centripetal") tearing a hole about the fovea.
OP	+	+	−	During true PVD abnormal vitreomacular adhesion about the fovea tears a hole with an operculum attached to the premacular vitreous cortex.
OPM	+	+	+	*Three possible mechanisms:* (a) Same as type OP, but PMM grew after PVD and is unrelated. (b) PVD occurred innocuously but PMM grew after PVD and tore a hole in perifoveal macula due to "centripetal" (toward the fovea) forces inducing inward contraction of the PMM. (c) PVD splits vitreous cortex ("vitreoschisis"). Outer layer of vitreous cortex exerts centripetal tangential traction, tearing an operculated hole. PMM is actually the outer layer of vitreoschisis cavity with hyalocytes ("hypocellular" PMM[119]).
P	−	+	−	*Two possible mechanisms:* (a) PVD not true but splits vitreous cortex leaving posterior layer attached to macula ("vitreoschisis"). Outward (away from the fovea) traction induces "centrifugal" forces opening a hole in the central macula which widens with domelike elevation of central macula. [Surgery effective] (b) PVD not complete but remains attached to macula (Fig. 9-21) and exerts antero-posterior traction, elevating a dome in the central macula, opening a hole centrally. [Surgery effective]
M	−	−	+	PMM grows in absence of PVD, causing "centripetal" (outward, away from the fovea) traction opening a hole in the central macula. [Surgery effective]

PVD = Posterior vitreous detachment
PMM = Premacular membrane
  O = operculated hole
 OM = operculated hole with PMM
 OP = operculated hole with PVD

OPM = operculated hole with PVD and PMM
  P = Non-operculated hole with PVD
  M = Non-operculated hole with PMM
  + = present
  − = absent

rection of tangential traction (centripetal versus centrifugal), there may be limitations in clinical utility. It is, nevertheless, valuable to consider these pathogenic mechanisms when selecting cases for surgery and delineating a surgical approach.

REFERENCES

1. Aguayo J, Glaser B, Mildvan A, et al: Study of vitreous liquefaction by NMR spectroscopy and imaging, Invest Ophthalmol Vis Sci 26:692, 1985.
2. Akiba J, Quiroz MA, Trempe CL: Role of posterior vitreous detachment in idiopathic macular holes, Ophthalmol 97:1610, 1990.
3. Akiya S, Uemura Y, Azuma N: Morphological study on the human developing vitreous collagen fibrils and persistent hyperplastic primary vitreous, Ophthalm Res 17:60, 1985.
4. Akiya S, Uemura Y, Saga U: Morphological study on glycosaminoglycans in the developing human vitreous, Ophthalm Res 16:145, 1984.
5. Akiya S, Uemura Y, Tsuchiya S, et al: Electron microscopic study of the developing human vitreous collagen fibrils, Ophthalm Res 18:199, 1986.
6. Ali S, Bettelheim FA: Distribution of freezable and non-freezable water in bovine vitreous, Curr Eye Res 3:1233, 1984.

7. Allen WS, Otterbein EC, Wardi AH: Isolation and characterization of the sulfated glycosaminoglycans of the vitreous body, Biochem Biophys Acta 498:167, 1977.

8. Anderson DR: Ultrastructure of the optic nerve head, Arch Ophthalmol 83:63, 1970.

9. Andley UP, Chapman SF: Effect of oxidation on the conformation of hyaluronic acid, Invest Ophthalmol Vis Sci 25(ARVO):318, 1984.

10. Andrews JS, Lynn C, Scobey JW, et al: Cholesterolosis bulbi: case report with modern chemical identification of the ubiquitous crystals, Br J Ophthalmol 57:838, 1973.

11. Appiah AP, Hirose T, Kado M: A review of 324 cases of idiopathic premacular gliosis, Am J Ophthalmol 106:533, 1988.

12. Araki M, Tokoro T, Matsuo C: Movement of the ciliary body associated to accommodation, Acta Ophthalmol Jpn 68:1852, 1964.

13. Arciniegas A, Amaya LE: Interaction between anterior and vitreous chambers, Ophthalmologica 179:119, 1979.

14. Arciniegas A, Amaya LE, Ruiz LA: Myopia—a bioengineering approach, Ann Ophthalmol 12:805, 1980.

15. Armand G, Balazs EA: Physical and chemical characterization of icthyosin-polysaccharides of fish eyes, Proc Intl Soc Eye Res 1:68, 1980.

16. Armand G, Chakrabarti B: Conformational differences between hyaluronates of gel and liquid human vitreous—fractionation and circular dichroism studies, Curr Eye Res 6:445, 1987.

17. Asakura A: Histochemistry of hyaluronic acid of the bovine vitreous body as studied by electron microscopy, Acta Soc Ophthalmol Jpn 89:179, 1985.

18. Atkins EDT, Phelps CF, Sheehan JK: The conformation of the mucopolysaccharides—hyaluronates, Biochem J 128:1255, 1972.

19. Atkins EDT, Sheehan JK: Structure for hyaluronic acid, Nature (New Biol) 235:253, 1972.

20. Auricchio G, Ambrosio A: Sul compartamento della riserva alcabina dei liquidi endoculari in condizioni normali e pathologiche, Bull Soc Ital Biol Sper 20:1172, 1953.

21. Avila MP, Jalkh AE, Murakami K, et al: Biomicroscopic study of the vitreous in macular breaks, Ophthalmol 90:1277, 1983.

22. Awan KJ, Thumayan M: Changes in the contralateral eye in uncomplicated persistent hyperplastic primary vitreous, Am J Ophthalmol 99:122, 1985.

23. Ayad S, Weiss JB: A new look at vitreous humour collagen, Biochem J 218:835, 1984.

24. Azuma N, Hida T, et al: Histochemical studies on hyaluronic acid in the developing human retina, Graefe Arch Clin Exp Ophthalmol 228:158, 1990.

25. Baker JR, Caterson B: The isolation of "link proteins" from bovine nasal cartilage, Biochem Biophys Acta 532:249, 1978.

26. Balazs EA: Structure of vitreous gel, Acta XVII Concilium Ophthalmologicum 11:1019, 1954.

27. Balazs EA: Studies on structure of vitreous body: absorption of ultraviolet light, Am J Ophthalmol 38:21, 1954.

28. Balazs EA: Acta XVIII Concilium Ophthalmologicum. 12:1296, 1958.

29. Balazs EA: Physiology of the vitreous body in retina surgery with special emphasis on reoperations, in Schepens CL, ed: Proceedings of the 11th Conference of the Retina Foundation, St Louis, CV Mosby, 1960, pp 29-48.

30. Balazs EA: Molecular morphology of the vitreous body, in Smelser GK, ed: The structure of the eye, New York, Academic Press, 1961, pp 293-310.

31. Balazs EA: Amino sugar-containing macromolecules in the tissues of the eye and the cap, in Balazs EA, Jeanloz RW, eds: The amino sugars—the chemistry and biology of compounds containing amino sugars, II, A, Distribution and biologic role, New York and London, Academic Press, 1965, pp 401-460.

32. Balazs EA: Sediment volume and viscoelastic behavior of hyaluronic acid solutions, Fed Proc 25:1817, 1966.

33. Balazs EA: Die Mikrostruktur und Chimie des Glaskörpers, in Jaeger W, ed: Bericht uber die 68 Zusammen Kunst der Deutschen Ophthalmologischen Gesellschaft, Heidelberg 1967, Munich, JF Bergmann Verlag, 1968, pp 536-572.

34. Balazs EA: The molecular biology of the vitreous, in McPherson A, ed: New and controversial aspects of retinal detachment, New York, Harper & Row, 1968, pp 3-15.

35. Balazs EA: The vitreous, in Zinn K, ed: Ocular fine structure for the clinician, Intl Ophthalmol Clin 13:169, 1973.

36. Balazs EA: Fine structure of developing vitreous, in Zinn K, ed: Ocular fine structure for the clinician, Int Ophth Clin 15:53, 1975.

37. Balazs EA: Functional anatomy of the vitreous, in Duane TD, Jaeger EA, eds: Biomedical foundations of ophthalmology, Philadelphia, Harper & Row, 1982, vol 1, ch 17, pp 6-12.

38. Balazs EA: The vitreous, in Davson H, ed: The eye, vol 1a, London, Academic Press, 1984, pp 533-589.

39. Balazs EA, Denlinger JL: Aging changes in the vitreous, in: Aging and human visual function, New York, Alan R. Liss, 1982, pp 45-57.

40. Balazs EA, Denlinger JL: The vitreous, in Davson H, ed: The eye, London, Academic Press, 1984, vol 1a, pp 533-589.

41. Balazs EA, Flood MT: Age-related changes in the physical and chemical structure of human vitreous, Third Intl Congress for Eye Research, Osaka, Japan, 1978.

42. Balazs EA, Gibbs DA: The rheological properties and biological function of hyaluronic acid, in Balazs EA, ed: Chemistry and Molecular Biology of the Intercellular Matrix, New York, Academic Press, 1970, pp 1241-1254.

43. Balazs EA, Laurent TC, Laurent UBG: Studies on the structure of the vitreous body, VI, Biochemical changes during development, J Biol Chem 234:422, 1959.

44. Balazs EA, Laurent TC, Laurent UBG, et al: Studies on the structure of the vitreous body, VIII, Comparative biochemistry, Arch Biochem Biophys 81:464, 1959.

45. Balazs EA, Sundblad L: Studies on the structure of the vitreous body, V, Soluble protein content, J Biol Chem 235:1973, 1960.

46. Balazs EA, Sundblad L, Toth LZJ: In vitro formation of hyaluronic acid by cells in the vitreous body and by comb tissue, Abstr Fed Proc 17:184, 1958.

47. Balazs EA, Toth LZ, Eckl EA, et al: Studies on the structure of the vitreous body, XII, Cytological and histochemical studies on the cortical tissue layer, Exp Eye Res 3:57, 1964.

48. Balazs EA, Toth LZ, Ozanics V: Cytological studies on the developing vitreous as related to the hyaloid vessel system, Graef Arch Clin Exp Ophthalmol 213:71, 1980.

49. Bard LA: Asteroid hyalitis—relationship to diabetes and hypercholesterolemia, Am J Ophthalmol 58:239, 1964.

50. Barraquer J: Totale Linsenextraktion nach aulosung der Zonula durch Chymotrypsin enzymatische Zonulyse, Klin Mbl Augenheilk 133:609, 1958.

51. Baurmann M: Untersuchungen ueber die Struktur des Glaskörpers bei Säugetieren, Alb v Graef Archiv f Ophthalmol 110:352, 1922.

52. Baurmann M: Über die Beziehungen der ultramikroscopischen Glaskörperstrucktur zu den Spaltlampenbefunden, Graef Archiv f Ophthalmol, 1926 (as cited by Redslob[454]).

53. Bay M: Water movement in the vitreous body evaluated experimentally and theoretically, Acta Pharmacol et Toxicol 34:174, 1974.

54. Beauchamp R, Mitchell B: Ultrasound measures of vitreous chamber depth during ocular accommodation, Am J Optom Physiol 62:523, 1985.

55. Beebe DC, Latker CH, Jebers HAH, et al: Transport and steady-state concentration of plasma proteins in the vitreous humor of the chicken embryo—implications for the mechanism of eye growth during early development, Dev Biol 114:361, 1986.

56. Bellhorn MB, Friedman AH, Wise GN, et al: Ultrastructure and clinicopathologic correlation of idiopathic preretinal macular fibrosis, Am J Ophthalmol 79:366, 1975.

57. Bembridge BA, Crawford CNC, Pirie A: Phase-contrast microscopy of the animal vitreous body, Br J Ophthalmol 36:131, 1952.

58. Benson AH: Diseases of the vitreous: a case of "monocular asteroid hyalitis," Trans Ophthalmol Soc UK 14:101, 1894.

59. Benson W, Spalter H: Vitreous hemorrhage: a review of experimental and clinical investigations, Surv Ophthalmol 15:297, 1971.

60. Berman ER: Studies on mucopolysaccharides in ocular tissues, I, Distribution and localization of various molecular species of hyaluronic acid in the bovine vitreous body, Exp Eye Res 2:1, 1963.

61. Berman ER, Gombos GM: Studies on the incorporation of U-14 C-glucose into vitreous polymers *in vitro* and *in vivo*, Invest Ophthalmol 18:521, 1969.

62. Berman ER, Michaelson IC: The chemical composition of the human vitreous body as related to age and myopia, Exp Eye Res 3:9, 1964.

63. Berman ER, Voaden M: The vitreous body, in Graymore CN, ed: Biochemistry of the eye, New York, Academic Press, 1970, pp 373-471.

64. Bettelheim FA, Balazs EA: Light scattering patterns of the vitreous humor, Biochim Biophys Acta 158:309, 1968.

65. Bettelheim FA, Christian S, Lee LK: Differential scanning calorimetric measurements on human lenses, Curr Eye Res 2:803, 1983.

66. Bettelheim FA, Wang TJY: Dynamic viscoelastic properties of bovine vitreous, Exp Eye Res 23:435, 1976.

67. Birk DE, Zycbard EI: Collagen fibrillogensis in situ: Fibril segments are intermediates in matrix assembly, Proc Natl Acad Sci USA 86:4549, 1989.

68. Bito LZ, Davson H: Steady state concentration of potassium in ocular fluids, Exp Eye Res 3:283, 1964.

69. Bleckmann H: Glycosaminoglycan metabolism of cultured fibroblasts from bovine vitreous, Graef Arch Clin Exp Ophthalmol 222:90, 1984.

70. Blix: Studier ofver glaskroppen, Medicinsk Archiv 14:1868.

71. Bloom GD, Balazs EA: An electron microscope study of hyalocytes, Exp Eye Res 4:249, 1965.

72. Bloom GD, Balazs EA, Ozanics V: The fine structure of the hyaloid arteriole in bovine vitreous, Exp Eye Res 31:129, 1980.

73. Boettner EA, Wolter JK: Transmission of the ocular media, Invest Ophthalmol 13:776, 1962.

74. Boeve MH, Stades FC: Glaucom big hond on Kat, Overzicht en retrospective evaluatie van 421 patienten, I, Patho biologische achtergronden, indehing en raspredispositie, Tijdschr Diergeneeskd 110:219, 1985.

75. Böhringer HR: Statistiches zur Häufigkeit und Riskio der Netzhautablösung, Ophthalmologica 131:331, 1956.

76. Boisdequin D, Croughs P, Regnier P, et al: Vitre et retinoschisis, Bull Soc Belge Ophthalmol 192:75, 1981.

77. Bowman: Observations on the structure of the vitreous humour, Dublin Quatr J Med Sci VI:102, 1848.

77a. Bradford JD, Wilkinson CP, Fransen SR: Pseudophakic retinal detachments—the relationships between retinal tears and the time following cataract surgery at which they occur, Retina 9:181, 1989.

78. Brandt HP, Leedhoff H: Biomicroscopie des Glaskorpers bei kindlicher myopie, Klin Monatsbl Augenheilkd 156:340, 1970.

79. Breen M, Bizzell JW, Weinstein MG: A galactosamine-containing proteoglycan in human vitreous, Exp Eye Res 24:409, 1977.

80. Bremer FM: Histochemical study on glycosaminoglycans in the developing mouse vitreous, Histochemistry 87:579, 1987.

81. Brewerton EW: Cysts in the vitreous, Trans Ophthalmol Soc UK 33:93, 1913.

82. Brownstein MH, Elliot R, Helwig EG: Ophthalmologic aspects of amyloidosis, Am J Ophthalmol 69:423, 1970.

83. Brubaker RF, Riley FC Jr: Vitreous body volume reduction in the rabbit, Arch Ophthalmol 87:438, 1972.

84. Brucke: Über den innern Bau des Glaskörpers, Archiv f Anat Physiol und Wissensch Med (Müller), 1843 (as cited by Redslob[454]).

85. Buckingham B, Perejda AJ, Sandborg C, et al: Skin, joint, and pulmonary changes in type I diabetes mellitus, Am J Dis Child 140:420, 1986.

86. Bullock JD: Developmental vitreous cysts, Arch Ophthalmol 91:83, 1974.

87. Burke J: An analysis of rabbit vitreous collagen, Conn Tiss Res 8:49, 1980.

88. Burke JM: Vitreal superoxide and superoxide dismutase after hemorrhagic injury: the role of invasive cells, Invest Ophthalmol Vis Sci 20:435, 1981.

89. Burke JM, Kower HS: Collagen synthesis by rabbit neural retina *in vitro* and *in vivo*, Exp Eye Res 31:213, 1980.

90. Burke JM, Sipos E, Cross HE: Cell proliferation in response to vitreous hemoglobin, Invest Ophthalmol Vis Sci 20:575, 1981.

91. Burke JM, Twining S: Vitreous macrophage elicitation-generation of stimulants for pigment epithelium in vitro, Invest Ophthalmol Vis Sci 28:1100, 1987.

92. Burns JJ: Overview of ascorbic acid metabolism, Am NY Acad Sci 258:5, 1975.

93. Busacca A: Observations biomicroscopiques sur le corps ciliaire normal et pathologique, Bull Soc Fr Ophtalmol 68:295, 1955.

94. Busacca A: La structure biomicroscopique du corps vitré normal, Ann D'Ocullist 91:477, 1958.

95. Busacca A, Goldmann H, Schiff-Wertheimer S: Biomicroscopie due corps vitré et du fond d'oeil, Paris, Masson, 1957.

96. Buschbaum G, Sternklar M, Litt M, et al: Dynamics of an oscillating viscoelastic sphere—a model of the vitreous humor of the eye, Biorheology 21:285, 1984.

97. Byer NE: Clinical study of retinal breaks, Trans Am Acad Ophthalmol Otolaryngol 71:461, 1967.

98. Byer NE: Lattice degeneration of the retina, Surv Ophthalmol 23:213, 1979.

99. Byer NE: The peripheral retina in profile, a stereoscopic atlas, Torrance, CA, Criterion Press, 1982.

100. Byer NE: Discussion of "Vitreous in lattice degeneration of retina," Ophthalmol 91:457, 1984.

101. Byer NE: Long-term natural history of lattice degeneration of the retina, Ophthalmol 96:1396, 1989.

102. Campochiaro PA, Gaskin HC, Vinores SA: Retinal cryopexy stimulates traction retinal detachment in the presence of an ocular wound, Arch Ophthalmol 105:1567, 1987.

103. Campochiaro PA, Glaser BM: Platelet-derived growth factor is chemotactic for human retinal pigment epithelial cells, Arch Ophthalmol 103:576, 1985.

104. Campochiaro PA, Jerdan JA, Glaser BM et al: Vitreous aspirates from patients with proliferative vitreoretinopathy stimulate retinal pigment epithelial cell migration, Arch Ophthalmol 103:1403, 1985.

105. Caterson B, Baker J: Interaction of link proteins with proteoglycan monomers in the absence of hyaluronic acid, Biochem Bioph Res Comm 80:496, 1978.

106. Caulfield JB: Medical progress in the application of the electron microscope to renal disease, N Engl J Med 270:183, 1964.

107. Chaine G, Shebag J, Coscas G: The induction of retinal detachment, Trans Ophthalmol Soc UK 103:480, 1983.

108. Chakrabarti B, Hultsch E: Owl monkey vitreous—a novel model for hyaluronic acid structural studies, Biochem Biophys Res Commun 71:1189, 1976.

109. Chakrabarti B, Park JW: Glycosaminoglycans: structure and interaction, CRC Crit Rev Biochem 8:255, 1980.

110. Chandler PA: Malignant glaucoma, Am J Ophthalmol 34:993, 1951.

111. Chatterjee IV: Evolution and the biosynthesis of ascorbic acid, Science 182:1271, 1974.

112. Chatzoulis D, Theodossiadis GP, Apostolopoulos M,

et al: Rezidivierende Glaskörperblutüngen infolge eines in die Glaskörperhohle hereingezogenen Netzhautgefalles, Klin Monatsbl Augenheilkd 183:256, 1983.

113. Chen CH, Chen SC: Studies on soluble proteins of vitreous in experimental animals, Exp Eye Res 32:381, 1981.

114. Chess J, Sebag J, et al: Pathologic processing of vitrectomy specimens, Ophthalmol 90:1560, 1983.

115. Chien JC, Chang EP: Dynamic mechanical and rheo-optical studies of collagen and gelatin, Biopolymers II:2015, 1972.

116. Christiansson J: Changes in mucopolysaccharides during alloxan diabetes in the rabbit, Acta Ophthalmol 36:141, 1958.

117. Chylack LT, Kinoshita JH: The interaction of the lens and the vitreous, I, The high glucose cataract in a lens-vitreous preparation, Exp Eye Res 14:58, 1972.

118. Cibis GE, Watzke RC, Chua J: Retinal hemorrhages: posterior vitreous detachment, Am J Ophthalmol 79:358, 1975.

119. Clarkson JG, Green WR, Massof D: A histopathologic review of 168 cases of preretinal membranes, Am J Ophthalmol 84:1, 1977.

120. Cleary PE, Ryan SJ: Histology of wound, vitreous and retina in experimental posterior penetrating eye injury in the rhesus monkey, Am J Ophthalmol 88:221, 1979.

121. Cockburn DM: Are vitreous asteroid bodies associated with diabetes mellitus? Am J Optom Physiol Opt 62:40, 1985.

122. Cohen AI: Electron microscopic observations of the internal limiting membrane and optic fiber layer of the retina of the rhesus monkey, Am J Anat 108, 1961.

123. Coleman DJ: Unified model for accommodative mechanism, Am J Ophthalmol 69:1063, 1970.

124. Combs JL, Welch RB: Retinal breaks without detachment—natural history, management, and long-term follow up, Trans Am Ophthalmol Soc 80:64, 1982.

125. Comper WD, Laurent TC: Physiological functions of connective tissue polysaccharides, Physiol Rev 58:255, 1978.

126. Constable IJ, Swann DA: Biological vitreous substitutes, inflammatory response in normal and altered animal eyes, Arch Ophthalmol 88:544, 1972.

127. Constable IJ, Tolentino FI, Donovan RH, et al: Clinico-pathologic correlation of vitreous membranes, in Pruett RC, Regan CDJ, eds: Retina Congress, New York, Appleton-Century Crofts, 1974, p 245.

128. Cooper WC, Holbert SP, Manski WJ: Immunochemical analysis of vitreous and subretinal fluid, Invest Ophthalmol 2:369, 1963.

129. Coull BM, Cutler RWP: Light-evoked release of endogenous glycine into the perfused vitreous in the intact rat eye, Invest Ophthalmol 17:682, 1978.

130. Coull BM, Owens DK, Cutler RWP: The release of endogenous amino acids into the vitreous of the intact eye of the albino rat; effect of light, potassium and ouabain, Brain Res 210:301, 1981.

131. Coulombe AJ: The role of introcular pressure in the development of the chicken eye, J Exp Zool 133:211, 1956.

132. Coulombre AJ, Steinberg SN, Coulombre JL: The role of intraocular pressure in the development of the chick

eye, V, Pigmented epithelium, Invest Ophthalmol 2:83, 1963.

133. Reference deleted in proofs.

134. Cox MS, Schepens CL, Freeman HM: Retinal detachment due to ocular contusion, Arch Ophthalmol 76:678, 1966.

135. Crawford JB: Cotton wool exudates in systemic amyloidosis, Arch Ophthalmol 78:214, 1967.

136. Criswell MH, Goss DA: Myopia development in nonhuman primates—a literature review, Am J Optom Physiol Optics 60:250, 1983.

137. Curtin BJ: The myopias—basic science and clinical management, Philadelphia, Harper & Row, 1985.

138. Daicker B: Sind die Symptome "Weiss Mit Druck" und weiss ohne Druck durch die Periphere Netzhautsklerose bedingt, Mod Probl Ophthalmol 15:82090, 1975.

139. Darzynkiewicz Z, Balazs EA: Effect of hyaluronic acid on lymphocyte stimulation, Exp Eye Res 66:113, 1971.

140. Davis M: Vitreous contraction in proliferative diabetic retinopathy, Arch Ophthalmol 75:741, 1965.

141. Davis MD: Natural history of retinal breaks without detachment, Arch Ophthalmol, 92:183, 1974.

142. Davson H: Physiology of the ocular and cerebrospinal fluids, Boston, Little, Brown, 1956.

143. Davson H, Luck CD: A comparative study of the total carbon dioxide in the ocular fluids, cerebrospinal fluid and plasma of some mammalian species, J Physiol (Lond) 132:454, 1956.

144. Deiter P, Wolf E, Geer S: Glare and the scatter of light in the vitreous—effect in postoperative retinal detachment patients, Arch Ophthalmol 87:12, 1972.

145. De Juan E, Dickson J, Hatchell DL: Interaction of retinal glial cells with collagen matrices—implications for pathogenesis of cell-mediated vitreous traction, Graef Arch Clin Exp Ophthalmol 227:494, 1989.

146. Delaney WV: Prepapillary hemorrhage and persistent hyaloid artery, Am J Ophthalmol 90:419, 1980.

147. Delori FC, Pomerantzeff O, Cox MS: Deformation of the globe under high-speed impact—its relation to contusion injuries, Invest Ophthalmol 8:290, 1969.

148. Delpech B, Halavent C: Characterization and purification from human brain of a hyaluronic acid-binding glycoprotein, hyaluronectin, J Neurochem 36:855, 1981.

149. Demours: Observations anatomiques sur la structure cellulaire du coprs vitre, Memoires de Paris, 1741 (as cited by Redslob[454]).

150. Denlinger JL, Eisner G, Balazs EA: Age-related changes in the vitreous and lens of rhesus monkeys (macaca mulatta), Exp Eye Res 31:67, 1980.

151. DeRosa L: Il Fosfaro del Vitreo nel corso della degenerazione pigmentaria esperimentale al iodato da sodio, Rass Ital Ottamol 24:114, 1955.

152. DiMattio J: A comparative study of ascorbic acid entry into aqueous and vitreous humors of the rat and guinea pig, Invest Ophthalmol Vis Sci 30:2320, 1989.

153. Disalvo J, Schubert M: Interaction during fibril formation of soluble collagen with cartilage protein polysaccharides, Biopolymers 4:247, 1966.

154. Doft BH, Rubinow A, Cohen AS: Immunocytochemical demonstration of prealbumin in the vitreous in heredofamilial amyloidosis, Am J Ophthalmol 97:296, 1984.

155. Doft BH, Weiskopf J, Nilsson-Ehle I, et al: Amphotericin clearance in vitrectomized versus nonvitrectomized eyes, Ophthalmol 92:1601, 1985.

156. Doncan H: De corporis vitrei structura, Utrecht, 1854, Nederlandisch Lancet 3; ser 8, jabrg, 1854.

157. Duke-Elder WS: Anomalies in the vitreous body, in System of ophthalmology, vol 3, London, Henry Kimpton, 1964, pt 2, pp 763-770.

158. Duke-Elder WS, MacFaul PA: Concussion changes in the vitreous, in Duke-Elder WS, ed: System of ophthalmology, vol 14, London, Henry Kimpton, 1972, p 197.

159. Edelhauser HF, Van Horn DL, Aaberg TM: Intraocular irrigating solutions and their use for vitrectomy, in Irvine AR, O'Malley C, eds: Advances in vitreous surgery, Springfield, IL, Charles C Thomas, 1976, pp 265-287.

160. Eisner G: Biomicroscopy of the peripheral fundus, New York, Springer-Verlag, 1973.

161. Eisner G: Zur Anatomie des Glaskörpers, Alb v Graef Arch Klin Exp Ophthalmol 193:33, 1975.

162. Eisner G: Licht Koagulation und Glaskörperbildung— zur Frage der Glaskörperenntstehung, Graef Arch Clin Exp Ophthalmol 206:33, 1978.

163. Eisner G, Bachmann E: Vergleichend morphologische Spaltlampenuntersuchung des Glaskörpers, Alb v Graef Arch Klin Exp Ophthalmol 191:329, 1974.

164. Eisner G, Bachmann E: Vergleichend morphologische Spaltlampenuntersuchung des Glaskörpers, Alb v Graef Arch Klin Exp Ophthalmol 192:1, 1974.

165. Elschnig A: Über Glaskörperablösung, Klin Mbl Augenheilkd 42:529, 1904.

166. Engel HA, Green WR, Michels RG, et al: Diagnostic vitrectomy, Retina 1:121, 1981.

167. Enoch JM, Birch DG: Evidence for alteration in photoreceptor orientation, Ophthalmol 87:821, 1980.

168. Epstein DL, Hashimoto JM, Anderson PJ, et al: Experimental perfusions through the anterior and vitreous chambers with possible relationships to malignant glaucoma, Am J Ophthalmol 88:1078, 1979.

169. Erggelet H: Klinische Befunde bei focaler Belechtung mit der Gullstrandischen Nernst-spalt Lampe, Klin Mbl Augenheilk 53:449, 1914.

170. Eyre DR, Apon S, et al: Collagen type IX: evidence for covalent linkages to type II collagen in cartilage, Federation of European Biochemical Societies, vol 220, 2:337, 1987.

171. Falbe-Hansen I, Ehlers N, Degn JK: The development of the human foetal vitreous body, I, Biochemical changes, Acta Ophthalmol 47:39, 1969.

172. Fatt I: Flow and diffusion in the vitreous body of the eye, Bull Math Biol 37:85, 1975.

173. Fatt I: Hydraulic flow conductivity of the vitreous gel, Invest Ophthalmol Vis Sci 16:565, 1977.

174. Fatt I, Hedbys BO: Flow of water in the sclera, Exp Eye Res 10:243, 1970.

175. Faulborn J, Bowald S: Combined macroscopic, light microscopic, scanning and transmission electron microscopic investigation of the vitreous body, II, The anterior viterous cortex, Ophthalmol Res 14:117, 1982.

176. Faulborn J, Bowald S: Microproliferations in proliferative diabetic retinopathy and their relation to the vitreous—corresponding light and electron microscopic

studies, Graef Arch Clin Exp Ophthalmol 223:130, 1985.

177. Faulborn J, Topping TM: Proliferations in the vitreous cavity after peforating injuries—a histopathological study, Alb v Graef Arch Clin Exp Ophthalmol 205:157, 1978.

178. Fessler JH: A structural function of mucopolysaccharide in connective tissue, Biochem J 76:124, 1960.

179. Fewan SM, Straatsma BR: Cyst of the posterior vitreous, Arch Ophthalmol 91:328, 1974.

180. Fincham EF: The mechanism of accommodation, Br J Ophthalmol 8:70, 1937.

181. Fine BS, Tousimis AJ: The structure of the vitreous body and the suspensory ligaments of the lens, Arch Ophthalmol 65:95; 119, 1961.

182. Fisher RF: The vitreous and lens in accommodation, Trans Ophthalmol Soc UK 102:318, 1982.

183. Fisher RF: Is the vitreous necessary for accommodation in man? Br J Ophthalmol 67:206, 1983.

184. Fledelius HC: Prematurity and the eye, Acta Ophthalmol (Kbh), (Suppl) 128 (Thesis), 1976.

185. Fledelius HC: Ophthalmic changes from age of 10 to 18 years, a longitudinal study of sequels to low birth weight, IV, Ultrasound oculometry of vitreous and axial length, Acta Ophthalmologica 60:403, 1982.

186. Foersch HC, Forman DT, Vye MV: Measurement of potassium in vitreous humor as an indication of the post-mortem interval, Am J Clin Pathol 72:651, 1979.

187. Font RL, Yanoff M, Zimmerman LE: Intraocular adipose tissue and persistent hyperplastic primary vitreous, Arch Ophthalmol 82:43, 1969.

188. Foos RY: Posterior vitreous detachment, Trans Am Acad Ophthalmol Otolaryngol 76:480, 1972.

189. Foos RY: Vitreoretinal juncture: topographical variations, Invest Ophthalmol 11:801, 1972.

190. Foos RY: Vitreous base, retinal tufts and retinal tears pathogenic relationships, in Pruett RC, Regan CDJ, eds: Retinal congress, New York, Appleton-Century-Crofts, 1974.

191. Foos RY: Vitreoretinal juncture, epiretinal membranes and vitreous, Invest Ophthalmol Vis Sci 16:416, 1977.

192. Foos RY, Gloor BP: Vitreoretinal juncture; healing of experimental wounds, Alb v Graef Arch Klin Exp Ophthalmol 196:213, 1975.

193. Foos RY, Roth AM: Surface structure of the optic nerve head, 2, Vitreopapillary attachments and posterior vitreous detachment, Am J Ophthalmol 76:662, 1973.

194. Foos RY, Simons KB: Vitreous in lattice degeneration of retina, Ophthalmol 91:452, 1984.

195. Foos RY, Wheeler NC: Vitreoretinal juncture—synchisis senilis and posterior vitreous detachment, Ophthalmol 89:1502, 1982.

196. Forrester JV, Balazs EA: Effect of hyaluronic acid and vitreous on macrophage phagocytosis, Trans Ophthalmol Soc UK 97:554, 1977.

197. Forrester JV, Balazs EA: Inhibition of phagocytosis by high molecular weight hyaluronate, Immunology 40:435, 1980.

198. Forrester JV, Docherty R, Kerr C, et al: Cellular proliferation in the vitreous—the use of vitreous explants as a model system, Invest Ophthalmol Vis Sci 27:1085, 1986.

199. Forrester JV, Grierson I: The cellular response to blood in the vitreous: an ultrastructural study, J Pathol 129:43, 1979.

200. Forrester JV, Grierson I, Lee WR: The pathology of vitreous hemorrhage, II, Ultrastructure, Arch Ophthalmol 97:2368, 1979.

201. Forrester JV, Lee WR: Cellular composition of post-haemorrhagic opacities in the human vitreous, Graef Arch Clin Exp Ophthalmol 215:279, 1981.

202. Foulds WS: Do we need a retinal pigment epithelium (or choroid) for the maintenance of retinal apposition? Br J Ophthalmol 69:237, 1985.

203. Foulds WS: Is your vitreous really necessary? The role of the vitreous in the eye with particular reference to retinal attachment, detachment and the mode of action of vitreous substitutes, Eye 1:641, 1987.

204. Foulds WS, Allan D, Moseley H, et al: Effect of intra-vitreal hyaluronidase on the clearance of tritiated water from the vitreous to the choroid, Br J Ophthalmol 69:529, 1985.

205. Francois J: Pre-papillary cyst developed from remnant of the hyaloid artery, Br J Ophthalmol 34:365, 1950.

206. Francois J, Victoria-Troncoso V, Albarran E: The histochemical structure of the vitreous fibers studied by phase contrast microscopy, Am J Ophthalmol 69:763, 1970.

207. Francois J, Victoria-Troncoso V: Transplantation of vitreous cell culture, Ophthalm Res 4:270, 1973.

208. Francois J, Victoria-Troncoso V, Maudgal PC: Immunology of the vitreous body, Mod Probl Ophthalmol 16:196, 1976.

209. Frangieh GT, Green WR, Engel HM: A histopathologic study of macular cysts and holes, Retina 1:311, 1981.

210. Freeman MI, Jacobson B, Toth LZ, et al: Lysosomal enzymes associated with vitreous hyalocyte granules, I, Intracellular distribution pattern of enzymes, Exp Eye Res 7:113, 1968.

211. Friedenwald JS, Bushke W, Michel HO: Role of ascorbic acid (vitamin C) in secretion of intraocular fluid, Arch Ophthalmol 29:535, 1944.

212. Friedenwald JE, Stiehler RD: Structure of the vitreous, Arch Ophthalmol 14:789, 1935.

213. Gardner-Medwin AR: Retinal physiology—a foot in the vitreous fluid, Nature 309:113, 1984.

214. Gartner J: Vitreous electron microscopic studies on the fine structure of the normal and pathologically changed vitreoretinal limiting membrane, Surv Ophthalmol 9:291, 1964.

215. Gartner J: Photoelastic and ultrasonic studies on the structure and senile changes of the intervertebral disc and of the vitreous body, Mod Probl Ophthalmol 8:136, 1969.

216. Gartner J: Electron microscopic observations on the cilio-zonular border of the human eye with particular reference to the aging changes, Z Anat Entwickl Gesch 131:263, 1970.

217. Gartner J: The fine structure of the vitreous base of the human eye and the pathogenesis of pars planitis, Am J Ophthalmol 71:1317, 1971.

218. Gartner J: Electron microscopic study on the fibrillar network and fibrocyte-collagen interactions in the vitreous cortex at the ora serrata of human eyes with special regard to the role of disintegrating cells, Exp Eye Res 42:21, 1986.

219. Gass JDM: Vitreous traction maculopathies, in Gass JDM, ed: Steroscopic atlas of macular disease, St Louis, CV Mosby 1987, pp 676-713.

220. Gelman RA, Blackwell J: Collagen-mucopolysaccharide interaction at acid pH, Biochem Biophys Acta 342:254, 1974.

221. Gelman RA, Blackwell J, Kefalides NA, et al: Thermal stability of basement membrane collagen, Biochim Biophys Acta 427:492, 1976.

222. Gerlach V: Beiträge zur normalen Anatomie des menschlichen Auges, 1880 (as cited by Redslob[454]).

223. Gersh I, Catchpole HR: The organization of ground substance and basement membrane and its significance in tissue injury, disease and growth, Am J Anat 85:457, 1949.

224. Gherezghiher T, Koss MC, Nordquist RE, Wilkinson CP: Analysis of vitreous and aqueous levels of hyaluronic acid—application of high-performance liquid chromatography, Exp Eye Res 45:347, 1987.

225. Gibbs DA, Merrille EW, Smith DA, et al: The rheology of hyaluronic acid, Biopolymers 6:777, 1968.

226. Glaser BM: Extracellular modulating factors and the control of intraocular neovascularization, Arch Ophthalmol 106:603, 1988.

227. Gloor BP: Zur Entwicklung des Glaskörpers und der Zonula, II, wahrend Entwicklung und Ruckbildung der Vasa Hyaloidea und der Tunika Vasculosa Lentis, Graef Arch Klin Exp Ophthalmol 186:311, 1973.

228. Gloor BP: Zur Entwicklung Des Glaskörpers und der Zonula, III, Henkunft, Lebenszeit und Ersatz der Glaskörpezellen beim Kaninchen, Alb v Graef Arch Klin Exp Ophthalmol 187:21, 1973.

229. Gloor BP: Zur Entwicklung des Glaskörpers und der zonula, VI, Autoradiographische Untersuchungen Zur Entwicklung der Zonula der Mays mit H-Markierten Aminosauren und H-Glucose, V Graefe Arch Ophthalmol 169:105, 1974.

230. Gloor BP: The vitreous, in Moses RA, ed: Adler's physiology of the eye, St Louis, CV Mosby, 1975, pp 252-274.

231. Gloor BP: Radioisotopes for research into vitreous and zonule, Adv Ophthalmol 36:63, 1978.

232. Gloor BP, Daicker BD: Pathology of the vitreo-retinal border structures, Trans Ophthalmol Soc UK 95:387, 1975.

233. Goedbloed J: Studien am Glaskörper 1. Die Struktur des Glaskörpers, Albrecht von Graefs Arch Ophthalmol: 323, 1934.

234. Goldmann H: Senescenz des Glaskörpers, Ophthalmologica 143:253, 1962.

235. Goodnight R, Nagy AR, Ryan SJ: Differential distribution of laminin in rabbit and monkey retinas, Invest Ophthalmol Vis Sci 29 (ARVO):203, 1988.

236. Gorevic PD, Rodrigues MM: Prealbumin—a major constituent of vitreous amyloid, Ophthalmol 94:792, 1987.

237. Goss DA, Ciswell MH: Myopia development in experimental animals—a literature review, Am J Optom Physiol Optics 58:859, 1981.

238. Grabner G, Baltz G, Forster O: Macrophage-like properties of human hyalocytes, Invest Ophthalmol Vis Sci 19:333, 1980.

239. Reference deleted in proof.

240. Green RL, Green WR: Vitreoretinal juncture, in Ryan SJ, ed: Retinal disease, St Louis, CV Mosby, 1989, vol 3, pp 13-69.

241. Green RL, Byrne SF: Diagnostic ophthalmic ultrasound, in Ryan SJ, ed: Retinal disease, St. Louis, CV Mosby, 1989, Ch 17.

242. Grierson I, Forrester JV: Vitreous hemorrhage and vitreal membranes, Trans Ophthalmol Soc UK 100:40, 1980.

243. Grierson I, Rahi AHS: Structural basis of contraction in vitreous fibrous membranes, Br J Ophthalmol 65:737, 1981.

244. Gross J: Comparative biochemistry of collagen, in Florkin M, Mason HS, eds: Comparative biochemistry, vol. V, New York, Academic Press, 1963, pp 307-347.

245. Grossniklaus HE, Frank KE, Farbi DC, et al: Hemoglobin spherulosis in the vitreous cavity, Arch Ophthalmol 106:961, 1988.

246. Gulati AK, Reyer RW: Role of neural retina and vitreous body during lens regeneration—transplantation and autoradiography, J Exp Zool 214:109, 1980.

247. Gullstrand A: Die Nernspaltlampe in der ophthalmologischen Praxis, Klin Monatsbl f Augenheilk 50:483, 1912.

248. Guyer DR, Sunness JS, Fine SL, et al: Idiopathic macular holes and cysts—a scanning laser ophthalmoscope analysis, Invest Ophthalmol Vis Sci 31 (ARVO):464, 1990.

249. Haddad A, Almeida JC, Laicine EM, et al: The origin of the intrinsic glycoproteins of the rabbit vitreous body—an immunohistochemical and autoradiographic study, Exp Eye Res 51:555, 1990.

250. Hageman GS, Johnson LV: Lectin-binding glycoproteins in the vertebrate vitreous body and inner limiting membrane—tissue localization and biochemical characterization, J Cell Biol 99:179a, 1984.

251. Hageman GS, Johnson LV: Identification and localization of vitreous body glycoproteins using lectin probes, Invest Ophthalmol Vis Sci 25(ARVO):317, 1984.

252. Hamlin CR, Kohn RR: Evidence for progressive age-related structural changes in post mature human collagen, Biochem Biophys Acta 236:458, 1971.

253. Hamming NA, Apple DJ, Geiser DK, et al: Ultrasound of hyaloid vasculature in primates, Invest Ophthalmol Vis Sci 16:408, 1977.

254. Hannover A: Endekung des Baues des Glaskörpers, Müller Archiv, 1845, pp 467-477.

255. Hansson HA: Scanning electron microscopy of the vitreous body in the rat eye, Z Zellforsch 101:323, 1969.

256. Hardingham TE: The role of link-protein in the structure of cartilage proteoglycan aggregates, Biochem J 177:237, 1979.

257. Harris M, Herp A, Pigman W: Metal catalysis in the depolymerization of hyaluronic acid by autoxidants, J Am Chem Soc 94:7570, 1972.

258. Hatfield RE, Gastineau CF, Rucke CW: Asteroid bodies in the vitreous—relationship to diabetes and hypercholesterolemia, Mayo Clin Proc 37:513, 1962.

259. Heergaard S, Jensen OA, Prause JU: Structure of the vitread face of the monkey optic disc (macacca mulatta)—SEM on frozen resin-cracked optic nerve heads supplemented by TEM and immunohistochemistry, Graef Arch Clin Exp Ophthalmol 226:377, 1988.

260. Heinegard D, Hascall VC: Aggregation of cartilage proteoglycans, III, Characteristics of proteins isolated from trypsin digests of aggregates, J Biol Chem 249:4250, 1974.

261. Helmholtz H von: Über die Akkomodation des Auges, Graef Arch Ophthalmol 1:2, 1924.

262. Henle J: Algemeine Anatomie, Leipzig, 1894.

263. Reference deleted in proof.

264. Hilton GF, Grizzard WS: Pneumatic retinopexy; a two-step outpatient operation without conjunctival incision, Ophthalmol 93:626, 1986.

265. Hirokawa H, Jalkh AE, Takahashi M: Role of vitreous in idiopathic preretinal macular fibrosis, Am J Ophthalmol 101:166, 1986.

266. Hirokawa H, Takahashi M, Trempe CL: Vitreous changes in peripheral uveitis, Arch Ophthalmol 103:1704, 1985.

267. Hirschel BJ, Gabbiani G, Ryan GB, et al: Fibroblasts of granulation tissue immunofluorescent staining with anti-smooth muscle serum, Proc Soc Exp Biol Med 138:466, 1971.

268. Hitchings RA, Triparthi RC: Vitreous opacities in primary amyloid disease, a clinical, histochemical, and ultrastructural report, Br J Ophthalmol 60:41, 1976.

269. Hoffmann K, Baurweig H, Riese K: Uber Gehalt und Verteilung niederund hoch molekularer Substanzen in Glaskörper, II, Hoch molekulare Substanzen (LDH, MDH, GOT), Graef Arch Clin Exp Ophthalmol 191:231, 1974.

270. Hogan MJ: The vitreous, its structure, and relation to the ciliary body and retina, Invest Ophthalmol 2:418, 1963.

271. Hogan MJ: The normal vitreous and its ultrastructure, in Irvine AR, O'Malley P, eds: Advances in vitreous surgery, Springfield, IL, Charles C Thomas, Publisher, 1974, pp 5-16.

272. Hogan MJ, Alvarado JA, Weddel JE: Histology of the human eye: an atlas and textbook, Philadelphia, WB Saunders, 1971, p 607.

273. Honda Y, Negi A, Kawano S: Mode of ion movements into vitreous—equilibration after vitrectomy, Arch Ophthalmol 101:105, 1983.

274. Hong BS, Davison DF: Identification of type II procollagen in rabbit vitreous, Ophthalm Res 17:162, 1985.

275. Hosoda Y, Okada M, Matsumura M, et al: Immunohistochemical study on epiretinal membrane of proliferative diabetic retinopathy, Invest Ophthalmol Vis Sci 31 (ARVO):128, 1990.

276. Hovland KR: Vitreous findings in fellow eyes of aphakic retinal detachment, Am J Ophthalmol 86:350, 1978.

277. Hruby K: Spaltlampenmikroskopie des hinterin augenabschnittes, Vienna, Urban & Schwarzenberg, 1950.

278. Hsu T, Dorey CK, Sorgente N, et al: Surgical removal of vitreous—its effect on intraocular fibroblast proliferation in the rabbit, Arch Ophthalmol 102:605, 1984.

279. Hui YN, Goodnight R, Zhang X-J, et al: Glial morphological studies, Arch Ophthalmol 106:1280, 1988.

280. Hui YN, Sorgente N, Ryan SJ: Posterior vitreous separation and retinal detachment induced by macrophages, Graef Arch Clin Exp Ophthalmol 225:279, 1987.

281. Hultsch E: Peripheral uveitis in the owl monkey—experimental model, Mod Probl Ophthalmol 18:247, 1977.

282. Hultsch E: Vitreous structure and ocular inflammation, in Silverstein S, O'Connor R, eds: Immunology and immunopathology of the eye, New York, Masson, 1979, pp 97-102.

283. Hultsch E: The vitreous of the baby owl monkey, Dev Ophthlalmol 2:1, 1981.

284. Hultsch E, Balazs EA: In vitro synthesis of glycosaminolglycans and glycoproteins by cells of the vitreous, Invest Ophthalmol 14 (Suppl):43, 1973.

285. Hultsch E, Freeman MI, Balazs EA: Transport and regeneration of hyaluronic acid in extracellular ocular compartments, Invest Ophthalmol (Suppl) 11:97, 1974.

286. Hyams SW, Newmann E: Peripheral retina in myopia with particular reference to retinal breaks, Br J Ophthalmol 53:300, 1969.

287. Hyams SW, Newmann E, Friedman Z: Myopia-aphakia, II, Vitreous and peripheral retina, Br J Ophthalmol 59:483, 1975.

288. Ichinonasama J: Influence of metabolic disorder in the vitreous induced by experimental uveitis on the rabbit lens, Nippon Ganka Gakkai Zasshi 83:1225, 1979.

289. Irvine SR: A newly-defined vitreous syndrome following cataract extraction, Am J Ophthalmol 36:599, 1953.

290. Ishizaki T: Immunochemical quantitative study of soluble proteins in the human vitreous, Acta Soc Ophthalmol Jpn 88:1487, 1985.

291. Iuvone PM, Tigges M, Fernandez A, et al: Dopamine synthesis and metabolism in rhesus monkey retina, Vis Neuro Sci 2:465, 1989.

292. Iwanoff AI: Beitrage zur normalen und pathologischen anatomie des Auges. A: Zur pathologischen Anatomie der retinal. B: Zur normalen und pathologischen Anatomie des Glaskörpers, Graef Arch Ophthalmol 11:135, 1865.

293. Iwanoff AI: Le corps vitré, in Stricker's Handbuch der Lehre von den Geweben, Leipzig, 1872 (as cited by Redslob[454]).

294. Jack RL: Regression of the hyaloid artery system, An ultrastructural analysis, Am J Ophthalmol 74:261, 1972.

295. Jack RL: Ultrastructure of the hyaloid vascular system, Arch Ophthalmol 87:555, 1972.

296. Jackson DS: Chondroitin sulphuric acid as a factor in the stability of tendon, Biochem J 54:638, 1953.

297. Jacobson B: Degradation of glycosaminoglycans by extracts of calf vitreous hyalocytes, Exp Eye Res 39:373,

298. Jacobson B: Identification of sialyl and galactosyl transferase activities in calf vitreous hyalocytes, Curr Eye Res 3:1033, 1984.

299. Jacobson B, Basu P, Hasany SM: Vascular endothelial cell growth inhibitor of normal and pathologic human vitreous, Arch Ophthalmol 102:1543, 1984.

300. Jacobson B, Dorfman T, Basu PK, et al: Inhibition of vascular endothelial cell growth and trypsin activity by vitreous, Exp Eye Res 41:581, 1985.

301. Jacobson B, Osterlin S, Balazs EA: A soluble hyaluronic acid synthesizing system from calf vitreous, Proc Fed Am Soc Exp Biol 25:588, 1966.

302. Jaffe NS: Macular retinopathy after separation of vitreoretinal adherence, Arch Ophthalmol 78:585, 1967.

303. Jaffe NS: Vitreous traction at the posterior pole of the fundus due to alterations in the vitreous posterior, Trans Am Acad Ophthalmol Otolaryngol 71:642, 1967.

304. Jaffe NS: Complications of acute posterior vitreous detachment, Arch Ophthalmol 79:568, 1968.

305. Jerdan JA, Pepose JS, Michels RG, et al: Proliferative vitreoretinopathy membranes—an immunohistochemical study, Ophthalmol 96:801, 1989.

306. Johnson RN, Gass JDM: Idiopathic macular holes—observations, stages of formation and implications for surgical intervention, Ophthalmol 95:917, 1988.

307. Jones H: Hyaloid remnants in the eyes of premature babies, Br J Ophthalmol 47:39, 1963.

308. Jongebloed WL, Humalda D, Worst JFG: A SEM correlation of the anatomy of the vitreous body—making visible the invisible, Doc Ophthalmol 64:117, 1986.

309. Jongebloed WL, Worst JFG: The cisternal anatomy of the vitreous body, Doc Ophthalmol 67:183, 1987.

310. Junqueria LCU, Montes GS: Biology of collagen-proteoglycan interaction, Arch Histol Jpn 46:589, 1983.

311. Kaczurowski MI: The surface of the vitreous, Am J Ophthalmol 63:419, 1967.

312. Kador PE, Akagi V, Terubayashi H, et al: Prevention of pericyte ghost formation in retinal capillaries of galactose-fed dogs by aldose reductase inhibitors, Arch Ophthalmol 106:1099, 1988.

313. Kain HL: Proliferative vitreoretinopathy—a role of lysosomal enzymes, Invest Ophthalmol Vis Sci 30 (ARVO):13, 1989.

314. Kamei A, Totani A: Isolation and characterization of minor glycosaminoglycans in the rabbit vitreous body, Biochem Biophys Res Comm 109:881, 1982.

315. Kampik A, Green WR, Michels RG, et al: Ultrastructural features of progressive idiopathic epiretinal membranes removed by vitreous surgery, Am J Ophthalmol 90:797, 1980.

316. Kampik A, Kenyon KR, Michels RG: Epiretinal and vitreous membranes—a comparative study of 56 cases, Arch Ophthalmol 99:1445, 1981.

317. Kanski JJ: Complications of acute posterior vitreous detachment, Am J Ophthalmol 80:44, 1975.

318. Kantarjian AD, DeJong RN: Familial primary amyloidosis with nervous system involvement, Neurology 3:399, 1953.

319. Katami C, Raymond LA, Lipman MJ, et al: Change in the synthesis of glycosaminoglycans by fibrotic vitreous induced by erythrocytes, Biochim Biophys Acta 880:40, 1986.

320. Kaufman HE: Primary familial amyloidosis, Arch Ophthalmol 60:1036, 1958.

321. Kawano SI, Honda Y, Negi A: Effects of biological stimuli on the viscosity of the vitreous, Acta Ophthalmologica 60:977, 1982.

322. Kayazawa F, Tamura S, Tsuji T, et al: The influence of aging on vitreous fluorophotometry, Nippon Ganka Gakkai Zasshi 87:380, 1983.

323. Kearns TP: Discussion of "Asteroid hyalitis and diabetes mellitus," Trans Am Acad Ophthalmol Otolaryngol 69:277, 1965.

324. Kefalides NA: The biology and chemistry of basement membranes, in Kefalides, NA, ed: Proceedings of the first international symposium on the biology and chemistry of basement membranes, New York, Academic Press, 1978, pp 215-228.

325. Khodadoust AA, Stark WJ, Bell WR: Coagulation properties of intraocular humors and cerebrospinal fluid, Invest Ophthalmol Vis Sci 24:1616, 1983.

326. Kim JO, Cotlier E: Phospholipid distributions and fatty acid composition of lysophosphatidylcholine in rabbit aqueous humor, lens and vitreous, Exp Eye Res 22:569, 1976.

327. Kinsey VE: Transfer of ascorbic acid and related compounds across the blood aqueous barrier, Am J Ophthalmol 30:1262, 1947.

328. Kinsey VE, Reddy DVN: An estimate of the ionic composition of the fluid secreted into the posterior chamber inferred from a study of aqueous humor dynamics, Doc Ophthalmol 137:7, 1959.

329. Kinsey VE, Reddy DVN, Skrentny BA: Intraocular transport of C-labelled urea and the influence of diamox on its rate of accumulation in the aqueous humours, Am J Ophthalmol 50:1130, 1960.

330. Kinsey VW, Grant WM, Cogan DC: Water movement and the eye, Arch Ophthalmol 27:242, 1942.

331. Kirchoff B, Kirchoff E, Ryan SJ, et al: Vitreous modulation of migration and proliferation of retinal pigment epithelial cells in vitro, Invest Ophthalmol Vis Sci 30:1951, 1989.

332. Kishi S, Demaria C, Shimizu K: Vitreous cortex remnants at the fovea after spontaneous vitreous detachment, Intl Ophthalmol 9:253, 1986.

333. Kishi S, Shimizu K: Posterior precortical vitreous pocket, Arch Ophthalmol 108:979, 1990.

334. Kitchen RG: Diffusion in model connective tissue systems (Thesis), Clayton, Victoria, Australia, Monash University, 1975.

335. Kloti R: Experimental occlusion of retinal and ciliary vessels in owl monkeys, I, Technique and clinical observations of selective embolism of the central retinal artery system, Exp Eye Res 6:393, 1967.

336. Knobloch WH: Inherited hyaloideoretinopathy and skeletal dysplasia, Trans Am Ophthalmol Soc 73:417, 1975.

337. Knudsen LL: Binding of fluorescein to vitreous in vitro, Acta Ophthalmol 65:352, 1987.

338. Koeppe L: Clinical observations with the slit lamp, Arch f Ophthalmol XC and XCVI:232, 1917.

339. Kohn RR, Rollerson E: Relationship of age to swelling properties of human diaphragm tendon in acid and alkaline solutions, J Gerontol 13:241, 1958.

340. Koretz JF, Handelman GH: Model of the accommodative mechanism in the human eye, Vision Res 22:917, 1982.

341. Kuhn W, Hargitay B, Katchalsky M, et al: Reversible dilation and contraction by changing the state of ionization of high polymer acid networks, Nature 165:514, 1956.

342. Kuwabara T, Cogan DG: Studies of retinal vascular patterns, I, Normal architecture, Arch Ophthalmol 64:904, 1960.

343. Lacqua H, Machemer R: Clinico-pathologic correlation in massive periretinal proliferation, Am J Ophthalmol 80:913, 1975.

344. Lacqua H, Machemer R: Glial cell proliferation in retinal detachment (massive periretinal proliferation), Am J Ophthalmol 80:602, 1975.

345. Lamba PA, Shukla KM: Experimental asteroid hyalopathy, Br J Ophthalmol 55:279, 1971.

346. La Nauze JH, Hembry RM, Jacobson W, Watson PG: Chemotaxis in vitreous haemorrhage—an experimental study, Exp Eye Res 34:803, 1982.

347. Larsen G: The hyaluronic acid in the rabbit vitreous variations following hormonal treatment, AMA Arch Ophthalmol 60:815, 1971.

348. Larsen JS: The sagittal growth of the eye, III, Ultrasonic measurement of the posterior segment from birth to puberty, Acta Ophthalmol (Kbh) 49:441, 1971.

349. Larsson L, Osterlin S: Posterior vitreous detachment—a combined clinical and physicochemical study, Graef Arch Clin Exp Ophthalmol 223:92, 1985.

350. Laurent TC, Bjork I, Pietruszkiewicz A, et al: On the interaction between polysaccharides and other macromolecules, II, The transport of globular particles through hyaluronic acid solutions, Biochim Biophys Acta 78:351, 1963.

351. Laurent TC, Obrink B: On the restriction of the rotational diffusion of proteins in polymer networks, Eur J Biochim 28:94, 1972.

352. Laurent TC, Pietruszkiewicz A: The effect of hyaluronic acid on the sedimentation rate of other substances, Biochim Biophys Acta 49:258, 1961.

353. Laurent TC, Preston BN, Pertoft, M, et al: Diffusion of linear polymers in hyaluronate solutions, Eur J Biochem 53:129, 1975.

354. Laurent TC, Ryan M, Pietruszkiewicz A: Fractionation of hyaluronic acid; the polydispersity of hyaluronic acid from the vitreous body, Biochim Biophys Acta 42:476, 1960.

355. Laurent UBG, Fraser JRE: Turnover of hyaluronate in aqueous humor and vitreous body of the rabbit, Exp Eye Res 36:493, 1983.

356. Laurent UBG, Granath KA: The molecular weight of hyaluronate in the aqueous humour and vitreous body of rabbit and cattle eyes, Exp Eye Res 36:481, 1983.

357. Laurent UBG, Laurent TC, Howe AF: Chromatography of soluble proteins from the bovine vitreous body on DEAE-cellulose, Exp Eye Res 1:276-285.

358. Laurent UBG, Tengblad A: Determination of hyaluronate in biological samples by a specific radioassay technique, Annal Biochem 109:386, 1980.

359. Liang JN, Chakrabarti B: Stereoscopic studies on pepsin-solubilized vitreous and cartilage collagens, Curr Eye Res 1:175, 1981.

360. Likar LJ, Likar IN, Robinson RW: Levels of acid mucopolysaccharides of the bovine aorta at different stages of the sexual cycle, J Atheroscl Res 5:388, 1965.

361. Lin T, Stone RA, Laties AM, et al: Altered dopamine metabolism and form-deprivation myopia, Invest Ophthalmol Vis Sci 29 (ARVO):33, 1988.

362. Lincoff H, Kreissig I, Richard G: Treating avulsed vessels with a temporary balloon buckle, Am J Ophthalmol 101:90, 1986.

363. Lindner B: Acute posterior vitreous detachment and its retinal complications, Acta Ophthalmol 87 (Suppl):1, 1966.

364. Lindner K: Zur Klinik des Glaskörpers, III, Glaskorper und Netzhautabehung, Alb V Graef Arch Ophthalmol 137:157, 1937.

365. Linsenmeyer TF, Gibney E, Little CD: Type II collagen in the early embryonic chick cornea and vitreous: immunoradiochemical evidence, Exp Eye Res 34:371, 1982.

366. Linsenmeyer TF, Little CD: Embryonic neural retina collagen: in vitro synthesis of high molecular weight forms of type II plus a new genetic type, Proc Natl Acad Sci USA 75:3235, 1978.

367. Lisch W, Rochels R: Zur Pathogenese kongenitaler glaskörperzystem, Klin Monatsbl Augenheilkd 195:375, 1989.

368. Lucas BC, Coleman DJ, Lizzi FL et al: Dating the age of vitreous hemorrhages—a histopathologic correlation with ultrasonic tissue characterization in the rabbit eye, Invest Ophthalmol Vis Sci 29:220, 1988.

369. Lutty GA, Mello RJ, Chandler C et al: Regulation of cell growth by vitreous humor, J Cell Sci 76:53, 1985.

370. Lutty GA, Thompson DC, Gallup JY, et al: Vitreous—an inhibitor of retinal extract-induced neovascularization, Invest Ophthalmol Vis Sci 24:52, 1983.

371. Luxenberg M, Sime D: Relationship of asteroid hyalosis to diabetes mellitus and plasma lipid levels, Am J Ophthalmol 406, 1969.

372. Luyckx-Bacus J, Weekers JF: Etude biometrique de l'oeil humain par ultrasonographie, Bull Soc Belge Ophthalmol 143:552, 1966.

373. Machemer R, Norton EWD: Experimental retinal detachment in the owl monkey, I, Methods of production and clinical picture, Am J Ophthalmol 66:388, 1968.

374. Maguire AM, Smiddy WE, Green WR, et al: Idiopathic epiretinal membranes—ultrastructural characteristics and clinicopathological correlations, Invest Ophthalmol Vis Sci 29 (ARVO):289, 1988.

375. Majno G: The story of the myofibroblasts, Am J Surg Pathol 31:535, 1979.

376. Mann I: The vitreous and suspensory ligament of the lens, in: The development of the human eye, New York, Grune & Stratton, 1964, p 150.

377. Manschot WA: Persistent hyperplastic primary vitreous, Arch Ophthalmol 59:188, 1958.

378. March WF, Shoch D: Electron diffraction study of asteroid bodies, Invest Ophthalmol 14:399, 1975.

379. Margherio RR, Schepens CL: Macular breaks, I, Diagnosis, etiology, and observations, Am J Ophthalmol 74:219, 1972.

380. Mark K von der, Rimpl R, Trelstad RL: Immunofluorescent localization of collagen types I, II, and III in the embryonic chick eye, Dev Biol 59:75, 1977.

381. Marsh-Tootle WL, Norton TT: Refractive and structural measures of lid-suture myopia in tree shrew, Invest Ophthalmol Vis Sci 30:2245, 1989.

382. Mathews MB: The interaction of collagen and acid mucopolysaccharides, a model for connective tissue, Biochem J 96:710, 1965.

383. Matolstsky AG, Gross J, Grignolo A: A study of the fibrous components of the vitreous body with the electron microscope, Proc Soc Exp Biol Med 76:857, 1951.

384. Maumenee AE: Further advances in the study of the macula, Arch Ophthalmol 78:151, 1967.

385. Maumenee IH: Vitreoretinal degeneration as a sign of generalized connective tissue diseases, Am J Ophthalmol 88:432, 1979.

386. Maurice DM: The exchange of sodium between the vitreous body and the blood and aqueous humour, J Physiol 137:100, 1957.

387. McBrien NA, Norton TT: Experimental myopia in tree

shrew is increased by treatment with lathyritic agents, Invest Ophthalmol Vis Sci 29 (ARVO):33, 1988.

388. McCord J: Free radicals and inflammation—protection of synovial fluid by superoxide dismutase, Science 185:529, 1974.

389. McCulloch C: The zonule of Zinn: its origin, course, insertion and relation to neighboring structures, Trans Am Ophthalmol Soc 52:525, 1954.

390. McDonnel PJ, Fine SL, Hillis AI: Clinical features of macular cysts and holes, Am J Ophthalmol 93:777, 1980.

391. McGahan MC: Ascorbic acid levels in aqueous and vitreous humors of the rabbit—effects of inflammation and cerruloplasmin, Vis Res 41:291, 1985.

392. McGahan MC, Fleisher LN: Antioxidant activity of aqueous and vitreous humor from the inflamed rabbit eye, Curr Eye Res 5:641, 1986.

393. McLaughlin PS, McLaughlin BG: Chemical analysis of bovine and porcine vitreous humors—correlation of normal values with serum chemical values and changes with time and temperature, Am J Vet Res 48:467, 1987.

394. Messner KH: Spontaneous separation of preretinal macular fibrosis, Am J Ophthalmol 83:9, 1977.

395. Meyer FA, Koblenz M, Silberberg A: Structural investigation of dextran fractions as non-interacting macromolecular probes, Biochem J 161:285, 1977.

396. Meyer K: Chemical structure of hyaluronic acid, Fed Proc 17:1075, 1958.

397. Meyer K, Palmer JW: The polysaccharide of the vitreous humor, J Biol Chem 107:629, 1934.

398. Miller H, Miller B, Rabinowitz H: Asteroid bodies—an ultrastructural study, Invest Ophthalmol Vis Sci 24:133, 1983.

399. Miyake K: Experimental and clinical studies on the active transport of substances from the vitreous cavity, Acta Soc Ophthalmol Jpn 92:909, 1988.

400. Monnier VM, Vasaroth, Vishwamath BA, et al: Relation between complications of type I diabetes mellitus and collagen-linked fluorescence, N Engl J Med 314:403, 1986.

401. Moore RF: Subjective "lightning streak," Br J Ophthalmol 19:545, 1935.

402. Morgan CM, Schatz H: Involutional macular thinning—a pre-macular hole condition, Ophthalmol 93:153, 1986.

403. Morner CT: Untersuchung der Proteinsubstanzen in der lichtbrechenden Medien des Auges, Z f Physiol Chem 18:223, 1894.

404. Morse PH: Symptomatic floaters as a clue to vitreoretinal disease, Am J Ophthalmol 7:865, 1975.

405. Mosely H: Mathematical model of diffusion in the vitreous humour of the eye, Clin Phys Physiol Meas 2:175, 1981.

406. Mueller-Jensen J, Machemer R, Azuronia R: Autotransplantation of retinal pigment epithelium in intravitreal diffusion chamber, Am J Ophthalmol 80:530, 1975.

407. Murakami K, Jalkh AE, Avila MD, et al: Vitreous floaters, Ophthalmol 90:1271, 1983.

408. Mutlu F, Leopold IH: Structure of the human retinal vascular system, Arch Ophthalmol 71:93, 1964.

409. Neumann E, Hyams S, Brakai S: Natural history of retinal holes with specific reference to the development of retinal detachment and time factor involved, in Michaelson IC, Berman ER, eds: Causes and prevention of blindness, New York/London, Academic Press, 1972.

410. Newman EA: Regional specialization of retinal glial cell membrane, Nature 309:155, 1984.

411. Newsome DA, Linsemayer TF, Trelstad RJ: Vitreous body collagen; evidence for a dual origin from the neural retina and hyalocytes, J Cell Biol 71:59, 1976.

412. Novak MA, Welch RB: Complications of acute symptomatic posterior vitreous detachment, Am J Ophthalmol 97:308, 1984.

413. Obrink B, Laurent TC: Further studies on the rotation of globular proteins in polymer solutions, Eur J Biochem 41:83, 1974.

414. Oegama TR Jr, Brown M, Dziewiatkowski DD: The link protein in proteoglycan aggregates from the swarm rat chondrosarcoma, J Biol Chem 252:6470, 1977.

415. Ogston AG, Phelps CF: The partition of solutes between buffer solutions containing hyaluronic acid, Biochem J 78:827, 1961.

416. Ogston AG, Sherman TF: Effects of hyaluronic acid upon diffusion of solutes and flow of solvents, J Physiol (Lond) 156:67, 1961.

417. Oksala A: Ultrasonic findings in the vitreous body at various ages, Alb v Graef Arch Klin Exp Ophthalmol 207:275, 1978.

418. Okubo A, Okubo Y, Ohara K, et al: Vitreous as tamponade in healing of rhegmatogenous retinal detachment, Jpn J Ophthalmol 34:36, 1990.

419. O'Malley P: The pattern of vitreous syneresis—a study of 800 autopsy eyes, in Irvine AR, O'Malley P, eds: Advances in vitreous surgery Springfield, IL, Charles C Thomas, Publisher, 1976, pp 17-33.

420. Orellara J, O'Malley P, et al: Pigmented free floating vitreous cysts in two young adults, electron microscopic observations, Ophthalmol 92:297, 1985.

421. Organisciak DT, Tiang Y-L, Wang H-M, et al: The protective effect of ascorbic acid in retinal light damage of rats exposed to intermittent light, Invest Ophthalmol Vis Sci 31:1195, 1990.

422. Orlidge A, D'Amore PA: Inhibition of capilliary endothelial cell growth by pericytes, Invest Ophthalmol Vis Sci 28(ARVO):56, 1987.

423. Osterlin SE: The synthesis of hyaluronic acid in the vitreous, III, In vivo metabolism in the owl monkey, Exp Eye Res 7:524, 1968.

424. Osterlin SE: The synthesis of hyaluronic acid in the vitreous, IV, Regeneration in the owl monkey, Exp Eye Res 8:27, 1969.

425. Osterlin SE: Changes in the macromolecular composition of the vitreous after removal of the lens, in: Proc XXI Int Congress, Mexico DF, Int Congr Ser No 222, Excerpta Medica, Amsterdam, 1971, p 1620.

426. Osterlin S: Changes in the vitreous with age, Trans Ophthalmol Soc UK 95:372, 1975.

427. Osterlin S: On the molecular biology of the vitreous in the aphakic eye, Acta Ophthalmologica 55:353, 1977.

428. Osterlin S: Macromolecular composition of the vitreous in the aphakic owl monkey eye, Exp Eye Res 26:77, 1978.

429. Osterlin SE, Balazs EA: Macromolecular composition

and fine structure of the vitreous in the owl monkey, Exp Eye Res 7:534, 1968.

430. Pajor R: Freeze-cleaved replicas of rabbit vitreous, Exp Eye Res 14:292, 1972.

431. Palm E: On the phosphate exchange between the blood and the eye—experiments on the entrance of radioactive phosphate into the aqueous humour, the anterior uvea and the lens, Acta Ophthalmol 32:1, 1948.

432. Pederson JE, Cantrill HL: Experimental retinal detachment, V, Fluid movement through the retinal hole, Arch Ophthalmol, 1984.

433. Pedler C: The inner limiting membrane of the retina, Br J Ophthalmol 45:423, 1961.

434. Perera: Bilateral cyst of the vitreous, Report of a case, Arch Ophthalmol 16:1015, 1936.

435. Pilkerton AR, Rao NA, Marak GE, et al: Experimental vitreous fibroplasia following perforating ocular injuries, Arch Ophthalmol 97:1707, 1979.

436. Pirie A, Schmidt G, Waters JW: Ox vitreous humor, I, The residual protein, Brit J Ophthalmol 32:321, 1948.

437. Pischel KD: Detachment of the vitreous as seen by slit lamp examination, Am J Ophthalmol 36:1497, 1952.

438. Podrazky V, Stevens FS, Jackson DS, et al: Interaction of tropocollagen with protein-polysaccharide complexes; an analysis of the ionic groups responsible for interaction, Biochim Biophys Acta 229:690, 1971.

439. Porte A, Stockel MD, Brini A, et al: Structure et differentiation du corps ciliare et du feuillet pigmente de la retine chez le poulet, Arch Ophthalmol 28:259, 1968.

440. Prager TC, Chu HH, Garcia CA, et al: The influence of vitreous change on vitreous fluorophotometry, Arch Ophthalmol 100:594, 1982.

441. Preston BN, Davies M, Ogston AG: The composition and physicochemical properties of hyaluronic acids prepared from synovial fluid and from a case of mesothelioma, Biochem J 96:449, 1965.

442. Preston BN, Obrink B, Laurent TC: The rotational diffusion of albumin in solutions of connective-tissue polysaccharides, Eur J Biochem 33:401, 1973.

443. Preston BN, Snowden J McK: Diffusion properties in model extracellular systems, in Kulonen E, Pillarainen J, eds: Biology of fibroblast, New York, Academic Press, 1973, pp 215-230.

444. Pruett RC, Schepens CL: Posterior hyperplastic primary vitreous, Am J Ophthalmol 69:535, 1970.

445. Rankin JA, Matthay RA: Pulmonary renal syndromes, II, Etiology and pathogenesis, Yale J Biol Med 55:26, 1982.

446. Raviola G: The fine structure of the ciliary zonule and ciliary epithelium, Invest Ophthalmol 10:851, 1971.

447. Raymond LA, Jacobson B: Isolation and identification of stimulatory and inhibiting growth factors in bovine vitreous, Exp Eye Res 34:267, 1982.

448. Raymond LA, Chromokos E, Bibler LW, et al: Change in vitreous collagen after penetrating injury, Ophthalm Res 17:102, 1985.

449. Raymond MC, Thompson JT: RPE-mediated collagen gel contraction inhibition by colchicine and stimulation by TGF-beta, Invest Ophthalmol Vis Sci 31:1079, 1990.

450. Reddy DV, Kinsey VE: Composition of the vitreous humor in relation to that of plasma and aqueous humors, Arch Ophthalmol 63:715, 1960.

451. Reddy DVN, Rosenberg C, Kinsey VE: Steady state distribution of free amino acids within aqueous humour, vitreous body and plasma of the rabbit, Exp Eye Res 1:175, 1961.

452. Reddy TS, Birkle DL, Packer AJ, et al: Fatty acid composition and arachidonic acid metabolism in vitreous lipids from canine and human eyes, Curr Eye Res 5:441, 1986.

453. Reddy VN: Dynamics of transport systems in the eye, Invest Ophthalmol Vis Sci 18:1000, 1979.

454. Redslob E: Le corps vitre, Société Francaise d'Ophtalmologie Mongr, Paris, Masson, 1932, pp 174-178.

455. Reese AB: Persistent hyperplastic primary vitreous, Am J Ophthalmol 40:317, 1955.

456. Reeser FH, Aaberg T: Vitreous Humor, in Records PE, ed: Physiology of the human eye and visual system. Hagerstown, Harper & Row, 1979, Ch 11, pp 1-31.

457. Reeser FH, Van Horn DL: Experimental vitreous membranes, Invest Ophthalmol Vis Sci (ARVO):84, 1976.

458. Regnault FR: Vitreous hemorrhage—an experimental study, Arch Ophthalmol 83:458, 1970.

459. Rentsch FJ, Van der Zypen E: Altersbedingte Veranderungen der Sog Membrana limitans interna des Ziliarkörpers im menschlichen Auge, in Bredt H, Rohen TW, eds: Altern und Entwicklung, Stuttgart, Schattaurer Verlag, 1971, pp 70-94.

460. Renz B, Vygantas C: Hyaloid vascular remnants in human neonates, Ann Ophthalmol 9:179, 1977.

461. Retina Society Terminology Committee: The classification of retinal detachment with proliferative vitreoretinopathy, Ophthalmol 90:121, 1983.

462. Retzius: Om membrana limitans retinae interna, Nordisk Archiv III 2:1, 1871.

463. Rhodes RH: A comparative study of vitreous body and zonular glycoconjugates that bind to the lectin from ulex europaeus, Histochemistry 78:349, 1983.

464. Rhodes RH: An ultrastructural study of complex carbohydrates in the posterior chamber and vitreous base of the mouse, Histochem J 17:291, 1985.

465. Rhodes RH, Mandelbaum SH, Minckler DS, et al: Tritiated fucose incorporation in the vitreous body, lens and zonules of the pigmented rabbit, Exp Eye Res 34:921, 1982.

466. Rieger M: Über die Bedeutung der Aderhautsveranderungen fur die Erstehung der Glaskörperabhebung, Alb v Graef Arch Ophthalmol 136:119, 1936.

467. Ringvold A: Aqueous humor and ultraviolet radiation, Acta Ophthalmologica 58:69, 1980.

468. Robertson DM, Curtin VT, et al: Avulsed retinal vessels with retinal breaks—a cause of recurrent vitreous hemorrhage, Arch Ophthalmol 85:669, 1971.

469. Robins SP, Bailey AJ: Age-related changes in collagen—the identification of reducible lysine-carbohydrate condensation products, Biochem Biophys Res Commun 48:76, 1972.

470. Rodman HI, Johnson FB, Zimmerman LH: New histopathological and histochemical observations concerning asteroid hyalitis, Arch Ophthalmol 66:552, 1961.

471. Rosenbloom AL, Silverstein JM, Lezotte DC, et al: Limited joint mobility in childhood diabetes mellitus indicates increased risk for microvascular disease, N Engl J Med 305:191, 1981.

472. Rosengren B, Osterlin S: Hydrodynamic events in the vitreous space accompanying eye movements—significance for the pathogenesis of retinal detachment, Ophthalmologica 173:513, 1976.

473. Roth AM, Foos RY: Surface wrinkling retinopathy in eyes enucleated by autopsy, Trans Am Acad Ophthalmol Otolaryngol 75:1047, 1971.

474. Roth AM, Foos RY: Surface structure of the optic nerve head, I, Epipapillary membranes, Am J Ophthalmol 74:977, 1972.

475. Ruby AJ, Jampol LM: Nd: YAG treatment of a posterior vitreous cyst, Am J Ophthalmol 110:428, 1990.

476. Rutnin U, Schepens CL: Fundus appearance in normal eyes, III, Peripheral degenerations, Am J Ophthalmol 64:1040, 1967.

477. Saga T, Tagawa Y, Takeuchi T, et al: Electron microscopic study of cells in vitreous of guinea pig, Jpn J Ophthalmol 28:239, 1984.

478. Saga U: Histochemical study on the developing vitreous and internal retina, Ann Rep Mitsukoshi Res Funds, 1977, pp 100-103.

479. Sakaue H, Akira N, Honda Y: Comparative study of vitreous oxygen tension in human and rabbit eyes, Invest Ophthalmol Vis Sci 30:1933, 1989.

480. Sanna G, Nervi I: Statistical research on vitreous changes in dependence on age and errors of refraction, Ann Ophthalm 91:322, 1965.

481. Sato K, Tsunakawa N, Inaba K, et al: Fluorescein angiography on retinal detachment and lattice degenerations, I, Equatorial degeneration with idiopathic retinal detachment, Acta Soc Ophthalmol Jpn 75:635, 1971.

482. Schachat AP, Sommer A: Macular hemorrhages associated with posterior vitreous detachment, Am J Ophthalmol 102:647, 1986.

483. Scheiffarth OF, Kampik A, Gunther H, et al: Proteins of the extracellular matrix in vitreo-retinal membranes, Graef Arch Clin Exp Ophthalmol 226:357, 1988.

484. Schepens CL: Subclinical retinal detachments, Arch Ophthalmol 47:593, 1952.

485. Schepens CL: Ophthalmoscopic observations related to the vitreous body, in Schepens CL, ed: Importance of the vitreous body in retina surgery with special emphasis on degeneration, St Louis, CV Mosby, 1960, p 94.

486. Schepens CL: Retinal detachment and allied diseases, Philadelphia, WB Saunders, 1983.

487. Schepens CL, Avila MP, Jalkah AE, et al: Role of the vitreous in cystoid macular edema, Surv Ophthalmol 28(52):499, 1984.

488. Schmut O, Mallinger R, Paschke E: Studies on a distinct fraction of bovine vitreous body collagen, Graef Arch Clin Exp Ophthalmol 221:286, 1984.

489. Schnider SL, Kohn RR: Effects of age and diabetes mellitus on the solubility of collagen from human skin, tracheal cartilage, and dura mater, Exp Gerontol 17:185, 1982.

490. Schuyler MR, Niewoehner DE, Inkley SR, et al: Abnormal lung elasticity in juvenile diabetes mellitus, Am Rev Resp Dis 113:37, 1976.

491. Schwalbe G: In Engelmann W, ed: Von Graefe-Sämisch's Handbuch der Gesammten Augenheilkunde, Leipzig, 1874, vol 1, p 457.

492. Schwalbe G: Lehrbuch der Anatomie des Auges, Erlangen, E Besold, 1887, p 288.

493. Schwartz MF, Green WR, Michels RG, et al: An unusual case of ocular involvement in primary systemic non-familial amyloidosis, Ophthalmol 89:394, 1982.

494. Schwarz W: Electron microscopic observations on the human vitreous body, in Smelser GK, ed: Structure of the eye, New York, Academic Press, 1961, pp 283-291.

495. Schwarz W: Electron microscopic study on the gel of the central part of the corpus vitreum in the ox, Cell Tiss Res 168:271, 1976.

496. Scott JD: Treatment of massive vitreous retraction, Trans Ophthalmol Soc UK 95:429, 1975.

497. Sebag J: Age-related changes in human vitreous structure, Graef Arch Clin Exp Ophthalmol 225:89, 1987.

498. Sebag J: Vitreo-retinal interface and the role of vitreous in macular disease, in Brancato R, Coscas G, Lumbroso B, eds: Proceedings of the retina workshop, Amsterdam, Kugler & Ghedini, 1987, pp 3-60.

499. Sebag J: Vitreous anatomy and dynamics during pneumatic retinopexy, in Tornambe P, Grizzard WS, eds: Pneumatic retinopexy: a clinical symposium, Des Plaines, IL, Ocular Resources, 1989, Ch 2.

500. Sebag J: The vitreous—structure, function, pathobiology, New York, Springer-Verlag, 1989.

500a. Sebag J: Letter to the editor, Arch Ophthalmol 109:1059, 1991.

500b. Sebag J: Age-related differences in the human vitreoretinal interface, Arch Ophthalmol 109:966, 1991.

501. Sebag J, Albert DM, Craft JS: The Alstrom syndrome—ocular histopathology and retinal ultrastructure, Br J Ophthalmol 68:494, 1984.

502. Sebag J, Balazs EA: Human vitreous structure in childhood, VI Congress of the International Society for Eye Research, Alicante, Spain, 1984.

503. Sebag J, Balazs EA: Pathogenesis of CME—anatomic consideration of vitreo-retinal adhesions, Surv Ophthalmol 29(Suppl):493, 1984.

504. Sebag J, Balazs EA: Human vitreous fibres and vitreoretinal disease, Trans Ophthalmol Soc UK 104:123, 1985.

505. Sebag J, Balazs EA: Morphology and ultrastructure of human vitreous fibers, Invest Ophthalmol Vis Sci 30:1867, 1989.

506. Sebag J, Balazs EA, Eakins KE, et al: The effects of Na-Hyaluronate on prostaglandin synthesis and phagocytosis by mononuclear phagocytes in vitro, Invest Ophthalmol Vis Sci 20 (ARVO):33, 1981.

506b. Sebag, J, Buzney SM, Belyea DA, et al: Posterior vitreous detachment following panretinal laser photocoagulation, Graef Arch Klin Exp Ophthalmol 228:5,1990.

507. Sebag J, McMeel JW: Diabetic retinopathy—pathogenesis and role of retina-derived growth factor in angiogenesis, Surv Ophthalmol 30:377, 1986.

508. Sebag J, Reiser K, Buckingham B, et al: Non-enzymatic glycosylation of human vitreous collagen in proliferative diabetic retinopathy, Invest Ophthalmol Vis Sci 31(ARVO):127, 1990.

509. Sen A, Roy R, Mukherjee KL: Ascorbic acid concentration in developing human fetal vitreous humor, Ind J Ophthalmol 31:73, 1983.

510. Shaeffer RN: The role of vitreous detachment in a

phakic and malignant glaucoma, Trans Am Acad Ophthal Otoaryngol 58:217, 1954.

511. Shimakado K, Raines E, Madtes D, et al (1985): A significant part of macrophage-derived growth factor consists of at least two forms of kPDGF, Cell 43:277, 1985.

512. Shires TK, Faeth JA, Pulido JS: Non-enzymatic glycosylation of vitreous proteins in vitro and in the streptozotocin-treated diabetic rat, Retina 10:153, 1990.

513. Sidd RJ, Fine SL, Owens SL, et al: Idiopathic preretinal gliosis, Am J Ophthalmol 94:44, 1982.

514. Sigelman J: Vitreous base classification of retinal tears clinical application, Surv Ophthalmol 25:59, 1980.

515. Singh A, Paul SD, Singh K: A clinical study of the vitreous body in emmetropia and refractive errors, Orient Arch Ophthalmol 8:11, 1970.

516. Singh AK, Glaser BM, Lemor M, et al: Gravity-dependent distribution of retinal pigment epithelial cells dispersed into the vitreous cavity, Retina 6:77, 1986.

517. Sirek OV, Sirek A, Fikar K: The effect of sex hormones on glycosamingoglycan content of canine aorta and coronary arteries, Atherosclerosis 27:227, 1977.

518. Smiddy WE, Michels RG, de Bustros S, et al: Histopathology of tissue removed during vitrectomy for impending idiopathic macular holes, Am J Ophthalmol 108:360, 1989.

519. Smiddy WE, Michels RG, Glaser BM, et al: Vitrectomy for macular traction caused by incomplete vitreous separation, Arch Ophthalmol 106:624, 1988.

520. Smith D: Structure of the adult human vitreous humour, The Lancet 11:365, 1868.

521. Smith GN, Linsenmayer TF, Newsome DA: Synthesis of type II collagen in vitro by embryonic chick neural retina tissue, Proc Natl Acad Sci USA 73:4420, 1976.

522. Smith GN, Newsome DA: The nature and origin of the glycosaminoglycans of the embryonic chick vitreous body, Dev Biol 62:65, 1978.

523. Smith HL: Asteroid hyalitis—incidence of diabetes mellitus and hypercholesterolemia, JAMA 168:891, 1958.

524. Smith TJ: Dexamethasone regulation of glycosaminoglycan synthesis in cultured human skin fibroblasts—similar effects of glucocorticoid and thyroid hormones, J Clin Invest 74:2157, 1984.

525. Smith TJ, Murata Y, Horwitz AL, et al: Regulation of glycosaminoglycan synthesis by thyroid hormone *in vitro*, J Clin Invest 70:1066, 1982.

526. Snowden JM: The stabilization of *in vivo* assembled collagen fibrils by proteoglycans/glycosaminoglycans, Biochim Biophys Acta 703:21, 1982.

527. Snowden JM, Eyre DR, Swann DA: Age-related changes in the thermal stability and crosslinks of vitreous, articular cartilage and tendon collagens, Biochem Biophys Acta 706:153, 1982.

528. Snowden JM, Swann DA: Vitreous structure, V, The morphology and thermal stability of vitreous collagen fibers and comparison to articular cartilage (type II) collagen, Invest Ophthalmol Vis Sci 19:610, 1980.

529. Spencer LM, Foos RY: Paravascular vitreoretinal attachments: role in retinal tears, Arch Ophthalmol 84:557, 1970.

530. Spencer WH: Vitreous, in Spencer WH, ed: Ophthalmic pathology: an atlas and textbook, Philadelphia, WB Saunders, 1985, pp 548-588.

531. Spitznas M, Koch F, Phols I: Ultrastructural pathology of anterior persistent hyperplastic primary vitreous, Graef Arch Clin Exp Ophthalmol 228:487, 1990.

532. Sramek SJ, Wallow IH, Stevens TS, et al: Immunostaining of preretinal membranes for actin, fibronectin, and glial fibrillary acidic protein, Ophthalmol 96:835, 1980.

533. Stefansson E, Novack RL, Hatchell DL: Hypoxia in branch retinal vein occlusion is prevented by vitrectomy, Invest Ophthalmol Vis Sci 29(ARVO):220, 1988.

534. Steinmetz RL, Straatsma BR, Rubin ML: Posterior vitreous cyst, Am J Ophthalmol 109:295, 1990.

535. Stephens RJ, Richards RG: Vitreous humor chemistry—the use of potassium concentration for the prediction of the postmortem interval, J Forensic Sci 32:503, 1987.

536. Stickler GB, Belau PG, Farrell FJ, et al: Hereditary progressive arthroophthalmopathy, Mayo Clin Proc 40:443, 1965.

537. Stilling: Eine Studie über den Bau des Glaskörpers, Arch Ophthalmol 15, 1869 (as cited by Redslob[454]).

538. Stone RA, Laties AM, Raviola E, et al: Increase in retinal vasoactive intestinal polypeptide after eyelid fusion in primates, Proc Natl Acad Sci USA 85:257, 1988.

539. Stone RA, Lin T, Laties AM, et al: Retinal dopamine and form-deprivation myopia, Proc Natl Acad Sci USA 86:704, 1989.

540. Straatsma BR, Allen RA: Lattice degeneration of the retina, Trans Am Acad Ophthalmol Otolaryngol 66:600, 1962.

541. Streeten BA (1982): Disorders of the vitreous, in Garner A, Klintworth GK, eds: Pathobiology of ocular disease—a dynamic approach, New York, Basel, Marcel Dekker, 1982, part B, Ch 49, pp 1381-1419.

542. Streeten BW, Licari PA, Marucci AA, et al: Immunohistochemical comparison of ocular zonules and the microfibrils of elastic tissue, Invest Ophthalmol Vis Sci 21:130, 1981.

543. Stroemberg: Zur Frage nach dem Bau des Glaskörpers, Acta Soc Med Suecanae, vol 57, 1931 (as cited by Redslob[454]).

544. Stuart JM, Cremer MA, Dixit SN, et al: Collagen-induced arthritis in rats—comparison of vitreous and cartilage-derived collagens, Arthritis and Rheumatism 22:347, 1979.

545. Sturner WO, Dowdey ABC, Putnam RS, et al: Osmolality and other chemical determinations in postmortem human vitreous humor, J Forensic Sci 17:387, 1972.

546. Sugita G, Tauo Y, Machemer R, et al: Intravitreal autotransplantation of fibroblasts, Am J Ophthalmol 89:121, 1980.

547. Swann DA: On the integrity of vitreous structure, in Freeman HM, Hirose T, Schepens CL eds: Vitreous surgery and advances in fundus diagnosis and treatment, New York, Appleton-Century Crofts, 1977, p 3.

548. Swann DA: Chemistry and biology of vitreous body, Int Rev Exp Pathol 22:1, 1980.

549. Swann DA: Biochemistry of the vitreous, in Schepens CL, Neetens A, eds: The vitreous and vitreoretinal interface, New York, Springer-Verlag, 1987, pp 59-72.

550. Swann DA, Caulfield JB: Studies on hyaluronic acid, V, Relationship between the protein content and viscosity of rooster comb dermis hyaluronic acid, Conn Tiss Res 4:31, 1975.

551. Swann DA, Caulfield JB, Broadhurst JB: The altered fibrous form of vitreous collagen following solubilization with pepsin, Biochim Biophys Acta 427:365, 1976.

552. Swann DA, Chesney C, Constable IJ, et al: The role of vitreous collagen in platelet aggregation in vitro and in vivo, J Lab Clin Med 84:264, 1974.

553. Swann DA, Constable IJ: Vitreous structure, II, Role of hyaluronate, Invest Ophthalmol Vis Sci 11:164, 1972.

554. Swann DA, Constable IJ, Caulfield JB: Vitreous structure, IV, Chemical composition of the insoluble residual protein fraction from the rabbit vitreous, Invest Ophthalmol 14:613, 1975.

555. Swann DA, Sotman SS: The chemical composition of bovine vitreous-humour collagen fibres, Biochem J 185:545, 1980.

556. Sweeney DB, Balazs EA: Fate of collagen and hyaluronic acid gels and solutions injected into the vitreous of the owl monkey, Invest Ophthalmol 3:473, 1964.

557. Swift PGF, Worthy E, Emery JL: Biochemical state of the vitreous humour of infants at necropsy, Arch Dis Childhood 49:680, 1974.

558. Szent-Gyorgi, A: Untersuchungen über die Struktur des Glaskörpers des Menschen, Archiv F Mikroscop Anat 89:324, 1917.

559. Szilly A von: Zur Glaskörperfrage, eine vorlaufige Mitteilung, Anat Anz 24:417, 1904.

560. Szirmai JA, Balazs EA: Studies on the structure of the vitreous body, III, Cells in the cortical layer, AMA Arch Ophthalmol 59:34, 1958.

561. Takei Y, Smelser GK: Electron microscopic studies on zonular fibers, II, Changes of the zonular fibers after the treatment with collagenase, alpha-chymotrypsin and hyaluronidase, Alb v Graef Arch Clin Exp Ophthalmol 194:153, 1975.

562. Tanioka A, Jojima E, Miyasaka J, et al: Effect of water on the mechanical properties of collagen fibers, J Poly Sci 11:1489, 1973.

563. Reference deleted in proof.

564. Tasman WS: Posterior vitreous detachment and peripheral retinal breaks, Trans Am Acad Ophthalmol Otolaryngol 72:217, 1968.

565. Tasman WS: Diabetic vitreous hemorrhage and its relationship to hypoglycemia, Mod Probl Ophthal 20:413, 1979.

566. Taylor CM, Weiss JB: Partial purification of a 5.7 K glycoprotein from bovine vitreous which inhibits both angiogenesis and collagenase activity, Biochem Biophys Res Comm 133:911, 1985.

567. Teng CC: An electron microscopic study of cells in the vitreous of the rabbit eye, Part I, The macrophage, The Eye, Ear, Nose and Throat Monthly 48:91, 1969.

568. Teng CC, Chi HH: Vitreous changes and the mechanism of retinal detachment, Am J Ophthalmol 44:335, 1957.

569. Theodossiadis GP, Kousandrea CN: Avulsed retinal vessels with and without retinal breaks, Trans Ophthalmol Soc UK 104:887, 1985.

570. Theodossiadis GP, Velissawfopoulos P, Magouritsas N, et al: Behandling und Nachuntersuchung Von Net-

zhautrissen ohne Netzhautablosung mit den Riss uberlagerndem abgehobenem Netzhautgefass, Klin Monatsbl Augenheilkd 170:411, 1977.

571. Theopold DH, Faulborn J: Scanning electron microscopy of the vitreous body, Massive retraction after perforating injury, Graef Arch Clin Exp Ophthalmol 211:259, 1979.

572. Thompson JT, Nguygen-Tan JO, Hillstrom MM: The diffusion of tracers in isolated vitreous body, Invest Ophthalmol Vis Sci 29 (ARVO):222, 1988.

573. Tigges M, Tigges J, Fernandez A, et al: Postnatal axial eye elongation in normal and visually deprived rhesus monkeys, Invest Ophthalmol Vis Sci 31:1035, 1990.

574. Tokita M, Fujiya Y, Hikichi K: Dynamic viscoelasticity of bovine vitreous body, Biorheology 21:751, 1984.

575. Tokl A: Vergleichende Untersuchungen über den Bau und Entwicklung des Glasköpers und seinem Inhaltsgebilde bei Wirbeltieren and Menschen, (Thesis) Stockholm, Almquist Wiksell, 1927.

576. Toledo DMS, Dietrich CP: Tissue specific distribution of sulfated mucopolysaccharides in mammals, Biochim Biophys Acta 498:114, 1977.

577. Tolentino FI, Schepens CL, Freeman HM, et al: Vitreoretinal disorders, Philadelphia, WB Saunders, 1976.

578. Toole BP, Trelstad RL: Hyaluronate production and removal during corneal development in the chick, Dev Biol 26:28, 1971.

579. Topping TM, Abrams GW, Machemer R: Experimental double-perforating injury of the posterior segment in rabbit eyes, The natural history of intraocular perforation, Arch Ophthalmol 97:735, 1979.

580. Tornambe PE: Pneumatic retinopexy, Surv Ophthalmol 32:270, 1988.

581. Tsukamota Y, Heisel W, Wabl S: Macrophage production of fibronectin, a chemoattractant for fibroblasts, J Immunol 127:673, 1981.

582. Ueno N, Sebag J, Hirokawa H, et al: Effects of visible-light irradiation on vitreous structure in the presence of a photosensitizer, Exp Eye Res 44:863, 1987.

583. Uga A: Some structural features of the retinal Müllerian cells in the juxtaoptic nerve region, Exp Eye Res 19:105, 1974.

584. Ussman BH, Cleary PE, Blanks JC, et al: Morphologic evaluation of vitreous collagen after penetrating ocular injury, Curr Eye Res 3:395, 1984.

585. Ussman BH, Lazarides E, Ryan SJ: Traction retinal detachment, A cell-mediated event, Arch Ophthalmol 99:869, 1981.

586. Reference deleted in proof.

587. Van Alphen GWHM: On emmetropia and ametropia, Int J Ophthalmol 142:1, 579.

588. Van Bockxmeer FM, Martin CE, Constable IJ: Iron-binding proteins in vitreous humour, Biochim Biophys Acta 758:17, 1983.

589. Van der Rest M: Type IX collagen, in Structure and function of collagen types, New York, Academic Press, 1987, pp 195-221.

590. Vidaurri-Leal J, Hohman R, Glaser BM: Effect of vitreous on morphologic characteristics of retinal pigment epitheal cells—a new approach to the study of proliferative vitreoretinopathy, Arch Ophthalmol 102:1220, 1984.

591. Vinores SA, Campochiaro PA, Conway BP: Ultrastruc-

tural and electron-immunocytochemical characterization of cells in epiretinal membranes, Invest Ophthalmol Vis Sci 31:14, 1990.

592. Virchow H: Die morphologische Natur des Glaskörpergewebes, Der 17, Ophthalmol Gesellschaft, Heidelberg, Klin Monatsbl f Augenh, 1885 (as cited by Redslob[454]).

593. Virchow R: Notiz über den Glaskörper, Arch Pathol Anat Physiol 4:468, 1852.

594. Voerhoeff FH: Microscopic findings in a case of asteroid hyalitis, Am J Ophthalmol 4:155, 1921.

595. Voerhoeff FH: Are Moore's lightning streaks of serious portent, Am J Ophthalmol 41:837, 1956.

596. Von der Mark K: Localization of collagen types in tissues, Int Rev Connect Tissue Res 9:265, 1981.

597. Von Haller: Elementa physiologiae corporis humani, Lausanne, 1763 (as cited by Redslob[454]).

598. Von Noorden GK, Crawford MCJ: Lid closure and refractive error in macaque monkeys, Nature 272:53, 1978.

599. Von Pappenheim A: Die Spezielle Gewebelehre des Auges, 1842, pp 179-184 (as cited by Redslob[454]).

600. Von Pflug KA: Mome wege zur Enforschung der Lehrever der Akkommodation; der Glaskörper in akkommodierenen Auge, Arch Ophthalmol 133:545, 1935.

601. Walker F, Patrick RS: Constituent monosaccharides and hexosamine concentration of normal vitreous humor, Exp Eye Res 6:227, 1967.

602. Wallman J, Gottlieb MD, Rajaram R, et al: Local retinal regions control local eye growth and myopia, Science 237:73, 1987.

603. Wallow IHL, Stevens TS, Greaser ML, et al: Actin filaments in contracting preretinal membranes, Arch Ophthalmol 102:1370, 1984.

604. Wallow IHL, Tso MOM: Proliferation of the retinal pigment epithelium over malignant choroidal tumor, Am J Ophthalmol 73:914, 1972.

605. Wasano T, Hirokawa H, Tagewa H, et al: Asteroid hyalosis posterior vitreous detachment and diabetic retinopathy, Am J Ophthalmol 19:255, 1987.

606. Wassilewa P, Hockwin O, Korte I: Glycogen concentration changes in retina, vitreous body and other eye tissues caused by disturbances of blood circulation, Graef Arch Clin Exp Ophthalmol 199:115, 1976.

607. Watzke RC: The ophthalmoscopic sign "white with pressure"—a clinicopathologic correlation, Arch Ophthalmol 66:812, 1961.

608. Weber H, Landuehr G, Kilp H, et al: Mechanical properties of the vitreous in pig and human donor eyes, Ophthlamol Res 14:335, 1982.

609. Webster EH, Silver AF, Gonsalves NI: Histochemical analysis of extracellular matrix material in embryonic mouse lens morphogenesis, Dev Biol 100:147, 1983.

610. Weisel TN, Raviola E: Myopia and eye enlargement after neonatal lid fusion in monkeys, Nature 266:66, 1977.

611. Weiss H: The carbohydrate reserve in the vitreous body and retina of the rabbit eye during and after pressure ischaemia and insulin hypoglycemia, Ophthalm Res 3:360, 1972.

612. Weller M, Heimann K, Wiedemann P: Demonstration of mononuclear phagocytes in a human epiretinal membrane using a monoclonal anti-human macrophage antibody, Alb V Graef Arch Clin Exp Ophthalmol 226:252, 1988.

613. Wiedemann P, Ryan SJ, Novak P, et al: Vitreous stimulates proliferation of fibroblasts and retinal pigment epithelial cells, Exp Eye Res 41:619, 1985.

614. Wiederhielm CA, Black LL: Osmotic interaction of plasma proteins with interstitial macromolecules, Am J Physiol 231:638, 1976.

615. Wiesinger AM, et al: The transmission of light through the ocular media of the rabbit eye, Am J Ophthalmol 42:907, 1956.

616. Wildsoet CF, Pettigrew JD: Lid-suture induced myopia in chickens is not dependent upon ganglion cell activity, Invest Ophthalmol Vis Sci 30:31, 1989.

617. Reference deleted in proof.

618. Williams DF, Burke JM: Modulation of growth in retina-derived cells by extracellular matrices, Invest Ophthalmol Vis Sci 31:1717, 1990.

619. Williams RN, Patterson CA, Eakins KE, et al: Ascorbic acid inhibits the activity of polymorphonuclear leukocytes in inflamed ocular tissue, Exp Eye Res 39:261, 1984.

620. Winthrop SR, Cleary PE, Minckler DS, et al: Penetrating eye injuries—a histopathological review, Br J Ophthalmol 64:809, 1980.

621. Wise GN: Relationship of idiopathic preretinal macular fibrosis to posterior vitreous detachment, Am J Ophthalmol 79:358, 1975.

622. Wise GM, Dollery CT, Henkind P: The retinal circulation, New York, Harper & Row, 1971, p 403.

623. Wiznia RA: Posterior vitreous detachment and idiopathic preretinal macular gliosis, Am J Ophthalmol 102:196, 1986.

624. Wolf E, Gardiner JS: Studies on the scatter of light in the dioptric media of the eye as a basis of visual glare, Arch Ophthalmol 74:338, 1965.

625. Wolter JR: Pores in the internal limiting membrane of the human retina, Acta Ophthalmologica 42:971, 1964.

626. Wolter JR, Flaherty NW: Persistent hyperplastic vitreous, Am J Ophthalmol 47:491, 1959.

627. Wong D, Restori M: Ultrasonic Doppler studies of the vitreous, Eye 2:87, 1988.

628. Wong HC, Schmiks H, McLeod D: Abortive neovascular outgrowths discovered during vitrectomy for diabetic vitreous haemorrhage, Graef Arch Clin Exp Ophthalmol 227:237, 1989.

629. Wong VG, McFarlin DE: Primary familial amyloidosis, Arch Ophthalmol 78:208, 1967.

630. Worst JGF: Cisternal systems of the fully developed vitreous body in the young adult, Trans Ophthalmol Soc U.K. 97:550, 1977.

631. Reference deleted in proof.

632. Xiong H, Cheng H-M: Change of vitreous tonicity in "sugar" cataracts, Invest Ophthalmol Vis Sci 29 (ARVO):149, 1988.

633. Yamada E: Some structural features of the fovea centralis in the human retina, Arch Ophthalmol 82:151, 1969.

634. Yamashita H, Hori S: A new model of neovascularization caused by tractional force, Invest Ophthalmol Vis Sci 29 (ARVO):177, 1988.

635. Reference deleted in proof.

636. Yannas IV: Collagen and gelatin in the solid state, J Macromol Sci Rev Macromol Chem CF:49, 1972.

637. Yanoof M, Rahn ED, Zimmerman LE: Histopathology of juvenile retinoschisis, Arch Ophthalmol 79:49, 1968.

638. Yinnon U: Myopia induction in animals following alteration of the visual input during development—a review, Curr Eye Res 3:677, 1984.

639. Young RA: The ground substance of connective tissue, J Physiol 16:325, 1894.

640. Young RG, Williams HH: Biochemistry of the eye—gelatinous protein of the vitreous body, Arch Ophthalmol 51:593, 1954.

641. Yu SY, Blumenthal HT: The calcification of elastic tissue, in Wagner BM, Smith DE, eds: The connective tissue, Baltimore, Williams & Wilkins, 1967 pp 17-49.

642. Zhu ZR, Goodnight R, Sorgente N, et al: Cellullar proliferation induced by subretinal injection of vitreous in the rabbit, Arch Ophthalmol 106:406, 1988.

643. Zimmerman LE, Straatsma BR: Anatomic relationships of the retina to the vitreous body and to the pigment epithelium, in Schepens CL, ed: Importance of the vitreous body in retina surgery with special emphasis on reoperation, St. Louis, CV Mosby, 1960, pp 15-28.

644. Zimmerman RL: *In vivo* measurements of the viscoelasticity of the human vitreous humor, Biophys J 29:539, 1980.

645. Zinn: Descriptio anatomica oculi humani, Göttingen, 1780 (as cited by Redslob[454]).

The Lens

CHRISTOPHER A. PATERSON, Ph.D., D.Sc.
NICHOLAS A. DELAMERE, Ph.D.

The crystalline lens of the eye is positioned behind the iris with its posterior aspect embedded in the vitreous body (Fig. 10-1). The lens plays a passive role in the process of accommodation by which light rays, which have passed through the cornea and aqueous humor, are focused upon the retina. It is the remarkable transparency of the lens that allows it to play this important role in normal vision. Apart from its transparency, the lens has several other special features. The lens, even at birth, is completely without blood supply and has no innervation; the lens grows in size and weight throughout life, since no cells are shed. The mass of lens cells, at various stages of development and maturation, is completely surrounded by an elastic acellular capsule that has a smooth outer surface.

The molecular makeup of the lens is also unique in that it is two-thirds water with one-third protein; other constituents represent only about 1% of the total lens wet weight. This high protein content is necessary for the lens to have a high refractive index, allowing it to bend light rays into focus onto the retina.

The metabolism of the lens is directed entirely toward the maintenance of transparency. A particularly intriguing aspect of lens metabolism is the role of an extensive system of low-resistance junctions between all the cellular components of the lens. These low-resistance gap junctions allow the lens to function as a syncytium, permitting more efficient exchange between the dense interior lens and its surroundings.

Since the lens does not shed any of its cells, all the cellular components from embryonic development onward are retained. The older cells of the lens, which are displaced toward the center of the lens, experience aging; consequently, there are a considerable number of post-translational molecular changes that take place in the lens throughout life. With aging, the lens often loses some of its transparency. When transparency is reduced to the point where visual acuity is impaired, the condition of cataract exists. Cataract is also associated with a number of other clinical conditions (such as diabetes) and environmental stresses (such as radiation).

The purpose of this chapter is to provide an overview of the lens in terms of its development, structure, biochemistry, physiology, and the mechanisms thought to lead to cataract. Adequate reference is given to more extensive texts

ACKNOWLEDGMENTS

We thank Elizabeth Paterson for outstanding editorial assistance and preparation of the manuscript. Dr. Ziad Husseini assisted in the development of several sections of this chapter. Support for preparing this manuscript was derived from USPHS research grant EY06916, The Kentucky Lions Eye Research Foundation, and an unrestricted award from Research to Prevent Blindness.

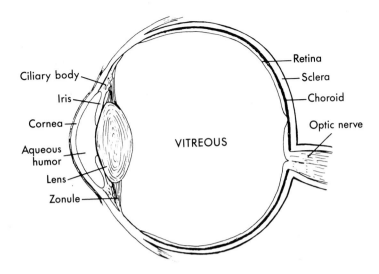

FIG. 10-1   Diagrammatic section of the human eye.

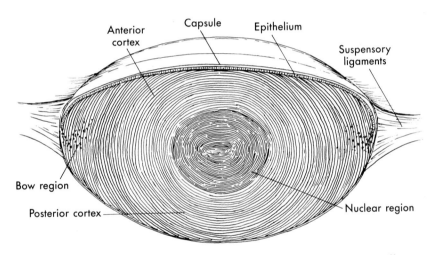

FIG. 10-2   Diagram of section through the lens. (Redrawn from Lerman,[150] p 72.)

for those readers who wish to explore the lens in greater detail.

STRUCTURE OF THE LENS
Overview

At birth the transparent human lens is already devoid of blood supply and innervation. Composed entirely of epithelial cells at various stages of maturation and enveloped in an acellular capsule, the lens is held in place by fine zonules running from the ciliary body and inserting into the capsule. The lens is also stabilized by contact with the vitreous body. Perpetual cell division in the outer equatorial zone of the lens gives rise to epithelial cells that differentiate into long fiber cells reaching toward the anterior and posterior poles of the lens. As a result of further cell division and fiber development, lens fibers are displaced toward the center of the lens to form the nuclear region. Cells in the outer region of the lens form the cortex. The end result is a tightly packed mass of lens fiber cells with a single layer of relatively cuboidal epithelium at the anterior surface just below the capsule (Fig. 10-2).

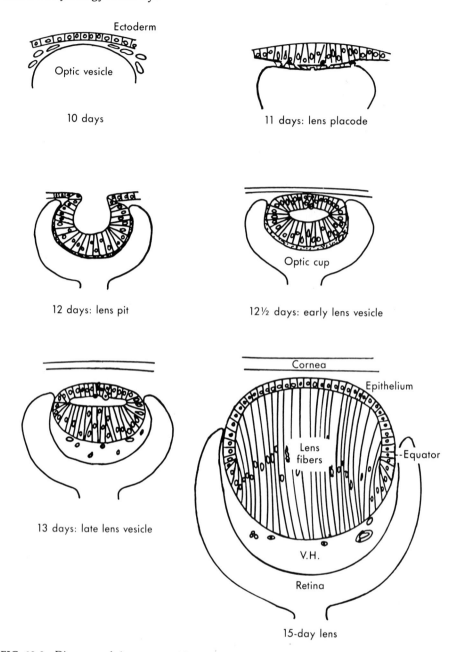

Ectoderm

Optic vesicle

10 days

11 days: lens placode

12 days: lens pit

Optic cup

12½ days: early lens vesicle

13 days: late lens vesicle

Cornea

Epithelium

Lens
fibers

Equator

V.H.

Retina

15-day lens

FIG. 10-3 Diagram of the stages of lens morphogenesis in the rat (V.H., vitreous humor). (From McAvoy,[170] p 16.)

Embryology

The vertebrate lens develops from the head ectoderm overlying the optic vesicle (Fig. 10-3). Comprehensive discussions of lens morphogenesis have been written by several authors.[145,163,170,244] At the 4 mm stage in human embryos the association between the surface ectoderm and the optic vesicle induces the development of the lens plate, or placode, as the cells of the optic vesicle elongate. By the 5 mm stage the lens placode begins to invaginate, forming the lens pit. The optic vesicle also invaginates, forming the optic cup in which the embryonic lens sits. The lens pit further invaginates and finally separates from the ectoderm to form the lens vesicle at the 9 mm stage. The cells in the posterior portion of the lens vesicle elongate to fill the vesicle; the elongated cells are the primary lens fibers. Eventually the primary lens fibers lose their nuclei and subsequently become the embryonic nucleus of the adult lens. Meanwhile, the cells in the anterior part of the vesicle continue to divide actively and become elongated, forming the secondary lens fibers. The secondary lens fibers elongate toward the anterior and posterior poles of the embryonic lens surrounding the embryonic nucleus. The equatorial zone of the lens epithelium continues to divide throughout life, producing the cells that differentiate into the long lens fibers.

While the cellular development of the lens is taking place, the lens capsule is also formed. At the 9 to 10 mm stage, a thin basal lamina is synthesized, representing the embryonic lens capsule. The embryonic lens is also surrounded by blood vessels, the tunica vasculosa lentis. This vascular supply is most prominent at the 60 mm stage and is designed to meet the nutritional demands of the developing lens. At about the 240 mm stage the vascular system regresses and it is absent shortly before birth, leaving the lens without a blood supply for the rest of its life.

The fine suspensory ligaments that support the lens (see Fig. 10-2), the zonules of Zinn, are seen at the 65 mm stage, when the ciliary body and iris develop from the optic vesicle. The zonules develop from the neuroepithelium, running from the inner surface of the ciliary body and fusing into the lens capsule.

The factors that govern lens morphogenesis have been the subject of interest for many years. In fact, the lens has been used as a model for the study of inductive mechanisms in developmental biology. A number of excellent reviews of lens induction have been written.[47,170,244] Recent studies have suggested the involvement of specific chemical factors in lens development. Recent studies by Chamberlain et al.[34] indicate that fibroblastic growth factor (FGF) might play an important role in lens differentiation. Also, Beebe et al.[9] found that lentropin, later identified as insulinlike growth factor, enhanced events in fiber differentiation.

Several forms of cataract result from an aberration of lens development; congenital cataracts are thoroughly discussed elsewhere.[47,214]

Lens growth and physical characteristics

One of the unique features of the lens is that it continues to grow throughout life as the germinative zone of the epithelium divides and new lens fibers are laid down. The pattern of lens growth can be readily appreciated both in terms of increasing weight and alterations in overall dimensions. The thickness of the human lens increases by 0.02 mm each year, although there is considerable variation in lens thickness among individuals.[32,255] Female lenses appear to be slightly thicker than male lenses, but Harding et al.[111] have published data indicating that male lenses are heavier than female lenses by about 8%. Figure 10-4 shows the growth of the lens based on the findings of Scammon and Hesdorffer[218] and of Brown.[32] The anterior-posterior diameter of the lens ranges from 3.5 mm in the newborn to 5 mm in nonagenarians. The equatorial diameter in the infant is about 6.5 mm, increasing to 9 mm in the mid-teenage years with little further increase. The anterior surface of the human lens has less curvature than the posterior surface; the radius of curvature anteriorly is from 8 to 14 mm, while posteriorly it is 4.5 to 7.5 mm. All of these cited values depend greatly on the measurement techniques and the state of accommodation of the lens. Useful reviews of lens dimensions are written by Rafferty[208] and Weekers et al.[254]

Since the role of the lens is to focus light upon the retina, it is important to consider its refractive power. The refractive power of the lens is related to two factors, the curvature of the anterior and posterior surfaces and the refractive index of the lens material itself. The refractive

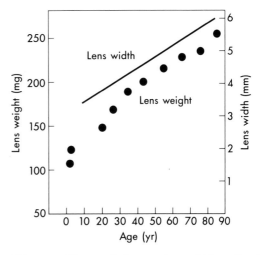

FIG. 10-4 Changes in human lens width and weight from birth to 90 years of age. (Data taken from Scammon and Hesdorffer[218] and Brown.[31])

index of the lens is higher than that of 1.336 determined in both the aqueous and vitreous humor;[146] Lerman reports that the average refractive index of the lens is 1.420.[150] Bettleheim, who gives an excellent description of the optical properties of the lens,[16] determined that at the surface of the lens the refractive index is higher in the central anterior part. Thus the part of the lens surface that has the least curvature apparently compensates by having the highest refractive index.

Microscopic structure

The lens can be readily separated into distinct morphologic regions: the acellular capsule, the lens epithelium, and the lens fiber cells of the outer cortex and inner nuclear zone (see Fig. 10-2). In-depth descriptions of the ultrastructure of the lens are available in several texts.[120,162,208]

Capsule

The lens capsule is an acellular and elastic structure that contains the growing mass of developing and differentiating lens cells. The inner surface of the anterior capsule is in immediate contact with the lens epithelium, while at the posterior region it contacts the most superficial lens fiber cells. The capsule is analogous to basement membrane and stains positively with periodic acid-Schiff's reagent; it is the thickest basement membrane in the body.[97] The principal composition of the capsule is type IV collagen together with about 10% glycosaminoglycans.[70,197,236] The capsule is synthesized by the epithelium and most superficial lens fiber cells at the posterior.[266] The rate of capsular growth appears to differ at the anterior and posterior lens surface;[181,208] synthesis of capsular material at the posterior surface appears to cease earlier in life. For example, the studies of Fisher and Wakely,[79] using rabbits, showed that holes placed in the capsule of 2-month-old rabbits remained open even at 3 years after the injury; a similar injury placed in the anterior capsule healed rapidly.

Electron microscopy of the capsule shows a fibrillar structure with the outer layers appearing more dense, referred to as the zonular lamella. Zonules, running from the ciliary processes, fuse into the outer layer of the capsule (Fig. 10-5). The zonular fibers are very similar in structure and composition to the elastic microfibrils described in other tissues.[234]

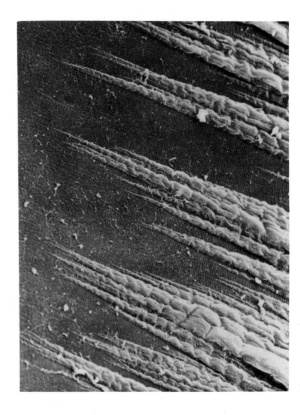

FIG. 10-5 Scanning electron micrograph showing bundles of zonular fibers tapering to their points as they insert into the dark anterior lens capsule (× 780). (From Streeten BW: Invest Ophthalmol Vis Sci 16:364, 1977.)

The capsule is freely permeable to low-molecular-weight compounds but restricts the movement of larger colloidal material.[85] The main function of the capsule then is to mold the shape of the lens in response to the tension on the zonules, which is altered during the process of accommodation.

Epithelium

The lens epithelium can be functionally divided into two zones. The cells located in the equatorial zone are those that actively divide and differentiate into lens cell fibers.[170] The remaining epithelium, which does not normally divide, plays an important role in transporting a variety of solutes between the lens and the aqueous humor; it also secretes the capsular material. These nondividing epithelial cells are some 5.5 to 8.0 μm high and 7 to 11 μm wide.[120] Electron microscopic studies show rich interdigitation of the lateral surfaces (Fig. 10-6). In a flat mount preparation the epithelial cells appear generally hexagonal in shape. The actively dividing cells in the equatorial zone are more cylindrical in cross-section and show less complex interdigitation (Fig. 10-6). All the cells of the epithelium are nucleated and the cytoplasm contains ribosomes, smooth and rough endoplasmic reticulum, Golgi figures, mitochondria, centrioles, and numerous vesicular structures.[120,208] The presence of key enzymes has also been demonstrated in the lens epithelium by cytochemical methods.[117] The sodium pump enzyme, Na,K-ATPase, is present at the lateral and apical surface membranes.[180,242]

There are several junctional relationships between the cells of the lens epithelium. The lateral and apical aspects of the plasma membranes have desmosomes for cell adhesion. It is not clear whether the epithelium is an effective barrier to the diffusion of solutes between aqueous humor and the lens fibers. From their observations of diffusion of tracer molecules between the epithelial cells, Gorthy et al.[96] and Rae and Stacey[207] drew the conclusion that the epithelial sheet is not a tight barrier. However, in a more recent study, Lo and Harding[157] suggested that there were zonulae occludentes between epithelial cells in both the frog and human lens and that these junctions could restrict the passage of high-molecular-weight solutes between the cells. There are, however, low-resistance gap

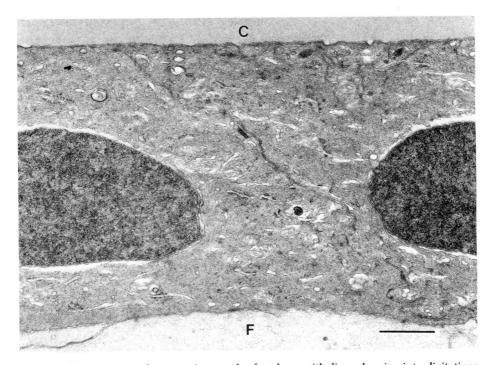

FIG. 10-6 Transmission electron micrograph of rat lens epithelium showing interdigitations between lateral cell membranes, particularly evident at the basal end. C = capsule; F = fiber cells; bar represents 1 μm. (Courtesy of W.-K. Lo.)

junctions between the epithelial cells allowing for cell-to-cell communication (see review by Kistler and Bullivant[143]). There may also be a small number of gap junctions between the lens epithelial cells and the underlying lens fibers, although these may be different from junctions between fiber cells.[30] By electron microscopy, gap junctions appear as regions of narrowed intercellular space; the normal intercellular space is some 15 to 20 nm, whereas in the region of the gap junction the space is reduced to 2 to 4 nm. There is also physiologic evidence for cell-to-cell communication in that dyes rapidly pass between adjacent epithelial cells.[173]

It should be evident to the most casual observer that the metabolic and synthetic activity of the lens epithelium must be critical for the survival of the entire lens.

Cortex

The differentiation of epithelial cells in the equatorial zone into adult lens cell fibers is accompanied by myriad molecular and structural changes. The newly formed lens cell elongates, with one end of the cell moving anteriorly and the other end moving toward the posterior (Fig. 10-7). As the fiber elongates, it becomes hexagonal in cross-section, ultimately becoming a lens fiber cell some 8 to 12 mm long at maturity (Fig. 10-8). These fiber cells are some 10 μ wide and 4.5 μ thick. The ends of each fiber meet the ends of similarly elongated fibers at the anterior and posterior regions of the lens, giving rise to a pattern called suture lines (Fig. 10-9). Thus a new lens fiber will have its center at the equator and its ends reaching toward the anterior and posterior poles of the lens. The development of lens suture pattern is discussed in depth elsewhere.[120]

In a specialization apparently directed toward the transparency of the lens cortex and nucleus, mature lens fibers do not have the normal cellular organelles such as nuclei and mitochondria. Only the young, most superficial lens fibers still contain cytoplasmic inclusions similar to those of epithelial cells. With time, as these fi-

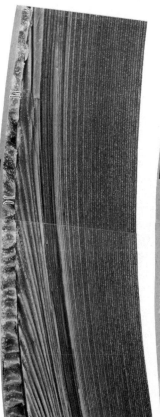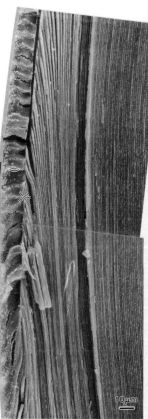

FIG. 10-7   SEM photomicrograph montage of the epithelial-fiber cell interface, the EFI, between pre-germinative (squiggly brackets), germinative (square brackets) and early transitional zone cells, and late transitional cells' (meridional rows; curved brackets) and the onset of fiber cells' elongation at the bow region (asterisk) in a juvenile frog lens. In this montage the upper portion of the figure on the right is a continuation of the lower portion of the figure on the left ($\times$ 780). (Courtesy of J. Kuszak.)

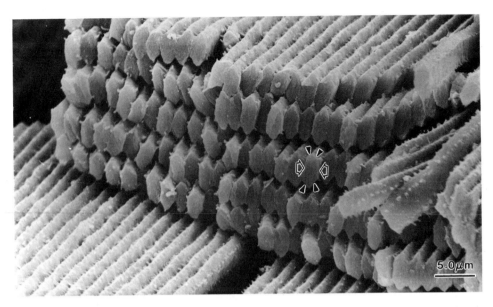

FIG. 10-8   Scanning electron micrograph showing the characteristic hexagonal cross sectional profiles of vertebrate lens fiber cells. (Courtesy J. Kuszak.)

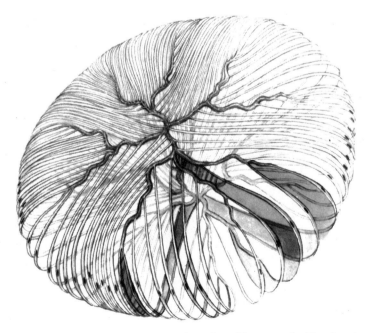

FIG. 10-9   Pattern of lens sutures resulting from lens fiber growth. The drawing shows the suture line in a single plane, but it should be noted that the suture extends throughout the thickness of the lens cortex and nucleus. (From Hogan, Alvarado, and Weddell,[120] p 642.)

bers mature and are displaced toward the center of the lens, the nucleus and other organelles disintegrate, leaving the lens fiber cells with a cytoplasm that is very low in particulate inclusions. This time-dependent loss of the nucleus as cells move toward the center of the lens creates a pattern of nuclei, seen in whole lens histological section, called the lens bow. At the same time that cytoplasmic organelles are lost, there is an increase of fibrillar material within the cell. The change in lens cell shape and displacement is accompanied by marked alteration in the pattern of lens protein synthesis. As will be discussed later, certain proteins are synthesized only in the lens fibers while other proteins are found in both the epithelium and the lens fibers. With maturation and aging of the lens fibers, the proteins undergo considerable posttranslational changes.

Microscopic studies show that within the lens cortex the long hexagon-shaped cells are densely packed, with an extracellular space of only about 20 nm. Transmission and scanning electron microscope studies show considerable interdigitation between lens fibers (Fig. 10-10).[144,149,208] Fibers lying most superficially have fingerlike projections into adjacent fibers. As the fibers move further into the lens, the interdigitations attain a ball-and-socket configuration. Those fibers lying more deeply in the lens also show an arrangement of ridges. There is no doubt that these interdigitations serve to stabilize the cells of the lens during accommodation.

Another unique feature of the lens is the extensive system of low-resistance gap junctions between the lens fiber cells. The dense packing of lens fibers connected by low-resistance gap junctions allows the tissue to function like a syncytium rather than a collection of individual cells. This arrangement has considerable impact on the metabolism and physiology of the tissue.

In some regions of the lens gap junctions account for some 30 to 60% of the plasma membrane surface[80] compared to only 3 to 4% as observed in most tissues (Fig. 10-11). The abundance of gap junctions in the lens reflects the need to enhance communication between the very large bulk of cells in the interior of the lens and the relatively tiny number of metabolically active cells at the lens surface. The morphologic characteristics of gap junctions can be

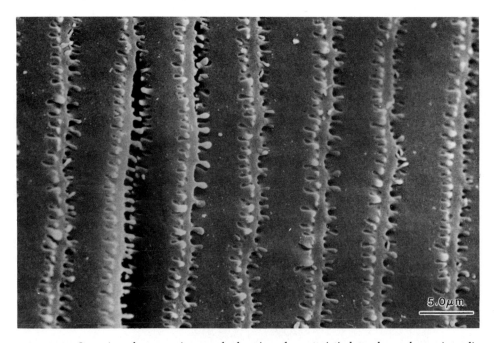

FIG. 10-10 Scanning electron micrograph showing characteristic lateral membrane interdigitations that arise at the acute angles formed by broad and narrow faces of lens fiber cells, and their complementary imprint made on adjacent cells. The lateral interdigitations are regularly arrayed along the entire length of lens fiber cells. (Courtesy J. Kuszak.)

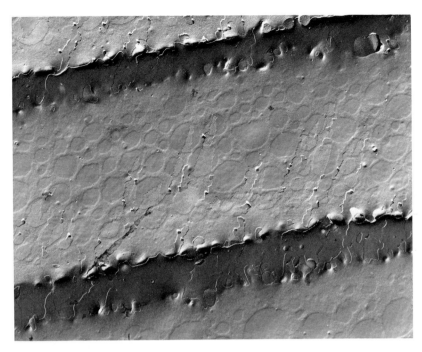

FIG. 10-11 Scanning electron micrograph demonstrating extensive distribution of gap junctions on surface of rat lens cortical fiber cells × 270,000. (From FitzGerald et al,[80] p 1204.)

seen clearly with both conventional transmission electron microscopy and freeze-fracture techniques. The outer surface of one cell has a pattern of fine particles while the opposing membrane surface has a corresponding pattern of pits (Fig. 10-12). Typically, lens fiber junctions show disordered arrays of particles within the junctional plaques, signifying that the junctions might allow the cell-cell communication apparent from dye diffusion and electrophysiologic studies of the lens.[206] In general, increased levels of calcium and hydrogen ions can close gap junctions,[192] and indeed calcium ions have been reported to influence lens fiber gap junctions.[193] However, it has been postulated that the crystallization of lens fiber junctions may be related to calcium-activated proteolysis of the gap junction protein.[143]

While there are distinct differences between the fiber-fiber junctions of the lens and gap junctions found in other tissues (see Kistler and Bullivant[143]) it has been shown that the major intrinsic membrane protein of the lens, MIP, is able to form channels in liposomes[94,193] and lipid bilayers.[267] Although this appears to be convincing evidence that the 26 kDa protein MIP may be the lens "gap junction protein," other membrane proteins such as MP70 have also been identified as possible components of fiber-fiber junctions.[143,144] Furthermore, the lack of homology between MIP and gap junction proteins in other tissues, together with differences in the dimensions of the fiber-fiber junctions, has led Ehring and his colleagues to propose that intercellular communication via MIP may take place by a mechanism that is quite distinct from the communication via gap junctions of other tissues.[77]

Nucleus

At the very center of the lens are those cells that formed the embryonic lens. The cells of the nuclear region of the lens have therefore been retained throughout life and have consequently experienced aging. The retention of cells within the lens from embryogenesis to death has attracted considerable attention of scientists wishing to study aging. As will become apparent later in this chapter, significant molecular changes take place as the lens cells mature and become displaced toward the center of the lens. Nevertheless, the cells in the nuclear region retain plasma membranes (Fig. 10-13) with physiologic integrity, even though the metabolism of the older lens cells is quite minimal.

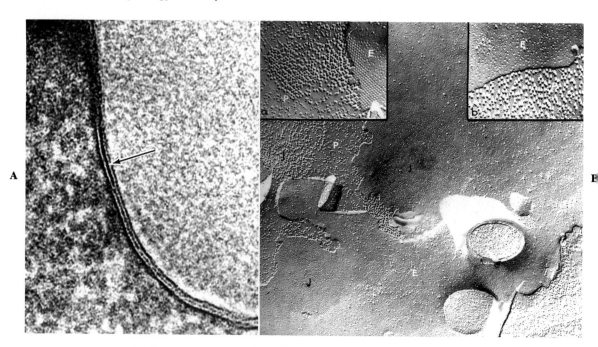

FIG. 10-12   **A,** Thin section profile of a junction between lens fiber cells fixed in the presence of lanthanum hydroxide. Lanthanum stain is seen between the two junctional membranes *(arrow),* showing the existence of an extracellular gap × 270,000. **B,** Freeze fracture replica of calf lens fiber junctions (*J*). The junctions contain loose and disordered particle arrays. Most, but not all, particles fracture with the protoplasmic leaflet (*P*). Inset A shows a typical gap junction of the lens surface epithelium. E = face E × 90,000; insets × 160,000. (From Peracchia et al,[193] pp 1156-1157.)

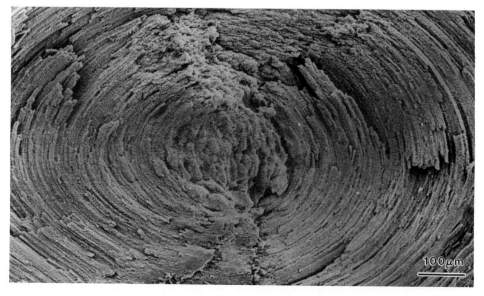

FIG. 10-13   Scanning electron micrograph showing the embryonic nuclear lens fiber cells from an 80-plus-year-old human lens. Note that while these lens fiber cells are among the most senescent cells of the body, they are still essentially intact. (Courtesy of J. Kuszak.)

Cytoskeleton

The structural framework of lens cells, as in other tissues, is composed of cytoskeleton, a complex system of intracellular filaments. The components of the cytoskeleton of the lens are listed in Table 10-1. One of the components, beaded-chain filaments, is unique to the lens. A full description of the current understanding of lens cytoskeleton is available from several sources.[1,12,208]

Actin is found in a soluble form and the polymerized form that constitutes the filaments. Actin microfilaments are about 5 nm in diameter; the polypeptide component of actin has a molecular weight of about 42 kDa. The microfilaments are thought to contribute to the maintenance of lens shape during accommodation. Stress fibers in the lens also contain actin; these structures are seen in cells migrating during wound repair in the lens.[95]

The intermediate filaments, composed of vimentin, have a diameter in the range of 7 to 11 nm. Vimentin has a molecular weight of 57 kDa. The role of intermediate filaments is not known at present, but they are found only in the epithelium and outer cortex of the lens. Microtubules are similarly limited to the epithelium and outer cortex and have a diameter of about 25 nm. The microtubules are a complex structure containing two subunits of tubulin with a molecular weight of approximately 50 kDa. Microtubules are thought to be involved in developmental events and also the maintenance of lens cell shape.

Beaded-chain filaments consist of globular proteins, 12 to 15 nm in diameter, attached to a backbone filament 7 to 9 nm in diameter. These are only found in the cortex and nucleus and are thought to be primarily associated with the integrity of the cell membrane.

A number of changes take place in the cytoskeleton of the lens with aging and cataract development. For example, there is almost complete loss of vimentin intermediate filaments in the lens cortex and nucleus in old age. Also, it has recently been shown that oxidative stress can result in damage to the cytoskeleton.[201]

Cataract morphology

The beautiful architecture of the lens undergoes considerable disruption in the process of cataract development.

Obviously there are a great many types of cataracts, and it follows that the range of morphologic changes is quite diverse. The disruption in cellular architecture, seen in the cataractous lens at both the light and electron microscopic level, is reviewed in detail elsewhere.[107,263] Harding and his associates, using scanning and transmission electron microscopy, also documented the cellular damage that takes place during cataract formation (Fig. 10-14). They took their studies one step further by correlating the structural changes with alterations in composition determined by energy dispersive x-ray analysis.[107] Since transparency of the lens depends greatly upon the cellular arrangement, it is not difficult to understand why such structurally damaged tissue loses its transparency.

TABLE 10-1 Cytoskeletal Components and Proteins of Lens Cells*

Cytoskeletal component	Cytoskeletal protein
Microfilaments	Actin
Intermediate-sized filaments	Vimentin
Microtubules	Tubulin
Beaded-chain filaments	Backbone protein
Stress fibers†	Myosin, α-actinin, tropomyosin
Membrane skeleton	Spectrin

*From Alcala and Maisel,[1] p 197.
†Also contain actin.

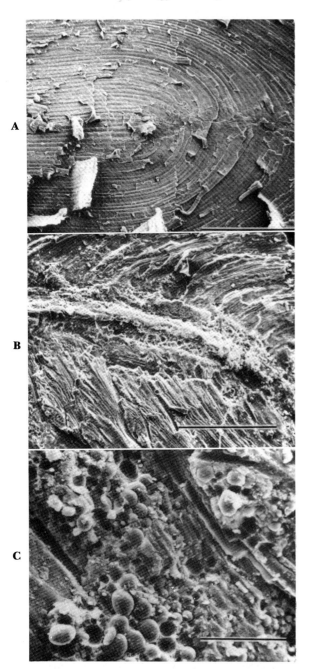

FIG. 10-14   A, Normal structure of suture system (bar = 200 μm). **B**, Abnormal suture system in cataractous lens (bar = 250 μm). **C**, Extensive cellular breakdown (at higher magnification) at the suture region (bar = 30 μm). (From Harding et al,[107] p 372.)

COMPOSITION OF THE LENS

Compared to most other tissues, the lens has a particularly high protein content and a low water content, as shown below. The high protein concentration is necessary for the lens to maintain a high refractive index. Protein accounts for over one third of the lens, the remaining two thirds being water. The other constituents of the lens, including lipids, amino acids, electrolytes and a variety of peptides and carbohydrates, account for only about 1% of the lens wet weight. The lens also contains many trace elements,[75,237] some of which have been carefully studied in the lens.[13,101–104]

Composition of the lens

Water	66% of wet weight
Protein	33% of wet weight
Sodium	17 mEq per kg lens water
Chloride	30 mEq per kg lens water
Potassium	125 mEq per kg lens water
Calcium	0.4 mEq per kg lens water
Glucose	1.0 mM
Lactic acid	14.0 mM
Gluthatione	12.0 mM
Ascorbic acid	1.6 mM
Inositol	5.9 mM
Lipids	28 mg/g wet weight

The constituents of the lens are discussed later in this chapter in the context of the biochemistry and physiology of the lens.

The pH of the lens has been measured by intracellular ion-sensitive microelectrodes[7] to yield a value of 6.9, which is in excellent agreement with the value determined by NMR studies.[100] Relatively little is known about the regulation of lens pH, but because of its high protein content, the lens should have considerable buffering capacity.

TRANSPARENCY

The sheer bulk of the lens and its high content of protein would seem to make it an unlikely candidate for transparency. Nevertheless, in order to focus an image on the retina, the lens, in addition to being highly refractile, must obviously be transparent. The theory and physical basis of transparency has attracted the attention of mathematicians and biophysicists for a long time, dating back to Brewster in 1816.[26] Over the years a number of explanations for transparency have unfolded. These have been dealt with in detail by Benedek[11] and Bettelheim.[16]

The transparency of the lens is largely the result of the highly ordered arrangement of the macromolecular components of the lens cells and the small differences in refractive index between light-scattering components. The regular arrangement of lens fibers is also important to transparency, and Kuszak et al.[148] have proposed that the arrangement of fibers depends strongly on the ability of newly formed cells to elongate in a pattern that corresponds with the underlying cells. The predominantly lamellar, rather than helical, conformation of lens proteins might also contribute to lens transparency. In 1962 Trokel[240] proposed that the even distribution of proteins and regularity of lens structure alone could account for lens transparency; however, in 1971[11] Benedek showed that transparency could be accounted for if changes in refractive index occurred over distances less than the wavelength of light. In a model of uniform light scattering Bettelheim[16] demonstrated that light scattering is markedly reduced by destructive interference. Delaye and Tardieu[65,238] studied small-angle x-ray scattering in calf lens cortex and also concluded that the short-range order of crystallins in the lens contributed to transparency.

The normal lens is not perfectly transparent but scatters about 5% of the light falling upon it. Over half of this light scattering is due to lens cell membranes. Although the cell membranes represent a volume fraction of only 0.05, their refractive index is considerably higher than that of the surrounding cytoplasm. Thus the remaining light scatter is caused by components within the cytoplasm. One source of light scattering may be the cytoskeleton.

Since transparency of the lens is so highly dependent on protein order and structural integrity, it is not surprising that relatively small changes in any of these parameters might lead to the development of opacification leading to cataract. Such changes in the lens might include aggregation, changes in tissue hydration, phase separation of molecular components, breakdown of cell membranes, and changes in the structure of the cytoskeleton. Most, if not all, of these changes can and do take place during aging and cataract development.

OVERVIEW OF LENS METABOLISM

The metabolism of the lens is entirely directed toward the maintenance of transparency. Cell division, protein metabolism, cellular differentiation, and maintenance of cellular homeostasis result in the maintenance of characteristics that support transparency. Regulation of lens electrolyte balance serves to maintain the normal hydration of the lens, another critical feature in lens transparency. Electrolyte balance is maintained by permeability properties of the lens cell membranes together with specialized active transport mechanisms. Protection of the lens from oxidative damage also seems to be critical to the lens and consequently there is a sophisticated set of biochemical pathways to preserve the oxidative status of the lens. There is no doubt that the main location of lens metabolism is in the lens epithelium. It is the elaborate system of gap junctions that allows cells deep within the lens to communicate with the outer cell layers. As will become apparent in the following sections, the composition and metabolism of the lens undergo significant changes as the lens ages. Certain of these changes might either contribute to the development of cataract or at least render the lens more susceptible to cataractogenic stresses.

CARBOHYDRATES AND ENERGY METABOLISM

Synthesis of the structural components and the active transport of a variety of materials across cell membranes relies on a continual source of metabolic energy. In the lens energy production is almost entirely dependent upon the metabolism of glucose. The history of the exciting discoveries that have led up to our present understanding of glucose metabolism has been reviewed recently by Chylack and Friend[39] and van Heyningen.[247]

Glucose and a number of other sugars enter the lens by simple diffusion assisted by a mediated transfer process, also called facilitated diffusion. It is not known whether or not the glucose transport system is affected by insulin. The mechanisms of sugar transport by the lens are the subject of a review by Kern.[136] Glucose transport appears to take place across both surfaces of the lens, and recent evidence suggests that the lens possesses a specific glucose transporter.[160] Glucose entering the lens is rapidly metabolized so that the level of free glucose in the lens is less than one tenth of that in aqueous humor. The lens is in a privileged position for the supply of glucose, since newly formed aqueous humor flows immediately across the anterior surface of the lens. It has been reported that the rabbit lens,[252] in organ culture, metabolizes about 3 to 4 mg of glucose a day.

The lens derives more than 70% of its energy through anaerobic glycolysis. The aerobic metabolism of glucose by the Krebs cycle is limited to the lens epithelium (Fig. 10-15).

Glycolysis

In anaerobic glycolysis one mole of glucose is metabolized to generate two moles of ATP. Op-

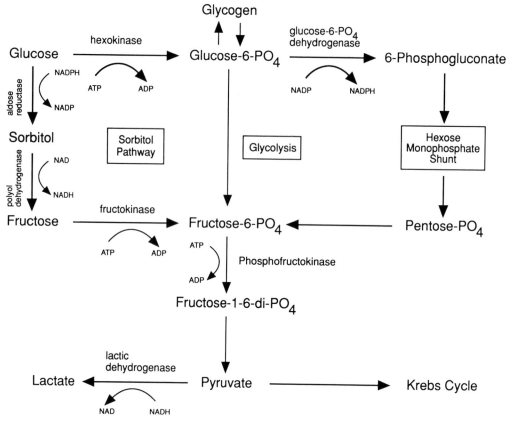

FIG. 10-15 Simplified scheme of glucose metabolism in the lens.

eration of the glycolytic pathway is regulated to a large extent by hexokinase, phosphofructokinase, and pyruvate kinase. While the glycolytic pathway in the lens does not differ from that in other tissues, several characteristics of the enzymes in the lens do impact upon the lens, particularly with respect to aging and cataract development. Hexokinase, the first enzyme of the glycolytic pathway, which catalyzes the conversion of glucose into glucose 6-phosphate, is found only at low levels.[245] The rate of glycolysis becomes limited by the amount of hexokinase present.[99] Although mammalian tissues express at least four isoforms of hexokinase, only types I and II are found in the lens.[36] The type I isoform has a lower K_m for glucose than type II and is thus preferentially extruded at physiologic glucose levels. However, the type II isoform might be more abundant in the lens, possibly being held in reserve until glucose levels increase. As will be discussed later, when excess glucose is present, it enters the sorbitol pathway with damaging consequences. There is a substantial loss of hexokinase in the cortex of the

aging lens.[36,37] This decrease in hexokinase might well impact upon the supply of energy, thereby impairing the synthesis of critical molecules and compromising the active control of electrolyte balance.

Although anaerobic glycolysis is not as efficient as the aerobic metabolism of glucose, its preponderance in the lens does avoid the problem of oxygen starvation. This is significant in the lens, since it is devoid of a blood supply and derives its oxygen from the aqueous humor, which has a rather low oxygen tension. Interestingly, it has been shown that lenses maintained in organ culture can survive in competely anaerobic conditions if there is an adequate glucose supply. However, the lens is unable to survive without glucose; when endogenous glucose sources are rapidly consumed and the supply of energy is reduced, resulting in pronounced alteration of the cytoplasmic composition of the lens, cellular deterioration and eventual loss of transparency occur.

Some of the lactic acid generated by anaerobic glycolysis is further metabolized by the

Krebs cycle. However, the majority of lactic acid diffuses from the lens into the aqueous humor to leave the eye through conventional pathways.

Aerobic metabolism of glucose

The production of ATP in the lens via the Krebs cycle is limited to the epithelium. The aerobic metabolism of glucose is much more efficient than glycolysis, since it produces 38 moles of ATP from each mole of glucose. Only about 3% of lens glucose is metabolized by the Krebs cycle; however, because of the efficiency of the Krebs cycle, this generates up to 20% of the total ATP needs of the lens.[116] Utilization of oxygen by the Krebs cycle has been demonstrated in the organ-cultured rabbit lens where oxygen is utilized at about 8 μl/g/hr. The carbon dioxide produced by the Krebs cycle enters the aqueous humor by simple diffusion.

Hexosemonophosphate shunt

In addition to glycolysis and the Krebs cycle the lens also metabolizes glucose via the hexosemonophosphate shunt.[139] Although the hexosemonophosphate shunt does not generate a large quantity of ATP in the lens, it is an important source of NADPH, which is critical to a number of other metabolic pathways, including the sorbitol pathway and the enzyme glutathione reductase. Thus the hexosemonophosphate shunt is linked to sugar cataract (through aldose reductase) and the oxidative status of the lens through glutathione metabolism.

In the rabbit lens about 14% of the glucose is metabolized by the hexosemonophosphate shunt in which hexoses are converted to pentoses (e.g., D-ribose (Fig. 10-15)). In addition to the generation of NADPH from NADP, this pathway is also important because the pentoses it generates are employed in the synthesis of nucleic acids. Some of the pentoses are recycled to reenter the glycolytic pathway.

Sorbitol pathway

The sorbitol pathway of the lens converts glucose to sorbitol using the enzyme aldose reductase and then to fructose using polyol dehydrogenase (see Fig. 10-15).[246] Under normal conditions the sorbitol pathway accounts for only some 5% of the metabolism of glucose by the lens. The role of the sorbitol pathway might simply be a secondary or tertiary mechanism for the lens to metabolize glucose, generating NADPH. However, it is also possible that the pathway is a means of protecting the lens from osmotic stress.[36]

Beginning in 1959 with a series of elegant studies by van Heyningen,[247] it became apparent that the polyols generated by the sorbitol pathway could be damaging to the lens. Later studies compared these findings and established the prominent role of the sorbitol pathway in the development of sugar cataracts.[140] As previously noted, there is a limited amount of the glycolytic pathway enzyme hexokinase so that when glucose levels are elevated glucose enters the sorbitol pathway. The K_m of aldose reductase, the first enzyme in the sorbitol pathway, is such that it is readily activated when there is only a moderate increase in glucose levels in the lens. Aldose reductase together with NADPH converts glucose to sorbitol, which accumulates within the cells of the lens. Since the cell membranes are relatively impermeable to sorbitol, it cannot diffuse out. This sets up an osmotic gradient that induces an influx of water and results in lens swelling and ultimate loss of lens transparency. However, sorbitol is slowly converted to fructose by polyoldehydrogenase, and fructose can slowly diffuse out of the cell. When galactose enters the aldose reductase pathway, it is converted to dulcitol, which is not further metabolized by polyoldehydrogenase; therefore, more rapid swelling of lens cells occurs.

The link between aldose reductase and the development of sugar cataract resulted in the search for inhibitors of aldose reductase[134] to prevent the development of sugar cataracts. The subject is discussed later in this chapter.[21]

WATER AND ELECTROLYTE BALANCE

Maintenance of lens hydration is critical to lens transparency. As in other tissues, cellular hydration is kept in equilibrium by the regulation of the electrolyte composition. The permeability properties of cell membranes coupled with active transport mechanisms maintain the intracellular ion concentrations in such a way as to counterbalance the natural tendency of water to enter both the epithelial and fiber cells.

Water

The adult human lens is approximately 65% water, a very low water content. The lens capsule is about 80% water, and the water content of the dense nuclear region of the lens is less than that of the outer cortex. There is no significant alteration in lens hydration with aging, but in many forms of cataract lens hydration is dramatically increased.

Much of the lens water is closely associated with molecular structures, particularly protein, and therefore not freely diffusible. Several studies have examined the proportions of bound versus free water. Early studies tackled the problem by examining the distribution of radioactively labeled water,[33,124] while later investigators have used nuclear magnetic resonance (NMR) techniques.[178,202] Both approaches confirmed that a substantial part of lens water was in an ordered nondiffusible state. Stankeiwicz et al.[231] have recently suggested that about half of the lens water may be associated with lens protein and that there may be two pools of this water: strongly bound and weakly bound. The proportion of bound water has been reported to decrease during the maturation of human cortical cataracts.[200]

Because the cells of the lens are tightly packed, there is only a very small extracellular space. The volume of extracellular water has been estimated by determining the distribution of tracer materials that do not penetrate cell membranes. The inulin space of the lens has been reported to be approximately 5%, but nearly a quarter of that space is thought to represent the space of the capsule.[183] Regulation of intercellular water is determined largely by the distribution of monovalent cations.

Monovalent cation balance

The sodium and potassium of the whole lens is similar to that of a single cell in that the normal potassium level is about 140 mEq/kg lens water, while sodium is in the range 14 to 26 mEq/kg lens water. Studies on the exchangeability of lens potassium with radioactive potassium and microelectrode experiments suggest that most of the potassium is freely diffusible.[188] On the other hand, about 15% of lens sodium appears to be bound and unavailable for exchange.[185]

The low sodium level and high potassium level in the lens were at one time explained by considering the cellular barriers to be impermeable. Changes in the concentration of these ions within the lens were thought to be the result of alterations in lens membrane permeability alone. However, numerous experiments have demonstrated that sodium, potassium, chloride, and many other small molecules freely enter and leave the lens.[185] Forty years ago Harris and Gehrsitz[112] demonstrated that the sodium-potassium balance of the lens was regulated by energy-dependent transport mechanisms. These authors showed that when rabbit lenses were cooled they lost potassium and gained sodium. When these same lenses were rewarmed to 37°C in the presence of glucose, the potassium content rose and the sodium level fell back

toward the control level. The phenomenon, referred to as the temperature reversible cation shift of the lens, could be abolished by a variety of metabolic insults. What we now know is that the electrolyte balance of the lens is governed principally by an active cation transport system located in the lens epithelium, although some functional cation transport probably does take place within the cells of the cortex.[177]

The most important transport mechanism is the sodium pump, which moves sodium out of the lens and at the same time allows potassium to accumulate within the lens cells. Not only does this pump regulate the amount of sodium and potassium in the cells of the lens, but the resulting ion gradients between the lens cytoplasm and the external environment provide the necessary energy for other membrane transport processes such as sodium-calcium exchange, sodium-bicarbonate co-transport, and amino acid transport. The sodium pump mechanism is, of course, the sodium potassium adenosine triphosphatase, Na,K-ATPase. This enzyme, which is embedded in the lens plasma membrane, uses the energy from one molecule of ATP to pump 3 molecules of sodium outward and 2 molecules of potassium inward. The action of Na,K-ATPase as the sodium pump has been well documented.[93]

The delicate balance between the active sodium pump and the passive permeability properties of the lens cell membranes has been described as a pump leak system[141] (Fig. 10-16). The major site of active cation transport is in the anteriorly located epithelium; consequently anterior-to-posterior electrolyte gradients are set up, with potassium being more concentrated anteriorly and sodium more concentrated posteriorly. These gradients have been clearly demonstrated by the studies of Paterson.[185] Ouabain, an inhibitor of Na,K-ATPase, causes the lens to gain sodium and lose potassium, with the resultant loss of osmotic balance and an increase in lens hydration. Since derangement of cation and water balance is a common feature in human cortical cataract,[73,164] a number of investigators have explored whether the cation transport system is altered in cataract. While some studies have shown that Na,K-ATPase activity is reduced in cataract,[4,105,179] a number of other investigators have presented convincing evidence that the activity of this enzyme is not substantially altered in most common types of cataracts.[182,186] It must be remembered, however, that the electrolyte balance of the lens depends not only upon the active transport mechanism but also upon the permeability properties of the

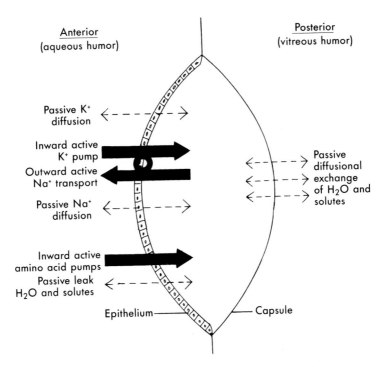

FIG. 10-16 Pathways of solute movement in the lens. The major site of active transport mechanisms is in the anterior epithelium, while passive diffusion occurs over both surfaces. There is also evidence (see text) for transport mechanisms at the level of lens cell fibers.

lens cell membrane. Recent studies by Gandolfi et al.[87] suggest that the human cataractous lens might have quite a high cation permeability. Even though the pump activity might be normal, an increased permeability might cause the transport capability of the pump to be exceeded.

Membrane permeability, ion channels, and electrical phenomena

The permeability properties of lens cell membranes have been studied by evaluation of their electrical properties and also by studying the flux of ions into and out of lens cells. Most of these studies have been fully reviewed elsewhere.[72,189] As with most cell membranes, those of the lens are more permeable to potassium than to sodium. The permeability properties of membranes are the result of ion channels, some of which are quite specific for certain ions and others that are regulated by membrane voltage. The detailed studies of Rae[204] have helped to uncover the types and characteristics of ion channels in lens membranes.

The permeability properties of the plasma membrane, together with the nonequilibrium distribution of sodium, potassium, and chloride

between the cytoplasm and the exterior, give rise to an electrical potential difference between the inside of the cells and their surrounding medium. In the lens microelectrode studies demonstrate a potential difference of about 70 mv negative with respect to the bathing medium. Alteration in membrane permeability or inhibition of the sodium pump reduces the magnitude of the lens potential.

In addition to the transmembrane electrical phenomenon, extracellular currents can be detected around the surface of the lens. The extracellular currents, which are measured using a vibrating electrode,[259] appear to be the result of electrical loops set up by the asymmetry of the properties of the membranes in different regions of the lens.

Calcium homeostasis

Calcium, a divalent cation, is present at about 0.3 mEq/kg lens water.[74] This level is more than 50 times less than that found in aqueous humor, suggesting that there must be a special transport mechanism to exclude calcium from the lens. Increased concentrations of calcium are cytotoxic in the lens and thought to contribute to the development of cataract. The intercellular concentration of free diffusible calcium is only 10^{-7} to 10^{-6} M, as demonstrated by microelectrode studies;[129] thus much of the intracellular calcium is in some way bound. Considerable attention has been given recently to the maintenance of lens cell calcium levels. There is strong evidence for a calcium ATPase in the lens.[22,23] Using isolated membrane vesicles prepared from lens cortex, a close association has been shown between calcium ATPase and the ability of these vesicles to actively transport calcium.[62] It is not yet known whether the calcium transport system is impaired during cataract development. However, the studies of Borchman et al.[24] have suggested that calcium ATPase is very sensitive to oxidative damage in vitro.

Another prominent cation in the lens is magnesium, found at a concentration of about 4 mEq/kg lens water.[6,73] Magnesium functions as a cofactor in a number of enzyme reactions. However, the level of magnesium in the lens changes little in human or experimental cataract. It has also been demonstrated that magnesium cannot substitute for calcium in maintaining lens cell membrane permeability properties.[64]

Cell-to-cell communication

The presence of an extensive gap junction system within the lens has been illustrated by morphologic studies. This extensive cellular coupling enables the lens epithelium to take care of many, if not all, of the metabolic needs of the lens cells lying deeper within the lens. If such low-resistance gap junctions did not exist, exchange of solutes between the lens and its environment would be severely limited by the diffusion pathways within the lens. Paterson[187] demonstrated in 1971 the limited diffusion within the lens. Later Rae and associates[203,205] confirmed those findings using both dye diffusion and also electrophysiological techniques. Thus solutes, rather than crossing a series of lens cell membranes or diffusing through the tortuous extracellular space, can move relatively quickly from cell to cell through the gap junctions.

The rather unusual properties of gap junctions of the lens and MIP, the 26 kDa putative gap junction protein, are discussed elsewhere in this chapter. Unlike several other tissues, the cell-cell junctions observed between adjacent lens fibers are found most often in a noncrystalline, low-resistance state. However, it seems likely that the lens might require some mechanism to "close off" regions of the fiber mass, particularly if groups of fibers become damaged, and so there is an intense search for the possible mechanisms of closing the fiber-fiber junction. To date, pH has been shown to uncouple lens cells in several species.[7,220]

NON-ELECTROLYTE TRANSPORT MECHANISMS
Amino acids

For uninterrupted protein synthesis the lens must have a continual supply of amino acids. It has been adequately demonstrated that amino acids are actively transported into the lens such that their concentration in the lens generally exceeds that in the aqueous humor (Fig. 10-17). The site of amino acid transport seems to be the lens epithelium. There are three separate transport mechanisms: one for alanine, another for leucine, and yet another for glycine and a number of small amino acids. The subject of amino acid transport in the lens has been reviewed by Kern.[136] Amino acid transport in the lens appears to be dependent upon the sodium gradient generated by Na,K-ATPase, but Marcantonio and Duncan[166] have suggested that the high sodium content found in human cataracts markedly interferes with amino acid uptake. Reduced amino acid transport accompanies aging and several forms of experimental cataract.[136]

There also appears to be a specialized transport mechanism for the amino acid taurine,[211] which can also be generated in the lens from methionine.[53] This amino acid is strongly acidic and is not one of the constituents of lens proteins. The taurine concentration in the human lens, 6.7 mg/100 g wet weight,[67] is higher than most other free amino acids, yet its function in the lens is not known. Reduction in taurine levels with cataract has been reported.[4]

Ascorbic acid

Studies with lenses of several species have suggested that the lens possesses a carrier-mediated transport system to accumulate ascorbic acid.[69,125,137] There is, however, some uncertainty as to whether the transport system is limited to the epithelium or is present also in the cells of the cortex. Kern and Zolot[137] have suggested that the carrier-mediated system is specific for dehydro-L-ascorbic acid, there being little transport of the reduced form, L-ascorbate.

The role of ascorbic acid in the lens has been recently reviewed by Varma.[248] Ascorbic acid might participate in the modulation of the hexosemonophosphate shunt. Of particular interest is the role of ascorbic acid as a scavenger of free radicals. However, ascorbic acid can also be pro-oxidant, since together with light and the presence of a metal ion, it will generate hydrogen peroxide.

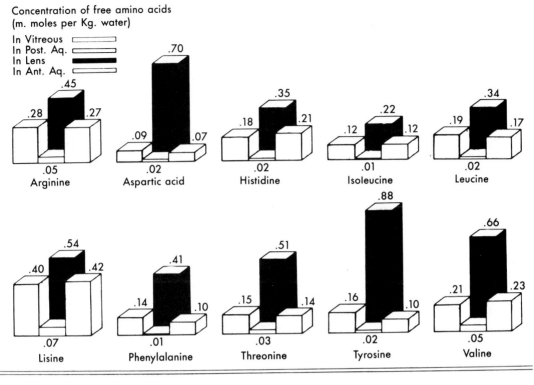

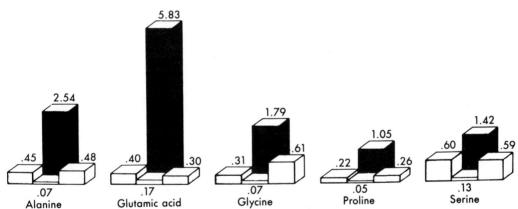

Concentration of free amino acids
(m. moles per Kg. water)

In Vitreous
In Post. Aq.
In Lens
In Ant. Aq.

FIG. 10-17   Relative concentrations of free amino acids in lens, aqueous humor, and vitreous of the rabbit eye. (From Reddy DVN, Kinsey VE, Invest Ophthalmol 1:635, 1962).

Choline

Normal rat lenses accumulate choline by a carrier-mediated transport mechanism.[132] Choline in the lens is quickly phosphorylated by choline kinase to P-choline, which is a precursor of membrane phospholipids. The normal human lens contains about 1 mM P-choline, but this is substantially lower in cataractous lenses, perhaps due to increased membrane permeability.[158] Recent studies by Lou et al.[158] showed that

treatment of experimental diabetic rats with an aldose reductase inhibitor to prevent osmotic changes prevented the fall in lens P-choline levels.

Inositol

Myoinositol, the most abundant isomer of inositol, is actively transported into the lens by a sodium-dependent carrier-mediated mechanism.[51,250] Levels of myoinositol in the lens, about 400 mg/100 g wet weight, are some 65 to 95 times greater than those in aqueous humor. In several forms of cataract, particularly diabetic cataract, myoinositol levels are significantly reduced. The precise role of myoinositol in the lens is uncertain. However, myoinositol is a precursor for membrane phophoinositides, which are involved in Na,K-ATPase function. There is also evidence for participation of myoinositol in ascorbic acid transport. Dickerson and Lou[66] have explored a number of other roles for inositol in the lens.

LENS PROTEINS

Protein accounts for about 35% of the wet weight of the lens, nearly double that found in other tissues. Lens proteins can be separated into two classes based upon their solubility in water. The water-soluble lens crystallins account for nearly 90% of the total lens proteins. The water-insoluble proteins consist of membrane proteins, cytoskeletal proteins, and aggregated crystallins. The lens crystallins are a heterogeneous group of structural proteins identified as alpha, beta, and gamma crystallin. In avian and reptilian species there is a fourth crystallin called delta crystallin. The original separation of lens proteins into three soluble fractions and an insoluble fraction was accomplished almost a hundred years ago by Morner.[174] Excellent reviews of lens protein composition and metabolism are available.[20,21,57,119,155]

Lens crystallins
Alpha crystallin

The alpha crystallin fraction has an average molecular weight of approximately 1×10^3 kDa. Although alpha crystallin is the largest of the crystallins, it accounts for only about 35% of total lens protein. It has been known for some time that alpha crystallin is not a single protein but is composed of variably sized aggregates of four polypeptide subunits. The subunits are identified as alpha A1, alpha A2, alpha B1, and alpha B2, each having a molecular weight of about 20 kDa. These polypeptide chains are held together by hydrogen bonding and hydrophobic forces. The three-dimensional structure of the α crystallin polypeptides is mainly a β-chain configuration, with some random coil arrangement but no helical structure.[154,219] It has been shown that the subunits A2 and B2 are primary products of gene translation, while A1 and B1 are post-translational products of A2 and B2. A2 and B2 are found only in the epithelium, while A1 and B1 are found only in the lens fibers. The combination of A and B chains in making up the aggregates is quite variable. However, at the time of synthesis α crystallin is homogenous, with a molecular weight of about 7×10^2 kDa. The amino acid sequences of the α crystallin polypeptides reveal approximately 55% homology between the A and B chains (Fig. 10-18).

As the lens ages, larger aggregates are formed with molecular weights as high as 50×10^3 kDa. These high-molecular-weight aggregates can become water insoluble and are thought to contribute to light scattering. More significant protein modification occurs with cataract, as will be discussed later.

Beta crystallin

The beta crystallins are the most abundant water-soluble protein, representing about 55%. The molecular weight of beta crystallins ranges from 40 to 250 kDa, making them the most heterogenous group of crystallins. The beta crystallins consist of four distinct subgroups of aggregates based upon their molecular weights. Two larger species with molecular weights of about 250 kDa and 130 kDa are called β high with the smaller species, 60 kDa and 37 kDa, being labeled β low. These subgroups of β crystallins each contain two subunits. The major subunit is a polypeptide chain, labeled βBp, and has a molecular weight of approximately 24 kDa. This polypeptide chain is a characteristic component of β crystallin in a wide number of mammalian species. Like α crystallins, the three-dimensional structure of β crystallin is largely β sheet conformation.

Gamma crystallin

With a molecular weight of about 20 to 27 kDa, gamma crystallin is not only the smallest crystallin but also the least abundant, representing only about 1 to 2% of the total. Gamma crystallins are found as monomers rather than aggregates, and they can be separated into at least five components. Like the other crystallins, gamma crystallin has little α helical structure, being mainly β sheets and some random coil.[121] The gamma crystallin has been shown to separate and precipitate when the temperature of the intact lens is lowered to less than 10°C; this results in opacification and is referred to as cold cataract. Rewarming of the lens permits solubilization of the protein and transparency.[122]

Water-insoluble protein

The lens proteins that are insoluble in water can be further separated on the basis of their solubility in 7 M urea. That fraction that is soluble in

α-CRYSTALLIN SEQUENCE : HOMOLOGY BETWEEN αA₂ AND αB₂ POLYPEPTIDE CHAIN

αA₂ ac-Met-Asp-Ile-Ala-Ile|Gln|His-Pro-Trp|Phe-Lys|Arg|Thr-Leu-Gly|Pro-Phe| -Tyr|Pro-Ser-Arg-Leu-Phe-Asp-Gln-Phe-Phe-Gly-Glu|
αB₂ ac-Met-Asp-Ile-Ala-Ile|His|His-Pro-Trp|Ile-Arg|Arg|Pro-Phe-Phe|Pro-Phe|His-Ser|Pro-Ser-Arg-Leu·Phe-Asp-Gln-Phe-Phe-Gly-Glu|

-Gly|Leu|Phe|Glu|Tyr|Asp-Leu|Leu|Pro|Phe-Leu|Ser|Ser-Thr-Ile|Ser-Pro|Tyr|Tyr| |Arg|Gln-| |Ser|Leu-Phe|Arg| -Thr-Val-
-His|Leu|Leu|Glu|Ser|Asp-Leu|Phe|Pro| -Ala|Ser|Thr-Ser-Leu|Ser-Pro|Phe|Tyr|Leu|Arg|Pro-Pro|Ser|Phe-Leu|Arg|Ala-Pro-Ser-Trp-

-Leu|Asp|Ser|Gly|Ile|Ser-Glu|Val|Arg|Ser-Asp-Arg|Asp|Lys|Phe|Val-Ile-Phe|Leu|Asp|Val-Lys-His-Phe-Ser-Pro-Glu|Asp|Leu|Thr|Val-
-Ile|Asp|Thr|Gly|Leu|Ser-Glu|Met|Arg|Leu-Glu-Lys|Asp|Arg|Phe|Ser-Val-Asn|Leu|Asn|Val-Lys-His-Phe-Ser-Pro-Glu|Glu|Leu|Lys|Val-

-Lys-Val|Gln-Glu|Asp|Phe-Val|Glu|Ile|His-Gly-Lys-His|Asn|Glu-Arg-Gln-Asp|Asp|His-Gly|Tyr|Ile-Ser-Arg-Glu-Phe-His-Arg|Arg|Tyr-
-Lys-Val|Leu-Gly|Asp|Val-Ile|Glu|Val|His-Gly-Lys-His|Glu|Glu-Arg-Gln-Asp|Glu|His-Gly|Phe|Ile-Ser-Arg-Glu-Phe-His-Arg|Lys|Tyr-

-Arg|Leu|Pro|Ser-Asn|Val-Asp|Gln-Ser|Ala|Leu-Ser-Cys|Ser-Leu-Ser|Ala|Asp-Gly|Met|Leu-Thr|Phe-Ser|Gly-Pro|Lys-Ile-Pro-Ser-Gly-
-Arg|Ile|Pro|Ala-Asp|Val-Asp|Pro-Leu|Ala|Ile-Thr-Ser|Ser-Leu-Ser|Ser|Asp-Gly|Val|Leu-Thr|Val-Asp|Gly-Pro|Arg-Lys-Gln-

-Val-Asp|Ala|Gly-His-Ser|Glu-Arg|Ala|Ile-Pro|Val-Ser|Arg-Glu-Glu-Lys-Pro| -Ser-Ser|Ala-Pro|Ser-Ser-COOH   173 RESIDUES
|Ala|Ser-Gly-Pro|Glu-Arg|Thr|Ile-Pro|Ile-Thr|Arg-Glu-Glu-Lys-Pro|Ala-Val-Thr-Ala|Ala-Pro|Lys-Lys-COOH   175 RESIDUES

HOMOLOGY : 55 %

FIG. 10-18 The primary structure of the α crystallin subunits αA₂, and αB₂. (From Bloemendal,[20] p 13.)

urea contains cytoskeletal proteins and modified crystallins. Most of the urea-insoluble fraction is composed of membrane protein.

Membrane proteins

Approximately 20 to 30% of the water-insoluble fraction of lens proteins is comprised of protein derived from cell membranes. Proteins that are an integral part of the lens cell membrane are called intrinsic membrane proteins, while those associated only with the membrane surface are called extrinsic membrane proteins. The main intrinsic membrane protein is a 26 kDa polypeptide, which is thought to be a principal component of lens gap junctions. There is evidence that the MP26 is degraded to 22 kDa molecular weight species, MP22, with aging. The gap junction structure is composed of the protein MP26 together with membrane lipids. Gap junctions isolated from membranes have been shown to contain a high cholesterol and sphingomyelin content.

Extrinsic membrane proteins include glycoproteins such as fibronectin.[217] In general, the extrinsic membrane proteins have been less well studied.

There are many important enzymes associated with the cell membrane, including the transport enzymes (ATPases), adenyl cyclase, and alkaline phosphatase.[1,21]

Cytoskeletal proteins

It is this component of insoluble lens proteins that is soluble in 7 M urea. The composition of the cytoskeleton proteins has been discussed earlier in this chapter (see Table 10-1).

Protein synthesis, proteolysis, and aging

The biosynthesis of proteins in the lens, as in all tissues, involves the transfer of genetic information contained within DNA via messenger RNA to the ribosomes of the cells that generate the polypeptide chains. The necessary energy is supplied in the form of ATP derived from carbohydrate metabolism. In the lens protein synthesis can be considered in three phases: initiation of synthesis, changes in synthesis that accompany cellular elongation, and finally termination of synthesis as cells are displaced inward away from the lens surface. Protein synthesis, therefore, takes place predominantly in the lens epithelium and the outer cell layers that contain the necessary intracellular organelles. After protein synthesis is complete, further structural modification can take place as a result of aggregation or proteolysis.

The rate of protein synthesis and distribution throughout the lens has been followed in rat lenses, where the radioactively labeled amino acid methionine is incorporated into outer cortex within one day.[52,265] After 1 month, the radioactivity is found deeper within the lens cortex, largely associated with all the soluble protein fractions. After 7 weeks, about half of the radioactivity was found in the insoluble fraction, indicating that protein aggregation had occurred.

Using immunofluorescence techniques, McAvoy[169] studied the pattern of rat lens protein synthesis in some detail, suggesting two synthetic compartments, one an anterior prolifera-tion compartment and the second an elongation compartment. Only α crystallin was detected in the epithelial cells of the proliferative compartment, while all three crystallins were found in the elongating compartment (Fig. 10-19). McAvoy[169] showed that β and gamma crystallin synthesis was turned on only when the cells began to elongate and that the trigger for this might depend on factors released from the retina. More recently, Chamberlain and McAvoy[34] have identified fibroblastic growth factor as a promoter of lens cell differentiation. Protein synthesis is also modulated by lens electrolyte balance, since inhibition of the sodium pump by ouabain slows protein synthesis[196,222] as does loss of calcium balance.[166]

The lens proteins undergo substantial molecular modification with aging, a subject of several reviews.[119] Much attention has been focused on the aggregation of the soluble lens proteins (crystallins), thereby generating high-molecular-weight species that become water insoluble. Young lenses contain little insoluble

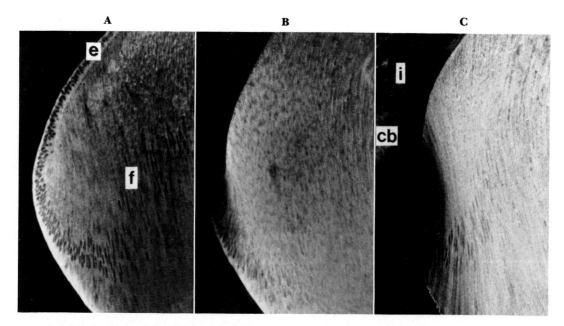

FIG. 10-19 Typical distribution of crystallins in sections of the neonatal lens. **A,** Alpha crystallin is detected in all lens epithelial (e) and fiber (f) cells. **B,** Beta crystallin is first detected in elongating fiber cells just below the lens equator and is not detected in the lens epithelium. **C,** Gamma crystallin is first detected in young fiber cells in the lens cortex and is not detected in the lens epithelium. Crystallins are not detected outside the lens, e.g., in iris (i) or ciliary body (cb). Scale bar represents 500 μm. (From McAvoy JW: The role of fibroblast growth factor in eye lens development, in "Proceedings of the Fibroblast Growth Factor Family," La Jolla, CA, 1991, NY Acad Sci, in press.

protein. By the age of 20, some 15% of the protein has become insoluble, and by the sixth decade this has increased to 50%.[2,91] The protein aggregates involve all three crystallins and can have molecular weights varying from several million up to 50 million Daltons. The aggregates in normal lenses are linked by noncovalent bonds. As will be seen later, in cataract another type of aggregate appears, resulting from the covalent binding of oxidized thiol groups, i.e., disulfide bonds. Oxidation of thiol groups in normal lenses appears to be minimal and confined to proteins associated with the membrane.[226]

The amino acids of lens proteins also can undergo racemization with aging.[90,168] Racemization is the transformation of the L-isomer form to the D-isomer form. The significance and impact of this process are not well understood. With aging, the proteins might also undergo nonenzymatic glycosylation,[109] by which carbohydrate molecules attach directly to the protein amino acids to eventually form carbonyl groups that favor protein aggregation.

Lens proteins also undergo proteolysis.[91] A number of low-molecular-weight polypeptides accumulate in the lens with aging. Both exopeptidases and endopeptidases have been demonstrated in the lens.[55,224,241] Calpain, a protease activated by calcium, has generated considerable interest in recent years. Proteases are probably responsible for the degradation of proteins that become damaged during aging. With aging, many synthetic and metabolic enzymes undergo changes in activity and distribution, a subject comprehensively reviewed by Hockwin and Ohrloff.[117]

Recent studies by Wistow and Piatigorsky have revealed that some lens crystallins are closely related to certain enzymes.[195,260] This close relationship is thought to result from gene sharing; however, there is little evidence for actual enzymatic activity of the crystallins in the mammalian lens.

LENS LIPIDS

Since most of the lens lipids are associated with cell membranes, they are found in a protein lipid complex. The lens lipids include cholesterol, phospholipids, and glycosphingolipids. About 50 to 60% of the lens lipid is cholesterol. The concentration of cholesterol in the lens is extraordinarily high, so that the ratio of cholesterol to phospholipid in the human lens is the greatest known.[28] The major phospholipid associated with the human lens cell membrane is sphingomyelin, while in the rabbit and bovine

lens phosphatidylethanolamine is the principal phospholipid.[28] The pattern of phospholipid distribution in the human lens is shown in Table 10-2. The high cholesterol content coupled with sphingomyelin makes the lens cell membranes quite rigid. Borchman et al.[25] have measured the lens cell membrane lipid fluidity by Fourier transform infrared spectroscopy, confirming the rigid nature of lens cell membranes; the rigidity appears to increase with aging. Glycosphingolipids, also present in the lens, are generally associated with the outer layers of the membrane and are thought to be involved in cell differentiation and cell-to-cell interactions.[28] There is no direct evidence for the presence of arachidonic acid in lens cell membranes, although it has been shown that lens epithelium can metabolize arachidonic acid via the cyclooxygenase pathway to prostanoid compounds[81]; there is no evidence for a lipoxygenase pathway.[257]

Lipid metabolism and breakdown have been investigated by determining the incorporation of radioactive precursors into lens lipids.[28,270] Using ^{32}P-orthophosphate and ^3H-myoinositol, Broekhuyse[27,29] has been able to demonstrate that the precursors are rapidly incorporated into phospholipids, both in the human and bovine lens. Studies on chick lens[268,269] have suggested that the half-life of phosphatidylcholine, phosphatidylinositol, and phosphatidylethanolamine is on the order of several days in lens fibers. The biosynthesis of sphingomyelin has been studied by Roelfzema et al.,[215] who determined that the enzymes necessary for sphingomyelin synthesis are present in the lens epithelium and perhaps also in the equatorial lens fibers. In order for the lens to synthesize lipids, it needs to accumulate the necessary precursors. Transport mechanisms for the precursors apparently depend upon the sodium gradient between the cytoplasm and extracellular fluid.[250] In the lens there is a specific mechanism for accumulating choline; in the rat lens choline accumulation exhibits the characteristics of a specific carrier mediated mechanism.[132]

In addition to their role as the principal constituents of lens cell membranes, lipid metabolites may be linked to regulatory functions. For example, phosphatidylinositol turnover appears to parallel lens epithelial cell division and phosphatidylethanolamine methylation seems to correlate with lens fiber cell formation.[269]

With aging, substantial changes take place in lipid composition and distribution; these studies have been nicely reviewed by Broekhuyse.[28] From about age 25 to 75 there is a doubling of

TABLE 10-2 Phospholipid Composition of Human Lens

	% of Total Phospholipid Present in Lens			
	Cortex	Nucleus	Cortex	Nucleus
	(20 years)		(66 years)	
Sphingomyelin	40.7	56.6	58.0	66.4
Phosphatidylcholine	9.4	1.1	5.5	0.1
Phosphatidylethanolamine	21.8	8.2	11.7	1.3
Phosphatidylserine	5.7	6.8	6.2	2.2
Phosphatidylinositol	0.8	0.4	0.1	0.5
Lysophosphatidylethanolamine	8.6	16.6	7.6	17.1
Lysophosphatidylcholine	3.4	1.2	1.3	2.1
Diphosphatidylglycerol	1.4	0.2	0.3	0.2
Unidentified component	5.2	5.0	5.8	6.1
Other phospholipids	3.0	3.9	3.5	4.0

Data from Broekhuyse.[27]

lens cholesterol and a concomitant increase in sphingomyelin. On the other hand, phosphatidylethanolamine and phosphatidylcholine decrease with aging. These changes, which reflect alteration in cell membrane structure, might be expected to have a considerable impact upon lens cell membrane function as the lens ages.

GLUTATHIONE AND OXIDATION-REDUCTION PATHWAYS

Oxidation-reduction mechanisms have special importance in the lens. Oxidative damage can result in a number of molecular changes that contribute to the development of cataract. The lens must therefore possess efficient reducing systems, as well as detoxification enzymes such as catalase and superoxide dismutase. These mechanisms are reviewed in greater detail by Spector,[226] Augusteyn,[3] and Reddy and Giblin.[212]

Glutathione plays a central role in protecting the lens from oxidative insult. Glutathione is a tripeptide (glycine-leucine-glutamic acid) that is synthesized in the lens.[212] An active transport mechanism for glutathione has also been described.[213] The enzymes responsible for glutathione synthesis have been shown to decrease in human senile cataract.[210]

Nearly all the glutathione in the lens is to be found in the reduced form (GSH). The level of both reduced glutathione and oxidized glutathione (GSSG) in the rabbit lens epithelium is 64 μmol/g.[212] There is five times less glutathione in the cortex and even less in the nucleus of the lens. The turnover of glutathione in the lens is

approximately 1.4% per hour.[213] It has also been estimated that the synthesis of glutathione uses about 11% of the ATP generated by glycolysis. The concentration of glutathione falls in virtually all forms of cataract, both human and experimental, thus leaving the lens more vulnerable to oxidative insult.

A number of critical roles have been assigned to glutathione. It has been suggested that glutathione is responsible for protecting the thiol groups on proteins, thereby preventing the generation of protein aggregation through disulfide bonds. Glutathione might also protect sulfhydryl groups at the membrane level, where they are essential for normal cation transport. There is also evidence for the involvement of glutathione in amino acid transport. Finally, glutathione is intimately involved with the detoxification of hydrogen peroxide.

For glutathione to fulfil its varied roles in the lens, it must be maintained in its reduced state. First of all, glutathione is not alone in protecting the lens from oxidative insult. There are small amounts of catalase in the lens that converts hydrogen peroxide to water and oxygen.[17] Hydrogen peroxide is also detoxified by glutathione peroxidase, a reaction in which glutathione serves as a cofactor. The enzyme superoxide dismutase is also present in the lens to detoxify superoxide radicals.[18] Nevertheless, glutathione plays a critical role in the oxidative defense mechanisms, and in the process glutathione is converted into its oxidized form (Fig. 10-20). In the mechanism by which glutathione acts as a cofactor to the enzyme glutathione peroxidase

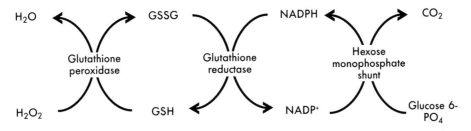

FIG. 10-20   Simplified scheme of glutathione metabolism in the lens.

the oxidized glutathione is reduced back to GSH by glutathione reductase, a mechanism in which NADPH is used as a cofactor. The principal source of NADPH in the lens is the hexosemonophosphate shunt, which therefore plays a major role in keeping glutathione in its reduced form.

There are two other mechanisms that contribute to the protection of thiol groups in the lens. Protein disulfide bonds can be reduced by the thio-redoxin system and a family of enzymes called thiol transferases, which involve glutathione as a cofactor. Relatively little attention has been given to these mechanisms, which are reviewed by Spector.[226]

PHOTOBIOLOGY

The lens is exposed to a considerable amount of ultraviolet radiation. Light with wavelengths less than about 300 nm is absorbed by the cornea, but almost all light between 300 and 400 nm is transmitted by the cornea to reach the lens. The lens absorbs much of the light between 300 and 400 nm but above 400 nm light is transmitted, passing onto the retina. Absorption of light by the lens can result in a number of chemical reactions, including the development of various fluorophores and pigments that contribute to the yellowing of the lens as it ages (Fig. 10-21). The neonatal lens is colorless but a pale yellow coloration develops, progressing to a deep yellow and sometimes dark brown as in brunescent cataract. There seems to be a direct relationship between aging and lens coloration. Pigmentation of the lens probably serves as a filter to protect the retina from ultraviolet light damage; the absorption maxima of the lens are 370 and 280 nm. The yellow coloration also corrects for chromatic aberration. The photobiology of the lens has been extensively discussed by a number of authors.[68,150,271,273]

The absorption of light by the lens is due to the reactivity of amino acid residues on lens proteins and also the presence of pigments and fluorophores that accumulate in the lens. The impact of ultraviolet light upon the lens is further influenced by the level of oxygen in the lens and surrounding fluids, and the presence of any quenching or photosensitizing molecules. The specific reaction site within the lens is also important; epithelial cells may be expected to differ from nonnucleated fiber cells in their response to ultraviolet light.

The intrinsic fluorescence of the lens is due to the protein amino acid residues, which contain aromatic side chains; these are phenylalanine, tyrosine, and tryptophan. Nearly all of the intrinsic lens fluorescence is attributed to tryptophan, because it has the highest quantum efficiency, i.e., the highest fluorescence yield. The chemistry of tryptophan fluorescence is described in detail by Lerman.[150]

Extrinsic fluorescence is generated by a variety of chromophores within the lens. The chromophores are named after the color of their fluorescent emission; green, orange, red, and blue chromophores have been described, although there are probably a number of chromophores responsible for the blue fluorescence. Several of the chromophores are derived from tryptophan. The precise origin of the yellow chromophore is not known, but appears to be tightly bound to the lens proteins.

A relationship is thought to exist between increased lens fluorescence and insolubilization of lens protein; it is hypothesized that the chromophores can contribute to protein cross linking and aggregation, thus contributing to cataract development.[68] Chromophores might also act as sensitizers of photooxidation of lens proteins. Photooxidation of lens components is, however, modulated by the presence of several antioxidant systems such as ascorbic acid, glutathione, and vitamin E.

Ultraviolet light may also interact with and damage lens lipids, a variety of enzymes and DNA, leading to altered lens function and cataractogenesis; this will be described later.

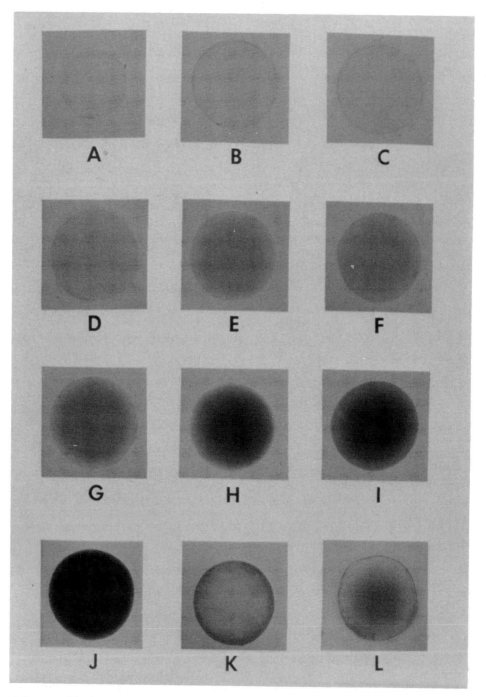

FIG. 10-21   The increasing yellow brown color of the normal lens as it ages from six months (*a*), through 8 years (*b*), 12 years (*c*), 25 years (*d*), 47 years (*e*), 60 years (*f*), 70 years (*g*), 82 years (*h*), and 91 years (*i*). Seventy-year-old brown nuclear cataract (*j*), 68-year-old cortical cataract (k), and 74-year-old mixed nuclear and cortical cataract (*l*). (From Lerman,[150] Plate 3-1.)

CATARACT—GENERAL CONSIDERATIONS

From a clinical standpoint, cataract is defined as visual impairment as a result of a disturbance of lens transparency. However, although small opacities that do not fall within the visual axis have little effect on visual acuity, any source of significant light scattering can be considered a cataractogenic lesion from a biochemical standpoint. The etiology of cataract is very diverse and there are many different forms of cataract, involving all regions of the lens. The precise cause of cataract is unknown but it is unlikely that there is a single precipitating event leading to opacification of the lens. It is more likely that a multitude of factors can influence various aspects of lens metabolism leading to the development of light-scattering centers and loss of transparency.

Epidemiology

It is estimated that 400,000 persons develop cataract each year in the United States; cataract is responsible for about 35% of existing visual impairment.[176] There are approximately 31,000 people legally blind as a result of cataract.[232] The global impact of cataract is quite astounding. Cataract is responsible for visual impairment in 30 to 45 million people and is the largest single cause of blindness worldwide.[262]

The incidence of cataract in the United States is not well documented. Data generated from the Framingham eye study in 1977[135] demonstrated that lens changes were observed in 70% of all individuals above the age of 65 and cataract was diagnosed in 18% of that group. In individuals aged 75 to 85, the incidence of lens changes was greater than 90%, with nearly half of those being diagnosed as clinical cataract. Unfortunately, however, the Framingham eye study was restricted to only a small regional population and the data cannot be reliably extrapolated. More reliable data is available on the incidence of congenital cataracts showing that there are 1.6 cataracts per 10,000 live births.[50]

Etiology and risk factors

There is no doubt that the development of cataract is associated with aging, diabetes, and exposure to a variety of environmental stresses, including all forms of radiation. Several studies have attempted systematically to evaluate risk factors for cataract development. Much of the earlier literature was reviewed by Clayton et al.[48] These same authors suggested a relationship between cataract development and a variety of factors, including diabetes, cardiovascular disease, cigarette smoking, and the use of topically applied ophthalmic drugs. Jahn et al.[131] focused their study on the metabolic risk factors for the development of posterior subcapsular cataract and suggested association of this form of cataract with hyperlipidemia and hyperglycemia. Other studies, including those of Chen et al.[35] and Harding,[110] have proposed a linkage between cataract development and a variety of clinical diseases and environmental factors. In 1991 Leske et al.[152] published the results of a case-controlled study involving 1380 individuals. The study confirmed that cataract is related to low socioeconomic and nutritional status; diabetes was confirmed as a risk factor for all cataract types except nuclear cataract. Nuclear cataract appeared to be associated with cigarette smoking, occupation, and exposure to sunlight. This excellent study confirmed the multifactorial etiology of cataractogenesis.

Classification of cataract

The uncertain etiology of cataract coupled with the diverse clinical and morphologic pathology of cataractous lenses has presented a major challenge to the development of a cataract classification system. There are three major approaches to classification: (1) etiology, (2) evaluation of lens changes in vivo, and (3) description of pathology of intact cataractous lenses after removal from the eye.

Classification of cataract based on etiology allows only for separation into broad categories such as age, radiation exposure, underlying metabolic disease, congenital anomalies, trauma, and the side effect of medical therapy. Such a classification system is valuable in helping us understand some of the stresses imposed on the lens and predicting molecular targets within the lens. Clinical evaluation of the cataractous lens in vivo has led to a broad range of cataract descriptions that, in most simple terms, encompass cortical cataract, nuclear cataract, brunescent cataract, posterior subcapsular cataract, and anterior cortical cataract.[161] These clinical descriptions lacked objectivity, and there was clearly a need to develop a reliable system to document cataractous changes in vivo.[175,256] A number of sophisticated optical techniques have been developed to address that need. For example, the Scheimpflug slit lamp camera system (Fig. 10-22) has been extensively employed by Hockwin[118] and evaluated by a number of other investigators.[54,76] Brown[31] has also developed a slit lamp photography system that has proved valuable in describing lens changes in vivo. Most recently, in the United

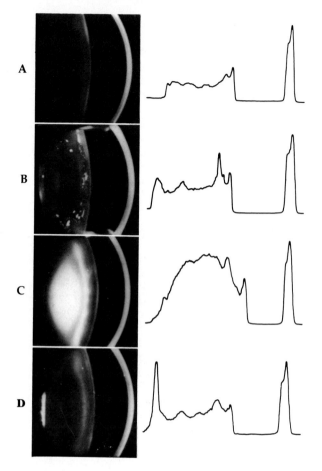

well as color. An elaborate scheme to classify human cataractous lenses that had been extracted from the eye was established in 1978 by Chylack.[41,43,45] The Coordinated Cataract Research Group Classification System, as Chylack's system was called, provided for an accurate description of opacity, precise location, and lens coloration. This system was widely used for a number of years but has become essentially obsolete with the advent of extracapsular cataract extraction, which does not deliver an intact lens for examination.

The range of cataract pathology is paralleled by a spectrum of biochemical changes. From the outset it is important to recall that many biochemical changes take place in the aging lens, but these do not necessarily result in significant opacification and cataract development. It must be assumed, therefore, that certain biochemical events, superimposed on the aging process, take place that result in cataractogenesis. In addition, a number of specific biochemical changes can occur to cause cataract. In sugar cataract (as in diabetes), a specific biochemical pathway contributes to osmotic derangement of the lens. Also, certain drugs can elicit cataractogenic mechanisms. The following sections will therefore examine some of the biochemical and physiologic events associated with several forms of

FIG. 10-22 Scheimpflug photographs of the anterior portion of the eye. **A**, Normal lens, **B** to **D**, three different forms of cataract with the corresponding curves of a linear densitometer. (From Hockwin et al,[118] p 289.)

States Chylack and associates[42,151] have developed a lens opacities classification system (LOCS), which grades the presence or absence of opacification in all the zones of the lens (Fig. 10-23). LOCS was used in the case-control study of Leske et al.[152] referred to above. There is no doubt that these reproducible and objective measuring systems will be valuable not only in describing and following the development of cataract but also in evaluating the impact of drugs that might be used in the future for the medical therapy of cataract.

A systematic approach to classifying excised human lenses was pioneered by Pirie[199] using a system based upon lens coloration. A later scheme, introduced by Marcantonio et al.,[167] took into account electrolyte levels in the lens as

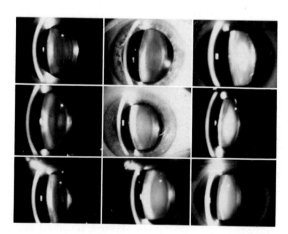

FIG. 10-23 Slit lamp photographs of different types of human cataracts showing varying degrees of nuclear opalescence (N) and coloration (nc), parameters by which the Lens Opacity Classification System can, in part, grade the cataracts. For example, cataract A would be classified N_0, nc_0, while cataract I would be rated N_2, nc_2, where the subscript refers to the intensity of opalescence or color in comparison to a standard. (From Chylack et al,[42] p 333.)

cataract. The possible mechanism of cataract will also be discussed.

SENILE CATARACT

The human lens is exposed to a variety of stresses throughout life, and the relative risk factors for the development of cataract have been discussed previously. Thus cataract developing with age probably represents the result of exposure to a variety of cataractogenic stresses coupled with a lessening of the ability of the lens to protect itself.

Despite the broad pathology, senile cataract can be divided into those lenses with principal changes in the cortex and those with principal changes in the nucleus. About two thirds of all senile cataracts exhibit primary changes in the cortex; however, most senile cataracts will manifest some changes in both cortical and nuclear regions. Cortical cataracts always manifest derangement of electrolyte and water balance, while the nuclear cataracts are associated more with protein modification and insolubilization, and increased coloration, sometimes even browning, as in brunescent cataract.

The disruption of electrolyte and water balance in cortical cataract is extensively documented.[189] There is a marked increase in lens sodium and chloride coupled with a decrease in potassium; substantial increases in lens calcium levels also take place. The electrolyte imbalance results in cellular hydration, lens cell swelling,

and rupture. Since lens electrolyte distribution is dependent upon membrane transport and permeability properties, several studies have examined these parameters in cataractous lenses. Physiological measurements have demonstrated marked increases in lens permeability in cataract,[159,165] but Maraini and Pasino[165] suggested that the active transport mechanisms were largely unimpaired in many forms of cataract. Direct measurements of the transport enzyme Na,K-ATPase in human cataractous lenses have led to conflicting data, some suggesting reduction of activity with cataract and other results indicating no change. Paterson et al.[186] examined Na,K-ATPase activity in human cortical, nuclear, and posterior subcapsular cataracts and found no significant difference between cataractous lenses and clear eye bank lenses (Fig. 10-24). Such data would appear to agree with the physiologic findings of Maraini and Pasino[165] discussed above. Thus a marked increase in lens membrane permeability might result in such excessive leakage of ions that the active transport mechanisms are unable to compensate. Similar alterations in membrane permeability might lead to the increase in lens calcium in cataract. Whether or not Ca-ATPase activity is altered in human cataract is not known. The extensive disruption of membrane permeability properties also leads to a loss of smaller molecules such as carbohydrates, amino acids, and small peptides from the lens.

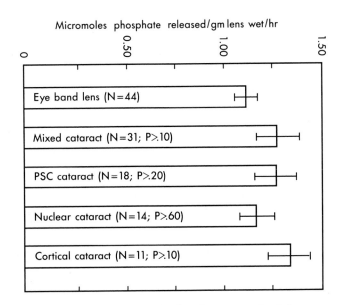

FIG. 10-24 Levels of Na,K-ATPase activity in clear human eye bank lenses compared to different types of human cataractous lenses. (Data redrawn from Paterson et al.[186])

The modification of lens proteins in both lens cortex and nucleus in senile cataract has been extensively studied and is the subject of excellent reviews.[3,108,226] The hallmark of protein modification in cataract is the dramatic increase in the water-insoluble fraction. The formation of high-molecular-weight protein aggregates accompanies aging, but the process is greatly accelerated in cataract development, involving cortex and nucleus. It is, however, unlikely that insolubilization of protein alone results in the extensive lens opacification, since some cataracts contain less insoluble protein than normal aged lenses.[226] Further studies on cataractous lens proteins reveal that some of the high-molecular-weight protein aggregates are different from those in normal old lenses. In cataract there is a high-molecular-weight aggregate characterized by linkage of the polypeptide chains through disulfide bonds, which are formed as a result of oxidation of thiol groups on the protein. As will be discussed later, oxidative modification of lens proteins is rarely observed in noncataractous lenses, suggesting a critical role of oxidation in cataract development. The high-molecular-weight aggregates appear to contain 43 kDa, 20 kDa, and 10 kDa polypeptides.[229] The smaller polypeptide units appear to be derived from the crystallins, but the 43 kDa polypeptide is characteristically found in all disulfide-linked protein aggregates and is probably derived from gamma crystallin.[88] This aggregate has also been shown to be associated with the surface of lens cell membranes, perhaps the site of early oxidative insult. Detailed analysis of the disulfide-linked protein aggregates has shown that they also contain intrinsic membrane protein (for example, MP26), suggesting considerable disruption of normal membrane organization.

Along with lens electrolyte imbalance, protein modification, and lipid disturbances, cataractous lenses manifest a number of other changes. Increased proteolysis leads to the formation of small polypeptide species, which can leak out of the lens. Many of the critical enzymes are reduced in activity or modified; ATP production is certainly reduced.[8] Glutathione levels are also greatly lowered. Several investigators have generated convincing evidence that oxidative damage can lead to many of the molecular events associated with cataract development.

Oxidative damage and cataract

There is an abundance of evidence to suggest an intimate relationship between oxidative damage and the development of cataract. Most forms of cataract manifest reduced glutathione levels, which might indicate a loss of the ability of the lens to withstand oxidative stress or that the protective mechanisms have been overcome.[190,212] Particular interest has been focused on the modification of lens proteins by oxidation and the impact of oxidation on membrane transport and permeability. Some more recent yet preliminary studies have also examined the direct effect of oxidative damage on cellular DNA[19] and lens cytoskeleton.[201]

The precise nature of the oxidizing agents responsible for molecular damage in the lens is uncertain. There are a number of potential sources of oxidants in the lens and these have been comprehensively reviewed by Augusteyn.[3] The cytotoxicity of oxygen is well established.[83,84] The damaging species of oxygen are superoxide, hydrogen peroxide, and the hydroxyl radical. Oxygen radicals can be produced within the eye as a result of photooxidation and ionizing radiation. The effects of ultraviolet light and ionizing radiation on the lens will be discussed later in this chapter.

The lens, like other tissues, possesses a number of mechanisms to protect itself against oxidation. The glutathione system, which has been discussed earlier, superoxide dismutase, catalase, and glutathione peroxidase, all play important roles. An additional source of protection is ascorbic acid, although ascorbic acid itself can lead to the generation of oxidant species.[198] In vitro studies have demonstrated a huge capacity of the lens epithelium to detoxify hydrogen peroxide.[92] For the lens to fall prey to oxidation, these antioxidant mechanisms must be overcome or suppressed. Elevated levels of hydrogen peroxide have been determined in the aqueous humor of some cataract patients.[228] In 7 of 17 patients the level of hydrogen peroxide was greater than the normal average of 26 μM; one of the patients was reported to have a hydrogen peroxide level in the aqueous humor of 663 μM. Further careful evaluation of this parameter would seem warranted. Whatever the source of oxidative species in the eye is, the potential for insult to the lens is substantial.

Modification of lens protein structure by oxidation has been studied extensively. The young lens shows little evidence of protein oxidation, and only relatively minor oxidative changes are seen in the proteins of older clear lenses. In cataractous lenses, however, there is extensive oxidative modification of proteins.

The amino acids methionine and cysteine are most vulnerable to oxidation, particularly in the proteins associated with the cell membranes. In cataractous lenses, it is not unusual to find greater than 50% of the methionine group oxidized to methionine sulfoxide and even 100% of the cysteine groups oxidized to form disulfide groups.[225] There is also evidence that oxidation of the accessible amino acid groups leads to an unfolding of the protein molecule and the exposure of buried cysteine groups to oxidation. The disulfide groups generated by oxidation link to each other, forming disulfide bonds that cause the protein to aggregate into very-high-molecular-weight insoluble molecules. A major component of these aggregates is a 43 kDa polypeptide that is attached to the cell membrane (Fig. 10-25).[78,227] It is thought that the divalent calcium ion can stabilize this 43 kDa peptide; thus elevation of calcium, as seen in cortical cataract, might enhance or contribute to the protein aggregation process. The linkage of protein aggregates to the membrane by the 43 kDa polypeptide component might interfere with normal membrane function. While membrane disruption following protein modification would be expected to impair transport and permeability properties, there is also evidence that the transport enzymes might be directly damaged by oxidation. Lenses incubated in the presence of

hydrogen peroxide certainly demonstrate electrolyte imbalance, increased permeability, and reduced transport ability by oxidation.[63,86] Several studies have demonstrated inhibition of isolated Na,K-ATPase by hydrogen peroxide.[63,89,230] More recently, Borchman et al.[24] have shown that Ca-ATPase might be even more sensitive to oxidative damage; however, when Na,K-ATPase and Ca-ATPase are isolated from lenses incubated for 20 hours in hydrogen peroxide, the activity of these enzymes seems little different from that in control lenses.[61] It would appear, therefore, that the ATPase function within the lens is in some way modified by hydrogen peroxide such that ion transport is impaired; however, after only a short-term exposure of the lens to hydrogen peroxide, the enzyme is essentially undamaged.

Oxidation could also impact directly on the membrane lipids that directly contribute to membrane permeability and form part of the membrane domain for the transport enzymes and ion channels. Modification of membrane lipids in other biological systems has been shown to directly alter cation pump activity.[264]

The accumulated evidence certainly favors a role for oxidative damage in the development of cataract. Whether oxidative damage is the single

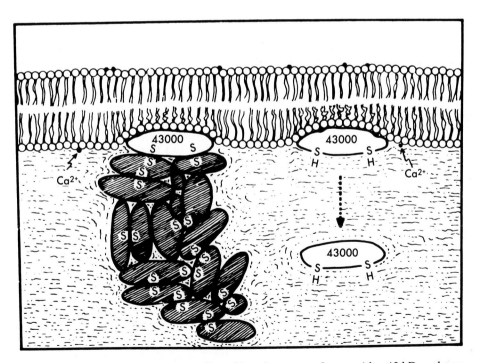

FIG. 10-25 Schematic representation of lens fiber plasma membrane with a 43 kDa polypeptide bound to the inner surface of the membrane. (From Spector,[225] p 137.)

initiating factor in the development of senile cataract is not known. It remains to be seen whether targeted antioxidant therapy will ultimately become a medical approach to treating cataracts.

Calcium and cataract

The elevation of calcium levels in cortical cataract is fully documented.[74] Loss of calcium homeostasis can lead to cell death.[223] Increased intracellular calcium levels can have a most deleterious effect on lens metabolism (for review, see Hightower[113]), including depressed glucose metabolism, inhibition of protein synthesis, induction of high-molecular-weight protein aggregates, and the activation of proteases, such as calpain. This elevation of lens calcium might lead to a cascade of cataractogenic events. Elevation of cellular calcium may also be linked directly to loss of transparency.[46,115]

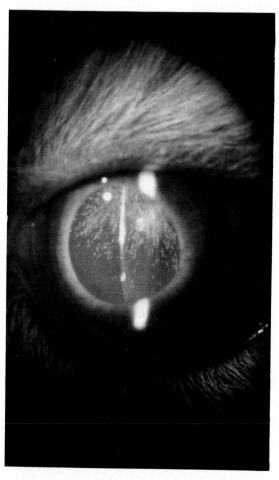

FIG. 10-26 Slit lamp photograph of hypocalcemic cataract induced in a juvenile rabbit.

Calcium might directly inhibit the lens sodium pump.[106,114] Intracellular levels of calcium have been shown to modulate lens gap junction structure and coupling.[14,130,191] Elevated calcium results in the activation of certain proteases;[56,126,216] in other systems it has been shown that a variety of proteases can modify ATPase function and membrane integrity.[10,142,171] Similarly, calcium-induced alteration of specific kinases might be expected to impact upon membrane function. Elevated calcium levels might also activate calmodulin to trigger a sequence of metabolic events in the lens.[128] Thus calcium might play a significant role in eliciting molecular changes that would contribute to the loss of lens transparency.

Cataract can also develop as a consequence of systemic hypocalcemia.[60] Depressed levels of serum calcium can result from a variety of pathological conditions and are frequently characterized by tetany. Hypocalcemic cataract is seen as numerous punctate opacities in the outer cortex that later spread out and merge to give a flaky appearance. Juvenile rabbits placed on a calcium-deficient diet develop lens opacities within several weeks (Fig. 10-26). The cause of hypocalcemic cataract is almost certainly related to the dependence of lens cell membrane permeability upon extracellular levels of calcium.[58,59] In vitro studies demonstrate marked electrolyte and water imbalance in lenses maintained in a low calcium environment.

DIABETIC AND GALACTOSEMIC CATARACT (SUGAR CATARACT)

Cataract is a complication of diabetes and galactosemia. Human diabetic cataract can develop rapidly in uncontrolled diabetes mellitus. Beginning as small superficial vacuoles, the opacity spreads into the cortex. Resolution, or effective early control of the diabetic event, can lead to isolated snowflakelike opacities in the cortex. In both cases an underlying mechanism is the conversion of glucose (in the case of diabetes) and galactose (in the case of galactosemia) to their respective sugar alcohols or polyols via the sorbitol pathway. As will be recalled from the earlier section on carbohydrate metabolism, when the level of glucose exceeds the capacity of the glycolytic pathway enzyme hexokinase, it spills over into the sorbitol pathway to be metabolized via the enzyme aldose reductase. Glucose is converted by aldose reductase into sorbitol, which is only slowly metabolized by polyoldehydrogenase. Sorbitol cannot readily diffuse out of the intracellular compartment and therefore accumulates within the lens, creating an os-

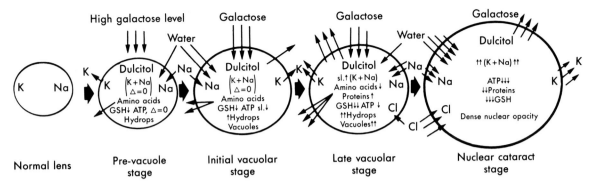

FIG. 10-27 Representation of changes occurring during the development of galactose cataract. (From Kinoshita,[139] p 786.)

motic gradient favoring the movement of water into the cells, which swell and ultimately rupture. The additional influx of glucose into the lens takes place in diabetes when the aqueous humor glucose level rises along with the blood level. In the case of galactosemia, elevated plasma levels of galactose are caused by a deficiency of galactose-1-phosphate-uridyl-transferase or galactokinase. Galactose enters the lens and is metabolized via aldose reductase to dulcitol, which accumulates within the lens fibers. Dulcitol is not further metabolized, and therefore results in cellular osmotic disturbance that is even more pronounced than that seen with sorbitol accumulation.

Our understanding of the osmotic mechanism of sugar cataract development has been made possible by extensive studies using animal models. The induction of experimental diabetes or feeding a galactose-rich diet results in characteristic changes in the lens leading to opacification. These events were diagrammed in the classic study of Kinoshita[138] (Fig. 10-27). The osmotic swelling induced by polyol accumulation leads to leakage of essential lens constituents, disruption of electrolyte balance, and depressed metabolism. Of considerable interest is the fact that the development of sugar cataract in animals can be inhibited by the use of several inhibitors of aldose reductase.[40,123,134,194,251] Such compounds have been shown to interfere effectively with the production of sorbitol or dulcitol, thereby preventing the osmotic imbalance. Unfortunately, the efficacy of aldose reductase inhibitors in man has been less significant, perhaps due to specific differences in the kinetics of human aldose reductase.[235]

While the accumulation of polyols would seem to be a major factor in the cataractogenic process, there is also evidence that sugars might directly interact with lens proteins by a process called glycosylation, leading to protein aggregation and ultimately cataract formation.[233] Glycosylation is a nonenzymatic process by which glucose attaches to certain amino acid residues on lens proteins; this ultimately results in the formation of carbonyl groups that can cross link, causing protein aggregation. It has also been suggested that glycosylation of proteins might cause conformational changes, increasing the chance of oxidation and formation of disulfide bonds and subsequent aggregation.[15] Aspirin has been suggested as an anticataract agent on the basis of its ability to block protein glycosylation.[209] More recently, Lewis and Harding[153] have demonstrated specific blockade of glycosylation by aminoguanidine. The relative role of protein glycosylation in sugar cataract development remains an open question. In fact, Chiou et al.[38] claim that glycosylation plays an insignificant role, since the same degree of glycosylation was evident in both cataractous and noncataractous (sorbinil-treated) lenses from rats fed a high galactose diet.

Cataract also occurs in hypoglycemia.[44] Neonatal hypoglycemia occurs in approximately 20% of newborn infants and the incidence is significantly increased in premature infants. The cataract is almost certainly due to inadequate availability of glucose and the consequent inability of the lens to produce sufficient metabolic energy.

ULTRAVIOLET LIGHT AND CATARACT

The cornea absorbs about 45% of light with wavelengths below 280 nm. Between 320 and 400 nm only 12% is absorbed by the cornea.[150] Thus the unprotected lens is exposed to a considerable amount of long-wave ultraviolet light, mainly from sunlight.

The relationship between cataract development and exposure to ultraviolet light has been suspected for many years.[71] Early epidemiologic studies suggested that the higher incidence of cataract in certain countries might be related to the greater exposure to sunlight. Zigman[272] has reviewed many of these early studies, concluding that exposure to sunlight does indeed increase the risk for cataract. Weale, also in 1983,[253] supported the relationship between sunlight and senile cataract. In more recent epidemiologic studies[49,152] the role of ultraviolet light as a major risk factor for cataract has been strongly supported and the value of eye protection has been reinforced. Taylor demonstrated the relationship between cataract development and ultraviolet light exposure in a class of fisherman regularly exposed to direct and reflected sunlight.[239]

The precise mechanism by which ultraviolet light results in metabolic damage to the lens is not entirely understood; however, there is a relationship between exposure of the lens to ultraviolet light and the oxidative mechanisms involved in cataract development. There is evidence that long-wave ultraviolet light can result in the formation of oxygen radicals and hydrogen peroxide within the eye, and also increase the production of fluorophores within the lens.[3] These issues have been more fully covered in the section on Photobiology.

IONIZING RADIATION AND MICROWAVE CATARACT

Cataractogenesis following exposure to ionizing radiation has been established for a long time.[172] Studies in animals have demonstrated substantial morphologic damage following x-irradia-

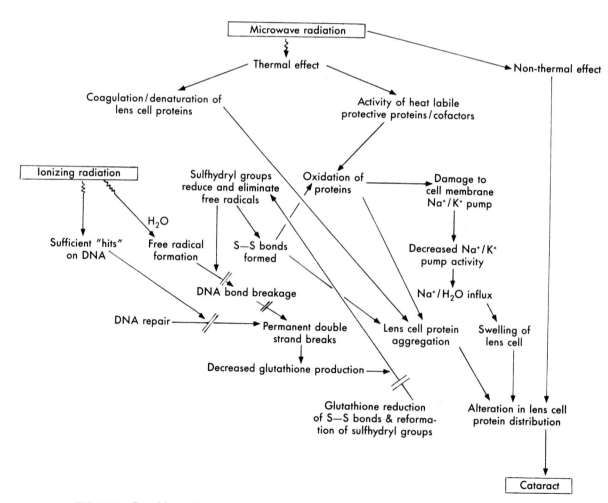

FIG. 10-28 Possible mechanisms of cataractogenesis following exposure of the lens to microwave and ionizing radiation. (From Lipman et al,[156] p 208.)

tion, including vacuolization in the anterior and posterior cortex, swollen epithelial cells, liquefaction of lens fiber cells, and posterior subcapsular opacities. Many of the significant morphologic studies have been summarized by Lipman et al.[156] The dose of radiation necessary to induce x-ray cataract is quite variable, depending upon the species of animal employed and the amount of lens that is exposed to radiation; the threshold for cataractogenesis would seem to be in the range of 1000 rads. The threshold for humans appears to be somewhat less, since the data of Merriam and Focht[172] suggest that some individuals can develop cataract after receiving only 200 rads in a single dose. A large single dose of radiation appears to be more cataractogenic than the additive effect of smaller doses.

The mechanism of ioinizing radiation induced cataract involves several factors, including oxidative damage resulting from free radical formation, changes in membrane permeability, and direct damage to cellular DNA.[261] The proposed mechanisms are summarized in Fig. 10-28. Shortly after radiation damage there is a marked decrease in lens glutathione levels and ascorbate, suggesting a loss of antioxidant protection.

The use of microwave radiation has grown considerably over the years, including the use of microwave ovens in the home. There is now ample evidence that microwave radiation can cause cataracts in experimental animals (see Lipman et al.[156] for review). Evidence for microwave-induced cataract in humans is less certain but there is no question that the potential does exist. Morphologic changes in microwave cataract are rather similar to those following ionizing radiation. After the development of anterior vacuoles within hours of microwave exposure, the lesion spreads to the posterior lens within days. The threshold for microwave-induced cataract is uncertain, but in experimental animals it would appear that microwave radiation doses in the range of 200 mW/cm² are definitely cataractogenic. There is no doubt that the temperature elevation following microwave injury contributes to the development of cataract (see Fig. 10-28). Temperatures above 41°C certainly result in considerable lens pathology; however, some of the pathology is probably the result of damage other than that induced by increased temperature.

DRUG-INDUCED CATARACT

Cataract is seen as a complication of systemic and topical delivery of a variety of chemical substances, including prescription drugs. The subject of drug-induced cataract has been covered in several lengthy reviews[147,184] and texts.[82,98]

Of principal interest is the cataract induced by corticosteroids, a topic reviewed by Urban and Cotlier.[243] The opacities observed as a result of systemic or topical corticosteroid therapy are initially confined to the posterior subcapsular region of the lens, later spreading into the cortex. The incidence of lens changes is dependent upon the total dosage of steroid, the age of the patient, and the nature of the underlying disease requiring corticosteroid therapy. The cataractogenic mechanism of corticosteroids is not clearly understood. There is some evidence that corticosteroids might impair electrolyte transport and permeability function. It has also been suggested that corticosteroids might modify lens proteins in such a way as to promote aggregation.

The role of phenothiazines in increasing the risk for cataract has recently been reaffirmed by Isaac et al.[127] Phenothiazines can act as photosensitizers, and there the cataractogenic effect is likely associated with exposure to ultraviolet light. Phenothiazine cataracts also manifest anterior pigmentation. Laboratory studies have revealed altered electrolyte transport following exposure of the lens to chlorpromazine.[258]

A number of miotics have been implicated as being cataractogenic, including the irreversible cholinesterase inhibitors such as echothiophate and phospholine iodide.[5]

TREATMENT OF CATARACT

In the United States treatment of cataract is restricted to surgical removal of the opaque lens. New surgical techniques reduce the risk and improved vision is brought about by the use of intraocular lenses. The rate of cataract surgery has increased more than threefold over the last 20 years. Presently there is no medical therapy to prevent the formation and progression of cataract. In a number of other countries a number of medications, including aspirin and antioxidants, are claimed to delay cataract formation. Several very informative reviews on the various medications and their supposed mode of action are available.[133,221,249] It would seem that there is very little strong evidence to support claims of efficacy.

REFERENCES

1. Alcala J, Maisel H: Biochemistry of lens plasma membranes and cytoskeleton, in Maisel H, ed: The ocular lens: structure, function, and pathology, New York, Marcel Dekker, 1985, pp 169-222.
2. Anderson EI, Spector A: The state of sulfhydryl groups

in normal and cataractous human lens proteins, I, Nuclear region, Exp Eye Res 26:407, 1978.

3. Augusteyn RC: Protein modification in cataract: possible oxidative mechanisms, in Duncan G, ed: Mechanisms of cataract formation in the human lens, London, Academic Press, 1981, pp 71-115.

4. Auricchio G, Rinaldi E, Savastano S, et al: The Na-K-ATPase in relation to the Na, K and taurine levels in the senile cataract, Metabol Ped Ophthalmol 4:15, 1980.

5. Axelson U: Miotic-induced cataract, in: The human lens—in relation to cataract, Ciba Foundation Symposium 19, pp 25-43, Amsterdam, Elsevier, 1973.

6. Baldwin GF, Bentley PJ: Some observations on the magnesium metabolism of the amphibian lens, Exp Eye Res 31:665, 1980.

7. Bassnett S, Duncan G: The influence of pH on membrane conductance and intercellular resistance in the rat lens, J Physiol (Lond) 398:507, 1988.

8. Beaulieu CF, Clark JI: ^{31}P nuclear magnetic resonance and laser spectroscopic analyses of lens transparency during calcium-induced opacification, Invest Ophthalmol Vis Sci 31:1339, 1990.

9. Beebe DC, Feagans DE, Jebens HA: Lentropin: a factor in vitreous humor which promotes lens fiber cell differentiation, Proc Nat Acad Sci 77:490, 1980.

10. Benaim G, Zurini M, Carafoli E: Different conformational states of the purified Ca^{2+}-ATPase of the erythrocyte plasma membrane revealed by controlled trypsin proteolysis, J Biol Chem 259:8471, 1984.

11. Benedek GB: Theory of transparency of the eye, Applied Optics 10:459, 1971.

12. Benedetti L, Dunia I, Ramaekers, FCS, et al: Lenticular plasma membranes and cytoskeleton, in Bloemendal H, ed: Molecular and cellular biology of the eye lens, New York, John Wiley, 1981, pp 137-188.

13. Bentley PJ, Chin B, Grubb B: Some observations on the zinc metabolism of the rabbit lens, Exp Eye Res 38:497, 1984.

14. Bernardini G, Peracchia C: Gap junction crystallization in lens fibers after an increase in cell calcium, Invest Ophthalmol Vis Sci 21:291, 1981.

15. Beswick HT, Harding JJ: Conformational changes induced in lens α-and gamma-crystallins by modification with glucose-6-phosphate; implications for cataract, Biochem J 246:761, 1987.

16. Bettelheim FA: Physical basis of lens transparency, in Maisel H, ed: The ocular lens: structure, function and pathology, New York, Marcel Dekker, 1985, pp 265-300.

17. Bhuyan K, Bhuyan D: Regulation of hydrogen peroxide in eye humors; effect of 3-amino-1H-1,2,4-triazole on catalase and glutathione peroxidase of rabbit eye, Biochim Biophys Acta 497:641, 1977.

18. Bhuyan KC, Bhuyan DK: Superoxide dismutase of the eye: relative functions of superoxide dismutase and catlase in protecting the ocular lens from oxidative damage, Biochim Biophys Acta, 542:28, 1978.

19. Block AL, Frederikse P, Kleiman NJ, et al: Oxidative damage to DNA transfected into bovine lens epithelial cells as a function of transcriptional activity, Invest Ophthalmol Vis Sci 31(Suppl):204, 1990.

20. Bloemendal H: Biosynthesis of lens crystallins, in Bloe-

mendal H, ed: Molecular and cellular biology of the eye lens, New York, John Wiley, 1981, pp 189-220.

21. Bloemendal H: The lens proteins, in Bloemendal H, ed: Molecular and cellular biology of the eye lens, New York, John Wiley, 1981, pp 1-47.

22. Borchman D, Delamere NA, Paterson CA: Ca-ATPase activity in the rabbit and bovine lens, Invest Ophthalmol Vis Sci 29:982, 1988.

23. Borchman D, Paterson CA, Delamere NA: Ca^{2+}-ATPase activity in the human lens, Curr Eye Res 8:1049, 1989.

24. Borchman D, Paterson CA, Delamere NA: Oxidative inhibition of Ca^{2+}-ATPase in the rabbit lens, Invest Ophthalmol Vis Sci 30:1633, 1989.

25. Borchman D, Yappert MC, Herrell P: Structural characterization of human lens membrane lipid by infrared spectroscopy, Invest Ophthalmol Vis Sci, 32:2404, 1991.

26. Brewster D: On the structure of the crystalline lens in fishes and quadrupeds, as ascertained by its action on polarised light, Phil Trans Roy Soc Lond 106:311, 1816.

27. Broekhuyse RM: Phospholipids in the tissues of the eye, III, Composition and metabolism of phospholipids in human lens in relation to age and cataract formation, Biochim Biophys Acta 187:354, 1969.

28. Broekhuyse RM: Biochemistry of membranes, in Duncan G, ed: Mechanisms of cataract formation in the human lens, London, Academic Press, 1981, pp 151-191.

29. Broekhuyse RM, Veerkamp JH: Phospholipids in the tissues of the eye, II, Composition and incorporation of $^{32}P_i$ of phospholipids of normal rat and calf lens, Biochim Biophys Acta 152:316, 1968.

30. Brown HG, Pappas GD, Ireland ME, et al: Ultrastructural, biochemical, and immunologic evidence of receptor-mediated endocytosis in the crystalline lens, Invest Ophthalmol Vis Sci 31:2579, 1990.

31. Brown NAP: Slit-image photography and measurements of the eye, Med Biol Illus 23:192, 1973.

32. Brown N: Dating the onset of cataract, Trans Ophthalmol Soc UK 96:18, 1976.

33. Cagianut B, Verrey F: An attempt to elucidate the water metabolism in the transparent media of the human eye by injection of heavy water into the anterior chamber, Ann Ocul 182:649, 1949.

34. Chamberlain CG, McAvoy JW: Evidence that fibroblast growth factor promotes lens fibre differentiation, Curr Eye Res 6:1165, 1987.

35. Chen TT, Hockwin O, Dobbs R, et al: Cataract and health status: a case-control study, Ophthalmic Res 20:1, 1988.

36. Cheng H-M, Chylack LT Jr: Lens metabolism, in Maisel H, ed: The ocular lens: structure, function, and pathology, New York, Marcel Dekker, 1985, pp 223-264.

37. Cheng H-M, Chylack LT Jr, von Saltza I: Supplementing glucose metabolism in human senile cataracts, Invest Ophthalmol Vis Sci 21:812, 1981.

38. Chiou SH, Chylack LT Jr, Bunn HF, et al: Role of nonenzymatic glycosylation in experimental cataract formation, Biochem Biophys Res Commun 95:894, 1980.

39. Chylack LT Jr, Friend J: Intermediary metabolism of

the lens: a historical perspective, 1928-1989, Exp Eye Res 50:575, 1990.

40. Chylack LT Jr, Henriques HF III, Cheng HM, et al: Efficacy of alrestatin, an aldose reductase inhibitor in human diabetic and non-diabetic lenses, Ophthalmol 86:1579, 1979.

41. Chylack LT Jr, Lee MR, Tung WH, et al: Classification of human senile cataractous change by the American Cooperative Cataract Research Group (CCRG) method, I, Instrumentation and technique, Invest Ophthalmol Vis Sci 24:424, 1983.

42. Chylack LT Jr, Leske MC, Sperduto R, et al: Lens opacities classification system, Arch Ophthalmol 106:330, 1988.

43. Chylack LT Jr, Ransil BJ, White O: Classification of human senile cataractous change by the American Co-operative Cataract Research Group (CCRG) method, III, The association of nuclear color (sclerosis) with extent of cataract formation, age, and visual acuity, Invest Ophthalmol Vis Sci 25:174, 1984.

44. Chylack LT Jr, Schaefer FL: Mechanism of "hypoglycemic" cataract formation in the rat lens, II, Further studies on the role of hexokinase instability, Invest Ophthalmol 15:519, 1976.

45. Chylack LT Jr, White O, Tung WH: Classification of human senile cataractous change by the American Co-operative Cataract Group (CCRG) method, II, Staged simplification of cataract classification, Invest Ophthalmol Vis Sci 25:166, 1984.

46. Clark JI, Mengel L, Bagg A, et al: Cortical opacity, calcium concentration and fiber membrane structure in the calf lens, Exp Eye Res 31:399, 1980.

47. Clayton RM: Developmental genetics of the lens, in Maisel H, ed: The ocular lens: structure, function, and pathology, New York, Marcel Dekker, 1985, pp 61-92.

48. Clayton RM, Cuthbert J, Seth J, et al: Epidemiological and other studies in the assessment of factors contributing to cataractogenesis, in Nugent J, Whelan J, eds: Human cataract formation, Ciba Foundation Symposium 106, London, Pitman, 1984, pp 25-47.

49. Collman GW, Shore DL, Shy CM, et al: Sunlight and other risk factors for cataracts: an epidemiologic study, Am J Public Health, 78:1459, 1988.

50. Congenital Malformations Surveillance Report, July 1978-June 1979, US Department of Health and Human Services, Centers for Disease Control, 1980.

51. Cotlier E: Myo-inositol: active transport by the crystalline lens, Invest Ophthalmol 9:681, 1970.

52. Coulter JB III, Swanson AA, Bond TJ: Metabolism of rat lens proteins, Ophthalmic Res 2:322, 1971.

53. Dardenne U, Kirsten G: Presence and metabolism of amino acids in young and old lenses, Exp Eye Res 1:415, 1962.

54. Datiles MB, Edwards PA, Trus BL, et al: In vivo studies on cataracts using the Scheimpflug slit lamp camera, Invest Ophthalmol Vis Sci 28:1707, 1987.

55. David LL, Shearer TR: Role of proteolysis in lenses: a review, Lens Eye Toxic Res 6:725, 1989.

56. David LL, Varnum MD, Lampi KJ, et al: Calpain II in human lens, Invest Ophthalmol Vis Sci 30:269, 1989.

57. de Jong WW: Evolution of lens and crystallins, in Bloemendal H, ed: Molecular and cellular biology of the eye lens, New York, John Wiley, 1981, pp 221-278.

58. Delamere NA, Paterson CA: The influence of calcium-free EGTA solution upon membrane permeability in the crystalline lens of the frog, J Gen Physiol 272:167, 1977.

59. Delamere NA, Paterson CA: The influence of calcium-free solutions upon permeability characteristics of the rabbit lens, Exp Eye Res 28:45, 1979.

60. Delamere NA, Paterson CA: Hypocalcaemic cataract, in Duncan G, ed: Mechanisms of cataract formation in the human lens, London, Academic Press, 1981, pp 219-236.

61. Delamere NA, Paterson CA, Borchman DB, et al: Alteration of lens electrolyte transport parameters following transient oxidative perturbation, Curr Eye Res 7:969, 1988.

62. Delamere NA, Paterson CA, Borchman D, et al: Studies on calcium transport, Ca-ATPase and lipid order in rabbit ocular lens membranes, Am J Physiol, in press, 1991.

63. Delamere NA, Paterson CA, Cotton TR: Lens cation transport and permeability changes following exposure to hydrogen peroxide, Exp Eye Res 37:45, 1983.

64. Delamere NA, Paterson CA, Duncan G, et al: Relative roles of Ca^{2+}, Sr^{2+}, Ba^{2+} and Mg^{2+} in controlling lens permeability characteristics, Cell Calcium 1:81, 1980.

65. Delaye M, Tardieu A: Short-range order of crystallin proteins accounts for eye lens transparency, Nature, 302:415, 1983.

66. Dickerson JE, Lou MF: Micro-quantitation of lens myo-inositol by anion exchange chromatography, Curr Eye Res 9:201, 1990.

67. Dickinson JC, Durham DG, Hamilton PB: Ion exchange chromatography of free amino acids in aqueous fluid and lens of the human eye, Invest Ophthalmol 7:551, 1968.

68. Dillon J: Photochemical mechanisms in the lens, in Maisel H, ed: The ocular lens: structure, function, and pathology, New York, Marcel Dekker, 1985, pp 349-366.

69. DiMattio J: Active transport of ascorbic acid into lens epithelium of the rat, Exp Eye Res 49:873, 1989.

70. Dische Z, Zelmenis G: The content and structural characteristics of the collagenous protein of rabbit lens capsules at different ages, Invest Ophthalmol 4:174, 1965.

71. Duke-Elder WS: The pathological action of light upon the eye, II, Action upon the lens: theory of the genesis of cataract, Lancet 1:1188, 1926.

72. Duncan G: Role of membranes in controlling ion and water movements in the lens, in: The human lens—in relation to cataract, Ciba Foundation Symposium 19, Amsterdam, Elsevier, 1973, pp 99-116.

73. Duncan G, Bushell AR: Ion analyses of human cataractous lenses, Exp Eye Res 20:223, 1975.

74. Duncan G, Jacob TJC: Calcium and the physiology of cataract, in Nugent J, Whelan J, eds: Human cataract formation, Ciba Foundation Symposium 106, London, Pitman, 1984, pp 132-152.

75. Eckhert CD: Elemental concentrations in ocular tissues of various species, Exp Eye Res 37:639, 1983.

76. Edwards PA, Datiles MB, Green SB: Reproducibility study on the Scheimpflug cataract video camera, Curr Eye Res 7:955, 1988.

77. Ehring GR, Zampighi G, Horwitz J, et al: Properties of

channels reconstituted from the major intrinsic protein of lens fiber membranes, J Gen Physiol 96:631, 1990.

78. Farnsworth PN, Spector A, Lozier JR, et al: The localization of a 43K polypeptide in normal and cataractous lenses by immunofluorescence, Exp Eye Res 32:257, 1981.

79. Fisher RF, Wakely J: Changes in lens fibres after damage to the lens capsule, Trans Ophthalmol Soc UK 96:278, 1976.

80. FitzGerald PG, Bok D, Horwitz J: The distribution of the main intrinsic membrane polypeptide in ocular lens, Curr Eye Res 4:1203, 1985.

81. Fleisher LN, McGahan MC: Endotoxin-induced ocular inflammation increases prostaglandin E_2 synthesis by rabbit lens, Exp Eye Res 40:711, 1985.

82. Fraunfelder FT: Drug-induced ocular side effects and drug interactions, Philadelphia, Lea and Febiger, 1976.

83. Fridovich I: Oxygen radicals, hydrogen peroxide and oxygen toxicity, in Pryor WA, ed: Free radicals in biology, vol 1, New York, Academic Press, 1976, pp 239-271.

84. Fridovich I: Oxygen: aspects of its toxicity and elements of defense, Curr Eye Res 3:1, 1984.

85. Friedenwald JS: The permeability of the lens capsule to water, dextrose and other sugars, Arch Ophthalmol 4:350, 1930.

86. Fukui HN: The effect of hydrogen peroxide on the rubidium transport of the rat lens, Exp Eye Res 23:595, 1976.

87. Gandolfi SA, Tomba MC, Maraini G: 86-Rb efflux in normal and cataractous human lenses, Curr Eye Res 4:753, 1985.

88. Garner WH, Garner MH, Spector A: Gamma-crystallin, a major cytoplasmic polypeptide disulfide linked to membrane proteins in human cataract, Biochem Biophys Res Commun 98:439, 1981.

89. Garner WH, Garner M, Spector A: H_2O_2-induced uncoupling of bovine lens Na^+,K^+-ATPase, Proc Nat Acad Sci USA 80:2044, 1983.

90. Garner WH, Spector A: Racemization in human lens: evidence of rapid insolubilization of specific polypeptides in cataract formation, Proc Nat Acad Sci USA 75:3618, 1978.

91. Garner WH, Spector A: A preliminary study of the dynamic aspects of age dependent changes in the abundances of human lens polypeptides, Doc Ophthalmol 81:91, 1979.

92. Giblin FJ, McCready JP, Reddy VN: The role of glutathione metabolism in the detoxification of H_2O_2 in rabbit lens, Invest Ophthalmol Vis Sci 22:330, 1982.

93. Glynn IM: The Na^+,K^+-transporting adenosine triphosphatase, in Martonosi AM, ed: The enzymes of biological membranes, vol 3, New York, Plenum, 1985, pp 35-114.

94. Gooden M, Rintoul D, Takehana M, et al: Major intrinsic polypeptide (MIP26K) from lens membrane: reconstitution into vesicles and inhibition of channel forming activity by peptide antiserum, Biochem Biophys Res Commun 128:993, 1985.

95. Gordon SR, Essner E, Rothstein H: In situ demonstration of actin in normal and injured ocular tissues using 7-nitrobenz-2-oxa-1,3-diazole phallacidin, Cell Motility 2:343, 1982.

96. Gorthy WC, Snavely MR, Berrong ND: Some aspects of transport and digestion in the lens of the normal young adult rat, Exp Eye Res 12:112, 1971.

97. Grant ME, Heathcote JG: A comparative study of lens capsule assembly, in Kuehn K, Schoene H-H, Timpl R, eds: Workshop Conference Hoechst, vol 10, New trends in basement membrane research, New York, Raven Press, 1982, pp 195-202.

98. Grant WM: Toxicology of the eye, 2nd ed, Springfield, IL, Charles C Thomas, Publisher, 1974.

99. Green H, Bocher CA, Leopold IH: Anaerobic carbohydrate metabolism of the crystalline lens, Am J Ophthalmol 40:237, 1955.

100. Greiner JV, Kopp SJ, Sanders DR, et al: Organophosphates of the crystalline lens: a nuclear magnetic resonance spectroscopic study, Invest Ophthalmol Vis Sci 21:700, 1981.

101. Grubb BR, Bentley PJ: The biology of strontium: interactions with the mammalian crystalline lens, Exp Eye Res 39:107 1984.

102. Grubb BR, Bentley PJ: Accumulation and toxicity of gold in the rabbit lens in vitro, Exp Eye Res 46:637, 1988.

103. Grubb BR, Driscoll SM, Bentley PJ: Exchanges of lead in vitro by the rabbit crystalline lens, Exp Eye Res 43:259, 1986.

104. Grubb BR, Driscoll SM, Bentley PJ: Mercury exchanges and toxicity in the crystalline lens in vitro, Ophthalmic Res 19:101, 1987.

105. Gupta JD, Harley JD: Decreased adenosine triphosphatase activity in human senile cataractous lenses, Exp Eye Res 20:207, 1975.

106. Hamilton PM, Delamere NA, Paterson CA: The influence of calcium on lens ATPase activity, Invest Ophthalmol Vis Sci 18:434, 1979.

107. Harding CV Jr, Maisel H, Chylack LT Jr, et al: The structure of the human cataractous lens, in Maisel H, ed: The ocular lens: structure, function, and pathology, New York, Marcel Dekker, 1985, pp 367-404.

108. Harding JJ: Changes in lens proteins in cataract, in Bloemendal H, ed: Molecular and cellular biology of the eye lens, New York, John Wiley, 1981, pp 327-365.

109. Harding JJ: Nonenzymatic covalent posttranslational modification of proteins in vivo, Adv Prot Chem 37:247, 1985.

110. Harding JJ: Case-control studies and risk factors for cataract: discussion paper, J Roy Soc Med 81:585, 1988.

111. Harding JJ, Rixon KC, Marriott FHC: Men have heavier lenses than women of the same age, Exp Eye Res 25:651, 1977.

112. Harris JE, Gehrsitz LB: Significance of changes in potassium and sodium content of the lens: a mechanism for lenticular intumescence, Am J Ophthalmol 34:131, 1951.

113. Hightower KR: Cytotoxic effects of internal calcium on lens physiology: a review, Curr Eye Res 4:453, 1985.

114. Hightower KR, Hind D: Cytotoxic effects of calcium on sodium-potassium transport in the mammalian lens, Curr Eye Res 2:239, 1982/83.

115. Hightower KR, Reddy VN: Ca^{++}-induced cataract, Invest Ophthalmol Vis Sci 22:263, 1982.

116. Hockwin O, Blum G, Korte I, et al: Studies on the citric

acid cycle and its portion of glucose breakdown by calf and bovine lenses in vitro, Ophthalmic Res 2:143, 1971.

117. Hockwin O, Ohrloff C: Enzymes in normal, aging and cataractous lenses, in Bloemendal H, ed: Molecular and cellular biology of the eye lens, New York, John Wiley, 1981, pp 367-413.

118. Hockwin O, Sasaki K, Lerman S: Evaluating cataract development with the Scheimpflug camera, in Masters BR, ed: Noninvasive diagnostic techniques in ophthalmology, New York, Springer-Verlag, 1991, pp 281-318.

119. Hoenders HJ, Bloemendal H: Aging of lens proteins, in Bloemendal H, ed: Molecular and cellular biology of the eye lens, New York, John Wiley, 1981, pp 279-326.

120. Hogan MJ, Alvarado JA, Weddell JE: Histology of the human eye, Philadelphia, WB Saunders, 1971, pp 638-677.

121. Horwitz J, Kabasawa I, Kinoshita JH: Conformation of gamma-crystallins of the calf lens: effects of temperature and denaturing agents, Exp Eye Res 25:199, 1977.

122. Horwitz J, Robertson NP, Wong MM, et al: Some properties of lens plasma membrane polypeptides isolated from normal human lenses, Exp Eye Res 28:359, 1979.

123. Hu TS, Datiles M, Kinoshita JH: Reversal of galactose cataract with sorbinil in rats, Invest Ophthalmol Vis Sci 24:640, 1983.

124. Huggert A, Odeblad E: Studies on the water of the crystalline lens, I, The exchangeable water of the cattle lens in different ages, Acta Ophthalmol 36:885, 1958.

125. Hughes RE, Hurley RJ: In vitro uptake of ascorbic acid by the guinea-pig lens, Exp Eye Res 9:175, 1970.

126. Ireland M, Maisel H: Evidence for a calcium activated protease specific for lens intermediate filaments, Curr Eye Res 3:423, 1984.

127. Isaac NE, Walker AM, Jick H, et al: Exposure to phenothiazine drugs and risk of cataract, Arch Ophthalmol 109:256, 1991.

128. Iwata S: Calcium-pump and its modulator in the lens: a review, Curr Eye Res 4:299, 1985.

129. Jacob TJC: A direct measurement of intracellular free calcium within the lens, Exp Eye Res 36:451, 1983.

130. Jacob TJC: Raised intracellular free calcium within the lens causes opacification and cellular uncoupling in the frog, J Physiol 341:595, 1983.

131. Jahn CE, Janke M, Winowski H, et al: Identification of metabolic risk factors for posterior subcapsular cataract, Ophthalmic Res 18:112, 1986.

132. Jernigan HM Jr, Kador PF, Kinoshita JH: Carrier mediated transport of choline in rat lens, Exp Eye Res 32:709, 1981.

133. Kador PF: Overview of the current attempts toward the medical treatment of cataract, Ophthalmol, 90:352, 1983.

134. Kador PF, Robison WG, Kinoshita JH: The pharmacology of aldose reductase inhibitors, Ann Rev Pharmacol Toxicol 25:691, 1985.

135. Kahn HA, Leibowitz HM, Ganley JP, et al: the Framingham eye study, I, Outline and major prevalence findings, Am J Epidemiol 106:17, 1977.

136. Kern HL: Transport of organic solutes in the lens, Curr Topics Eye Res 1:217, 1979.

137. Kern HL, Zolot SL: Transport of vitamin C in the lens, Curr Eye Res 6:885, 1987.

138. Kinoshita J: Cataracts in galactosemia, Invest Ophthalmol 4:786, 1965.

139. Kinoshita JH: Pathways of glucose metabolism in the lens, Invest Ophthalmol 4:619, 1965.

140. Kinoshita JH: A thirty year journey in the polyol pathway, Exp Eye Res 50:567, 1990.

141. Kinsey VE, Reddy DVN: Studies on the crystalline lens, XI, The relative role of the epithelium and capsule in transport, Invest Ophthalmol 4:104, 1965.

142. Kirchberger MA, Borchman D, Kasinathan C: Proteolytic activation of the canine cardiac sarcoplasmic reticulum calcium pump, Biochemistry 25:5484, 1986.

143. Kistler J, Bullivant S: Structural and molecular biology of the eye lens membranes, CRC Crit Rev Biochem Mol Biol 24:151, 1989.

144. Kistler J, Gilbert K, Brooks HV, et al: Membrane interlocking domains in the lens, Invest Ophthalmol Vis Sci 27:1527, 1986.

145. Kronfeld PC: The gross anatomy and embryology of the eye, in Davson H, ed: The eye, vol 1, 2nd ed, New York, Academic Press, 1969, pp 1-66.

146. Kuck JFR Jr: Chemical constituents of the lens, in Graymore CN, ed: Biochemistry of the eye, New York, Academic Press, 1970, pp 183-260.

147. Kuck JFR Jr: Drugs influencing the lens, in Dikstein S, ed: Drugs and ocular tissues, Basel, S Karger, 1977, pp 433-523.

148. Kuszak JR, Ennesser CA, Bertram BA, et al: The contribution of cell-to-cell fusion to the ordered structure of the crystalline lens, Lens Eye Tox Res 6:639, 1989.

149. Kuszak JR, Rae JL: Scanning electron microscopy of the frog lens, Exp Eye Res 35:499, 1982.

150. Lerman S: Radiant energy and the eye, New York, Macmillan, 1980.

151. Leske MC, Chylack LT Jr, Sperduto R, et al: Evaluation of a lens opacities classification system, Arch Ophthalmol 106:327, 1988.

152. Leske MC, Chylack LT Jr, Wu S-Y: The lens opacities case-control study; risk factors for cataract Arch Ophthalmol 109:244, 1991.

153. Lewis BS, Harding JJ: The effects of aminoguanidine on the glycation (non-enzymic glycosylation) of lens proteins, Exp Eye Res 50:463, 1990.

154. Li L-K, Spector A: Circular dichroism and optical rotatory dispersion of the aggregates of purified polypeptides of alpha-crystallin, Exp Eye Res 19:49, 1974.

155. Lindley PF, Narebor ME, Summers LJ, et al: The structure of lens proteins, in Maisel H, ed: The ocular lens: structure, function, and pathology, New York, Marcel Dekker, 1985, pp 123-168.

156. Lipman RM, Tripathi BJ, Tripathi RC: Cataracts induced by microwave and ionizing radiation, Surv Ophthalmol 33:200, 1988.

157. Lo WK, Harding CV: Structure and distribution of gap junctions in lens epithelium and fiber cells, Cell Tissue Res 244:253, 1986.

158. Lou MF, Garadi R, Thomas DM, et al: The effect of an aldose reductase inhibitor on lens phosphorylcholine under hyperglycemic conditions: biochemical and NMR studies, Exp Eye Res 48:11, 1989.

159. Lucas VA, Duncan G, Davies P: Membrane perme-

ability characteristics of perfused human senile cataractous lenses, Exp Eye Res 42:151, 1986.

160. Lucas VA, Zigler JS Jr: Transmembrane glucose carriers in the monkey lens, Invest Ophthalmol Vis Sci 28:1404, 1987.

161. Luntz MH: Clinical types of cataract, in Tasman W, Jaeger EA, eds: Duane's clinical ophthalmology, Philadelphia, JB Lippincott, 1990, Chap 73, pp 1-20.

162. Maisel H, Harding CV, Alcala JA, et al: The morphology of the lens, in Bloemendal H, ed: Molecular and cellular biology of the eye lens, New York, John Wiley, 1981, pp 49-84.

163. Mann I: The development of the human eye, New York, Grune and Stratton, 1950.

164. Maraini G, Mangili R: Differences in proteins and in water balance of the lens in nuclear and cortical types of senile cataract, in: The human lens—in relation to cataract, Ciba Foundation Symposium 19, Amsterdam, Elsevier, 1973, pp 79-97.

165. Maraini G, Pasino M: Active and passive rubidium influx in normal human lenses and in senile cataracts, Exp Eye Res 36:543, 1983.

166. Marcantonio J, Duncan G: Amino acid transport and protein synthesis in human normal and cataractous lenses, Curr Eye Res 6:1299, 1987.

167. Marcantonio JM, Duncan G, Bushell AR, et al: Classification of human senile cataracts by nuclear colour and sodium content, Exp Eye Res 31:227, 1980.

168. Masters PM, Bada JL, Zigler JS Jr: Aspartic acid racemisation in the human lens during ageing and in cataract formation, Nature 268:71, 1977.

169. McAvoy JW: Cell division, cell elongation and distribution of α-, β- and gamma-crystallins in the rat lens, J Embryol Exp Morphol 44:149, 1978.

170. McAvoy JW: Developmental biology of the lens, in Duncan G, ed: Mechanisms of cataract formation in the human lens, London, Academic Press, 1981, pp 7-46.

171. Mellgren RL: Calcium-dependent proteases: an enzyme system active at cellular membranes? FASEB J 1:110, 1987.

172. Merriam GRJ, Focht EF: A clinical study of radiation cataracts and the relationship to dose, Am J Roentgenol 77:759, 1957.

173. Miller TM, Goodenough DA: Evidence for two physiologically distinct gap junctions expressed by the chick lens epithelial cell, J Cell Biol 102:194, 1986.

174. Morner CT: Untersuchungen der Proteinsubstanzen in den lichtbrechended medien des Auges, Hoppe-Seylers Z Physiol Chem 18:61, 1894.

175. National Advisory Eye Council, Cataract Panel: Vision research—a national plan: 1983–1987, vol 1, National Institutes of Health publication 83-2470, Washington DC, 1983.

176. National Society to Prevent Blindness: Vision problems in the US: a statistical analysis prepared by the operational research development, New York: the Society, 1980.

177. Neville MC, Paterson CA, Hamilton PM: Evidence for two sodium pumps in the crystalline lens of the rabbit eye, Exp Eye Res 27:637, 1978.

178. Neville MC, Paterson CA, Rae JL, et al: Nuclear mag-

179. Nordmann J, Klethi J: L'activité Na,K-ATPaseque dans le cristallin normal viellissant et dans la cataracte senile, Arch d'Ophthalmol 36:523, 1976.

180. Palva M, Palkama A: Electronmicroscopical, histochemical and biochemical findings on the Na,K-ATPase activity in the epithelium of the rat lens, Exp Eye Res 22:229, 1976.

181. Parmigiani CM, McAvoy JW: A morphometric analysis of the development of the rat lens capsule, Curr Eye Res 8:1271, 1989.

182. Pasino M, Maraini G: Cation pump activity and membrane permeability in human senile cataractous lenses, Exp Eye Res 34:887, 1982.

183. Paterson CA: Extracellular space of the crystalline lens, Am J Physiol 218:797, 1970.

184. Paterson CA: Effects of drugs on the lens, in Ellis PP, ed: Side effects of drugs on the eye, Int Ophthalmol Clin 11:63, 1971.

185. Paterson CA: Distribution and movement of ions in the ocular lens, Doc Ophthalmol 31:1, 1972.

186. Paterson CA, Delamere NA, Mawhorter L, et al: Na,K-ATPase in simulated eye bank and cryoextracted rabbit lenses, and human eye bank lenses and cataracts, Invest Ophthalmol Vis Sci 24:1534, 1983.

187. Paterson CA, Maurice DM: Diffusion of sodium in extracellular space of the crystalline lens, Am J Physiol 220:256, 1971.

188. Paterson CA, Neville MC, Jenkins RM II, et al: Intracellular potassium activity in frog lens determined using ion specific liquid ion-exchanger filled microelectrodes, Exp Eye Res 19:43, 1974.

189. Patmore L, Duncan G: The physiology of lens membranes, in Duncan G, ed: Mechanisms of cataract formation in the human lens, London, Academic Press, 1981, pp 193-217.

190. Pau H, Graf P, Sies H: Glutathione levels in human lens: regional distribution in different forms of cataract, Exp Eye Res 50:17, 1990.

191. Peracchia C: Calcium effects on gap junction structure and cell coupling, Nature 271:669, 1978.

192. Peracchia C: Cell coupling, in Martonosi A, ed: The enzymes of biological membranes, vol 1, New York, Plenum, 1985, pp 81-130.

193. Peracchia C, Girsch SJ, Bernardini G, et al: Lens junctions are communicating junctions, Curr Eye Res 4:1155, 1985.

194. Peterson MJ, Sarges R, Aldinger CE, et al: CP-45,634: a novel aldose reductase inhibitor that inhibits polyol pathway activity in diabetic and galactosemic rats, Metabolism 28(Suppl 1):456, 1979.

195. Piatigorsky J: Molecular biology: recent studies on enzyme crystallins and Á-crystallin gene expression, Exp Eye Res 50:725, 1990.

196. Piatigorsky J, Fukui HN, Kinoshita JH: Differential metabolism and leakage of protein in an inherited cataract and in normal lens cultured with ouabain, Nature 274:558, 1978.

197. Pirie A: Composition of ox lens capsule, Biochem J 48:368, 1951.

198. Pirie A: Glutathione peroxidase in lens and a source of

hydrogen peroxide in aqueous humour, Biochem J 96:244, 1965.

199. Pirie A: Color and solubility of the proteins of human cataracts, Invest Ophthalmol 7:634, 1968.

200. Pope JM, Chandra S, Balfe JD: Changes in the state of water in senile cataractous lenses as studied by nuclear magnetic resonance, Exp Eye Res 34:57, 1982.

201. Prescott AR, Stewart S, Duncan G, et al: Diamide induces reversible changes in morphology, cytoskeleton and cell-cell coupling in lens epithelial cells, Exp Eye Res 52:83, 1991.

202. Racz P, Tompa K, Pocsik I: The state of water in normal human, bird and fish eye lenses, Exp Eye Res 29:601, 1979.

203. Rae JL: The electrophysiology of the crystalline lens, Curr Topics Eye Res 1:37, 1979.

204. Rae JL: The application of patch clamp methods to ocular epithelia, Curr Eye Res 4:409, 1985.

205. Rae JL, Kuszak JR: The electrical coupling of epithelium and fibers in the frog lens, Exp Eye Res 36:317, 1983.

206. Rae JL, Mathias RT: The physiology of the lens, in Maisel H, ed: The ocular lens: structure, function, and pathology, New York, Marcel Dekker, 1985, pp 93-121.

207. Rae JL, Stacey T: Lanthanum and procion yellow are extracellular markers in the crystalline lens of the rat, Exp Eye Res 28:1, 1979.

208. Rafferty NS: Lens morphology, in Maisel H, ed: The ocular lens: structure, function and pathology, New York, Marcel Dekker, 1985, pp 1-60.

209. Rao GN, Lardis MP, Cotlier E: Acetylation of lens crystallins: a possible mechanism by which aspirin could prevent cataract formation, Biochem Biophys Res Commun 128:1125, 1985.

210. Rao GN, Sadasivudu B, Cotlier E: Studies on glutathione s-transferase, glutathione peroxidase, and glutathione reductase in human normal and cataractous lenses, Ophthalmic Res 15:173, 1983.

211. Reddy DVN: Studies on intraocular transport of taurine, II, Accumulation in the rabbit lens, Invest Ophthalmol 9:206, 1970.

212. Reddy VN, Giblin FJ: Metabolism and function of glutathione in the lens, in Nugent J, Whelan J, eds: Human cataract formation, Ciba Foundation Symposium 106, London, Pitman, 1984, pp 65–87.

213. Reddy VN, Varma SD, Chakrapani B: Transport and metabolism of glutathione in the lens, Exp Eye Res 16:105, 1973.

214. Renie WA (ed): Goldberg's genetic and metabolic eye disease, Boston, Little Brown, 1986.

215. Roelfzema H, Broekhuyse RM, Veerkamp JH: Lipids in tissues of the eye, XI, Synthesis of sphingomyelin in the calf lens, Exp Eye Res 22:85, 1976.

216. Roy D, Chiesa R, Spector A: Lens calcium activated proteinase: degradation of vimentin, Biochem Biophys Res Commun 116:204, 1983.

217. Russell P, Robison WG Jr, Kinoshita JH: A new method for rapid isolation of the intrinsic membrane proteins from lens, Exp Eye Res 32:511, 1981.

218. Scammon RE, Hesdorffer MB: Growth in mass and volume of the human lens in postnatal life, Arch Ophthalmol 17:104, 1937.

219. Schachar RA, Solin SA: The microscopic protein structure of the lens with a theory for cataract formation as determined by Raman spectroscopy of intact bovine lenses, Invest Ophthalmol 14:380, 1975.

220. Scheutze SM, Goodenough DA: Dye transfer between cells of the embryonic chick lens becomes less sensitive to CO_2 treatment with development, J Cell Biol 92:694, 1982.

221. Seddon JM, Christen WG, Manson JE, et al: Low-dose aspirin and risks of cataract in a randomized trial of US physicians, Arch Ophthalmol 109:252, 1991.

222. Shinohara T, Piatigorsky J: Regulation of protein synthesis, intracellular electrolytes and cataract formation in vitro, Nature 270:406, 1977.

223. Siesjö BK: Historical overview; calcium, ischemia, and death of brain cells, Ann NY Acad Sci 522:638, 1988.

224. Spector A: Lens aminopeptidase, I, Purification and properties, J Biol Chem 238:1353, 1963.

225. Spector A: The search for a solution to senile cataracts, Invest Ophthalmol Vis Sci 25:130, 1984.

226. Spector A: Aspects of the biochemistry of cataract, in Maisel H, ed: The ocular lens: structure, function, and pathology, New York, Marcel Dekker, 1985, pp 405-438.

227. Spector A, Garner MH, Garner WH, et al: An extrinsic membrane polypeptide associated with high molecular weight protein aggregates in human cataract, Science 204:1323, 1979.

228. Spector A, Garner WH: Hydrogen peroxide and human cataract, Exp Eye Res 33:673, 1981.

229. Spector A, Roy D: Disulfide-linked high molecular weight protein associated with human cataract, Proc Nat Acad Sci USA 75:3244, 1978.

230. Sredy J, Spector A: Phosphorylation of H_2O_2 treated lens Na^+,K^+-ATPase, Exp Eye Res 39:479, 1984.

231. Stankeiwicz PJ, Metz KR, Sassani JW, et al: Nuclear magnetic resonance study of free and bound water fractions in normal lenses, Invest Ophthalmol Vis Sci 30:2361, 1989.

232. Statistics on Blindness in the Model Reporting Area, 1969–70, US DHEW Publication No (NIH) 73-427, 1973.

233. Stevens VJ, Rouzer CA, Monnier VM, et al: Diabetic cataract formation: potential role of glycosylation of lens crystallins, Proc Nat Acad Sci USA 75:2918, 1978.

234. Streeten BW: The nature of the ocular zonule, Trans Am Ophthalmol Soc 80:823, 1982.

235. Stribling D: Clinical trials with aldose reductase inhibitors, Exp Eye Res 50:621, 1990.

236. Sundar-Raj CV, Freeman IL: Structure and biosynthesis of rabbit lens capsule collagen, Invest Ophthalmol Vis Sci 23:743, 1982.

237. Swanson AA, Truesdale AW: Elemental analysis in normal and cataractous human lens tissue, Biochem Biophys Res Commun 45:1488, 1971.

238. Tardieu A, Delaye M: Eye lens transparency analyzed by x-ray and light scattering, in Duncan G, ed: The lens: transparency and cataract, Proceedings of the Symposium, Eurage, Rijswijk, The Netherlands, 1986, pp 49-56.

239. Taylor HR, West SK, Rosenthal FS, et al: Effect of ul-

traviolet radiation on cataract formation, N Engl J Med 319:1429, 1988.

240. Trokel S: The physical basis for transparency of the crystalline lens, Invest Ophthalmol 1:493, 1962.

241. Tse SS, Ortwerth BJ: Activation and release of a trypsin-like proteinase from bovine lens α-crystallin, Exp Eye Res 34:659, 1982.

242. Unakar NJ, Tsui JY: Sodium-potassium-dependent ATPase, I, Cytochemical localization in normal and cataractous rat lenses, Invest Ophthalmol Vis Sci 19:630, 1980.

243. Urban RC Jr, Cotlier E: Corticosteroid-induced cataracts, Surv Ophthalmol 31:102, 1986.

244. van Doorenmaalen WJ: The developmental mechanics of the lens, in Bloemendal H, ed: Molecular and cellular biology of the eye lens, New York, John Wiley, 1981, pp 415-435.

245. van Heyningen R: Some glycolytic enzymes and intermediates in the rabbit lens, Exp Eye Res 4:298, 1965.

246. van Heyningen R: The lens: metabolism and cataract, in Davson H, ed: The eye, vol 1, 2nd ed, New York, Academic Press, 1969, pp 381-488.

247. van Heyningen R: Sorbitol pathway—reminiscences, Exp Eye Res 50:583, 1990.

248. Varma SD: Ascorbic acid and the eye with special reference to the lens, in Burns JJ, Rivers JM, Machlin LJ, eds: Third Conference on Vitamin C, Annals NY Acad Sci New York, NY Academy of Sciences, 1987, pp 280-306.

249. Varma SD: Scientific basis for medical therapy of cataracts by antioxidants, Am J Clin Nutr 53:335S, 1991.

250. Varma SD: Chakrapani B, Reddy VN: Intraocular transport of myoinositol, II, Accumulation in the rabbit lens in vitro, Invest Ophthalmol 9:794, 1970.

251. Varma SD, Mizuno A, Kinoshita JH: Diabetic cataracts and flavonoids, Science 195:205, 1977.

252. Wachtl C, Kinsey VE: Studies on the crystalline lens, VIII, A synthetic medium for lens culture and the effects of various constituents on cell division in the epithelium, Am J Ophthalmol 46:288, 1958.

253. Weale RA: Senile cataract; the case against light, Ophthalmol 90:420, 1983.

254. Weekers R, Delmarcelle Y, Luyckx J: Biometrics of the crystalline lens, in Bellows JG, ed: Cataract and abnormalities of the lens, New York, Grune and Stratton, 1975, pp 134-147.

255. Weekers R, Delmarcelle Y, Luyckx-Bacus J, et al: Morphological changes of the lens with age and cataract, in The human lens—in relation to cataract, Ciba Foundation Symposium 19, Amsterdam, Elsevier, 1973, pp 25-43.

256. West SK, Taylor HR: The detection and grading of cat-

aract: an epidemiologic approach, Surv Ophthalmol 31:175, 1986.

257. Williams RN, Delamere NA, Paterson CA: Generation of lipoxygenase products in the avascular tissues of the eye, Exp Eye Res 41:733, 1985.

258. Wilson CC, Delamere NA, Paterson CA: Chlorpromazine effects upon rabbit lens water and electrolyte balance, Exp Eye Res 36:559, 1983.

259. Wind BE, Walsh S, Patterson JW: Equatorial potassium currents in lenses, Exp Eye Res 46:117, 1988.

260. Wistow G, Piatigorsky J: Recruitment of enzymes as lens structural proteins, Science 236:1554, 1987.

261. Worgul BV, Merriam GR Jr, Medvedovsky C: Accelerated heavy particles and the lens, II, Cytopathological changes, Invest Ophthalmol Vis Sci 27:108, 1986.

262. World Health Organization Programme Advisory Group: report of the eighth meeting of the WHO programme advisory group on the prevention of blindness WHO publication 89.17, World Health Organization, Geneva, Switzerland, 1989.

263. Yanoff M: Pathology of cataract, in Bellows JG, ed: Cataract and abnormalities of the lens, New York, Grune and Stratton, 1975, pp 155-189.

264. Yeagle PL: Lipid regulation of cell membrane structure and function, FASEB J 3:1833, 1989.

265. Young RW, Fulhorst HW: Regional differences in protein synthesis within the lens of the rat, Invest Ophthalmol 5:288, 1966.

266. Young RW, Ocumpaugh ED: Autoradiographic studies on the growth and development of the lens capsule in the rat, Invest Ophthalmol 5:583, 1966.

267. Zampighi GA, Hall JE, Kreman M: Purified lens junctional protein forms channels in planar lipid films, Proc Nat Acad Sci USA 82:8468, 1985.

268. Zelenka PS: Changes in phosphatidylinositol metabolism during differentiation of lens epithelial cells into lens fiber cells in the embryonic chick, J Biol Chem 255:1296, 1980.

269. Zelenka PS: Phosphatidylcholine and phosphatidylethanolamine metabolism during lens fiber cell formation, Biochim Biophys Acta 752:145, 1983.

270. Zelenka PS: Lens lipids, Curr Eye Res 3:1337, 1984.

271. Zigman S: Photochemical mechanisms in cataract formation, in Duncan G, ed: Mechanisms of cataract formation in the human lens, London, Academic Press, 1981, pp 117-149.

272. Zigman S: The role of sunlight in human cataract formation, Surv Ophthalmol 27:317, 1983.

273. Zigman S: Photobiology of the lens, in Maisel H, ed: The ocular lens: structure, function, and pathology, New York, Marcel Dekker, 1985, pp 301-347.

CHAPTER 11

Accommodation and Presbyopia: Neuromuscular and Biophysical Aspects

PAUL L. KAUFMAN, M.D.

Accommodation is a complex constellation of sensory, neuromuscular, and biophysical phenomena by which the overall refracting power of the eye changes rapidly to image objects at different viewing distances clearly on the retina. In the abstract one can envision a variety of optical strategies for accomplishing this task: (1) changing the corneal curvature, (2) changing the distance between the cornea and retina, (3) placing another lens system between the cornea and retina whose effective refracting power can be varied by changing its surface curvatures or its position within the globe (Figs. 11-1 and 11-2), (4) changing the index of refraction of one or more components of the ocular media, (5) having two or many separate optical pathways of different refracting power.

All of these mechanisms save (4) are represented among the vertebrates, and every vertebrate class has at least some species capable of significant amounts of accommodation.[22,93] Interestingly, relatively few terrestrial mammalian species have this capability. Carnivores generally can accommodate a few diopters, but only the raccoon, which can accommodate ~20 diopters, has an amplitude equivalent to that of humans or subhuman primates.[79] The carni-

vores, including the raccoon, increase their ocular refractive power by moving the lens anteriorly toward the cornea without changing lens thickness. Primates reshape their lens without translating it; i.e., the lens thickens and its an-

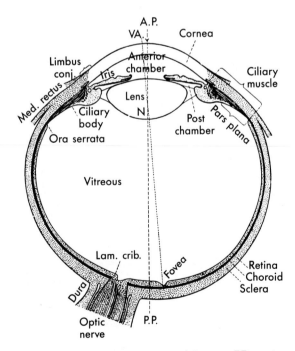

FIG. 11-1 Mid-sagittal section of the eye. PP, posterior pole; AP, anterior pole; VA, visual axis. (From Warwick RB: Eugene Wolff's anatomy of the eye and orbit, Philadelphia, WB Saunders, 1976, p 30.)

ACKNOWLEDGMENTS

Preparation of this chapter was supported in part by NIH grant EY02698 and aided by B'Ann Gabelt, Bernadette Bull, and William Hubbard.

FIG. 11-2 Crystalline lens and zonular ligaments. (From Cotlier E, in Moses RA, Hart WM Jr, eds: Adler's physiology of the eye, St Louis, CV Mosby, 1987, p 268.)

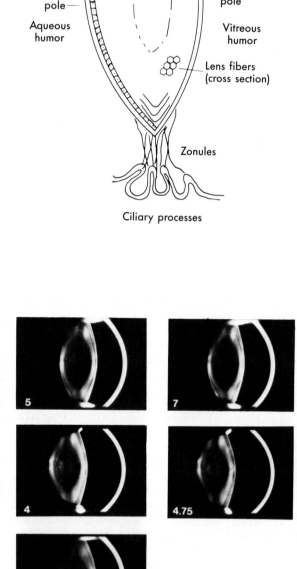

FIG. 11-3 Composite of axial slit-lamp Scheimpflug photographs of human lenses. The corneal section is at the right of each panel. *First row:* 21-year-old subject; *left to right,* unaccommodated, 2, 5, and 7 diopters of accommodation. *Second row:* 28-year-old subject; unaccommodated, 2, 4, and 4.75 diopters of accommodation. *Third row:* 39-year-old subject; unaccommodated, 2 and 4.25 diopters of accommodation. *Fourth row:* 57-year-old subject; unaccommodated and 1.25 diopters of accommodation. In each row the final panel is the maximum accommodation for that subject. Diopters of accommodation are given in the lower left hand corner of each panel. Lens thickness and curvature increase with increasing age and accommodation. Zones of discontinuity increase in number and prominence with age; after ~45 years the zones tend to merge.

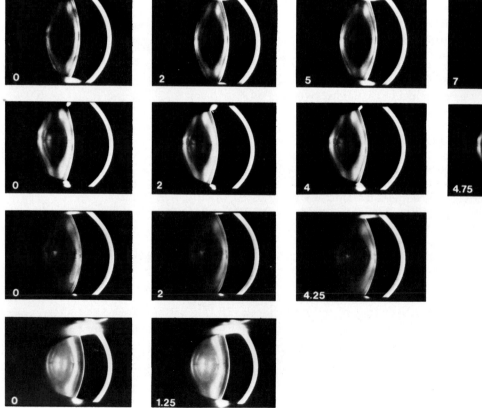

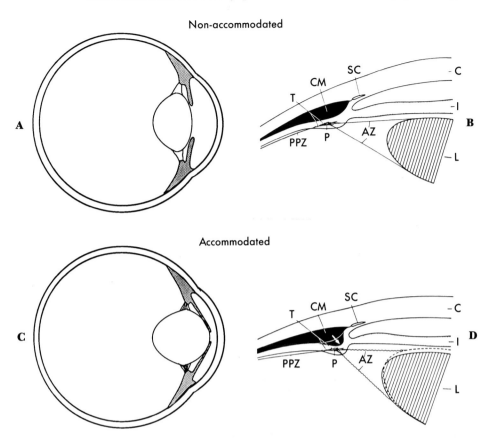

Non-accommodated

Accommodated

FIG. 11-4   Schematic representation of ocular geometry and cilio-zonular mechanisms at rest (**A,B**) and during accommodation (**C,D**). Ciliary muscle contracted (**D**), forming an inner edge; the tension fiber system (T) is stretched, taking up the traction from posterior zonular fibers and the choroid. Thus the anterior zonular fibers become relaxed and the lens more spherical (dotted lines). P, zonular plexus; I, iris; C, cornea, SC, Schlemm's canal. Arrow indicates direction of ciliary muscle movement during accommodation. (**A,C**, from Crawford KS, Kaufman PL, Bito LZ: Invest Ophthalmol Vis Sci 31:2189, 1990; **B,D** from Rohen, JW: Invest Ophthalmol Vis Sci 18:142, 1979.)

terior, posterior, and internal refracting surfaces become more sharply curved (Figs. 11-3 and 11-4).[52,54,61]

The primates accomplish lenticular rounding and flattening (accommodation and disaccommodation) through the action of the parasympathetically dominated ciliary smooth muscle. This muscle is attached anteriorly by means of true tendons to the scleral spur and trabecular meshwork,[78] and posteriorly to the elastic network of Bruch's membrane of the choroid.[41,75] The latter is in turn anchored to the scleral canal encasing the optic nerve at the back of the globe.[41] Consequently, when the outer longitudinally oriented muscle fibers contract under stimulation by parasympathetic motor neurons or local application of cholinomimetic drugs, the main mass of the muscle slides forward along the curved inner wall of the sclera (against which it is held by the intraocular pressure and to which it is loosely attached by collagenous bands)[41] toward the scleral spur.[76] By sliding away from the equator along the curved surface of the spherical globe, diametrically opposite points on the muscle are actually moving toward one another, i.e., the ring formed by the inner apex of the muscle narrows (see Fig. 11-4). This narrowing may be further augmented by contraction of other more circularly oriented muscle fibers, analogous to the action of a true sphincter muscle.[41,65,68,75]

Internal to the ciliary muscle and separated from it by a condensed connective tissue ground plate is the looser, highly vascularized connective tissue stroma of the ciliary processes, and internal to the stroma lies the double-layered ciliary epithelium.[41] The cells of the innermost nonpigmented epithelial (NPE) layer are structurally adapted for two distinct functions: the active secretion of aqueous humor into the posterior chamber and mechanical anchoring of the zonular fibers that attach to the lens anteriorly and Bruch's membrane posteriorly. The NPE cells at the anterior crests of the processes appear to be primarily concerned with secretion, while those in the valleys between the processes appear to harbor the zonular attachments.[14,39,41]

The zonule of Zinn is a complex arrangement of elasticlike fibers[88,89] that connect the ciliary processes and the lens (Figs. 11-5 and 11-6). The posterior component forms a meridionally oriented mat extending forward from the ora serrata between the cortical vitreous and the ciliary NPE of the pars plana.[50,76] These fibers arise from the basement membrane of the NPE (the internal limiting membrane).[43] Anteriorly, they travel into the valleys between the ciliary processes of the pars plicata, to which they are anchored by a set of finer "tension" fibers.[76] These "tension fibers" in effect form a fulcrum at which the main zonular fibers make a nearly right-angle turn centripetally to attach to the lens capsule in three distinct sets. The two major sets attach respectively to the anterior and posterior capsule approximately 1.5 mm axipetal to the equator. The third less numerous and finer set attaches to the equator itself (Fig. 11-7).[41,43,59]

With this arrangement it is immediately apparent that when the ciliary muscle contracts and the fulcrum formed by the tension fibers moves forward and inward, the pars plana zonules will stretch while the fibers attaching to the

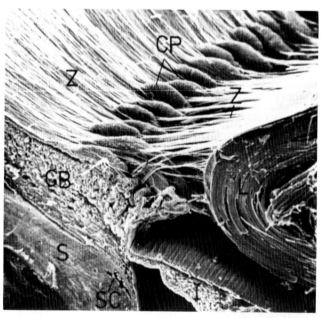

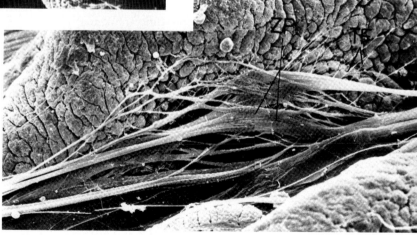

FIG. 11-5 **A**, Survey of the entire accommodative apparatus. **B**, Zonular plexus (ZP) located within a ciliary valley. Note the tension fibers (TF) spreading to the lateral wall of the ciliary process (CP). Z, zonule; CB, ciliary body (ciliary muscle); L, lens; I, iris; S, sclera; SC, Schlemm's canal. (SEM, cynomolgus monkey; **A**, × 50; **B**, × 500). (From Rohen JW: Invest Ophthalmol Vis Sci 18:136, 1979.)

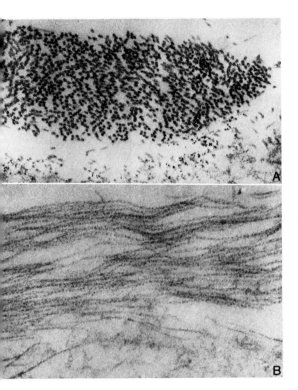

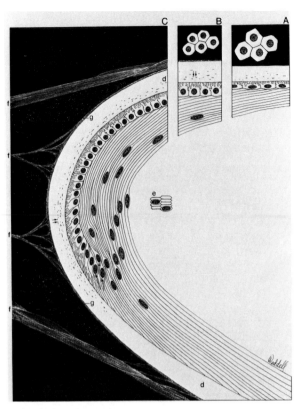

FIG. 11-6 Electron micrographs of zonular fibers. **A,** Cross-section of a zonular fiber. The fibrils are round and measure 100 to 120 Å in diameter. They appear to have a dense rim and a lucent core. (×112,000.) **B,** Longitudinal section of a zonular fiber that is composed of numerous fibrils. The banding is about 125 Å, and the fibrils have a diameter of around 83 Å (× 120,000.) (From Hogan MJ, Alvarado JA, Weddel JE in Histology of the human eye, Philadelphia, WB Saunders, 1971, p 675.)

FIG. 11-7 A composite drawing of the lens cortex, epithelium, capsule, and zonular attachments. At (**A**) is the anterior central lens epithelium, seen in flat and cross-section. The size and shape of these cells can be compared with those of the cells in (**B**), the intermediate zone, and (**C**) the equatorial zone. At the equator the dividing cells are elongating (*arrows*) to form lens cortical cells. As they elongate they send processes anteriorly and posteriorly toward the sutures, and their nuclei migrate somewhat anterior to the equator to form the lens bow. At the same time the nuclei become more and more displaced into the lens as new cells are formed at the equator. The lens capsule (d) is thicker anterior and posterior to the equator than it is at the equator itself. The anterior and equatorial capsule contains fine filamentous inclusions (*double arrows*); these are not present posteriorly. Zonular fibers (f) attach to the anterior, posterior, and equatorial capsule, forming the pericapsular or zonular lamella of the lens (g). (From Hogan MJ, Alvarado JA, Weddell JE, in Histology of the human eye, Philadelphia, WB Saunders, 1971, p 649.)

lens will become flaccid.[41,43,59] Thus liberated from the centrifugal pull of the zonular fibers, the lens approaches its less stressed, more spherical equilibrium shape. The relative roles of the lens capsule and internal substance in determining the unstressed equilibrium are debated, but in any event the lens thickens axially (and consequently narrows equatorially) and its anterior, posterior, and internal surfaces become more sharply curved (see Fig. 11-2).[52,54,61] The posterior lens surface remains in a fixed anterior-posterior location,[52,54] prevented from moving posteriorly probably by the noncompressible vitreous humor against which it abuts[16,17] and by the anterior translation of the fulcrum formed by the zonular plexus. Consequently, the increase in axial thickness of the lens is exactly equal to the forward movement of its anterior pole and the shallowing of the an-

terior chamber.[52,54] Optically, each of these changes (increased lenticular thickness and convexity and closer proximity of the cornea to the anterior lenticular refracting surface) serves individually to increase the refracting power of the entire system[52,55,61]; i.e., the eye accommodates.

When viewing shifts from near to distant objects, the sequence is reversed. Parasympathetic input to the ciliary muscle decreases and the muscle relaxes. The elastic Bruch's membrane pulls the muscle posteriorly and outward along the inner scleral surface, widening the ciliary ring. The pars plana zonules slacken while the anterior zonules stretch, pulling the elastic lens capsule centrifugally and posteriorly. As a consequence, the equatorial diameter of the lens increases, the axial thickness decreases, and the anterior, posterior, and internal surfaces become less sharply curved. The anterior surface recedes from the cornea (the anterior chamber deepens), while the posterior surface still remains in place relative to the cornea and retina, braced by the vitreous.[52,54,61] These changes decrease the refractive power of the entire optical system,[52,54,61] and the eye "disaccommodates."

This description of the events occuring during accommodation and disaccommodation is greatly oversimplified, and it is worthwhile to consider the workings of the various components of the system and the effects of aging on them in more detail.

The resting state of the accommodative apparatus does not leave the retina conjugate with the far point of the eye. Rather, the position of rest is about 1 to 1.5 diopters accommodated.[35] The resting state is attained when there is no definite object of regard; i.e., during sleep, general anesthesia, darkness, entrancement, and has been variously termed tonic accommodation, dark focus, night myopia.[34,81] It seems due to a balance of resting sympathetic and parasympathetic tone to the ciliary muscle, with the latter predominating. Thus tonic accommodation can be completely reversed by topical anticholinergic drugs, but only partially by β-adrenergic agonists,[35] and is slightly enhanced by β-adrenergic antagonists.[36] The purpose of sympathetically mediated "negative accommodation" is not clear. It could serve an internal antagonistic function to smooth out parasympathetically mediated ciliary muscle contraction, since there is no separate antagonist for the ciliary muscle.

The sensory stimulus to accommodation or disaccommodation is a blurred retinal image of the object of regard, the "sensation" or "consciousness" of an object of interest being at distance or near, based on various other sensory cues (e.g., sound, touch), or both.[71] Via central connections, excitatory or inhibitory impulses are sent to the Edinger-Westphal nucleus at the rostral portion of the midbrain, which contains the first-order parasympathetic motor neurons

to the ciliary muscle (Fig. 11-8).[96,98] Traveling with the branch of the oculomotor nerve supplying the inferior oblique muscle,[95] their axons synapse with the second-order neurons in the ciliary ganglion,[95] which lies adjacent to the optic nerve and the central retinal artery within the extraocular muscle cone in the orbit, approximately 1 cm behind the globe.[95] Some investigators find electrophysiologic[98] and anatomic[44,74] evidence that some fibers mediating the accommodative responses reach the ciliary muscle without synapsing, but this is probably not a major functional pathway.[23] The axons of the second-order neurons travel from the ciliary ganglion to the globe as several lightly myelinated trunks[82,83,95] (short posterior ciliary nerves, SPCN).[42] These splay out to enter the posterior pole of the globe, surrounding the optic nerve as a ring of about 6 to 10 smaller fiber bundles.[42] Two additional trunks, the long posterior ciliary nerves (LPCN), travel from the ganglion to enter the globe farther anteriorly at the 3 and 9 o'clock positions.[42] From their entry points into the globe both the short and long posterior ciliary nerves travel anteriorly to provide parasympathetic and sensory innervation to the choroid and to the ciliary and iris sphincter muscles.[42] Another source of parasympathetic innervation to the eye travels by way of the facial nerve and probably uses vasoactive intestinal polypeptide (VIP) as a transmitter; this pathway may be primarily concerned with the uveal vasculature.[4,73,82]

The distribution of parasympathetic nerves subserving accommodation between the short and long posterior ciliary nerves and their precise pathways within the eye is not entirely clear. LPCN do not preferentially carry the parasympathetic efferents to the ciliary muscle, but may carry some of them.[51] The majority of the fibers appear to travel with the SPCN, losing their myelin and arborizing posteriorly in the choroid to travel forward diffusely.[51] The sympathetic innervation appears to follow the typical hypothalamic-brainstem-spinal cord-superior cervical ganglion-cervical-carotid plexus route into the orbit, where the axons of the third-order neurons, which originate in the superior cervical ganglion, eventually reach the globe in the company of the SPCN and LPCN and travel forward to the ciliary muscle (Fig. 11-8).[42] The intracranial coordination or communication between the sympathetic and parasympathetic outflow subserving accommodation is not known.

The ciliary muscle is a very complex and in many ways atypical smooth muscle, and sub-

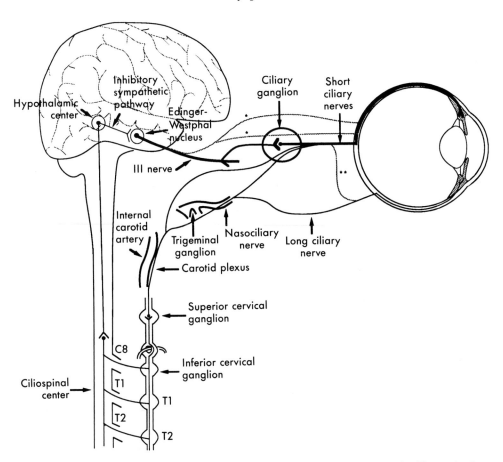

FIG. 11-8 Parasympathetic and sympathetic pathways to the ciliary muscle. The major innervation to the ciliary muscle is parasympathetic and follows the pathway shown by the thick solid bold lines. The parasympathetic pathway originates in the Edinger-Westphal nucleus and courses with the third nerve, whence the fibers travel to and synapse in the ciliary ganglion. The majority of the postganglionic parasympathetic fibers travel to the ciliary muscle via the short ciliary nerves, but some postganglionic fibers (double asterisk) also travel with the long ciliary nerves. There is also evidence for a direct pathway of uncertain functional significance (single asterisks) to the internal eye structures from the Edinger-Westphal nucleus. The sympathetic supply to the ciliary muscle (thin solid lines) originates in the diencephalon and travels down the spinal cord to the lower cervical-upper thoracic segments, to synapse in the spinociliary center of Budge in the intermediolateral tract of the cord. From there second-order nerves leave the cord by the last cervical and first two thoracic ventral roots; these preganglionic fibers run up the cervical sympathetic chain to synapse in the superior cervical ganglion. The third-order fibers continue up the sympathetic carotid plexus and enter the orbit with the first division of the trigeminal nerve (following the nasociliary division) or independently, whence they join the long and short ciliary nerves, in the latter instance passing through the ciliary ganglion without synapsing. (Adapted from Duke-Elder S, in System of ophthalmology, vol XII, St Louis, CV Mosby, 1971, pp 600, 602; Parelman JJ, Fay MT, Burde RM, Trans Am Ophthalmol Soc 82:371, 1984; Warwick R, in Eugene Wolff's anatomy of the eye and orbit, Philadelphia, WB Saunders, 1976, pp 308-312.)

serves multiple functions. In addition to its accommodative role, the ciliary muscle plays a major role in the outflow of aqueous humor via both the trabecular and the uveoscleral routes.[3,45] By virtue of its intimate anatomic connections to the trabecular meshwork and inner wall of Schlemm's canal,[78,80] contraction of the muscle expands the meshwork, widening the intertrabecular spaces and dilating the canal, thus facilitating the outflow of aqueous humor from the anterior chamber into the canal and thence into the general circulation.[46] Since the anterior chamber shallows and decreases in volume during accommodation, due to the thickening of the lens,[52,54] this accommodation-linked enhancement of aqueous outflow is essential to maintain normal IOP and to rid the eye of some noncompressible fluid and provide "room" for the expanding lens.[17,77] Aqueous humor also leaves the eye via a more posteriorly directed route, the uveoscleral pathway.[3,45] Since there is no epithelial or endothelial bridge extending from the trabecular meshwork across the anterior part of the ciliary muscle and the iris root, the intertrabecular spaces communicate freely with the spaces between the ciliary muscle bundles. Aqueous humor can therefore flow through these spaces into the supraciliary and suprachoroidal regions and then leave the eye through the sclera into the orbit. Along this pathway aqueous mixes with the tissue fluid of the ciliary body and choroid, and thus provides a vehicle for the elimination of large protein molecules and other tissue wastes. This is analogous to lymphatic drainage in other tissues,[3,45] and indeed the eye has no true lymphatics.[3,70] When the ciliary muscle contracts, the intermuscular spaces are obliterated,[1] obstructing uveoscleral outflow.[2] However, under typical near and distance viewing conditions the degree and duration of the contraction do not cause total or long-term interruption of uveoscleral outflow. In general, the enhancement of aqueous drainage via the trabecular route exceeds its interruption via the uveoscleral route, so the IOP and chamber volume decrease consequent to accommodation.[3,45]

The ultrastructure of primate ciliary muscle cells differs from that of gut or vascular smooth muscle. The almost parallel myofibrils, Z-band-like extensions of the dark bands, and dense innervation all resemble striated skeletal muscles, as does the ciliary muscle's ability to contract and relax rapidly. Additionally, among smooth muscles the large number of mitochondria compared to the myofibrils is unique to ciliary muscle cells.[67] The ciliary muscle (and iris) is also unique among smooth muscles in having its second-order parasympathetic neurons located at some distance, in the ciliary ganglion, rather than within the organ itself.[23] The neurons themselves are atypically large and reminiscent in other ways of somatic motor neurons.[67,82]

The primate ciliary muscle is described as having three regions, based on the orientation of the muscle bundles—longitudinal, reticular, and circular.[14,65,75] There has been considerable debate over their functional interrelationship in terms of accommodation. During accommodation the area occupied by the longitudinal and reticular portions decreases, while the circular portion enlarges, putatively consequent to a re-orientation of some fibers.[65,68] A long-held view that the outer longitudinal fibers are primarily concerned with deforming the meshwork and canal to facilitate aqueous outflow while the inner circular fibers are primarily concerned with accommodation by narrowing the ciliary ring[68] is resisted by investigators, who view the entire muscle as a unified system organized to accomplish various aspects of interrelated and complementary tasks.[41] The debate is further confused by recent observations suggesting that (1) pharmacologic dissociation of accommodative and outflow responses to certain cholinergic drugs may be possible under some conditions;[24,25] (2) different subtypes of muscarinic receptors may predominate in different regions of the ciliary muscle;[38] (3) ultrastructural and immunohistochemical-enzymatic differences exist between muscle cells in the different regions favoring different types of contractile dynamics.[30]

Structural and functional uncertainties notwithstanding, it is clear that the ciliary muscle is the engine powering the accommodative mechanism.

There is also universal agreement that the zonule transduces the various muscular and extralenticular elastic forces to the lens capsule. However, the precise geometric and vector analysis of this transduction is in some dispute. It is clear that the zonular system would have to be anchored relatively far anteriorly in the ciliary body to be effective, and indeed it is so anchored to the ciliary epithelium in the valleys between the ciliary processes of the pars plicata.[43,76] At first pass one could imagine that such a system could work with only a single row of zonular fibers attached precisely to the equatorial rim of the lens capsule and without the pars plana zonules. However, the presence of the pars plana zonules, the intricacy of the zonular plexus within the valleys of pars plicata, and the presence of three "rows" of zonular attachments to the peripheral lens capsule (anterior, equatorial, and posterior) argue for much more complex dynamics. Anteriorly, this may relate to a putative capsular component of lens reshaping and translation, where different magnitudes and vectors of forces are placed on the anterior and posterior aspects of the capsule,[16,17] which themselves differ in thickness and perhaps in other properties,[27] to produce specific changes in lenticular contour and position. Posteriorly, the pars plana zonules may allow for a smoother change and distribution of force on the capsule than would occur if anterior zonular anchorage were solely to the ciliary processes.[76] Additionally, since the entire choroid may slide forward and backward as the ciliary muscle contracts and relaxes,[71] it may be advantageous to have a comparable pull on the internal aspect of the retina. The pars plana zonules being continuous, at the ora serrata, with the internal limiting membrane of the retina may accomplish this.[41,43,76] Finally, such posterior traction could be relevant to retinal photoreceptor directional reorientation in terms of retinal imaging through the pupillary miosis that accompanies accommodation.[40]

The specifics of these functional relationships are poorly understood and beyond the scope of this presentation, but they point to the importance of the extralenticular elastic components

of the accommodative apparatus.[9] One can view the zonule and choroid as an elastic system or a giant rubber band, held against the curved sclera by the IOP, connecting the lens to the scleral canal of the optic nerve (Fig. 11-9). The rubber band is on stretch when the ciliary muscle is relaxed, and this force stretches the lens capsule and "disaccommodates" the eye. When the anteriorly anchored muscle contracts, the posterior portion of rubber band is stretched or tensed further, while the anterior portion, i.e., the part of the zonular complex between the ciliary processes and the lens, is relaxed, allowing lenticular-capsular elastic forces to alter the lens shape. Looked at in this manner, disaccommodation can be viewed as the active application of force to the lens by extralenticular elastic tissues, while accommodation represents an active neuromuscular process that releases or diverts such forces from the lens.[9] This concept is of some interest in considering various hypothetical pathophysiologies for presbyopia (see below).

The role played by the vitreous has also been debated considerably. In one view it serves at most as a support to stabilize the posterior surface of the lens, i.e., to prevent the lens from moving posteriorly as it changes shape.[16,17,56] Another view assigns the vitreous a much more important, "active" function by compressing the lens peripherally when the ciliary muscle

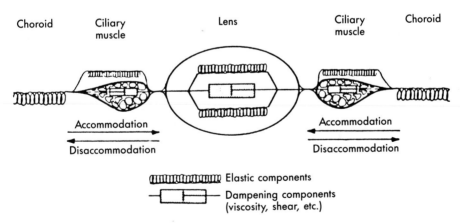

FIG. 11-9 The Helmholtz model of accommodation as modified from Bito and Miranda, 1987. Elastic components, depicted by coil springs, are shown in the lens and in parallel and in series with the ciliary muscle. Presbyopia may occur when the total force that can be developed by the extralenticular elastic components falls below that required to overcome the elastic components of the accommodated lens. At that point the capacity of force development by the ciliary muscle becomes irrelevant, since the system is "stuck" in the accommodated position. This linear model essentially ignores forces that are not delivered in the direction of displacements, and hence do not contribute to the energetics of accommodation and disaccommodation. (From Bito LZ, Miranda OC, in Reinecke RD, ed: Ophthalmology annual, New York, Raven Press, 1989, p 113.)

contracts, thereby aiding its sphericization.[16,17] This putative mechanism also has implications with regard to the development of presbyopia (see below).

As with other components of the system, the biophysical dynamics of the lens capsule and substance, and their optical consequences, are complex and incompletely understood. Optical analyses often treat the crystalline lens according to the mathematics of thin lens optics, but of course this structure constitutes a thick lens. Furthermore, its internal structure is not uniform and indeed comprises many refractive interfaces, or lenses within the lens.[52,58] Finally, the lens substance may well have its own elastic or viscoelastic properties, relevant to changing or maintaining shape, independent of the capsule.[28,29]

The primate lens is an oblate spheroid. In the nonaccommodated state its coronal diameter is approximately three times its anterior-posterior thickness. Its front and back surfaces at their intersection with the visual axis are respectively termed the anterior and posterior poles, and the peripheral rim is called the equator (see Fig. 11-2). The outermost envelope or capsule of the lens is a thick hyaline ectodermal basement membrane consisting of collagenlike glycoproteins.[18,42] It is thicker anteriorly than posteriorly and in the midperipheral as compared to the polar or equatorial regions. Underlying the capsule anteriorly and equatorially is the lens epithelium, a single layer of cuboidal cells. Mitoses in the equatorial epithelium produce elongated, flattened hexagonal cells that extend both anteriorly and posteriorly. These are the lens fibers, which comprise the substance of the lens (see Figs. 11-2, 11-3, and 11-7). The ends of different fibers meet to form the so-called suture lines. In the fetal lens these suture lines constitute biomicroscopically visible Y's. The anterior Y is erect and the posterior Y is inverted.[43] As the lens grows and more fibers are produced, the sutures become progressively more complex and stellate, extending throughout the entire thickness of the lens. However, the central infantile Y sutures are visible at the slit lamp well into adult life. As the newest fibers are laid down closest to the lens surface, the older fibers shrink, lose their nuclei, and become incorporated into the central part of the lens. This central region, called the lens nucleus, increases in size and firmness throughout life, and as cataract surgeons well know, becomes quite distinct and easily separable mechanically from the softer and more peripheral, or cortical, lens material. Proteins comprise approximately one third of the total lens weight and consist of soluble (85%) and insoluble (15%) fractions. The former are found primarily in the lens cortex, the latter primarily in the nucleus.[18,42]

From a functional anatomic standpoint, the lens can be divided into five zones from anterior to posterior: the anterior capsule, anterior cortex, nucleus, posterior cortex, and posterior capsule (see Figs. 11-2 and 11-3).[10] The center of the nucleus is bisected perpendicular to the optical axis by an optically lighter zone. The anterior and posterior cortical regions are of equal thickness and contain several nested parabolic refractive interfaces called zones of discontinuity.[10,52,54] The anatomic substrate for these curved internal structures is unclear.[53] However, there are equal numbers of them in the anterior and posterior cortex, and with age their number increases and they become more densely packed together.[54,60]

The physical basis for the lens discontinuity zones is currently unclear. Alpha crystallin, a major protein component of vertebrate lenses, exhibits increased heterogeneity in size and molecular weight with age;[85] this process leads to the formation of very-high-molecular-weight species, some of which are insoluble. The presence of these larger species results in decreased lens transparency[84,86] and increased glare effects through light scatter.[15] It is possible that the discontinuity zones are regions with especially high concentrations of these species; such an interpretation is consistent with the ability to discern the zones with the slit lamp, but raises the more fundamental question of why such aggregation is enhanced within these regions. Whatever is the true nature of the discontinuity zones, it is certain that an optical phenomenon that can be recorded on photographic film[10] or videotape[72] must have a real physical basis.[53]

The anterior and posterior lens surface curvatures both constitute paraboloids, with the sharpest curvature located centrally near the optical axis and the surfaces becoming progressively flatter toward the periphery.[52-54] Such a configuration, which is similar to that of the cornea,[37,94] tends to minimize spherical aberration, which is further reduced by having the iris cover the peripheral lens. When focus is most critical, as when examining small objects at near, the pupil constricts as part of the near reflex triad (accommodation, miosis, and convergence),[92] further reducing corneal and lenticular peripheral aberration, enhancing the depth of field and depth of focus, and providing a pinhole effect to further sharpen the image.[92]

In the unaccommodated state the anterior

lens surface is less sharply curved than the posterior surface.[12,52] Although both surface curvatures sharpen during accommodation, the anterior does so more rapidly, but its steepness never exceeds that of the posterior surface (see Fig. 11-3).[12,52] The central radius of curvature for both surfaces decreases approximately linearly with increasing accommodation, i.e., the same curvature change is required for the last diopter of accommodation as for the first, and for each diopter in between in a given eye at a given age. It remains to be determined whether this also applies to lens thickening and anterior chamber shallowing.[11,12] The internal curvatures mimic the behavior of their corresponding (anterior or posterior) surface curvatures.[54,60] Thus for each lens half a plot of the location of each internal curve relative to the cornea against its radius of curvature defines a straight line, and the lines so defined for the anterior and posterior halves have the same absolute slope. During accommodation both lines are shifted, but their slopes are unchanged. Although all the curvatures sharpen during accommodation, their parabolic state is maintained.[54,60] As a whole, the lens thickens axially (and thins coronally) during accommodation (see Fig. 11-3). In young adults (e.g., 20 years of age) overall axial thickness may increase from 3.5 to 5.0 mm, as measured by A-scan ultrasonography or Scheimpflug photography. This thickening occurs entirely in the nuclear region, with the axial dimensions of the anterior and posterior cortex remaining constant.[11,13,52,54,60,61] The axial position of posterior lens surface relative to the cornea[52,54] is essentially unchanged while the anterior lens surface approaches the cornea, indicating that the center of the lens mass (the central sulcus) is translated anteriorly by half the total lens thickening.[60,61]

The relative roles of capsular versus internal lens substance elastic and viscoelastic properties in determining lens shape under various levels of zonular tension, and the specific mechanisms involved, have been extensively debated[11,97] but the issue is largely unresolved, beyond the scope of this chapter, and unnecessary to conceptually understand the system as a whole.

Most reptile and bird species, and some amphibious mammals such as the otter, accommodate at least partly by iridogenic lenticonus, i.e., the iris pinches the lens to produce a more highly refracting anterior surface.[22] It has been generally felt that the only role of the iris in the human accommodative process is to narrow the pupillary aperture, improving depth of field and reducing spherical aberration so as to sharpen

the imaging of small near objects.[92] However, after unilateral total iridectomy, maximum accommodation as well as ultrasonographically measured anterior chamber shallowing and lens thickening inducible by corneal iontophoresis of carbachol in rhesus monkeys was approximately 40% less in the iridectomized than in the contralateral untouched eyes, regardless of age (Fig. 11-10). Neither submaximal accommodation induced by intramuscular pilocarpine infusion nor maximum accommodation inducible by midbrain electrical stimulation differed in iridectomized and intact eyes.[19] Although slit lamp examination of monkeys during maximal carbachol-induced accommodation does not reveal definite iridogenic lenticonus, that phenomenon cannot be excluded. An alternative hypothesis is that at maximum cholinomimetic

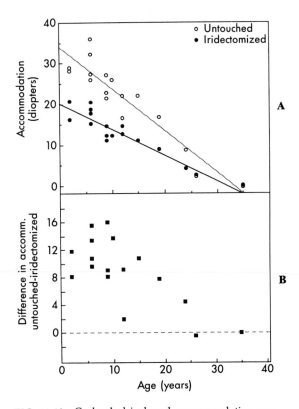

FIG. 11-10 Carbachol-induced accommodation versus age in intact and iridectomized eyes of 17 unilaterally iridectomized rhesus monkeys. Data are shown as (**A**) maximal accommodative amplitude in individual eyes, and (**B**) difference between accommodative amplitude in iridectomized and contralateral intact eyes of individual animals. (From Crawford KS, Kaufman PL, Bito LZ, Invest Ophthalmol Vis Sci 31:2187, 1990.)

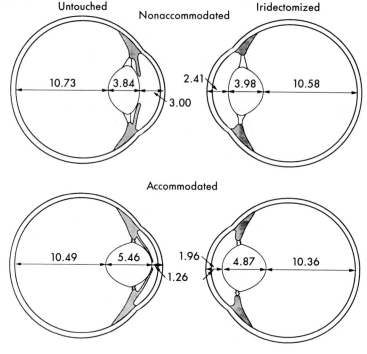

FIG. 11-11 Schematic representation of ocular geometry in the intact and iridectomized eye of a 2-year-old rhesus monkey at rest and 80 minutes after corneal iotophoresis of carbachol. Resting refraction was −0.8 diopters in both eyes; the maximum carbachol-induced accommodation was 28 and 16 diopters, in the intact and iridectomized eye, respectively. Intraocular distances (mm) were determined by A-scan ultrasonography immediately after coincidence refractometry and are illustrated proportionately; however, lens curvatures and iris and ciliary body configurations are schematic and theoretical. (From Crawford KS, Kaufman PL, Bito LZ: Invest Ophthalmol Vis Sci 31:2189, 1990.)

drug-induced contraction, the iris sphincter muscle, stretching the iris around the anteriorly bulging lens, pulls the ciliary body further forward and inward than does maximum ciliary muscle contraction alone, further narrowing the ciliary ring and thus allowing additional lens rounding and accommodative power (Fig. 11-11).[19] An influence of the iris on human accommodation therefore cannot be excluded.

AGING OF THE ACCOMMODATIVE MECHANISM: PRESBYOPIA

Human accommodative amplitude declines progressively, beginning in the second decade of life and perhaps earlier, so that it is completely gone by the age of 50 to 55 years.[21] Put another way, the near point of the eye recedes toward the far point, so that small objects must be held farther and farther from the eye to be clearly visualized. Although studies of accommodation measured subjectively (bring an object closer to the eye until it blurs, adding minus lenses of progressively increasing power until

blur) indicate that 1 to 1.5 diopters remains even into old age (> 65 years),[21] this residual probably does not represent "active" accommodation as described in the first part of this chapter. Rather, most of it probably represents depth of field and depth of focus of the optical system and retinal elements.[63] Under normal circumstances most near work is done at a distance of 25 to 40 cm. If the nonaccommodating eye is emmetropic (i.e., retina conjugate with infinity) or if any ametropia is corrected by spectacles or contact lenses, 2.5 to 4 diopters of accommodation is required to clearly image objects at this distance. By the middle of the fifth decade of life, the remaining accommodative amplitude is insufficient to do this,[21] so that near objects are blurred. Even if sufficient accommodative amplitude remains in some instances, the entire remaining amount must be employed, causing fatigue after some time (asthenopia).

The condition of insufficient accommodative amplitude for clear near vision is called presbyopia (literally, "old eye") and is the most common ocular affliction in the world. No individual appears exempt, although of course high myopes who remove their spectacles may have their far point close enough to the eye to function satisfactorily. Although certainly not a blinding condition, and correctable by various optical means (bifocal or reading spectacles), its cost in devices and lost productivity is probably in the order of tens of billions of dollars annually in the United States alone.[9]

The rate of decline of accommodative amplitude is said to occur with very little interindividual variability, even among heterogeneous or different populations.[9,21] Although the uniformity of the decline across any given population and even within a given individual has been questioned,[5,8,47] we must still consider this to be one of the most reliable biomarkers of human age known.

The pathophysiology of presbyopia is poorly understood, and alterations of every component of the accommodative mechanism have been proposed. Resolution of the issue has been hampered by lack of a suitable animal model. Although much useful and relevant information has been garnered from studies in living and postmortem human eyes, the invasive techniques required to answer some of the most critical questions cannot be employed in the living human. Subprimate species either do not accommodate or accommodate by mechanisms very different from that of the human.[22] The accommodative apparatus of the rhesus monkey is very similar to that of the human;[6,68,72] the rhesus lens grows throughout life, long after growth of the globe has ceased,[6,64] as does the human lens[62] (in marked contrast to other mammalian species where lens and eye growth both cease relatively early in the lifespan);[8] and rhesus accommodation declines on a time scale essentially identical to that of the human relative to species life span (Fig. 11-12).[6] Consequently, in recent years the rhesus monkey has contributed significant new information relevant to presbyopia pathophysiology, although the definitive mechanism remains elusive. We will summarize what is known about the aging of each component of the accommodative apparatus and how such aging changes might contribute to the loss of accommodative amplitude.

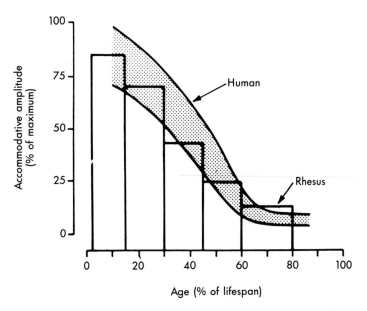

FIG. 11-12 The similarity of the patterns of age-dependent loss of accommodative amplitude in humans and rhesus monkeys expressed as percent of life span. The mean accommodative amplitude for each age group of rhesus monkey (bars) is superimposed on the time course of decrease in accommodative amplitude in humans, shown by the shaded area that includes most normal human cases as originally reported by Duane. It is assumed that the life spans of rhesus monkeys and humans are 35 and 80 years and that their maximum accommodative amplitudes are 40 and 16 D, respectively. (From Bito LZ, Miranda OC, in Stark L, Obrech G, eds: Presbyopia: recent research and reviews, from the Third International Symposium, New York, Churchill/Professional Press, 1987, p 418.)

Ciliary muscle

Presbyopia would be easily explained if with age the ciliary muscle lost its ability to contract, and most muscular systems do indeed lose strength as part of the aging process. However, loss of accommodative amplitude begins at least by the second decade of life in humans,[21] at a time when overall growth continues and overall muscular development and strength are just reaching their peak. Furthermore, no other muscular system loses its function so dramatically by the mid 40s and so completely by the age of 50 or 55 years. Although the ciliary muscle in very elderly humans indeed exhibits great loss of muscle fibers and replacement by connective tissue (hyalinization),[87] loss of accommodative ability occurs at a much earlier stage of life, when the muscle histologically appears quite healthy. Rhesus monkeys > 30 years of age are close to the end of their life span (probably equivalent to 75- or 80-year-old humans) and have completely lost their ability to accommodate (Fig. 11-12).[6] Although some ciliary muscle mass has been lost, by standard histologic (light microscopic) criteria the ciliary muscle appears extremely healthy, with little connective tissue replacement of the muscle, and one would never imagine such muscles to be incapable of contracting sufficiently to produce substantial accommodation (Fig. 11-13).[68] Some age-related neural and muscular alterations are visible at the electron microscopic level, but again these are minor and unlikely to be related to the complete functional loss.[67] Neither the overall number nor the affinity of muscarinic receptors, as measured by the specific binding of the non-subtype specific muscarinic antagonist quinuclidinyl benzilate (QNB), in the rhesus ciliary muscle changes with age.[33] Similarly the activity, as defined by K_D and V_{max}, of choline acetyltransferase and acetylcholinesterase, the biosynthetic and biodegradative enzymes for the cholinergic neurotransmitter acetylcholine, in the rhesus ciliary muscle remain constant with age.[33] While these morphologic and biochemical techniques are not specific enough to exclude a selective loss of muscle or nerve fibers, receptors, or enzymes especially critical to accommodation, this possibility seems rather remote.

Several reports have stated that the human ciliary muscle does not weaken or otherwise functionally decline with age,[29,90] and even that the contractile force of the ciliary muscle reaches its maximum at the very time in life when presbyopia becomes clinically manifest.[29] However, such studies utilized indirect methods, such as impedance cyclography in living eyes,[90] or in

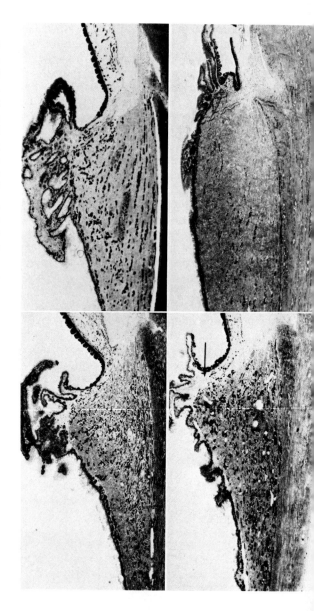

FIG. 11-13   A, Ciliary muscle of 8-year-old rhesus monkey treated topically with atropine (*left,* left eye) or pilocarpine (*right,* right eye) before enucleation. Note extremely anterior position of inner apex of ciliary muscle in pilocarpine-treated eye and absence of intramuscular connective tissue. **B,** Ciliary muscle of 34-year-old rhesus monkey was treated topically with atropine (*left,* left eye) or pilocarpine (*right,* right eye) before enucleation. Note similar position of inner apex of ciliary muscle, well posterior to scleral spur, in both eyes. In right eye, arrow indicates increased amount of connective tissue between ciliary muscle and iris root (ground plate) compared with younger animals; no increase in connective tissue is seen within muscle (Richardson's stain, original magnification × 120). (From Lütjen-Drecoll E, Tamm E, Kaufman PL: Arch Ophthalmol 106:1594, 1988.)

vitro passive stretch and lens deformation in postmortem eyes,[29] to make inferences about ciliary muscle function. Despite their unquestionable technical innovativeness and other merits, such studies do not provide direct and specific information about possible age-related changes in ciliary muscle position, configuration, and contractility. Thus impedance cyclography, which measures the electrical resistance across the ciliary muscle, reveals that the change in resistance when the eye attempts to accommodate does not decline with age; this finding has been interpreted to indicate that contractile force does not change with age.[90] However, it is not the *force* of muscle contraction but rather the *movement* of the muscle that provides the geometric alterations needed for accommodation to occur. Furthermore, contraction of the muscle not accompanied by muscle movement could easily alter blood flow within the muscle and anterior choroid, which might produce the impedance changes attributed to the muscle contraction itself.[9] In other words, impedance cyclography may tell us little about muscle configuration and position, but only that some type of contraction is occurring. The widely quoted passive stretch and deformation experiments of Fisher are ingenious, but only indicate

forces applied *to* the muscle consequent to forces on or configurational changes in the lens, not the other way around.[29] Furthermore, they were performed in postmortem eyes, so they really say nothing about the living muscle.

The concept of ciliary muscle contraction without configurational change was given credence by recent experiments in rhesus monkeys. If the anterior attachment to the scleral spur and the posterior attachment, via Bruch's membrane, to the scleral canal near the optic nerve are left intact, the ciliary muscle in freshly enucleated rhesus eyes exhibits an age-related loss in its positional and configurational responses to pilocarpine, using quantitative histological criteria (Fig. 11-14).[68] However, if the posterior attachments are cut, the response to pilocarpine is largely or completely restored, even in the oldest eyes.[68,69] In the living surgically iridectomized monkey the lens can be imaged by Scheimpflug videography, while the lens equator, zonule, and ciliary process can be imaged by goniovideography.[72] By electrically stimulating the Edinger-Westphal nucleus via an implanted electrode,[20] the movements and spacings of these structures can be visualized, recorded, and analyzed in real-time during accommodation and disaccommodation.[7,72] Caution must be ex-

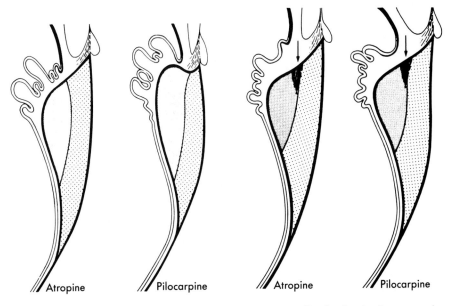

FIG. 11-14 Ciliary muscle topography and connective tissue distribution in rhesus monkeys. Representative sections based on histologic specimens from Figure 11-13 are depicted schematically. *Left,* 8-year-old rhesus monkey exhibits essentially no intramuscular connective tissue. *Right,* 34-year-old rhesus monkey exhibits connective tissue (*arrows*) only anteriorly between longitudinal and reticular zones. (From Lütjen-Drecoll E, Tamm E, Kaufman PL: Arch Ophthalmol 106:1593, 1988.)

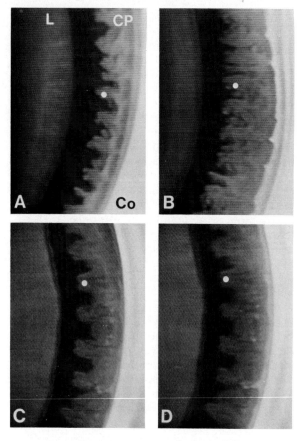

FIG. 11-15 Goniovideography of anterior segment 2 to 3 years following total iridectomy and midbrain electrode implantation in 4-year-old and 24-year-old rhesus monkeys. **A** and **B**, 4-year-old monkey, non-accommodating and maximally accommodating (17.3 diopters), respectively; **C** and **D**, 24-year-old monkey, nonaccommodating and maximally accommodating (1.5 diopters), respectively. L, lens; CP, ciliary processes (white dots indicate same ciliary process); and Co, cornea. Note centripetal excursion of ciliary processes during accommodation in young animal (**B** vs **A**) and virtual absence of such excursion in the old animals attempting to accommodate (**D** vs **C**). Angle of observation unchanged from **A** to **B**, or from **C** to **D**. (From Neider MW, Crawford K, Kaufman PL, Bito LZ: Arch Ophthalmol 108:73, 1990.)

ercised in quantifying such analyses because of optical distortion induced by the cornea and the gonioscopy lens, but it is qualitatively clear that both lenticular *and* ciliary body movement decline with age.[7,72] The loss of ciliary body movement is not due to restriction by the enlarged elderly lens, since at rest a circumlenticular space is always present, even in the most elderly animals (Fig. 11-15).[72] Ciliary body mobility is not

totally lost, and in an occasional elderly animal the circumlenticular space is noticeably narrowed or even obliterated during midbrain stimulation,[48] indicating that factors other than ciliary body hypomobility or immobility may be at least partly responsible for lenticular hypomobility or immobility (see below). Nonetheless, the histologic and videographic data in rhesus clearly raise the possibility that a loss of ciliary muscle excursion is involved in the pathophysiology of presbyopia.

Extralenticular elastic components

It seems unlikely that the neuromuscular apparatus itself is the culprit (see above). Loss of muscle movement and accommodative amplitude could be consequent to alterations in the elastic tissue of Bruch's membrane, which attaches the ciliary muscle posteriorly to the sclera near the optic nerve. If this tissue lost its elasticity, i.e., became more like a rigid steel cable than a rubber band, the ciliary muscle would not move forward when it contracted; it would be held in place by the "steel cable" anchoring it posteriorly (see Fig. 11-9).[68] Preliminary histochemical and ultrastructural studies of the connective tissue at the posterior aspect of the ciliary muscle are consistent with this concept.[91] Thus the posterior attachment of the ciliary muscle in young adult rhesus eyes normally consists exclusively of elastic tendons. Where the tendons and the muscle bundles join, the muscle cells stain more strongly for actin and desmin than in other parts of the muscle. These elastic tendons are continuous with the elastic network of Bruch's membrane. In old eyes the posterior insertion shows pronounced changes. The elastic fibers appear markedly thickened and contain increased amounts of associated microfibrils. There is also a marked increase in different types of collagen fibers that adhere to the elastic fibers. These increases in nonstretchable fibrillous material could cause stiffening of the elastic system and prevent ciliary muscle movement.[91]

Another hypothesis[9] has the posterior elastic tissue becoming not rigid, but, rather, flaccid. The muscle at rest would then be shorter, not being stretched posteriorly, and contraction would produce less anterior movement and less reduction in zonular force on the lens. This scenario would also predict that the lens in the elderly eye would always have an accommodated (more spherical) configuration (see Fig. 11-9). Although in some aspects the muscle[31,87] and the lenticular surface and internal cortical curvatures do indeed exhibit this "accommodated" topography, the lens nucleus maintains the same unaccommodated configuration throughout life.[57,68]

Lens

As human and rhesus eyes age, the anterior and posterior lens surfaces and internal curvatures become sharper (see Fig. 11-3), with the age-dependence being steeper for the anterior curves.[12,52,53,60,64] The lens also thickens due to the continual addition of new fibers to the anterior and posterior cortex; the adult nucleus does not thicken significantly with age.[6,53,61,63,64] The posterior surface of the lens remains fixed in position relative to the cornea, so that the anterior surface approaches the cornea—i.e., the anterior chamber shallows—and the main mass or center of the lens translates forward by about half this distance.[63,64] In the human the internal zones of discontinuity become more numerous and distinct up to 40 to 50 years of age; after that they seem to merge into fewer regions of still greater distinctness.[60,61] Slit lamp Scheimpflug photography also demonstrates that lenticular aging is accompanied by an increasing degree of high-angle light scattering. This is due not merely to the discontinuity zones, but occurs throughout the cortex and nucleus. Since this phenomenon occurs when particulate scatterers attain diameters roughly between 0.05 and 20 times the wavelength of light, the increased light scattering by the aging lens must be associated with an increase in size of suspended protein aggregates within the lens fibers. Since overall protein concentration within the lens remains essentially constant, the number of particles, and especially the number of soluble particles that contribute to the refractive index, must be decreasing. This may have important implications for the overall refractive power of the lens (see below). The increased light scattering is also the basis of the psychophysical phenomenon of glare.[15,53,61,84–86]

This age-related lenticular rounding and thickening closely mimics the events occurring during active accommodation, but these eyes are not accommodating—indeed, they cannot accommodate and remain focused at distance. This is surprising, since the changes indicated should all lead to a more powerfully refracting optical system, rendering the eye myopic. This constitutes the so-called lens paradox; the far point remains constant while the near point recedes, all in the presence of a lenticular geometry that would predict just the opposite.[58,61] To explain this requires the assumption that the refractive index of the lens itself must undergo an age-dependent change that compensates for the sharpened lens curvatures and surface positional changes. This could occur in several ways; for instance, as lens protein aggregates increase in size with age, an increasing percentage of the protein would become insoluble and no longer contribute to the refractive power of the lens, which would therefore decrease.[53,58] Studies are under way to confirm or refute the various hypotheses predicting decreased lenticular index of refraction, but, as with so many aspects of accommodation, the issue is presently unresolved.

Another characteristic of lenticular aging relates to the change in curvature and thickness required to produce a given amount of accommodation. With increasing age in the human, the slope of the change in radius of curvature as a function of accommodation decreases for both surfaces and for the corresponding internal curvatures delineating the zones of discontinuity and the nucleus, i.e., the change in curvature per unit dioptric change increases with increasing age. A corollary of this is that in prepresbyopic eyes, the older the subject the more sharply curved is the lens for any given accommodative state (see Fig. 11-3).[11,13,55,57] The age-dependence of the relationship between lens thickening, anterior chamber shallowing, and accommodation has not yet been determined. In the rhesus monkey the spacing-accommodation and curvature-accommodation relationships are all linear, with slopes independent of animal age or maximum accommodative amplitude.[52,53]

Classical teaching attributes presbyopia to lenticular "sclerosis,"[9] a term both ill-defined and of uncertain biophysical meaning. Conceptually, it is taken to indicate that the lens capsule loses its elasticity or that the lens substance "hardens" so that even when zonular tension is relaxed by contraction of the ciliary muscle the lens does not change shape. A detailed critique of this concept is beyond the scope of this chapter. Suffice it to say that a loss of inherent lenticular deformability, independent of other factors, as a necessary and sufficient explanation for presbyopia is by no means proved and is undoubtedly an oversimplification and perhaps even a misstatement of the events leading to the development of presbyopia.[9] The primate lens unquestionably continues to grow throughout life.[12,43,59] This growth occurs not only during the 30 to 40 years that accommodative amplitude is slowly declining, but for another 30 to 40 years thereafter, i.e., for the half life span during which the eye has entirely ceased accommodating. Such growth could produce some compaction of the lens and, although precise physical measurements are not available, the clinical impression is that the elderly cataractous nucleus is harder than that in the noncataractous younger lens. The only direct measurement of lens elasticity was made by Fisher, and while he noted age-related changes in lens elasticity, the changes did not correlate well with the timetable for accommodative loss.[29] Increased lens mass through normal growth processes is not synonymous with lenticular hardening, but increased bulk without changes in elastic properties would itself necessitate an increased magnitude in the force required for a given amount of deformation of any material. Changes in lenticular deformability could occur consequent to dehydration, formation of various types of chemical or physical bonds within the lens, hyperpolymerization of proteins, or myriad other events. However, the concept of presbyopia as due to lens "hardening" or loss of lenticular "elasticity" must be viewed as just another hypothetical player in the pathophysiology of presbyopia, with no more and perhaps much less evidence to support it than the various other possibilities.[9]

One potentially relevant consequence of continued lens growth relates to altered zonulo-lenticular-ciliary body geometry and the consequent changes in magnitude and vector of the ciliary and choroidal forces applied to the lens. Since the axial posterior surface of the lens remains fixed in position relative to the cornea and the retina while the lens grows, the central sulcus bisecting the lens equatorially is translated anteriorly, as is the actual lens equator.[52] Growth of the lens equatorially reduces the space between the lens edge and the ciliary body, and age-related shifts in the position and geometry of the zonular insertion into the lens capsule have been reported.[26,59]

One can hypothesize many optical consequences of these changes. The anterior shift of the lens could increase zonular tension on the capsule, making accommodation more difficult. On the other hand, the smaller cilio-lenticular distance would favor decreased zonular tension, perhaps causing the lens to adopt a more "accommodated" configuration even when the system is not trying to accommodate (see Fig. 11-3). If the lens were already in the partially or fully accommodated configuration with the system at rest, activation of the system (i.e., ciliary muscle contraction) would produce correspondingly less change in lenticular configuration even if the elasticity and deformability of the lens remained normal. Thus in elderly rhesus monkeys even though ciliary body excursion in-

duced by electrical stimulation of the Edinger-Westphal nucleus is markedly reduced, the muscle still moves slightly, and the circumlenticular space is narrowed (see Fig. 11-15).[72] This indicates that extralenticular factors also may not entirely account for presbyopia. Of course, one would expect such an eye to be focused at near in the resting state, which is not the case. However, as we have seen earlier, other compensatory age-dependent changes, most likely in the overall refractive index of the lens, may occur to keep the "resting" eye focused at distance.

Vitreous

If one views the vitreous as having a more significant role in accommodation than merely providing support and stabilization for the posterior surface of the lens,[16,17] then it is reasonable to speculate that age changes in the vitreous may play a pathophysiologic role in the development of presbyopia. With age, the vitreous becomes progressively more liquid, which could affect its efficacy in peripheral compression of the lens. Alternatively, Coleman[17] reasons that growth of the lens itself places the vitreous at a geometric-mechanical disadvantage in subserving this accommodative function.

One must reluctantly conclude that although our knowledge of the events that accompany the aging of the accommodative mechanism has increased vastly over the past decade, we still do not completely understand the age-related changes in any of the components, nor how they interact to produce presbyopia. It is clear that the classical view of presbyopia as consequent to "lenticular hardening," with everything else remaining normal, can no longer be accepted. Rather, lenticular growth, and changes in external and internal lenticular geometry and optical properties, ciliary muscle mobility, extralenticular elastic tissue, and the vitreous may all converge and conspire to produce the phenomenon of age-related loss of accommodative amplitude. These processes may also play a role in the pathophysiology of other age-related ocular afflictions, such as senile cataractogenesis and primary open-angle glaucoma.[5,9,32,49,72]

REFERENCES

1. Bárány EH, Rohen JW: Localized contraction and relaxation within the ciliary muscle of the vervet monkey (*Cercopithecus ethiops*), in Rohen JW, ed: The structure of the eye, second symposium, Stuttgart, FK Schattauer Verlag, 1965, p 287.
2. Bill A: Effects of atropine and pilocarpine on aqueous

humour dynamics in cynomolgus monkeys *(Macaca irus)*, Exp Eye Res 6:120, 1967.

3. Bill A: Blood circulation and fluid dynamics in the eye, Physiol Rev 55:383, 1975.

4. Bill A, Anderson SE, Mandahl A, et al: Effects of neuropeptides in the uvea, Invest Ophthalmol Vis Sci 29 (ARVO Suppl):323, 1988.

5. Bito LZ: Presbyopia, Arch Ophthalmol 106:1526, 1988.

6. Bito LZ, DeRousseau CJ, Kaufman PL, et al: Age-dependent loss of accommodative amplitude in rhesus monkeys: an animal model for presbyopia, Invest Ophthalmol Vis Sci 23:23, 1982.

7. Bito LZ, Kaufman PL, Neider M, et al: The dynamics of accommodation (ciliary muscle contraction, zonular relaxation and lenticular deformation) as a function of stimulus strength and age in iridectomized rhesus eyes, Invest Ophthalmol Vis Sci 28(ARVO Suppl):318, 1987.

8. Bito LZ, Miranda OC: Presbyopia: the need for a closer look, in Stark L, Obrech G, eds: Presbyopia: recent research and reviews from the third international symposium, New York, Churchill/Professional Press, 1987, p 411.

9. Bito LZ, Miranda OC: Accommodation and presbyopia, in Reinecke RD, ed: Ophthalmology annual, New York, Raven Press, 1989, p 103.

10. Brown N: Quantitative slit-image photography of the lens, Trans Ophthalmol Soc UK 92:303, 1972.

11. Brown N: The change in shape and internal form of the lens of the eye on accommodation, Exp Eye Res 15:441, 1973.

12. Brown NP: The change in lens curvature with age, Exp Eye Res 19:175, 1974.

13. Brown NP: The shape of the lens equator, Exp Eye Res 20:571, 1974.

14. Calasans OM: The architecture of the ciliary muscle of man, Ann Fac Med Univ Sao Paolo 27:3, 1953.

15. Carter JH: The effects of aging upon selected visual functions: color vision, glare sensitivity, field of vision, and accommodation, in Sekuler R, Kline D, Dismukes K, eds: Aging and human visual function, New York, Alan R Liss, 1982.

16. Coleman DJ: On the hydraulic suspension theory of accommodation, Trans Am Ophthalmol Soc 84:846, 1986.

17. Coleman DJ: Unified model for accommodative mechanism, Am J Ophthalmol 69:1063, 1970.

18. Cotlier E: The lens, in Moses RA, Hart WM, eds: Adler's physiology of the eye, clinical application, St Louis, CV Mosby, 1987.

19. Crawford KS, Kaufman PL, Bito LZ: The role of the iris in accommodation of rhesus monkeys, Invest Ophthalmol Vis Sci 31:2185, 1990.

20. Crawford K, Terasawa E, Kaufman PL: Reproducible stimulation of ciliary muscle contraction in the cynomolgus monkey via a permanent indwelling midbrain electrode, Brain Res 503:265, 1989.

21. Duane A: Studies in monocular and binocular accommodation with their clinical applications, Am J Ophthalmol 5:867, 1922.

22. Duke-Elder S: In System of ophthalmology, the eye in evolution, vol 1, St Louis, CV Mosby, 1958.

23. Erickson-Lamy KA, Kaufman PL: Reinnervation of primate ciliary muscle following ciliary ganglionectomy, Invest Ophthalmol Vis Sci 28:927, 1987.

24. Erickson-Lamy KA, Kaufman PL: Effect of cholinergic drugs on outflow facility after ciliary ganglionectomy, Invest Ophthalmol Vis Sci 29:491, 1988.

25. Erickson-Lamy K, Schroeder A: Dissociation between the effect of aceclidine on outflow facility and accommodation, Exp Eye Res 50:143, 1990.

26. Farnsworth PN, Shyne SE: Anterior zonular shifts with age, Exp Eye Res 28:291, 1979.

27. Fincham E: The mechanism of accommodation, Br J Ophthalmol 8:7, 1937.

28. Fisher RF: The elastic constants of the human lens, J Physiol 212:147, 1971.

29. Fisher RF: Presbyopia and the changes with age in the human crystalline lens, J Physiol (Lond) 228:765, 1973.

30. Flugel C, Bárány EH, Lütjen-Drecoll E: Histochemical differences within the ciliary muscle and its function in accommodation, Exp Eye Res 50:219, 1990.

31. Fuchs E: Uber den Ciliarmuskel, Albrecht von Graefe's Arch Ophthalmol 120:733, 1928.

32. Gabelt BT, Crawford K, Kaufman PL: Outflow facility and its response to pilocarpine decline in aging rhesus monkeys, Arch Ophthalmol 109:879, 1991.

33. Gabelt BT, Kaufman PL, Polansky JR: Ciliary muscle muscarinic binding sites, choline acetyltransferase and acetylcholinesterase in aging rhesus monkeys, Invest Ophthalmol Vis Sci 31:231, 1990.

34. Gilmartin B: A review of the role of sympathetic innervation of the ciliary muscle in ocular accommodation, Ophthal Physiol Opt 6:23, 1986.

35. Gilmartin B, Hogan RE: The relationship between tonic accommodation and ciliary muscle innervation, Invest Ophthalmol Vis Sci 26:1024, 1985.

36. Gilmartin B, Hogan RE, Thompson SM: The effect of timolol maleate on tonic accommodation, tonic vergence, and pupil diameter, Invest Ophthalmol Vis Sci 25:763, 1984.

37. Girard LJ: Nomenclature of corneal contact lenses, in Girard LJ, ed: Corneal contact lenses, 2nd ed, St Louis, CV Mosby, 1970.

38. Gupta N, Cynader M: in Drance SM, Neufeld AH, Van Buskirk EM, eds: Applied pharmacology of the glaucomas, Baltimore, Williams and Wilkins, in press.

39. Hara K, Lütjen-Drecoll E, Prestele H, et al: Structural differences between regions of the ciliary body in primates, Invest Ophthalmol Vis Sci 16:912, 1977.

40. Hart WM: Entoptic imagery, in Moses RA, Hart WM Jr, eds: Adler's physiology of the eye, clinical application, 8th ed, St Louis, CV Mosby, 1987.

41. Hogan MJ, Alvarado JA, Weddell JE: Ciliary body and posterior chamber, in Histology of the human eye, Philadelphia, WB Saunders, 1971.

42. Hogan MJ, Alvarado JA, Weddell JE: Eyeball, in Histology of the human eye, Philadelphia, WB Saunders, 1971.

43. Hogan MJ, Alvarado JA, Weddell JE: Lens, in Histology of the human eye, Philadelphia, WB Saunders, 1971.

44. Jaeger RJ, Benevento LA: A horseradish peroxidase study of the innervation of the internal structures of the eye; evidence for a direct pathway, Invest Ophthalmol Vis Sci 19:575, 1980.

45. Kaufman PL: Aqueous humor dynamics, in Duane TD, ed: Clinical ophthalmology, Philadelphia, Harper & Row, 1985, chap 45, p 1.

46. Kaufman PL, Bárány EH: Loss of acute pilocarpine effect on outflow facility following surgical disinsertion and retrodisplacement of the ciliary muscle from the scleral spur in the cynomolgus monkey, Invest Ophthal 15:793, 1976.

47. Kaufman PL, Bito LZ, De Rousseau CJ: The development of presbyopia in primates, Trans Ophthalmol Soc UK 102:323, 1983.

48. Kaufman PL, Crawford K, Neider M: Unpublished results.

49. Kaufman PL, Gabelt BT: Cholinergic mechanisms and aqueous humor dynamics, in Drance SM, Van Buskirk EM, Neufeld AH, eds: Applied pharmacology of the glaucomas, Baltimore, Williams & Wilkins, 1991, in press.

50. Kaufman PL, Rohen JW, Bárány EH: Hyperopia and loss of accommodation following ciliary muscle disinsertion in the cynomolgus monkey: physiologic and scanning electron microscopic studies, Invest Ophthalmol Vis Sci 18:665, 1979.

51. Kaufman PL, Rohen JW, Gabelt BT, et al: Parasympathetic denervation of the ciliary muscle following panretinal photocoagulation, Curr Eye Res, 10:437, 1991.

52. Koretz JF, Bertasso AM, Neider MW, et al: Slit-lamp studies of the rhesus monkey eye, II, Changes in crystalline lens shape, thickness and position during accommodation and aging, Exp Eye Res 45:317, 1987.

53. Koretz JF, Bertasso AM, Neider MW, et al: Slit-lamp studies of the rhesus monkey eye, III, The zones of discontinuity, Exp Eye Res 46:871, 1988.

54. Koretz JF, Bertasso AM, Neider MW, et al: Preliminary characterization of human crystalline lens geometry as a function of accommodation and age, in Non-invasive assessment of the visual system, 1988 Technical Digest Series, vol 3, p 130, Washington, DC, Optical Society of America, 1988.

55. Koretz JF, Handleman GH: Model of the accommodative mechanism in the human eye, Vision Res 22:917, 1982.

56. Koretz JF, Handelman GH: A model for accommodation in the young human eye: the effects of lens elastic anisotropy on the mechanism, Vision Res 23:1679, 1983.

57. Koretz JF, Handelman GH: Internal crystalline lens dynamics during accommodation: age-related changes, Atti Fondazione G Ronchi 40:409, 1985.

58. Koretz JF, Handelman GH: The "lens paradox" and image formation in accommodating human eyes, in Duncan G, ed: The lens: transparency and cataract, vol 6, p 57, Rijswijk, Topics in Aging Research in Europe, 1986.

59. Koretz JF, Handelman GH: How the human eye focuses, Scientific American 259:92, 1988.

60. Koretz JF, Handelman GH, Brown NP: Analysis of human crystalline lens curvature as a function of accommodative state and age, Vision Res 24:1141, 1984.

61. Koretz JF, Kaufman PL: Scheimpflug slit-lamp photographic characterization of the aging of the human crystalline lens and the development of presbyopia, in Non-invasive assessment of the visual system, 1990 Technical Digest Series, vol 3, p 160, Washington, DC, Optical Society of America, 1990.

62. Koretz JF, Kaufman PL, Neider MW, et al: Accommodation and presbyopia in the human eye, I, Evaluation of in vivo measurement techniques, Applied Optics 28:1097, 1989.

63. Koretz JF, Kaufman PL, Neider MW, et al: Accommodation and presbyopia in the human eye, II, Aging of the anterior segment, Vision Res 29:1685, 1989.

64. Koretz JF, Neider MW, Kaufman PL, et al: Slit-lamp studies of the rhesus monkey eye, I, Survey of the anterior segment, Exp Eye Res 44:307, 1987.

65. Lütjen E: Histometrische Untersuchungen über den Ziliarmuskel der Primaten, Albrecht von Graefes Arch Klin Exp Ophthalmol 171:121, 1966.

66. Lütjen-Drecoll E: Functional morphology of the ciliary epithelium, in Lütjen-Drecoll E, ed: Basic aspects of glaucoma research, Stuttgart, FK Schattauer, 1982.

67. Lütjen-Drecoll E, Tamm E, Kaufman PL: Age changes in rhesus monkey ciliary muscle: light and electron microscopy, Exp Eye Res 47:885, 1988.

68. Lütjen-Drecoll E, Tamm E, Kaufman PL: Age-related loss of morphologic responses to pilocarpine in rhesus monkey ciliary muscle, Arch Ophthalmol 106:1591, 1988.

69. Tamm E, Croft MA, Jungkunz W, et al: Age-related loss of ciliary muscle mobility in the rhesus monkey; role of the choroid, Arch Ophthalmol, in press.

70. McGetrick JJ, Wilson DG, Dortzbach RK, et al: A search for lymphatic drainage of the monkey orbit, Arch Ophthalmol 107:255, 1989.

71. Moses RA: Accommodation, in Moses RA, Hart WM, eds: Adler's physiology of the eye, clinical application, 8th ed, St Louis, CV Mosby, 1987.

72. Neider MW, Crawford K, Kaufman PL, et al: In vivo videography of the rhesus monkey accommodative apparatus, Arch Ophthalmol 108:69, 1990.

73. Nilsson SF, Sperber GO, Bill A: Effects of vasoactive intestinal polypeptide (VIP) on intraocular pressure, facility of outflow and formation of aqueous humor in the monkey, Exp Eye Res 43:849, 1986.

74. Parelman JJ, Fay MT, Burde RM: Confirmatory evidence for a direct parasympathetic pathway to internal eye structures, Trans Am Ophthalmol Soc 82:371, 1984.

75. Rohen J: Das Auge und seine Hilfsorgane, in Mollendorf WV, Bargmann W, eds: Handbuch der mikroskpischen Anatomie des Menschen, vol 3, part 4, New York, Springer-Verlag, 1964.

76. Rohen JW: Scanning electron microscopic studies of the zonular apparatus in human and monkey eyes, Invest Ophthalmol Vis Sci 18:133, 1979.

77. Rohen JW: The evolution of the primate eye in relation to the problem of glaucoma, in Lütjen-Drecoll E, ed: Basic aspects of glaucoma research, Stuttgart, Schattauer, 1982, p 3.

78. Rohen JW, Futa R, Lütjen-Drecoll E: The fine structure of the cribriform meshwork in normal and glaucomatous eyes as seen in tangential sections, Invest Ophthalmol Vis Sci 21:574, 1981.

79. Rohen JW, Kaufman PL, Eichhorn M, et al: Functional morphology of accommodation in the raccoon, Exp Eye Res 48:523, 1989.

80. Rohen JW, Lütjen E, Bárány E: The relation between the ciliary muscle and the trabecular meshwork and its importance for the effect of miotics and aqueous outflow resistance, Albrecht von Graefes Arch Klin Exp Ophthalmol 172:23, 1967.

81. Rosenfield M, Gilmartin B, Cunningham E, et al: The influence of alpha-adrenergic agents on tonic accommodation, Curr Eye Res 9:267, 1990.

82. Ruskell GL: Innervation of the anterior segment of the eye, in Lütjen-Drecoll E, ed: Basic aspects of glaucoma research, Stuttgart, Schattauer, 1982.

83. Ruskell GL, Griffiths T: Peripheral nerve pathway to the ciliary muscle, Exp Eye Res 28:277, 1979.

84. Sigelman J, Trokel SL, Spector A: Quantitative biomicroscopy of lens light back-scatter in aging and opacification, Arch Ophthalmol 92:437, 1974.

85. Spector A: Aging of the lens and cataract formation, in Sekuler R, Kline D, Dismukes K, eds: Aging and human visual function, New York, Alan R Liss, 1982.

86. Spector A, Li S, Sigelman J: Age-dependent changes of human lens proteins and their relationship to light scatter, Invest Ophthalmol 13:795, 1974.

87. Stieve R: Uber den Bau des menschlichen Ciliarmuskels, seine Veranderungen wahrend des Lebens und seine Bedeutung fur die Akkommodation, Anat Anz 97:69, 1949.

88. Streeten BW, Gibson SA: Identification of extractable proteins from bovine ocular zonule: major zonular antigens of 32 kD and 250 kD, Curr Eye Res 7:139, 1988.

89. Streeten BW, Licari PA, Marucci AA, et al: Immunohistochemical comparison of ocular zonules and the microfibrils of elastic tissue, Invest Ophthalmol Vis Sci 21:130, 1981.

90. Swegmark G: Studies with impedance cyclography on human ocular accommodation at different ages, Acta Ophthalmologica 47:1186, 1969.

91. Tamm E, Lütjen-Drecoll E, Jungkunz W, et al: Posterior attachment of the ciliary muscle in young, accommodating old, presbyopic rhesus monkeys, Invest Ophthalmol Vis Sci 32:1678, 1991.

92. Thompson HS: The pupil, in Moses RA, Hart WM, eds: Adler's physiology of the eye: clinical application, 8th ed, St Louis, CV Mosby, 1987.

93. Walls GL: The vertebrate eye and its adaptive radiation, Bloomfield Hills, MI, Cranbook Institute of Science, 1942.

94. Warwick R: The eyeball, in Eugene Wolff's anatomy of the eye and orbit, 7th ed, Philadelphia, WB Saunders, 1976.

95. Warwick R: The orbital nerves, in Eugene Wolff's anatomy of the eye and orbit, 7th ed, Philadelphia, WB Saunders, 1976.

96. Warwick RB: The ocular parasympathetic nerve supply and its mesencephalic sources, J Anat 88:71, 1954.

97. Weale R: Presbyopia toward the end of the 20th century, Surv Ophthalmol 34:15, 1989.

98. Westheimer G, Blair SM: The parasympathetic pathways to internal eye muscles, Invest Ophthalmol 12:193, 1973.

The Pupil

H. STANLEY THOMPSON, M.D.

This chapter is chiefly concerned with the application of pupillary signs to clinical diagnosis. After a brief review of pupillary neuroanatomy, physiology, and pharmacology, the reader is asked to consider afferent and efferent pupillary defects, tonic pupils, light-near dissociation, anisocoria, and Horner's syndrome.

ANATOMY
Muscles of the iris

The iris contains two muscles, the sphincter iridis and the dilator pupillae. They are among the very few muscles of the body derived from the neural ectoderm. At about the beginning of the fourth month of gestation, the rim of the optic cup differentiates into a circular band of muscle, the sphincter iridis (Fig. 12-1). When fully formed, the sphincter is typical smooth muscle and lies anterior to the neuroectodermal pigment epithelium in the iris stroma. The dilator muscle arises from the outer layer of the primitive optic cup at about the seventh month by elongation of the cells in a radial direction. The myoid elongations of the dilator cells lie anterior to their pigmented cell bodies; the cell bodies remain in apposition to the pigmented inner wall of the optic cup. As can be seen in Figure 12-1, the inner, retinal layer of the optic cup becomes the single, deeply pigmented cell layer of the posterior iris epithelium, whereas the outer layer of the optic cup, corresponding to the pigment epithelium of the retina, gives rise to a pigmented myoepithelium, the dilator of the iris.

The excursion of the pupil can be extraordinarily large. When maximally contracted, the diameter of the human pupil may be less than 1 mm; when maximally dilated, it may be more than 9 mm. The iris sphincter shortens about 87% of its length, an amount seldom seen in other smooth or striated muscles in the body. It is generally believed that those muscles that move their insertions through large distances have long fibers.

The spincter muscle does not move freely in the iris like a pajama string; its fibers are intimately connected with the iris stroma and with the dilator muscle to such an extent that constriction of the pupil is possible even after part of the sphincter has been cut—that is, following spincterotomy or sector iridectomy.

Innervation of the iris muscles

The muscles of the iris are innervated by the autonomic nervous system. The sympathetic innervation of the dilator muscle is shown in Figure 12-16 and is described on p. 434, where Horner's syndrome is discussed. The parasympathetic innervation of the iris sphincter muscle is the efferent (outflow) arm of the light reflex arc.

Afferent pathway of the light reflex. There can be little question that the receptors for the pupillary light reflex are identical to those concerned with vision. The question arises as to whether two separate sets of optic nerve fibers are used to carry the pupillary and the visual impulses or whether these messages, going to quite different parts of the brain, originate in the same

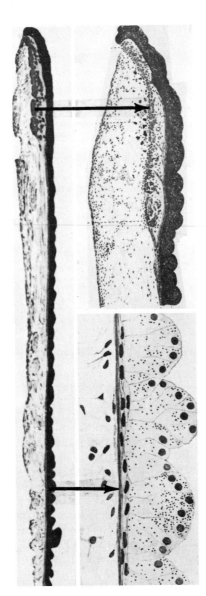

even though this has not been established with certainty in primates. In support of this assumption is the observation that damage to an optic nerve produces roughly comparable loss of pupillary function and loss of visual field.[71] If there are indeed separate pupillary fibers, they msut follow the visual fibers *very* closely because a fully convincing case of the clinical dissociation of these two functions has yet to be reported. In any event, the pupillary impulses part company with the visual impulses in the posterior third of the optic tract and enter the dorsal midbrain, where they stimulate the cells of the pretectal nucleus. The axons from this nucleus travel around the periaqueductal gray matter and connect to the cells of the Edinger-Westphal group of the oculomotor nucleus.

In humans the intercalated neurons from each side of the pretectum are distributed in a balanced fashion to the oculomotor nuclei of both sides. There are probably more crossed than uncrossed fibers in this hemidecussation. The intercalated fibers destined for the opposite third nerve parasympathetic nucleus (of Edinger-Westphal) cross dorsal to the cerebral aqueduct in the posterior commissure; then, in company with axons arising on that side, they arch ventrally to reach the Edinger-Westphal nucleus. Thus each optic tract carries pupillary fibers from both eyes (Fig. 12-2), and the pupillary fibers synapse with intercalated neurons that distribute the impulses of each tract in such a way that both third nerve nuclei usually receive the same number of pupil constriction impulses.

Pupilloconstrictor responses are obtained from stimulation of the optic chiasm, the optic tract on the lateral surface of the brainstem and ventral to the lateral geniculate body, the brachium of the superior colliculus, the pretectal region, the posterior commissure, and fibers arching ventrally around the central gray matter at the level of transition between the third ventricle and cerebral aqueduct (Fig. 12-2).

Efferent pathway to sphincter and ciliary muscle. The intraocular muscles are controlled by the Edinger-Westphal nucleus, which is part of the oculomotor nucleus (see Chapter 5). The third nerve leaves the midbrain in the interpeduncular fossa carrying near its epineurium the small-caliber fibers that serve the intraocular muscles. The synapse in this typical two-neuron parasympathetic outflow path is in the ciliary ganglion, deep in the muscle cone of the orbit (Fig. 12-11). The postganglionic fibers follow the short ciliary nerves to the anterior segment of the globe.

FIG. 12-1   Cross section of iris. Upper arrow points to sphincter muscle drawn in higher magnification; lower arrow points to dilator muscle of bleached specimen drawn in higher magnification. (From Saltzmann M: Anatomy and histology of the human eyeball, Chicago, The University of Chicago Press, 1912.)

retinal ganglion cell and travel along the same axon in the optic nerve. In cats the axons of the retinal ganglion cells, on their way to the lateral geniculate nucleus, are known to send branches into the midbrain along the brachium of the superior colliculus; thus it is generally assumed that the optic nerve axons of these ganglion cells convey both visual and pupillary impulses—

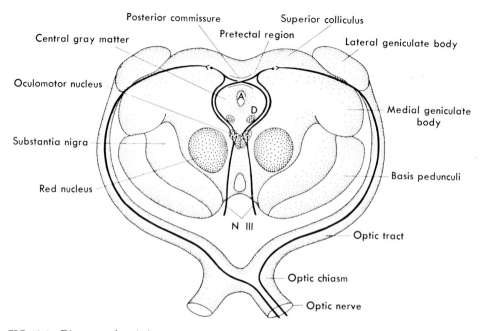

FIG. 12-2   Diagram of path for pupillary light reflex. A, Aqueduct; D, nucleus of Darkschewitsch; N III, oculomotor nerve. (Modified from Ranson.)

PHYSIOLOGY
The normal pupil

Normally, the pupil is placed not quite at the center of the iris but slightly nasally and inferiorly. The size of the pupil varies with age. A premature baby has no pupillary light reaction until 31 weeks of gestational age. The amplitude of the light response gradually increases until it is almost 2 mm at term.[20] This may be due to the gradual arrival of parasympathetic nerves at the iris sphincter muscle. Sympathetic innervation reaches the dilator muscle at full term, as evidenced by the fact that the pupils of premature infants do not dilate to hydroxyamphetamine but do dilate to phenylephrine.[29] The miosis of the newborn is due in part to the fact that the baby is asleep or sleepy 22 hours out of every 24 and partly because the eyeball is far from gull-grown. In adolescence the pupils are at their largest. They then become steadily smaller until about age 60, when the size levels off (Fig. 12-3).[34]

Pupillary unrest and hippus

A healthy iris is moving most of the time, even when illumination and accommodation are constant. This physiologic pupillary unrest is presumed to be due to fluctuations in the activity of the sympathetic and parasympathetic innervation of the iris muscles, which have reached an unsteady sort of equilibrium. The movements of the iris are largest in moderately bright light, and the frequency of the oscillation increases with the light intensity (Fig. 12-4). This pupillary instability is most apparent in young people and may be unhesitatingly accepted as a normal phenomenon and called "physiologic pupillary unrest" or "hippus." The word hippus has a long and interesting history. For the last 200 years it has meant a pupillary unrest "of abnormal degree," a tremor of the iris muscles. It was thought during the nineteenth century to be a sign of various neurologic diseases but has gradually become accepted as a normal phenomenon.[67]

Simple anisocoria

A small amount of pupillary inequality is common. Roughly one fifth of the normal population has an anisocoria in dim light of 0.4 mm or more.[27,33] It is interesting that this pupillary inequality is not constant in a given individual; it may increase or decrease or even reverse sides within days or hours. It has been called a "see-saw" anisocoria when these changes are dramatic.

This is an anisocoria that decreases slightly in bright light; it has not been associated with any disease process, it produces no symptoms, it is common, it is benign. For these reasons it has

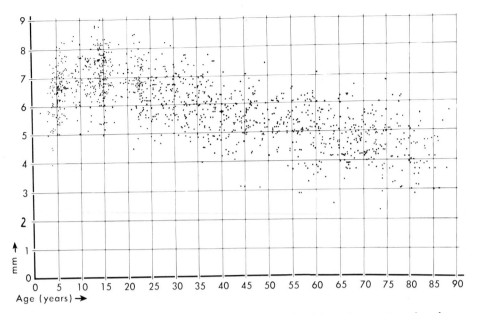

FIG. 12-3 Pupillary size in darkness at various ages. 1263 subjects chosen at random from a population survey. Each point represents the average diameter of the two pupils taken together. The ordinate shows horizontal diameters (in millimeters); the abscissa shows age in years. Note the wide scatter among individuals and the obvious age trend. (From Loewenfeld IE: Pupillary changes related to age, in Thompson HS, ed: Topics in neuro-ophthalmology, © [1979], The Williams & Wilkins Co., Baltimore.)

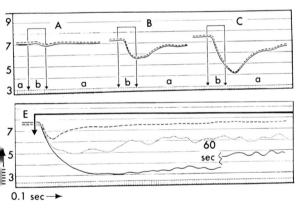

FIG. 12-4 *A, B,* and *C,* Dark-adapted normal subject. Light flashes, *b,* of increasing intensity produce increasing pupillary constriction. Latent period decreases with intensity of flash. Right eye *(solid line)* was stimulated; left eye *(broken line)* remained in darkness. Reactions are equal on two sides. *E,* Reaction of pupil to prolonged light of different intensities. (From Löwenstein O, Loewenfeld IE: in Davson H, ed: The eye, vol 3, New York, Academic Press, 1962.

been called a "simple" anisocoria. The terms "physiologic anisocoria" and "essential anisocoria" are also in use, but the former implies normalcy and the latter is deliberately obfuscatory. In any case, the peripheral innervation of the iris muscles is normal in both eyes and no further workup is called for.

Tournay's phenomenon

In 1917 Tournay said that it was normal to have unequal pupils in lateral gaze—with the larger pupil in the abducting eye. It has recently been established that this is not the case[35,55]; almost everyone has equal pupils in all directions of gaze. Lateral gaze induced an anisocoria of more than 0.5 mm in less than 5% of a population studied.[35] It is to these rare cases that Tournay's name is now attached, and it is interesting to speculate that, in some people there might be an anomalous co-innervation of the iris sphincter and the medial rectus muscle, so that both muscles are inhibited in abduction.

Pupillary reaction to light

The pupil seems easy to observe, but it is also easy to introduce artifacts into the observation and thus to reach false conclusions because of these artifacts. Through the years a vast and confusing literature on the pupil has accumulated. Löwenstein and Loewenfeld[31,43] have sorted through this tangle of conflicting opinion and have tested the evidence with their own observations. Their development and extensive use of techniques for the measurement of the human pupil in infrared light have been helpful to our understanding of pupillary response in health and disease. Much of the following section on the behavior of the pupils in healthy subjects has been drawn from their work.*

Effect and intensity of the stimulus

When the dark-adapted eye is exposed to light flashes of short duration, the pupillary threshold is found to be very low. With the use of appropriate recording techniques, small but distinct pupillary reactions usually can be obtained well within the first log unit of stimulus luminance above the subject's scotopic visual threshold. The intensity and the duration of the stimulus are interchangeable only for very short flashes (less than 100 msec.).

When the intensity of the light is increased over a range of approximately 3 log units, the pupillary contractions gradually become stronger and less variable. Throughout the low-intensity range of luminance the pupillary responses are, however, typically shallow; the contraction is preceded by a long latency, and it is slow and of low amplitude and short duration. When the light intensity is further increased, the reflexes begin to grow markedly in amplitude, speed of movement, and duration of contraction until maximal values are reached at about 7 to 9 log units above the scotopic visual threshold. There is a sudden increase in the effectiveness of the light stimuli when the cone threshold is exceeded.

Very powerful light flashes fail to add further to the amplitude and speed, and they do not reduce the latency of the reactions but they greatly prolong the contraction; after such stimuli the pupil may remain in spastic miosis for several seconds. There is no doubt that the afterimage contributes to this delayed redilation.

Modifying effects of fatigue and emotional excitement

Fatigue and emotional excitement are so much a part of everyday life and their modifying influence on pupillary diameter and reactions is so profound that their effects must be well understood and constantly borne in mind when considering the pupillary reaction to light.

The light reflex is not independent of the subject's level of consciousness. While the subject is alert, the central synapse of the pupillomotor reflex arc in the Edinger-Westphal nucleus is subject to supranuclear inhibitory influences. Simultaneously, hypothalmic discharges are brought into play by sensory or emotional stimuli provided by the environment or, at least in humans, by spontaneous thoughts or emotions; they travel via the brainstem, cervical cord, and peripheral sympathetic chain to the dilator muscle of the iris. Under the influence of these mechanisms the pupil in healthy alert subjects is relatively large and quiet in darkness, and this condition may be maintained for long periods of time. But when the subject becomes tired, the pupils gradually become smaller and begin to oscillate. In the moments immediately preceding sleep, the pupils are quite small, but a psychosensory stimulus such as a sudden sound will restore the waking condition and redilate the pupils.[42]

As the subject drifts toward sleep, cerebral and diencephalic centers shut down in an orderly sequence. Supranuclear inhibition of the Edinger-Westphal nucleus decreases, and sympathetic activity is gradually lost. The consequent relative preponderance of parasympathetic outflow results in miosis.[39] At the moment of spontaneous or reactive awakening, the sympathetic activity and supranuclear inhibition of the sphincter nucleus cooperate in dilating the pupil.[30]

Pupillary light reflexes are superimposed on this constantly shifting equilibrium of autonomic innervation of the iris, which can be further modified by humoral adrenergic mechanisms and influenced by the mechanical limitations of the iris.

Latent period of the light reflex

The latent period of the light reaction is relatively long, as is to be expected in a reflex with a smooth muscle effector. With a very bright light the latent period can be approximately 0.2 second, and as the stimulus is dimmed the latent period is prolonged until it may approach 0.5 second.[40] Because the response is slow, contraction to light flickering at the low rate of 5 Hz is fused into a steady contraction.

Spectral sensitivity of the light reaction

The pupillomotor effectiveness of a colored light simulus is related to its apparent brightness; for each color, the threshold of pupillary reactions is almost as low as the corresponding visual

---

*Loewenfeld's major two-volume text, *The Pupil*, should be available from the Iowa State University Press, Ames, IA, early in 1992.

threshold. This is true for all areas of the retina and in the dark-adapted as well as the light-adapted eye. In other words, the Purkinje shift and the rod-cone break also can be seen in dark-adapted pupillary responses. (These visual phenomena are discussed in Chapters 16 and 22.)

Pupillomotor sensitivity of various parts of the retina

The retinal periphery is far less efficient than the fovea for the production of large pupillary contractions, and if the amplitude of the light reaction were used as a measure of retinal sensitivity, the pupillomotor responsiveness of the fovea would seem to be far greater than that of the periphery. However, with light stimuli of low intensity, the periphery of the retina has a much lower pupillomotor threshold and is thus much more sensitive than the fovea, although the light reactions produced by stimulating the periphery are of low amplitude. The pupillary sensitivity of the retina is thus remarkably similar to the visual sensitivity.

Consensual light reflex

The stimulation of one retina by light produces a contraction of the pupil in the opposite eye in all animals in which there is partial decussation of both the optic nerve fibers in the chiasm and the pupillary fibers in the midbrain. In primates the hemidecussation in the dorsal midbrain seems to be functionally 50-50 when a full field stimulus is used. Unfortunately, any bright focal stimulus becomes a full field stimulus because of the intraocular scatter of light, and therefore stimulates both pretectal nuclei. This hides the predominately crossed midbrain hemidecussation of the pupillary light reflex pathway.

Consensual deficits

It has been suggested by careful observers that in humans this wiring is not as precise as it seems and that a large number of normal subjects will have a slightly smaller consensual reaction than direct reaction.[5] However, most of these difference are of the order of 0.1 mm, and clinically visible consensual deficits (0.4 mm or more) are rare (probably less than 5% of the population). Unilateral consensual deficits are more common than bilateral consensual deficits ("alternating contraction of anisocoria" of Löwenstein).[38]

Cats, phylogenetically lower than primates, normally have a bilateral consensual deficit because the pupillary pathways in the midbrain and chiasm are much more crossed than uncrossed. Birds have chiasms that are entirely crossed. An owl illuminated from the left will have an anisocoria, with the left pupil smaller than the right. This kind of anisocoria is rarely seen in humans and in monkeys, and even when present to a clinically visible degree it is seldom recognized. An impaired consensual pupillary reaction is not yet of any known clinical significance except as a potential source of confusion when a clinician looks carefully at the pupillary light reactions (Fig. 12-5). If you are going to look carefully, it is worth knowing

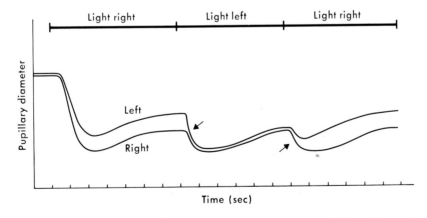

FIG. 12-5 Pupillographic tracing of a patient with a left consensual deficit. Notice that an anisocoria is present only when the right eye is stimulated and the left eye is in darkness. Since in the usual alternating light test you look only at the illuminated eye, you may not be aware that you are producing an anisocoria; all you see is the larger initial constriction in the eye with the impaired consensual reaction (*arrows*). A unilateral consensual deficit presents itself clinically during the alternating light test as asymmetric initial pupillary constriction in the two eyes without the usual accompanying asymmetric pupillary escape seen in relative afferent defects. (From Thompson HS: Trans Ophthalmol Soc UK 96:377, 1976.)

about.[5,59] A consensual deficit can be readily seen in flash photographs taken with one eye in bright light and the other in darkness.

Accommodation-convergence reaction (near reflex)

When gaze is directed at an object held close to the face, the pupils contract. This contraction is independent of any change in illumination and depends on a supranuclear connection between the neurons serving the sphincter pupillae and the ciliary muscle and the medial recti. It is not a true reflex but an associated movement. These three muscles work together in a common cause: they all serve to sharpen the image of a near object. The medial recti move the images onto the fovea of each eye, the ciliary muscle focuses the image, and the pupillary sphincter improves the depth of field. Since the amount of pupillary constriction varies with the nearness of the object of regard, this part of the synkinesis is best called the "near-point reaction," the "near reaction of the pupil," or the "pupillary constriction to near."

The contraction of the pupil "at near" does not depend on either the accommodation or the convergence any more than does the convergence or accommodation depend on others of the triad. All three must be looked on as being associated in a common function. Normally they work together, but one may be dissociated from the others. Thus it is possible to have contraction of the pupil with convergence of the visual axes without accommodation by placing plus lenses in front of each eye to take the place of the accommodation needed for the near point. Likewise, convergence can be prevented by placing base-in prisms in front of each eye. When a person is asked to read fine print under both these circumstances, the pupil will contract. The near pupillary contraction exists in uncorrected myopic persons and in very old people who have lost all accommodation. The constriction of the pupil takes place equally in both eyes, although one is covered. This is true even though the vision in one eye is considerably impaired.

When a near effort is difficult to obtain, the "lid closure reaction" may be used.[62] The patient is asked to read the chart at distance while trying to close his or her eyes. One eye is held open by the examiner. This often brings out an involuntary "near reaction."

PHARMACOLOGY OF THE PUPIL

The parasympathetic and sympathetic neural impulses to the iris muscles can be modified by drugs at the snyapses and at the effector sites be-

cause it is at these locations that the transmission of the impulse depends on chemical mediators. Drugs also can have central actions that affect the pupils. These drugs and their various modes of action are summarized in Figure 12-6 and in the following paragraphs, where they are grouped according to the site and mechanism of their action.

A few cautionary words should first be said about the interpretation of pupillary responses to topically instilled drugs. There are large interindividual differences in the responsiveness of the iris to topical drugs. This becomes most evident when weak concentrations are used. For example, 0.25% pilocarpine will produce a minimal constriction in some patients and an intense miosis in others. This means that the most secure clinical judgments stem from comparisons with the action of the drug on the other, normal eye.

It also should be remembered that the general status of the patient will influence the size of the pupils. If the patient becomes uncomfortable or anxious while waiting for the drug to act, both pupils may dilate. If the patient becomes drowsy, both pupils will constrict. Thus, if a judgment is to be made about the dilation or contraction of the pupil in response to a drug placed in the conjunctival sac, one pupil should be used as a control whenever possible.

If only one eye is involved, the drug should be put in both eyes so that the response of the normal and abnormal eye can be compared. When the condition is bilateral, no such comparisons are possible, but an attempt should be made to make sure that the observed response is indeed caused by the instilled drug. Thus, if both eyes are involved, the drop should be put in one eye only so that the responses of the medicated and unmedicated eyes can be compared.

Parasympatholytic (anticholinergic) drugs

The belladonna alkaloids occur naturally. They can be found in various proportions in deadly nightshade (Atropa belladonna), henbane (Hyoscyamus niger), and jimsonweed (Datura stramonium). Potions made from these plants were the tools of professional poisoners in ancient times. The word "belladonna" ("beautiful lady") was derived from the cosmetic use of these substances as mydriatics in sixteenth-century Venice. Youth and excitement have always dilated the pupils, and age and boredom still constrict them. The mischief caused by the ubiquitous jimsonweed is typical of this group of plants.[57] Jimsonweed has been used as a poison, has been taken as a hallucinogen, and has caused accidental illness and death, and it can cause an

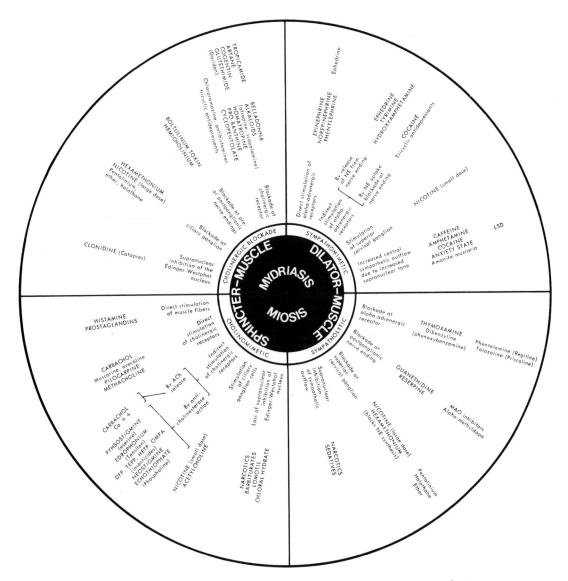

FIG. 12-6 Drugs that affect the size of the pupil and their mechanism of action.

alarming accidental mydriasis. These solanaceous plants, which are related to the tomato, potato, and eggplant, are still cultivated for medicinal purposes.

Atropine and scopolamine block parasympathetic activity by competing with acetylcholine at the effector cells of the iris sphincter and ciliary muscle, thus preventing depolarization. After conjunctival instillation of atropine (1%), mydriasis begins within about 10 minutes and is fully developed at 35 to 45 minutes; cycloplegia is complete within 1 hour. The pupil may stay dilated for several days, but accommodation usually returns in 48 hours. Scopolamine (0.2%) causes mydriasis that lasts, in an uninflamed

eye, for about 2 days; it is a less effective cycloplegic than atropine.

Homatropine and eucatropine (Euphthalmine) are synthetic anticholinergic drugs that were introduced into ophthalmology late in the nineteenth century. Homatropine (2% to 5%) causes mydriasis that lasts for 1 to 2 days, but repeated applications are necessary for effective cycloplegia. Eucatropine mydriasis (2% to 10%) lasts for less than 12 hours and is accompanied by only slight cycloplegia.

Tropicamide (Mydriacyl) and cyclopentolate (Cyclogyl) are more recently developed synthetic parasympatholytics with a short duration of action. Tropicamide (1%) is an effective, short-acting mydriatic (3 to 6 hours), which results in only a very transient paresis of accommodation. Compared with tropicamide, cyclopentolate (1%) seems to be a more effective cycloplegic and a slightly less effective mydriatic, especially in dark eyes; accommodation takes about half a day to return and the pupil still may not be working perfectly after more than 24 hours.

Botulinum toxin blocks the release of acetylcholine, and hemicholinium interferes with the synthesis of acetylcholine both at the preganglionic and at the postganglionic nerve endings, thus interrupting the parasympathetic pathway in two places. The outflow of sympathetic impulses is also interrupted by systemic doses of these drugs, since the chemical mediator in sympathetic ganglia is also acetylcholine (Fig. 12-7).

Parasympathomimetic (cholinergic) drugs

Pilocarpine and methacholine (Mecholyl) are structurally similar to acetylcholine and are capable of depolarizing the effector cell, thus causing miosis and spasm of accommodation. Mecholyl is still sometimes used in a weak (2.5%) solution to test for cholinergic supersensitivity of the sphincter muscle. It is being replaced by weak pilocarpine (0.1%).

Arecoline is a naturally occurring substance with an action similar to that of pilocarpine and methacholine; its chief advantage is that it acts quickly, producing a full miosis in 10 to 15 minutes rather than 20 to 30 minutes.

Carbachol (carbamylcholine, Doryl) acts chiefly at the postganglionic cholinergic nerve ending to release the stores of acetylcholine. There is also some direct action of carbachol on the effector cell. A 1.5% solution causes intense miosis, but the drug does not penetrate the cornea easily and is therefore usually mixed with a wetting agent (1:3500 benzalkonium chloride).

Acetylcholine is liberated at the cholinergic nerve endings by the neural action potential and is promptly hydrolyzed and inactivated by cholinesterase. Cholinesterase, in turn, can be inactivated by any one of many anticholinesterase drugs. These drugs either block the action of cholinesterase or deplete the stores of the enzyme in the tissue. They are thus able to potentiate the action of the chemical mediator by preventing its destruction by cholinesterase. It follows from their mode of action that these drugs will lose their cholinergic activity after the nerve supply has been completely blocked.

Physostigmine is a classic anticholinesterase. Along the Calabar coast of West Africa the native tribes once conducted trials "by ordeal" using a poison prepared from the bean of the plant *Physostigma venenosum*. The local name for this big bean was the "esere nut." If justice was ever served at these trials it was surely for the wrong reasons. The guilty man can be imagined, lingering at the poison cup, sipping slowly, aware that this was the end; he might thus take the time to absorb a fatal dose. However, the innocent man, knowing that the potion could not harm him, would cheerfully quaff it down, and his stomach would respond to this assualt by vomiting it all back up.

A paper published by Argyll Robertson helped to introduce the miotic Calabar extract into clinical ophthalmology. Physostigmine (eserine) was first used to stretch out the iris so that a peripheral iridectomy could be done more easily.[25]

The organic phosphate esters (echothiophate [Phospholine], isofluorphate [diisopropyl fluorophosphate—DFP], tetraethyl pyrophosphate, hexaethyltetraphosphate, parathion), many of which are in widespread use as insecticides, cause a much longer lasting miosis than the other anticholinesterases, but even this potent effect, thought to be due to interference with cholinesterase synthesis, can be reversed by pralidoxime chloride (P-2-AM).

Sympathomimetic drugs

Epinephrine (Adrenalin) is capable of direct stimulation of the receptor sites of the dilator cell. When applied to the conjunctiva, the 1:1000 solution does not penetrate into the normal eye in sufficient quantity to have an obvious mydriatic effect. If, however, the receptors have been made supersensitive by previous denervation, this concentration of epinephrine usually dilates the pupil. Phenylephrine (Neo-Synephrine) in the 10% solution has a powerful mydriatic effect. Its action is almost exclusively a direct alpha stimulation of the effector cell. The pupil recovers in 8 hours and shows a "rebound miosis" lasting several days.[13] Both 5% and 2.5% solutions are now commonly used. Ephedrine acts chiefly by releasing endogenous norepinephrine from the nerve ending, but it also has a definite direct stimulating effect on the dilator cells. Tyramine and hydroxyamphetamine act adrenergically by releasing norepinephrine from the stores in the postganglionic nerve endings; as far as is known this is their only effective mechanism. Cocaine (5% to 10%) is applied to the conjunctiva as a topical anesthetic, a mydriatic, and a test for Horner's syndrome. Its mydriatic effect is the result of an accumulation of norepinephrine at the receptor sites of the dilator cells. The amount of transmitter substance builds up at the neuroeffector

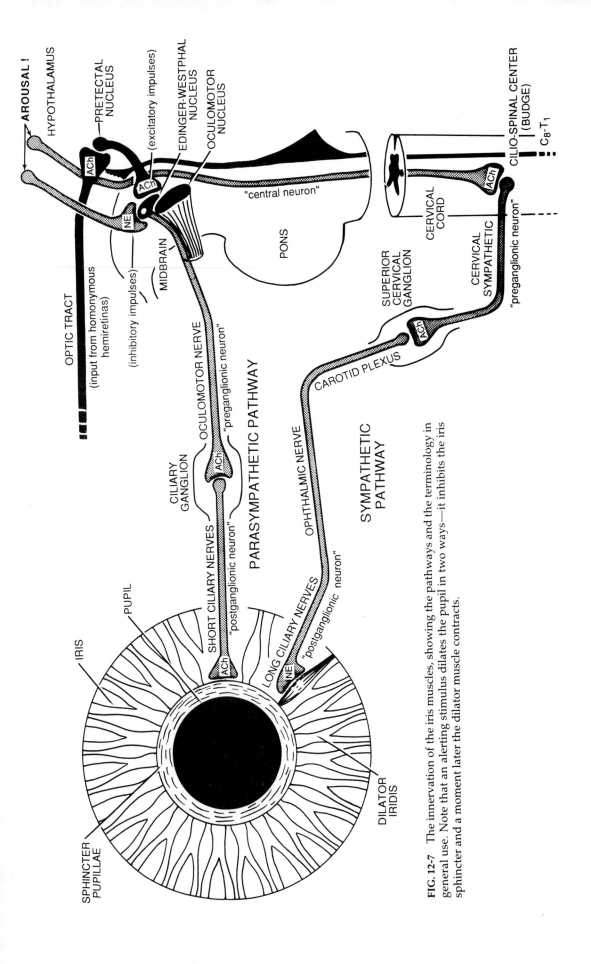

FIG. 12-7 The innervation of the iris muscles, showing the pathways and the terminology in general use. Note that an alerting stimulus dilates the pupil in two ways—it inhibits the iris sphincter and a moment later the dilator muscle contracts.

junction because cocaine prevents the reuptake of the norepinephrine back into the cytoplasm of the nerve ending. The action of cocaine is thus analogous to the action of the anticholinesterases at the cholinergic junction in that it interferes with the mechanism for prompt disposition of the chemical mediator.

Cocaine itself has no direct action on the effector cell nor does it serve to release norepinephrine from the nerve ending. Furthermore, it does not block the physiologic release of norepinephrine from the stores in the nerve ending. Since the reuptake mechanism is blocked, the norepinephrine accumulates at the junction until it throws the muscle cell of the iris dilator into spasm. If the nerve action potential in the sympathetic pathway is interrupted, as in Horner's syndrome, the transmitter substance will not accumulate and the pupil will not dilate. The duration of cocaine mydriasis is quite variable; it may last more than 24 hours. It does not show "rebound miosis."[13]

Sympatholytic drugs

Thymoxamine and dapiprazole are alpha-adrenergic blockers that will reverse phenylephrine mydriasis by taking over the alpha-receptor sites on the iris dilator muscle. The other drugs producing alpha-receptor blockage are less precise in their modes of action and are no longer used in clinical ophthalmology. These include dibenzyline (phenoxybenzamine), phentolamine (Regitine), and tolazoline (Priscoline).

Guanethidine (Ismelin) and reserpine interfere with the normal release of norepinephrine from the nerve ending and deplete the norepinephrine stores. When applied to the eye, they cause Horner's syndrome complete with ptosis, miosis, and supersensitivity to adrenergic drugs.

Other drugs that affect the pupil

Substance P affects the sphincter fibres directly; it will constrict the pupil of a thoroughly atropinized eye.

The chief pupillary action of *morphine* is to cut off cortical inhibition of the Edinger-Westphal nuclei with resultant miosis. It also may have a direct central stimulating action on the sphincter nucleus. Topical morphine, however, even in strong solutions (5%) has a minimal miotic effect on the pupil.

Nalorphine (Nalline) and levallorphan (Lorfan) are antinarcotic agents that, when given subcutaneously, reverse the miotic action of morphine.

Intravenous heroin seems to produce miosis in proportion to its euphoric effect. Dependent heroin users require larger doses than nonde-pendent users to produce the same amount of pupillary constriction. The plasma drug concentration and the pupil diameter in darkness should indicate a measure of the degree of physical dependence in a given individual.[72]

During the induction of anesthesia the patient may be in an excited state and the pupils are often dilated. As the anesthesia deepens, supranuclear inhibition of the sphincter nuclei is cut off and the pupils become small. If the anesthesia becomes dangerously deep and begins to encroach on the midbrain, the pupils become dilated and fail to react to light.

The concentration of *calcium and magnesium* ions in the blood may affect the pupil. Calcium facilitates the release of acetylcholine, and when calcium levels are abnormally low, the amount of acetylcholine liberated by each nerve impulse drops below the level needed to produce a postsynaptic potential, thus effectively blocking synaptic transmission. Magnesium has an opposite effect; thus a *high* concentration of magnesium can block transmission and may dilate the pupil.

Topical dexamethasone (Decadron) not only tends to increase the intraocular pressure but at the same time acts as a mild mydriatic. The reaction of the pupil to light does not, however, appear to be blocked. The mechanism of this mydriasis is not yet understood.

Maximal mydriasis

Full mydriasis can be obtained with eyedrops. Topical anesthetic is put in the conjunctival sac (because 10% cocaine stings) and the patient lies supine for 10 minutes so that gravity will retard lacrimal drainage. During the first minute 1 drop of 10% cocaine is given, during the third minute 1 drop of cyclopentolate 1%, and during the sixth minute 1 drop of viscous 10% phenylephrine. The peak effect occurs in 1 hour. The cocaine increases the corneal penetration of the other drugs and adds to the tightening of the dilator muscle and numbs the eye, thus diminishing the reflex tearing that might dilute the medication. The cyclopentolate takes the iris sphincter out of action in 20 to 30 minutes so that when the phenylephrine reaches the dilator muscle a few minutes later, a maximal mydriasis can occur.

Iris pigment and pupillary response to drugs

In general, the more pigment in the iris, the more slowly the drug takes effect and the longer its action lingers. This is probably due to the drug being bound to iris melanin and then slowly released. It should be noted that there are wide individual differences in pupillary responses to topical drugs. There is probably a greater range of responses among blue eyes than there is between the average response of blue eyes and the average response of dark-brown eyes. Some of these individual differences are due to corneal penetration of the drug.[4]

AFFERENT PUPILLARY DEFECTS

The pupil of an eye that is blind from retinal or optic nerve disease will fail to react directly to light but will constrict consensually when the other, healthy, eye is stimulated. The blind eye is said to show a "relative afferent pupillary defect," because the pupillomotor stimulus reaching the brain from the blind eye is diminished relative to the seeing eye.

Alternating light test

Relative afferent pupillary defects are best seen by moving a hand-held light from one eye to the other (the so-called "swinging flashlight test" of Levatin[28]). Understanding and making use of this sign is of the greatest clinical importance. The pupils are clinically more useful as indicators of optic nerve disease than they are as indicators of the integrity of iris innervation.

The patient looks into the distance while the examiner shines a bright hand-held light first into one eye and then the other. After illuminating one eye for about 1 second, the light is quickly moved across to the other eye. As the light shifts from the "good" eye to the "bad" eye, the direct light stimulus is no longer sufficient to keep the pupils small; thus they both dilate (Fig. 12-8). It is also possible to simply compare the initial constriction of each pupil as the light is switched from one eye to the other. If this end point is used, then the swing can be faster—about 1 second on each eye. This test is quick and easy to do, and it will reveal subtle differences in the photomotor input of the two eyes. For example, a definite relative afferent pupillary defect usually is seen in an eye that has recovered to 20/20 after an attack of optic neuritis.[66]

Only one visible and working iris sphincter is required to test for afferent defects. The test can be done in the presence of a third nerve palsy, corneal opacity, or posterior synechia by observing the direct and consensual responses of the intact pupil as each eye is alternately stimulated (Fig. 12-9).

If a bright hand-held light is used in a darkened room, the pupillary excursions are amplified; this makes the test more sensitive. The light should not be left longer on one eye than on the other because the increased exposure would

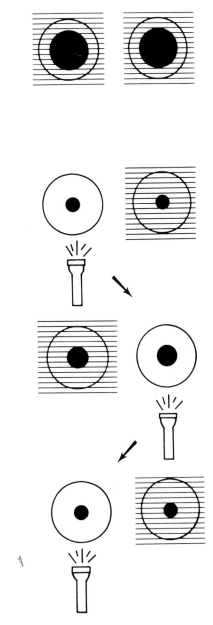

FIG. 12-8 "Alternating light test" done in dim light in a patient with a moderate relative afferent pupillary defect.

tend to bleach one retina more than the other. This tends to create a small afferent defect in the eye in which the examiner is expecting a defect.

Measuring afferent pupillary defects

It is possible simply to record the afferent defect as present or absent for each eye without having to mumble about "direct and consensual responses." The great advantages of the alternating light test are that it automatically checks the

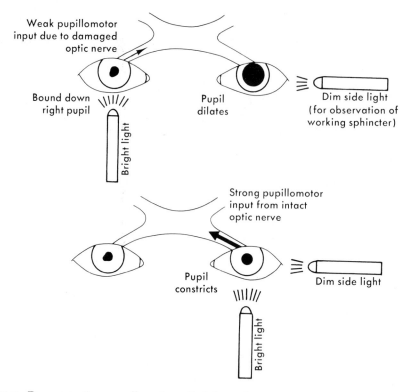

Weak pupillomotor
input due to damaged
optic nerve

Bound down
right pupil

Bright light

Pupil
dilates

Dim side light
(for observation of
working sphincter)

Strong pupillomotor
input from intact
optic nerve

Pupil
constricts

Dim side light

Bright light

FIG. 12-9 Demonstrating an afferent pupil defect when one eye has an immobile pupil. When one pupil (OD) is immobilized by posterior synechiae, it is still possible to demonstrate an afferent defect by observing the direct and consensual response of the intact pupil. The side light must be kept very dim or it will induce an afferent defect.)

consensual response and that it can be quickly and simply recorded.

An effort is sometimes made to refine the test by estimating the amount of relative input defect and making a comment on the patient's chart, for example, "obvious afferent defect" or "mini-afferent." Some careful observers have tried to judge the relative defect on a scale of 1+ to 4+, but two competent observers may score the afferent defect differently. Young pupils are bigger and move better than the pupils of the elderly. This makes small input differences seem larger in the young (Fig. 12-10).

Kestenbaum suggested in 1946 that the strength of the direct light reaction of each eye could be estimated by simply measuring the size of each pupil while the other eye was in darkness. This can be done with a pupil guage and a hand light and, provided there is nothing wrong with the innervation of any of the iris muscles in either eye, the difference in diameter of the two pupils (each measured in millimeters with the other eye in darkness) comes very close to the relative afferent pupil defect (measured in log units of neutral density filter required to balance the light reactions in the two eyes). This mea-

surement of "Kestenbaum's number" may seem a little rough, but there are situations in which a rough measure is better than none at all.[16,21]

It is possible to quantify the relative afferent pupillary defect by putting neutral density filters over the good eye until the defect disappears. The stimulus to the good eye must be dimmed by a certain number of log units before a balance point is reached at which no relative afferent defect can be seen. This number (in log units of neutral density filter) is a *measure* of the relative pupillomotor input deficit in the bad eye.

Using this technique, certain clinical rules of thumb have emerged.

Optic neuritis. More than 90% of patients with an optic neuritis (past or present) have a relative afferent pupillary defect. If a patient with a "unilateral" optic neuritis does *not* have a pupillary defect, then bilateral disease should be suspected. A fresh optic neuritis may have a relative afferent pupillary defect of almost any size—from 0.3 to 3 whole log units, depending on how much damage has been done to the optic nerve. The average relative afferent pupillary defect in fresh cases of optic neuritis is in the

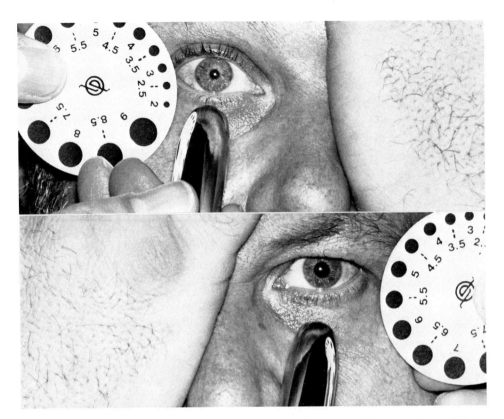

FIG. 12-10 Measurement of Kestenbaum's number. The direct pupillary response to light is measured in each eye and the two pupillary diameters are compared. (From Jiang MQ, Thompson HS, Lam BL: Kestenbaum's number as an indicator of pupillomotor input asymmetry, Am J Ophthalmol 107:528, 1989.)

1.0 to 1.5 log unit range. On the other hand, most patients with an old "recovered" optic neuritis have a relative afferent pupillary defect in the 0.3 to 0.9 log unit range.

Amblyopia. The clinician should *expect* a small relative afferent pupillary defect in an amblyopic eye. It is not always there, but a careful look will reveal a relative afferent pupillary defect in about half the cases. The pupillary defect in the amblyopic eye is generally less than 0.5 log units. If, in an amblyopic eye the relative afferent pupillary defect is between 0.5 and 1.0 log units, this should be considered suspiciously large and only reluctantly accepted as due to the amblyopia. The size of the relative afferent pupillary defect does not correlate well with the acuity of the amblyopic eye.[10,14,23,51] This apparent afferent defect may be due to the inability of some amblyopes to take up fixation under any circumstances with their amblyopic eye. The study has not yet been done that records pupillary responses while fixation is shifted from one eye to the other in a way that does not itself influence pupillary function.

Macular disease. In pure macular disease (for example, disciform) there *is* a rough correlation between the relative afferent pupillary defect and the visual acuity. This is because, in the macula, both of these functions (pupil and acuity) are related to the size of the macular lesion and to the size of the central scotoma. If the visual acuity is no worse than 20/200, a relative afferent pupillary defect bigger than 0.5 log units should not be expected. It is difficult to get a relative afferent pupillary defect larger than 1 log unit with a lesion confined to the macula. When unilateral macular disease causes a relative afferent pupillary defect of 1.2 log units, the central scotoma is generally large enough to include the blind spot.

Central serous retinopathy. The relative afferent pupillary defect is very small in central serous retinopathy, as would be expected in a macular disease producing very little field loss. Initially there may be as much as 0.3 log units of relative afferent pupillary defect, but when the subretinal fluid disappears, so usually does the pupillary defect.

Retinal detachment. One quadrant of fresh retinal detachment (with the macula on) produces approximately 0.3 log units of relative afferent pupillary defect, and two quadrants produces 0.6, etc.[9] As might be expected, when the macula comes off, the relative afferent pupillary defect jumps by about 0.7 log units.[12] Thus a recent complete retinal detachment would be expected to have a relative afferent pupillary defect of more than 2 log units.

An anisocoria in bright light that is larger than 2 mm (that is, a very large anisocoria) will tend to produce a small afferent defect because one retina is being shaded by the iris more completely than the other. I usually add 0.1 log units of relative afferent pupillary defect to the eye with the smaller pupil for every millimeter of anisocoria in bright light.

As a rule, a cataract does not cause an afferent pupillary defect; in fact, a dense unilateral cataract will usually induce a small (0.4 log units) "afferent defect" *in the other eye*.[26] If an afferent pupillary defect is present in a cataractous eye, there is usually something else going on back there, and the prognosis for sharp aphakic vision is not good.[8,59] It is however possible to have a pupillary defect from an ischemic optic neuropathy or glaucoma and still retain central acuity. It is not fully understood why "don't blame the pupil defect on the cataract" is such a good clinical rule. Surely a brunescent lens must block most of the light entering the pupil. Is it because the shaded retina is more sensitive? Is this due to a change in the orientation of the receptors, or does the cataract simply scatter the light onto more retinal elements?

Functional visual loss. Functional visual loss does *not* produce a relative afferent pupillary defect. If an eye with functional visual loss shows a relative afferent pupillary defect, then some other event is occurring in addition to the functional visual loss.

Afferent defects in tract lesions

Consider the patient with (1) an incongruous homonymous field loss, (2) nothing to suggest superimposed optic nerve or retinal disease, and (3) an afferent pupillary defect in the eye with the greater field loss. In this patient the field loss is more likely to be due to a tract lesion than to a suprageniculate lesion because, as would be expected in a tract lesion, the pupillary fibers seem to be damaged to the same extent that the visual fibers are damaged. The patient with a complete tract lesion, a total homonymous hemianopia with 20/20 vision in each eye, and a band pallor (or "bowtie atrophy") of the contralateral disc fits into this description, since a temporal field has been lost in one eye and a nasal field in the other. These patients also have a small afferent defect (0.3 to 0.6 log units) in the eye with the greater field loss.[1,48]

The other pupillary signs of tract lesions, Behr's anisocoria and Wernicke's pupillary hemiakinesia, are hard to demonstrate in the office because focal retinal stimulation requires special care.

Pupil cycle time

A small beam or slit of light focused at the pupillary margin induces regular, persistent oscillations of the pupil. These oscillations can be timed with a stopwatch. The period of the average complete cycle is called the "pupil cycle time." The pupil cycle time, as measured at the slit lamp,[47] tends to be prolonged in optic neuritis and in compressive optic neuropathy, but this may, in part, be an artifact of the testing situation.[73] In any case, the pupillary cycle time has proved to be a weak and uncertain indicator of optic nerve disease.[6,64]

PUPIL PERIMETRY

It may soon be possible to plot a map of pupillary responsiveness in the central 30 degrees of the visual field, using an automated perimeter as the source of stimuli and the pupil reactions as the patient's response.[22] This has never been easy to do,[17,56] but modern computer techniques have overcome some of the difficulties.

EFFERENT PUPILLARY DEFECTS

When the parasympathetic innervation to the iris sphincter is impaired, the pupil reacts poorly to light and may appear to be fixed in the dilated position.

"Fixed" dilated pupil

The differential diagnosis of a "fixed" dilated pupil is summarized here (Fig. 12-11):

I. Midbrain damage—vascular accidents, tumors, degenerative and infectious diseases, etc.
   A. Dorsal midbrain (the Edinger-Westphal nucleus and its light reflex input)
      1. Relatively rare
      2. Usually involves both pupils
      3. Pupillary near-vision reaction often retained
      4. Often associated with supranuclear vertical gaze palsy
   B. Ventral midbrain (fascicular portion of third nerve)
      1. Often associated with other neurologic deficits, for example, Nothnagel's, Benedikt's, or Weber's syndromes
      2. Unlikely to spare the extraocular components of the third nerve (the reverse seems to be more common)

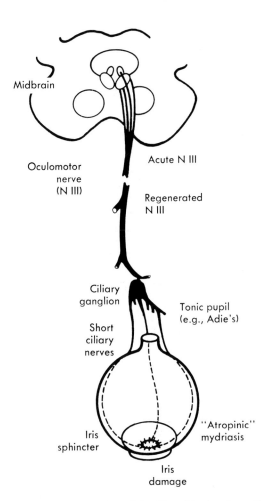

FIG. 12-11 Innervation of the iris sphincter, from the Edinger-Westphal nucleus via oculomotor nerve, ciliary ganglion, and short ciliary nerves, with some of the causes of a fixed dilated pupil.

II. Damage to the third nerve (from interpeduncular fossa to ciliary ganglion)
   A. Basal aneurysms
   B. Supratentorial space-occupying masses
      1. Cause displacement of the brainstem or transtentorial herniation of the uncus
      2. Patient is usually stuporous or comatose
   C. Basal granulomatous meningitis—often causes bilateral internal ophthalmoplegia
   D. Ischemic oculomotor palsy ("diabetic ophthalmoplegia")—usually spares the pupillary fibers
   E. Parasellar tumor (for example, pituitary adenoma, meningioma, craniopharyngioma, nasopharyngeal carcinoma, or distant metastases)
   F. Parasellar inflammation (for example, "Tolosa-Hunt" syndrome, temporal arteritis, herpes zoster)

III. Damage to the ciliary ganglion or short ciliary nerves—results in "tonic pupil"
   A. Local tonic pupil
      1. Viral ciliary ganglionitis (for example, herpes zoster)
      2. Orbital or choroidal trauma, tumor, or injury
      3. Blunt trauma to the globe; may injure branches of the short ciliary nerves at the iris root (traumatic iridoplegia)
   B. Neuropathic tonic pupil—part of the picture of peripheral neuropathy
   C. Idiopathic tonic pupil with benign areflexia (Adie's syndrome)
IV. Damage to the iris
   A. Degenerative or inflammatory diseases of the iris
   B. Posterior synechiae
   C. Acute rise of intraocular pressure (hypoxia of sphincter)
   D. Blunt injury to the globe with sphincter damage (traumatic iridoplegia)
V. Drug-induced mydriasis
   A. Anticholinergic blockage at the sphincter muscle (for example, atropine)
   B. Adrenergic stimulation of the dilator muscle (for example, phenylephrine, cocaine, hydroxyamphetamine)

Of all the possible causes of a poor light reaction in one eye in an outpatient clinic, Adie's syndrome is probably the most common. About 90% of Adie's pupils have a sector of residual light reaction when examined at the slit lamp. However, a patient who walks into an ophthalmologist's office with a dilated and absolutely unresponsive pupil of recent onset probably has been exposed to an atropinic drug; intracranial aneurysm and Adie's tonic pupil are less likely possibilities. Nurses and pharmacists who handle these drugs may get them on their hands and inadvertently rub them into the eye. Farmers and others who work outside may be exposed to plants that are rich in belladonna alkaloids, and an occasional patient will deliberately use a mydriatic drop or ointment and then deny it. There is a simple way for the ophthalmologist to recognize the pupil dilated because of pharmacologic blockade and to distinguish it from a paralytic mydriasis such as a partial third nerve palsy or Adie's tonic pupil. One drop of a weak pilocarpine solution (0.5% to 1.0%) will contract the normal pupil. It also will contract the pupil in cases of paralytic mydriasis due to preganglionic or postganglionic nerve damage. In fact, an interruption of the parasympathetic innervation of the iris tends to cause supersensitivity of the sphincter to cholinergic drugs. However, when the iris sphincter has been blocked by atropine or other anticholineric drugs, 1 drop of a weak pilocarpine solution will not constrict the pupil.

Atropinic drugs are successful competitive antagonists of pilocarpine; they use up the available cholinergic receptor sites on the sphincter muscle cell. The pilocarpine test clearly distinguishes parasympathetic denervation from pharmacologic blockade, because denervation can only increase the sensitivity of the iris to pilocarpine, whereas atropine drugs decrease pilocarpine miosis.[69]

The Edinger-Westphal nucleus is at the rostral end of the oculomotor group, and the parasympathetic fibers for the pupil and accommodation are at the upper edge of the third nerve as it emerges into the interpeduncular fossa. These smaller fibers stay at the periphery of the bundle and gradually move to a more medial position. When the third nerve enters the cavernous sinus, the pupillary fibers have worked their way around to the lower edge of the nerve, so that when the nerve separates into superior and inferior divisions, the pupillary fibers are always in the lower bundle.

Basal meningitis, especially tubercular or syphilitic, was once a common cause of bilateral internal ophthalmoplegia. This was considered to be due to the peripheral and hence vulnerable location of the parasympathetic fibers in the subarachnoid course of the oculomotor nerve. The third nerve can be stretched or compressed by an adjacent aneurysm, and this usually produces a complete oculomotor palsy but occasionally the first sign is a dilated pupil—usually soon followed by ptosis or diplopia.

In the obtunded or comatose patient, unilateral pupillary dilation is an important sign of transtentorial herniation of the uncus. This is also due to stretching and compression of the third nerve. Again, the pupillary fibers may be damaged early but are soon followed by impairment of fibers serving the extraocular muscles.

Aberrant regeneration of the third nerve

After a third nerve palsy caused by an aneurysm, the fibers start to grow again, and in 6 to 8 weeks there appears to be some recovery. The lid lifts, but the pupillary light reaction seldom recovers,[19] and there is usually a residual diplopia in various directions of gaze.

Nerves, like the oculomotor nerve and the facial nerve, which carry fibers bound for several different destinations in a single bundle, are particularly subject to aberrant regeneration. If there has been scar formation or structural damage to the nerve, the signs of aberrant regeneration are to be expected.

A patient with an ischemic oculomotor palsy (a pupil-sparing third nerve palsy) usually has recovered completely in 2 months without signs of aberrant regeneration. In fact, if any of the following signs of aberrant regeneration appear as the third nerve is recovering, the possibility of aneurysm should be reconsidered.

1. Inappropriate lid retraction on adduction or depression (pseudo-von Graefe's sign)
2. Pupil constriction on adduction, elevation, or depression, especially up and in
3. Segmental constriction of parts of the iris sphincter with eye movements—a slit-lamp sign[7]

It is common for fibers originally destined for the extraocular muscles to innervate the pupil during the recovery of a third nerve palsy. This results in a pupillary constriction when an effort is made to turn the eye in one of the directions served by the third nerve. Because the pupil fails to react to light but may constrict on convergence, this apparent light-near dissociation has been called a "pseudo-Argyll Robertson pupil," but the pupil in such a case will constrict with any adduction movement of the eye.

With the magnification provided by the slit lamp, it can be seen that this aberrant reinnervation of the iris sphincter is sometimes segmental and of a degree insufficient to produce an obvious pupillary constriction.[7]

It has long been accepted that some supersensitivity of the pupillary sphincter is produced when the denervating lesion is in the preganglionic neuron, but more supersensitivity is said to be in evidence when the lesion involves the postganglionic neuron.[53] Recently it has been suggested that lesions in both locations produce a comparable degree of supersensitivity and that methacholine therefore cannot be used to distinguish a fresh Adie's tonic pupil from a pupil dilated because of pressure on the oculomotor nerve by an intracranial aneurysm.[50] This dilemma seldom comes up in office practice because the extraocular muscles are usually involved when the third nerve is damaged.

Cyclic oculomotor spasms

Patients with a congenital oculomotor palsy will sometimes show an intermittent spasm of all the components of the third nerve. These cyclic spasms on a background of paresis ("cyclic oculomotor palsy") may well be a mixture of aberrant regeneration of the peripheral nerve and an abnormality of the oculomotor nucleus that results from damage to the immature nervous system.[37]

Iris damage

Blunt injury to the globe will cause a traumatic iridoplegia. There seem to be several factors at work: (1) the chamber angle can be recessed, tearing the branches of the short ciliary nerves that serve the iris muscles; (2) the sphincter muscle itself can be injured so that it will not constrict to pilocarpine; (3) the short ciliary nerves may be damaged as the choroid is ruptured. These injuries may produce a segmental palsy of the sphincter, a light-near dissociation, and an undersensitivity or oversensitivity of the sphincter to pilocarpine, depending on the exact nature of the damage. An attack of acute angle-closure glaucoma often produces a pupil of moderate size that fails to react to light or to pilocarpine. This is due to hypoxia of the iris muscles.

TONIC PUPIL

Damage to the ciliary ganglion or short ciliary nerves produces a very characteristic combination of signs:

1. A poor pupillary reaction to light, which, at the slit lamp, can be seen to be a regional palsy of the iris sphincter
2. Accommodative paresis
3. Cholinergic supersensitivity of the denervated muscles
4. Often a pupillary response to near vision that is unusually strong and tonic

Patients who show these signs are said to have "tonic pupils." That is, a tonic pupil is any postganglionic, parasympathetic denervation of the intraocular muscles. This can, of course, occur because of a local infection or injury (for example, chickenpox, orbital surgery), or it may be part of a widespread peripheral neuropathy (for example, diabetes, alcoholism).

ADIE'S SYNDROME

Adie's syndrome is a form of tonic pupil in which no local cause for the denervation is evident and there is no peripheral neuropathy to account for the tendon areflexia.

The typical patient with Adie's syndrome is a woman, aged 20 to 40, with one pupil reacting poorly to light. Less than 30% of the patients are men. The mean age of onset is 32 years for both men and women. When first seen, only 10% of the patients have involvement of both eyes.[60]

Light reaction in Adie's syndrome

When examined at the slit lamp, some response of the sphincter to light can be seen in 90% of the affected eyes. This residual reaction is always a segmental contraction of the iris sphincter. Most of these pupils have lost more than half of the sphincter function and continue to lose more with the passage of time. The loss of light reaction in the denervated pupils seems to occur randomly around the sphincter without any clear predilection for one quadrant.[61]

Cholinergic supersensitivity in Adie's syndrome

In 1905, Markus[2] suggested that a very weak solution of eserine could be used as a diagnostic test to localize the lesion causing a denervation of the iris sphincter; a good constriction put the lesion in the ciliary ganglion or in the short ciliary nerves. This recommendation was based on the work of Anderson, who had shown differences in the behavior of the sphincter, depending on the location of the lesion. But it was not until Cannon and Rosenblueth had sorted out all of these observations into a "law of denervation supersensitivity" that these phenomena were understood. Scheie and Adler, in 1940, clearly showed that Adie's tonic pupils were supersensitive to cholinergic substances. They chose a concentration (2.5%) of methacholine hydrochloride (Mecholyl) that would not contract a normal pupil, and they showed that most Adie's pupils constricted to this cholinergic stimulus, some quite dramatically.

It was soon recognized that some tonic pupils failed to constrict with 2.5% methacholine. At first this was blamed on an instability of the methacholine solution, and it was recommended that a fresh solution be prepared for each use. It was finally concluded that an aqueous solution of methacholine hydrochloride is reasonably stable but that there are large interindividual variations in the ability of the drug to penetrate a normal cornea. In addition, there appear to be large variations from one tonic pupil to another in the sensitivity of the denervated iris sphincter.

Methacholine has not been available as a commerical eyedrop for a number of years and has become increasingly difficult to find. This has prompted a search for substitutes, and the most readily available one is pilocarpine, which is known to be stable and is cheap and always at hand.

Pilocarpine 0.125% (⅛%) constricts most normal pupils slightly, with a degree of miosis differing among individuals from just noticeable to about 2 mm (mean = 1 mm), whereas methacholine 2.5% has no consistent miotic effect. There are some advantages to using a concentration of the cholinergic substance sufficient to bring the normal pupil down a small amount. If neither pupil constricts to methacholine 2.5%, as often happens, it could be because the drug has not penetrated the patient's cornea, in which case the absence of a cholinergic supersensitivity has not been demonstrated. However, when the normal pupil shows a drug effect and constricts slightly and the Adie's pupil does not constrict more than the normal pupil, it can be said confidently that the affected sphincter is not supersensitive.

Pilocarpine 0.1% or 0.0625% also will serve to demonstrate supersensitivity of the sphincter. These concentrations of pilocarpine are not only adequate substitutes for methacholine 2.5%; they are also more sensitive testing substances in unilateral cases simply because they have a slightly stronger miotic action.[2]

Near reaction in Adie's syndrome

The near response of the pupil generally exceeds the light reaction in Adie's syndrome. The near response is slow and steady, and on looking back into the distance it tends to hold the contraction for a few seconds (that is, it is "tonic"). The reasons for this behavior are not fully understood. The slowness of the tonic pupil might be due to the diffusion of acetylcholine through the aqueous to the supersensitive receptors of the iris sphincter, but the light-near dissociation cannot be so easily explained.

Tonicity. The tonic behavior of an Adie's pupil might result from the diffusion of acetylcholine released from remaining or regenerated nerve endings through the aqueous to the nearby supersensitive receptors of the iris sphincter.[7,36,53] This behavior might also be due to the lack of acetylcholinesterase in the collateral sprouts of regenerating nerves.

Light-near dissociation. The near reaction is not spared in Adie's syndrome; it is restored. Its strength is best explained by postulating aberrant regeneration of fibers that were originally destined for the ciliary muscle into the iris sphincter, so that with every effort to focus the eye on a near object, impulses spill into the spincter, constricting the pupil. Accommodative fibers in the short ciliary nerves outnumber sphincter fibers by 30 to 1. This means that the ciliary muscle will probably receive appropriate reinnervation, but the odds against the iris sphincter receiving the right fibers are very high. Thus with random regeneration of fibers the power of accommodation is likely to recover, whereas the light reaction will not; at the same time the sphincter is likely to be served by aberrant accommodative impulses that constrict the pupil firmly with every near effort.[36,68,76]

Tendon reflexes in Adie's syndrome

About 90% of the patients with Adie's tonic pupil have diminished or absent tendon reflexes. This is a "benign areflexia," in that it is not due to a sensory or motor deficit; there is no peripheral neuropathy. The reflex impairment is widespread, affecting the arms as well as the legs, and it is bilaterally symmetric in half the cases. In the patients with asymmetric tendon reflex loss it cannot be predicted from the distribution of the defect which eye is most likely to have the tonic pupil.[65]

Corneal sensation in Adie's syndrome

Many patients with Adie's syndrome have a mild regional impairment of corneal sensation.[52] This is thought to result from damage to the sensory afferent nerves from the cornea, which travel with the short ciliary nerves and pass through the ciliary ganglion.

Natural history of Adie's syndrome

The onset of Adie's syndrome seems to be abrupt and is marked by new symptoms of anisocoria or blurred near vision, yet patients will occasionally say that their tendon reflexes have been weak for years and that physicians always have had trouble eliciting knee jerks. The accommodative paresis soon starts to recover; reading glasses that have been prescribed are quickly discarded. The dilated pupil slowly comes down until the anisocoria is hardly noticeable. In darkness the tonic pupil does not dilate fully and is now the smaller pupil. Tonicity of accommodation sometimes develops.

There is a strong tendency for the second eye to be affected by a similar process some years later, but the onset is seldom noticed by the patient. This may be because near vision is already disturbed and presbyopia is approaching. Eventually both pupils are small and react poorly to light. The characteristic tonic near response, light-near dissociation, and cholinergic supersensitivity are still present but are much harder to demonstrate because both pupils are involved and both are miotic. Fig. 12-12 plots the fluctuating anisocoria in just such a typical case.

Many patients believe that they have recovered from their Adie's syndrome because after 2 years accommodation has improved and the pupil is no longer dilated. But the light reaction has not recovered; in fact, further segments of the sphincter are likely to be palsied. The tendon reflexes are just as bad, and the second eye may now be involved. The patients have actually lost more function through progressive loss of ganglion cells than they have regained through regeneration of nerve fibers.

Etiology of Adie's syndrome

It has been suggested that a viral ciliary ganglionitis is the cause of the denervated intraocular

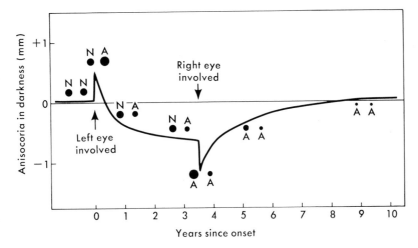

FIG. 12-12   Changing anisocoria of Adie's syndrome. First one pupil is involved and then the other. Both pupils gradually become smaller and smaller until it is hard to recognize them as Adie's tonic pupils. N, Normal; A, Adie's. (From Thompson HS, ed: Topics in neuro-ophthalmology, © [1979] The Williams & Wilkins Co., Baltimore.)

muscles. A search was made for viral antibodies in the serum of patients with Adie's syndrome, but nothing much was found.[45] In results from an autopsied patient, Harriman[18] discovered that the ciliary ganglion on the affected side seemed to be suffering from an indolent degenerative process such as might occur with a "slow virus" infection. A similar process may be going on in the dorsal columns of the spinal cord to account for the impaired deep tendon reflexes.[54] There has not been a systematic search for evidence of an auto-immune process affecting the ciliary ganglia and dorsal root ganglia.

PUPILLARY LIGHT-NEAR DISSOCIATION

Wilson,[32] in 1921, wrote an important paper entitled "The Argyll Robertson Pupil." It was about pupils that react better to near than to light—pupils that we would now say showed a "light-near dissociation." Today Argyll Robertson pupils are thought of as pupils with a light-near dissociation due to syphilis. Any time the pupillary light reaction seems impaired a light-near dissociation should be looked for.

How to test for a pupillary near response

The near response should be tested in good room light so that the patient's pupils are mid-sized and the near object is clearly visible. The patient is given an accommodative target to look at, something of interest or with fine detail on it. Sometimes a better response is obtained if some other sensory input is added to the stimulus: for example, *auditory*—a ticking watch or clicking fingernails—or *proprioceptive*—the patient's own thumbnail can be held up in front of him or her, perhaps with something drawn on it.

Watching for convergence helps the physician judge how hard the patient is trying. Remember that the near response, although it may be triggered by blurred or disparate imagery, has a large volitional component and the patient may need encouragement. If, for some reason, the patient has not been making a near effort recently—for example, because stereopsis is not achieved at near—then the patient may need a few practice runs. Often the third or fourth try will be a good one. When a near response is not obtained, it is usually because the patient (or the physician) has not been trying hard enough.

A patient who is completely blind and has no pupillary reaction to light will still sometimes do a good near response if asked to deliberately cross the eyes or pretend there is a fly on the nose. If the patient cannot achieve a near response, the "lid closure reflex"[62] may work: the patient looks at the physician and squeezes the eyes shut while the physician tries with both hands to hold one of the patient's eyes open. This often will produce a surprisingly strong near response.

Recognizing a light-near dissociation

Sometimes, in a doubtful case, it is hard to know where to draw the line. When is the near response clearly greater than the light reaction? When the physician faces the patient, with pocket light in hand, there are usually three levels of light available: darkness, with a side light on the pupils, room light, and room light plus a

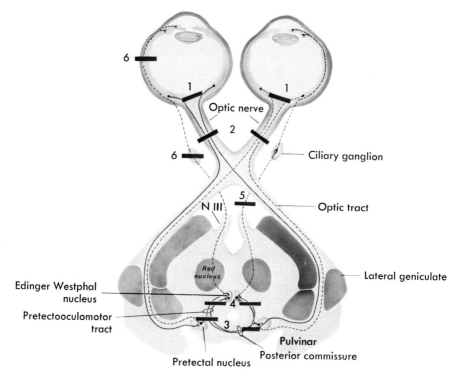

FIG. 12-13   Possible sites of isolated damage to pupillary light reflex pathway, which may result in light-near dissociation. *1* and *2,* Lesion in retina or optic nerve (e.g., optic neuritis). *3,* Lesion in midbrain (e.g., pinealoma). *4,* Lesion in intercalated neuron (e.g., Argyll Robertson's pupils). *5,* Lesion in third nerve (e.g., aneurysm). *6,* Lesion in ciliary ganglion or short ciliary nerves (e.g., tonic pupil). The "near" input to the Edinger-Westphal nuclei is thought to approach from the ventral side because it is spared in Parinaud's syndrome.

bright light in the eyes. With the patient looking in the distance, shine the bright light in the eye three or four times, each time for only 1 or 2 seconds. This tells how small the pupils will go with just a light stimulus. Never judge the near response by adding a near stimulus to a bright light stimulus; this almost always produces an apparent light-near dissociation because the *near* stimulus always adds something to the *light* stimulus. A real light-near dissociation is present only if the near response (tested in moderate light) exceeds the best constriction that bright light can produce.

Causes of light-near dissociation

It is very difficult to discuss the differential diagnosis of a light-near dissociation unless some assumptions are made: (1) in a light-near dissociation it is always the near response that is stronger than the light response because most weak near responses are simply due to a weak near effort; (2) all light-near dissociations are due to some failure of the light reaction, which

somehow "spares" the near reaction; therefore (3) there are no light-near dissociations due *only* to a hyperactive near response.

These assumptions allow us to simply trace the light reflex pathway and consider the ways in which the light reaction might be damaged and the near reaction spared (Fig. 12-13, *1-6*).

Lesions of the afferent pathway

Lesions of the afferent pathway (see Fig. 12-13, *1-4*) produce a light-near dissociation by sparing the near reaction.

1, The lesion is in the retina. If both eyes are blind—for example, from diabetic retinopathy or old retinal detachment—there will be no light perception and no pupillary response to light, but if the iris and the sphincter innervation remain intact, there may be a good near response.

2, The lesion is in the anterior visual path (optic nerves, tracts, or chiasm). Once again, if both eyes are blind from optic nerve disease (for example, temporal arteritis), there will be no light reaction, but the near response should be preserved—if the patient can remember how to cross his or her eyes.

3, The lesion is in the midbrain. The light reflex path can be interrupted here in the pretectal area without damaging the more ventrally located input for the near reflex. Tumors are the most common cause for this kind of light-near dissociation. Pinealomas classically cause Parinaud's syndrome, which includes poor light reaction and light-near dissociation; this is also called the sylvian aqueduct syndrome. Vascular disease in this area can cause a light-near dissociation, for example, occlusion of a posterior choroidal artery. Encephalitis and demyelinization are rare causes of light-near dissociation.

4, Argyll Robertson's pupils deserve a category of their own, although the defect is most likely a variation of the midbrain defects presented in this list.

Lesions of the efferent pathway

Lesions of the efferent pathway (see Fig. 12-13, 5-6) produce a light-near dissociation by *restoring* the near reaction with new, aberrantly regenerating, fibers.

5, The lesion is in the third nerve. How is it possible to damage the light reflex and spare the pupillary near reaction with a lesion in the outflow pathway when the fibers serving the two functions are identical? It is not possible. The near reaction is not actually spared; it appears to be restored in some cases because of aberrant regeneration of medial rectus innervation into the spincter innervation pathway. This has been called the "pseudo-Argyll Robertson pupil associated with abberrant regeneration of the third nerve.[74] It is a false light-near dissociation; the pupil (which fails to react to light because of the third nerve damage) constricts not only on convergence but also any time the medial rectus is innervated, for example, with horizontal gaze (p. 428).

6, The lesion is in the ciliary ganglion or short ciliary nerves. Why do Adie's tonic pupils almost always show a light-near dissociation, when the "light" and "near" innervation of the iris sphincter follow an identical final common pathway? This is another example of aberrant regeneration in a mixed nerve. This time it is the accommodative impulses that find their way into the innervation of the iris sphincter; thus every time an effort is made to focus the lens, ciliary muscle innervation spills over into the sphincter and constricts the pupil (p. 429).

A pupillary light-near dissociation has been observed with various peripheral neuropathies (amyloidosis, diabetes, alcoholism, Charcot-

Marie-Tooth disease, Déjérine-Sottas disease). This light-near dissociation probably is produced by a similar mechanism—the regrowth of damaged fibers.

Argyll Robertson pupils

In 1869, Douglas Argyll Robertson published two papers in which he described some patients with tabes dorsalis who showed the following characteristics:

1. The retina was sensitive to light.
2. The pupil did not respond on exposure to light.
3. There was pupillary contraction during act of accommodation for near objects.
4. The pupils contracted further with extracts of the Calabar bean (physostigmine), but they dilated poorly with atropine.
5. The pupils were very small.

This curious finding of pupils that failed to respond to light despite good vision, yet contracted well on accommodation to near stimuli, attracted immediate attention and soon became the most famous of all pupillary phenomena. One reason for the great interest in the Argyll Robertson syndrome was the fact that it was found in a high percentage of patients suffering from tabes dorsalis, general paresis, and "lues cerebri" and in very few other diseases. About 30 years after Argyll Robertson's publications, when Wassermann helped establish that these three conditions were actually only different manifestations of central nervous system syphilis, the Argyll Robertson pupil became widely accepted as being virtually pathognomonic of neurosyphilis.

After all these years, the pathogenesis of this kind of light-near dissociation is still not clearly understood. The reader is referred to Loewenfeld's monograph for an authoritative discussion of this question. She concludes that the classic Argyll Robertson pupil is the result of neuronal damage in the rostral midbrain near the sylvian aqueduct, interfering with the light reflex fibers and the supranuclear inhibitory fibers as they approach the Edinger-Westphal nucleus.[32]

Argyll Robertson pupils today

There is no doubt that neurosyphilis still produces pupillary abnormalities, including in many cases small, poorly reactive pupils with a light-near dissociation (Argyll Robertson's pupils). But there has always been a large group of patients with peripheral neuropathies of all kinds that tend to denervate both iris sphincters as part of the generalized neuropathy. Denervated sphincters eventually become miotic. Even Adie's tonic pupils tend to become bilateral and miotic with time.

Flagrant neurosyphilis (tabes dorsalis and general paresis) has become uncommon, and therefore a smaller percentage of miotic, light-palsied pupils can be proved to be related to syphilis. In making the diagnosis of syphilis, more weight is now put on the serologic, rather than the clinical, signs. A quick look at the pupils used to give the right answer 90% of the time. Nowadays, if we say "syphilis" when we see "Argyll Robertson pupils," we are often wrong; the patient is just as likely to have a diabetic or an alcoholic neuropathy. Since Argyll Robertson's pupils are not quite as firm a diagnostic sign as they used to be, we are not as careful to look for them as we used to be. If we do not look for something, we seldom see it.

I suspect that the same percentage of patients with neurosyphilis have Argyll Robertson's pupils as ever did, but far fewer patients with Argyll Robertson's pupils have neurosyphilis.

Argyll Robertson's pupils have not vanished—we just do not bother to look for them anymore. This is too bad, because Argyll Robertson's pupils are still strongly suggestive of neurosyphilis. Any patient with both pupils abnormal (small, large, irregular, or reacting poorly to light) should at least have a serum fluorescent treponemal antibody test.

HORNER'S SYNDROME

Horner's syndrome is due to ipsilateral interruption of the sympathetic outflow to the head and neck. Bilateral Horner's syndrome is very hard to diagnose because most of the signs are recognized only by comparison with the normal eye on the other side.

Horner's syndrome can result from lesions in the brainstem or spinal cord, damage at the apex of the lung or in the supraclavicular space, or interruption of the fibers in the carotid plexus along the internal carotid artery all the way up to the cavernous sinus. Any defect in this long pathway produces the same kind of clinical picture; thus the combination of miosis and ptosis is by itself of little localizing value. However, the lesion causing Horner's syndrome often affects neighboring structures, producing signs and symptoms suggesting the site of the problem.

J. F. Horner (1834 to 1886) was a Swiss ophthalmologist. In 1869 he described a patient who showed a ptosis, miosis, and facial anhidrosis and reminded his readers that this combination of signs pointed to damage to the ipsilateral cervical sympathetic pathway. The features of sympathetic denervation and irritation had been thoroughly described many times during the preceding 140 years by Pourfour du Petit, 1727; Claude Bernard, 1852; Brown-Sequard, 1854; John W. Ogle, 1858; S. Weir Mitchell, 1864; and many others. However, it was Horner's name that stuck. Modern usage seems to allow Horner's eponym for any oculosympathetic paresis, wherever the lesion, even though Horner's case was presumably a neck lesion. Thus we speak of "central Horner's syndrome" when the lesion is in the cord or brainstem and "postganglionic Horner's syndrome" when the lesion is in the head, even though the anhidrosis of Horner's clinical triad is missing. The term "Horner's syndrome" will be used in this way throughout this section. I admit that this is both careless and historically unjust.

Clinical signs of Horner's syndrome

Ptosis. There is a moderate droop of the upper lid because of the paralysis of Müller's muscle. When the patient's eyes are wide open, this ptosis almost disappears.

There are also sympathetically innervated retractor fibers in the lower lid. In Horner's syndrome the lower lid rises slightly ("upside-down ptosis"), contributing to narrowing the palpebral fissure and the apparent enophthalmos.

Miosis. There is a moderate decrease in pupil size because of paralysis of the dilator muscle. In bright light both pupils are nearly equal. The anisocoria is much more evident in dim light because the sphincter relaxes in both eyes, leaving a tight dilator muscle in the normal eye and a flaccid one in the affected eye. Self-developing flash photographs taken in darkness and in bright light help to quickly confirm this observation (Fig. 12-14).

Facial anhidrosis. Impairment of sweating on the ipsilateral face and neck is characteristic of preganglionic Horner's syndrome, but in an air-conditioned office this may not be a helpful sign. The sudomotor fibers to the face follow the branches of the *external* carotid artery; thus a Horner's syndrome caused by damage to the postganglionic fibers along the *internal* carotid plexus is not associated with any anhidrosis of the face, except in a small patch on the forehead where sudomotor fibers may reach the face via the supraorbital artery or nerve.

Ocular hypotony and conjunctival hyperemia. Ocular hypotony and conjunctival hyperemia are transient signs in acute Horner's syndrome and cannot be depended on to be present after the first few weeks.

Dilation lag. When the lights are turned out,

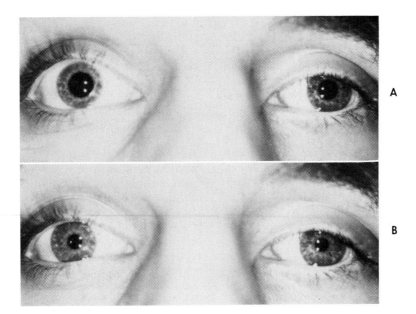

FIG. 12-14   Horner's syndrome in darkness and in light. **A**, Taken in darkness shows more anisocoria than **B**, which was taken in bright light.

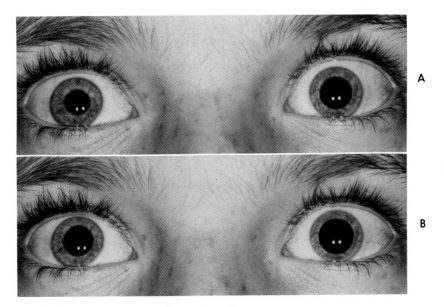

FIG. 12-15   "Dilation lag" in Horner's syndrome. **A**, Taken in darkness 5 seconds after the lights went out. **B**, Taken after 15 seconds of darkness. The Horner's pupil (the patient's right eye) is slow to dilate because it lacks dilator tone.

the Horner's pupil dilates more slowly than the normal pupil does because it lacks the pull of the dilator muscle. This characteristic behavior of the sympathetically denervated iris is best seen with an infrared-sensitive video camera but in a young person it also can be seen clinically. In addition, it can be documented with self-developing flash photographs taken 5 seconds after

the lights go out and again after 15 seconds of darkness.[49] In Horner's syndrome there will be more anisocoria in the 5-second photograph than in the 15-second photograph (Fig. 12-15). This is a useful and highly specific sign for Horner's syndrome, and the diagnosis often can be made with certainty at this point without proceeding to the cocaine test.

Cocaine test

Cocaine will dilate the pupil only when the sympathetic pathway is intact and norepinephrine is being released from the nerve endings in the dilator muscle. One drop of a 5% or 10% solution is placed in each eye and repeated a minute or two later. The anisocoria of Horner's syndrome will increase after cocaine instillation because the Horner's pupil dilates less than the normal pupil. This can be estimated in room light with a pupil gauge, or measured from a Polaroid photograph. All Horner's pupils, no matter where the defect in the pathway is located, will dilate poorly in response to cocaine. This means that cocaine helps to confirm the diagnosis and establishes that the miosis is caused by a sympathetic innervation deficit, but it does not help much in localizing the lesion. If the post-cocaine anisocoria is 0.8 mm or more, it is almost certainly a Horner's syndrome.[22,46-47]

Localizing the lesion

When it has been determined that the patient does have Horner's syndrome, the next step is to find out where the lesion is in the sympathetic pathway. The pathway is long and complex, but it is usually thought of as falling into three divisions, each separated by a synapse (Fig. 12-16).

The *central neuron* is in the brainstem and cervical cord (from hypothalamus to the ciliospinal center of Budge at C8 to T2). The *preganglionic neuron* is in the chest and in the neck (from cervical cord via stellate ganglion at the pulmonary apex to the superior cervical ganglion at the carotid bifurcation). The *postganglionic neuron* penetrates the base of the skull and passes through the cavernous sinus to enter the orbit (from the superior cervical ganglion at the angle of the jaw, via the carotid plexus, the cavernous sinus, and the long ciliary nerves to the iris).

It is necessary and important to understand this neuroanatomy; without it the differential diagnosis of Horner's syndrome is meaningless.

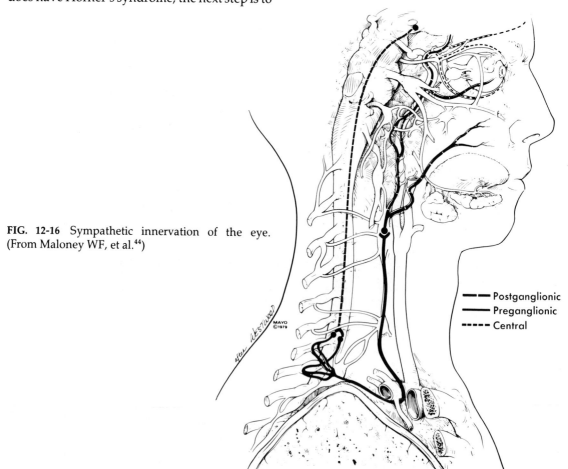

FIG. 12-16 Sympathetic innervation of the eye. (From Maloney WF, et al.[44])

— — Postganglionic
—— Preganglionic
----- Central

It is into these three categories (central, preganglionic, and postganglionic) that Horner's syndrome can be divided by making use of associated signs and symptoms and the hydroxyamphetamine test.

Associated signs and symptoms

A patient with a *central* neuron lesion often has had the sudden onset of vertigo and sensory deficits caused by a medullary infarction, or the signs may point to cervical cord disease. The sweating deficit extends over more of the body than just the head and neck.

The patients with an isolated *preganglionic* Horner's syndrome may have a lung or breast malignancy that has spread to the thoracic outlet. There may be a history of surgery or injury to the neck, chest, or cervical spine. The anhidrosis involves the face and neck.

The patient with a *postganglionic* lesion most commonly has an ipsilateral vascular headache syndrome. There may have been a skull fracture or intraoral or retroparotid trauma; anything that gets the carotid artery into trouble may damage the carotid plexus. Occasionally a tumor of the middle cranial fossa or the cavernous sinus will involve some parasellar cranial nerves and affect the sympathetic fibers to the eye. Isolated Horner's syndrome due to orbital lesions is rare.

Although the history and physical examination can tell much about the location of the lesion in Horner's syndrome, sometimes despite our best efforts there are no clues to help us decide whether the lesion causing the Horner's syndrome is in the chest or in the head. It is at this point that the hydroxyamphetamine test can be extremely helpful.

Hydroxyamphetamine test

Hydroxyamphetamine hydrobromide 1% (Paredrine) eye drops have been commercially available since 1938. The solution has full FDA approval as a mydriatic. It is an indirectly acting adrenergic mydriatic that acts by releasing norepinephrine from the nerve endings in the dilator muscle. If there are no nerve endings because there are no postganglionic nerves, the drug will have no effect. This is the best drug test for identifying a postganglionic lesion.* Tyramine hydrochloride 2% has the same mode of

---

*Paredrine has been off the market for 2 years, but Allergan Pharmaceuticals has now decided to make Paredrine available. For more information, contact Janet K. Cheetham, Pharm D, Allergan Pharmaceuticals, 2525 Dupont Drive, Irvine, CA 92713-9534 (714-752-4463).

action and can be used if Paredrine is not available, and in Germany "Pholedrin" is available. There is no drug test that will clearly separate central from preganglionic lesions.[58]

Drug tests making use of the principle of denervation supersensitivity (epinephrine 1:1000, phenylephrine 1%) also are helpful in identifying postganglionic lesions, but the drugs must be placed on strictly untouched corneas so that approximately the same dose reaches each iris. If this precaution is not taken, the tests are useless. The hydroxyamphetamine test does not suffer from these limitations, since hydroxyamphetamine mydriasis is limited by the amount of norepinephrine available in the nerve endings for release rather than by the amount of the drug that penetrates the cornea (see Table 12-1).

As can be seen in Tables 12-2 and 12-3, the diagnosis of Horner's syndrome is divided into two stages: (1) the recognition of the sympathetic deficit and (2) the localization of the lesion. The second step is of vital importance in the management of the patient with Horner's syndrome. In the patient with an isolated preganglionic lesion there may be an occult malignancy[44]; in Pancoast's syndrome there is an associated pain in the arm. If the lesion is postganglionic, it most likely is due to a benign vascular headache syndrome affecting the internal carotid artery.

Raeder's syndrome

The term "Raeder's syndrome" has been applied to many types of painful postganglionic Horner's syndrome, thus blurring its meaning and weakening its clinical usefulness. Most of Raeder's own cases had a parasellar syndrome of multiple cranial nerve palsies. Unfortunately, Raeder's name has been attached to the benign syndrome of cluster headaches with Horner's syndrome. Cluster headaches are easily recognizable by history and are not associated with cranial nerve palsies. "Raeder's paratrigeminal syndrome" is a term that should probably be limited to the occasional middle fossa mass that produces trigeminal nerve involvement with pain and a postganglionic Horner's syndrome.[15]

Congenital Horner's syndrome

When the sympathetic ocular innervation is interrupted early in life, the pigment of the iris stroma fails to develop. This produces an iris heterochromia. It is unusual nowadays to see a Klumpke's palsy associated with congenital Horner's syndrome, but birth trauma is still a significant cause (stretching of the pathway, forceps injury, skull fracture). Many of these chil-

TABLE 12-1 Adrenergic Mydriasis in Horner's Syndrome: Sympathetic Defect

Drug	Normal	Central lesion	Preganglionic lesion	Postganglionic lesion
Cocaine 5% to 10% (2 drops)	Mydriasis	Impaired dilation	No dilation*	No dilation*
Hydroxyamphetamine HBr 1% (2 drops) (or tyramine HCl 5%)	Mydriasis	Normal dilation; pupils became equal	At least normal dilation; Horner's pupil often becomes the larger one	No dilation*
Supersensitivity tests		Least dilation	Some dilation	Most dilation
Epinephrine 1:1000 (several drops)	No dilation	No dilation	Moderate dilation	Dramatic dilation
Phenylephrine 1% (2 drops)	Slight dilation	Slight dilation	Slight to moderate dilation	Moderate to dramatic dilation

From Thompson HS: Bristol Med Chir J **90**:37, 1976.
*Partial dilation suggests a partial defect.

TABLE 12-2 The Diagnosis of Acquired Horner's Syndrome: Is It a Horner's Syndrome?

History and physical examination	Pupillary drug test
Ptosis Miosis More anisocoria in darkness Facial anhidrosis Upside-down ptosis Pupillary dilation lag Hyperemia of conjunctiva Apparent enophthalmos	Cocaine 5%: all Horner's pupils dilate poorly to cocaine (compared to the full dilation of the normal pupil)

From Grimson BS, Thompson HS: Horner's syndrome, overall view of 120 cases, in Thompson HS, ed: Topics in neuro-ophthalmology, © (1979), The Williams & Wilkins Co., Baltimore.

TABLE 12-3 The Diagnosis of Acquired Horner's Syndrome: What Kind of Horner's Syndrome Is It?

History	Physical examination	Pupillary drug tests
Central Sensory deficits Vertigo	Brainstem signs Cervical cord signs Syringomyelia	Hydroxyamphetamine in both eyes; both pupils dilate Phenylephrine in both eyes; both pupils dilate
Preganglionic Lung or breast tumor Thoracotomy Neck injury or surgery Brachial plexus injury	Facial anhidrosis Brachial plexus palsy Pancoast's syndrome	Hydroxyamphetamine in both eyes; both pupils dilate Phenylephrine in both eyes; both pupils dilate
Postganglionic Ipsilateral vascular headache Head trauma Intraoral or retroparotid trauma	Normal facial sweating Parasellar cranial nerve involvement Signs of internal carotid artery (contralateral hemiplegia, etc.)	Hydroxyamphetamine 1%—little or no dilation of Horner's pupil; full dilation of normal pupil Phenylephrine 1%—Horner's pupil dilates more than the normal pupil does (denervation supersensitivity)

From Grimson BS, Thompson HS: Horner's syndrome, overall view of 120 cases, in Thompson HS, ed: Topics in neuro-ophthalmology, © (1979), The Williams & Wilkins Co., Baltimore.

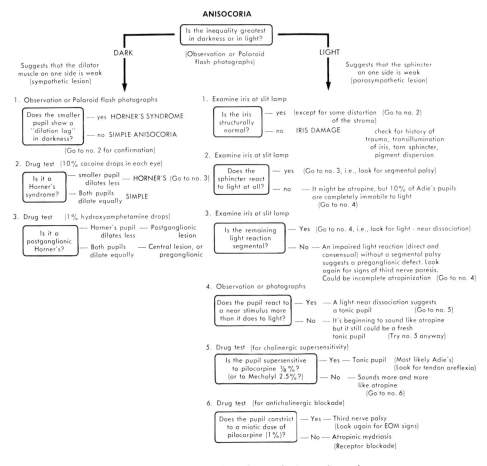

FIG. 12-17 Flow chart for analyzing anisocoria.

dren have sweating and vasomotor abnormalites of the entire side of the face (suggesting a preganglionic lesion), yet the pupil fails to dilate to hydroxyamphetamine (suggesting a loss of postganglionic fibers). This paradox is probably due to a transynaptic dysgenesis of the postganglionic neuron following a preganglionic injury.[75] This same process of transynaptic dysgenesis is thought to account for the heterochromia iridis of congenital Horner's syndrome.[75]

Sympathetic irritation

When the sympathetic outflow suddenly fires, the pupil dilates, the lid lifts, and the conjunctiva blanches. This has been called the Pourfour du Petit syndrome.[3] It may occur intermittently against a background of ipsilateral Horner's syndrome in cervical cord disease.[24] This can give the appearance of an alternating Horner's syndrome on the other side.

Intermittent spasm of a dilator segment may occur with or without Horner's syndrome, re-sulting in a distorted, tadpole-shaped pupil.[70] Intermittent Horner's syndrome in an otherwise normal eye occurs during cluster headaches.

ANISOCORIA

When you see a patient with unequal pupils you naturally suspect a denervation of one of the iris muscles. If both pupils react reasonably well to light, you have gone a long way toward ruling out a sphincter denervation and your attention turns to the smaller pupil. However, sometimes it is hard to be sure whether one sphincter is slightly weaker than the other. At this point a camera that takes self-developing flash photographs is very useful: take one photograph after 5 seconds of darkness and one in bright light; since the weaker sphincter falls behind, there is more anisocoria in bright light than in darkness. This test is good only for fresh denervations. The most common exception is an Adie's tonic pupil that has grown small with age, dilates poorly in darkness, and still constricts poorly in light.

Having decided that sphincter function is not impaired, the next problem is to distinguish between simple anisocoria (p. 414) and Horner's syndrome (p. 434). The patient with unequal pupils brings to the physician a problem in differential diagnosis. There are so many factors that might produce an anisocoria that it is sometimes hard to think of them in a logical order. Fig. 12-17 summarizes the steps that are helpful in analyzing an anisocoria.

REFERENCES

1. Behr C: Die Lehre von den Pupillenbewegungen, Berlin, Springer Verlag, 1924, p 65.
2. Bourgon P, Pilley SFJ, Thompson HS: Cholinergic supersensitivity of the iris sphincter in Adie's tonic pupil, Am J Ophthalmol 85:373, 1978.
3. Byrne P, Clough CA: A case of Pourfour de Petit syndrome following parotidectomy, J Neurol Neurosurg and Psych 53:1014, 1990.
4. Carlson D, Tychsen L: Touching the cornea enhances pharmacologic dilation of the pupil, mainly in the dark iris, Aviat Space Environ Med 60:994, 1989.
5. Cox TA, Drewes CP: Contraction anisocoria resulting from half field illumination, Am J Ophthalmol 97:577, 1984.
6. Cox TA, et al: Visual evoked potential and pupillary signs: a comparison in optic nerve disease, Arch Ophthalmol 100:1603, 1982.
7. Czarnecki JSC, Thompson HS: The iris sphincter in aberrant regeneration of the third nerve, Arch Ophthalmol 96:1606, 1978.
8. DeLacey PH, ed and trans: On the doctrines of Hippocrates and Plato by Galen, 2nd ed, Berlin, Akadem Verlag, 1981.
9. Fineberg E, Thompson HS: Quantitation of the afferent pupillary defect, in Smith JL, ed: Neuroophthalmology update, New York, Masson, 1980, pp 25–29.
10. Firth AY: Pupillary responses in amblyopia, Br J Ophthalmol 74:676, 1990.
11. Folk JC, et al: Visual function abnormalities in central serous retinopathy, Arch Ophthalmol 102:1299, 1984.
12. Folk JC, Thompson HS, Farmer SG, et al: Relative afferent pupillary defect in eyes with retinal detachment, Ophthal Surg 18:757, 1987.
13. Gillum WN: Sympathetic stimulators and blockers, Ophthalmic Semin 2:283, 1977.
14. Greenwald MJ, Folk ER: Afferent pupillary defects in amblyopia, J Pediatr Ophthalmol Strabismus 20:63, 1983.
15. Grimson BS, Thompson HS: Raeder's syndrome, a clinical review, Surv Ophthalmol 24:199, 1980.
16. Gruber H, Lessel MR: Modifikation des Swinging Flashlight Tests, Klin Mbl f Augenheilk 181:402, 1982.
17. Hamann KU, Hellner KA, Müller-Jensen A, et al: Videopupillographic and VER investigations in patients with acquired lesions of the optic radiations, Ophthalmologica 178:348, 1979.
18. Harriman DGF: Pathological aspects of Adie's syndrome, Adv Ophthalmol 23:55, 1970.
19. Hepler RS, Cantu RC: Internal carotid aneurysms and third nerve palsies: ocular status of survivors, Surg Forum 17:436, 1966.
20. Isenberg SJ, Molarte A, Vasquez M: The fixed and dilated pupils of premature neonates, Am J Ophthalmol 110:168, 1990.
21. Jiang MQ, Thompson HS, Lam BL: Kestenbaum's number as an indicator of pupillomotor input asymmetry, Am J Ophthalmol 107:528, 1989.
22. Kardon RH, Denison CE, Brown CK, et al: Critical evaluation of the cocaine test in Horner's syndrome, Arch Ophthalmol 108:384, 1990.
23. Kase M, et al: Pupillary light reflex in amblyopia, Invest Ophthalmol Vis Sci 25:467, 1984.
24. Kline LB, McCluer SM, Bonikowski FP: Oculosympathetic spasm with cervical spinal cord injury, Arch Neurol 41:61, 1984.
25. Kronfeld PC: Eserine and pilocarpine: our 100 year old allies, Surv Ophthalmol 14:479, 1970.
26. Lam BL, Thompson HS: A unilateral cataract produces a relative afferent defect in the contralateral eye, Ophthalmol 97:334, 1989.
27. Lam BL, Thompson HS, Corbett JJ: The prevalence of simple anisocoria, Am J Ophthalmol 104:69, 1987.
28. Levatin P: Pupillary escape in disease of the retina or optic nerve, Arch Ophthalmol 62:768, 1959.
29. Lind N, et al: Adrenergic neurone and receptor activity in the iris of the neonate, Pediatrics 47:105, 1971.
30. Loewenfeld IE: Mechanisms of reflex dilatation of the pupil: historical review and experimental analysis, Doc Ophthalmol 12:185, 1958.
31. Loewenfeld IE: Pupillary movements associated with light and near vision: an experimental review of the literature, in Whitcomb M, ed: Recent developments in vision research, Publ. no. 1272, Washington, DC, 1966, National Research Council, National Academy of Sciences, pp 17–105.
32. Loewenfeld IE: The Argyll Robertson pupil, 1869–1969: a critical survey of the literature, in Schwartz B, ed: Syphilis and the eye, Baltimore, Williams & Wilkins, 1970 (reprinted from Surv Ophthalmol 14:199, 1969).
33. Loewenfeld IE: "Simple, central" anisocoria: a common condition, seldom recognized, Trans Am Acad Ophthalmol Otolaryngol 83:832, 1977.
34. Loewenfeld IE: Pupillary changes related to age, in Thompson HS, ed: Topics in neuroophthalmology, Baltimore, Williams & Wilkins, 1979.
35. Loewenfeld IE, Friedlaender RP, McKinnon PF: Pupillary inequality associated with lateral gaze (Tournay's phenomenon), Am J Ophthalmol 78:449, 1974.
36. Loewenfeld IE, Thompson HS: The tonic pupil: a reevaluation, Am J Ophthalmol 63:46, 1967.
37. Loewenfeld IE, Thompson HS: Oculomotor paresis with cyclic spasms: a critical review of the literature and a new case, Surv Ophthalmol 20:81, 1975.
38. Löwenstein O: Alternating contraction anisocoria, Arch Neurol Psychiatry 72:742, 1954.
39. Löwenstein O, Feinberg R, Loewenfeld IE: Pupillary movements during acute and chronic fatigue: a new test for the objective evaluation of tiredness, Invest Ophthalmol 2:138, 1963.
40. Löwenstein O, Kawabata H, Loewenfeld IE: The pupil as an indicator of retinal activity, Am J Ophthalmol 57:569, 1964.

41. Löwenstein O, Levine AS: Pupillographic studies, V, Periodic sympathetic spasm and relaxation and role of sympathetic nervous system in pupillary innervation, Arch Ophthalmol 31:74, 1944.

42. Löwenstein O, Loewenfeld IE: The pupil, Chap 9 in Davson H, ed: The eye, New York, Academic Press, 1962, p 246.

43. Löwenstein O, Loewenfeld IE: The pupil, in Davson H, ed: The eye, 2nd ed, vol 3, Muscular mechanisms, New York, Academic Press, 1969.

44. Maloney WF, et al: Evaluation of the causes and accuracy of pharmacologic localization in Horner's syndrome, Am J Ophthalmol 90:394, 1980.

45. Meek ES, Thompson HS: Serum antibodies in Adie's syndrome, in Thompson HS, ed: Topics in neuro-ophthalmology, Baltimore, Williams & Wilkins, 1979, p 119.

46. Miller SD, Thompson HS: Edge-light pupil cycle time, Br J Ophthalmol 62:495, 1978.

47. Moster ML: Cocaine test and Horner's syndrome (letter), Arch Ophthalmol 108:1667, 1990.

48. Newman SA, Miller NR: The optic tract syndrome: neuro-ophthalmologic considerations, Arch Ophthalmol 101:1241, 1983.

49. Pilley SJF, Thompson HS: Pupillary dilatation lag in Horner's syndrome, Br J Ophthalmol 50:731, 1975.

50. Ponsford JR, Bannister R, Paul EA: Methacholine pupillary responses in third nerve palsy and Adie's syndrome, Brain 105:583, 1982.

51. Portnoy JZ, et al: Pupillary defects in amblyopia, Am J Ophthalmol 96:609, 1983.

52. Purcell JJ, Krachmer JH, Thompson HS: Corneal sensation in Adie's syndrome, Am J Ophthalmol 84:496, 1977.

53. Scheie HG: Site of disturbance in Adie's syndrome, Arch Ophthalmol 24:225, 1940.

54. Selhorst JB, Madge G, Ghatak N: The neuropathology of the Holmes-Adie syndrome, Ann Neurol 16:138, 1984.

55. Sharpe JA, Glaser JS: Tournay's phenomenon, a reappraisal of anisocoria in lateral gaze, Am J Ophthalmol 77:250, 1974.

56. Sugita K, Sugita Y, Mutsuga N, et al: Pupillary reflex perimetry for children and unconscious patients, J Clin Ophthalmol (Japan): 24:517, 1970.

57. Thompson HS: Cornpicker's pupil: jimson weed mydriasis, J Iowa Med Soc 71:475, 1971.

58. Thompson HS: Diagnostic pupillary drug tests, in Blodi FC, ed: Current concepts in ophthalmology, vol 3, St Louis, CV Mosby, 1972, Ch 6.

59. Thompson HS: Pupillary signs in the diagnosis of optic nerve disease, Trans Ophthalmol Soc UK 96:377, 1976.

60. Thompson HS: Adie's syndrome: some new observations, Trans Am Ophthalmol Soc 75:587, 1977.

61. Thompson HS: Segmental palsy of the iris sphincter in Adie's syndrome, Arch Ophthalmol 96:1615, 1978.

62. Thompson HS: Book review: illustrated medical dictionaries, Stedman's 24th edition and Dorland's 26th edition, Am J Ophthalmol 93:668, 1982.

63. Thompson HS: Light-near dissociation of the pupil, Ophthalmologica 189:21, 1984.

64. Thompson HS: Editorial: the pupil cycle time, J Clin Neuro-Ophthalmol 7:38, 1987.

65. Thompson HS, Bourgon P, Van Allen MW: The tendon reflexes in Adie's syndrome, in Thompson HS, ed: Topics in neuro-ophthalmology, Baltimore, Williams & Wilkins, 1979, p 96.

66. Thompson HS, Corbett JJ: Asymmetry of pupillomotor input, Eye 5:36, 1991.

67. Thompson HS, Franceschetti AT, Thompson PM: Hippus, Am J Ophthalmol 71:1116, 1971.

68. Thompson HS, Hurwitz J, Czarnecki JSC: Aberrant regeneration and the tonic pupil, in Glaser JS, ed: Neuro-ophthalmology, Symposium of the University of Miami and the Bascom Palmer Eye Institute, vol 10, St Louis, CV Mosby, 1980.

69. Thompson HS, Newsome DA, Loewenfeld IE: The fixed dilated pupil, sudden iridoplegia or mydriatic drops? A simple diagnostic test, Arch Ophthalmol 86:21, 1971.

70. Thompson HS, Zackon DH, Czarnecki JSC: Tadpole-shaped pupils caused by segmental spasm of the iris dilator muscle, Am J Ophthalmol 96:467, 1983.

71. Thompson HS, et al: The relationship between visual acuity, pupillary defect and visual field loss, Am J Ophthalmol 93:681, 1982.

72. Tress KH, El-Sobky AA: Pupil responses to intravenous heroin (diamorphine) in dependent and non-dependent humans, Br J Clin Pharmacol 7:213, 1979.

73. Ukai K, Higashi J, Ishikawa S: Edge-light pupil oscillation of optic neuritis, Neuro-ophthalmology 1:33, 1980.

74. Walsh FB: Third nerve regeneration: a clinical evaluation, Br J Ophthal 41:577, 1957.

75. Weinstein JM, Zweifel TJ, Thompson HS: Congenital Horner's syndrome, Arch Ophthalmol 98:1074, 1980.

76. Wirtschafter JD, Volk CR, Sawchuk RJ: Transaqueous diffusion of acetylcholine to denervated iris sphincter muscle: a mechanism for the tonic pupil syndrome (Adie's syndrome), Ann Neurol 4:1, 1978.

CHAPTER

13

Radiometry and Photometry

WILLIAM M. HART, Jr., M.D., Ph.D.

Light is the visible portion of the spectrum of electromagnetic radiation. Although radiant energy is a physical phenomenon, vision is said to be psychophysical or subjective in nature. Thus, although radiant energy has well defined and physically measurable properties, vision can be measured only by subjective techniques. Some objectively recordable biologic responses, such as pupillary constriction or electrical events arising from the retina or cerebral cortex, are closely associated with vision. But these represent relatively crude and distant parallel events when compared to the exquisitely sensitive and richly diverse complexity of the visual experience. Although objectively recordable physiologic events are occasionally helpful in evaluating the status of the visual system, the most sensitive measures of visual function are psychophysical in nature. They depend on subjective responses, in which human subjects are used as if they were instruments of measurement. Typical examples of such tests include absolute thresholds for perception of light, comparison of test lights to standard lights, and detection of just noticeable differences when test lights are altered in some fashion. Some functions of the human visual system are extraordinarily sensitive. The dark-adapted human eye can detect a flash of light when the retina absorbs as few as a dozen

photons. This threshold rivals the sensivity of the best photographic emulsions.

Stimuli for visual sensation may be divided into two types, adequate and inadequate. Light is the adequate stimulus for vision and is that portion of the electromagnetic spectrum falling in the range of wavelengths of approximately 400 to 750 nm. Inadequate stimuli include any nonlight events that yield any sensation of vision. Such stimuli generally produce unformed visual sensations called "phosphenes" or "photopsias." (See Chapter 15.) The pressure phosphene appears as a patch of contrasting light and dark when mechanical pressure is applied to the exterior of the eye. The appearance of such a phosphene depends on whether it is observed in the light or in the dark; it will appear dark in the light-adapted eye and light in the dark-adapted eye. Movement phosphenes are seen in the dark-adapted eye following rapid eye movements. Circles or sheaves of light may appear in the visual field corresponding to the position of the optic disc or the positions of the rectus muscle insertions. Movement phosphenes are thought to be the result of distortion of the retina by the inertial drag of the optic nerve or vitreous, or the tug of the extraocular muscles. Electrical phosphenes are observed with the passage of weak alternating electrical currents through the eye. Radiation phosphenes appear with the passage of ionizing radiation through the retina. Phosphenes presumed to be due to cosmic rays have been reported by orbiting astronauts.

This work was supported in part by Research Grant EY 06582 from the National Eye Institute, National Institutes of Health.

There are two different ways in which light may be detected and measured. The first involves the use of physical measuring techniques (radiometry), whereas the second employs psychophysical methods, in which human subjects are used to detect and compare the visual sensations produced by light (photometry). Radiometric measures of electromagnetic radiation involve the characterization of its frequency, its energy content, and its distribution in time and space. Photometric measures involve the detection and comparison of lights by the color and brightness sensations that they produce.

The brightness observed by human observers is not a simple function of the energy content of light. Differing wavelengths of light have differing efficiencies for the production of visual sensations. Wavelengths subjectively identifiable as green are most efficient in stimulating a visual sensation, whereas those that produce the sensations of blue or red require much higher levels of energy to produce equivalent levels of subjective brightness.

This chapter first considers the physical properties of light and the means at our disposal to detect and measure these properties—radiometry. The latter part of the chapter considers psychophysical techniques of light measurement—photometry.

PHYSICAL PROPERTIES OF LIGHT

Electromagnetic radiation is produced (emitted and propagated from a source) when the distribution of electrical charge in a physical system is altered. For example, such radiation is produced around a conductor carrying an electrical current. Radio waves are generated about an antenna by such techniques. Oscillation of electrons within the atoms of a substance produces electromagnetic radiation varying from the infrared, through the visible portions of the spectrum, and into the ultraviolet. Abrupt deceleration of rapidly moving electrons impacting a dense target produces x-rays. Pulsating nuclear charges generate gamma rays.

The propagation of electromagnetic radiation may be thought of as occurring as waves and/or particles. All forms of such radiation have properties that may be best described by a wavelike character. The phenomena of interference and refraction are understood best when thinking of light as propagated in waves. However, such radiation also may be considered as being emitted in discrete units, which are called quanta. Phenomena such as the photoelectric effect and the detection of low levels of light by the retina are best explained by quantum detec-

tion theory. A quantum is the smallest unit of energy of which electromagnetic radiation is composed. The energy content of a single quantum is proportional to its frequency: it is greatest at the short wavelength end of the spectrum, and it is lowest at the long wavelength end. In a vacuum all radiation is propagated at a constant velocity of 3×10^{10} cm/sec, or 186,000 miles/sec. The velocity of electromagnetic radiation in a vacuum is a universal constant, symbolized by the letter c. The fundamental characteristic that distinguishes different portions of the electromagnetic radiation spectrum is the frequency of radiation, symbolized by the letter ν. Frequency is expressed in cycles per second or hertz (Hz). Since the velocity of radiation in a vacuum is a constant, the frequency of radiation is inversely related to its wavelength. Radio waves are of low frequency and long wavelength, whereas light waves have a higher frequency and shorter wavelength (Fig. 13-1). The frequency of an electromagnetic wave is constant regardless of the medium in which it is traveling. However, the velocity of light varies with the medium through which it is traveling. It is slowed when passing through any optically transmitting medium other than a vacuum. The ratio of the velocity of light in a vacuum, c, to the velocity in an optical medium, v_m, is called the index of refraction, n_m, of the medium:

$$n_m = c/v_m$$

The velocity of electromagnetic radiation in air is nearly the same as that in a vacuum. As a convenience, the index of refraction of air is usually approximated at a value of 1. Because the velocity of light in air is always greater than that in a denser medium, the index of refraction of substances such as glass and water is always greater than 1.

The reciprocal relationship between wavelength and frequency of radiation varies for light when passing through media whose index of refraction is greater than 1. If radiation of frequency ν (in cycles per second) is propagated in a medium with a velocity of v_m, in 1 second ν waves, or cycles, will pass a given point. During this second, the first wave will travel v cm from that point. There will then be v centimeters for ν cycles or v/ν centimeters for one cycle. The distance occupied by one cycle is the wavelength λ:

$$\lambda = v/\nu$$

Note that, although the frequency of light is a constant, its wavelength varies with the index

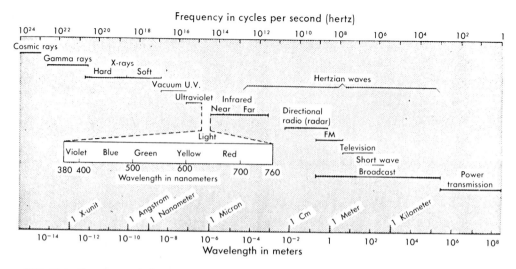

FIG. 13-1 Spectrum of electromagnetic radiation. (From Illuminating Engineering Society: IES lighting handbook, 4th ed, New York, The Society, 1966.)

of refraction of the medium through which it is traveling. Light having a wavelength of 510 nm in air will have a wavelength of approximately 382 nm* at the level of the retina (while passing through a largely aqueous medium). This is illustrated as follows. In a vacuum (or as a close approximation in air) radiation of any wavelength, λ_a, and frequency, ν, travels at a constant velocity, c:

$$\lambda_a = c/\nu \text{ or } \lambda_a\nu = c$$

In a medium with a higher index of refraction the velocity of propagation is less, v_m. Since the frequency of the light remains constant, the wavelength in the medium, λ_m, is less than in air:

$$\lambda_m\nu = \nu_m$$

The change in wavelength is then proportional to the change in velocity:

$$\frac{\lambda_a\nu}{\lambda_m\nu} = \frac{\lambda_a}{\lambda_m} = \frac{c}{v_m}$$

The index of refraction of a medium, n, is the ratio of speed of light in a vacuum, c, to its speed in the medium, v_m. Consequently,

$$\lambda_a/\lambda_m = n_m \quad \text{or} \quad \lambda_m = \lambda_a/n_m$$

The wavelength of light in a medium is its wavelength in air divided by the refractive index of the medium in which it is traveling.

The refractive index of the vitreous body is about that of water, 1.336; thus green light having a wavelength of 510 nm in air will have a wavelength of

$$\lambda_{vit} = \frac{510 \text{ nm}}{1.336} = 382 \text{ nm}$$

in vitreous.

The refractive index of an optical medium is constant only for a constant frequency of light. Actually, each optical medium has a different refractive index for each frequency of light. Higher frequency light (the blue end of the spectrum) is slowed more by passage through an optical medium than is a lower frequency light (the red end of the spectrum). Thus the refractive index for blue light is greater than that for red light. A simple convex lens will bring blue light to a focus closer to it than the focus for a red light (Fig. 13-2). This phenomenon is termed "chromatic aberration." The chromatic aberration of the eye is put to use in the practice of refraction in the familiar red-green or duochrome test.

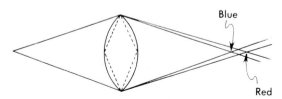

FIG. 13-2 Chromatic aberration. Distance of image from lens is proportional to wavelength. Prismatic effect of lens is suggested by dotted lines.

---

*1 nanometer (nm) is 10^{-9} m (.000,000,001 m). The wavelength of light has in the past also been expressed in angstrom units (1 nm = 10 Å), or in millimicrons (1 nm = 1 mμ).

When Snellen chart letters illuminated with green light and letters illuminated with red light are seen to be equally blurred, it can be inferred that the green image is in focus to the anterior side of the point of detection on the retina, while the red portion of the image is in focus on the posterior side.

Energy content of light

As already mentioned, some of the physical properties of electromagnetic radiation are best explained in terms of particle theory. Electromagnetic radiation is thought of as being emitted in discrete packets of energy called "quanta" or "photons." The energy, U, of a photon is directly proportional to its frequency, ν:

$$U = h\nu$$

The proportionality constant, h, is Planck's constant, which has a value of 6.62×10^{-27} erg sec.*

Since the wavelength of radiation in air, λ, is related to frequency, ν, by

$$\nu = c/\lambda$$

the energy of quanta also can be calculated on the basis of wavelength:

$$U = hc/\lambda$$

Since the energy of a photon is inversely proportional to its wavelength in a given medium, the energy of a photon of wavelength 400 nm (violet) is twice as great as that of a photon of wavelength 800 nm (red). The energy of a photon can be calculated by means of the formula $U = hc/\lambda$; for example, the energy of a quantum of radiation of 500 nm:

$$U = \frac{(6.62 \times 10^{-27} \text{ erg sec}) (3 \times 10^{10} \text{ cm/sec})}{5 \times 10^{-5} \text{ cm}}$$
$$= 3.97 \times 10^{-12} \text{ erg}$$

where

$\lambda = 500 \text{ nm} = 5 \times 10^{-5} \text{ cm}$
$h = 6.62 \times 10^{-27} \text{ erg sec}$
$c = 3 \times 10^{10} \text{ cm/sec}$

The probability that a quantum of light of a given wavelength will be absorbed by the retina is determined by its wavelength, and by the absorption spectrum of photopigments in the retina. However, once absorbed, quanta of differing wavelengths are indistinguishable to the visual system. They appear as if they were equally effective in the production of a visual

sensation. Differences in the energy of quanta that have been absorbed have no bearing on their effectiveness as visual stimuli.

UNITS OF RADIOMETRIC MEASURE

Terms for expressing the physical dimensions of electromagnetic radiation specify both the temporal and spatial distributions of quantities of radiant energy. Quantities of radiant energy (U) are measured in basic units of ergs or joules. In the centimeter-gram-second system of physical units a dyne is defined as the force necessary to accelerate a mass of 1 g at a rate of 1 cm/sec². An erg (a very small amount of energy) is defined as a force of 1 dyne acting through a distance of 1 cm:

1 erg = 1 dyne cm

In the meter-kilogram-second system of units a newton is defined as the force necessary to accelerate a mass of 1 kg at a rate of 1 m/sec². A joule is defined as a force of 1 newton acting through a distance of 1 m:

1 joule = 1 newton m

One joule is equal to 10^7 (10 million) ergs.

Quantities of radiant energy alone are, however, insufficient to describe the distribution of radiant energy in any system. The rate of transfer (flux) of energy also must be specified. Energy flux per unit time (t) is called power (P), and the standard unit of radiant power is the watt. A watt is defined as 1 joule of energy flux per second:

$$P = U/t = \text{joules/sec} = \text{watts}$$

Expressions for instantaneous values of continuously varying functions require the use of symbols of the differential calculus. An approximation of an instantaneous rate of change can be thought of as the slope of a straight line (a differential ratio), when the line is approximately tangent to the curve of a variable, x, as a function of time: $\Delta x/\Delta t$. The exact instantaneous rate of change is then the limiting value approached by the differential ratio, as the time differential (Δt) approaches zero at the time of interest. The instantaneous value of energy flux (power) at some point in time can be expressed as the limiting value approached by the differential ratio of energy flux per unit time, as the time differential approaches zero:

$$P = \lim_{\Delta t \to 0} \frac{\Delta U}{\Delta t} = \frac{dU}{dt} \text{ watts}$$

Having defined power, we must also specify the spatial dimensions within which the energy flux occurs. Radiant intensity (J) is a measure of

---

*The erg and other physical units of measure are defined in the box on p. 458.

TABLE 13-1   Radiometric Quantities*

Radiometric term	Symbol	Derivation	Units
Radiant energy	U	force · distance	Joules or ergs
Radiant flux	P	$\dfrac{dU}{dt}$	Watts
Radiant intensity	J	$\dfrac{dP}{d\omega}$	Watts/ steradian
Irradiance	H	$\dfrac{dP}{dA}$	Watts/m^2
Radiant excitance (emittance)	M	$\dfrac{dP}{dA}$	Watts/m^2
Radiance	N	$\dfrac{dM}{d\omega}$	Watts/m^2 steradian

*See box on p. 458 for definitions of symbols, constants, and units used in radiometry and photometry.

radiation propagated in a given direction. It is the flux of energy, or radiant power, emitted from a point source and propagated in a specified direction. For uniformly emitting sources of light, cross sections of a solid angle with its apex at the source will show a uniform energy distribution. That is, the ratio of power to cross-sectional area of the solid angle will be a constant. The steradian (ω) is the metric unit used for expression of the solid angle. Radiant intensity is defined as the limit of the ratio of power to the solid angle in which it is contained, as the angle approaches a value of zero in the direction of interest:

$$J = \frac{dP}{d\omega} \text{ watts/steradian}$$

Irradiance (H) is the radiant power incident on a unit surface. It is directly proportional to the intensity of the light source and is inversely proportional to the square of the distance between the source and the surface on which the energy is incident. For a given point on the surface, and in the same manner as for radiant intensity, irradiance is defined as the limit of the ratio of radiant power to area (A), as area approaches a value of zero at the point of interest:

$$H = \frac{dP}{dA} \text{ watts/m}^2$$

Radiant excitance (M), sometimes called "emittance," is closely related to irradiance and is expressed in the same units of watts per square meter. It is the radiant power per unit area that is emitted from a point on a surface, whether it is a primary source (an emitter of light) or a secondary source (a reflector of light).

Radiance (N) is the radiant power emitted from a point on an extended surface and in a specified direction. It is expressed in units of watts per unit solid angle and unit area. Since extended surfaces are either imperfectly emitting or imperfectly reflecting sources of light, energy emitted from points on such surfaces will vary with the direction of propagation. Radiance (N) is defined as the limit of the ratio of power to the cross-section of solid angle and area of surface, as the latter two dimensions approach a value of zero at the point and in the direction of interest. It also can be expressed as the radiant excitance (M) from a given point on a surface and in a specified direction:

$$N = \frac{dM}{d\omega} \text{ watts/steradian/m}^2$$

Radiometric terms and their units are outlined in Table 13-1.

RADIOMETRY

The methodology of physical detection and quantification of electromagnetic radiation constitutes the field of radiometry. This is to be distinguished from the use of the eye as a detection instrument for the measurement of the visible portion of the electromagnetic spectrum. The latter, termed "photometry," will be discussed later.

A variety of instruments is available for measuring the physical properties of electromagnetic radiation. Two basic types of detectors are used: thermal detectors and quantum detectors. With thermal detectors the radiant energy to be measured is absorbed in a blackened chamber, converting the radiation to heat. The heat in turn generates an electrical current at the bimetallic junction of a thermocouple. The heat produced per unit time is a direct measure of the power in the beam. Quantum detectors, which are much more sensitive measuring devices, use the photoelectric effect. Photons are absorbed by a negatively charged surface (cathode). Electrons that are excited by the energy absorption are emitted from the surface and are subsequently captured at an oppositely charged interface (anode). A series of such electrodes can be arranged to produce a cascade effect, multiplying the number of electrons excited at each charged surface. Such a device is called a "photomultiplier."

The spectral sensitivities of the two types of detectors are quite different. That of the thermal detector is broad and uniform. Photomultipliers have highly variable spectral sensitivities, being most sensitive to higher energy (short wavelength) photons. The spectral sensitivity curve of a photomultiplier must be known if it is to be used to measure the spectral distribution of radiant energy. Both types of radiometric detectors are nonspecific; they measure total power but not the spectral distribution of power. For the spectral distribution of power in a beam of radiant energy to be measured, it first must be spread into its component parts by a prism or diffraction grating such as those found within analytic spectrophotometers. The power contained within narrow regions of the electromagnetic spectrum then must be separately measured.

For complete characterization of radiant energy it is not enough to know the total power available and its spectral distribution; one must also know something about the spatial distribution of the power falling on (or being emitted from) a given area. The power per unit area is termed the "energy density." The physical specification of a light source, whether it is a primary source, such as an electric lamp, or secondary source, such as an illuminated object, must give

the area of the source, the energy density of the source, the spectral distribution of the energy, and the directional distribution of the radiation.

Radiant energy considerations in clinical ophthalmology

Radiometry is of practical significance for the clinical ophthalmologist. When a projected image of a Snellen test chart is used for visual acuity testing, the reflective projection screen becomes a secondary source of radiation. The light arriving at the patient's eye is actually diverging from multiple points on the projection screen. Thus the light available to the patient cannot be measured by simply recording the amount of light arriving at the screen, but rather the light reflected from the screen must be measured (Fig. 13-3). Since most projection screens for Snellen charts are highly directional reflectors, it is also necessary to measure the light radiating from the screen in the specific direction of the patient being tested. The spectral distribution of the light reflected from the screen also can be of some consequence. If significant portions of ultraviolet or infrared radiation are produced by the projector bulb, a photographic light meter might indicate more radiant energy reflected from the screen than the eye can see.

A second example of common importance is in the use of hemispheric bowl perimeters for examination of the visual field. Here the subject is required to report visual detection of a luminous test object (spot of light) projected onto the diffusely illuminated, featureless, matte-white internal surface of the hemisphere. Again, we are not interested in the characteristics of the light actually falling on the surface as much as we are in the amount of light being reflected from it. If the reflecting surface of the hemisphere becomes soiled, or if dirt enters the projection system for the test objects, the adapting background luminance and/or the projected test objects may be of lower energy than expected. Thus hemisphere perimeters must be re-

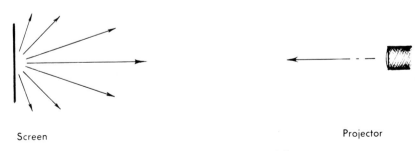

Screen   Projector

FIG. 13-3 Reflection from imperfectly diffusing screen.

peatedly recalibrated to confirm both the level of light being produced by the incandescent bulb of the projector, as well as the efficiency of reflection of the light from the reflecting surface of the hemisphere.

A third example of adequate characterization of the radiant energy from light sources involves the use of reflective colored objects in testing the color vision attributes of hue discrimination and saturation discrimination, such as in the Farnsworth-Munsell 100 hue test. Unless these standardized objects are presented under a light of defined spectral composition, the test can be quite misleading. For example, incandescent light is rich in the longer wavelength end of the visible spectrum and is relatively deficient in the blue. Manufacturers provide a blue filter that can be placed over an incandescent bulb to adjust its spectral composition to that of a standard illuminant.

The total amount of energy absorbed by a surface depends on the extent of the area exposed to radiant energy, the energy density arriving at the area, and the duration of exposure to the radiant source. The incident energy may be absorbed, transmitted, or reflected. Photocoagulators that use xenon arcs or argon lasers have been designed with careful consideration of these factors. The radiant energy emitted by them is transmitted through the transparent media of the eye but is absorbed by the pigmented tissues. The absorbed energy is in turn converted to heat, creating the burn lesions characteristic of surgical photocoagulation.

Reflection of light within the eye can occur where the refractive index changes abruptly between adjacent tissues. Reflection from such a surface increases with the angle of incidence (Fig. 13-4). The greatest difference in refractive index is found at the air-cornea interface, which is where the greatest degree of light reflection occurs. Reflections from the posterior surface of the cornea and the surfaces of the lens and retina also may decrease the amount of light arriving at photoreceptors. For a beam of light whose incidence is normal to a reflecting surface, the intensity of the reflected portion of the beam is

$$I_r = I \left(\frac{n_1 - n}{n_1 + n} \right)^2$$

where

I = Intensity of incident beam
I_r = Intensity of reflected beam
n = Index of refraction of surrounding medium (for air, $n = 1$)
n_1 = Index of refraction of reflecting medium (for cornea, $n_1 = 1.336$)

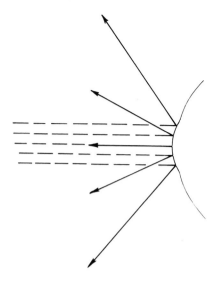

FIG. 13-4 Reflection of light parallel to optic axis from cornea. Peripheral rays are more reflected than axial rays because of greater angle of incidence.

At the anterior surface of the cornea

$$I_r = I \left(\frac{1.336 - 1}{1.336 + 1} \right)^2$$

Thus I_r is 0.02, or 2% of the light incident normal to the cornea is reflected. The intensity of the light reflected from the surface of a cornea will increase with increasing angles of incidence away from normal, until at a grazing incidence a majority of the light will be reflected. Illumination of the retina by a perimetric test object presented in the periphery of the visual field is considerably reduced (Fig. 13-5), not only because of the oblique aspect of the pupillary aperture, but also because of reflection of test object light by the surfaces of the cornea and lens.

The lens is responsible for much of the absorption of radiant energy in the ocular media. Its optical density is greatest for short wavelengths. The aphakic eye can be stimulated by ultraviolet light, which is ordinarily invisible to the normal eye, because it is blocked from the retina by the lens. Light absorption by the lens, particularly in the blue portions of the spectrum, increases with age.[6] If colored test objects are to be used for perimetric testing, this phenomenon has to be taken into consideration.

Considerable short wavelength radiation is absorbed by the yellow macular pigment, xanthophyll, which lies in crystals between the elongated fibers of the outer plexiform layer of the macula (Henle's fiber layer). The partially

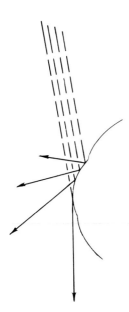

FIG. 13-5   Reflection of light obliquely incident to cornea. At grazing incidence, large proportion of light is reflected.

oriented xanthophyll crystals polarize light so that sheaflike patterns are seen entoptically in a uniform field of polarized light. This phenomenon, called "Haidinger's brushes," is discussed in Chapter 15.

In addition to reflection and absorption, scattering also produces light loss in the normal passage of radiant energy through the eye.[1] The difference between total transmission (Fig. 13-6, *A*) and direct transmission (Fig. 13-6, *B*) is the result of light scatter. The net light actually reaching the receptors is shown in Figure 13-7. The optical sections of the cornea and other transparent media seen with the slit-lamp are the result of light being scattered from within cellular structures in the media. Scattering of light by submicroscopic particles, the so-called Tyndall effect, is ordinarily not seen in the aqueous humor. Thus visibility of the slit-lamp beam within the aqueous is usually pathologic and is caused by accumulation of soluble proteins, so-called flare. Larger particles within the aqueous, such as cells, appear as bright points of light.

RADIANT ENERGY DISTRIBUTION IN A RETINAL IMAGE

The units for radiant energy that have been outlined may be used to express the amount of radiation reaching the retina from a given source. If the radiant excitance (M) of a point source of light is W watts per cm^2, at a distance d from the source, the power will be spread over a spherical surface (Fig. 13-8). If the pupil of an observing eye is made a portion of the sphere, the proportion of the radiant excitance entering the pupil from the unit area of source is

$$W \times \frac{A_{pupil}}{A_{sphere}}$$

The radiant flux passing through the pupil of the eye is focused on an area of retina, A_{ret} (Fig. 13-9):

$$\frac{A_{source}}{d^2} = \frac{A_{ret}}{f^2}$$

in which f is the posterior focal length of the eye.

The area of the retinal image is

$$A_{ret} = \frac{A_{source} \times f^2}{d^2}$$

The radiant flux falling on the pupil from 1 cm^2 of the source

$$W \times \frac{A_{pupil}}{A_{sphere}}$$

is distributed over the retinal area (f^2/d^2) cm^2. The radiant power per unit area of retinal image is

$$H = \frac{W \times (A_{pupil}/A_{sphere})}{f^2/d^2} \ watts/cm^2$$

The area of the pupil is πr^2. The area of the spherical surface, including the pupil, is $4\pi d^2$.

The irradiance of the image at the retina then reduces to

$$H = \frac{W \times r^2_{pupil}}{4f^2}$$

The result, surprising at first, is that the irradiance in the image at the retina is independent of the distance of the eye from the source of light. However, consider the fact that as the eye recedes from the light source and the light that enters the pupil diminishes as the square of the distance, the area of the retinal image also diminishes as the square of the distance. This phenomenon of power distribution in a retinal image explains in part how the appearance of brightness of a spot of light can seem to be relatively independent of the distance at which it is viewed.

Assumptions in this first-order estimate include the following:

1. All the radiation is transmitted, none is reflected, and none is absorbed or scattered.
2. A sharp image is formed on the retina.
3. The source is uniformly emitting.

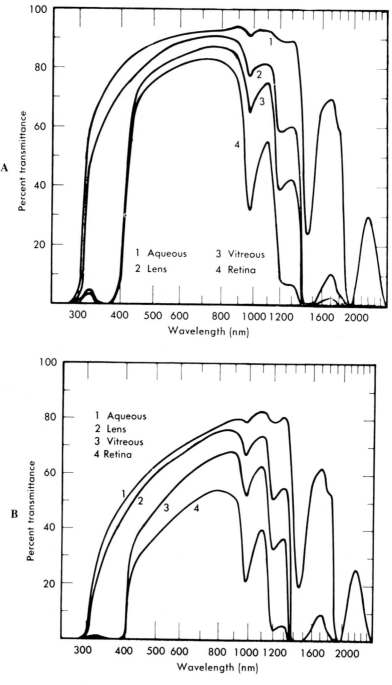

FIG. 13-6 Transmission of visible light and near infrared by ocular media. **A**, Total transmittance through entire eye. **B**, Direct transmittance through entire eye. (From Boettner EA, Wolter JR: Invest Ophthalmol 1:776, 1962.)

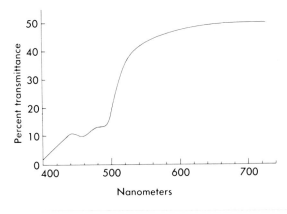

FIG. 13-7 Transmission of light of visible range by ocular media. Low transmission of short wavelengths is due largely to lens. Irregular dip in blue region (440 to 500 mm) is due to absorption by yellow macular pigment, xanthophyll. (From Wyszecki G, Stiles WS: Color science, New York, John Wiley, 1967.)

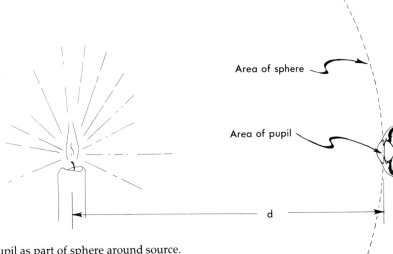

FIG. 13-8 Pupil as part of sphere around source.

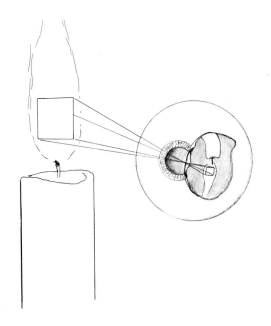

FIG. 13-9 Projection of unit area of source on retina.

SURGICAL USES OF LIGHT ENERGY

Aside from being a stimulus for vision, light also is used therapeutically as a source of energy for photocoagulation and photodisruption within the eye. Lasers that are used for ocular surgery are calibrated in units of radiometric measure, and the energy they deliver to the eye is expressed in these terms.[3] For example, a typical Q-switched Neodymium-YAG laser delivers a focal spot of light having a diameter of 60 μm, containing 5 millijoules of energy, with an extremely short pulse duration of 10 nsec. The energy density at the delivery site will be approximately 180 joules per cm². Since, however, the 5 millijoules (total) of energy are delivered within the short time span of 10 nsec, the radiant flux (power) of the laser pulse at the energy site will be one half megawatt (5 × 10⁵ watts)! Perhaps even more impressive is that irradiance at the delivery site of the YAG laser will be 18 gigawatts per cm² (18 × 10⁹ watts/cm²). Thus relatively small amounts of energy delivered to small areas for extremely short durations can achieve truly impressive heights of power density. These extraordinarily high levels of power density are responsible for the generation of a zone of optical breakdown at the focus of the laser beam. This event in turn generates a mechanical shock wave that is propagated through the surrounding medium, producing the surgically useful photodisruptive effect. By contrast, a continuous laser, such as the argon laser, may deliver as much as 50 millijoules over a period of one tenth of a second for a power output of 500 milliwatts. Due to the longer time span of delivery, power densities obtained with such lasers are 1 million times less than those obtained with Q-switched YAG lasers, even though the total amount of energy delivered may be 10 times as great. The irradiance or power density, assuming a 60 μm spot size, would be 17.8 kilowatts per cm². Unlike the disruptive effect generated by the Q-switched YAG laser, the energy of the argon laser, when absorbed by pigmented tissue, is converted directly into heat, producing a thermal burn.

UNITS OF PHOTOMETRIC MEASURE

Corresponding to each term of radiometric measure is an analogous dimension of photometric measure (Table 13-2). Photometric quantities may be derived directly from their radiometric equivalents by multiplying the radiometric quantity by V_λ, the photopic luminosity coefficient. The function V_λ is represented by the standard photopic luminous efficiency curve shown in Fig. 13-10, B. Note that calculations of photometric quantities based on their radiometric equivalents must be made on a wavelength-dependent basis. This is because the photopic luminosity coefficient varies continuously with wavelength.

The photometric equivalents of radiometric measure require integration across the spectrum of visible wavelengths and depend on complete spectral characterization of the radiometric quantities from which the photometric measures are being derived. The radiometric measure of radiant energy (U) has its photometric equivalent in "luminous energy" (Q), a psycho-

TABLE 13-2   Photometric Quantities*

Photometric term	Symbol	Derivation	Units
Luminous energy	Q	$Q = 685 \int_{400}^{750} V_\lambda U_\lambda d_\lambda$	Lumen seconds
Luminous flux	F	$\dfrac{dQ}{dt}$	Lumens
Luminous intensity (candlepower)	I	$\dfrac{dQ}{dt}$	Lumens/steradian (candelas)
Illuminance	E	$\dfrac{dQ}{dA}$	Lumens/m² (lux)
Luminance (photometric brightness)	L	$\dfrac{dI}{dA}$	Candelas/m² (nits)

*Compare to analogous radiometric terms in Table 13-1. See box on p. 458 for definitions of symbols, constants, and units used in radiometry and photometry.

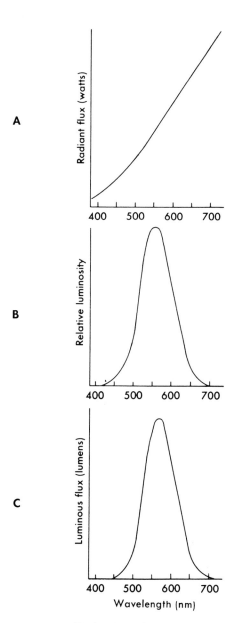

FIG. 13-10 Evaluation of spectroradiometric data in terms of luminosity. **A**, Power distribution in incandescent light (standard illuminant). **B**, Standard photopic luminous efficiency curve. Luminous flux of light source is calculated by multiplying power ordinates of **A** by efficiency ordinates of **B**, giving curve **C**. Area under curve **A** is watts; are under curve **C** is lumens.

physical measure of the quantity of light rated according to its ability to produce a visual sensation of brightness. Whereas radiant energy is expressed in units of ergs or joules, which are units of physical measurement, luminous energy is expressed in the psychophysical units of lumen seconds. This value can be derived from the spectral distribution of radiant energy (U) by integration:

$$Q = 685 \int_{400}^{750} V_\lambda U_\lambda d_\lambda$$

where V_λ is the photopic luminosity coefficient function. V_λ is a dimensionless coefficient, which has a maximum value of 1.0 at 555 nm. The number 685 is a conversion constant: the value of lumens per watt at the same wavelength (555 nm).

Luminous flux (F) is the photometric equivalent of radiant flux (P). It represents the rate of transfer (flux) of energy, evaluated according to its ability to produce a visual sensation. Since luminous energy is measured in units of lumen seconds, F, which is luminous energy per unit time, is expressed in units of lumens.

Luminous intensity (I) is the photometric equivalent of radiant intensity (J). It represents the luminous flux emitted per unit solid angle in a specified direction. It is expressed in units of candelas, which in turn are calculated as lumens per steradian.

Illuminance (E) is the photometric equivalent of irradiance (H). It is the luminous flux incident on a surface per unit area and is expressed in units of lux, which in turn have the dimensions of lumens per m². An alternative unit of illuminance is the "foot candle," measured as lumens per square foot.

Perhaps the most commonly used photometric measures are those of luminance. Luminance (L) is the photometric equivalence of radiance (N) and is the luminous intensity (I) per unit of visible area of a surface source of light (whether emitting or reflecting). Its units are those of luminous intensity per unit area of surface source expressed as candelas per unit area, for example, candelas per m². A large and bewildering variety of names and units of luminance have been used in the past. All of these units can, however, be reduced to some measure of the number of candelas of luminous intensity per unit of apparent area of source of light. Such units include the stilb (candelas per cm²), the nit (candelas per m²), the foot lambert (candelas per area of circle with radius of 1 foot), the lambert (candelas per area of circle with radius of 1 cm), and the apostilb (candelas per area of circle with radius of 1 m). The terms of photometric and radiometric measure and their various symbols are summarized in Tables 13-1 and 13-2. The key for definitions of symbols, constants and units is shown in the box on p. 458.

PHOTOMETRY AND THE SPECTRAL SENSITIVITY OF THE EYE

Although the visible portions of the electromagnetic spectrum can be characterized physically by their wavelength and energy content, these physical measures do not in any way specify the subjective sensation of vision they induce. Although color and the sensation of brightness are related to the wavelength and energy content of light, the relationship is very complex and actually varies from one individual to the next. The efficiency of light in producing a sensation of vision changes with its wavelength in a fashion that is not proportional to its energy content. Green light is most effective in producing a visual sensation: fewer watts of green light are needed to produce a given sensation of brightness than for any other spectral color. The wavelength of light to which the retina is most sensitive depends on whether the determination is made in the presence of relatively high or low levels of ambient light. When the eye has become accustomed to a high ambient level of light it is said to be light-adapted and to have photopic vision. An eye that has become accustomed to a prolonged period of darkness is said to be dark-adapted and to have scotopic vision.

To measure the relative efficiency of a light to produce a sensation of brightness, one can conveniently compare it with another source of light (of the same or different spectral composition) to be used as a standard. If a field of view is divided in half such that one half is illuminated by the standard light, the intensity of the light to be tested (presented in the other half of the bipartite field) can be adjusted until the apparent brightness or luminosity of the two fields is equal (Fig. 13-11). This process is called "heterochromatic brightness matching." The number of watts per unit area of each light required to make the two halves appear equally luminous is a measure of the relative efficiency of the wavelengths to produce a subjective sensation of brightness. If the most efficient wavelength is given the value of 1.0 and the efficiencies of other wavelengths are rated as fractions of the most efficient wavelength, a normalized curve of relative efficiencies can be generated. If such a process is applied to the light-adapted eye, the most efficient wavelength is found to be 555 nm; under scotopic conditions the efficiency curve will shift such that the most efficient wavelength is found to be 510 nm (Fig. 13-12). This shift in the efficiency or luminosity curve was first described by Purkinje.

Different observers and different conditions will produce somewhat varying luminosity curves. Such curves are important to commercial and industrial processes (such as paint and dye manufacture), as well as to ophthalmologists. Color standards and standard curves of the visual efficiency of the visible spectrum have been established by the International Committee on Illumination (in French, CIE, or Commission Internationale de l'Éclairage). These stan-

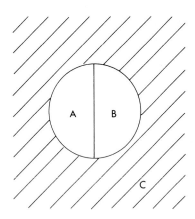

FIG. 13-11 Bipartite field. A and B, Fields presented for comparison. Surround, C, may be dark or of other specified characteristics.

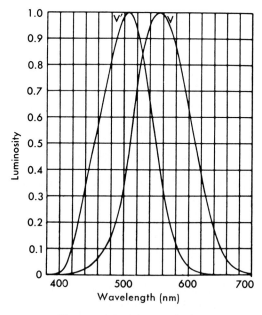

FIG. 13-12 Photopic, V, and scotopic, V', luminous efficiency curves. Most efficient wavelength in light-adapted eye is 555 nm, in dark-adapted eye is 510 nm. Efficiency of other wavelengths given as decimal fraction of most efficient wavelength.

dards have been established using a so-called standard observer for photopic and scotopic luminosity curves, as shown in Figure 13-12. The "standard observer" is actually an average of several subjects with normal trichromatic vision.

The standard luminosity curves allow the weighting of each narrow region of wavelengths (for any light of given spectral composition) in accordance with its ability to excite a visual sensation. The radiant power of each narrow region, multiplied by its efficiency, defines the luminous flux density of that region of wavelength. The sum of luminous flux densities for a series of spectral bands is the luminous flux density of the composite illuminant. Figure 13-10 illustrates how a given spectroradiometric curve for an illuminant can be evaluated with respect to the eye. Curve *A* represents standard illuminant A (an incandescent light source at color temperature 2854°). Curve *B* is the photopic luminosity curve, and curve *C* was obtained by multiplying the ordinants of *A* by the corresponding values of *B* for each wavelength. The area under curve *A* is expressed in watts, whereas the area under curve *C* is expressed in lumens or equivalent units. The link between the physical measurements of radiometry and the effect of light as a stimulus is the luminosity curve for the standard observer, as established by the International Commission.

ADDITIVITY OF LUMINANCE

The integration of luminance across wavelengths illustrated in Figure 13-10 implicitly assumes that the value of luminance obtained at one wavelength is equivalent to that obtained at another. If this is true, total luminance values for any source of light can be determined by simply adding together or summing the separate effects of the different wavelengths. The general principle that the total luminance of a light should be equal to the sum of its separate parts is termed "Abney's law." Ordinarily, when the spectral composition of two lights is approximately the same, Abney's law is found to be largely valid. Thus if two lights are equated in luminance, they may be added to one another to produce a third light having twice the level of luminance. Alternatively, they may be proportionately added to one another (*x*% of one light plus a quantity equal to 100% minus *x*% of the other) to produce a third light of identical luminance to either of the first two. However, when the spectral composition of the two lights differs to the extent that they are noticeably different in color, brightness matches between the two

sources do not always obey the predictions of Abney's law. The photopic luminosity function (V or V_λ), set up as a standard by the CIE, generally yields valid results for additivity, closely approximating the predictions of Abney's law. However, direct subjective brightness matching of lights of differing spectral composition yields results that differ significantly from the predictions of additivity. This phenomenon, termed "brightness matching errors," was largely unexplained as a psychophysical phenomenon until it was realized that the visual system behaves as if it separately and independently assigns brightness values to colored (chromatic) and uncolored (achromatic) components of lights.[2,4] Therefore a distinction between brightness (the chromatic component) and luminance (the achromatic component) has developed, following the discovery of photometric techniques that allow distinctions to be made between the two (see the following discussion).

Brightness matching errors can be demonstrated with experiments that use heterochromatic brightness matching techniques.[2] If a red light is matched in subjective brightness to a green light, subsequent addition of 50% of the luminance of the red light to 50% of the luminance of the green light (by use of suitable neutral density filters and optical mixing) will produce a yellow light having a distinctly lower subjective brightness than either the red or green lights that were originally matched to one another. Such failures of Abney's law of additivity are most dramatically demonstrable using spectrally different lights near the threshold of visibility.[4] Failures of additivity at threshold are most pronounced for lights that are widely separated from one another in the visible spectrum. For example, a green light, adjusted to be just barely suprathreshold, can actually be rendered invisible by the addition of a small amount of red light! Conversely, if a red light is attenuated to one half of its threshold value by the insertion of a neutral density filter, the intensity of green light necessary to bring the combination back to visibility is actually greater than 50% of its threshold value, as would be predicted by Abney's law. Such failures of additivity are found to be greatest for complementary pairs of colors, such as red and green or yellow and blue.

Two psychophysical (photometric) techniques have been discovered that can be used to eliminate the additivity errors obtained with heterochromatic brightness matching. One technique uses the adjustment of a heterochromatic bipartite field to a criterion of a minimally distinct border (MDB) separating the two spectrally different lights. The second technique uses heterochromatic flicker photometry, a technique in which the two spectrally different lights to be matched in luminance are flickered in alternation at a constant frequency while the luminance of one of the two is varied to an end point of minimum flicker perception. Although the visual system can perceive achromatic luminance flicker at frequencies exceeding 30 Hz, the critical flicker fusion frequency for the purely chromatic component of flicker is much lower, approximately 10 Hz.[7] By choosing an intermediate frequency of flicker (for example, 15 to 20 Hz), adjustment to a criterion of minimum flicker between two heterochromatic lights matches the achromatic components of the two. Luminance matches made in either of these two ways, minimally distinct border matches or minimum flicker end points of heterochromatic flicker photometry, produce results that essentially obey Abney's law of additivity. Thus if two lights are matched to one another using the minimally distinct border criterion, algebraic addition of their components (x% of one plus 100% minus x% of the other) will produce a third light, which also will have a minimally distinct border when juxtaposed against either of the first two. When either minimally distinct border matching or flicker photometry is used, the relative luminous efficiency function of the visual system differs from that obtained by direct brightness matching as illustrated in Figure 13-13. The two curves being compared in the figure are normalized at 570 nm. When examined in this fashion, the data show that the visual system assigns a greater subjective value for brightness to colored lights toward either end of the visible spectrum. These are the colors (red or blue) that subjectively appear to be the most saturated. Less saturated lights, such as green or yellow, show a lesser degree of difference between subjective brightness and achromatic luminance values obtained by the two alternate methods of heterochromatic brightness matching.

A number of theoretic schemes have been advanced to explain why additivity failures occur for heterochromatic brightness matching but not when the minimally distinct border criterion or minimum flicker criteria are used. One of the more easily understood theories is that advanced by Boynton.[2] He assumed that elements of visual perception exist in two main classes: chromatic and achromatic. The chromatic elements of perception are those that indicate perception of red, yellow, green or blue, whereas the achromatic elements signal the per-

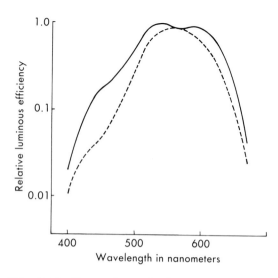

FIG. 13-13 Comparison of relative luminous efficiency function measured by direct brightness matching *(solid curve)* and by flicker photometry or minimally distinct border criterion *(dashed curve)*. Curves have been normalized at 570 nm, which is the wavelength of minimum color saturation. (From Boynton RM: J Opt Soc Am 63:1037, 1973.)

ception of white. A key assumption of the theory is that the elements indicating the perception of chromaticism (brightness) and whiteness (luminance) can respond more or less independently and luminance matching occurs (minimally distinct border is obtained) when the numbers of activated achromatic elements are equal in the two halves of a bipartite field. The reason that a colored field appears to be brighter than its white neighbor when matched by the minimally distinct border criterion is that extra chromatic elements are being activated in the case of the colored light. The excess of activated chromatic elements causes a perception of extra brightness. Figure 13-14 illustrates an experiment comparing heterochromatic brightness matching with minimally distinct border matching. If the subjective brightness of a yellow field is matched to that of a white field, 100 achromatic elements may have been activated on the white side, and 90 white (W) elements and 10 yellow (Y) elements may have been activated on the other. The two fields would appear to be equally bright because the total number of elements active in each is the same. Suppose the experiment is repeated for the matching of white and blue fields, and 100 achromatic elements are matched by the apparent brightness of a combination of 70 achromatic elements with 30 blue (B) elements. If the stimulus hem-

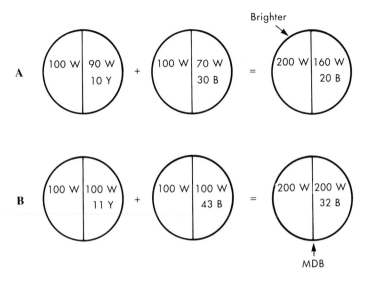

FIG. 13-14   Theoretic scheme to explain how additivity failures occur for heterochromatic brightness matching (**A**) but not for criterion of minimally distinct border (**B**). See text for explanation. (From Boynton, RM: J Opt Soc Am 63:1037, 1973.)

ifields of the two prior results are then superimposed, 200 achromatic elements would now be activated in the left hemifield, but because of an opponent colors cancellation at the retina of blue and yellow elements, a total of only 20 chromatic elements (30 B minus 10 Y) would be activated in conjunction with 160 (90 plus 70) achromatic elements. The result would be a right (blue) hemifield somewhat less in brightness than the left (white) hemifield. This is an example of the failure of additivity of heterochromatic brightness matching.

The theory explains the additivity of minimally distinct border matches by assuming that an equal number of achromatic elements in the two hemifields will be activated when the minimally distinct border criterion is used for matching. In the second half of the figure, matching of yellow and white hemifields is found to produce activation of 100 achromatic elements on the left side and 100 on the right in conjunction with 11 yellow (Y) elements. Although the border is minimally distinct at this end point, because of the extra activation of chromatic elements in the right hemifield it appears to be subjectively brighter. If a similar experiment is done for a minimally distinct border match of white and blue hemifields, 100 achromatic elements would be matched with 100 achromatic (W) elements and 43 blue (B) elements. The sum of these two matching experiments would produce two hemifields that have equal numbers of achromatic elements activated (200

W), but the right blue hemifield would appear subjectively brighter because of its excess of blue elements. The result, however, would be one in which the border was already minimally distinct. Summation for subjective brightness of achromatic and chromatic elements by the visual system explains why, at the minimally distinct border setting, a chromatic field will appear brighter than a white one.

It should be noted that the CIE photopic luminous efficiency curve was experimentally established by means of flicker photometry and that the additivity of luminances predicted by this function is valid, as long as flicker photometry or minimally distinct border matching is used to verify the results.

A neurophysiologic correlate of the human photopic luminosity function (V$_\lambda$)

Lee et al. have studied the responses of *macaque* retinal ganglion cells to stimulation by heterochromatic flicker.[5] The responses of phasic ganglion cells (those cells that respond transiently to changes in luminance and send their axons into the magnocellular layers of the lateral geniculate body) were found to go through a minimum at the relative radiances for equal luminance described by the human photopic luminosity function. The responses were even found to obey the laws of additivity and transitivity that are characteristic of equal luminance heterochromatic flicker photometric matches. Tonic ganglion cells (spectrally opponent cells having tonic re-

Symbols, Constants, and Units Used in Radiometry and Photometry

Units of force

1 dyne = force to accelerate a mass of 1 g at 1 cm/sec^2

1 newton = force to accelerate a mass of 1 kg at 1 m/sec^2

Units of energy

1 erg = 1 dyne cm

1 joule = newton meter = 10^7 ergs

Units of power

1 watt = 1 joule/sec

Units of solid angle

ω = 1 steradian = ¼ π sphere

Equivalents

c = Velocity of light in vacuum

= 2.9976×10^{10} cm/sec

V_m = Velocity of light in medium = $\dfrac{c}{n_m}$ cm/sec

n_m = Refractive index of medium = $\dfrac{c}{v_m}$ cm/sec

v = Frequency of light = $\dfrac{v}{\lambda}$ hertz (Hz)

λ = Wavelength of light = $\dfrac{v}{v}$ nanometers (nm)

h = Planck's constant = 6.624×10^{-27} erg sec

V_λ = Relative photopic luminous efficiency (a dimensionless coefficient)

V'_λ = Relative scotopic luminous efficiency (a dimensionless coefficient)

Units of luminous intensity (I)

candela = lumens/steradian

Units of illuminance (E)

lux (also called the meter candle) = lumens/m^2

foot candle = lumens/square foot

Units of luminance (L)

nit	= candela/m^2
stilb	= candela/cm^2
apostilb	= candela/π m^2 (area of circle of radius 1 m)
footlambert	= candela/π ft^2 (area of circle of radius 1 foot)
lambert	= candela/π cm^2 (area of circle of radius 1 cm)

1 nit = 0.3142 millilambert

1 nit = 0.2919 footlambert

1 lambert = 929 footlambert

1 lambert = 10,000 apostilb

1 lambert = 0.318 stilb

1 lambert = 3183 nit

Unit of retinal illuminance

troland = illuminance at retina for an eye viewing a surface with a luminance of 1 candela/m^2 through an artificial pupil with an area of 1 mm^2

sponses to spectrally shifting stimulus pairs and sending their axons to the parvocellular layers of the lateral geniculate body) could not be correlated with the V_λ function in any way. Noting that behavioral measures of photopic luimous efficiency in the macaque indicate a close identity with the same function in humans, Lee et al. concluded that the phasic, magnocellular ganglion cell system of the primate visual pathway mediates the psychophysical behavior found in heterochromatic flicker photometry.

REFERENCES

1. Boettner EA, Wolter JR: Transmission of the ocular media, Invest Ophthalmol 1:776, 1962.
2. Boynton RM: Implications of the minimally distinct border, J Optical Soc Am 63:1037, 1973.
3. Gaasterland DE: Fundamental aspects of light and lasers for the opthalmologist, in Aron-Rosa D, ed: Pulsed YAG laser surgery, Thorofare, NJ, Charles B. Slack, 1983, pp 11-17.
4. Guth SL, Lodge HR: Heterochromatic additivity, foveal spectral sensitivity, and a new color model, J Optical Soc Am 63:450, 1973.
5. Lee BB, Martin PR, Valberg A: The physiological basis of heterochromatic flicker photometry demonstrated in the ganglion cells of the macaque retina, J Physiol (Lond) 404:323, 1988.
6. Pirie A: Color and solubility of the proteins of human cataracts, Invest Ophthalmol 7:634, 1968.
7. Regan D, Tyler CW: Some dynamic features of colour vision, Vision Res 11:1307, 1971.

GENERAL REFERENCES

Committee on Colorimetry of the Optical Society of America: The science of color, Washington, DC, The Optical Society of America, 1966.

Enoch JM: Physiology, vision, in Sorsby A, ed: Modern ophthalmology, vol 1, New York, Appleton-Century-Crofts, 1963.

Graham CH, ed: Vision and visual perception, New York, John Wiley, 1965.

LeGrand Y: Light, colour and vision, London, Chapman & Hall, 1968.

Padgham CA: Subjective limitations on physical measurements, Philadelphia, Franklin Publishing, 1965.

Pirenne MH: Vision and the eye, 2nd ed, London, Science Paperbacks and Chapman & Hall, 1967.

Wyszecki G, Stiles WS: Color science, New York, John Wiley, 1967.

The Biochemistry of Sensory Transduction in Vertebrate Photoreceptors

JOHN C. SAARI, Ph.D.

The apparent simplicity of the layered neuronal array of the retina has attracted a number of investigators to study sensory transduction and neuronal function in this tissue. An overwhelming literature has developed dealing with the organization, development, and function of the retina, much of it describing a molecular level of inquiry. A review of this burgeoning field is clearly impossible so the more limited topic of photoreceptor cell function and metabolism will serve as the theme of this chapter. Even in this relatively restricted area, enormous advances in our comprehension of retinal metabolism, phototransduction, and regeneration of bleached visual pigment have occurred in recent years. Recombinant DNA methodology has brought about a molecular understanding of the genetic defects in several inherited retinal diseases and conditions and has provided structural information for proteins such as cone visual pigments that have not yet been isolated. The literature is too extensive to allow citation of all pertinent references. Reviews have been cited following the section headings. The interested reader is encouraged to refer to these articles for a more thorough coverage.

CARBOHYDRATE METABOLISM[83,129,181,205]

Visual excitation is the unique function of the retina. Associated with this process are substantial demands for energy to fuel the active transport processes necessary for electrical activity of the retina and to maintain a considerable adenine and guanine nucleotide turnover in the outer segment. Superimposed on these specialized demands for energy are the ATP requirements of other, more common physiologic activities of the retina such as biosynthesis of cellular constituents that must be replaced as a result of turnover, synthesis of neurotransmitters, axonal transport, and photoreceptor outer segment renewal.

Early studies revealed an unusually active metabolism for retinal tissue. Rat retinas consumed oxygen at a rate substantially higher than that observed in any other tissue.[199] Subsequent studies confirmed that observation, placing the rate of oxygen utilization at 1.5 μmol/mg dry wt/hr, approximately twice that of brain cortex.[205] About 70% of the oxygen uptake is due to glucose oxidation by the classical pathways of glycolysis, the tricarboxylic cycle, and oxidative phosphorylation,[38] with oxidation of other endogenous substrates (e.g., pyruvate-lactate, or glutamine-glutamate) accounting for the remainder. Glucose is clearly the major fuel for retinal metabolism.

Despite the high rate of respiration in retinal tissue, the oxidation of pyruvate in mitochon-

ACKNOWLEDGMENT

The author is grateful for helpful discussions with Drs. James Hurley, James Kinyoun, Ann Milam and Robert Rodieck, and for preparation of the figures and manuscript by Gregory Garwin and Julie Seng, respectively. Research in the author's laboratory was supported in part by grants from the National Institutes of Health (EY02317, EY01730, EY07031) and by an award from Research to Prevent Blindness, Inc.

dria does not keep pace with pyruvate production from glucose[199] and excess pyruvate is reduced to lactate. Many other tissues, including muscle, heart, kidney, and liver, show lactate accumulation only under conditions sufficiently anaerobic to reduce mitochondrial metabolism and release inhibition of glycolysis by the presence of abundant oxygen (a phenomenon known as the Pasteur effect). Retina, in common with embryonic tissues, leukocytes, brain, and some tumors, shows a net accumulation of lactate even when it is adequately supplied with oxygen.

Oxidation of glucose by the pentose phosphate pathway accounts for approximately 23% of its utilization, although the pathway has a capacity for considerably more than this under oxidative stress.[205] This pathway supplies pentoses for synthesis of nucleotides and is a major source of NADPH in the cell.[184] Reduction of all-*trans*-retinaldehyde in the photoreceptor outer segments requires NADPH, emphasizing the importance of this pathway in retinal metabolism[75,77] (see the section entitled Visual Cycle).

About half of the in vitro respiration and lactate production in adult rabbit retina is attributable to the photoreceptor cells.[38] Recent observations that the glycolytic enzyme glyceraldehyde phosphate dehydrogenase is abundant in rod outer segment preparations[140] suggests that anaerobic glycolysis in the outer segment may supply some of the energy requirements of phototransduction. Quantitative microanalyses of the distribution of the activities of mitochondrial enzymes or cytoplasmic glycolytic enzymes at various depths in the retina of rabbit and monkey have been made.[131] These, together with early electron-microscopic examinations, revealed the dense accumulation of mitochondria in the ellipsoid region of photoreceptor cells and confirmed that the photoreceptors are largely responsible for the high rate of metabolism of the retina.

A limited amount of glycogen is present in retinal tissue, localized primarily in Müller cells.[113] It is somewhat less abundant in the highly vascularized rat, mouse, and human retinas than in the poorly vascularized retinas of rabbit and guinea pig. Müller cells also appear to contain glucose-6-phosphatase activity[117] and are likely to be able to convert their stores of glycogen to glucose for use by neighboring neuronal cells. Glycogenolysis in brain cortical glial cells is stimulated by vasoactive intestinal peptide (VIP) and a number of other neurotransmitters.[132] An effector coordinating glycogenolysis in retinal Müller cells with glucose availability has not yet been identified.

The metabolic requirements for visual excitation were determined in early studies employing in vitro conditions that allow measurement of a counterpart of the a-wave of the electroretinogram (ERG).[6,181] In the absence of glucose in the external medium endogenous energy stores were insufficient to sustain retinal function, and within approximately 10 minutes the amplitude of the light-evoked electrical response fell to a fraction of the initial amplitude (Fig. 14-1). The loss in electrical response was even more rapid when the preparation was made anaerobic by substituting nitrogen as the gas phase. After brief oxygen deprivation, virtually complete recovery of the amplitude of the electrical response was generally observed. These studies emphasize that the retina does not possess a large store of glycogen, that it cannot function anaerobically even when abundantly supplied with glucose, and that it does not require insulin for glucose uptake.[204,205]

Glucose and oxygen metabolized by the inner layers of the retina are largely supplied by the retinal capillaries, whereas photoreceptor cells receive glucose and oxygen from the choroidal circulation. The high metabolic rate of the

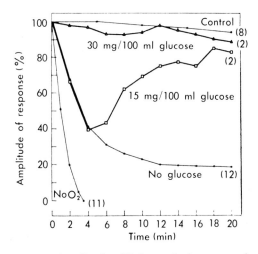

FIG. 14-1 Amplitude of light-evoked compound action potentials recorded from optic nerve and plotted relative to control response recorded at zero time. Various curves show change in amplitude during incubation in control medium and in media containing normal glucose but no O_2; normal O_2 but no glucose; normal O_2 and two intermediate levels of glucose as shown. (With permission of Ames A III: Studies with isolated retina in Graymore CN, ed: Biochemistry of the retina, London, 1965, copyright by Academic Press, Inc [London], Ltd.)

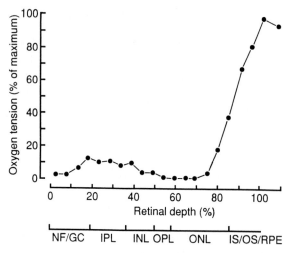

FIG. 14-2   Profile of PO_2 as a function of retinal depth in a dark-adapted cat retina obtained by penetration with an O_2 microelectrode. Under normoxic conditions the PO_2 at the choroid (100% retinal depth) is 69 $\pm$ 19 mmHg (mean and SD, 135 measurements). The lower abscissa shows the approximate position of the retinal layers: NF/GC, nerve fiber/ganglion cell; IPL, inner plexiform layer; INL, inner nuclear layer; OPL, outer plexiform layer; IS/OS/RPE, inner segment/outer segment/retinal pigment epithelium. (Modified with permission, from Linsenmeier RA: J Physiol (Lond) 88:521, 1986.)

photoreceptors and the clusters of mitochondria in the inner segment predict a steep gradient in oxygen tension (PO_2) between the retinal pigment epithelium and the inner segments. Recent studies (Fig. 14-2) employing double-barreled microelectrodes capable of measuring oxygen tension and electrical responses have confirmed the existence of this gradient[127] and suggest that the inner segments experience a PO_2 of less than 5 mm Hg in the dark, a mild hypoxia.[182] Perhaps as a consequence, human dark adaptation is particularly sensitive to effects of hypoxia, with delays observable at PO_2 values experienced at an elevation of 5000 feet.[182] This finding also suggests that photoreceptor cells will be highly susceptible to disease processes that affect delivery of oxygen to the retina, such as retinal detachments, choroidal ischemia, or increased intraocular pressure.[127,182,209]

The changes in metabolism caused by light have been the subject of intense interest. Recent studies in cat retina have demonstrated that illumination causes an approximate 50% reduction in oxygen consumption,[126] in keeping with earlier results[104,181,221] (Fig. 14-2). Recent biophysical and biochemical studies lead to a complex picture of the known changes that occur in energy metabolism following illumination.

These processes are discussed in more detail in the section dealing with phototransduction but may be summarized here. The maintenance of ionic gradients across cell membranes requires a constant utilization of ATP, and it is likely that a major function of the ellipsoid mitochondria is to provide ATP for the cation pumping in the visual cell associated with the maintenance of the dark current. Light is known to suppress the dark current, suggesting that energy demand should be diminished following illumination. However, light also induces turnover of cGMP in the outer segment, hydrolysis of GTP, and phosphorylation of rhodopsin, processes that ultimately consume ATP. It appears that the reduced demand for ATP by ion pumps is large relative to the light-induced turnover of guanine and adenine nucleotides in the photoreceptor outer segment and the energetic requirements of neural signal processing.

VISUAL PIGMENTS[8,54,65,142]

Visual pigments are distinguished by their spectral properties. An example of the absorption spectrum of rhodopsin dissolved in detergent is shown in Figure 14-3. The light-sensitive pigments of the human retina[198] include rhodopsin, the well-known rod pigment employed for dim light vision, and three cone pigments responsible for color discrimination and normal daylight

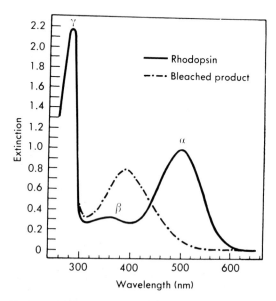

FIG. 14-3   Absorption spectrum of rhodopsin from bullfrog retinas in solution in 2% aqueous digitonin at pH 5.6 showing three absorption bands. Bleaching replaces the α and β bands with absorption spectrum of retinal, but alters the protein γ band only very slightly. (From Wald G: J Opt Soc Am 41:949, 1951.)

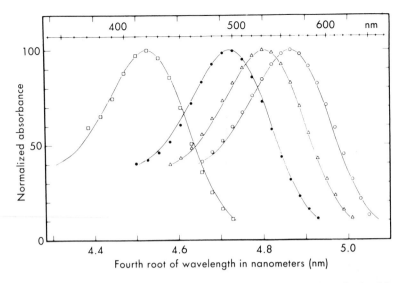

FIG. 14-4 Mean absorbance spectra of the four human visual pigments obtained by micro-spectrophotometry. *Squares*, blue-sensitive cones (λ_{max} = 419 nm); *filled circles*, rods (λ_{max} = 496 nm); *triangles*, green-sensitive cones (λ_{max} = 531 nm); *open circles*, red-sensitive cones (λ_{max} = 558 nm); *solid lines*, curves calculated using a nomogram. The curves are all exactly the same shape when plotted in this format. Note the more conventional units for the abscissa (nm) at the top of the graph. (From Dartnall HJA, Bowmaker JK, Mollon JD: Microspectrophotometry of human photoreceptors, in Mollon JD, Sharpe LT, eds: Colour vision, 1983, copyright by Academic Press, Inc. [London] Ltd.)

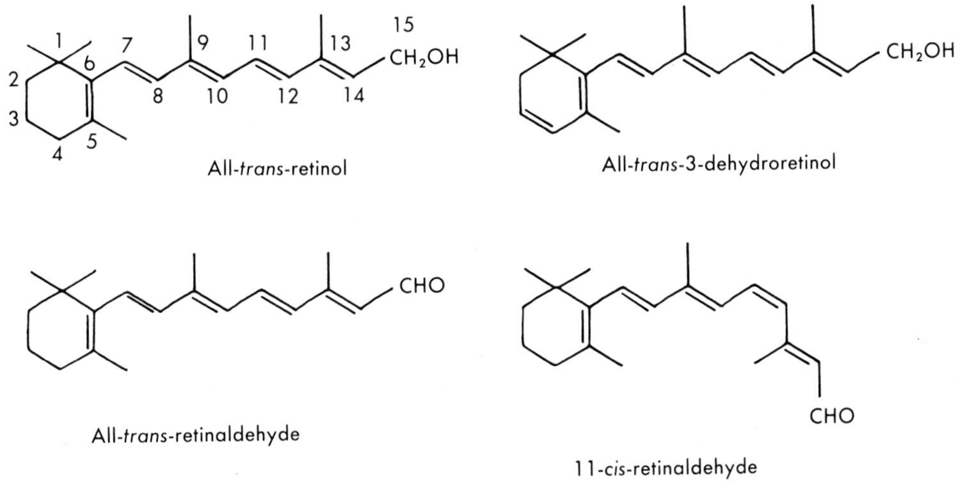

FIG. 14-5 Vitamin A and structurally related compounds are now classified as retinoids. The figure gives the structures of retinoids important in visual physiology.

vision (Fig. 14-4). All known visual pigments consist of an apo-protein, opsin, to which is attached the chromophore molecule 11-*cis*-retinaldehyde, derived from vitamin A_1, or 11-*cis*-3-dehydroretinaldehyde, derived from vitamin A_2 (Fig. 14-5). The latter is a constituent of porphyropsins that serve as visual pigments in some fish and amphibians. The retinas of these species are apparently able to convert retinaldehyde to the 3-dehydro derivative. This capacity may be regulated largely by the properties of the light available in the natural environment and in other species may be under hormonal control.[31]

The curve reflecting the spectral sensitivity of the dark-adapted human matches almost perfectly the absorption spectrum of rhodopsin (Fig. 14-6) with peak sensitivity occurring at 500 nm, providing the appropriate corrections are made for partial absorption of shorter wavelengths by the slightly yellow human lens. The photopic luminosity curve of normal trichromats (persons with normal color vision) matches reasonably well the composite absorption spectrum representing the three cone pigments (Fig. 14-7).

A detailed picture of the structure and orientation of rhodopsin with respect to the disc membrane has emerged from studies over the last decade. Early biochemical studies had established that the pigment is an integral membrane protein associated with the discs of the photoreceptor outer segment.[8,54] It is now apparent that rhodopsin is asymmetrically oriented across the phospholipid bilayer of the disc membrane (Figs. 14-8 and 14-9).[71] A considerable amount of rhodopsin is within the hydrophobic portion of the membrane, consistent with results from x-ray and neutron diffraction analyses[34] and thus interacts directly with phos-

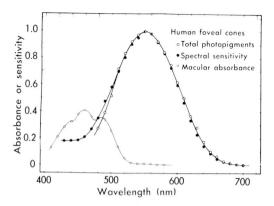

FIG. 14-7 Difference spectrum of total photopigments of human fovea (average of five), compared with spectral sensitivity of foveal vision, measured as at level of cones. To obtain the latter function average photopic luminosity curve was converted to quantum basis and corrected for ocular and macular transmission. Spectrum of a human macula is shown at left. Corrected luminosity curve agrees with difference spectrum of foveal photopigments down to about 510 nm. Below this wavelength difference spectrum falls off, owing to formation of colored products of bleaching. (From Wald G, Brown PK: Cold Spring Harbor Symp Quant Biol 30:345, 1965.)

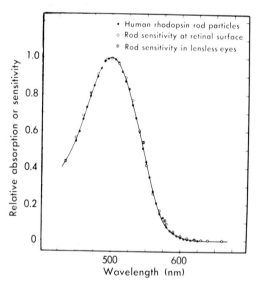

FIG. 14-6   Absorption spectrum of human rhodopsin, measured in a suspension of rod outer segments, compared with the spectral sensitivity of human rod vision, measured as at the retinal surface. The latter data involve either average scotopic luminosity corrected for ocular transmission or uncorrected measurements of spectral sensitivity of rod vision in an aphakic (lensless) eye. (From Wald G, Brown PK: Cold Spring Harbor Symp Quant Biol 30:345, 1965.)

pholipids of the membrane.[3] The amino acid sequence of the protein has been completed, allowing detailed structure-function studies to be pursued.[89,145,152] Secondary structure algorithms predict that the polypeptide chain traverses the membrane bilayer in seven α-helical segments (Fig. 14-8)[10,54] generating three cytoplasmic and three intradiscal loops. A fourth, putative cytoplasmic loop is generated by insertion of the palmitoyl residues of cysteines 322 and 323 into the lipid bilayer[152] (Fig. 14-8). The cytoplasmic loops are associated with binding of transducin (discussed in the section entitled Phototransduction), since synthetic peptides corresponding to these regions block the interaction[107] and deletion or modification of key amino acids by mutagenesis results in a visual pigment that can be bleached but that fails to activate transducin.[69] The two glycosylation sites are close to the amino terminus, localized to the intradiscal side of the membrane, whereas the carboxyl terminus, the site of multiple, reversible phosphorylation, is on the cytoplasmic side of the disc membrane.

The chromophore, 11-cis-retinaldehyde, is located close to the center of the bilayer with the long axis of the π-electron system oriented approximately parallel to the plane of the disc

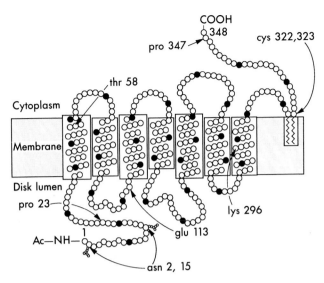

FIG. 14-8 Predicted orientation of the linear sequence of opsin with respect to the disc membrane. Each circle in the string represents an amino acid in the sequence of bovine opsin; darkened circles indicate every tenth residue. Seven α-helical regions (shown in boxes) of the polypeptide are predicted to traverse the membrane resulting in three cytoplasmic and three intradiscal loops. A putative fourth cytoplasmic loop results from association of palmitoylated cysteines 322 and 323 with the membrane. The two palmitoyl residues are depicted by wavy lines. The amino terminal residue (#1) is depicted with its acetyl modification (Ac). Oligosaccharide chains are shown on asparagines 2 and 15. Amino acid residues with functional significance are denoted with arrows: lysine 296, site of attachment of 11-*cis*-retinaldehyde; glutamate 113, counterion for the charged Schiff base; proline 23, threonine 58, and proline 347, sites of known point mutations in autosomal dominant retinitis pigmentosa, as of January, 1991.[23]

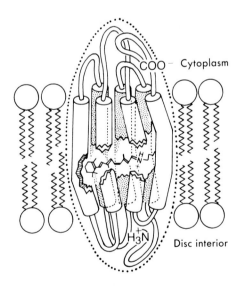

FIG. 14-9 Depiction of rhodopsin and its topology with respect to the disc membrane. Helical regions are likely to surround the 11-*cis*-retinaldehyde chromophore. Phospholipids are depicted as circles with 2 wavy lines. (Modified from Dratz EA, Hargrave PA: Trends Biochem Sci 8:128, 1983.)

membrane.[186] Although a three-dimensional structure for rhodopsin is not available, it is likely that the transmembrane helices surround the chromophore, an orientation that has been observed in bacteriorhodopsin[92] (Fig. 14-9). In rhodopsin and probably all other visual pigments the chromophore is covalently linked to a lysine (lysine 269 in bovine rhodopsin) as a protonated Schiff base (Fig. 14-10).[30,61] Systematic conversion of each negatively charged amino acid within the putative transmembrane spanning regions to its neutral amide (i.e., aspartate to asparagine or glutamate to glutamine) demonstrated that the counterion for the positively charged, protonated Schiff base is provided by the carboxylate of glutamate 113[143,176,219] (Fig. 14-10). Schiff base formation and protonation account for a portion of the bathochromic spectral shift observed when 11-*cis*-retinaldehyde interacts with opsin (380 nm → 440 nm). An additional component of the bathochromic shift is believed to result from a perturbation of the π-electron system in 11-*cis*-retinaldehyde by a polar or polarizable group of the protein (440

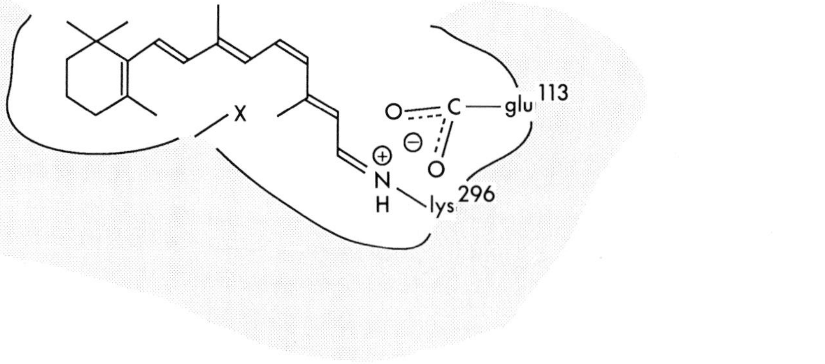

FIG. 14-10   A depiction of the 11-*cis*-retinaldehyde-binding site of rhodopsin. Regions of protein structures forming a pocket are represented by shading. All known visual pigments are composed of 11-*cis*-retinaldehyde (or the 3-dehydro derivative) covalently linked to a protein by Schiff base formation. In bovine rhodopsin the Schiff base involves condensation of the ε-amino group of lysine (lys) 296 and the aldehyde of 11-*cis*-retinaldehyde. The absorption maximum of a visual pigment results, in part, from protonation of the Schiff base. The counter ion is provided by glutamate (glu) 113. The absorption maximum is further adjusted by interaction of a polar or polarizable group from the protein (−X) with the π-electron system of the chromophore. This model can account for the wide variation in spectral sensitivity observed in visual pigments.

nm → 500 nm for bovine rhodopsin).[144] The mutagenesis studies mentioned above ruled out participation of a negatively charged residue predicted from theoretical studies.[94]

Rhodopsin undergoes several postribosomal modifications of its structure. Glycosylation in the endoplasmic reticulum and subsequent processing in the Golgi apparatus produces short oligosaccharide chains on asparagines 2 and 15.[8,119] Enzymatic palmitoylation of cysteines 322 and 323[150,152] produces a hydrophobic domain at this locus and has been postulated to generate a fourth cytoplasmic loop (see Fig. 14-8). Finally, phosphorylation of opsin at several theonines and serines near the carboxyl terminus by rhodopsin kinase generates affinity for arrestin and is important in terminating the photoresponse[110,111,203] (discussed further in the Phototransduction section).

Cone visual pigments, being much less abundant than rod opsin and less stable, were difficult to study using traditional methods of protein isolation and chemistry. The advent of molecular cloning techniques, which can yield structural information for proteins that have never been isolated, has opened inquiry into this problem and provided a wealth of structural information (see also the section on Molecular Genetics). The fundamental assumption made was that rod and cone visual pigments would belong to a family of proteins with similar amino acid sequences. Once a cDNA for rod opsin was obtained,[145,146] human retinal cDNA and genomic libraries could be screened at low stringency to identify clones coding for proteins of similar structure. Sequences encoding three proteins were obtained,[148] and assigned to the red-, green-, and blue-sensitive opsins with criteria that will be described in the Medical Genetics section. The predicted secondary structures for the cone visual pigment opsins are remarkably similar to that already described for rod opsin. Each polypeptide crosses the membrane bilayer seven times, generating the cytoplasmic and extracellular loops seen with rod opsin (see Fig. 14-9). The amino acid sequences for the red- and green-sensitive opsins are very similar, differing only by 4%. The sequence of the blue-sensitive opsin is no more related to the red- and green-sensitive opsins than it is to rod opsin, suggesting that evolutionary divergence of blue-sensitive, long wavelength (red-, green-) sensitive, and rod opsins occurred early, whereas divergence of red- and green-sensitive opsins was relatively recent. The similarity of the three cone visual pigments to one another and to rod opsin points out the likelihood that the fundamental molecular mechanism of phototransduction is the same in these photoreceptors.

BLEACHING OF VISUAL PIGMENTS[9,18,20]

Nineteenth-century physiologists recorded the loss of color (bleaching) that occurs when an isolated retina is exposed to light, assuming the phenomenon to be directly related to vision.[112]

Attempts to understand the process in more detail followed many years later when it was appreciated that bleaching intermediates could be stabilized and characterized at low temperatures.[217,218] The introduction of picosecond spectroscopy (1 psec = 10^{-12} sec) allowed the rates of formation and decay of such transient intermediates as bathorhodopsin to be estimated at room temperature[9] and considerably expanded our knowledge of the bleaching pathway. Although the outline of bleaching intermediates shown in Figure 14-11 would be accepted by most investigators, active research and controversy continues.

The early studies of Wald established that 11-*cis*-retinaldehyde was isomerized to all-*trans*-retinaldehyde at some point in the bleaching process.[196,218] However, modern spectroscopic techniques were needed to establish the configurations of the bleaching intermediates and how rapidly all-*trans*-retinaldehyde was formed. Even though bathorhodopsin forms within 30 psec after the absorption of a photon, resonance Raman spectroscopy demonstrated that a twisted form of all-*trans*-retinaldehyde is already present in this intermediate.[60,61] Thus the only reaction in vision involving light is over in a few picoseconds, and all the remaining reactions are dark, thermally driven processes. Some question remains as to whether bathorhodopsin is really the primary photoproduct, i.e., the first intermediate generated after the absorption of a photon. Hypsorhodopsin, once considered to be an intermediate, has been shown to result from the absorption of two photons.[20] The reader is encouraged to consult the review by Birge[20] for further details.

Interaction of 11-*cis*-retinaldehyde and opsin appears to sensitize the retinoid to photoisomerization, since the quantum efficiency of photoisomerization of rhodopsin is 0.69, whereas that of 11-*cis*-retinaldehyde in methanol is 0.04.[193] It is interesting to note that approximately 32 kcal/mol, or about 60% of the energy of the absorbed photon, is stored in the primary photoproduct as conformational distortion and charge separation.[45,178] Conformational changes of the protein that occur during the formation of subsequent intermediates are driven by this stored energy.

Metarhodopsin II is the last of the intermediates that forms rapidly enough to precede the electrophysiologic response and has been established to couple the absorption of light to the activation of phosphodiesterase (see Liebman[121] for a discussion of the evidence). Hydrolysis of the N-retinylidene-opsin Schiff base occurs at metarhodopsin II or metarhodopsin III.[23]

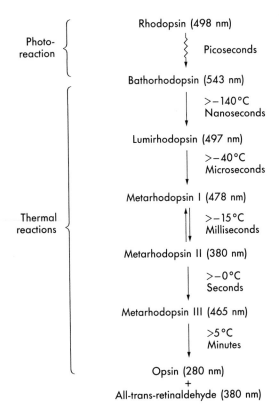

FIG. 14-11 Stages in the bleaching of bovine rhodopsin. The photoreaction is indicated by a wavy line and thermal reactions by straight lines. The times are approximate decay times of intermediates at physiologic temperatures. Temperatures are those employed in trapping intermediates. The wavelengths in parentheses are the absorption maxima of the intermediates. A change in color occurs on going from metarhodopsin I to metarhodopsin II (purple to yellow). Color is lost by reduction of all-*trans*-retinaldehyde to all-*trans*-retinol, a reaction not shown.

The high activation energy necessary to generate R* befits a molecule whose thermal isomerization rate determines the psychophysical "dark noise." The frequency of these thermal events is approximately one per 160 sec in monkey rods, corresponding to a half-life of rhodopsin of 420 years.[17]

PHOTOTRANSDUCTION[12,96,109,115,121,135,159,192,210]

One of the central problems in molecular visual physiology concerns the coupling of the absorption of a photon by rhodopsin in disc membranes with the closure of cation channels in the plasma membrane of the outer segment, a process termed "phototransduction." The results of the last 5 years have provided a satisfying broad outline of both the excitation and recovery phases of this process. Following a statement of the electrophysiologic response of the cell and a brief historical outline, which will be presented to provide continuity for readers familiar with the earlier literature, this elegant mechanism will be described in some detail along with an indication of areas that remain unsettled.

In the dark a potential difference between the inner retina (positive) and the tips of the outer segments (negative) can be measured with extracellular electrodes. The resulting ionic flow, termed the dark current, is carried primarily by Na^+, which enters the outer segment via light-sensitive cation channels in the plasma membrane (Fig. 14-12).[84,85] Sodium returns to the

inner segment via the cytoplasm of the connecting cilium. While the outward positive current of the inner segment is primarily carried by K^+, gradients of K^+ (high inside the cell) and Na^+ (low inside the cell) are maintained by an ATP-dependent Na^+/K^+ pump of the inner segment.[183] The dark current has been calculated to turn over all the cations of the cell every 47 seconds and to consume 5×10^6 ATP molecules $rod^{-1} sec^{-1}$. This process accounts, in part, for the high oxidative metabolism of the retina.

A bleaching flash of light results in a transient decrease in the dark current due to a reduction in the Na^+ conductance (g_{Na}) of the outer segment plasma membrane.[187] Reduction of g_{Na} shifts the transmembrane potential of the pho-

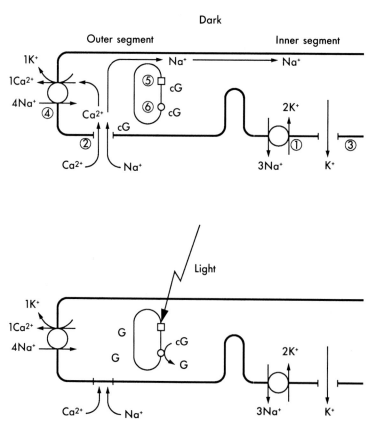

FIG. 14-12 Schematic depicting key events in the rod photoreceptor cell associated with phototransduction. In the dark Na^+ extruded from the inner segment by a Na^+/K^+ pump (1) flows into the outer segment through cation channels (2) in the outer segment that are open when cGMP (cG) is bound. Na^+ returns to the inner segment where the main outward current is carried by K^+ (3). Ca^{2+} also enters the outer segment via the cation channel (2). Its cytoplasmic concentration is kept low by a $Na^+/Ca^{2+}:K^+$ exchanger (4). Following absorption of a photon by rhodopsin (5) a phosphodiesterase (6) is activated that reduces the cytoplasmic concentration of cGMP, allowing a fraction of the cation channels to close. Ca^{2+} extrusion by the exchanger (4) continues even though its entry is blocked by the closed cation channels, producing a transient decrease in cytoplasmic Ca^{2+} concentration following a flash.

toreceptor cell toward the K^+ equilibrium potential (approximately -75 mvolts) and produces a transient hyperpolarization. Photoreceptors respond to light not with action potentials but with graded hyperpolarizations whose magnitude is proportional to the intensity of the illumination over a range of about 3.5 log units. The dynamic range of the photoreceptor is extended to 5 to 6 log units of intensity by processes of adaptation[163,180] (see next section). Passive transmittance of this electrical response to the synaptic terminus of the photoreceptor cell reduces its output of excitatory amino acids, thereby passing on the signal to second-order neurons of the inner retina.[46,139]

Since the disc membrane and the plasma membrane involved in phototransduction are separate in the rod cell, it is apparent that a substance, termed an "internal transmitter," must traverse the physical gap between the two in order to communicate the signal (see Fig. 14-12). An additional component of the response is the enormous amplification of the signal that occurs. Absorption of a single photon stops the flow of approximately 10^6 cations.[135] Analysis of the kinetics of the response of the photoreceptor cells suggests that the process involves several slow steps.[14–16] The identity of the internal transmitter and these slow, thermally driven processes has occupied the attention of vision scientists for many years and has generated a fair share of controversy.

Baylor and Fuortes[13] suggested a model in which light released an internal transmitter whose direct interaction with Na-channels caused their closure. In the dark low cytoplasmic concentrations of internal transmitter would be maintained, allowing a fraction of the channels to be open. Following absorption of a photon, the concentration of the internal transmitter was postulated to increase, closing the channels. Subsequently, a large body of indirect evidence was produced[39,81,84,86,216] showing that Ca^{2+} appeared to have the properties expected of an internal transmitter. A direct test of the calcium hypothesis was not possible until refined electrophysiologic techniques were applied in the mid eighties. Patch clamping techniques then allowed the direct application of putative internal transmitters to the cytoplasmic side of a patch of plasma membrane that was sealed over the end of a recording pipette. Unexpectedly, experiments using this technique clearly demonstrated that Ca^{2+} is not the internal transmitter, since its application had no effect on the conductance of the patch.[64] This result was subsequently borne out by others employing modifications of the patch clamp technique, allowing access to the interior of whole photoreceptors or isolated outer segments or techniques in which the outer segment itself was sucked into the orifice of the recording pipette.[12,135,212]

While it is now clear that Ca^{2+} is not the internal transmitter, it nonetheless plays an important role in phototransduction and its concentration does change following a flash, but in the opposite direction of what was originally proposed. Approximately 10% of the current through the cation channels[212] is carried by Ca^{2+}. This inward flow of Ca^{2+} in the dark is opposed by an outflow mediated by an Na/Ca:K exchanger (see Fig. 14-12). The stoichiometry of this exchanger, originally thought to be 3 Na in for each Ca out,[212] has been determined to be 4 Na in for each Ca and K out.[135] Light-induced closure of cation channels thus results in decreased influx of Ca^{2+}, whereas the Na-mediated efflux of Ca^{2+} continues unabated, producing a transient decrease in cytoplasmic Ca^{2+} concentration.[162] As will be discussed later, the level of cytoplasmic Ca^{2+} determines the activity of guanylate cyclase, the enzyme responsible for synthesis of cGMP and is likely to be involved in light adaptation. Na/Ca:K exchange activity is associated with a 220 kDa protein of the rod outer segment plasma membrane.[42]

While the calcium hypothesis was under investigation, an independent approach yielded evidence for a vigorous nucleotide metabolism in the outer segment that was affected by light. The concentration of guanine nucleotides in the outer segment is about 5 mM and cyclic GMP (cGMP) concentration is about 60 μM,[37,103,206] higher than in other tissues. Studies in the early seventies characterized a cGMP specific phosphodiesterase (Fig. 14-13) of the rod outer segment that was activated by light.[138] An additional protein called transducin (T) was found to act as an intermediary in transmitting the signal from rhodopsin to the phosphodiesterase.[72,73,80] The pathway was completed when patch clamping experiments demonstrated that application of cGMP directly opened the cation channels of the plasma membrane.[64] There is now considerable evidence that cGMP is the internal transmitter for phototransduction. The proposed cGMP model differs from the calcium model in that cGMP concentration is high in the dark, keeping channels open. The signal that a photon has been absorbed by rhodopsin is thus a decrease in cGMP concentration, not an increase (see Fig. 14-12).

The mechanism of phototransduction, as it is

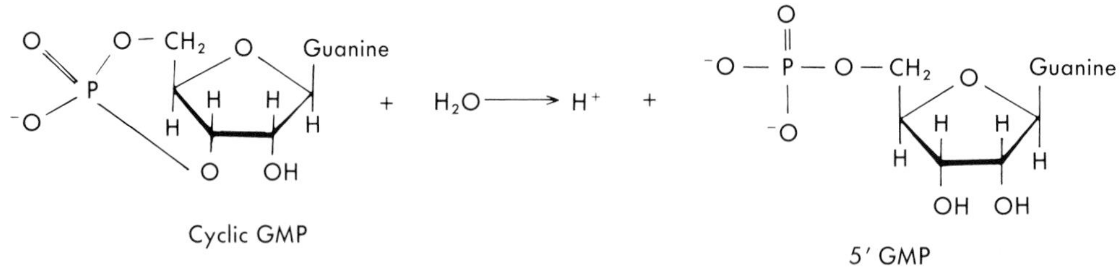

FIG. 14-13 Reaction depicting the hydrolysis of cyclic GMP (cGMP).

now understood, is shown in detail in Figure 14-14. The biochemistry is complex; however, the phototransduction cascade is more easily understood if one appreciates that it involves the successive interconversion of inactive and active states of several proteins, analogous to the activation of glycogenolysis in muscle.[184] Thus light activates rhodopsin, which produces sequential activation of transducin and phosphodiesterase. The enzymatic activity of the latter enzyme decreases the cGMP concentration, allowing channels to close. Recovery following a flash must involve a means of shutting off the processes that had been turned on and restoring the cGMP concentration to a dark level.

At least two of the important proteins of phototransduction are made up of several different subunits in their inactive states and dissociation into smaller complexes is likely to be involved in their activation. Transducin is a complex of three proteins, termed the α-, β-, and γ-subunits ($T_{\alpha,\beta,\gamma}$). The amino acid sequence of each has been determined and cDNAs have been cloned.[63,70,76] The presence of the γ-subunit keeps transducin in an inactive state. Rod phosphodiesterase is larger than transducin and is a tetrameric protein composed of one α-, one β-, and two γ-subunits ($PDE_{\alpha,\beta,\gamma2}$).[11,50,97,137] Again the presence of the γ-subunits keeps the protein in an inactive state.[97]

The biochemistry will now be explained in more detail, emphasizing the role of protein-protein interactions and pointing out steps where amplification occurs (Fig. 14-14). Following absorption of a photon by rhodopsin, meta-rhodopsin II (R*)[59,158] binds to a complex of transducin and GDP ($T_{\alpha\beta\gamma}\cdot GDP$) and promotes the exchange of bound GDP for GTP.[72,73,80] Binding of GTP allows the dissociation of the $\beta\gamma$-subunits, leaving $T_{\alpha}\cdot GTP$ in an active state. R* also dissociates and is free to interact with and activate another transducin molecule. One R*, by completing many rounds of activation, can catalyze the exchange of GTP on about 500

transducins, producing a considerable amplification of the original signal.[72,73] Wald,[194,195] in his early studies, considered the possibility that rhodopsin might be a light-activated enzyme whose function would govern the electrical activity of the photoreceptor. Although R* is not an enzyme in the strict sense of the term, since it does not catalyze a chemical reaction, it does catalyze the rate of exchange of guanine nucleotides on transducin.

Activated transducin ($T_{\alpha}\cdot GTP$) is now free to activate the phosphodiesterase by binding the γ-subunits and releasing their inhibitory constraint.[50] Whether the PDE γ-subunits are actually removed by $T_{\alpha}\cdot GTP$ has not been unequivocally demonstrated. Since there are two γ-subunits per phosphodiesterase, full activation of the enzyme requires two $T_{\alpha}\cdot GTPs$.[74,200,207] A further amplification of the original signal occurs on activation of the phosphodiesterase,[11,214] since each active enzyme molecule can catalyze the hydrolysis of approximately 800 cGMP molecules second^{-1}. Thus the linear amplification through these two steps is a factor of approximately 10^5.

It has been difficult to measure a decrease in cGMP concentrations in retina and photoreceptor cells in response to a flash. At low Ca^{2+} levels, which result in elevated cGMP levels, a light-mediated decrease in cGMP concentration that preceded the changes in membrane conductance was noted with frog and mammalian photoreceptors.[22,47] It is now appreciated that much of the cGMP of the outer segment is bound to proteins—e.g., the noncatalytic binding sites of phosphodiesterase[79,208]—reducing the level of free cGMP from an apparent 60 μM to less than 10 μM.[211]

Each of the three proteins discussed thus far is associated with the disc membrane: rhodopsin as an integral membrane protein, and transducin and phosphodiesterase as peripheral membrane proteins. Following absorption of light, R* activates each transducin it encounters

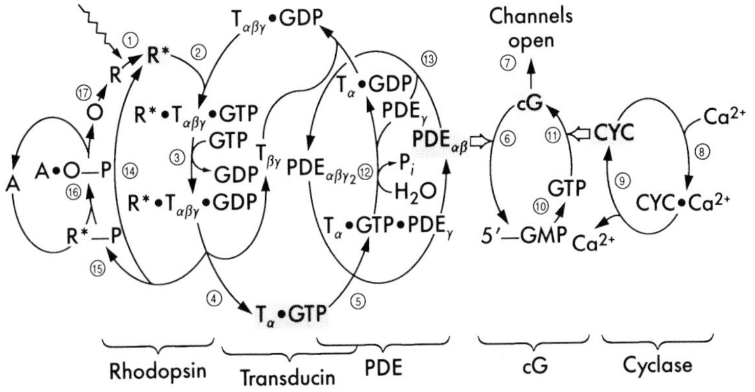

FIG. 14-14 Biochemical events in the photoreceptor outer segment linking photon absorption and cation channel closure. The schematic is organized as a set of cycles in which species (denoted in brackets below) alternate between active (*shaded*) and inactive states. Events associated with excitation (channel closure) and recovery (channel opening) are depicted. *Activation Reactions. 1*, Absorption of a photon by rhodopsin generates metarhodopsin II (R*). *2*, Collision of R* with inactive transducin induces *3*, exchange of bound GDP for GTP by transducin. *4*, R* and the $\beta\gamma$-subunits of transducin dissociate, leaving the active α-subunit with bound GTP. *5*, The active α-subunit of transducin removes an inhibitory γ-subunit from phosphodiesterase. *6*, The enzymatic activity of PDE hydrolyzes cyclic GMP to 5'-GMP. *7*, The cation channel is open when cyclic GMP is bound and closes in its absence. Lowering the cyclic GMP concentration by active phosphodiesterase results in a larger proportion of closed channels. *8*, Calcium complexes with guanylate cyclase, producing an inactive enzyme. *Recovery Reactions. 9*, Lowering of the free calcium concentration results in its dissociation from guanylate cyclase and activation of the enzyme. *10*, 5'-GMP is converted to GTP in several enzymatic steps. *11*, Activated guanylate cyclase converts GTP to cyclic GMP. *12*, An intrinsic GTPase activity of transducin hydroloyzes bound GTP to bound GDP, releasing the phosphodiesterase γ-subunit. *13*, The γ-subunit of phosphodiesterase binds to the α,β-subunits, inactivating the phosphodiesterase. R* either undergoes additional rounds of transducin activation, *14*, or, *15*, is phosphorylated by rhodopsin kinase. *16*, Phosphorylated opsin complexes with arrestin. *17*, Regeneration of rhodopsin. Abbreviations used are cG, cyclic 3',5' guanosine monophosphate; CYC, guanylate cyclase; O, opsin; PDE, phosphodiesterase; P_i, inorganic phosphate; R, rhodopsin; R*, metarhodopsin II; T, transducin.

in its random, diffusional walk within the plane of the disc membrane.[121,123,192,214] Activated transducin, in turn, activates the phosphodiesterase molecules it encounters on the membrane surface. Rhodopsin has been demonstrated to undergo rotational and translational brownian diffusion in the disc membrane.[120,160]

The focus of this cascade of reactions is the cation channel in the plasma membrane of the outer segments, which must close in response to photon absorption. Electrophysiologic evidence indicates that cGMP interacts directly with cation channels, keeping them open. Binding of cGMP is cooperative with a Hill coefficient of approximately 2.5 and an apparent $K_{1/2}$ of 15 to 45 μM, depending on the species.[135,212] Only a small fraction of the channels is estimated to be open in the dark. A reduction in cGMP levels in the cytoplasm of the outer segment would result

in its dissociation from binding sites on the channel and an additional increment of the channels would close. Closure of the channels represents the final stage of gain in phototransduction, since each channel allows the flow of approximately 10^4 Na^+ sec^{-1}. Water-soluble cGMP thus bridges the gap between the disc and plasma membrane systems and is the internal transmitter. The initial signal is enormously amplified by the catalytic properties of R*, $PDE_{\alpha\beta}$, and the flux of the cation channel.

Several laboratories attacked the problem of defining the molecular structure of the cGMP-sensitive cation channel in the mid eighties. Kaupp's laboratory was successful in purifying a protein with a subunit molecular mass of 63 kDa that displayed channel activity on reconstitution in liposomes except for a lack of inhibition by Diltiazem.[42,44,88] Based on a partial amino acid sequence obtained from this preparation, oligonucleotide probes were prepared and used to search for a hybridizing cDNA in a library derived from retinal mRNA. Subsequent cloning and sequencing of the cDNA revealed that it encoded a protein whose sequence contained several typical membrane-spanning α-helical segments and a region similar in sequence to other cGMP binding proteins.[102] Expression of the cDNA in *Xenopus* ococytes generated cGMP-sensitive cation channel activity with properties similar to those reported for membrane patches. Recent reports of the isolation of an 80 kDa subunit that demonstrates channel activity and Diltiazem inhibition suggests that the cloned cDNA may encode a truncated subunit of the channel.[98] The cGMP-gated channel of rod outer segments belongs to a superfamily of ion channels that includes the voltage-gated NA^+, K^+, and Ca^{2+} channels.[99] It is also interesting to note that a cAMP-gated ion channel of olfactory neurons is structurally related to the cGMP-gated channel of rod outer segments.[51]

Restoration of the dark condition following a flash involves inactivating those active species generated in response to the flash and resynthesizing dark levels of cGMP. Activated transducin ($T_\alpha \cdot GTP$) is capable of turning itself off by virtue of an intrinsic GTPase activity of the protein.[159,214] Thus $T_\alpha \cdot GTP$ is converted to $T_\alpha \cdot GDP$, a complex that no longer has an affinity for the inhibitory γ-subunits of PDE (see Fig. 14-14). The released subunits reassociate with $PDE_{\alpha\beta}$, returning it to its inactive dark state. In a similar fashion $T_\alpha \cdot GDP$ will now avidly bind its $\beta\gamma$-subunits, returning it to the dark state.

R* is inactivated in a complex process involving its phosphorylation by rhodopsin kinase,[110] an enzyme that transfers phosphate from ATP to 7 to 8 seryl residues near the C-terminus of rhodopsin.[203] Phosphorylated opsin is avidly bound by an additional protein called arrestin (or 48 K, or S-antigen), preventing it from undergoing further rounds of transducin activation.[111,122,123,202,222] The sequence of events involving dissociation of all-*trans*-retinaldehyde, binding of arrestin and its eventual release, the hydrolysis of phosphate by protein phosphatase 2A,[155] and regeneration of rhodopsin has not been unequivocally determined. The enzymatic processing of retinoids required for regeneration of rhodopsin is discussed in more detail in the section entitled Visual Cycle.

Synthesis of cGMP is carried out by guanylate cyclase, an axonemal enzyme[66] that also cycles between active and inactive states.[52,106] The effector that determines the state of activity of the enzyme is Ca^{2+}, which as we have seen, decreases in concentration following a flash. Ca^{2+} inhibition of guanylate cyclase is mediated by Ca^{2+}-sensitive protein called "recoverin."[52] The biochemical properties of guanylate cyclase predict that the enzyme will be relatively inactive in the dark when Ca^{2+} levels are elevated. However, cation channel closure during the phase of falling cGMP concentration will also decrease the Ca^{2+} concentration, as discussed earlier, relieve inhibition of guanylate cyclase, and result in cGMP synthesis. Thus both guanylate cyclase and phosphodiesterase should be partially active for a brief time, generating a futile cycle. This scenario is likely to explain results obtained with whole retina indicating that cGMP turnover (hydrolysis and resynthesis) increases dramatically following a flash.[82]

While phototransduction in cones has not been studied as thoroughly as in rods, several findings suggest the process is very similar in the two types of photoreceptors. Electrophysiologic studies with fish and mammalian cones have demonstrated cGMP-sensitive channels that respond similarly to those of rods.[90,118] Isozymes of phosphodiesterase[78,87] and transducin[116] have been detected in cones with properties similar to their rod counterparts. Cone opsins have conserved sequences in regions known to be associated with function (e.g., phosphorylation).[148] However, cones are about two orders of magnitude less sensitive and respond to a flash more rapidly than rods, allowing them to function at higher levels of illumination.[12] Biochemical studies of the enzymes of cone phototransduction have been pursued with the aim of providing a molecular explanation for the noted differences in the photoresponses of the two types of photoreceptors. cDNA for a human cone transducin T_α has been cloned and found to encode a protein 78% homologous to rod T_α.[116,128] A bovine cone phosphodiesterase has been isolated and found to differ from the rod enzyme in subunit size and composition, to bind about tenfold more cGMP than the rod enzyme and to require only 1/60 as much rod transducin for half maximal activation.[78] Though interesting, these differences do not explain the differences in rod and cone photoresponses in vivo.

LIGHT ADAPTATION[62,163]

The visual system is able to adjust the sensitivity of its response to the ambient illumination, enabling humans to detect contrast over an enormous range of about 10 log units of intensity.[180] This phenomenon of background adaptation is distinguished from bleaching adaptation by the

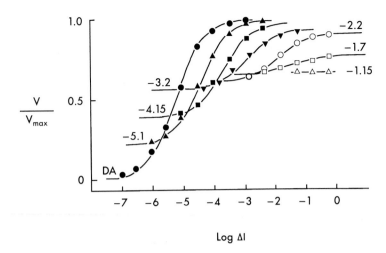

Log ΔI

FIG. 14-15 Background adaptation of an isolated gecko rod photoreceptor. The fractional voltage response (V/V_{max}) is shown as a function of the stimulus flash intensity (ΔI) at several background intensities. As the intensity of the background light increases (numbers on the curves are the logs of the intensity of the background light; DA, dark adapted), the response to a flash is attenuated and the midpoint shifted to a higher intensity. The dynamic range of the photoreceptor is shifted from approximately 3 log units of stimulus intensity to approximately 7. (Modified with permission, from Kleinschmidt J, Dowling JE, J Physiol (Lond) 66:717, 1975.)

rapidity of its onset and by the low levels of illumination at which it occurs.[165,180] It is generally accepted that mechanisms at several levels of organization are involved in background adaptation.[165,166] This topic is covered in detail in Chapter 16 and remarks here will be directed toward recent results that point toward a molecular mechanism for the portion of the process that occurs in rod photoreceptors. Although it has been well established that isolated rod photoreceptors of lower vertebrates are capable of adaptation,[105] not until recently has a similar process been demonstrated in mammalian rods (for contrasting views see Baylor et al.[17] and Tamura et al.[185]). The molecular mechanisms of adaptation at the photoreceptor level remain sketchy and several processes may be at work within the photoreceptor. Nontheless, recent experiments demonstrate that Ca^{2+} is involved.[62]

Background adaptation involves, in part, decreasing the gain of the response to a flash as the intensity of ambient illumination is increased (Fig. 14-15). Recently it has been shown that introduction of BAPTA, a Ca^{2+} chelator, into the photoreceptor cell or low external Ca^{2+} conditions produce responses that are consistent with a role for the ion in adaptation.[62,133,134,188] Since Ca^{2+} is known to affect the rate at which cGMP

levels recover after a flash (see Phototransduction section), it seems likely that its role in adaptation occurs at this step. Background illumination would decrease the concentration of Ca^{2+} in the outer segment by closing a larger fraction of the cation channels (see Fig. 14-12). The decreased Ca^{2+} would result in an increase in the basal level of cGMP synthesis, resulting in a faster recovery from a flash and a reduced incremental response. While this mechanism is plausible and quantitatively accounts for the kinetics and sensitivity modulation of adapation,[62,68] one can not rule out interaction of Ca^{2+} with other components of the phototransduction cascade.

VISUAL CYCLE[161,167]

The cyclical nature of the bleaching and regeneration of visual pigments was recognized in the early studies of Wald.[194,195] The term "visual" or "regeneration cycle" is currently used to describe the metabolic reactions of vitamin A known to be involved in the regeneration of visual pigment. Collectively vitamin A (all-*trans*-retinol) and structurally related compounds are now called retinoids. Readers of the early literature in this field should note that the retinoid bound to opsin was formally referred to as neo-b retinene and the product of bleaching as all-

trans-retinene.[95] The recommended names for these compounds are 11-*cis*-retinaldehdye and all-*trans*-retinaldehyde, respectively. Structures of retinoids important in the visual cycle are shown in Figure 14-5.

The involvement of photoreceptor and retinal pigment epithelium in the regeneration of bleached visual pigment was implicit in the earliest representation of the visual cycle.[194,195] The flow of retinoids between these two cells during bleaching and dark adaptation, evident in early fluorescence studies,[100] was firmly established by the biochemical studies of Dowling[53] and later of Zimmerman[220] and Bridges.[32] Recent studies have demonstrated that most of the reactions of the mammalian cycle, including the isomerization regenerating the 11-*cis*-configuration, occur in retinal pigment epithelium, establishing a rationale for the observed intercellular retinoid transport.

The known reactions of the mammalian visual cycle and their compartmentation in mammalian retina are shown in Figure 14-16. Each of these reactions has been shown to take place *in vitro*; however, their integration into a cycle has not been unequivocally demonstrated *in vivo*. The cycle begins with the photoisomerization of 11-*cis*-retinaldehyde, bound to opsin, to all-*trans*-retinaldehyde, the event that triggers the electrophysiologic response of the photoreceptor cell to light. All-*trans*-retinaldehyde is reduced to all-*trans*-retinol by a retinol dehydrogenase of the outer segment[197] and never accumulates to any extent, perhaps because of its general toxicity. This dehydrogenase, unlike the soluble alcohol dehydrogenase of retina, is associated with photoreceptor membranes and shows a preference for long-chain aldehydes. Nicotinamide adenine dinucleotide phosphate (NADPH) generated by the pentose cycle ap-

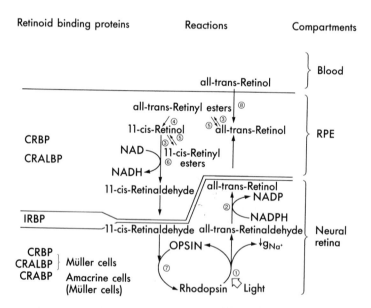

FIG. 14-16 Reactions of the visual cycle in mammalian rod photoreceptors. Reactions 3 to 6 occur within retinal pigment epithelium (RPE), whereas reactions 1, 2, and 7 occur within the rod photoreceptor. There is evidence to suggest that modifications of this pathway occur in amphibian rods and mammalian cones (see text for details). *1*, Absorption of a photon by rhodopsin produces all-*trans*-retinaldehyde, which is reduced to all *trans*-retinol in reaction *2*, is reduced by a dehydrogenase of the outer segment. *3*, Retinol is esterified by lecithin:retinol acyltransferase (LRAT) of RPE. *4*, The 11-*cis*-configuration is generated from all-*trans*-retinyl ester by a "hydroisomerase." *5*, Retinyl esters are hydrolyzed by retinyl ester hydrolase. *6*, 11-*cis*-retinol is oxidized by a specific dehydrogenase of RPE. *7*, 11-*cis*-retinaldehyde and opsin associate nonenyzmatically to regenerate visual pigment. Uptake of plasma retinol by retinal pigment epithelium, *8*, appears to be receptor-mediated. Retinoid-binding proteins and their localizations are depicted on the left. CRBP, cellular retinol-binding protein; CRABP, cellular retinoic acid-binding protein; CRALBP, cellular retinaldehyde-binding protein; IRBP, interphotoreceptor retinoid-binding protein.

pears to be the exclusive reducing agent for retinaldehyde in the photoreceptor.[75,77]

Retinol produced during bleaching diffuses out of the photoreceptor outer segment and moves to the retinal pigment epithelium for further processing. Intercellular transfer of retinol across the subretinal space (or interphotoreceptor matrix) is mediated by a protein of the interphotoreceptor space named interphotoreceptor retinoid-binding protein (IRBP).[2,33,35,114,125] The relatively weak affinity of IRBP for retinoids (K_d = 10^{-6} M),[2] its abundance in interphotoreceptor matrix,[1,33,67,173,175] and its broad specificity suggest a role in which it simply provides binding sites for 11-*cis*-retinol and 11-*cis*-retinaldehyde; transport is likely to occur by aqueous diffusion,[93] driven by the concentration gradients of the two retinoids.[167] At present there is no evidence for receptor-mediated uptake of retinol bound to IRBP. However, recent studies have demonstrated that release of 11-*cis*-retinaldehyde from cultured retinal pigment cells is facilitated by IRBP,[151] suggesting that more than a binding site for retinaldehyde is required.

Esterification of all-*trans*-retinol in the retinal pigment epithelium[108] generates the substrate for the isomerization reaction and perhaps also protects the retina from sustained exposure to high concentrations of retinol, which are well known to affect adversely the stability of membranes. Palmitate and smaller amounts of stearate and oleate[76] are transferred from phosphatidyl choline (lecithin) to retinol to generate retinyl esters in this reaction catalyzed by lecithin: retinol acyl transferase (LRAT).[169,170]

The key isomerization reaction regenerating the 11-*cis*-configuration has recently been shown to involve the conversion of all-*trans*-retinyl ester to 11-*cis*-retinol and the corresponding fatty acid (primarily palmitate).[49,191] In this reaction the energy for isomerization to the 11-*cis*-configuration (4 kcal/mol) is produced by the concerted hydrolysis of the retinyl ester bond.[161] The unique localization of this enzyme in retinal pigment epithelium[19] provides an explanation for the observation that bleached neural retina will regenerate its visual pigment only when placed in apposition to retinal pigment.[112] LRAT of retinal pigment epithelium will readily esterify 11-*cis*-retinol, leading to the buildup of 11-*cis*-retinyl ester in the dark.[169]

Since mammalian retina will not regenerate bleached rod opsin when provided with 11-*cis*-retinol,[156,215] this alcohol must be oxidized to 11-*cis*-retinaldehyde by 11-*cis*-retinol dehydrogenase[124] before leaving the retinal pigment epithelium. There is evidence that cellular retinaldehyde-binding protein (CRALBP), a retinoid-binding protein that binds either 11-*cis*-retinol or 11-*cis*-retinaldehyde,[172] acts as a substrate carrier for this dehydrogenase.[168] Release of 11-*cis*-retinaldehyde from retinal pigment epithelium in vitro has been reported.[151] Its translocation to outer segments is likely to be mediated by IRBP, which has the ability to bind this retinoid as well as all-*trans*-retinol.[2,67,175]

The association of 11-*cis*-retinaldehyde and opsin to regenerate rhodopsin completes the cycle and occurs nonenzymatically in the outer segment. This process remains poorly characterized. It is known that neither phosphorylation of opsin nor binding of arrestin affect the rate of regeneration in vitro.[203]

Several retinoid-binding proteins have been discovered in retina and there is evidence for the participation of three of these in visual cycle reactions. The role of IRBP has already been mentioned in the translocation of retinoids between photoreceptors and retinal pigment epithelium. The role of CRALBP as a substrate carrier protein for 11-*cis*-retinol dehydrogenase of retinal pigment epithelium has also been mentioned. In addition, this protein enhances oxidation of 11-*cis*-retinol relative to esterification in vitro and is likely to play a role in reaction control.[171] Finally, cellular retinol-binding protein (CRBP) is found in retinal pigment epithelium and neural retina[26,174,201] and may be involved in intracellular retinol transport or substrate presentation. The distribution of these proteins is shown in Figure 14-16.

It should be stressed that there are several variations of the visual cycle among vertebrates. Recent evidence[101] that mammalian cones will regenerate with 11-*cis*-retinol suggests that variations of the cycle will be found within the same retina. A dehydrogenase specific for cis-retinols is present in neural retina of frog and toad.[156] Mammalian retinas tested do not have this activity and are unable to use exogenous 11-*cis*-retinol for visual pigment synthesis.[156,215] Retinyl esters are present in relatively large amounts in avian but not mammalian retina.[164]

While the broad outlines of the visual cycle now appear clear, many interesting questions remain. 11-*cis*-retinyl ester hydrolase[21] appears to play a key role in mobilizing stores of 11-*cis*-retinyl esters, yet we know little of this enzyme. Release of 11-*cis*-retinaldehyde from retinal pigment epithelium has been demonstrated[48,151] but remains uncharacterized. Control processes that govern substrate flow at the branch point in the cycle where 11-*cis*-retinol can either be oxidized to 11-*cis*-retinaldehyde or esterified to 11-*cis*-retinyl ester have not been thoroughly examined.[171] The presence of retinoid-binding proteins in Müller cells and the role of these cells in retinoid processing remain enigmatic.[26,33] Uptake of plasma retinol by retinal pigment epithelium is apparently receptor-mediated,[24,25,91,157] but molecular details are lacking.

MEDICAL GENETICS[7,27,56,141,142]

The application of the techniques of molecular biology to inherited retinal degenerations has produced startling advances in our understanding of these conditions. In this section results recently obtained in four inherited retinal conditions will be summarized: color vision defects and autosomal dominant retinitis pigmentosa in humans, and the *rd* and *rds* mutations in mice. These examples have been chosen because they illustrate the power of the methods and involve mutations that affect gene products expressed uniquely in photoreceptor cells.

Color vision defects

Cloning the cDNA encoding bovine rod opsin[145] opened the pathway to a molecular understanding of human color defects and anomalies. The hybridization techniques that led to the cloning of cDNA and genomic DNA coding for human cone visual pigments have already been described in the section dealing with Visual Pigments. Two of the genes identified, which encoded remarkably similar proteins (97% amino acid sequence identity), were localized to the X chromosome and one or the other was absent in protanopes or deuteranopes.[148] By these criteria these two genes were proposed to code for the red and green visual pigments. The third visual pigment gene mapped to chromosome 7 and was assigned to code for the blue-sensitive visual pigment, the only human cone pigment gene that maps to an autosome. A gene cluster on the X chromosome of males with normal color vision was proposed to consist of a tandem array of one red pigment gene and from one to five copies (usually <3) of the green pigment gene (Fig. 14-17).[55]

Attention was then directed toward elucidation of the molecular defects in X linked human color deficiencies.[147] Oligonucleotide probes derived from various regions of normal red and green pigment genes allowed investigators to determine the stoichiometries of the genes and whether rearrangements had occurred. The genomic structures of 25 males with color deficiences of varying severity showed rearrangements and several different genotypes were

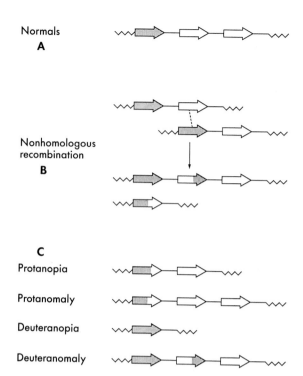

FIG. 14-17 Representation of the cluster of genes on the X-chromosome coding for red- and green-sensitive visual pigments. Structural genes are represented by an arrow (*filled*, red-sensitive; *open*, green-sensitive), connecting regions of DNA by straight lines. Wavy lines represent extraneous DNA. **A**, Males with normal color vision have a single copy of the red-sensitive pigment gene and one or more copies of the green-sensitive pigment gene. One example is shown. **B**, A mechanism for the generation of hybrid genes is shown. The close similarity of the red- and green-sensitive gene sequences results in their pairing. Crossing over leads, in this example, to one chromosome with a normal red-sensitive gene, one red-green hybrid, and a normal green-sensitive gene plus a second chromosome with only a red-green hybrid gene. An individual with the upper chromosome would likely be an anomalous trichromat, whereas an individual with the lower chromosome would likely be a dichromat. **C**, Examples of hybrid genes in a group of males with color deficiencies of varying severity. (Adapted from Nathans et al: Science 232:203, 1986.)

found to produce the same general phenotype. The simplest cases were the six deuteranopes or green-blind individuals (R^+G^-) who possessed a single red pigment gene and no green pigment genes. Six protanopes or red-blind individuals (R^-G^+) were more complicated, as their genotypes were all different (one genotype is shown in Figure 14-17). All had a single copy of a hybrid red-green pigment gene and either no, one, or two copies of green pigment genes.

Examples of anomalous trichromacy also showed clearly that gene rearrangement was the main underlying genetic mechanism. A protanomolous phenotype ($R''G^+$) was associated with one or more normal green pigment genes and a hybrid red-green gene (Fig. 14-17), whereas a deuteranomalous phenotype (R^+G'') was associated with an intact red pigment gene and at least one red-green hybrid gene. The mechanism for production of the hybrid genes was suggested to be recombination following pairing of the closely similar red and green pigment genes (nonhomologous recombination)[147] (Fig. 14-17). This mechanism predicts a family of hybrid genes in color-defective individuals and provides an interesting explanation for the psychophysical observation that five deuteroanopes produced different anomolous matches.[4,5]

The hypothesis presented in these elegant studies will require modification since it is not in accord with some psychophysical data.[149] Nonetheless, it has already stimulated additional research, and the result is certain to be a more coherent description of color deficiencies at the molecular level. Several interesting questions related to expression of visual pigment genes are also raised by the study: How many of the green pigment genes are active? What determines the cell-specific expression of the visual pigments? If several copies of green genes are transcriptionally active, how is the ratio of red to green visual pigment maintained? In dichromats is the gene for the remaining opsin expressed in cone cells originally programmed for the missing opsin?

Autosomal dominant retinitis pigmentosa (ADRP)

Retinitis pigmentosa encompasses a group of inherited retinal degenerations of varying severity and rapidity of onset.[154] The dominantly inherited form of the disease has a relatively slow progression. Mapping of the defective gene to human chromosome 3q[136] suggested a possible involvement of rhodopsin, since the gene for the rod photopigment maps to the same region of that chromosome. Dryja and coworkers[57,58] employed the polymerase chain reaction to amplify DNA corresponding to each of the four exons of rhodopsin in samples obtained from patients with ADRP. Four different mutations in the rhodopsin gene were found in 27 of the 148 patients examined. Each of the mutations resulted in a single amino acid substitution in res-

idues that are invariant or highly conserved in mammalian opsins, suggesting that an important structural determinant was perturbed. The amino acids mutated are noted by arrows in the two-dimensional display of the opsin sequence (see Fig. 14-8). Continued analysis of additional patients is likely to reveal other point mutations in the opsin sequence that produce the same phenotype. These results are important for genetic counseling of affected individuals, but the mechanism of photoreceptor degeneration in ADRP remains unknown and it remains impossible to predict phenotype from genotype. Substitutions at amino acids 23 and 58 conceivably could disrupt the tertiary structure of rhodopsin, leading to, perhaps, a disc membrane of reduced stability. However, a substitution at the penultimate residue is surprisingly deleterious to photoreceptor integrity. A three-dimensional structure of this protein will be instructive.

Retinal degeneration mutant (rd) mice

This autosomal recessive mutation results in retinal degeneration characterized by early onset and rapid progression. Photoreceptor outer segment abnormalities can be detected by postnatal day 7 and by 28 days photoreceptor degeneration is complete. A candidate gene was identified in early biochemical studies that noted diminished activity of photoreceptor cGMP phosphodiesterase.[179] Cloning strategy relied on the knowledge that the defect mapped to mouse chromosome 5 and appeared to have a primary effect only in photoreceptor cells. Thus a retinal cDNA was identified that was present in normal retina and absent in rd/rd animals and mapped to mouse chromosome 5.[28] The results of an unrelated study were key to identifying the gene product, as the candidate cDNA was found to have an amino acid sequence that was 93% identical to that of the β-subunit of bovine cGMP phosphodiesterase.[29] Elevated cGMP levels are present in the rd mice retinas, and an increased cGMP level produced experimentally by a phosphodiesterase inhibitor has been shown to mimic the disease by causing rod death in vitro.[130] The mechanism of cGMP toxicity has not been determined but may be associated with the metabolic demands that result from the increased proportion of open cation channels (see the section on Phototransduction).

Retinal degeneration, slow (rds) mutant mice

This autosomal recessive condition is characterized by a slow, progressive degeneration of the retina. However, aberrant photoreceptor cell maturation is evident as early as 14 days post-natal, since outer segments fail to appear from the cilium extending from the inner segments.[177] Cohen[36] noted an "ability to form, but not retain, membranes associated with the photoreceptor cilium." The strategy used to localize the molecular defect of this condition was based on prior knowledge that the defect was localized to mouse chromosome 17 and was expressed exclusively in photoreceptors.[189] The investigators first employed the *rd/rd* mutation in mice to generate photoreceptorless animals and screened for a cDNA that was present in normals and absent in older *rd/rd* animals. One of the photoreceptor cDNAS obtained was localized to chromosome 17 and its mRNA was abnormal in size and amount in retinas of *rds* mice. Analysis of its sequence revealed that it encoded a transmembrane protein. The *rds* mutation was determined to result from an insertion of a 10 kilobase segment of extraneous DNA into an exon of the *rds* gene, precluding expression of a normal protein.

A standard method of gaining information about a novel protein if one has only its sequence is to search a protein sequence data base for proteins of similar structure. This approach was not immediately productive, as the sequence of the *rds* gene product did not resemble any known proteins. Subsequently, other investigators, examining an unrelated question, found that the amino acid sequence of bovine peripherin, a structural protein of the outer segment, was 92% identical to that of the mouse *rds* gene product.[40,41] A recent study employing immunocytochemistry demonstrates that the *rds* gene is a glycoprotein associated with outer segment disc membranes.[190] Although the function of peripherin has not yet been determined, this result suggests it plays a role in outer segment assembly or stability.

These studies demonstrate the interplay of multiple approaches and occasional serendipity in identification of defective gene products in the retina. What was apparent from morphologic studies is emphasized by the results of molecular cloning; the photoreceptor cell is delicately poised on a line between health and death and defects in several apparently unrelated gene products result in a common phenotype of photoreceptor cell death. We can anticipate continued excitement in this pursuit as one by one the defects in other inherited ocular conditions are revealed by the application of the techniques of molecular biology.

REFERENCES

1. Adler AJ, Evans CD, Stafford WF III: Molecular properties of bovine interphotoreceptor retinol-binding protein, J Biol Chem 260:4850, 1985.
2. Adler AJ, Martin KJ: Retinol-binding proteins in bovine interphotoreceptor matrix, Biochem Biophys Res Commun 108:1601, 1982.
3. Albert AD, Yeagle PL: Phospholipid domains in bovine retinal rod outer segment disc membranes, Proc Natl Acad Sci 80:7188, 1983.
4. Alpern M: Color blind color vision, Trends Neurosci 4:131, 1981.
5. Alpern M, Pugh EN Jr: Variation in the action spectrum of erythrolabe among deuteranopes, J Physiol 266:613, 1977.
6. Ames A III: Studies of morphology, chemistry and function in isolated retina, in Graymore CN, ed: Biochemistry of the retina, New York, Academic Press, 1965, p 22.
7. Applebury ML: Insight into blindness, Nature 343:316, 1990.
8. Applebury ML, Hargrave PA: Molecular biology of the visual pigments, Vision Res 26:1881, 1986.
9. Applebury ML, Rentzepis PM: Picosecond spectroscopy of visual pigments, Methods Enzymol 81:354, 1982.
10. Argos P, Ras JKM, Hargrave PA: Structural prediction of membrane-bound proteins, Eur J Biochem 128:565, 1982.
11. Baehr W, Devlin MJ, Applebury ML: Isolation and characterization of cGMP phosphodiesterase from bovine rod outer segments, J Biol Chem 254:11669, 1979.
12. Baylor DA: Photoreceptor signals and vision, Invest Ophthalmol Vis Sci 28:34, 1987.
13. Baylor DA, Fuortes MGF: Electrical responses of single cones in the retina of the turtle, J Physiol 207:77, 1970.
14. Baylor DA, Hodgkin AL: Detection and resolution of visual stimuli by turtle photoreceptors, J Physiol (Lond) 242:163, 1973.
15. Baylor DA, Hodgkin AL: The electrical response of turtle cones to flashes and steps of light, J Physiol (Lond) 242:685, 1974.
16. Baylor DA, Lamb TD, Yau, K-W: The membrane current of single rod outer segments, J Physiol (Lond) 288:589, 1979.
17. Baylor DA, Nunn BJ, Schnapf JL: The photocurrent, noise and spectral sensitivity of rods of the monkey *Macaca fascicularis*, J Physiol (Lond) 357:575, 1984.
18. Becker RS: The visual process: Photophysics and photoisomerization of model visual pigments and the primary reaction, Photochem Photobiol 48:369, 1988.
19. Bernstein PS, Law WC, Rando RR: Isomerization of all-*trans*-retinoids to 11-*cis*-retinoids *in vitro*, Proc Nat'l Acad Sci USA 84:1849, 1987.
20. Birge RR: Nature of the primary photochemical events in rhodopsin and bacteriorhodopsin, Biochim Biophys Acta 1016:293, 1990.
21. Blaner WS, et al: Hydrolysis of 11-*cis*- and all-*trans*-retinyl palmitate by homogenates of human retinal epithelial cells, J Biol Chem 262:53, 1987.
22. Blazynski C, Cohen AI: Rapid decline in cyclic GMP of

rod outer segments of intact frog photoreceptors after illumination, J Biol Chem 261:14142, 1986.

23. Blazynski C, Ostroy SE: Pathways in the hydrolysis of vertebrate rhodopsin, Vision Res 24:459, 1984.

24. Bok D: Autoradiographic studies on the polarity of plasma membrane receptors in retinal pigment epithelial cells, in Hollyfield JG, ed: The structure of the eye, New York, Elsevier North-Holland, 1982, p 248.

25. Bok D, Heller J: Transport of retinol from the blood to the retina: an auto-radiographic study of the pigment epithelial cell surface receptor for plasma retinol-binding protein, Exp Eye Res 22:395, 1976.

26. Bok D, Ong DE, Chytil F: Immunocytochemical localization of cellular retinol-binding protein in the rat retina, Invest Ophthalmol Vis Sci 25:877, 1984.

27. Botstein D: The molecular biology of color vision, Science 232:142, 1986.

28. Bowes C, Danciger M, Kozak CA, et al: Isolation of a candidate cDNA for the gene causing retinal degeneration in the *rd* mouse, Proc Natl Acad Sci USA 86:9722, 1989.

29. Bowes C, Li T, Danciger M, et al: Retinal degeneration in the *rd* mouse is caused by a defect in the beta-subunit of rod cGMP phosphodiesterase, Nature 347:677, 1990.

30. Bownds D: Site of attachment of retinal in rhodopsin, Nature 216:1178, 1967.

31. Bridges CDB: The rhodopsin-porphyropsin visual system, in Dartnall HFA, ed: Handbook of sensory physiology, vol 7/1, New York, Springer-Verlag, 1972, p 417.

32. Bridges CDB: Vitamin A and the role of the pigment epithelium during bleaching and regeneration of rhodopsin in the frog eye, Exp Eye Res 22:435, 1976.

33. Bunt-Milam AH, Saari JC: Immunocytochemical localization of two retinoid-binding protein in vertebrate retina, J Cell Biol 97:703, 1983.

34. Chabre M, Worcester DL: X-ray and neutron diffraction of retinal rod outer segments, Meth Enzymol 81:593, 1982.

35. Chader GJ, Wiggert B, Lai Y-L, et al: Interphotoreceptor retinol-binding protein: a possible role in retinoid transport to the retina, in Osborne N, Chader GJ, eds: Progress in retinal research, vol 2, Oxford, Pergamon Press, 1982, p 163.

36. Cohen AI: Some cytological and initial biochemical observations on photoreceptors in retinas of *rds* mice, Invest Ophthalmol Vis Sci 24:832, 1983.

37. Cohen AI, Hall, IA, Ferrendelli JA: Calcium and cyclic nucleotide regulation in incubated mouse retinas, J Gen Physiol 71:595, 1978.

38. Cohen LH, Noell WK: Glucose metabolism of rabbit retina before and after development of visual function, J Neurochem 5:253, 1960.

39. Cone RA: The internal transmitter model for visual excitation: some quantitative implications, in Langer H, ed: Biochemistry and physiology of the visual pigments, New York, Springer-Verlag, 1973, p 275.

40. Connell G, Boscom R, Molday L, et al: Photoreceptor peripherin is the normal product of the gene responsible for retinal degeneration in the *rds* mouse, Proc Natl Acad Sci USA 88:723, 1991.

41. Connell GJ, Molday RS: Molecular cloning, primary structure, and orientation of the vertebrate photoreceptor cell protein peripherin in the rod outer segment disc membrane, Biochemistry 29:4691, 1990.

42. Cook NJ, Hanke W, Kaupp UB: Identification, purification and functional reconstitution of the cyclic GMP-dependent channel from rod photoreceptors, Proc Natl Acad Sci USA 84:585, 1987.

43. Cook NJ, Kaupp UB: Solubilization, purification and reconstitution of the sodium-calcium exchanger from bovine retinal rod outer segments, J Biol Chem 261:11382, 1988.

44. Cook NJ, Zeilinger C, Koch K-W, et al: Solubilization and functional reconstitution of the cGMP-dependent cation channel from bovine rod outer segments, J Biol Chem 261:17033, 1986.

45. Cooper A: Energy uptake in the first step of visual excitation, Nature 282:531, 1979.

46. Copenhagen DR, Jahr CE: Release of endogenous excitatory amino acids from turtle photoreceptors, Nature 341:537, 1989.

47. Cote RH, et al: Light-induced decreases in cGMP concentration preceded changes in membrane permeability in frog rod photoreceptors, J Biol Chem 259:9635, 1984.

48. Das SR, Ghardwaj N, Gouras P: Synthesis of retinoids by human retinal pigment epithelium and transfer to rod outer segments, Biochem J 2678:201, 1990.

49. Deigner PS, Law WC, Canada FJ, et al: Membranes as the energy source in the endergonic transformation of vitamin A to 11-*cis*-retinol, Science 244:968, 1989.

50. Deterre P, Bigay J, Forquet F, et al: cGMP phosphodiesterase of retinal rods is regulated by two inhibitory subunits, Proc Natl Acad Sci USA 85:2424, 1988.

51. Dhallan RS, Yau K-Y, Schrader KA, et al: Primary structure and functional expression of a cyclic nucleotide-activated channel from olfactory neurons, Nature 347:185, 1990.

52. Dizhoor AM, Ray S, Kumar S, et al: Recoverin, a calcium-sensitive activator of retinal rod guanylate cyclase, Science 251:915, 1991.

53. Dowling JE: Chemistry of visual adaptation in the rat, Nature 163:114, 1960.

54. Dratz EA, Hargrave PA: The structure of rhodopsin and the rod outer segment disc membrane, Trends in Biochem Sci 8:128, 1983.

55. Drummond-Borg M, Deeb SS, Motulsky AG: Molecular patterns of X chromosome-linked color vision genes among 134 men of European ancestry, Proc Natl Acad Sci USA 86:983, 1989.

56. Dryja TP: Deficiencies in sight with the candidate gene approach, Nature 347:614, 1990.

57. Dryja TP, McGee TL, Hahn LB, et al: Mutations within the rhodopsin gene in patients with autosomal dominant retinitis pigmentosa, N Eng J Med 323:1302, 1990.

58. Dryja TP, McGee TL, Reichel EL, et al: A point mutation of the rhodopsin gene in one form of retinitis pigmentosa, Nature 343:364, 1990.

59. Emeis D, Kuhn H, Reichert J, et al: Complex formation between metarhodopsin II and GTP-binding protein in bovine photoreceptor membranes leads to a shift of

the photoproduct equilibrium, FEBS Lett 143:29, 1982.

60. Eyring G, Curry B, Mathies R, et al: Interpretation of the resonance Raman spectrum of bathorhodopsin based on visual pigment analogues, Biochemistry 19:2410, 1979.

61. Eyring G, Mathies R: Resonance Raman studies of bathorhodopsin: evidence for a protonated Schiff base linkage, Proc Natl Acad Sci USA 76:33, 1979.

62. Fain GL, Matthews HR: Calcium and the mechanism of light adaptation in vertebrate photoreceptors, Trends in Neuro Sci 13:378, 1990.

63. Falk JD, Applebury ML: The molecular genetics of photoreceptor cells, in Osborne N, Chader GJ, eds: Progress in retinal research, vol 7, Oxford, Pergamon Press, 1988, pp 89-112.

64. Fesenko EE, Kolensikov SS, Lyubarsky AL: Induction by cyclic GMP of cationic conductance in plasma membrane or retinal rod segment, Nature 313:310, 1985.

65. Findlay JBC, Pappin DC, Elipoulos EE: The primary structure, chemistry and molecular modelling of rhodopsin, in Osborne N, Chader GJ, eds: Progress in retinal research, vol 6, Oxford, Pergamon Press, 1987, pp 63-87.

66. Fleischman D, Denisevich M: Guanylate cyclase of isolated bovine retina rod axonemes, Biochemistry 18:5060, 1979.

67. Fong S-L, Liou GI, Landers RA, et al: Purification and characterization of a retinol-binding glycoprotein synthesized and secreted by bovine neural retina, J Biol Chem 259:6534, 1984.

68. Forti S, Menini A, Rispoli G, et al: Kinetics of phototransduction in retinal rods of the newt *Triturus cristatus,* J Physiol (Lond) 419:265, 1989.

69. Franke RR, Konig B, Sakmar TP, et al: Rhodopsin mutants that bind but fail to activate transducin, Science 250:123, 1990.

70. Fung BK-K: Transducin: structure, function and role in phototransduction, in Osborne NN, Chader GJ, eds: Progress in retinal research vol 7, Oxford, Pergamon Press, 1988, p 151.

71. Fung, BK-K, Hubell WL: Organization of rhodopsin in photoreceptor membranes, II, Transmembrane organization of bovine rhodopsin: evidence from proteolysis and lactoperoxidase-catalyzed iodination of native and reconstituted membranes, Biochemistry 17:4403, 1978.

72. Fung BK-K, Hurley JB, Stryer L: Flow of information in the light-triggered cyclic nucleotide cascade of vision, Proc Natl Acad Sci 78:152, 1981.

73. Fung BK-K, Stryer L: Photolyzed rhodopsin catalyzes the exchange of GTP for bound GDP in retinal rod outer segments, Proc Natl Acad Sci 77:2500, 1980.

74. Fung BK-K, Young JH, Yamane HK, et al: Subunit stoichiometry of retinal rod cGMP phosphodiesterase, Biochemistry 29:2657, 1990.

75. Futterman S: Metabolism of the retina, III, The role of reduced triphosphopyridine nucleotide in the visual cycle, J Biol Chem 238:1145, 1963.

76. Futterman S: Metabolism of the retina, IV, The composition of vitamin A ester synthesized by the retina, J Biol Chem 239:81, 1964.

77. Futterman S, Hendrickson A, Bishop PE, et al: Metabolism of glucose and reduction of retinaldehyde in retinal photoreceptors, J Neurochem 17:149, 1970.

78. Gillespie PG, Beavo JA: Characterization of a bovine cone photoreceptor phosphodiesterase purified by cyclic GMP-Sepharose chromatography, J Biol Chem 263:8133, 1988.

79. Gillespie PG, Beavo JA: cGMP is tightly bound to bovine retinal rod phosphodiesterase, Proc Natl Acad Sci USA 86:4311, 1989.

80. Godchaux W III, Zimmerman WF: Membrane-dependent guanine nucleotide-binding and GTPase activities of soluble protein from bovine rod cell outer segments, J Biol Chem 254:7874, 1979.

81. Gold GH, Korenbrot JI: Light-induced calcium release by intact retinal rods, Proc Natl Acad Sci USA 75:5557, 1980.

82. Goldberg ND, et al: Magnitude of increase in retinal cGMP metabolic flux determined by O^{18} incorporation into nucleotide α-phosphoryls corresponds with intensity of photic stimulation, J Biol Chem 258:9213, 1983.

83. Graymore CN: Biochemistry of the retina, in Graymore CN, ed: Biochemistry of the retina, New York, Academic Press, 1970, p 645.

84. Hagins WA: The visual process: excitatory mechanisms in the primary receptor cells, Ann Rev Biophys Bioeng 1:131, 1972.

85. Hagins WA, Penn RD, Yoshikami S: Dark current and photocurrent in retinal rods, Biophys J 10:380, 1970.

86. Hagins WA, Yoshikami S: A role for Ca^{2+} in excitation of retinal rods and cones, Exp Eye Res 18:299, 1974.

87. Hamilton SE, Hurley JB: A phosphodiesterase inhibitor specific to a subset of bovine retinal cones, J Biol Chem 265:11259, 1990.

88. Hanke W, Cook NJ, Kaupp UB: cGMP-dependent channel protein from photoreceptor membranes: single-channel activity of the purified and reconstituted protein, Proc Natl Acad Sci USA 85:94, 1988.

89. Hargrave PA, et al: The structure of bovine rhodopsin, Biophys Struct Mech 9:235, 1983.

90. Haynes L, Yau K-W: Cyclic GMP-sensitive conductance in outer segment membrane of catfish cones, Nature 317:61, 1985.

91. Heller J: Interactions of plasma retinol-binding protein with its receptor, J Biol Chem 250:3613, 1975.

92. Henderson R, et al: Model for the structure of bacteriorhodopsin based on high-resolution electron cyromicroscopy, J Molec Biol 213:899, 1990.

93. Ho M-TP, Massey JB, Pownall HJ, et al: Mechanism of vitamin A movement between rod outer segments, interphoto-receptor retinoid-binding protein and liposomes, J Biol Chem 264:928, 1989.

94. Honig B, Dinur U, Nakanishi K, et al: An external point-charge model for wavelength regulation in visual pigments, J Am Chem Soc 101:7084, 1979.

95. Hubbard R, Wald G: *Cis-trans* isomers of vitamin A and retinene in the rhodopsin system, J Gen Physiol 36:269, 1952.

96. Hurley JB: Molecular properties of the cGMP cascade of vertebrate photoreceptors, Ann Rev Physiol 49:793, 1987.

97. Hurley JB, Stryer L: Purification and characterization of the g regulatory subunit of the cyclic GMP phosphodiesterase from retinal rod outer segments, J Biol Chem 257:11094, 1982.

98. Hurwitz R, Holcombe V: Affinity purification of the photoreceptor cGMP-gated cation channel, J Biol Chem 266:7975, 1991.

99. Jan LY, Jan YN: A superfamily of ion channels, Nature 345:672, 1990.

100. Jansco Nv, Jansco Hv: Fluoreszenzmikroskopische beobachtungen der reversiblen vitamin A bildung in der netzhaut wahrend des sehaktes, Biochem Z 287:289, 1936.

101. Jones GJ, Crouch RK, Wiggert B, et al: Retinoid requirements for recovery of sensitivity after visual pigment bleaching in isolated photoreceptors, Proc Natl Acad Sci USA 86:9606, 1989.

102. Kaupp UB, Niidome T, Tanabe T, et al: Primary structure and functional expression from complementary DNA of the rod photoreceptor cyclic GMP-gated channel, Nature 342:763, 1989.

103. Kilbride P, Ebrey TG: Light-initiated changes of cyclic guanosine monophosphate levels in the frog retina measured with quick-freezing techniques, J Gen Physiol 74:415, 1979.

104. Kimble EA, Svoboda RA, Ostroy SE: Oxygen consumption and ATP changes of the vertebrate photoreceptor, Exp Eye Res 31:271, 1980.

105. Kleinschmidt J, Dowling JE: Intracellular recordings from Gecko photoreceptors during light and dark adaptation, J Gen Physiol 66:617, 1975.

106. Koch K-W, Stryer L: Highly cooperative feedback control of retinal rod guanylate cyclase by calcium ions, Nature 334:64, 1988.

107. Konig B, Arendt A, McDowell JH, et al: Three cytoplasmic loops of rhodopsin interact with transducin, Proc Natl Acad Sci 85:6878, 1989.

108. Krinsky NI: The enzymatic esterification of vitamin A, J Biol Chem 232:881, 1958.

109. Kühn H: Interactions between photoexcited rhodopsin and light-activated enzymes in rods, in Osborne N, Chader GJ, eds: Progress in retinal research, vol 3, Oxford, Pergamon Press, 1984, p 123.

110. Kühn H, Dreyer WJ: Light-dependent phosphorylation of rhodopsin by ATP, FEBS Lett 20:1, 1972.

111. Kühn H, Hall SW, Wilden U: Light-induced binding of 48-kDa protein to photoreceptor membranes is highly enhanced by phosphorylation of rhodopsin, FEBS Lett 176:473, 1984.

112. Kühne W: Chemische Vorgange in der Netzhaut, in Hermann L, ed: Handbuch der physiology, vol 3, part 1, Leipzig, Vogel FCW, 1879; Chemical processes in the retina (English trans) Vision Res 17:1269, 1977.

113. Kuwabara T, Cogan D: Retinal glycogen, Arch Ophthalmol 66:680, 1961.

114. Lai YL, Wiggert B, Liu YP, et al: Interphotoreceptor retinol-binding proteins: possible transport vehicles between compartments of the retina, Nature 298:848, 1982.

115. Lamb TD: Transduction in vertebrate photoreceptors: the roles of cyclic GMP and calcium, Trends in Neurosci 9:224, 1986.

116. Lerea CL, Somers DE, Hurley JB, et al: Identification of specific transducin α subunits in retinal rod and cone photoreceptors, Science 234:77, 1986.

117. Lessell S, Kuwabara T: Phosphatase histochemistry of the eye, Arch Ophthalmol 71:851, 1964.

118. Li T, Volpp K, Applebury ML: Bovine cone photoreceptor cGMP phosphodiesterase structure deduced from a cDNA clone, Proc Natl Acad Sci USA 87:293, 1990.

119. Liang, CJ, Yamashita K, Muellenberg CG, et al: Structure of the carbohydrate moieties of bovine rhodopsin, J Biol Chem 254:6414, 1979.

120. Liebman PA, Entine G: Lateral diffusion of visual pigment in photoreceptor disc membranes, Science 185:457, 1974.

121. Liebman PA, Parker KR, Dratz EA: The molecular mechanism of visual excitation and its relation to the structure and composition of the rod outer segment, Ann Rev Physiol 49:765, 1987.

122. Liebman PA, Pugh EN: ATP mediates rapid reversal of cyclic GMP phosphodiesterase activation in visual receptor membranes, Nature 287:734, 1980.

123. Liebman PA, Pugh EN Jr: Gain, speed and sensitivity of GTP-binding vs PDE activation in visual excitation, Vision Res 22:1475, 1982.

124. Lion F, Rotmans JP, Daemen FJM, et al: Biochemical aspects of the visual process, XXVII, Stereospecificity of ocular retinol dehydrogenases and the visual cycle, Biochim Biophys Acta 384:282, 1975.

125. Liou GI, Bridges CDB, Fong S-L, et al: Vitamin A transport between retina and pigment epithelium—an interstitial protein carrying endogenous retinol (interstitial retinol-binding protein), Vision Res 22:1457, 1982.

126. Linsenmeier RA: Effects of light and darkness on oxygen distribution and consumption in the cat retina, J Gen Physiol 88:521, 1986.

127. Linsenmeier RA, Yancey CM: Effects of hyperoxia on the oxygen distribution in the intact cat retina, Invest Ophthalmol Vis Sci 30:612, 1989.

128. Lochrie ML, Hurley JB, Simon MI: Sequence of the alpha subunit of photoreceptor G protein: Homologies between transducin, ras and elongation factors, Science 228:96, 1985.

129. Lolly RN: Metabolic and anatomical specialization within the retina, in Lajtha A, ed: Handbook of neurochemistry, vol 2, New York, Plenun Press, 1963, p 473.

130. Lolley RN, Farber DB, Rayborn ME, et al: Cyclic GMP accumulation causes degeneration of photoreceptor cells: simulation of an inherited disease, Science 196:664, 1977.

131. Lowry O, Roberts N, Lewis C: The quantitative histochemistry of the retina, J Biol Chem 220:879, 1956.

132. Magistretti PJ: Regulation of glycogenolysis by neurotransmitters in the central nervous system, Diabete & Metabolisme, Paris 14:237, 1988.

133. Matthews HR, Fain GL, Murphy RLW, et al: Light adaptation in cone photoreceptors of the salamander: a role for cytoplasmic calcium, J Physiol (Lond) 420:447, 1990.

134. Matthews HR, Murphy RLW, Fain GL, et al: Photore-

ceptor light adaptation is mediated by cytoplasmic calcium concentration, Nature 334:67, 1988.

135. McNaughton PA: Light response of vertebrate photoreceptors, Physiol Revs 70:847, 1990.

136. McWilliam P, Farrar GJ, Kenna P, et al: Autosomal dominant retinitis pigmentosa (ADRP): localization of an ADRP gene to the long arm of chromosome 3, Genomics 5:619, 1989.

137. Miki N, Baraban JB, Keirns JJ, et al: Purification and properties of the light-activated cyclic nucleotide phosphodiesterase of rod outer segments, J Biol Chem 250:6320, 1975.

138. Miki N, Keirns JJ, Marcus FR, et al: Regulation of cyclic nucleotide concentrations in photoreceptors: an ATP-dependent stimulation of cyclic nucleotide phosphodiesterase by light, Proc Natl Acad Sci USA 70:3820, 1973.

139. Miller RF, Slaughter MM: Excitatory amino acid receptors of the retina: diversity of subtypes and conductance mechanisms, Trends in Neurosci 9:211, 1986.

140. Molday RS, Hsu S-C: Glyceraldehyde-3-phosphate dehydrogenase is a major protein associated with the plasma membrane of retinal photoreceptor outer segments, J Biol Chem 265:13308, 1990.

141. Mollon JD: Questions of sex and colour, Nature 323:578, 1986.

142. Nathans J: Molecular biology of visual pigments, Ann Rev Neurosci 10:163, 1987.

143. Nathans J: Determinants of visual pigment absorbance: identification of the retinylidene Schiff's base counterion in bovine rhodopsin, Biochemistry 29:9746, 1990.

144. Nathans J: Determinants of visual pigment absorbance: role of charged amino acids in the putative transmembrane segments, Biochemistry 29:937, 1990.

145. Nathans J, Hogness DS: Isolation, sequence analysis, and intron-exon arrangement of the gene encoding bovine rhodopsin, Cell 34:807, 1983.

146. Nathans J, Hogness DS: Isolation and nucleotide sequence of the gene encoding human rhodopsin, Proc Natl Acad Sci 81:4851, 1984.

147. Nathans J, Piantanida TP, Eddy RL, et al: Molecular genetics of inherited variation in human color vision, Science 232:203, 1986.

148. Nathans J, Thomas D, Hogness DS: Molecular genetics of human color vision: the genes encoding blue, green and red pigments, Science 232:193, 1986.

149. Neitz J, Jacobs GH: Polymorphism in normal human color vision and its mechanisms, Vision Res 30:621, 1990.

150. O'Brien PJ, Zatz M: Acylation of bovine rhodopsin by [^{3}H]palmitic acid, J Biol Chem 259:5054, 1984.

151. Okajima T-I, Pepperberg DR, Ripps H, et al: Interphotoreceptor retinoid-binding protein promotes rhodopsin regeneration in toad photoreceptors, Proc Nat Acad Sci USA 87:6907, 1990.

152. Ovchinnikov YA, Abdulaev NG, Bogachuk AS: Two adjacent cysteine residues in the C-terminal cytoplasmic fragment of bovine rhodopsin are palmitylated, FEBS Letters 230:1, 1988.

153. Ovchinnikov YA, et al: The complete amino acid sequence of visual rhodopsin, Bioorg Khim 8:1011, 1982.

154. Pagon RA: Retinitis pigmentosa, Surv Ophthalmol 33:137, 1988.

155. Palczewski K, Hargrave PA, McDowell JH, et al: The catalytic subunit of phosphatase 2A dephosphorylates phosphoopsin, Biochemistry 28:415, 1989.

156. Perlman JI, Nodes BR, Pepperberg DR: Utilization of retinoids in the bullfrog retina, J Gen Physiol 80:885, 1982.

157. Pfeffer BA, Clark VM, Flannery JG, et al: Membrane receptors for retinol-binding protein in cultured human retinal pigment epithelium, Invest Ophthalmol Vis Sci 27:1031, 1986.

158. Pfister CL, Kuhn H, Chabre M: Interaction between photoexcited rhodopsin and peripheral enzymes in frog retinal rods, influence on the postmetarhodopsin II decay and phosphorylation rate of rhodopsin, Eur J Biochem 136:489, 1983.

159. Pober JS, Bitensky MW: Light-regulated enzymes of vertebrate retinal rods, in Greengard P, Robinson GA, eds: Advances in cyclic nucleotide research, vol 11, New York, Raven Press, 1979, p 265.

160. Poo M, Cone RA: Lateral diffusion of rhodopsin in the photoreceptor membrane, Nature 247:438, 1974.

161. Rando RR: The chemistry of vitamin A and vision, Angew Chem Int Ed Engl 29:461, 1990.

162. Ratto GM, Payne R, Owen WG, et al: The concentration of cytosolic free calcium in vertebrate rod outer segments measured with Fura-2, J Neurosci 8:3240, 1988.

163. Rodieck RW: The vertebrate retina, San Francisco, WH Freeman, 1973, p 316.

164. Rodriguez KA, Tsin ATC: Retinyl esters in the vertebrate neuroretina, Am J Physiol 256:R255, 1989.

165. Rushton WAH: The Ferrier Lecture, 1962, Visual adaptation, Proc R Soc London Ser B 162:20, 1965.

166. Rushton WAH: Light and dark adaptation of the retina, in Straatsma BR, et al, eds: The retina, morphology, function and clinical characterstics, Berkeley and Los Angeles, University of California Press, 1969, p 257.

167. Saari JC: Enzymes and proteins of the mammalian visual cycle, in Osborne N, Chader GJ, eds: Progress in retinal research, vol 9, Oxford, Pergamon Press, 1990, p 363.

168. Saari JC, Bredberg DL: Enzymatic reduction of 11-cis-retinal bound to cellular retinal-binding protein, Biochim Biophys Acta 716:266, 1982.

169. Saari JC, Bredberg DL: CoA- and non-CoA-dependent retinol esterification in retinal pigment epithelium, J Biol Chem 263:8084, 1988.

170. Saari JC, Bredberg DL: Lecithin: retinol acyltransferase in retinal pigment epithelial microsomes, J Biol Chem 264:8636, 1989.

171. Saari JC, Bredberg DL: Modulation of visual cycle enzyme reaction parameters by retinoid-binding proteins, Invest Ophthalmol Vis Sci 31 (Suppl):111, 1990.

172. Saari JC, Bredberg L, Garwin GG: Identification of the endogenous retinoids associated with three cellular retinoid-binding proteins from bovine retina and retinal pigment epithelium, J Biol Chem 257:13329, 1982.

173. Saari JC, Bunt-Milam AH, Bredberg D, et al: Properties

and immunocytochemical localization of three retinoid-binding proteins from bovine retina, Vision Res 24:1595, 1984.

174. Saari JC, Futterman S, Bredberg L: Cellular retinol- and retinoic acid-binding proteins of bovine retina, J Biol Chem 253:6432, 1978.

175. Saari JC, Teller DC, Crabb JW, et al: Properties of an interphotoreceptor retinoid-binding protein from bovine retina, J Biol Chem 260:195, 1985.

176. Sakmar TP, Franke RR, Khorana HG: Glutamic acid-113 serves as the retinylidene Schiff base counterion in bovine rhodopsin, Proc Natl Acad Sci USA 86:8309, 1989.

177. Sanyal S, De Ruiter A, Hawkins RK: Development and degeneration of retina in rds mutant mice: light microscopy, J Comp Neurol 194:193, 1980.

178. Schick GA, Cooper TM, Holloway RA, et al: Energy storage in the primary photochemical events of rhodopsin and isorhodopsin, Biochemistry 26:2556, 1987.

179. Schmidt SY, Lolley RN: Cyclic nucleotide phosphodiesterase; an early defect in inherited retinal degeneration of C3II mice, J Cell Biol 57:117, 1973.

180. Shapley R, Enroth-Cugell C: Visual adaptation and retinal gain controls, in Osborne NN, Chader GJ, eds: Progress in retinal research, vol 3, Oxford, Pergamon Press, 1984, p 263.

181. Sickel W: Retinal metabolism in dark and light, in Fuortes MGF, ed: Handbook of sensory physiology, vol 7/2, Heidelberg, Springer-Verlag, 1972, p 667.

182. Steinberg RH: Monitoring communications between photoreceptors and pigment epithelial cells: effects of "mild" systemic hypoxia, Invest Ophthalmol Vis Sci 28:1888, 1987.

183. Stirling CE, Lee A: [³H]Ouabain autoradiography of frog retina, J Cell Biol 85:313, 1980.

184. Stryer L: Biochemistry, 3rd ed, New York, WH Freeman, 1988, p 427.

185. Tamura T, Nakatani K, Yau K-W: Light adaptation in cat retinal rods, Nature 245:755, 1989.

186. Thomas DD, Stryer L: Transverse location of the retinal chromophore of rhodopsin in rod outer segment disk membranes, J Molec Biol 154:145, 1982.

187. Tomita T: Electrical activity of vertebrate photoreceptors, Q Rev Biophys 3:179, 1971.

188. Torre V, Matthews HR, Lamb TD: Role of calcium in regulating the cyclic GMP cascade of phototransduction, Proc Natl Acad Sci USA 83:7109, 1986.

189. Travis GH, Brennan MG, Danielson PE, et al: Identification of a photoreceptor specific mRNA encoded by the gene responsible for retinal degeneration slow (rds), Nature 338:70, 1989.

190. Travis GH, Sutcliffe JG, Bok D: The retinal degeneration slow (rds) gene product is a photoreceptor disc membrane-associated glycoprotein, Neuron 6:61, 1991.

191. Trehan A, Cañada FJ, Rando RR: Inhibitors of retinyl ester formation also prevent the biosynthesis of 11-cis-retinol, Biochemistry 29:309, 1990.

192. Uhl R, Wagner R, Ryba N: Watching G proteins at work, Trends Neurosci 13:64, 1990.

193. Waddell WH, Crouch R, Nakanishi K, et al: Quantitative aspects of the photochemistry of isomeric retinals and visual pigments, J Am Chem Soc 98:4189, 1976.

194. Wald G: Carotenoids and the vitamin A cycle in vision, Nature 134:65, 1934.

195. Wald G: Carotenoids and the visual cycle, J Gen Physiol 19:351, 1935.

196. Wald G: Molecular basis of visual excitation, Science 162:230, 1968.

197. Wald G, Brown PK: Human color vision and color blindness, Cold Spring Harbor Symp Quant Biol 30:345, 1965.

198. Wald G, Hubbard R: The reduction of retinene 1 to vitamin A1 in vitro, J Gen Physiol 32:367, 1949.

199. Warburg O: Uber die klassifizierung tierischer gewebe nach ihrem stoffwechsel, Biochem Z 184:484, 1927.

200. Wensel TG, Stryer L: Activation mechanism of retinal rod cyclic GMP phosphodiesterase probed by fluorescein-labeled inhibitory subunit, Biochemistry 29:2155, 1990.

201. Wiggert B, Chader GJ: A receptor for retinol in developing retina and pigment epithelium, Exp Eye Res 21:143, 1975.

202. Wilden U, Hall SW, Kuhn H: Phosphodiesterase activation by photoexcited rhodopsin is quenched when rhodopsin is phosphorylated and binds the intrinsic 48-kDa protein of rod outer segments, Proc Natl Acad Sci 83:1174, 1986.

203. Wilden U, Kuhn H: Light-dependent phosphorylation of rhodopsin: number of phosphorylation sites, Biochemistry 21:3014, 1982.

204. Winkler BS: Glycolytic and oxidative metabolism in relation to retinal function, J Gen Physiol 77:667, 1981.

205. Winkler BS: The intermediary metabolism of the retina: biochemical and functional aspects, in Anderson RE, ed: Biochemistry of the eye, American Academy of Ophthalmology, 1983, p 227.

206. Woodruff ML, Bownds MD: Amplitude, kinetics and reversibility of a light-induced decrease in guanosine 3',5'-cyclic monophosphate in frog photoreceptor membranes, J Gen Physiol 73:429, 1979.

207. Yamazaki A, Hayashi F, Tatsumi M, et al: Interactions between the subunits of transducin and cyclic GMP phosphodiesterase in Rana catesbiana rod photoreceptors, J Biol Chem 265:11539, 1990.

208. Yamazaki A, Sen I, Bitensky MW, et al: Cyclic GMP-specific, high affinity, noncatalytic binding sites on light-activated phosphodiesterase, J Biol Chem 255:11619, 1980.

209. Yancey CM, Linsenmeier RA: Oxygen distribution and consumption in the cat retina at increased intraocular pressure, Invest Ophthalmol Vis Sci 30:600, 1989.

210. Yau K-W, Baylor DA: Cyclic GMP-activated conductance of retinal photoreceptor cells, Ann Rev Neurosci 12:289, 1989.

211. Yau K-W, Nakatani K: Electrogenic Na-Ca exchange in retinal rod outer segment, Nature 311:611, 1984.

212. Yau K-W, Nakatani K: Light-induced reduction of cytoplasmic-free calcium in retinal rod outer segment, Nature 313:579, 1985.

213. Yau K-W, Nakatani K: Light-suppressible, cyclic GMP-sensitive conductance in the plasma membrane of a truncated rod outer segment, Nature 317:252, 1985.

214. Yee R, Liebman PA: Light-activated phosphodiester-

ase of the rod outer segment, kinetics and parameters of activation and deactivation, J Biol Chem 253:8902, 1978.

215. Yoshikami S, Noll GN: Isolated retinas synthesize visual pigments from retinol congeners delivered by liposomes, Science 200:1393, 1978.

216. Yoshikami S, George JS, Hagins WA: Light-induced calcium fluxes from outer segment layer of vertebrate retinas, Nature 286:395, 1980.

217. Yoshizawa T, Schichida Y: Low temperature spectrophotometry of intermediates of rhodopsin, Methods Enzymol 81:333, 1982.

218. Yoshizawa R, Wald G: Prelumirhodopsin and the bleaching of visual pigments, Nature 197:1279, 1963.

219. Zhukovsky EA, Oprian DD: Effect of carboxylic acid side chains on the absorption maximum of visual pigments, Science 246:928, 1989.

220. Zimmerman WF: The distribution and proportions of vitamin A compounds during the visual cycle in the rat, Vision Res 14:795, 1974.

221. Zuckerman R, Weiter JJ: Oxygen transport in the bullfrog retina, Exp Eye Res 30:117, 1980.

222. Zuckerman R, Cheasty JE: A 48 kDa protein arrests cGMP phosphodiesterase activation in retinal disc membranes, FEBS Letters 207:35, 1986.

CHAPTER
15

Entoptic Imagery

WILLIAM M. HART, Jr., M.D., Ph.D.

Entoptic imagery refers to visual perceptions that are produced or influenced by the native structures of one's own eye. The structures producing these images may be normal anatomic components of the eye, or they may be pathologic imperfections, such as opacities in the media of the eye. Images arising from or heavily influenced by the normal structures of the eye, such as the shadows of retinal blood vessels or the movement of blood cells in retinal capillaries, are not ordinarily visible to the casual observer. Rather, these images usually require special circumstances of illumination, as well as the direct visual attention of the observer. Using this concept of entoptic phenomena somewhat loosely, we may also include those visual experiences that result from stimulation of the retina by inadequate (nonlight) stimuli, including the unformed images produced by mechanical stimulation of the retina, so-called phosphenes.

An appreciation of entoptic phenomena and their origins is useful to clinicians and students as a means of improving their understanding of the physiology of vision. Occasionally the phenomena are of clinical utility by allowing a subjective confirmation of some capacity for visual function where objective findings may not be available. Because of their subjective nature, however, entoptic phenomena require skills of perception and articulate description of their appearance on the part of the observer before they can be clinically useful.

This chapter is arranged so that entoptic images are discussed in an order roughly corresponding to the anatomic distribution of the structures related to the images. The first phenomena to be considered are those arising from opacities in the media, including the cornea, lens, and vitreous. The latter part of the chapter deals with images determined by the structure of the retina.

IMPERFECTIONS IN THE OCULAR MEDIA

When the ocular fundus is illuminated by a focal source of light held close to the examiner's eye, and within 1 m or so distant from the eye being observed, the pupil of the eye will appear to be filled with a diffuse reddish glow. This phenomenon is commonly termed the "fundus reflex." (Do not confuse this term with the neurally mediated reactions of the pupil to light stimulation of the retina.) The reddish glow of the fundus reflex is the result of diffuse reflection of light by the retina and choroid. The reflected light exits from the eye through the pupil and serves to reveal in the ocular media any imperfections that prevent light from returning through the pupil toward the examiner's eye. Such imperfections are seen as dark areas within the otherwise diffusely illuminated pupil (Fig. 15-1). The imperfections need not be true opacities in the sense of blocking the passage of light completely, but they may only be local variations in the refractive index of the media. For example, a streak of mucus across the corneal surface will be seen as a dark line, because it refracts the light of the fundus reflex away from the examiner's view. Localized variations in the refractive index of

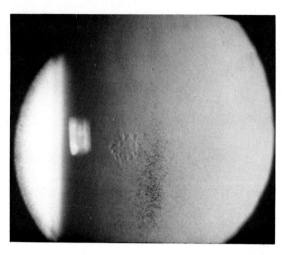

FIG. 15-1   Slit lamp view of the fundus reflex through dilated pupil. Illuminating beam enters pupil at left. In the center of the pupil a small central disc of a posterior subcapsular cataract is visible. To its right there is a vertical spindle-shaped pattern of dark particles where pigment granules have been deposited on the corneal epithelium (so-called Krukenberg's spindle).

the media are also commonly produced by surface irregularities in the corneal epithelium, by defects in Descemet's membrane, or by changes in the state of hydration of the lens.

Small discrete opacities of the cornea and lens reduce the optical clarity of the media by scattering light. They appear as fine dark specks when retroilluminated by the fundus reflex. Larger opacities produce dark areas in the red fundus reflection seen by the examiner. For example, clumps of pigmented cells on the anterior lens capsule may be torn loose from adhesions of the posterior iris surface to the lens (posterior synechias). These appear to the examiner as black spots within the pupillary aperture. This sort of opacity in the ocular media may significantly reduce the amount of light reaching the retina, but it will scatter only a small fraction of the light.

The various types of optical defects produce entirely different effects on the patient's vision. Translucent defects, which are local discontinuities in the index of refraction of the optical media, do not completely block the passage of light. They spread or scatter the light and are often damaging to vision by reducing the contrast of images at the retina. Numerous small opacities will produce the same effect. In an apparent paradox, a larger opacity may be completely inapparent to the patient if it is not too large. Although this type of opacity reduces the total amount of light reaching the retina, it does

not appreciably reduce the contrast of the image by light scatter. Prior to the development of corneal transplantation for the treatment of corneal scarring, an effective form of therapy was to convert an area of corneal translucency into a true opacity by means of tattooing. If an adequate aperture of clear tissue remained, considerable improvement in visual acuity often resulted.

ENTOPTIC IMAGES ARISING FROM THE TEAR FILM AND CORNEA

Opacities of the ocular media that are visible as defects within the fundus reflex can be visualized entoptically by using appropriate light sources. If a small pinhole (0.1 mm) in an opaque card or a disc is held before the eye and is illuminated from behind by a bright background such as the sky or a diffusely illuminated wall, the pinhole will be seen as a bright spot that grows in size as it approaches the eye. The pinhole thus acts as a small source of light. When it is brought to the anterior focal point of the eye (about 17 mm in front of the cornea), the refractive media of the eye add sufficient vergence to the light rays to make them parallel to one another within the vitreous cavity (Fig. 15-2). The observer then sees a patch of light, the border of which is actually the shadow of the pupillary margin of the iris. The patch will thus vary in size with changes in pupillary diameter. Optical discontinuities in the ocular media are then seen as shadows or bright areas within the circular patch. The shape, position, and movement of these light and dark areas correspond to their density and position within the eye.

Use of the pinhole method allows entoptic visualization of a number of both normal and pathologic phenomena arising from the anterior corneal surface and its tear film. Occasionally, horizontal bands of light apparently caused by folds in the corneal epithelium may be seen in the entoptic field. They course in unbroken lines across the entire width of the pupillary image and change their position as the margins of the eyelids are slowly approximated or separated. They can be distinguished easily from the entoptic image of the tear film. The tear film that adheres to the lid margins produces a longitudinal stripe that can be seen as the pupillary fissure is narrowed. This image appears first along the inferior portions of the pupillary image (note that since the retinal image of the pupil is erect, the image will appear to be inverted).

Droplets and threads of mucus on the surface of the tear film of the cornea likewise can be seen as bright spots surrounded by a dark ring.

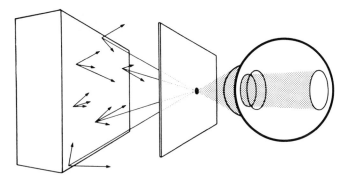

FIG. 15-2   Illuminated pinhole at anterior focus of eye acts as point source of light. Light entering eye is collimated by ocular refracting elements and casts sharp shadows on retina. (From Rubin ML, Walls GL: Studies in physiological optics, Springfield, IL, Charles C Thomas, Publisher, 1965.)

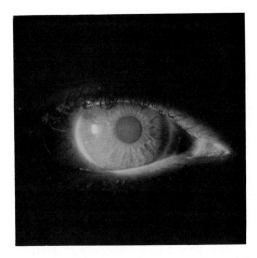

FIG. 15-3   Anterior corneal mosaic pattern stained with fluorescein dye. Pattern is most visible in pupillary area.

These move up and down in a slow swimming fashion as the palpebral fissure is widened or narrowed. Also, a variety of folds and channels may be seen. These consist of vertical lines that are gently curved in some locations while in other regions they may bend more angularly. The curved lines and the channels that separate them can be observed on repetitive examinations at different times, suggesting that they represent definite anatomic structures. Their origin is not certain, but they may represent vitreous membranes or folds in the surface of the corneal epithelium underlying the tear film. Staining of the tear film with fluorescein dye will sometimes show a mosaic pattern outlined by straight and curved lines in the corneal epithelium (Fig. 15-3). This anterior corneal mosaic pattern is easily produced by a brief period of gentle digi-

tal pressure on the cornea through the closed upper lid. Entoptic visualization of the mosaic pattern by the pinhole method was first reported by Esser.[10] The mosaic pattern is thought to be caused by the formation of shallow, linear channels in the corneal epithelium; these are produced by elevated ridges in Bowman's membrane that are created during the period of corneal flattening. Corneal flattening by hard contact lenses frequently produces this phenomenon.[8]

PHYSIOLOGIC AND PATHOLOGIC HALOS

Under some conditions colored halos can be seen to surround small white lights that are viewed from a distance. These rings are caused by chromatic dispersion of white light by the various layers of cells in the ocular media through which the light must pass on its way to the retina. Halos may occur either physiologically or as the result of pathologic conditions. The source of physiologic halo formation is thought to be in the radial arrangement of lens fibers, which act as a diffraction grating. Physiologic halos are not very bright when compared to those resulting from pathologic conditions. In addition, they have somewhat smaller angular diameters than pathologic halos, having a maximum size estimated at from 7 to 8 degrees (angular diameter). The colors of halos are arranged spectrally, with the short wavelength lights such as blue and violet being closest to the stimulating white source, while the long wavelength colors such as red lie toward the outermost portions of the halo ring.

Pathologic halos may be simulated by condensing a layer of steam on a piece of glass and then viewing a bright source of light through it. Pathologic halos can arise from several circumstances. Accumulation of mucus and debris in the corneal tear film in patients with conjunctivitis may result in the appearance of halos around lights. This is usually most evident to patients when first arising in the morning. This is also the time when intraocular pressure may be elevated in patients with glaucoma. Halos also are reported by patients suffering from the severe photophobia of ultraviolet radiation keratopathy, which results in damage to corneal epithelial cells. Similarly, persons with endothelial corneal dystrophies that result in corneal edema will frequently notice halos as a first symptom of their disorder.

In patients with otherwise normal endothelial function elevations of intraocular pressure can be sufficient to produce epithelial edema. In such individuals the appearance and disappearance of halos can be seen to parallel fluctuations in ocular pressure. When the intraocular pressure is elevated, microscopic spaces of fluid appear among the epithelial cells just anterior to Bowman's membrane. Light striking the cornea is broken into its spectral components by droplets of fluid in the epithelium in the same manner that light passing through suspended droplets of rain is broken up to a form a rainbow.

ENTOPTIC IMAGES ARISING FROM THE LENS

A point source of light such as a star does not appear to be a point, but rather it has the appearance of a blurred disc. Its appearance as a blurred circle of light is a consequence of the diffraction of light at the circular margin of the pupillary aperture. Star gazers from the time of early antiquity noted that the image of a star appears to have radiating lines extending from the central disc, evoking the familiar symbolic representation of the star: a pointed figure or asterisk. This image pattern is thought to be caused by the structure of the ocular lens, which breaks up the rays of light. Since the radiating line figures are apparent to the normal viewer, they probably are related to a normal component of lens anatomy, such as the suture lines. The pinhole method previously described for viewing opacities in the cornea and tear film will also very readily show defects in the optical qualities of the lens (Fig. 15-4).

Under ordinary circumstances observers are not consciously aware of the imperfections in the ocular media. Many people have small opacities in the lens that do not interfere in any way with vision. With the exception of the aqueous humor, no part of the ocular media is optically perfect. The cornea, lens, and vitreous body all

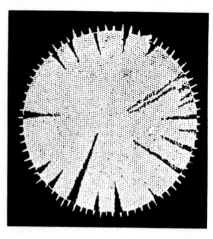

FIG. 15-4   Early cortical cataract as it appears entoptically in collimated light. (Modified from Darier.)

contain cellular elements with membranes and nuclei. Under ordinary circumstances one is quite unaware of these imperfections.

Even large opacities of the cornea or lens may not produce noticeable defects in the retinal image if they only block, rather than scatter, the light entering the eye. Shadows cast by objects that are illuminated by diffuse sources of light contain both umbral and penumbral portions. The umbral portion of a shadow is a cone that has its base at the position of the opacity and its apex at a point where the transition from total into partial shadow is created. The shadow is complete within the umbra. Lying outside the umbra is a penumbral cone, within which there is a partial shadow created by partial obstruction of the light source by the margin of the opacity. Smaller opacities may lie so far in front of the retina that their umbral shadows do not directly interfere with formation of the retinal image.

ENTOPTIC IMAGES PRODUCED WITHIN THE VITREOUS

Figure 15-5 shows that the effect of an opacity in the media is to reduce the total amount of light reaching the retina. The closer an opacity is to the retina, however, the more likely it is to interfere with formation of the retinal image by having its shadow fall directly on the retina. The size of the cross section of its umbral cone, intersected by the retina, will be inversely proportional to its distance from the retina. For a given location within the eye the larger the opacity the longer and broader will be its umbra. Thus a small opacity close to the retina may cast a noticeable shadow, whereas a more extensive opacity that happens to be farther from the ret-

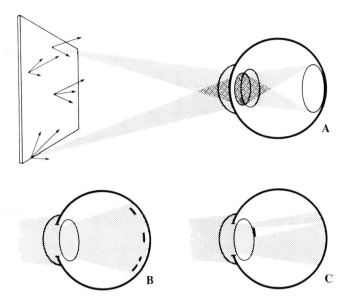

FIG. 15-5   A, Since light from any point in extended source can reach pupil, brightly illuminated field gives large brightly illuminated image, most of eyeball being filled with light. **B**, If opacity is near retina, shadows are sharply seen. **C**, Small opacity directly behind lens, for example, will not cast sharp shadow (umbra) on retina, since some light from extended source can still reach spot in retina where shadow should be, thus blotting it out. This explains severe annoyance caused by even very small opacities lying near retina (shadows cast being sharply defined), and "inconspicuousness" of much larger opacities situated more anteriorly in vitreous or lens, such as early cataractous changes—opacities within lens (shadow in latter case being only blurrily outlined, if at all visible). (From Rubin ML, Walls GL: Studies in physiological optics, Springfield, IL, Charles C Thomas, Publisher, 1965.)

ina may not cast a significant retinal shadow. Posteriorly located opacities that cast sharp umbral shadows on the retina will appear as positive scotomas when seen against an evenly illuminated white background. Uniformity of the background allows better detection of such scotomas by removing distracting details of contrasting borders within the image, which might interfere with their recognition. Although a small opacity located far from the retina may cause little or no visual disturbance, large numbers of small opacities may scatter enough light to reduce the contrast of the retinal image. This appears to the patient as glare, a problem that usually is aggravated by attempts to improve visibility by increasing the brightness of a scene.

The closer an opacity lies to the plane of the retina, the less evident is the penumbral portion of its shadow and the larger and more sharply defined is the umbral portion. To demonstrate this phenomenon, hold a small opaque object such as a coin or pencil between a source of light and a white piece of paper. The closer the object is held to the paper the larger and more clearly defined is the dense portion of its central

shadow and the less evident is the partially illuminated peripheral portion of the shadow. There is a much greater contrast between the dark central portion of the shadow and the rest of the illuminated surface when the umbra is at its maximum and the penumbra is at its minimum size. This phenomenon also applies to shadows cast on the retina and explains the extreme annoyance caused by even very small opacities located adjacent to the retinal surface. It likewise explains the occasional very large opacity lying in the anterior portion of the vitreous, which is, surprisingly, completely inapparent to the patient.

Patients frequently will complain of small specks or dots that can be seen against a bright background such as a diffusely illuminated wall or the blue sky. Such images can be seen to move about irregularly as the eye is moved. The dots may be seen as single round globules or sometimes chains of little bright spots of light resembling a string of pearls. Fine dark lines in amorphous masses that appear like pieces of dust or small branching twigs are also seen occasionally and may become annoying when they cross the center of the field of view. Although they usually do not interfere with vision, they may sometimes be a source of discomfort and alarm to the patient. They are called "muscae volitantes," because they seen to dart about like flies as the eye is moved.

Most of the vitreous opacities that are seen entoptically are entirely harmless, and in most cases patients who are alarmed by them need no more than reassurance. However, some vitreous opacities may be of serious consequence. When a sudden increase in opacities is noted in accompaniment with flashes of light, these symptoms may be caused by vitreoretinal traction and/or the creation of retinal breaks that may eventually lead to retinal detachment.

Occasionally, a large vitreous opacity may be seen with an ophthalmoscope as a disc-shaped structure floating in the posterior vitreous. This is probably caused by detachment of the posterior vitreous from the margin of the optic disc (separation of the so-called posterior vitreous base),[23] or it may represent a transverse tear across the posterior portion of the hyaloid canal. By itself, this finding is of little consequence. However, it should be emphasized that, despite the generally benign nature of vitreous floaters, a distinction should be made between those that develop slowly and those that appear abruptly. The latter variety are more likely to be related to retinal breaks or hemorrhage into the vitreous body. Patients should not be reassured about the generally benign nature of floaters until complications have been ruled out by appropriate examination for posterior vitreous separation, retinal breaks, and possible retinal detachment.

Perhaps the most striking demonstration of the relative insignificance of optical effects of vitreous opacities is provided by those patients who have asteroid hyalosis. Asteroid bodies in the vitreous are caused by local accumulations of calcium soaps. Patients with this disorder are rarely aware of the opacities, which serve only to reduce the total amount of light reaching the retina without degrading the image. Only rarely do such patients experience a reduction in their visual acuity. This is because the opacities themselves are small and dense. They cast very short umbral cones, which do not reach the retina, and they scatter only a small proportion of the light that strikes them. When seen with an ophthalmoscope, however, these structures reflect considerable light back toward the observer, creating the image of a swarm of brightly illuminated dots within the vitreous body. Indeed, the observer's view of the fundus may be ob-scured entirely and yet the patient may experience only a minor disturbance of vision.

VITREORETINAL SOURCES OF ENTOPTIC IMAGES: MOORE'S LIGHTNING STREAKS

Moore[18] originally described an entoptic phenomenon consisting of flashes of light that were likened to the appearance of flashes of lightning. These lightning streaks, which are now recognized as very common, are seen most often in the temporal visual field and are largely vertical in orientation. They are sometimes accompanied by the simultaneous development of a shower of small vitreous opacities and occur most often in middle-aged patients, more frequently among women than men. Moore originally believed that this phenomenon did not imply the presence of a serious underlying disorder. However, Berens[5] and others[29] have since stressed that this common syndrome is of more serious import than Moore originally believed. The phenomenon is thought to result from degenerative changes in the vitreous body that lead to detachment of the posterior vitreous from the surface of the retina. As a separation occurs between the posterior vitreous face and the internal limiting membrane of the retina, traction on the retina at some points produces phosphenes (flashes of light). The preference of these phosphenes for the temporal visual field may be a result of the asymmetry of retinal sensitivity. Traction on the temporal retina near the ora serrata (subserving nasal visual field) may not be noticed subjectively, since the periphery of the temporal retina is blind. Similar traction on the seeing portions of the peripheral nasal retina produces phosphenes that are seen in the temporal visual field.

Patients seeking attention for the sudden appearance of lightning flashes should be carefully examined, particularly if the symptom is recent or has been associated with the appearance of a large number of bothersome floaters. A dilated examination of the fundus by indirect ophthalmoscopy is required to rule out the presence of retinal breaks that might subsequently lead to the development of retinal detachment. Although a large majority of patients reporting such phosphenes do not develop serious retinal disease, a small but significant proportion do.

PHOSPHENES OF QUICK EYE MOVEMENT

Nebel[21] has described an entoptic phenomenon that appears to be related to, although distinct from, Moore's lightning streaks. He gave the phenomenon the term "flick phosphene." It is best seen in a completely dark-adapted eye, such as when awaking from sleep in a still darkened room. If the eyes are then rapidly moved from one side to the other, one can observe in the visual field of each eye a bright pattern having the general shape shown in Figure 15-6. Each eye produces its own individual phosphene, which lasts only a fraction of a second.

The retina seems to "fatigue" so that repeated observations produce a gradual fading of the phosphenes. The images (Fig. 15-7) are seen separately and simultaneously by the two eyes. Each image has the shape of a sheaf, the truncated apex of which points toward either the physiologic blind spot or the center of fixation.

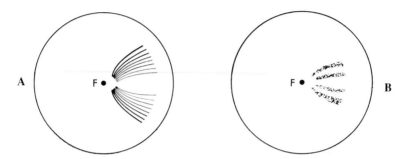

FIG. 15-6 Phosphene of right eye in right-to-left flick. **A,** Phosphene pattern in rested eye. **B,** Pattern after fatigue. F, fovea, as identified by afterimage of fixated inducing light. (From Nebel B: Arch Ophthalmol 58:236, 1957.)

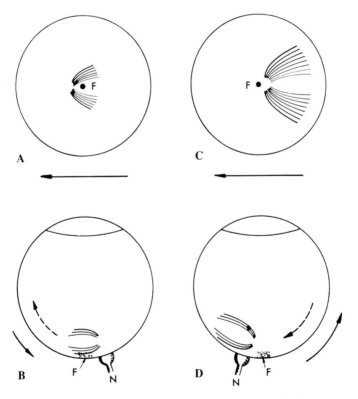

FIG. 15-7 Phosphenes of right-and-left flick and interpretation relating to topography of their origin. **A** and **C,** Phosphenes as seen by person. **B** and **D,** Nebel's projection of phosphenes back to retina. Opposing arrows, shearing forces set up by acceleration of wall of globe and inertial retardation of vitreous. N, nerve; F, fovea. Projected phosphene is tilted and displaced slightly to make it visible. (From Nebel B: Arch Ophthalmol 58:237, 1957.)

When first seen, the pattern is bright yellow or orange with sharp borders. Repeated attempts to elicit the images cause them to become indistinct, blurred, and less brightly colored. Nebel attributed these phosphenes to physical deformation of the retina by the posterior surface of the vitreous body. Abrupt saccadic motion of the eye causes the inertial drag of the vitreous body to be transmitted directly to the retina. The resulting deformation of the cellular structures within the retina results in a mechanical phosphene. Support for this interpretation lies in the observation that the images are more easily elicited in the eyes of individuals undergoing the early senescent changes of vitreous liquefaction (syneresis).

PURKINJE FIGURES: IMAGES OF THE RETINAL BLOOD VESSELS

As explained, illumination of the fundus by parallel light rays will allow visualization of small opacities located close to the retina. Since the columns of blood contained within retinal blood vessels are linear opacities situated in front of the retinal photoreceptors, it follows that the retinal blood vessels should be visible. In fact, this is true, although only with certain qualifications. If a focal source of light (such as a small penlight) is pressed firmly against the exterior of the eye through closed lids, the arborizing pattern of retinal blood vessels can be made briefly visible. This phenomenon was first described by Purkinje. Similarly, use of a pinhole source of light at the anterior focal plane of the eye will allow visualization of the branching pattern of retinal blood vessels. The image is, however, very transient and can be prolonged only by setting the source of light (the pinhole or the penlight) in constant motion. Stabilization of the position of the image of the blood vessels on the surface of the retina for periods of a few seconds causes it to disappear entirely. Patients often note during slit lamp examination that, as the beam of light sweeps over the anterior segment, the pattern of the retinal vessels appears as a black branching lacework against a reddish-orange background.

Contrasting images that are stabilized in position on the retinal surface by artificial means will fade rapidly from view, leaving only a diffusely illuminated field with no structural detail. Vitreous opacities are suspended within a partially liquid medium and tend to be freely mobile. The shadows they cast on the retina consequently change with each movement of the eye, producing entoptic images that are easily seen. The shadows cast by the internal structures of the retina itself remain fixed in position relative to the location of the photoreceptor cells. The shadows they cast on the photoreceptors remain fixed in position despite movements of the eye and are not subjectively apparent under ordinary circumstances. Since the blood vessels lie so close to the photoreceptors, only angular movements of focal sources of light close to the vessels themselves can cause significant shifts in their shadows to occur, allowing them to be seen.

When examining patients who have opacities of the media preventing visualization of the retina, entoptic images of the vascular pattern of the retina can be of clinical utility. The test is restricted in that it requires intelligent and perceptive patients who can accurately describe what they see. If a bright penlight is pressed over the closed upper eyelid and is vigorously and rapidly shifted from side to side, many patients can describe very accurately the image of the retinal vascular arborization. Some can even describe the presence of defects in the image such as those arising from macular scars. However, a surprisingly large proportion of patients seem incapable of recognizing or reporting accurately any image at all. The test is therefore of somewhat limited utility. Although a negative response is not conclusive evidence of retinal disease, an accurate description of an apparently normal pattern by the patient is reasonably good evidence that retinal function is grossly intact.

If pressure is applied to the eye, induced pulsations in the retinal vessels can sometimes be seen entoptically, especially after physical exercise.[14] Rapid expansions of the arteriolar vessels, synchronous with cardiac systole, can be observed. These are followed by a second, diastolic phase in which slower contractile movements are seen along the paths of the same vessels. If the subject has not exercised prior to this examination, the pulsations are usually too small to be entoptically apparent.

The explanation of all these phenomena must lie in the shadow cast by the retinal circulation, since all features of the retinal circulation—including the position and shape of the optic disc, as well as the avascular zone of the central macula—can be seen. Thus it is unlikely that the choroidal circulation is responsible for the Purkinje images.

THE BLUE FIELD ENTOPTIC PHENOMENON (FLYING SPOTS)

If one looks at a bright and diffusely illuminated surface with no contrasting features, a series of fast moving, luminous points or spots can be readily seen. The spots tend to move in a generally curved pattern, while trailing short, tapering segments behind them. The spots are best seen if the background is illuminated by blue light in the spectral region of 350 to 450 nm. Since this region contains the spectral absorption peak of hemoglobin, it has been suggested that the moving particles represent red blood cells passing through the retinal capillaries. Others have proposed that the flying spots represent the passage of leukocytes rather than erythrocytes. Two observations about the flying spots tend to support this point of view: (1) the spots are not sufficiently numerous to represent red blood cells and (2) the spots themselves actually appear as brighter or more luminous points. If a continuous chain of red cells in a capillary loop is occasionally broken by the passage of a leukocyte through the capillary, a small region of lower optical density moves through the capillary, allowing greater transmission of the blue light. This break in the blood column would appear as a fine, bright moving point. Thus it is argued that one sees passing zones of increased transmission of blue light accompanying the passage of white blood cells through the retinal capillaries. Since red light is almost equally well transmitted by erythrocytes and leukocytes, gazing at a monochromatic red background will make the flying spots inapparent.

There are two vascular beds that could be the source of the flying spot images. The blood cells may be passing through the precapillary arterioles of the nerve fiber layer, or they may actually lie in the capillary loops of the inner nuclear and outer plexiform layers. The patterns generated by the flying spots seem to correspond in position with the finest branchings of the retinal vessels, which can be seen on Purkinje images, suggesting that they might actually lie in the precapillary arterioles. However, Marshall has concluded that the corpuscles are not in the arterioles of the nerve fiber layer.[17] He based this conclusion on observations of the size and velocity of the flying luminous spots when seen dichoptically: one eye being illuminated by a diffuse blue source of light from a mercury lamp and the other eye being stimulated entoptically by eccentric rotation of the pinhole source of light. This allowed binocular comparison between the size and velocity of the flying corpuscles (seen with one eye) with the distribution of retinal vessels marked by the Purkinje figures (seen with the other eye). Marshall took these observations as evidence that the flying spots

are caused by the passage of cells through retinal vessels that are in layers of the retina more external than the nerve fiber and ganglion cell layers. This would correspond better to the distribution of capillaries than to precapillary arterioles.

Measurements have been taken of the area in the center of the visual field where entoptic visualization of the moving spots is inapparent. If the spots are indeed markers of the position of retinal capillaries, their distribution should correspond to the foveal avascular zone, and the size of the entoptically seen area of absence of flying spots should match the dimensions of the capillary-free zone of the fovea. Values experimentally determined by several investigators are given in Table 15-1. These figures for blood-free area of the foveal retina show reasonably good agreement with measurements taken from histologic preparations and fluorescein angiograms of the retina. The source of the blue field entoptic phenomenon has been studied in animal models, using microvascular preparations, viewed by video microscopy, and transilluminated with short wavelength light.[25] Leukocytes within capillaries were found to appear as moving bright spots that simulated the motion of the entoptic phenomenon and were found to be easily distinguishable from (and brighter than) plasma gaps within the capillary columns of red cells. Thus it has been reasonably well established that the flying spot phenomenon is associated intimately with the circulation of leukocytes in retinal capillary loops. In addition to following patterns that match those of the capillary architecture, the flying spots have a pulsatile movement that accelerates with an increase in heart rate.

TABLE 15-1 Blood-free Area of Retina Determined Entoptically*

Author	Measurement of blood-free area
Abelsdorff and Nagel	1 degree 30 minutes 0.410 mm (author's eye)
Gescher	1 degree 29 minutes 0.420 mm (author's eye)
Sperling, Miller and Adler	0.40-0.50 mm (38 normal eyes)

*Anatomic measurements of capillary free zone of fovea have been reported at 0.4 to 0.5 mm. (Salzmann M: The anatomy and histology of the human eye in the normal state; its development and senescence, Chicago, University of Chicago Press, 1912.)

Clinical application of vascular entoptic phenomena

Purkinje images and the flying spot phenomenon have been used to study the anatomy of the foveal avascular zone and autoregulation of retinal vascular perfusion in health and disease. Applegate et al.[3] have systematically determined the optimal parameters for observing the Purkinje images of the retinal vasculature in the close vicinity of the foveal avascular zone. They found some variations among normal individuals, including the apparent absence of an avascular zone in some, as had been previously reported by Bird and Weale.[6] They also found that the preferred point of fixation does not always correspond to the center of the avascular zone. In some individuals with an avascular zone the preferred locus of visual fixation (presumably the foveola) was found located directly under the path of a capillary, eccentrically positioned with respect to the avascular zone.[31] This observation is of practical importance when planning photocoagulation therapy in regions close to the foveal center, as in the management of diabetic retinopathy.

The velocity of blood flow in the perifoveal capillaries can be estimated by comparing the flying spot phenomenon to the apparent speed of motion of spots in an adjustable video display that mimics the flying spot appearance.[24] Autoregulation of macular blood flow has been studied by using this technique to estimate blood flow velocity in subjects (normal human adults) exposed to conditions of hypoxia and hyperoxia.[11] Isocapneic hypoxia (inspired pO_2 of 10.5%) induced a 38% increase in capillary flow velocity, while hyperoxia (inspired pO_2 of about 60%) resulted in an average 36% decrease in capillary flow velocity. A subsequent study using the same technique in patients with proliferative diabetic retinopathy found that conditions of hypoxia (inspired pO_2 of 10.5%) failed to result in the expected increase in macular capillary flow velocity.[12] This presumably was the result of antecedent, disease caused conditions of hypoxia in the diabetic retinas, causing them to have already fully expressed the autoregulatory response to oxygen deprivation.

CHORIOCAPILLARY CIRCULATION

Descriptive reports have been published of entoptic images that have been thought to arise from the choriocapillary circulation.[17] These images are seen under circumstances similar to those for visualizing the flying corpuscles, relying on intent examination of a uniform, brightly illuminated surface with no contrasting features. The images of the flying corpuscles are at length replaced by a darkened field in which a surging circulation in regular sinuses appears in a fanlike pattern. These observations have not been uniformly confirmed by others,[14] and it is somewhat difficult to understand how circulatory events external to the retina could account for sufficient alterations in light reaching photoreceptors to produce an entoptic image.

ENTOPTIC IMAGES INFLUENCED BY THE DISTRIBUTION OF RETINAL NERVE FIBERS: BLUE ARCS OF THE RETINA

During the nineteenth century Purkinje described numerous important visual phenomena. In addition to his observations on the shift of the spectral sensitivity of the eye during dark adaptation and his description of visualization of the retinal vascular tree, he was also the first to describe the phenomenon known as blue arcs. Moreland[19] refers to Purkinje's original description, in which he reported eliciting the presence of blue arcs in his visual field by using a glowing tinder taken from a fire. The effect was clearest when the glowing stimulus was on the nasal side of the field of view and was seen as two faint blue transient arcs bowed like a pair of horns around the point of fixation. These extended from the stimulus toward the position of the physiologic blind spot. On moving the stimulus farther from or closer to the point of fixation, the arcs drew apart or came together.

The level of light adaptation of the retina is important for the observation of the blue arcs. The eye must be partially light-adapted for the arcs to be visible, because with prolonged dark adaptation the arcs lose their blue color and become more difficult to see. The stimulating light may be of any color, but red has been found to be the most effective. This is probably because there is less scattering of the rays of long wavelength light. Moreland's extensive research on the phenomenon has shown that stimuli that are generally rectangular in shape are most effective.[19] When the long axis of the rectangle is parallel to the bundles of nerve fibers in the nerve fiber layer of the retina, the resulting arcs can be seen to extend in patterns exactly matching the shape of the nerve fiber bundles. Spreading or enlargement of the arcs proximal to the stimulus suggests spread of electrical excitation from nerve fibers to surrounding structures. However, the fact that the arcs do not extend from the stimulus back to the horizontal raphe argues that the electrical spread does not occur from fiber to adjacent fiber but rather from nerve fiber to underlying ganglion cell bodies

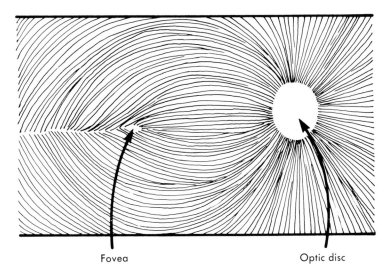

FIG. 15-8   Diagram of pattern created by nerve fiber bundles of retina in and around the macula and optic disc. Note horizontal raphe temporal to fovea and arcuate paths taken by fibers.

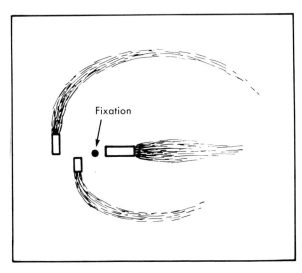

FIG. 15-9   Typical patterns created by blue arcs phenomenon. Rectangles represent shape and orientation of red stimuli most effective at eliciting the arcs. Patterns are for a right eye. Compare arcs to distribution of retinal nerve bundles in Figure 15-8. (Modified from Moreland JD, Vision Res 8:99, 1968.)

that are immediately adjacent to passing nerve fibers. When the rectangular stimulus is positioned in a horizontal orientation just temporal to the point of fixation, a blue spike appears, extending from the temporal side of fixation in a direct path toward the physiologic blind spot. Note that this image also parallels the distribution of nerve fiber bundles in the papillomacular bundle. A schematic diagram of the pattern of retinal nerve fibers surrounding the macula is shown in Figure 15-8. Patterns of blue arcs elicited by rectangular light stimuli in various portions of the central visual field are shown in Figure 15-9.

Numerous theories of the origin of the blue arc phenomenon have been proposed.* One of the best of these has been the explanation advanced by Ingling and Drum.[15] They use the phenomenon of the "silent surround" to explain what we know about the arc phenomenon. These authors used the simple experiment of partially dark adapting one portion of the visual field, while simultaneously light adapting another portion. When the arc phenomenon was then elicited across the border between dark-

*References 1, 2, 7, 13, 16, 20, 26.

and light-adapted portions of the retina, the arcs appeared dim gray in the dark-adapted portion of the visual field and bright blue in the light-adapted portion. There was a sharp zone between the two portions of the arc corresponding to the transition border between dark- and light-adapted portions of the retina. They concluded that the red-inducing stimulus somehow excites activity in cone and rod pathways underlying the nerve fiber bundles. Rod pathways are thought to provide a silent surround for the receptive fields of blue/yellow color opponent ganglion cells.

The term "silent surround" refers to a neurophysiologic property of some ganglion cell receptive fields. Stimulation of the surround portions of this type of receptive field produces a response from the cell only when the center of its receptive field is being simultaneously stimulated. Stimulation of the surround while the center of the receptive field is inactive (unstimulated) produces no response: the surround appears to be silent. There is thought to be a rod component input to the receptive fields of blue/yellow color opponent ganglion cells. This input is thought to provide a silent surround that inhibits a "yellow-on" response, but only when activity is present in the receptive field center. When the retina is partially light-adapted, tonic "yellow-on" neural activity is present in some color opponent cells. Electrical leakage of passing signals in overlying nerve fibers into the rod component of these cells produces a surround inhibition of the tonic yellow signal. In blue/yellow color opponent cells this is perceived as a blue sensation. The pattern of the blue sensation corresponds to that of the current leak from the overlying nerve fiber bundles. Where the retina has become dark-adapted and the tonic yellow signal has subsided, electrical leakage to the rod component produces only a scotopic response: a dim gray light, having no color.

ENTOPTIC IMAGES ARISING FROM THE OUTER PLEXIFORM LAYER: HAIDINGER'S BRUSHES

If one views a diffusely illuminated source of plane-polarized white or blue light, brushes or sheaves radiating from the point of fixation in the form of a Maltese cross can be seen. The brushes have contrasting yellow and blue hues. The darker portions of the Maltese pattern are yellow, whereas the brighter portions are blue. De Vries et al.[9] and Stanworth and Naylor[28] have demonstrated that the phenomenon is caused by variations in absorption of plane-polarized light by oriented molecules of xantho-

phyll pigment in the foveal retina. Stanworth found that the strength of the effect, measured by threshold measurements of the appearance of the brush effect as a function of the extent of polarization of the light, varied with the wavelength of light in a manner directly paralleling the optical density of carotenoid pigments such as xanthophyll. More recent studies by Snodderly et al.[27] of the anatomic distribution of carotenoid pigments in the foveal retina of primates have shown an appropriate density and orientation of pigment molecules in Henle's fiber layer of the macular retina to explain the Haidinger brush phenomenon. Figure 15-10 shows photomicrographs of the foveomacular portion of a monkey retina, transilluminated by green light and blue light. The yellow pigment preferentially blocked the blue light, producing a dark central spot in the inner layers of the fovea. Scanning densitometry of this section of tissue with plane-polarized light showed that the optical density of the tissue varied with the rotational orientation of the plane of polarization (Fig. 15-11). Assuming central symmetry in the orientation of the pigment molecules, this effect would explain the entoptic appearance of Haidinger's brushes.

Since the brush effect is determined by the orientation of the pigment molecules in front of the photoreceptor layer, any process that disturbs this orientation may lead to a loss of the brush image, even though the photoreceptor layer itself is normal. For this reason loss of the Haidinger brush image may indicate the presence of macular disease, such as edema, at a time when visual acuity is normal and the macula appears normal by direct ophthalmoscopy.

Two additional phenomena are closely related to the concentration of xanthophyll pigment in the macular retina: the presence of a physiologic scotoma for the detection of blue light at the fovea, as well as the phenomenon called Maxwell's spot. The latter phenomenon is seen as a dark circle surrounded by a brighter blue halo when a diffuse source of flickering blue light is observed. This has been observed frequently by subjects performing heterochromatic flicker photometry. The spot appears at the point of fixation, is approximately 2 to 3 degrees in angular size, is horizontally oval, and may also be associated with the appearance of a dark grain pattern within the spot. The physiologic scotoma for blue light is small and is centered at the point of fixation. It is not subjectively noticeable but is easily detected when using monochromatic blue lights to measure sensitivity across the center of the visual field.

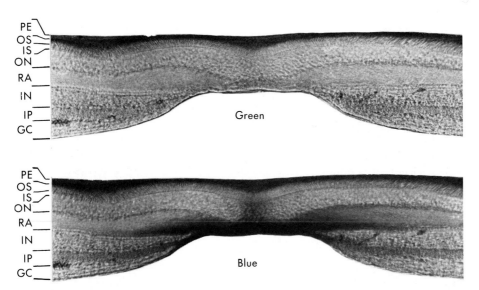

FIG. 15-10 Photomicrographs of foveal portion of macular retina of *M. mulatta* in green light *(top)* and blue light *(bottom)*. Macular xanthophyll pigment transmits green light but absorbs blue light, producing dark areas in bottom image. Pigment appears most concentrated in receptor axon (RA) layer of foveal retina. Retinal layers: PE, pigment epithelium; OS, receptor outer segments; IS, receptor inner segments; ON, outer nuclear layer; RA, receptor axons; IN, inner nuclear layer; IP, inner plexiform layer; GC, ganglion cell layer. Photomicrographs courtesy Dr. D.M. Snodderly. (From Snodderly, DM, et al: Invest Opthalmol Vis Sci 25:674, 1984.)

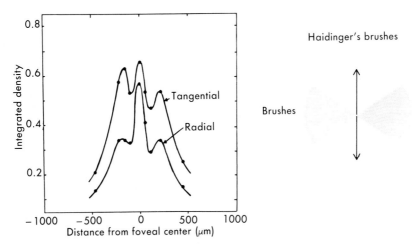

FIG. 15-11 Appearance of Haidinger's brushes is determined by differential absorption of plane polarized light by xanthophyll pigment molecules oriented about the center of the foveal macula. *Left,* Microdensitometry scans of tissue section in Figure 15-10 gave curves for tangentially and radially oriented plane polarized light. Absorption is lower for radially oriented plane of polarization. *Right,* Dark portion of brush pattern results from greater absorption of tangentially oriented light (vertically oriented plane of polarization). Courtesy Dr. D.M. Snodderly. (From Snodderly, DM, et al: Invest Opthalmol Vis Sci 25:674, 1984.)

ENTOPTIC PHENOMENA CAUSED BY PROPERTIES OF RETINAL PHOTORECEPTORS

Self-illumination of the retina

When the eye has become fully dark-adapted, one does not have a visual sensation of blackness, but rather of a definite grayness that is actually subjectively lighter in appearance than the sensation produced by looking at a matte black surface of near zero reflectance. This persistent sensation of light in a dark-adapted eye probably arises from spontaneous neural activity (noise), which has been termed the "dark light" or equivalent background of the dark-adapted retina.[4] In addition there are probably central (cerebral) origins of such sensations as well.

Phosphenes

Mechanical pressure on the eye will produce the impression of a dark circular spot in the visual field directly opposite the point of contact with the globe. This type of sensation, which is produced by inadequate retinal stimuli, is called a phosphene. Prolongation of the mechanical pressure against the globe will slowly generate the appearance of a contrasting ring of colored light in the form of a broad circular band of blue surrounding the central dark zone.[14] The pressure has to be strong enough to cause slight discomfort and, according to some authors, must be maintained for 3 minutes. Two areas of blue (one to either side of fixation) first appear and slowly expand to assume the form of a broad arc. The figure expands until the arcs coalesce into a blue circle, the center of which is oval and devoid of color. The cause of the phenomenon is unknown, but the location of the pressure oval corresponds roughly to the zone of maximum rod population described by Østerberg.[22]

Unlike the blue ring of prolonged pressure, a more transient phenomenon can be seen in a completely dark-adapted eye. An immediate bright blue ring appears after application of gentle pressure to the globe. This ring is transient and appears in the visual field opposite the point of pressure. Its onset is almost instantaneous, and it disappears rapidly even though the pressure is maintained. For maximal dark adaption the phenomenon is best elicited after a night's sleep, while the room is still completely dark.

Stiles-Crawford effect

The Stiles-Crawford effect is a phenomenon related to the directional sensitivity of retinal photoreceptors. Parallel rays of light entering the

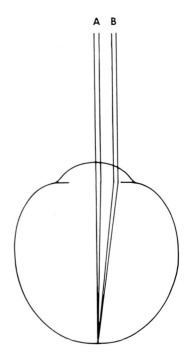

FIG. 15-12 Normal retinal directional sensitivity effect. Light in bundle entering through center of the pupil, A, is more effective in stimulating retinal cones than in bundle coming into eye near edge of dilated pupil and hence reaching retinal cones obliquely, B. (From Westheimer G: Arch Ophthalmol 79:584, 1968.)

pupil through its center are more effective in stimulating retinal cones than are those that enter the eye near the edge of a dilated pupil, reaching the retinal cones somewhat more obliquely (Fig. 15-12). If the strength of an adapting light beam is measured at various points of entry through the pupillary aperture, according to its ability to bring a constant brightness of flickering test light to the threshold of perception (Fig. 15-13), its effectiveness is found to vary in a systematic fashion. Its peak effectiveness is near the center of the pupillary aperture for the normal eye and falls steadily toward the periphery of the pupillary aperture in a symmetric fashion. Eyes that are not normal, such as those having irregular posterior staphylomas or myopia, may have an asymmetric arrangement of foveal cone receptors in relation to the pupillary aperture. In such eyes (Fig. 15-14) there may be marked asymmetry of the Stiles-Crawford effect. Westheimer[30] has demonstrated for his own eye that by deliberately throwing the image of a point source of light out of focus (Figs. 15-15 and 15-16), the brightness

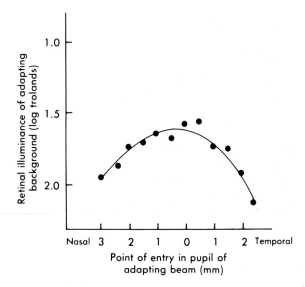

FIG. 15-13   Normal retinal directional sensitivity pattern. Abscissae: point of entry along horizontal meridian of pupil, of bundle of light providing background; ordinates: relative sensitivity of retina, measured by inverse of amount of light necessary in background field to bring constant ΔI stimulus to threshold. Background (7.5 degrees) was exposed continously and ordinates give its retinal illuminance in trolands of green light (tungsten source filtered by gelatin filter and neutral wedge). Incremental stimulus was circular field, 12 minutes of arc in diameter, 0.05 second in duration, 30 trolands of red light, and was placed at threshold by adjustment of wedge in background beam. (From Westheimer G: Arch Ophthalmol 79:584, 1968.)

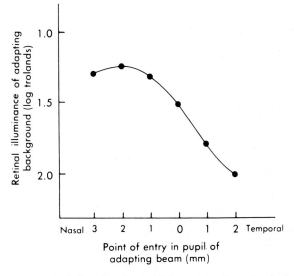

FIG. 15-14   Asymmetric retinal directional sensitivity pattern in author's right eye, foveal vision. Abscissae: point of entry of bundle of light providing background; ordinates: relative sensitivity of retina, measured by inverse of amount of light necessary in background field to bring constant ΔI stimulus to threshold. (From Westheimer G: Arch Ophthalmol 79:584, 1968.)

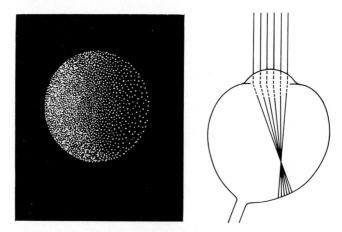

FIG. 15-15 *Left*, Appearance of foveal blue patch of bright star against dark sky seen with uncorrected myopic right eye with large pupil. Stiles-Crawford pattern of this eye, illustrated in Fig. 15-14, is asymmetric. *Right*, Schematic diagram illustrating path of rays making up blur patch. Fact that seen pattern is brightest near its left border implies that receptors in region of fovea point in direction of nasal edge of dilated pupil. (From Westheimer G: Arch Ophthalmol 79:584, 1968.)

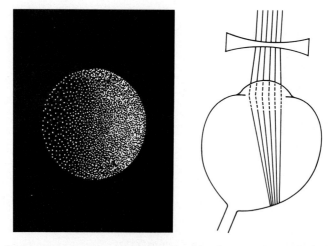

FIG. 15-16 *Left*, Appearance of foveal blur patch of bright star against dark sky seen under artificially hyperopic condition with large pupil in right eye with asymmetrical Stiles-Crawford effect (Figs. 15-14 and 15-15). *Right*, Schematic diagram illustrating path of rays making up blur patch. Right edge of seen pattern corresponds to nasal edge of retinal blur patch. Fact that it is brightest implies that receptors in foveal region are pointing to nasal edge of dilated pupil. (From Westheimer G: Arch Ophthalmol 79:584, 1968.)

of the foveal blur patch can itself be seen to be asymmetric. The asymmetry can be predicted from the known foveal cone tilt.

REFERENCES

1. Alpern M, Dudley D: The blue arcs of the retina, J Gen Physiol 49:405, 1966.
2. Amberson W: Secondary excitation in the retina, Am J Physiol 69:354, 1924.
3. Applegate RA, Bradley A, van Heuven WAJ: Entoptic visualization of the retinal vasculature near fixation, Invest Ophthalmol Vis Sci 31:2088, 1990.
4. Barlow HB: Dark adaptation: a new hypothesis, Vision Res 4:47, 1964.
5. Berens C, et al: Moore's lightning streaks, Trans Am Ophthalmol Soc 52:35, 1954.
6. Bird AC, Weale RA: On the retinal vasculature of the human fovea, Exp Eye Res 19:409, 1974.
7. Boehm G: The entoptic phenomenon of the "blue arcs" (observations on subjects affected with night blindness and total color blindness), Ophthalmologica 4-5:276, 1949.
8. Dangle ME, Kracher OD, Stark WJ: Anterior corneal mosaic in eyes with keratoconus wearing hard contact lenses, Arch Ophthalmol 102:888, 1984.
9. De Vries H, Spoor A, Jielff R: Properties of the eye with respect to polarized light, Physica 19:419, 1953.
10. Esser AAM: Mikroskopie der eigenen Hornhaut, Klin Monatsbl Augenheilk 76:389, 1926.
11. Fallon TJ, Maxwell D, Kohner EM: Retinal vascular autoregulation in conditions of hyperoxia and hypoxia using the blue field entoptic phenomenon, Ophthalmol 92:701, 1985.
12. Fallon TJ, Maxwell DL, Kohner EM: Autoregulation of retinal blood flow in diabetic retinopathy measured by the blue-light entoptic technique, Ophthalmol 94:1410, 1987.
13. Friedman B: The blue arcs of the retina, Arch Ophthalmol 6:663, 1931.
14. Friedman B: Observations on entoptic phenomena, Arch Ophthalmol 28:285, 1942.
15. Ingling CR Jr, Drum BA: Why the blue arcs of the retina are blue, Vision Res 17:498, 1977.
16. Ladd-Franklin C: Alternative theories to account for the reddish blue arcs and the reddish blue glow of the retina, J Opt Soc Am 16:333, 1928.
17. Marshall C: Entoptic phenomena associated with the retina, Br J Ophthalmol 19:177, 1935.
18. Moore RF: Subjective lightning streaks, Br J Ophthalmol 19:545, 1935.
19. Moreland JD: On demonstrating the blue arcs phenomenon, Vision Res 8:99, 1968.
20. Moreland JD: Threshold measurements of the blue arcs phenomenon, Vision Res 8:1093, 1968.
21. Nebel B: The phosphene of quick eye motion, Arch Ophthalmol 58:235, 1957.
22. Østerberg G: Topography of the layer of rods and cones in the human retina, Acta Ophthalmol 6(Suppl):1, 1935.
23. Pischel D: Detachment of the vitreous as seen with slit-lamp examination, Trans Am Ophthalmol Soc 50:329, 1952.
24. Riva CE, Petrig B: Blue field entoptic phenomenon and blood velocity in the retinal capillaries, J Opt Soc Am 70:1234, 1980.
25. Sinclair HS, et al: Investigation of the source of the blue field entoptic phenomenon, Inv Ophthalmol Vis Sci 30:668, 1989.
26. Snell P: The entoptic phenomenon of the blue arc, Arch Ophthalmol 1:475, 1929.
27. Snodderly DM, Auran JD, Delori FC: The macular pigment, II, Spatial distribution in primate retinas, Invest Ophthalmol Vis Sci 25:674, 1984.
28. Stanworth A, Naylor E: The measurement and clinical significance of the Haidinger effect, Trans Ophthalmol Soc UK 75:67, 1955.
29. Verhoeff F: Are Moore's lightning streaks of serious portent? Am J Ophthalmol 41:837, 1956.
30. Westheimer G: Entoptic visualization of Stiles-Crawford effect, Arch Ophthalmol 79:584, 1968.
31. Zeffren BS, Applegate RA, Bradley A, et al: Retinal fixation point location in the foveal avascular zone, Invest Ophthalmol Vis Sci 31:2088, 1990.

GENERAL REFERENCE

Rubin ML, Walls GL: Studies in physiological optics, Springfield, IL, Charles C Thomas, Publisher, 1965.

Visual Adaptation

WILLIAM M. HART, Jr., M.D., PH.D.

The vertebrate visual system is highly specialized for the detection and analysis of patterns of light distributed in time and space. Variations of radiant intensity in naturally occurring images cover an extremely large dynamic range of energies. To be capable of light detection at extremely low levels of energy and yet also be capable of analyzing the spatial distribution of light at very high energies, the visual system has the capacity to modify its behavior as needed. After exposure of the eye to a strong source of light, visual sensitivity decreases. However, at the same time the visual system also develops a more rapid response to changes in light (temporal acuity) and an increased level of spatial resolution (visual acuity). Conversely, the process is reversed in the dark; the sensitivity of the eye to light increases dramatically over a period of time, although at the expense of a reduction in temporal and spatial acuities. This complex set of phenomena is referred to as visual adaptation.

A useful but deceptively simplified analogy compares visual adaptation to the photographer's use of varying photographic emulsions, lens apertures, and shutter speeds to produce an image with maximal clarity. If an excessive quantity of light strikes a too-sensitive film, an "overexposure" results, in which the entire image is very bright but contains no contrasting detail. Conversely, an inadequate level of light in a dim image that strikes a film with too low a sensitivity results in an "underexposure," a dark image that also lacks sufficient contrasting detail. Suitable adjustments to the amount of light entering the camera, or the use of a photographic emulsion with an appropriate sensitivity, can produce an average level of light energy in the image that is near the midrange of sensitivity of the film. This allows capture of a photographic image of maximal clarity. However, as a practical matter, few living organisms have the time to make similar adjustments to their visual systems. There is little need to capture static images. Rather, the requirement is for near-instantaneous perception of surrounding objects whose appearance is continuously changing. Biologic visual systems have evolved to rely on automatic and nearly instantaneous adjustments to their visual sensitivities to extract the maximal amount of information from the images of their surrounding environments.

MECHANISMS OF VISUAL ADAPTATION

The variation of intensities of light from the threshold of light detection through the maximal operating range of the eye at the upper limit of photopic vision is truly enormous. Visual sensitivity varies to cover a dynamic range of more than one billion to one. Because of this tremendous disparity in sizes of numbers from the top to the bottom of the response range of the eye, it is customary to compress the scale of light in-

This work was supported in part by Research Grant EY 06582 from the National Eye Institute, National Institutes of Health.

tensities by expressing the values as the logarithms of the numbers involved.* If the range of intensity of illumination within which the eye can discriminate changes is from 1 to 1 billion, then expressed in logarithmic units the range is from 0 to 9. Across this broad variation of light levels, there are three kinds of sensitivity adjustment that the visual system can make. These include: (1) changes in the size of the pupil, (2) changes in the level of neural activity in the cellular elements of the afferent visual system, and (3) changes in the steady-state concentrations of photosensitive pigments in the retina. These three adapting mechanisms differ from one another in the rapidity and extent of their responses to changes in light. The size of the pupil can be altered in a period of approximately 1 second and can change the amount of light entering the eye by a factor of about 16. This is little more than a single log unit, which is only a small fraction of the total range within which the eye is capable of adjusting. Changes in neural activity in the retina occur within a few milliseconds and adjust the sensitivity of the retina to changes in light intensity over a range of more than 1000 to one, or 3 log units. Changes in the steady-state concentrations of photosensitive pigments require time periods of minutes, but can alter the sensitivity of the eye over the broadest range of light intensities: 100 million to one, or 8 log units.

SUBJECTIVE OBSERVATIONS

To illustrate the phenomenologic consequences of the differing mechanisms of adaptation, it is helpful to review some familiar observations of how our eyes respond to altering levels of illumination. Everyone is aware that it "takes time to become accustomed to the dark." The time course of change in sensitivity of the eye kept in the dark after a period of exposure to a high level of light is a protracted one, requiring many minutes. On entering a darkened movie theater on a sunlit day, at first one is completely blind, unable to distinguish any detail. However, during a period of approximately 8 to 10 minutes, dimly lit objects become gradually discernible. The sensitivity of the eye increases gradually, and after 20 to 30 minutes a maximal visual sensitivity is reached that allows one to move about with ease in the darkened room without stumbling over chairs or colliding with other people.

The reverse process, adaptation to a high level of illumination, is more rapid. On leaving the theater, initially one will be dazzled by bright sunlight, the intensity of which may be enough to cause a sensation of discomfort. However, within a period of 3 to 5 minutes, one becomes comfortably adapted to this very high level of light.

What may not be immediately apparent during the course of visual adaptation to extremely high or low levels of illumination is that the quality of vision is radically altered during the transition between the two extremes. The retina actually has a dual photoreceptor system. One of these is extremely sensitive, operates best at low levels of illumination, and depends on light detection by photoreceptor elements that are filled with rhodopsin. These cells are called rods. The other type of photoreceptors, called cones, are less sensitive to light and act most effectively in daylight. There are three separate types of cones, differing from one another by the spectral absorptions of the photosensitive pigments they contain. Dark-adapted or rod-dependent vision is termed "scotopic vision," while light-adapted or cone-dependent vision is termed "photopic vision." Scotopic vision is characterized by a high sensitivity to light, allowing visual detection of objects at extremely low levels of illumination. At the same time, scotopic vision is remarkable for a low level of visual acuity (poor discrimination of fine detail) and a complete absence of color perception.

As retinal illumination increases, there is a change from rod-dominated vision to cone-dominated vision. This is associated with a change in the spectral sensitivity of the eye. The wavelength of light at which the eye is maximally sensitive is longer for photopic than for scotopic vision (see Chapter 13). This change in spectral sensitivity first was noted in the nineteenth century by Purkinje, and for this reason is called the Purkinje shift. Anatomists were the first to propose the duplex theory of vision, based on their observations of the dominance of rods in the retinas of nocturnal animals and the presence or dominance of cones in the retinas of diurnal animals.

The shift from photopic to scotopic vision in the human is characterized by multiple changes in visual performance. The scotopically (dark) adapted retina is maximally sensitive to the lowest energies of available light. However, this form of vision is characterized by an absence of color perception and very poor spatial resolution (low visual acuity). On the other hand, photopic vision is characterized by relatively

---

*In a base 10 numbering system, the logarithm of a number is the power to which 10 must be raised to yield that number. Thus the logarithm of 1 is 0, of 10 is 1, of 100 is 2, etc.

low sensitivity to light, such that objects must be illuminated brightly to be perceived. However, in return for sacrificing threshold sensitivity for perception of light, there is an increase in both spatial and temporal acuities as well as the addition of color perception. These phenomena are easily demonstrable. If one becomes fully dark-adapted and attempts to read a book by very dim illumination, it will be observed that colors on the book cover cannot be distinguished and that, although the very largest type elements might be distinguishable, attempts to read the body of the text itself are hopeless. This in spite of the fact that the book itself is visible. In common terms it is said that the light is "not good enough." Simply turning on a lamp in the room will make the colors of the text cover immediately visible, and one will be capable of reading the finest print in the text.

The differences between rod and cone vision account for the phenomenon of a relative foveal depression of visual sensitivity in the fully dark-adapted retina. Anatomically, rods are absent from the very center of the retina, where there is a pure cone photoreceptor layer. For this reason, in the fully dark-adapted retina the maximal sensitivity for detection of light is present in the extrafoveal retina. If one gazes at a very dim point of light while fully dark-adapted (for example, a faint star on a moonless night), it can be demonstrated that the star is invisible when attempts are made to look directly at it. Diverting one's gaze to a point a few degrees to one side of the star's position will make it visible. The location of maximal rod density in the retina, and hence of maximal dark-adapted visual sensitivity, is approximately 7 degrees away from fixation in a zone concentric with the fovea.

Stars are visible at night but not during the day. This is in spite of the fact that the brightness of the stars is the same whether the sun appears in the overhead sky or is located on the opposite side of the earth. The fact that the stars become invisible during the day is caused by the higher levels of light to which the eye has become adapted in the presence of sunlight. The intensity of dispersed light in the daytime sky is many logarithmic units higher than that of the dim sources of light provided by the distant stars. Therefore the brightness of the stars would have to increase by several orders of magnitude (log units) to be visible during the day. The degree to which the brightness of a point source of light must be increased relative to its background describes a function known as the increment brightness sensitivity, or the threshold for brightness contrast perception.*

PSYCHOPHYSICAL OBSERVATIONS
Increment brightness sensitivity

Most of what we know about visual adaptation was first studied experimentally by the techniques of psychophysics. Such experiments use the human subject as an "instrument of measurement." Despite the use of what might seem a very subjective method, this approach has extraordinary sensitivity and specificity for the study of sensory systems. This presumes that adequate controls are used to fix the values of as many variables as possible and to allow changes in only one experimental variable at a time. One of the most important psychophysical experiments for studying visual adaptation has been the determination of increment brightness sensitivity. A general method for the determination of increment brightness sensitivity is as follows: a uniform field of light of luminance I (for intensity) is presented to the test subject. After a period of adaptation to this level of illumination, a spot of light is superimposed (projected) onto the background light as a short flash (Fig. 16-1). The luminance of the spot of light is the sum of the background luminance, I, plus the added luminance, ΔI, so that the total luminance of the test spot is $I + \Delta I$. If ΔI is too dim, the test flash will be invisible. If ΔI is sufficiently bright, the test flash will be seen with every presentation. Between these two extremes, the threshold in-

---

*Remember that sensitivity and threshold are inverse expressions of the same function: sensitivity = 1/threshold.

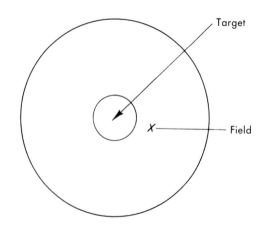

FIG. 16-1 Test target of light projected on background or adapting field of light.

tensity of the test flash generally will be seen with a probability greater than 0 but less than 1. Threshold intensity is defined arbitrarily as that brightness of test flash that will be seen with a probability of 0.5. ΔI is termed the "liminal brightness increment," when its intensity (added to the background) is just sufficient to reach threshold.

The Weber-Fechner relation

If ΔI is determined for a range of different background luminances, the results will vary with the location of retina being tested. Thus if the test spot of light is viewed foveally, a different result will be obtained than if it is viewed at a point 7 degrees from fixation. However, although absolute levels of sensitivity will vary from one point on the retina to another, the general behavior of changes in ΔI with variations in I remains remarkably similar. As shown in Figure 16-2, when the background adapting light intensity is low, very little additional light (ΔI) must be added to reach threshold. Over a range of background luminances that are very low, the increment ΔI stays much the same or may even decrease slightly. In this dark-adapted range in the peripheral retina (in this case, 7 degrees from fixation), the eye is a very efficient detector of light. Although the low background luminances may not be perceptible, the sum of $I + \Delta I$ is a constant. The slight decreases in ΔI, plotted 7 degrees from the fovea between -4 and -3 log units of adapting field intensity as one proceeds to the right, is an expression of the fact that when I is below threshold, $I + \Delta I$ is nearly constant. As the background intensity rises, ΔI increases and the function of ΔI versus I over a broad range above threshold is that of a straight line. Because the line is straight, its slope is a

constant. In this linear range ΔI is a constant fraction of I, which is to say

$$\Delta I / I = \text{constant} \tag{1}$$

This relationship is termed the "Weber fraction," and the constancy of this fraction is often termed the "Weber-Fechner relation." The phenomenon of relative constancy of the ratio of an increment stimulus to its adapting level is a feature that has been found to be common to almost all sensory receptors, including mechanoreceptors, thermoreceptors, and chemoreceptors.

In the middle of the graph of Figure 16-2 the curves flatten abruptly. It is at this adapting level of intensity that colors begin to be perceptible and visual acuity improves markedly. This region is the threshold intensity for cone function. The angulation of the curve is the transition zone between all rod and rod plus cone activity. Note that to the left side of the graph the function rises linearly, demonstrating a constant Weber fraction for the rod limb of the adaptation function. As the adapting intensity rises into the region of cone function and cones become more and more dominant, a second ascending limb of the function again shows a nearly straight line. This shows that the Weber fraction remains constant over a range of at least 3 logarithmic units for cone function. If data were to be collected at higher levels of adapting intensity than those shown in Figure 16-2, the curve would be found to again rise steeply far off to the right-hand side. The cone mechanism eventually becomes saturated at very high intensities of light and no longer functions effectively to detect differences between the test spot and its background. At these extremely high levels of radiant intensity energy transfer to the

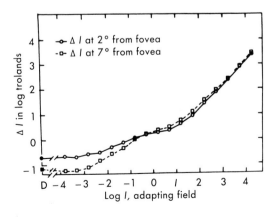

FIG. 16-2 Equilibrium relationships between absolute threshold *(black points on extreme left)* and difference threshold to various background luminances *(open points)* in one subject. (From Baker HD: Night vision and visual sensitivity in Whitcomb MA, Benson W, eds: The measurement of visual function, Washington, DC, Armed Forces NRC Committee on Vision, National Academy of Sciences, National Research Council, 1968.)

retina can become high enough to cause thermal damage, resulting in edema and eventually photocoagulation of the tissue.

Also shown in Figure 16-2 is the difference between the increment sensitivity function at points close to the fovea, as compared with those farther away. In the cone-dominated region of the retina close to the fovea the absolute threshold for vision is much higher, and the rod-cone transition between the two (left and right) portions of the curve is not so easily discernible.

Increment sensitivity and clinical perimetry

An understanding of increment sensitivity is basic to an appreciation of the techniques used in clinical perimetry to test visual sensitivity distributed in visual space: the visual field examination. The technique of static perimetry involves the use of diffusely illuminated adapting backgrounds, against which small test objects are projected at predetermined positions. The projected spots of light, of controlled intensity and size, represent the ΔI stimuli added to the intensity of the background adapting light, I. At any one location in the retina $\Delta I/I$ will be found to be a constant over a broad range of adapting luminances. In practice, a single adapting background intensity usually is selected for testing all regions of the retina. As shown in Figure 16-3, in the fully dark-adapted eye, where absolute thresholds are being measured, a small relative depression of visual sensitivity can be demonstrated at the fovea.[5] This is a physiologic scotoma (a focal depression of visual sensitivity) caused by the absence of rods from the foveal

retina. With adaptation to mesopic and photopic levels of background illumination, increment brightness sensitivity drops for all regions of the retina, but drops to a greater extent for the rod-dominated portions of the extrafoveal retina. Consequently, the profile shape of the visual field at mesopic and photopic adapting brightnesses no longer shows the presence of the foveal scotoma, but rather has the shape of a peak of visual sensitivity at the point of fixation with a steadily falling sensitivity as one moves away from the fovea into increasingly peripheral locations of the retina. By convention, the adapting luminance used with the Goldmann perimeter is 31.5 asb (10.0 candelas/m²).* This represents a so-called mesopic level of visual adaptation, at which rods and cones contribute nearly equally to visual sensitivity.

Lateral inhibition

In addition to the constancy of increment brightness sensitivity as a multiple of adapting luminance, other adaptation phenomena are of equal importance for the definition of visual images. These generally act to improve the contrast of adjacent but differing zones of brightness of images falling on the retina. Termed "lateral inhibition," these features of adaptation are thought to result from neural mechanisms. They are mediated by facilitation and inhibition of retinal neural activity in response to local variations in retinal illumination and respond rap-

---

*For definitions of apostilbs, candelas, and other units of luminance see Chapter 13, p. 458.

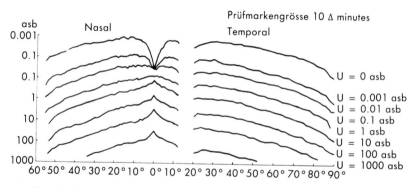

FIG. 16-3 Threshold static perimetry. Threshold luminances of 10-minute test objects (projected spots of light on a diffusely illuminated background) at different levels of adaptation (background luminances), U. Threshold values are plotted (ordinate) at various angular distances from fixation (abscissa) along the horizontal meridian. (From Aulhorn E: Graefes Arch Ophthalmol 167:4, 1964.)[5]

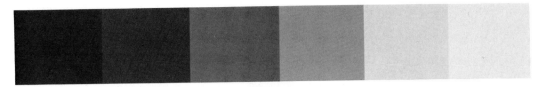

FIG. 16-4 Mach bands. *Rectangles,* Uniform shades of gray, separated by contrast borders. Dark band is seen on dark side of each contrast border and light band on each light side.

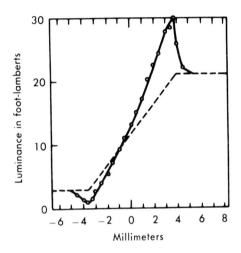

FIG. 16-5 Mach bands at junctions of brightness gradient with uniform field. *Broken line,* luminance distribution; *solid line,* subjective distribution. (From Lowry EM, DePalma JJ: J Opt Soc Am 51:740, 1961.)

idly to changes in illumination to adjust the apparent brightness of adjacent zones in the visual field. First characterized by psychophysical methods, the physiologic bases for these phenomena have been more difficult to define. By whatever mechanisms, stimulation of one portion of the retina can be shown to induce a depression of visual sensitivity in surrounding areas. This effect is responsible for the enhancement of contrasting borders. This enhancement can be demonstrated with images like that of Figure 16-4. This picture was produced with solid gray rectangles of differing brightness placed adjacent to one another. Although the central area of each rectangle appears to be uniform in brightness, at the right-hand border of each rectangle a band of relative darkness is seen, while a band of relative lightness can be seen at its left edge where it adjoins a darker neighbor. These are referred to as "Mach bands."[49] The dark and bright Mach bands may be separated from one another by broadening the junction of the two fields of differing brightness into a gradient of transition from one brightness level to the other (Fig. 16-5). Then

the dark and bright enhancement stripes appear at either side of the ramp.[40]

Another observation that can be attributed to lateral inhibition is shown in Figure 16-6. The gray squares at the center of the right and left halves of this image are identical in brightness (reflectivity). However, the part surrounded by a black border appears to be brighter than its counterpart, which is surrounded by a white border. The presence of the black frame around the square on the left serves to enhance its apparent brightness.

Yet another related illusion is that discovered by Dr. Kenneth Craik, shown in Figure 16-7. The inner half of the circular disc appears to be brighter than the outer half, although this is only an illusion. The reflectivity of each half is identical. The disc was formed by rapid rotation about its center of the structure shown in Figure 16-8. This disc has a black sector with an irregularity along one of its edges. When the disc is rotated rapidly, the irregularity along the edge of the black sector causes a small excess of darkness to appear on one side of a circular boundary and a small excess of brightness on the other

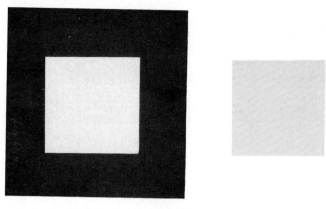

FIG. 16-6 A gray square looks lighter on a black background than it does on a white background.

FIG. 16-7 Disc shown in Fig. 16-8 spun fast and photographed. Except for discontinuity near midradius, whole disc is ⅚ white and ⅙ black, but outer half looks darker. (Courtesy Kenneth Craik.)

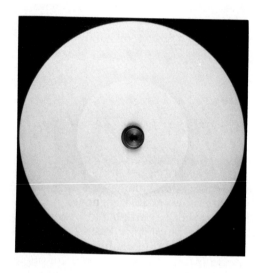

FIG. 16-8 White circular disc with 60-degree sector cut out of form shown. (Courtesy Kenneth Craik.)

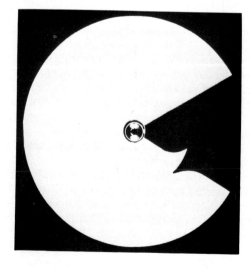

side. The circular boundary in the photograph of the spinning disc is located at the position of the irregularity. This boundary has the effect of producing a lateral spread of deceptive information across the entire surface of the disc. If the boundary on the image of the spinning disc is covered, such that the zone surrounding the boundary is selectively removed from view, the two remaining (inner and outer) portions of the spinning disc that remain visible will appear to be identically bright.

Troxler's phenomenon

A related phenomenon of contrasting borders is termed "Troxler's phenomenon." If a spot of light is presented in the peripheral visual field at a fixed increment above an adapting background light, and if the position of the spot remains unchanged for a period of several seconds, it will begin slowly to disappear from view. As soon as the spot of light is changed in position, or if the point of fixation of the eye is changed, the spot will reappear immediately. At first one might think that this phenomenon could be explained by local bleaching of photoreceptors at the position of the stabilized spot stimulus. However, the fact that the spot appears immediately on movement of the eye shows that recovery of sensitivity is nearly instantaneous and does not follow the time course of regeneration of photopigments. Rather, this appears to be a rapid mechanism that is presumably neural in its basis. The entoptic imagery of the Purkinje figures probably is a good example of the same phenomenon (see Chapter 15). As long as the shadows of the retinal vessels are superimposed in a constant position over the underlying photoreceptors, their contrasting borders on the retinal surface remain invisible. This would suggest that any image that was stabilized in position on the retinal surface would lose all contrasting detail. This has been found to be the case experimentally. If a suitable optical arrangement is used to fix the location of an image on the surface of the retina, its contrasting details fade slowly from view within a few seconds, to be replaced by a luminous brightness that contains no discernible features. However, minute displacement of the image on the surface of the retina results in an instantaneous reappearance of all contrasting features within the image. The motor system that controls eye position during steadily maintained visual fixation has a built-in mechanism that causes the eye to undergo constant and imperceptibly small movements. These consist of slow drifts and rapid flicks with angular amplitudes no greater than a fraction of a degree (see section on fixation maintenance system, p. 174). The effect of these involuntary movements is to prevent images from becoming fixed in position on the retina and to maintain visibility of contrast features within images in spite of attempts to hold steady visual fixation.

EARLY THEORIES OF VISION AND ADAPTATION

After the isolation of rhodopsin from rods, the cycle of photopigment bleaching by light and regeneration in the dark was identified. Early investigators proposed a "photochemical theory" of vision and adaptation.[36] This theory explained much of what was known at the time about visual performance on the basis of the bleach-regeneration kinetics of photopigments. Although the exact concentrations of photopigments in the receptors could not be measured, the best assumptions at the time concluded that there was a direct correspondence between photon capture by the pigments, accompanied by photochemical bleaching and the subjective sensations of vision. According to the theory, perception of light required photochemical bleaching of a fixed amount of pigment for a given subjective sensation of brightness. Bleaching of the pigment in turn resulted in its depletion, thus reducing visual sensitivity. Dark adaptation required complete regeneration of the photopigment to its light-sensitive state. Subsequent work has shown this theory to be grossly inadequate, however. Since then it has become apparent that only a very small fraction of the total available photopigment needs to be bleached to produce a very large reduction in visual sensitivity. The photochemical theory predicted that 50% bleaching of photopigment should double the visual threshold. In fact, threshold is raised by approximately 8 logarithmic units (a factor of 100 million) under these circumstances. The actual relation between bleaching and the rise of log threshold is closely approximated by

$$\log(\Delta I/\Delta I_0) = 10HB \qquad (2)$$

where

ΔI = threshold
ΔI_0 = fully dark threshold
B = fraction of rhodopsin still in bleached state
H = constant of about 2

H is the rise in log threshold as a result of 10% bleaching. This relationship first was determined in the human by a technique called reflection densitometry[13] and later was confirmed in experimental animals by recording changes in the threshold of the electroretinogram.[19,20]

If not photopigment depletion, then what does determine the relationship between the eye's prior exposure and its current sensitivity to light? It is apparent from our prior discussions that some changes in sensitivity are nearly instantaneous, having delay times of very small fractions of a second. Other changes in sensitivity may require many minutes, such as the prolonged dark adaptation required for complete regeneration of photopigment.

THE PSYCHOPHYSICS OF RAPID EVENTS IN VISUAL ADAPTATION

If a subject is allowed to adapt to a dimly lighted background and then is presented with a sequence of two flashes of light separated in time by a variable extent, the effect of these two flashes on one another follows a characteristic time course. If the first flash of light is thought of as an adapting light and the second flash is thought of as a test stimulus, it can be shown that the adapting flash will increase the threshold (reduce sensitivity) for detection of the test flash if it is presented near enough in time to the test flash. This sort of experiment, as reported by Crawford,[18] is illustrated in Figure 16-9. The data show the instantaneous changes in threshold for the detection of test flashes of light as a function of the timing of an adapting flash having a duration of 500 milliseconds. Data are shown for three different brightnesses of conditioning flash. On the left-hand side of the figure, threshold before presentation of the conditioning flash has a value of −1.5 logarithmic units. In a seeming paradox, threshold for the test spots of light is seen to rise prior to the actual time at which the bright conditioning flash is turned on. This "anticipation" effect is termed "backward masking." This phenomenon has been explained by assuming that the time required by the visual system to transmit information to the brain about a flash of light is inversely proportional to the brightness of the flash. The latency for perception of a dim threshold flash of light is greater than that for a bright flash. Even though the test flash may be presented prior to the bright flash, it arrives at cortical centers for visual perception at a later time than the adapting flash. Therefore threshold for detection of the test flash appears to be elevated even before presentation of the adapting flash.

Several other features of the tracings in Figure 16-9 are of interest. After an initial spike in threshold for detection of test flashes, the curves settle down into a gently sloping plateau. Near the termination of the adapting flash, there is another slight peak before the threshold values drop rapidly toward the original levels of adaptation. Note that these changes are rapid, and threshold fluctuates by as much as 4.5 logarithmic units in times of less than 50 milliseconds at the onset of the conditioning flash. Similarly, at the cessation of the conditioning flash, threshold falls by approximately 2.5 logarithmic units in less than 100 milliseconds. It is clear that these rapid changes in sensitivity need some explanation other than the regeneration of photopigments, a process that has a time constant of approximately 2 minutes.

THE PSYCHOPHYSICS OF SLOW EVENTS IN VISUAL ADAPTATION

If a subject is taken from a brightly illuminated environment and put into total darkness, the sensitivity of his or her vision will begin to recover in a slow and characteristic fashion, a process that is called "dark adaptation." This recov-

FIG. 16-9 Crawford's measurements of threshold luminance of test flash as affected by brief flash of conditioning (adapting) light. Duration of conditioning flash was 0.5 second in each case, beginning at time 0. (From Crawford BH: Proc Roy Soc 134:283, 1947.)[18]

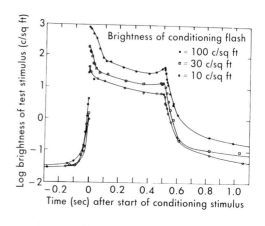

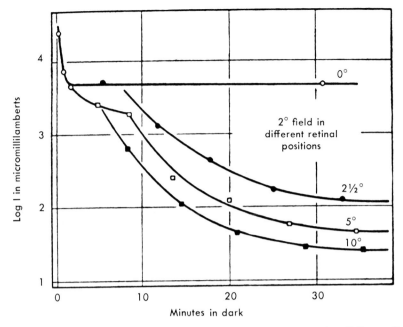

FIG. 16-10 Dark adaptation as measured with a 2-degree field placed at different distances from center. (From Hecht S, Haig C, Wald G: J Gen Physiol 19:321, 1935.)[35]

ery of sensitivity can be recorded by measuring the brightness of a dim flashing light necessary for achieving the threshold of perception. The brightness of the flashing test light at threshold is recorded as a function of time in the dark. Figure 16-10 shows a set of dark adaptation curves obtained by this technique.[35] Notice that the shape of the dark adaptation curves varies with the location of the retina where the test is performed. When the test flashes are presented at a location 5 degrees from the fovea, the curve is seen to have a biphasic characteristic. At time zero, threshold is very high. It then falls rapidly to nearly level out at about 1 log unit below its initial value. However, at approximately 9 minutes into the recording, the threshold again begins to fall more quickly, subsequently taking more than 30 minutes to reach its fully dark-adapted state at 3 logarithmic units (1000 times) more sensitive than the initial point of the curve.

It has been shown through a variety of experimental techniques that the upper branch of the biphasic dark adaptation curve measures the threshold of cone perception, whereas the lower portion of the biphasic curves represents the recovery of sensitivity of rods. Also shown in Figure 16-10 is that when the test light falls on the fovea (at the visual center of the retina) the lower branch of the biphasic curve is missing. This finding fits the duplex theory of the bi-

phasic (cone-rod) feature of dark adaptation curves, because the foveal population of photoreceptors is known to be devoid of rods and to consist entirely of cones. At more peripheral locations in the retina rods are the dominant type of photoreceptor, and the lower branch of the biphasic curve becomes correspondingly more prominent (see 10 degree eccentricity tracing in Fig. 16-10). Further evidence for the rod-cone theory of the biphasic adaptation curves is that during the upper first branch of the curve, the colors of test lights can be identified accurately, whereas along the lower branch of the threshold curve the test flashes have a colorless appearance no matter what their wavelength. Finally, the spectral sensitivity of the two branches of the biphasic curves can be measured independently. By using test flashes of varying wavelength and finding the threshold energy for each, it has been determined that the lower branch of the adaptation curve has a spectral sensitivity corresponding to the scotopic luminous efficiency of the eye, whereas the upper branch has a spectral sensitivity that matches that of photopic vision.

DARK ADAPTATION AND REGENERATION OF RHODOPSIN

Early suggestions that the slow recovery of rod sensitivity in the dark could be explained by the

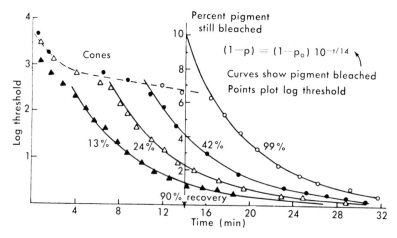

FIG. 16-11 Circles and triangles show dark adaptation curves. Log threshold plotted against time in the dark following a light that bleached away 99%, 42%, 24%, or 13% of rhodopsin, as labeled. Continuous lines show percent of rhodopsin still in bleached state (central scale) as measured by retinal densitometry. (From Rushton WAH, Powell DS: Vision Res 12:1073, 1972.)[54]

biochemical regeneration of rhodopsin pigment that had been bleached previously[36] subsequently was shown to be correct in the human when the course of bleaching and regeneration of pigments could be measured by reflection densitometry.[13] Figure 16-11 from Rushton and Powell[54] shows the correspondence in the human between the recovery of visual sensitivity in the dark and the simultaneous curves for regeneration of rhodopsin pigment. For this series of experiments a bleaching exposure of light was given that bleached 99%, 42%, 24%, or 13% of the total photopigment as labeled. After these exposures and at time zero, subjects subsequently responded to conventional test flashes of light at threshold during dark adaptation. Simultaneous retinal reflection measurements in the densitometer were recorded to demonstrate the percentage of pigment in the bleached state. Photopigment regeneration is plotted as the continuous lines with the ordinant scale shown in the middle of the illustration. After each bleaching exposure to light, rhodopsin regenerates along the same exponential curve. At each time along the curve points indicating the recovery of visual sensitivity coincide with the curves for regeneration of photopigment. This means that the logarithm of the threshold is elevated by some fixed multiple of the fraction of rhodopsin that has been converted to the bleached state. This is the relationship that is expressed in equation 2 (p. 509).[2]

The course of photopigment depletion by

bleaching also is a relatively slow phenomenon, taking several minutes to reach a maximum. The rate of depletion varies complexly with the brightness and duration of exposure to light, but generally has a time constant on the order of tens of seconds. This period of time is considerably longer than the millisecond response times to adapting flashes of light illustrated in Figure 16-9. Unlike the more rapid process of inhibitory neural adaptation, photochemical responses to light adaptation require many seconds or even minutes to reach their full extent.[52]

EQUIVALENT BACKGROUND

The fact that there is a direct, although not proportional, relationship between the extent of photopigment depletion by bleaching and the degree of elevation of threshold (measured during recovery from an exposure to light)[54] suggests that this important type of adaptation may be the basis for a stable level of neural activity in photoreceptors that is determined by the steady-state concentrations of one or more of the bleached products of photopigments. This steady-state level of adaptation has been referred to as "equivalent background." (The concept of equivalent background was first proposed by Crawford.[18]) An equivalent background level can be reached by either dark adaptation (waiting in the dark after full exposure to light to arrive at a given level of adaptation) or light adaptation (exposing the retina to a steady light so as to bleach that quantity of pig-

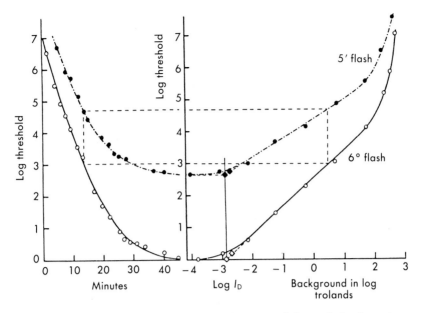

FIG. 16-12 Equivalent background experiment. Curves on left are dark adaptation curves, plotting log threshold against time in dark. Curves on the right show log increment threshold against log intensity of steady adapting background light. *Open circles:* Test flash size of 6 degrees; *closed circles:* 5 minutes. (From Blakemore CB, Rushton WAH: Dark adaptation and increment threshold in a rod monochromat, J Physiol (Lond) 181:612, 1965.)[12]

ment necessary to arrive at the same steady-state level of adaptation). This principle was tested in a rod monochromat, an individual with a congenital absence of retinal cone function.[11] As shown in Figure 16-12, the principle of equivalent background was found to apply over a range of more than 7 logarithmic units of rod sensitivity. The left-hand side of the figure shows recovery of threshold during dark adaptation, with flashing test spots of two different sizes. Note that the larger spots of light had the lower thresholds, because the effect of spatial summation made them more easily detectable. The right-hand side of the figure shows thresholds for increment perception of the same size of test flashes after steady-state adaptation to constant background levels of light. At any given time during the course of dark adaptation (curves on the left), the log threshold for either of the two sizes of test flashes can be compared with the log threshold for the same sizes of test flashes measured under conditions of steady-state adaptation (curves on the right). As indicated by the dotted lines, the equivalent background for a given time of dark adaptation may be read from the abscissa at the bottom right by dropping a vertical line from the corresponding points on the threshold curves on the right-hand side of the figure. This yields an experi-

mental determination of the equivalent background luminance reached after a given time of dark adaptation. The vertical solid line indicates the equivalent background level in the fully dark-adapted retina. This corresponds to the residual level of neural activity ("noise") in the retinal circuitry in the absence of light.

It can be shown by this method that the equivalent background corresponding to a given time of dark adaptation is a constant that is independent of the size or duration of the test flashes used to determine the equivalent background. This fact is illustrated by comparing the equivalent background for the two different sizes of test lights, as plotted in Figure 16-13. This figure shows the same data as that of Figure 16-12, replotted in a different form. The change of equivalent background with time is seen to be identical for the two different sizes of test spots used to determine visual threshold during the course of dark adaptation. The concept of equivalent background suggests that the mechanism that determines the level of rod sensitivity during a steady exposure to light is the same process that undergoes a gradual decay during the course of dark adaptation. Whether the equivalent background is determined by the extent of bleaching of rhodopsin into its various products or is set by the level of electrical activity in reti-

FIG. 16-13   Data of Figure 16-12 replotted to show that equivalent background is the same for different sizes of test flash used to measure increment threshold. Horizontal dotted lines in Figure 16-12 intercept left curves at time of dark adaptation and right curves at equivalent steady background luminance. The two values are plotted against one another in this figure. *Open circles:* Test flash size of 6 degrees; *closed circles:* 5 minutes. (From Blakemore CB, Rushton WAH: J Physiol (Lond) 181:612, 1965.)[11]

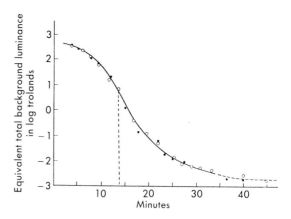

nal photoreceptors or other neural elements is not precisely known. However, evidence has been accumulated to suggest that both of these phenomena play an integral role in determining the level of retinal adaptation.

ADAPTATION IN PHOTORECEPTORS

By use of intracellular microelectrode techniques, the electrophysiologic behavior of individual photoreceptors can be measured. Most experiments of this type have been done in amphibian species, because the retinas of these animals contain photoreceptors that are relatively large and thus are easily impaled by recording microelectrodes.[29] Figure 16-14, from the work of Fain,[24] shows the responses of a single rod photoreceptor in the retina of a toad after stimulation by full-field adapting lights and individual flashes of test spots of light. When a microelectrode first penetrates the membrane of a rod photoreceptor, a negative resting potential is recorded. In the figure the resting potential is represented by the dashed lines. Stimulation of the rod by flashes of light can be shown to produce a hyperpolarization of the rod's membrane, indicated by a downward deflection in the tracings. In Fain's experiment three different levels of adaptation were used, as indicated by the log background intensities of 8.8, 9.7, and 10.7 for the three tracings from top to bottom of the figure. At each of these three levels of adaptation, test flashes of approximately 0.1 of a second at varying intensities produced recorded spikes of membrane hyperpolarization. The amplitudes of these spikes, as a function of log intensity of the inducing flashes, are shown in Figure 16-15 for a series of different levels of adaptation. The electrophysiologic responses are plotted on a logarithmic scale. Note that at low levels of flash intensity the magnitude of the photoreceptor response rises linearly with increasing intensity of flash until its response is saturated, as indicated by the formation of a plateau on the right-hand side of each curve. The plateau represents the maximal level of photoreceptor response for a given level of light adaptation. Increasing intensities of test flash produce no further increase in electrophysiologic response. This maximum-voltage response sometimes is referred to as V_{max}. Fain demonstrated that his data closely fit the expression

$$V/V_{max} = \frac{I}{I + \sigma} \qquad (3)$$

where

V = the increment response amplitude
V_{max} = the maximal amplitude
I = the increment flash intensity
σ = a constant respresenting the flash intensity at which one-half maximal response is obtained

Note that near the threshold for response of the rod, where the flash intensity is lowest, the amplitude of the response is proportional to the test intensity. With increasing levels of adaptation a family of curves is produced that is shifted progressively toward the right. There is a different sigma for each curve (a different flash intensity for one-half maximal response). When the rod was dark adapted, the log intensity for one-half maximal response was 8, whereas with adaptation to 10.8 log units of background intensity a nearly 3 log unit increase in flash intensity for one-half maximal response was recorded.

The use of plots, such as those shown in Figure 16-15, emphasizes the linearity of responses of photoreceptors over a wide range of stimulus intensities, covering several logarithmic units from threshold to saturation of the receptor.

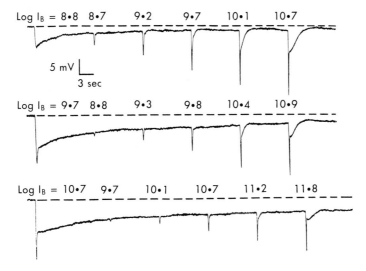

FIG. 16-14 Adaptation of rods to differing levels of background illumination. Intracellular recordings show responses of rod to brief flash stimuli (intensities given by numbers above each response spike) at three different levels of background illumination (log I_B). *Dashed lines:* Dark resting membrane potential. Hyperpolarization of membrane potential increases with increasing levels of adaptation. Higher levels of adaptation require greater stimulus intensities for response spikes to rise above resting potential. (From Fain GL: J Physiol 261:71, 1976.)

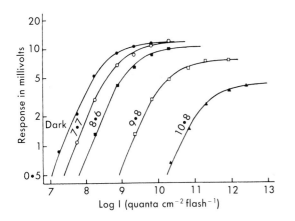

FIG. 16-15 Shifting of rod intensity-response curves by varying intensities of adapting background illumination. Curves generated using data like that of Figure 16-14. Spike response amplitudes plotted against log intensity of stimulus flash at five different levels of adaptation to steady background illumination. Background intensities given at left of each curve in same log units as stimulus intensities (log quanta cm^{-2} flash^{-1}). (From Fain GL: J Physiol 261:71, 1976.)[24]

However, it also has been customary to plot the results of such experiments so that V/V_{max} is shown as a function of log I, the test flash intensity. Figures 16-16 and 16-17 show the use of this type of plotting method to display the results for electrical recordings from single photoreceptors. The data of Figure 16-16 were obtained from rods in the excised eye of the axolotl,[29] whereas those of Figure 16-17 were recorded from single cones in the excised eye of the turtle.[10] The general shape of these curves is identical; the only differences are the dynamic range of test light intensities from threshold to

saturation and the intensity of light producing one-half maximal response (sigma). Note in Figure 16-16 that each sigmoid curve represents the responses of a rod at a single level of adaptation. At each level of adaptation electrical responses were recorded at multiple points along the sigmoid curve, with brief test flashes that did not change the shape or position of the curve. Any change in position of a curve would more closely parallel the slower processes of adaptation: the changes in steady-state concentrations of photosensitive pigments and their bleached products. Changes in electrical response along a

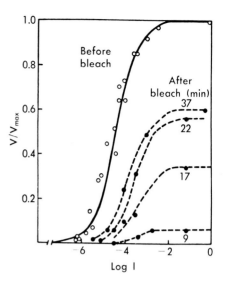

FIG. 16-16 Electrical response from single rod in excised eye of an axolotl resulting from flash of intensity (I). Intracellular recording. (From Grabowski SR, Pinto LH, Pak WL: Science 176:1240, 1972.)[29]

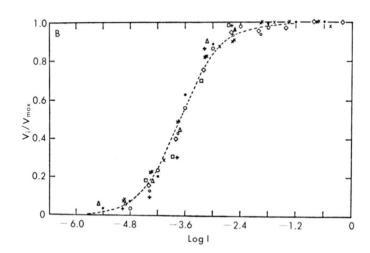

FIG. 16-17 Electrical response from single cone in excised eye of a turtle, resulting from flash of intensity (I). Intracellular recording. (From Baylor DA, Fuortes MGF: J Physiol [Lond] 207:77, 1970.)[10]

given curve more closely parallel the rapid processes of adaptation, such as those embodied in the psychophysical experiment of Crawford[18] (see Fig. 16-9).

A PSYCHOPHYSICAL CORRELATE OF PHOTORECEPTOR ELECTROPHYSIOLOGY

Although one cannot make similar recordings from the rods of the living human eye, psychophysical techniques have been used in which excitatory and inhibitory flashes were balanced against one another at varying levels of light adaptation to determine the magnitude of response (apparent brightness) as a function of I, the number of quanta in the test flash of light.[3] The same relationship was found:

$$N/N_{max} = \frac{I}{I + \sigma} \qquad (4)$$

where

N = the magnitude of psychophysical response and

σ = intensity of light for one-half maximal psychophysical response (a value of approximately 1000 quanta absorbed per rod per flash)

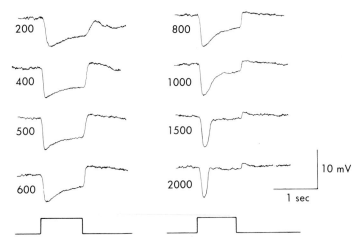

FIG. 16-18 Center-surround organization of bipolar cell receptive field. Graded potential responses of bipolar cell to stimulation by spots of light of increasing diameter. Numbers by each tracing specify stimulus diameter in μm. Initial peak response greatest at 400 μm; increasing spot sizes inhibit response up to diameter of 2000 μm. Diameter of receptive field excitatory center is 400 μm; inhibitory surround, 2000 μm. (From Werblin FS: Synaptic interactions mediating bipolar response in the retina of the tiger salamander, in Barlow HB, Fatt P, eds: Vertebrate photoreception, New York, Academic Press, 1977, pp 205-230.)[65]

In psychophysical experiments responses are measured at the highest degree of neural integration: the level of consciousness. We must assume that although the basic characteristics of responses as a function of stimulus intensity may parallel those measured at the receptor level, there must also be considerable alteration of the visual information between the point of receptor detection and the level of visual perception.

ADAPTATION IN BIPOLAR CELLS

Although most of the elements of the rapid and slow processes of adaptation can be recorded electrophysiologically at the level of the photoreceptor, there is extensive integration of information by the subsequent neural elements in the retina. Rod-mediated vision shows a high degree of neural convergence, for example. The signals from hundreds of rods may be pooled to determine the electrical responses of a single bipolar cell. An important feature that results from neural convergence is the formation of a spatial distribution of visual sensitivity for a retinal cell, termed its "receptive field." Werblin[65] has studied the receptive fields of bipolar cells by recording their electrophysiologic responses to stimulation by spot and anulus sources of light. His findings for the retina of the tiger salamander were similar to those reported for a variety of species. The bipolar receptive field is concentrically organized into antagonistic zones of center and surround. Stimulation of the center of the receptive field of the bipolar cell will cause hyperpolarization of its membrane, but simultaneous illumination of its concentric surround will inhibit responses to the central stimulus. Figure 16-18 shows the responses of a biplar cell to spots of light of varying diameter positioned over the center of its receptive field. As the diameter of the circular stimulus was increased from an initial size of 200 μm, the response first increased in amplitude. This held true up to a diameter of 400 μm, above which the maximum amplitude of response decreased slightly. There was also a more dramatic decrease in the plateau response measured approximately 150 milliseconds after the initiation of the stimulus. The level of the plateau continued to decrease for larger stimulus sizes, up to the maximum diameter of 2000 μm. Werblin interpreted these results as being consistent with a receptive field center of 400 μm in diameter, surrounded by an anular zone of antagonism extending out to a diameter of 2000 μm (2 mm on the retinal surface).

By plotting the maximum amplitude of the response of the bipolar cell as a function of the

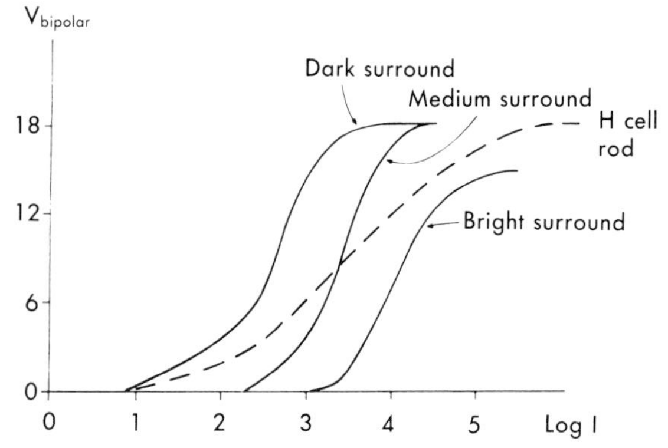

FIG. 16-19 Adaptation of bipolar cell responses to inhibitory surround stimulation. Responses of bipolar
cells (unbroken curves) to varying stimulus intensities
(log I) at three different levels of surround inhibition.
Central stimulus diameter 400 μm, in presence of surrounding inhibitory anulus of 700 μm inside diameter
and 2000 μm outside diameter. Anulus intensities: 0
(dark), 3.2 (medium), and 4.4 (bright) log units relative to stimulus intensity. Broken line, Response curve
of typical rod photoreceptor to spot stimulus. Bipolar
responses cover only portion of response range of
photoreceptor, but bipolar curves are shifted to different portions of photoreceptor range by varying
conditions of surround inhibition. (From Werblin FS:
Synaptic interactions mediating bipolar response in
the retina of the tiger salamander, in Barlow HB, Fatt
P, eds: Vertebrate photoreceptors, New York, Academic Press, 1977, pp 205-230.)[65]

log intensity of stimulus to the center of its receptive field (Fig. 16-19), a series of sigmoid response curves was obtained that closely mimics
the shape of those recorded for photoreceptor
responses (see Figs. 16-16 and 16-17). The test
conditions for the experiment of Figure 16-19
included central circular stimuli with a diameter
of 400 μm surrounded by an inhibitory anulus
with an internal diameter of 700 μm and an external diameter of 2000 μm. The effect of stimulation of the inhibitory surround is shown for
three different intensities: 0 (dark), 3.2 (medium), and 4.4 (bright) log units relative to the
center flash intensities. The test flash intensities
are plotted in log units on the abscissa. The
dashed curve in the figure shows for comparison the stimulus-response curve recorded from
rods in the same retina. Notice that although the
response curves of bipolar cells have the same
shape as those obtained from photoreceptors,
each one covers only a fraction of the response
range of the photoreceptors. Manipulation of
the inhibitory surround, a form of neurally mediated adaptation, causes the response curve of
the bipolar cell to be shifted or repositioned to
different parts of the range of stimulus intensities covered by the rod response.

The center-surround organization of receptive fields is widespread throughout the retina,
being found in many cell types, including ganglion cells.[7,9,34,39] The antagonistic organization
of receptive field center and surround provides
a plausible explanation for the phenomena of
lateral inhibition, such as the appearance of
Mach bands (see p. 507). Receptive fields falling
sufficiently close to highly contrasting borders
can be expected to have greater (or lesser) stim-

ulation of their inhibitory surrounds than those
that are illuminated uniformly. Cells whose receptive field centers are located just on the
bright side of such a border will consequently
have slightly less surround inhibition of their
signal strengths (because of overlap of their inhibitory surround zones by the dark side of the
border). Therefore they will transmit a greater
brightness signal than their uniformly illuminated neighbors on the same side of the border.
The converse situation will hold for cells located
on the opposite (dark) side of the border: weaker
signals will arise from cells located adjacent to
the contrast border than from those fully enveloped by the darker field. The result should be
the appearance of zones of exaggerated darkness and brightness that tend to enhance the
contrast of borders, such as those seen subjectively in Mach bands.

ADAPTATION IN GANGLION CELLS

The electrical responses recorded from photoreceptor cells, horizontal cells, and bipolar cells
are all graded, nonpropagated potentials. More
proximal neural elements in the retina, such as
ganglion cells, have electrical responses characterized by the formation of propagated spike
potentials. Enroth-Cugell and Shapley[22,23] have
studied extensively the adaptation properties of
retinal ganglion cells in the cat. Rather than
measuring the amplitudes of graded responses,
their experiments involved integration over
time of the number of membrane spikes (or "impulses") that occurred in response to stimulation of underlying photoreceptors by spots of
light. Figure 16-20 illustrates the results of an
experiment that measured the intensity of a spot

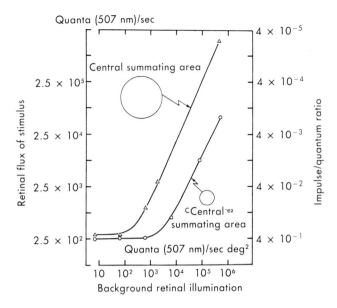

FIG. 16-20 Adaptation in ganglion cells: responses to small stimulus spots as a function of background illumination. Strength of stimulus spot (retinal flux of stimulus) needed to produce a criterion response from ganglion cells (a given number of impulses) is plotted against the log intensity of a steady background light. Results shown for two cells. Log stimulus intensity for criterion response rises linearly with log background intensity. (From Enroth-Cugell C, Shapley RM: J Physiol 233:311, 1973.)[23]

of light necessary to induce a predetermined number of impulses in the membrane of a ganglion cell. The stimulus strength required to induce this criterion response was determined as a function of the background illumination of the retina. Over a low range of adapting backgrounds, the strength of the retinal stimulus (expressed as the flux of photons per unit area of retina per second) was found to be constant. However, as background illumination rose, there was an abrupt increase in the luminous flux of the stimulus necessary to induce the criterion response. This is plotted as a linear increase in stimulus flux and a decrease in the ratio of membrane spike potentials to stimulus quanta, the impulse-quantum, or I/Q, ratio. (Note that the values of the right-hand ordinate in Figure 16-20 are inverted numerically.) Results are shown for two different cells, one with a large central summating area and one with a small central summating area. The area of central summation corresponds to the excitatory receptive field center of the cell. The cell with the larger central summating area required the greater stimulus flux to produce the criterion response. That the log stimulus versus log adapting illumination plot is linear represents an electrophysiologic parallel of Weber's law. The

slope of these straight lines (Δ stimulus flux/Δ background flux) is analogous to the constancy of the $\Delta I/I$ of equation 1.

Other electrophysiologic properties of ganglion cell responses are similar to psychophysical observations. Crawford's experiment[18] (Fig. 16-9), which demonstrated transient elevations of threshold for the detection of increment flashes of light superimposed on transient adapting pulses of light, has been mimicked by use of similar experimental stimulus conditions, while recording the electrophysiologic responses of ganglion cells. Figure 16-21 shows recordings of the rate of spike formation in a ganglion cell during stimulation by conditioning spot stimuli with superimposed test flashes. The conditioning spot was alternated at a fixed rate: 1.5 seconds on, 3.5 seconds off. Tracing A in the figure shows the response of a ganglion cell to this conditioning spot. There was a transient increase in firing activity when the conditioning spot was turned on, followed by a transient depression of spike activity after the spot was turned off. In tracings B through F on the left-hand side, 20 millisecond test flashes were superimposed on the conditioning stimulus at varying times after its onset. For each of the left-hand tracings B through F, the control tracing in

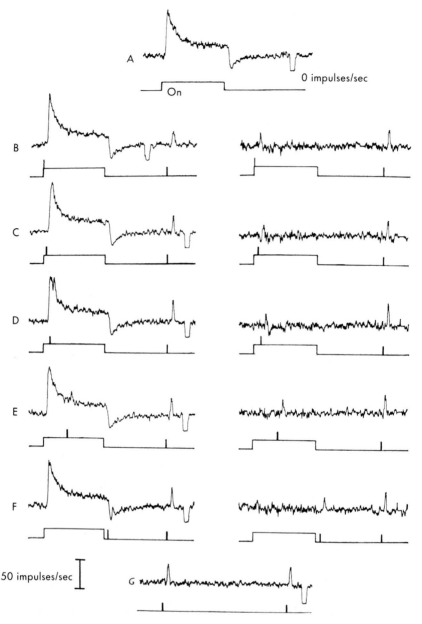

FIG. 16-21   Electrophysiology of adaptation in ganglion cell. Responses of cat ganglion cell to stimulation by conditioning and test spots of light (an electrophysiologic analogue of Crawford's experiment, Fig. 16-9). Spike formation rate (impulses/sec) recorded on time scale. Tracing A shows cell response to conditioning spot turned on for period of 1.5 sec. Tracings B through F on left-hand side show responses to test flashes of 20 ms duration superimposed over conditioning spot at varying latencies after onset of conditioning spot. Tracings B through F on right-hand side (obtained by numeric subtraction of tracing A) show estimated responses to test flash isolated from responses to conditioning spot. Tracing G shows control response to two test flashes in absence of conditioning spot. (From Enroth-Cugell C, Shapley RM: J Physiol 233:271, 1973.)[22]

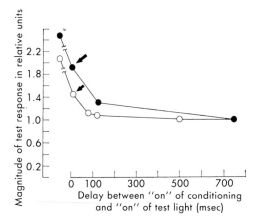

FIG. 16-22 Time course of decay of ganglion cell response after onset of conditioning light. Data calculated from recordings like those of Figure 16-21. Magnitude of test responses obtained by integration of area under tracings of spike formation rate. Results shown for two cells. Response magnitudes indicated by arrows coincide with each cell's maximum response to conditioning spot. (From Enroth-Cugell C, Shapley RM: J Physiol 233:271, 1973.)[22]

A was subtracted, producing the corresponding right-hand tracings for B through F. These show the change in the rate of impulse formation associated with presentation of the test flashes. The magnitudes of the cell's responses to the test flashes were computed by integrating the areas under the response curves, where brief increases in activity accompanied the presentation of the test pulses. In Figure 16-22, the magnitudes of the ganglion cell responses to the test flashes have been plotted as a function of the time delay between the onset of the conditioning stimulus and the onset of the test flash. Results are shown for two different cells. The two values on the extreme left were obtained in the absence of a conditioning stimulus. Although ganglion cell behavior mimicked the transient changes in threshold seen in the Crawford experiment, there were significant differences. Depression of the cells' responses to the test flashes coincided with the onset of the conditioning stimulus, as indicated by the dark arrows. However, there was a distinct time lag between onset of the conditioning spot and the maximum degree of test response depression. In addition, the adaptation effect (the test response depression) lasted beyond the time period of conditioning flash presentation, as indicated by the right-hand extreme of the curves in Figure 16-22.

AUTOMATIC GAIN CONTROL

As we have discussed, adaptation consists of both rapid and slow changes in visual sensitivity after exposure of the eye to changing levels of light. Photopigment bleaching and regeneration, which have time constants on the order of minutes, can satisfactorily explain the slow changes in visual sensitivity that occur with adaptation to varying levels of light. However, the rapid changes in visual sensitivity, such as those determined psychophysically in Crawford's experiment,[18] and the rapidly changing sensitivities recorded electrophysiologically in photoreceptors and other retinal neural elements in response to abrupt changes in illumination require some alternate explanation.

Rushton[53] has compared the rapid components of visual adaptation to the automated gain control circuits built into electronic imaging systems, such as those found in television cameras. Figure 16-23 shows a schematic model proposed by Rushton to explain how the eye could use a neural feedback mechanism to adjust the size of its output signal, N, which is sent to the brain in response to stimulation by a light of intensity, I. Stimulation of the photoreceptor elements results in a neural output, V. The electrical signal, V, then enters the automatic gain box, which is symbolized by the letter G. The output of the gain box in turn feeds back onto itself, attenuating the output signal, N, toward a fixed value, N_0, near the middle of the brain's operating range. In this way, if V remains steady at any one value, N soon becomes N_0. If V changes, G soon operates to again force N back toward the value N_0. Thus as V alters from moment to moment, N alters correspondingly while always drifting back toward the value N_0, which happens to be the value for optimal image contrast. Such a mechanism easily could account for the phenomenon of the Weber-Fechner relation (equation 1). A steady adapting light of intensity, I, will produce a steady rod output, V, proportional to it ($V = aI$), and the resulting G box output is GaI, where G is the signal gain in passing through the G box. As a result of the feedback, G soon changes to G_1, where $G_1aI = N_0$.

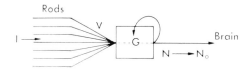

FIG. 16-23   Schematic automatic gain control for rod signals.

If to this state of equilibrium, which has been set up in response to background luminance I, we add a flash, ΔI, the increase of G box input will be $a\Delta I$ and the increase of output will be $G_1 a \Delta I$. However, we have just seen that $G_1 a = N_0/I$. The increase of output is therefore $N_0\Delta I/I$. If the condition for detection of a flash, ΔI, is that the resulting increase of output reaches some criterion level, K, then $N_0\Delta I/I = K$. Because N_0 is also a constant, it may be concluded that $\Delta I/I = $ a constant, which is the Weber-Fechner relation. Thus a feedback gain control model can be used to explain the physiologic property of the visual system that rapidly adjusts the strength of visual signals, keeping them properly scaled to the center of the eye's response range, where image contrast is optimal.

Stiles[61,62] used two-color methods for testing increment sensitivities in which one color of light was used as the adapting background and another was used as the increment stimulus. He found that the Weber-Fechner relation also holds true for vision mediated by individual types of cones. For example, the threshold of red cones is altered by adaptation of other surrounding red cones to background lights of appropriate color. This occurs in an independent fashion, such that red, green, and blue cone types seem to be isolated from one another. This suggests that each cone type has a separate and independent gain control mechanism.

Another aspect of retinal behavior that can be explained by the feedback gain control model is Troxler's phenomenon. If one assumes that a gain control mechanism is operating, it follows that stabilization of the image on the retina will cause the signal, N, to be driven toward a fixed value, N_0, in every nerve fiber, regardless of the value of the input, I. The result will be to produce a uniform level of apparent light intensity in the image with no contrasting borders. Thus the fading of stabilized images on the retina also can be explained adequately by assuming the presence of a gain control mechanism that has suitable time constants for adjusting output levels.

Automatic gain control and background adaptation

Equation 4 describes the magnitude of neural signals for various energies of stimulating light in the fully dark-adapted retina. If we suppose that a stimulating flash of light falls on a steady adapting background of intensity, Θ, that operates according to the mechanism of the automatic gain control model shown in Figure 16-23, the formula then becomes

$$N/N_{max} = \frac{I}{1 + \sigma} \times \frac{\Theta_D}{\Theta_D + \Theta} \quad (5)$$

where Θ_D is the "intrinsic light of the retina," or receptor noise.[8] The residual noise level of neural activity is the same conceptually as the equivalent background in the fully dark-adapted retina (I_D in Fig. 16-12). Although a single quantum of light may be sufficient to produce a neural response in the retina,[30] in general at least 6 quanta must be captured by the retinal photoreceptors within a restricted time and retinal area to be detected against the background noise.[36] Equation 5 is depicted graphically in Figure 16-24 from Alpern et al.[1,2] The curve marked H_1 for human rods plots N, the neural signal, against log I, the test flash intensity. This is the same relation plotted in Figure 16-16 for axolotl rods, and the curves are identical. Curve A in Figure 16-24 is the same as H_1, but the ordinate is scaled as the log of N (scale to left) instead of N/N_{max} (scale to right). Curve A has a linear portion with a slope of 45 degrees covering a 1000-fold range over which N is proportional to I.

The other curves in Figure 16-24 show the values of N when I falls on a steady background (Θ) of 0.3, 0.9, and 2.1 log trolands, respectively. As can be seen in the upper set of curves, a change of background simply displaces the curve vertically by an amount equal to log ($\Theta + \Theta_D$).

This is in accord with equation 5, which also may be written

$$\log N = \log N_{max} + \log \left(\frac{\Theta_D \times I}{i + \sigma} \right) - \log (\Theta + \Theta_D)$$

Consequently, a change in log ($\Theta + \Theta_D$) changes log N by a fixed amount for every point on the curve. That is, the curve is displaced vertically. In the curves plotted on the lower right portion of Figure 16-24 (with the N/N_{max} values on the ordinate to the right), the same effect is displayed as a change in the vertical scaling factor. The good fit between the experimentally determined points and the theoretic curves means

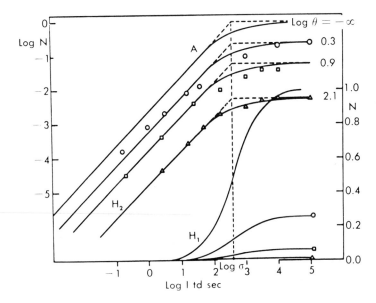

FIG. 16-24 Lower set of curves, H_1, Plot size of rod signals (scale right) resulting from flashes of intensity, I, projected on steady background θ indicated in log trolands by numbers on right, namely log θ = $-\infty$, 0.3, 0.9, and 2.1 for the four curves in descending order. Upper set of curves, H_2, are same results but with rod signals, N, plotted on log scale *(left)*. (From Alpern M, Rushton WAH, Torii S: J Physiol [Lond] 206:209, 1970.)

that equation 4 accurately represents the behavior of rods over a range of many log units of N, I, and Θ.

Where does automatic gain control occur?

Rushton[53,54] concluded that the main signal attenuation that underlies the Weber-Fechner phenomenon is likely to take place in the eye rather than in the brain. As we have seen, electrophysiologic recordings from bipolar cells and ganglion cells show evidence of the automatic gain control mechanism that underlies the basis of Weber's law. However, the basic elements of feedback inhibition are found in recordings from individual photoreceptors. Rushton felt that the horizontal cells of the retina played an integral role as feedback inhibitors of photoreceptor activity. Horizontal cell dendrites can be shown to spread across broad areas of the retina and have synaptic connections with multiple photoreceptors adjacent to their bipolar cell synapses. Horizontal cells are anatomically connected to photoreceptors in a manner ideally suited to the generation of feedback inhibition loops.[21] Moreover, studies of horizontal cell activity have shown that individual photoreceptors can be inhibited (depolarized) by injecting hyperpolarizing currents into horizontal cells. However, these findings have been limited to

studies of cone photoreceptors and their associated horizontal cells. It is interesting that horizontal cells appear to provide interconnections only for groups of cones of like pigment types. Thus input from red-sensitive cones should inhibit only red-sensitive cones. Enroth-Cugell and Shapely[22,23] have proposed a similar feedback loop of horizontal cells onto rods as a means of gain control. However, confirmatory evidence for this is not as good as that for cone vision.

What is the molecular basis for the gain control of photoreceptors?

We know that a means of automated gain control operates at the level of individual photoreceptors. (See above discussion on adaptation in photoreceptors, page 514, and Figures 16-14 through 16-16.) The molecular basis for this adaptation is not yet fully understood, but work over the past few years has begun to unravel the mystery. It appears that rapid, light-stimulation-induced changes in internal calcium ion concentration $[Ca^{2+}]_i$ modulate the response of photoreceptors, serving as an internal "messenger" for light adaptation (for a recent review see Fain and Mathews).[25]

Light stimulation of a photoreceptor initiates a complex cascade of enzymatically catalyzed events (see Chapter 14). Photon capture by a rhodopsin molecule results in a series of conformational changes that facilitate binding of the light-activated rhodopsin to the G protein *transducin,* in turn resulting in the exchange of bound GTP and GDP on the alpha subunit of transducin and liberation of the activated transducin subunit T_α-GTP. This intermediate then binds to and causes the release of an inhibitory subunit from the enzyme cGMP *phophodiesterase.* Activation of the phosphodiesterase accelerates the hydrolysis of cGMP, and the resulting drop in cGMP concentration closes ion conductance channels in the outer segment membrane of the photoreceptor. This is what causes the graded hyperpolarization of the photoreceptor's response to light stimulation.

Once initiated, light excitation must be followed by a countervailing recovery process to restore the resting level of cGMP. There are three phenomena that contribute to the recovery process: (1) photoactivated rhodopsin is phosphorylated by an enzyme *(rhodopsin kinase),* and the phosphorylated rhodopsin binds to a protein called *arrestin* that hinders the binding of rhodopsin to transducin; (2) the activated transducin subunit T_α-GTP, spontaneously hydrolyzes to T_α-GDP, causing it to disassociate from (and allow inactivation of) the phosphodiesterase, showing the hydrolsis of cGMP; and (3) cGMP concentrations are returned toward resting (dark) levels by the continued activity of the enzyme *guanylate cyclase,* which catalyzes the synthesis of cGMP.

It has long been thought that cytoplasmic concentrations of calcium, $[Ca^{2+}]_i$, play an integral role in the phototransduction of invertebrate photoreceptors, and at one time it was thought that calcium might be directly responsible for modulating membrane conductance. In vertebrate receptors this messenger is now known to be cGMP, but calcium also plays a central role in the sensitivity regulation of vertebrate rods and cones.[46] This regulation is not through a direct effect of calcium on membrane conductance, however, but rather by indirect effects on the enzymatic activities that control the concentration of cGMP.[67]

Calcium levels not only affect the activities of important enzymes in the phototransduction cascade, but light also has a profound effect on $[Ca^{2+}]_i$ in vertebrate rods and cones. Like Na^+ and K^+, Ca^{2+} is also in constant flux across the semi-permeable membrane of the photoreceptor outer segment. In fact Ca^{2+} flux accounts for about 10% of the dark current across the outer segment membrane. The light-induced decrease

in membrane conductance (mediated by a drop in cGMP levels) also reduces the rate at which Ca^{2+} enters the cell. There is, however, a constant rate, energy dependent pump across the outer segment membrane that counter-transports Ca^{2+} and K^+ out of the cell in return for an electro-equivalent number of Na^+ ions pumped into the cell. Closing of conductance channels for Ca^{2+} results in an immediate drop in $[Ca^{2+}]_i$, because the rate of calcium pumping is not affected by light exposure.[47] Thus the conditions are ideal for linking transient fluctuations in outer segment $[Ca^{2+}]_i$ to fluctuations in light stimulation.

Evidence that fluctuations in $[Ca^{2+}]_i$ are a necessary condition for adaptation has been obtained through experiments in which the cytoplasmic concentration of calcium in isolated photoreceptors has been artificially stabilized. This has been done chiefly by introducing chelating agents into the cytoplasm of outer segments, thus buffering the internal concentration of calcium,[63] or by bathing the outer segments in solutions with very low calcium and zero sodium concentrations, thereby eliminating the calcium influx contribution to the dark current and removing the sodium ions needed for the pumped transport of calcium out of the cell.[42,43] In both of these circumstances the usual phenomena of light adaptation in isolated photoreceptor preparations are completed erased; stimulation of such a preparation is followed by a loss of recovery from the stimulus. The photoreceptor simply sums the effects of multiple stimuli, behaving like a linear integrator. In this situation the dynamic range of a sensory receptor is radically reduced, since stimuli will lock it progressively into the "on" position, there being no further capacity to respond to additional changes in stimulus strength.

Several sources of evidence suggest that modulation of the activity of guanylate cylase is the principal means by which the changing levels of $[Ca^{2+}]_i$ account for photoreceptor adaptation. Although calcium concentrations as high as 10 μM can affect some of the steps of the excitatory cascade,[6] the dynamics of excitation are not affected by varying $[Ca^{2+}]_i$ within a physiologic range (approximately one tenth of the 10 μM concentration.[50] Mathematical modeling of the kinetics of cGMP production and hydrolysis indicate that modulation of guanylate cyclase activity can account for all of the known manifestations of light adaptation.[27] Steady illumination of photoreceptors results in an increased steady-state turnover rate for cGMP[4] (at constant cGMP levels), while decreases in $[Ca^{2+}]_i$

lead to immediate increases in cGMP levels.[16,41,66]

The story of adaptation, however, is not yet complete. Modulation of $[Ca^{2+}]_i$ is a necessary but probably not sufficient condition for photoreceptor adaptation. Internally dialyzed outer segments show no correlation between $[Ca^{2+}]_i$ and light sensitivity in the absence of an adapting background light. In other words, light must also be present for variations in $[Ca^{2+}]_i$ to express their adaptation effects.[51,55]

CLINICAL DISORDERS OF VISUAL ADAPTATION

Symptoms of defective visual adaptation are not uncommon among patients with ophthalmic diseases. There are two general types of abnormal adaptation seen clinically: hemeralopia and nyctalopia. Hermeralopia, or "day blindness," is characterized by selective impairment of cone function. Such patients have abnormal photopic vision, including poor visual acuity and poor or absent color vision. However, at the same time, scotopic vision is relatively preserved, so that final dark adaptation thresholds and peripheral visual field patterns are normal. When present congenitally, hemeralopia frequently is accompanied by nystagmus and photophobia (discomfort induced by exposure to photopic levels of light). Nyctalopia, often called "night blindness," is a selective or preponderant impairment of rod-mediated vision. Such patients may have normal visual acuity and relatively well-preserved color perception, but have very poor ability to distinguish even large objects at low (scotopic) levels of illumination. This usually is accompanied by a significant loss of the peripheral visual field, leaving only an island of central visual field, corresponding to the preserved function of macular cones.

Occasionally, nyctalopia or hemeralopia will be the presenting symptom or primary feature of ophthalmic disease. Patients with acquired progressive nyctalopia often will complain initially of visual problems in low-light environments, such as difficulty reading restaurant menus or driving a car after dusk. Diseases producing nyctalopia commonly are inherited disorders, although they may seem to be acquired, because they often become manifest in adult life and are not evident at birth. Diseases causing hemeralopia include both congenital (inherited) and acquired disorders of cone function.

Congenital disorders of adaptation

Inherited disorders of visual adaptation that are manifest from the time of birth include diseases

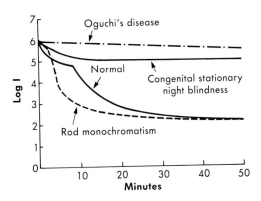

FIG. 16-25 Typical normal and abnormal clinical dark adaptation curves. Normal curve is biphasic with upper cone limb and lower rod limb. Abnormal curve appear monophasic. Curve for rod monochromatism is typical of hemeralopia: nearly absent cone function with rapidly falling curve to normal levels of rod adaptation. Curve for congenital night blindness is typical for nyctalopia: delayed cone limb with no evidence of rod function.

of both rod and cone function. Figure 16-25 shows typical dark adaptation curves for diseases characterized by congenitally abnormal visual adaptation. The primary distinction between normal and abnormal curves in this group of patients is that whereas the normal dark adaptation curve is biphasic and includes both an early cone limb and a later rod portion, the pathologic curves are generally monophasic, showing recovery of threshold in the dark for either rod or cone function in the absence of the other. The curves in Figure 16-25 are for three well-recognized congenital disorders of visual adaptation: rod monochromatism, congenital stationary night blindness, and Oguchi's disease.

Rod monochromatism

This disorder is a form of hemeralopia (day blindness). It is inherited as an autosomal recessive defect and is relatively rare, being found in only 0.003% of the population. Children born with rod monochromatism suffer from photophobia. A behavioral clue to their diagnosis is that they prefer to avoid the bright light of day. Additionally, they have nystagmus and poor visual acuity, usually of about 20/200. The photophobia may be so severe as to prevent examination of the eyes with an ophthalmoscope or slit lamp. A characteristic finding is that, after exposure to bright lights, visual sensitivity recovers rapidly in the dark. The speed of threshold recovery is greater than in those with normal vision, and final dark-adapted thresholds are normal. Pathologic studies of the retinas of these patients have shown many missing and abnormal cones.[26,31] The rods of the retina appear to be normal, and although the fovea may contain a normal number of cones, these photoreceptors show numerous morphologic abnormalities. Through an accident of nature, these people appear to have a nearly pure rod retina from a functional point of view, having normal scotopic vision and a nearly total absence of photopic visual function. Very dark glasses or contact lenses often are useful in treating the photophobia, allowing these patients to see more comfortably under ordinary levels of daytime illumination.

Congenital stationary night blindness

Congenital, nonprogressive nyctalopia is transmitted by all three forms of mendelian inheritance. Pedigrees have been found for X-linked recessive, autosomal recessive, and autosomal dominant types. Night blindness is the chief complaint in most of these patients, although some children are not initially aware of their difficulty, since they have no basis for comparison. The autosomal dominant type is uniformly associated with normal visual acuity.[48] The most famous pedigree of the dominantly inherited form (records cover 10 generations over three centuries) originated in seventeenth century France with a man named Jean Nougaret. The dominantly inherited disease is frequently termed the "Nougaret type." The X-linked form of the disease is usually associated with myopia and reduced visual acuity (20/30 to 20/100); color vision, however, remains largely normal.

The diagnostic finding in these individuals is that of a monofunctional dark adaptation curve (Fig. 16-25). The drop in visual threshold with dark adaptation may be no greater than 1 logarithmic unit and there is no secondary (rod) curve. The adaptation curve recorded for these individuals represents recovery of cone sensitivity only. Even the cone adaptation is not entirely normal, since it is both delayed and lesser in extent than that in normals.[38] The retina appears normal by ophthalmoscopy, save for nonspecific findings associated with myopia in the X-linked form. The peripheral visual field is usually constricted at mesopic levels of adaptation, and there is no spectral (Purkinje) shift in sensitivity during dark adaptation. Histologic studies of the retina have shown no abnormality by light microscopy, and the rod content of rhodopsin and the kinetics of rhodopsin bleaching and regeneration seem to be normal by fundus reflectometry.[15] Thus, although the pathogenesis of this defect in rod function is unknown, it most likely does not have a photochemical basis. There may be an abnormality of pigment epithelial or bipolar cell function. There is no known effective therapy.

Oguchi's disease

Also a congenital and nonprogressive form of nyctalopia, Oguchi's disease is inherited as in autosomal recessive trait. It is characterized by abnormal dark adaptation. There is also an unusual discoloration of the fundus that gradually disappears during prolonged dark adaptation over a period of 24 hours. Night blindness is the sole complaint in affected individuals. Visual acuity is not usually impaired. The abnormal fundus color has been described as having a golden yellow or grayish white appearance. Disappearance of this abnormal coloration following prolonged dark adaptation is called "Mizuo's phenomenon." Color perception is usually normal, even if visual acuity is mildly impaired. Dark recovery of rod function is extremely prolonged. Some patients require as short a period as 2 to 4 hours, whereas others need up to a full day. Recovery of rod sensitivity does not appear to be directly related to Mizuo's phenomenon. Following prolonged periods of dark adaptation, during which rod threshold may return to normal, a brief exposure to a photopic level of light will cause an immediate rise in visual threshold to the preadapted level and a reversal of Mizuo's phenomenon.[56]

Primary hereditary pigmentary retinopathy

Primary hereditary pigmentary retinopathy, also called rod-cone dystrophy and previously referred to as retinitis pigmentosa, is actually an allied group of inherited disorders that appear in pedigrees that include all three forms of mendelian inheritance. Abnormal dark adaptation is frequently the first symptom of the disease in an affected individual. The symptoms of acquired nyctalopia may occur before the presence of ophthalmoscopically visible changes in the fundus. Dark adaptation testing will show elevated thresholds for both cone and rod portions of the curves.[68] This group of diseases seems to preferentially involve rods more than cones. Consequently, there is a greater loss of peripheral visual field and impairment of dark adaptation early in the course of the disease, at a time when color perception and visual acuity have been relatively well preserved. The dark-adaptation curve may mimic that recorded for patients with congenital stationary night blindness, since the deflection in the curve separating the cone and rod limbs may be too small to be detectable.[59]

Hereditary cone degenerations

This group of disorders is most commonly passed in an autosomal dominant pattern of inheritance. Affected individuals appear normal at birth, but symptoms of hemeralopia characteristically are manifest within the first two decades of life. Loss of visual acuity is invariably the initial symptom, followed shortly by reduced color vision. Photophobia and an acquired fixation nystagmus may be found when the onset is early in life. A striking appearance of the fundus is typical in which a target or "bulls eye" lesion of the macula develops.[37] This mimics the appearance of the toxic maculopathy of chloroquine (see following discussion). Dark-adaptation curves are normal in the early stages of the disease, which distinguishes it from the large group of diffuse receptor degenerations known as the pigmentary retinopathies.

Later defects develop in the dark-adaptation curves, which then appear monophasic, very much like those obtained from patients with rod monochromatism. The rod-cone break, when recordable, occurs earlier than normal. The cone plateau may be elevated or entirely absent. The fall of threshold may be more rapid than normal, and the final values for dark-adapted threshold are usually normal.[37] Perimetry will demonstrate a dense central scotoma, although the peripheral visual field is usually normal. Therapy with darkly tinted contact lenses may be useful in treating the photophobia, improving visual performance at photopic levels of brightness.

Acquired disorders of visual adaptation
Toxic and metabolic disorders

A large number of drugs cause toxic retinopathies that lead to significant defects in visual adaptation. Quinine[28] and major tranquilizers like thioridazine[17] can result in profound defects in rod sensitivity, and subacute intoxication by ethyl alcohol has been shown to produce transient elevations of visual thresholds.[64] Chloroquine is an antimalarial drug frequently used in the treatment of connective tissue diseases. The more commonly used analog of the drug is hydroxychloroquine, which produces a characteristic retinopathy.

The rod limb of the dark-adaptation curve in people with chloroquine toxicity is remarkably unaffected. However, the drug appears to selectively destroy cone function. It has a cumulative effect when ingested over periods of months or years. This appears to be caused by very tight binding of the drug to pigment within the pigment epithelial cells of the retina. In the fully developed syndrome visual acuity is markedly reduced (20/200 or worse) and color vision is impaired. Small but dense central scotomas can be mapped by perimetry, and the fundus shows a characteristic macular lesion of pigment epithelial atrophy in the shape of a target or "bull's eye." Early in the course of the disease (even before visual acuity is damaged) defects in the cone limb of the dark-adaptation curve can be detected by using small test lights confined to the central macular area of the visual field.[14] This test is quite sensitive. In some cases of hydroxychloroquine toxicity focal depressions of visual sensitivity have been mapped in the central visual field in locations just superior to the point of fixation, before the development of decreased acuity or the appearance of visible changes in the retina.[33]

Systemic metabolic diseases can also result in significant impairment of dark adaptation. Profound vitamin A deficiency resulting from starvation, chronic alcoholism, sprue, celiac disease, intestinal paracytosis, or chronic hepatic disease can produce sufficient depletion of body stores of vitamin A as to affect retinal function. Hepatic stores of vitamin A are very generous, however, and depletion of the vitamin must be so complete as to have removed all hepatic stores before retinal function will be affected.[12,60] Vitamin A deficiency results in a reduced rhodopsin content within rods, which has been found to cause a reduction in the amplitude of the electroretinogram and elevated ERG thresholds in the rat.[20]

Similarly, any cause of general hypoxemia will result in elevated thresholds and dark-adaptation curves.[45] Thus pulmonary diseases and exposure to high altitudes can result in significant impairment of dark-adapted visual sensitivity.[44]

Primary ocular disorders

A variety of nonretinal primary ocular disorders is known to cause significant impairment of dark adaptation. Elevation of intraocular pressure produces a reversible impairment of sensitivity in all portions of the visual field.[32] This is usually not clinically significant, although some patients with markedly elevated intraocular pressure will notice improvement in their ability to see in poor light following adequate treatment of their glaucoma. Such alterations in visual sensitivity can be demonstrated in patients even in the absence of more specific forms of glaucomatous visual field defects.[69]

Loss of clarity of the ocular media or reductions in size of the pupil can, by reducing the amount of light striking the retina, produce generalized reductions in visual sensitivity (elevations in threshold). Patients with glaucoma who are placed on miotic agents frequently notice significant impairment of visual function, such as difficulty reading by incandescent lamp light during the evening.

Patients with myopia frequently complain of difficulty seeing at night. To some extent this is due to "night myopia," an increase in the apparent myopic refractive error attributed to the spectral shift of evening light toward the short end of the spectrum. Due to the chromatic aberration of the optical system of the eye, images formed with shorter wavelengths of light fall more anteriorly relative to the position of the retina. In patients with extreme myopia defects in retinal dark adaptation have been reported in the absence of ophthalmoscopically visible pathologic changes in the retina. Such patients may actually have one of the inherited forms of stationary night blindness.

A curious anomaly of retinal adaption, called erythropsia, is the symptom of seeing all images cast in a pink or reddish hue. This symptom is very disturbing to those patients who misinterpret what they see as evidence of intraocular bleeding. A common circumstance for this situation is the aphakic patient (one whose cataractous lens has been surgically removed) who has been outdoors in very high levels of sunshine, such as those found on the beach or a snow-covered landscape on a cloudless day. The shift in color perception toward the red is presumably caused by differentially greater bleaching of blue- and green-sensitive cones by high intensities of short wavelength light, leaving the red-sensitive cones to transmit a proportionally greater signal. Aphakic eyes are particularly prone to this phenomenon, since surgical extraction of the adult lens has also removed a yellow filter that normally would absorb a large proportion of light at the blue end of the spectrum. Erythropsia usually lasts at most a few hours after high-intensity light exposures.

Photo-stress testing of retinal adaptation in macular disease

Patients with degenerative diseases of the macula can frequently be found to have defects in cone adaptation that are clinically significant. In some instances this may occur at a time when the appearance of the macula is grossly normal.

For example, macular edema may produce significant impairment of central visual function and yet be very difficult to see without fluorescein angiography or careful examination by slit lamp biomicroscopy and the use of a contact lens. Photo-stress testing of macular function is a simple and very effective way of detecting this form of functional defect. The test is performed by first measuring visual acuity, using a brightly illuminated Snellen chart while the patient is adapted to the illumination level of the darkened refraction lane. A strong focal source of light (such as that from an electric ophthalmoscope) then is projected onto the macula for a period of 15 seconds. In all individuals visual acuity will be temporarily reduced by this maneuver. The rate of return of acuity to the preexposure level is a measure of foveal cone adaptation. In a normal eye recovery of acuity may require only 15 to 30 seconds, but many minutes or even hours may be needed in diseases such as central serous retinopathy, cystoid macular edema, or macular degeneration.[57,58]

REFERENCES

1. Alpern M, Rushton WAH, Torii S: The attenuation of rod signals by background, J Physiol (Lond) 206:209, 1970.
2. Alpern M, Rushton WAH, Torii S: The attenuation of rod signals by bleaching, J Physiol (Lond) 207:449, 1970.
3. Alpern M, Rushton WAH, Torii S: The size of rod signals, J Physiol (Lond) 206:193, 1970.
4. Ames A III, Walseth TF, Heyman RA, et al: Light-induced increases in cGMP metabolic flux correspond with electrical responses of photoreceptors, J Biol Chem 261:13034, 1986.
5. Aulhorn E: Uber die Beziehung zwischen Lichtsinn und Sehsharfe, Graefes Arch Ophthalmol 167:4, 1964.
6. Barkdoll AE III, Pugh EN Jr, Sitaramayya A: Calcium dependence of the activation and inactivation kinetics of the light-activated phosphodiesterase of retinal rods, J Gen Physiol 93:1091, 1989.
7. Barlow HB: Summation and inhibition in the frog's retina, J Physiol (Lond) 119:68, 1953.
8. Barlow HB, Sparrock JMB: The role of afterimages in dark adaptation, Science 144:1309, 1964.
9. Barlow HH: Action potentials from the frog's retina, J Physiol (Lond) 119:58, 1953.
10. Baylor DA, Fuortes MGF: Electrical responses of single cones in the retina of the turtle, J Physiol (Lond) 207:77, 1970.
11. Blakemore CB, Rushton WAH: Dark adaptation and increment threshold in a rod monochromat, J Physiol (Lond) 181:612, 1965.
12. Brenner S, Roberts L: Effects of vitamin A depletion in young adults, Arch Intern Med 71:474, 1943.
13. Campbell FW, Rushton WAH: Measurement of the scotopic pigment in the living human eye, J Physiol (Lond) 130:131, 1955.

14. Carr RE, Gouras P, Gunkel RD: Chloroquine retinopathy: early detection by retinal threshold test, Arch Ophthalmol 75:171, 1966.

15. Carr RE, et al: Rhodopsin and the electrical activity of the retina in congenital stationary night blindness, Invest Ophthalmol 5:497, 1966.

16. Cohen AI, Hall IA, Ferendelli JA: Calcium and cyclic nucleotide regulation in incubated mouse retinas, J Gen Physiol 71:595, 1978.

17. Connell MM, Poley BJ, McFarlane JR: Chorioretinopathy associated with thioridazine therapy, Arch Ophthalmol 71:816, 1964.

18. Crawford BH: Visual adaptation in relation to brief conditioning stimuli, Proc R Soc Lond (Biol) 134:283, 1947.

19. Dowling JE: The chemistry of visual adaptation in the rat, Nature 188:114, 1960.

20. Dowling JE: Night blindness, dark-adaptation and the electroretinogram, Am J Ophthalmol 50:875, 1960.

21. Dowling JE: The site of visual adaptation, Science 155:273, 1967.

22. Enroth-Cugell C, Shapley RM: Adaptation and dynamics of cat retinal ganglion cells, J Physiol 233:271, 1973.

23. Enroth-Cugell C, Shapley RM: Flux, not retinal illumination, is what cat retinal ganglion cells really care about, J Physiol 233:311, 1973.

24. Fain GL: Sensitivity of toad rods: dependence on wavelength and background illumination, J Physiol 261:71, 1976.

25. Fain GL, Mathews HR: Calcium and the mechanism of light adaptation in vertebrate photoreceptors. Trends in Neurosciences 13:378, 1990.

26. Falls HF, Wolter JR, Alpern M: Typical total monochromacy, Arch Ophthalmol 74:610, 1965.

27. Forti S, Menini A, Rispoli G, et al: Kinetics of phototransduction in retinal rods of the newt *Triturus cristatus,* J Physiol (Lond) 419:265, 1989.

28. Francois J, Verriest G, DeRouck A: Etude des fonctions visuelles dans deux cas d'intoxication par la quinine, Ophthalmologica 153:324, 1967.

29. Grabowski SR, Pinto LH, Pak WL: Adaptation in retinal rods of axolotl: intracellular recordings, Science 176:1240, 1972.

30. Hallett PE: Quantum efficiency and false positive rate. J Physiol (Lond) 202:421, 1969.

31. Harrison R, Hoefnagel D, Hayward JN: Congenital total color blindness: a clinicopathological report, Arch Ophthalmol 64:685, 1960.

32. Hart WM, Becker BB: Visual field changes in ocular hypertension, Arch Ophthalmol 95:1176, 1977.

33. Hart WM, et al: Static perimetry in chloroquine retinopathy: perifoveal patterns of visual field depression, Arch Ophthalmol 102:377, 1984.

34. Hartline HK: The receptive fields of optic nerve fibers, Am J Physiol 130:690, 1940.

35. Hecht S, Haig C, Wald G: Dark adaptation of retinal fields of different size and location, J Gen Physiol 19:321, 1935.

36. Hecht S, Shlaer S, Pirenne MH: Energy, quanta and vision, J Gen Physiol 25:819, 1942.

37. Krill AE, Deutman AF: Dominant macular degenerations: the cone dystrophies, Am J Ophthalmol 73:352, 1972.

38. Krill AE, Martin D: Photopic abnormalities in congenital stationary night blindness, Invest Ophthalmol 10:625, 1971.

39. Kuffler SW: Discharge patterns and functional organization of mammalian retina, J Neurophysiol 16:37, 1953.

40. Lowry EM, DePalma JJ: Sine-wave response of the visual system, I, The Mach phenomenon, J Opt Soc Am [A] 51:740, 1961.

41. Lolley RN, Racz E: Calcium modulation of cyclic GMP synthesis in rat visual cells, Vision Res 22:1481, 1982.

42. Matthews HR, Fain GL, Murphy RL, et al: Light adaptation in cone photoreceptors of the salamander: a role for cytoplasmic calcium, J Physiol (Lond) V420; N; P447-69; D1990.

43. Matthews HR, Murphy RL, Fain GL, et al: Photoreceptor light adaptation is mediated by cytoplasmic calcium concentration, Nature 334:67, 1988.

44. McDonald R, Adler F: Effects of anoxia on the dark adaptation of the normal and of the vitamin A deficient subject, Arch Ophthalmol 22:980, 1939.

45. McFarland RA, Evans JN: Alternations in dark adaptation under reduced oxygen tensions, Am J Physiol 127:37, 1939.

46. Miller WH: Ca^{2+} and cGMP, Cur Top Membr Trans 15:441, 1981.

47. Nakatani K, Yau KW: Calcium and magnesium fluxes across the plasma membrane of the toad rod outer segment, J Physiol (Lond) 395:695, 1988.

48. Nettleship E: A history of congenital stationary night blindness in nine consecutive generations, Trans Ophthalmol Soc UK 27:269, 1907.

49. Ratliff F: Mach bands: quantitative studies on neural networks in the retina, San Francisco, Holden Day, 1965.

50. Ratto GM, Payne R, Owen WG, et al: The concentration of cytosolic free calcium in vertebrate rod outer segments measured with fura-2, J Neurosci 8:3240, 1988.

51. Rispoli G, Detwiler PB: Light adaptation in gecko rods may involve changes in both initial and terminal stages of the transduction cascade, Biophys J 55:(Abstract Suppl) 380a, 1989.

52. Rushton WAH: Effect of instantaneous flashes on adaptation of the eye, Nature 199:971, 1963.

53. Rushton WAH: Bleached rhodopsin and visual adaptation, J Physiol 181:645, 1965.

54. Rushton WAH, Powell DS: The rhodopsin content and the visual thresholds of human rods, Vision Res 12:1073, 1972.

55. Sather WA, Rispoli G, Detwiler PB: Effect of calcium on light adaptation in detached gecko rod outer segments, Biophys J 53(Abstract Suppl): 390a, 1988.

56. Sato T, Baba K: Appearance and disappearance of the fundus disturbance in Oguchi's disease, Am J Ophthalmol 51:243, 1961.

57. Severin SL, Tour RL, Kershaw RH: Macular function and the photo-stress test, part 1, Arch Ophthalmol 77:2, 1967.

58. Severin SL, Tour RL, Kershaw RH: Macular function and the photo-stress test, part 2, Arch Ophthalmol 77:163, 1967.

59. Sloan LL: Light sense in pigmentary degeneration of the retina, Arch Ophthalmol 28:613, 1942.

60. Steffins L, Blair, H, Sheard C: Dark adaptation and di-

etary deficiency in vitamin A, Am J Ophthalmol 23:1325, 1940.

61. Stiles WS: Increment thresholds and the mechanisms of colour vision, Doc Ophthalmol 3:138, 1949.

62. Stiles WS: Colour vision: the approach through increment threshold sensitivity, Proc Natl Acad Sci USA 45:100, 1959.

63. Torre V, Matthews HR, Lamb TD: Role of calcium in regulating the cyclic GMP cascade of phototransduction in retinal rods, Proc Natl Acad Sci USA 83:7109, 1986.

64. Verriest G, Laplasse D: New data concerning the influence of ethyl alcohol on human visual thresholds, Exp Eye Res 4:95, 1965.

65. Werblin FS: Synaptic interactions mediating bipolar response in the retina of the tiger salamander, in Barlow HB, Fatt P, eds: Vertebrate photoreception, New York, Academic Press, 1977.

66. Woodruff ML, Fain GL: Ca^{2+}-dependent changes in cyclic GMP levels are not correlated with opening and closing of the light-dependent permeability of toad photoreceptors, J Gen Physiol 80:537, 1982.

67. Yau KW, Baylor DA: Cyclic GMP-activated conductance of retinal photoreceptor cells, Ann Rev Neurosci 12:289, 1989.

68. Zeavin BH, Wald G: Rod and cone vision in retinitis pigmentosa, Am J Ophthalmol 42:253, 1956.

69. Zuege P, Drance SM: Studies of dark adaptation of discrete paracentral retinal areas in glaucomatous subjects, Am J Ophthalmol 64:56, 1967.

GENERAL REFERENCES

Cornsweet TN: Visual perception, New York, Academic Press, 1970.

For clinical methods of dark adaptation testing:
Krill AE: Hereditary retinal and choroidal diseases, vol I, evaluation, New York, Harper & Row, 1972.

For hereditary disorders of visual adaptation:
Krill AE, Archer DB: Hereditary retinal and choroidal diseases, vol II, Clinical characteristics, Hagerstown, Harper & Row, 1977.

Visual Acuity

GERALD WESTHEIMER, Ph.D., F.R.S.

Visual acuity refers to the spatial limit of visual discrimination. It is surely the single most significant measure of functional integrity of the biologic apparatus to which the eye professions are dedicated. If restricted to expressing a patient's visual status in only one number, most practitioners would opt for one of the form 20/20.

Technically speaking, a visual acuity measurement involves the determination of a threshold, and therefore our discussion will have to deal with the problems typically associated with sensory thresholds: specification of the physical stimulus, transduction in the sense organ, anatomic and physiologic substrates, criteria and scales of measurements, techniques of obtaining threshold values, and influence of interacting variables.

Fechner,[13] who claimed to have invented his psychophysical law on Oct. 22, 1850 (in the morning, in bed), made the distinction between outer and inner psychophysics. By "outer psychophysics," he meant the relationship between the physical stimulus outside the body and the associated mental state; he applied the term "inner psychophysics" to the relationship between the physiologic state at the level of the sense cells and the mental state. Leaving aside the emphasis Fechner placed on the mental, or psychologic, aspect, the distinction between outer and inner psychophysics focuses attention on the role of transduction of the physical stimulus in the sense organ. Nowhere does this distinction assume greater significance than in spatial vision. Later generations of students of sensation have used the terms "distal" and "proximal" stimulus, the former denoting in our case the light distribution in object space, as a physicist might describe it, and the latter the pattern of photon absorption in retinal receptors. The intervening processes of optical image formation, including refraction, diffraction, absorption, and scattering, are at least as important in understanding visual acuity and what can interfere with it as any of the succeeding stages: photochemical transduction in the retinal receptors, sorting and transmission of neural signals in the retina and visual pathways, and higher cortical processing. There is no need at present to define the end stage of visual acuity. Depending on the situation, we may seek a patient's verbal response, a "voluntary" motor response such as a gesture or a button press, or an "involuntary" response such as pupil contraction or optokinetic nystagmus, or we may be satisfied with a set of electric signals from some part of the central nervous system.

SPECIFICATION OF THE STIMULUS (PHYSICAL BASIS)

The retinal receptor cells are not exposed directly to the light from the objects, but rather to the energy distribution in the image formed by the eye's optical system. The first step in dealing with visual acuity then is the specification of the relationship between objects and their retinal images.

The schema for this relationship has two aspects: the relative spacing of the images of sequential object points and the light spread in the image of each point. The discussion is facilitated by choosing the chief ray as the reference.

Of the light emanating from any object, only the bundle that is admitted by the pupil matters as far as the retinal image is concerned. To save the effort of tracing all the rays through the cornea and checking which are intercepted by the iris, we employ the artifice of finding the image of the iris formed by the cornea: the entrance pupil. Any ray from any object that passes through the entrance pupil also will end up in the retinal image. The ray from the object to the center of the entrance pupil is called the chief ray because it will identify the center of the light bundle from that particular object. To examine the situation in any region of the retina in which reasonable homogeneity of imagery applies, it suffices to study the locations of the intercept of the chief rays with the retina because the light spread associated with the image of each point is centered around the chief ray.

The entrance pupil is situated about 3 mm behind the corneal vertex. When one looks at an eye and measures the pupil size, one is in reality measuring the size of the entrance pupil, which is about 10% larger. Each chief ray uniquely defines a retinal position. Therefore it is a satisfactory procedure to transfer specification of retinal distances (in linear measure along the retina) into the measure of angular separation of object-sided chief rays. In a typical emmetropic eye a retinal distance of 1 mm corresponds to angular separation of chief rays of about 3.5 degrees. The convention of expressing retinal distance in angular measure of chief rays in object space is almost universal.

A significant feature of the chief-ray method of specifying retinal image position is that, be-cause the bundle of rays converging onto the image plane is centered on the chief ray, the method retains its validity even in the presence of focus changes due to lenses or accommodation (so long as the pupil center stays put). The image patch may change size with focus changes, but the location of its center (the chief ray intercept) does not move. If the eye were an ideal optical instrument without diffraction or aberrations, no more need be said about imagery than what angle the chief rays of the objects make with each other and where the objects are situated with respect to the plane conjugate to the retina. In actual practice, additional considerations center on the extent of departure of the image quality from the ideal of a point image for a point object.

In optical instrument design, it is customary to partition the deviations from point imagery into a variety of classes. However, the significant datum is the total effect of all of them, that is, the actual light spread in the image of a point object or the point-spread function. Once this basic information is available, it is possible to describe the light distribution in any object merely by superposing the spread functions centered on all the elements making up the object.

It is difficult to ascertain the value for the light spread in the retinal image of a given eye, but indirect measurements have shown it to have the general shape shown in Figure 17-1. Several factors contibute to the spread.

1. Diffraction. According to the wave theory of light, limitation of the aperture causes a spread of light even in a fully focused system. The Fraunhofer diffraction image of a point object by a circular aperture has the familiar bell shape with oscillating fringes shown in textbooks of physics (Fig. 17-2). It comes to its first

FIG. 17-1 Line-spread function, i.e., light distribution in the image of a very thin line object, for a human eye in best focus and moderate pupil diameter.

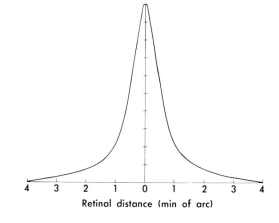

Retinal distance (min of arc)

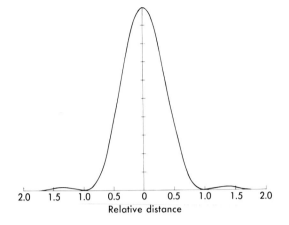

2.0 1.5 1.0 0.5 0 0.5 1.0 1.5 2.0
Relative distance

FIG. 17-2 Fraunhofer's diffraction pattern for a point object. Abscissae are in normalized coordinates, where 1.00 is equal to an angle of 1.22 λ/a radians in object space. Pupil diameter = a, wavelength of light = λ.

zero at a radial distance of 1.22 λ/a radians (angle in object space), where λ is the wavelength of the light and a is the diameter of the entrance pupil. The central patch of the pattern is called Airy's disc and contains most of the light energy; the height of the first ring is only 1.75% of the central peak. Whenever the eye's pupil is less than 2 mm in diameter, the actual image spread is equal to the diffraction image, and the other factors (below) can usually be ignored.

2. Aberrations. Because of a variety of factors that may vary from one eye to the next, rays entering through the periphery of the pupil may not converge on the geometric image point, therefore contributing to the spread of light in the image beyond that caused by diffraction. These effects become more prominent as the pupil widens, more or less offsetting the resulting reduction of the diffraction effects. As a consequence, the image quality usually does not improve much beyond that of a diffraction-limited instrument with a 2.5 mm pupil diameter. For pupil diameters larger than 5 mm, there usually is an incease of the spread, because the peripheral regions of the cornea and lens are often afflicted with optical aberrations while contributing heavily to the total light entering the eye. For example, enlarging of the pupil from 6 to 7 mm contributes 6.5 times more additional light than enlarging it from 2 to 3 m.. For cone vision, the Stiles-Crawford effect would reduce this to a factor of about 2.

3. Scatter. Because the ocular media have some microscopic and ultramicroscopic structure, light is scattered in its passage from the cornea to the retina. Backward scatter is used by an examiner when examining an eye with the slit lamp, but forward scatter can be more serious.

Its effect can be quite extensive, spreading light from even a narrow incident beam over a considerable portion of the retina. Complaints of glare can have their origin in scattered light, which increases in prominence with age. Shielding the eyes from the direct rays of intense light sources (wearing the green eyeshades of older days) is good advice, although not easily put into effect for automobile headlights at night.

4. Absorption. The media are not uniformly transparent to incoming light. In general, the shorter the wavelength of the entering light, the smaller the proportion that reaches the retinal receptors.

5. Focus factors. The effect of defocus on visual acuity will be dealt with separately and has been characterized adequately. However, it must be remembered that when a person has active accommodation, it cannot be taken for granted that the accommodative stance will always be appropriate to the stimulus distance. This is a problem especially when no sharply delineated targets are available to anchor accommodation. Night and instrument myopia are well-known instances of the phenomenon, but it also can occur when "fogging" during a refractive examination.

Altogether, it is only a conjecture to assume that a given eye under a given set of circumstances will display the optimal point-spread function.

The procedures needed to deduce the light spread in images other than points have been outlined elsewhere.[43] They have to be followed for each particular target when the relative effect of the various factors on visual acuity is being determined. Light spread, the first in a sequence of transformations, needs special attention, lest phenomena be assigned to complex neural interaction when, for example, they may have a simple explanation in light scatter or accommodation instability.

RETINAL ANATOMY

One unavoidable bottleneck in the processing of spatial information in the retina is the finite size of the retinal receptors. In the fovea the cones are packed approximately two to the linear minute of arc,[7,8] and each cone's local sign is indivisible. Therefore, in principle it is not possible to resolve patterns whose spacing demands separate sampling of intensity at intervals smaller than half a minute of arc (Fig. 17-3).

Other limits are set by the neural connectivity of retinal cells at their various layers.[6] This applies particularly in the retinal periphery, where many rod connections converge on a ganglion cell. Although the rods themselves are small, the fact that summation of their signals takes place over areas up to several degrees in diameter sets upper bounds to the partitioning of spatial information.

Although there is no question of the role played by the elements of the retinal mosaic in limiting resolution, certain spatial distinctions can be made that appear to have a finer grain— the hyperacuities. Since the diameter of the retinal receptors constitutes an unavoidable limitation to partitioning spatial information except

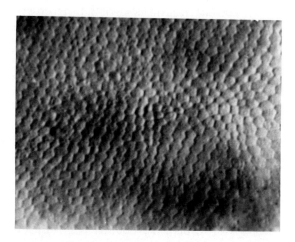

FIG. 17-3 Optical section through the cone inner segments of the human fovea. Width of section is about 55 μ, i.e., it covers a substantial fraction of the rod-free area. (From Curcio CA, Sloan KR, Packer O, et al: Distribution of cones in human and monkey retina: Individual variability and radial symmetry, Science 236:579, 1987.)

at defined intervals, just as does the extended dimension of the image of a point object, there must be sophisticated neural processing that interrelates signals from adjoining cells to provide the information as to location.

PHYSIOLOGIC FACTORS

Because visual acuity is conceptually and operationally well anchored in psychophysics, the detailed dissection of its physiologic substrates is not an issue central to its discussion. In fact, current electrophysiology has not yet demonstrated neural processing mechanisms that approach the best human thresholds.

Nevertheless, spatial differentiation is inevitably coupled to light difference detection. If for any reason this is deficient, spatial resolution suffers. Thus one finds that visual acuity follows *pari passu* intensity discrimination sensitivity for the small stimulus areas that are involved.[34] For example, the detection of a double star as composed of two separate stimuli requires that the trough between the two light peaks be deep enough that an intensity discrimination ($\Delta I/I$) for such a small stimulus area can be carried out. Because $\Delta I/I$ has to be larger when the luminance gets lower, resolution deteriorates; that is, the peaks have to be separated further to create a trough that delivers a $\Delta I/I$ value sufficiently large to be detected for that area at the prevailing luminance.

Many other variables that influence visual acuity, for example, adaptation and exposure duration, exert their effect predominantly on the light discrimination sense and only through it on resolution. In many cases the effects can be traced for some distances through the optical, anatomic, and physiologic stages and the threshold identified by a prevailing limitation along the way.

Before returning to a brief survey of some of these interacting variables, we need to outline the procedures involved in actual measurements of visual acuity.

ACUITY CRITERIA

Within the general definition of visual acuity, that is, thresholds in which spatial dimension is the variable, some obvious subdivions can be recognized, and they are outlined best by the different criteria set for the response of the observer (Table 17-1):

1. The criterion of the presence of a single feature ("minimum visible")
2. The criterion of the presence, or internal

TABLE 17-1 Classification of Visual Acuity According to Criteria

Criterion	Minimum visible	Minimum resolvable (ordinary visual acuity)	Minimum discriminable (hyperacuity)
Task	Determine presence or absence of a target	Determine presence of, or distinguish between more than one, identifying feature in a visible target	Determine relative location of two or more visible features with respect to each other
Typical forced choice psychophysical question	Is there a line in this field? If there was a line in the field, was it horizontal or vertical?	Is this a "C" or an "O"? Is the gap in the C up, down, right, or left?	Is the upper line to the right or the left of the lower line?
Physiologic basis	Local brightness difference threshold (ΔI)	Detection of brightness differences between several adjoining small areas	Assignment of relative local signs to two or more suprathreshold visual features
Method of measurement	Vary object size	Vary object size or spacing between object components	Vary relative location of features
Magnitude of best threshold	~1 second of arc	~30 seconds of arc	~3 seconds of arc
Effect of image degradation	Moderate	Serious	Slight (except in stereoacuity)

arrangement, of identifying features in a visible target ("minimum resolvable" or ordinary visual acuity)

3. The criterion of the relative location of visible features (the "spatial minimum discriminable" or hyperacuity)

Minimum visible

What is involved in minimum visibility is the detection of the presence of a visual stimulus, but the stimulus variation is carried out by manipulating the contrast of the target through the medium of varying its size. The most typical example of this remains the experiments in which one measures the minimum width of a telegraph wire that can be seen against a uniform sky. The threshold value is of the order of 1 second of arc, that is, a very small fraction of the diameter of a retinal receptor. However, the situation is not as startling as it sounds, because it has a simple basis in the variation of the physical stimulus. The retinal light spread for a single, thin dark line seen against a uniform bright background is a dimple with the cross-sectional outline of the line-spread function. In the human eye this has a width at half height of at least 1 minute of arc. For all targets that have a

width of about this value or less, the shape of the light distribution remains about the same; variations of target width will manifest themselves purely as variations of dimple depth. Threshold measurements for the minimum visible (for example, where a dark line is widened progressively until its presence is detected) in reality are merely ΔI thresholds for a more or less fixed retinal light distribution whose contrast is varied by varying the target width (Fig. 17-4). The situation is analogous to one in the time domain, when one can let a light pulse reach threshold by increasing either the intensity of a stimulus or its duration, so long as the pulse length remains within the limits of the critical duration of the Bunsen-Roscoe-Bloch law (see Chapter 18).

In a definitive study Hecht and Mintz[17] showed that variations in contrast sensitivity as a function of luminance, for example, can fully account for variations in the minimum visible spatial threshold.

Although the stimulus change is effected in the dimension of space, the minimum visible threshold really does not approach the essence of visual acuity, because the subject's judgment does not demand the making of any spatial dif-

FIG. 17-4 Schematic diagram to illustrate that the *minimum visible* is a brightness rather than a spatial visual threshold. A single dark line seen against a uniform background is widened until it can be detected. As the line is widened, the retinal image pattern, which has the outline of the complement of the eye's line-spread function, increases in contrast but remains invariant in shape. Detection occurs when the ΔI threshhold is reached for the prevailing adaptation level. Although the object is changed in a spatial dimension, detection is purely that of a brightness change. For threshold line width (∼1 second of arc) the retinal image contrast is just a few percentage points. (From Westheimer G: Invest Ophthalmol 18:893, 1979.)

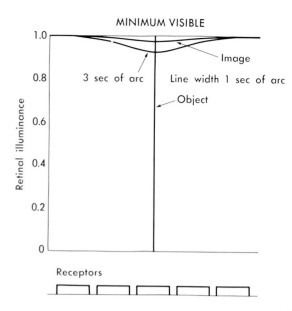

ferentiations, except in the trivial sense of whether a field is uniform. However, the other two subdivisions of visual acuity demand just that differentiation.

Minimum resolvable or ordinary visual acuity

Most commonly associated with visual acuity is the concept of Snellen's letters or Landolt's C's. A high-contrast, clearly visible target is shown, and the subject has to make a spatial judgment best exemplified by the distinction between a P or an F, a B or an R, and a C or an O. That is, either the presence of a gap or the relative arrangement of components of a letter has to be detected. Because we are dealing with a resolution task, there are more pointed tests of this capacity than Snellen's letters: for example, a double star that is being separated until seen double or a grating whose spatial frequency is being reduced until its structure becomes apparent. However, Snellen's letters have the virtue of not requiring a binary decision that is subject to guessing; they belong to a moderately sized ensemble of well-known patterns and optimize information transfer between patient and examiner.

Conceptually, the simplest situation is one in which members of a point or line pair are moved apart until the observer can judge them to be separate. Each of the two bright points or lines would be imaged on the retina with the light distribution of the point- or line-spread function. Initially, the two spread functions will overlap thoroughly, but as the target pair is sep-

arated, overlap will be only partial. A pattern emerges, characterized by two humps with an intervening trough (Fig. 17-5). Resolution, that is, correct judgment of doubleness, can be achieved when the peak-trough ratio of retinal illuminance is accommodated by the ΔI/I ratio of the visual system for the stimulus area involved at the prevailing level of adaptation. In addition, the effective grain of the visual system has to be small enough for the peaks and trough to fall in separate detecting units, regardless of whether they are defined by the limitations of retinal anatomic structure or synaptic organization.

In a normal observer in best focus the resolution limit or, as it is usually called, the minimum angle of resolution (MAR) is between 30 seconds of arc and 1 minute of arc.

There is remarkable concordance between the observed minimum angle of resolution, the expected resolving capacity of the eye's optics, and the predicted performance of a system that has a manifest visual acuity of 20/20 or better; the requirements are good optical imagery, foveal fixation, intact receptor structure and function, photopic luminance levels, and, of course, full integrity of the involved neural pathways.

For the actual determination of the resolution limit in a clinical or physiologic setting, the most widely used procedure involves gratings. The period of a high-contrast grating is reduced, i.e., the spatial frequency increased, until the observer can no longer resolve it. It is perfectly acceptable to use a square-wave grating, because at the resolution limit it will not differ in practice

TWO-POINT RESOLUTION

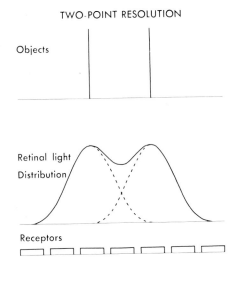

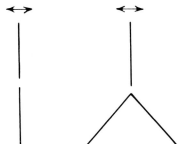

FIG. 17-5 Example of ordinary visual acuity is the detection of doubleness for a stimulus consisting of two points, each of which is imaged on the retina as a point-spread function. The amount of overlap depends on point separation. The essential elements for detecting doubleness, i.e., for resolution, are (1) an underlying retinal image pattern with two peaks separated by a trough, (2) a retinal illuminance difference between the peaks and the trough that is within the ΔI capability of the visual system in the prevailing state of adaptation, and (3) separate localization of the differentially stimulated regions.

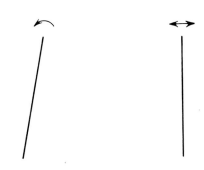

FIG. 17-6 Typical target configurations, which demonstrate the hyperacuity capability of the visual system, i.e., the detection of very small differences in relative localization of features. Arrows indicate the direction of displacement, which in each case can be judged to a few seconds of arc under optimal conditions. From left to right, vernier offset detection of two vertical lines; offset detection of the tip of a chevron from a line; detection of orientation change of a line; detection of lateral displacement of a target.

from a sinusoidal grating; the third-harmonic component, which is present in a square-wave grating, will by definition be already beyond the resolution limit.

In most clinical situations conceptually pure tests such as two-line or grating resolution are not practicable and one prefers to have a patient read letters or numerals. It must be realized, however, that factors other than resolution enter into a discrimination between letters of the alphabet. These are generally classed as belonging to form perception,[47] about which very little is known as yet at the physiologic and psychophysical levels. As will be seen later in this chapter, in some abnormalities of visual acuity the decrement in letter acuity is higher than in grating resolution, implying that in the end a distinction must be made between these two kinds of tasks.

Minimum discriminable or hyperacuity

Certain spatial distinctions can be made by a normal observer when the threshold is much lower than ordinary acuity, and therefore these must have a fundamentally different basis. The best known of these is alignment or vernier acuity.[55] The tasks share with ordinary acuity the presence of a clearly delineated target and therefore should never be confused with the threshold for the minimum visible, where merely the presence or absence of a target is being judged. However, in a hyperacuity test the subject is asked to make a judgment as to location of an element, usually relative to another element of the same target. Typical examples of hyperacuity configurations are shown in Figure 17-6. They all share the property of allowing spatial judgments whose thresholds in normal observers are 2 to 10 seconds of arc.

The mechanism subserving hyperacuity is still being explored,[45] but so much is clear: no contradiction is involved with the optical and receptor mosaic factors that limit ordinary visual acuity. Localization of a feature can be achieved with arbitrary precision so long as enough light quanta are available. However, the neural processing that is required for these judgments must be quite sophisticated.

Stereoscopic acuity also has a threshold of a few seconds of arc and therefore may be included under this heading, but its processing probably differs somewhat from that in ordinary hyperacuity.

MEASUREMENT OF ORDINARY VISUAL ACUITY (MINIMUM ANGLE OF RESOLUTION)

A variety of patterns have been employed to ascertain a patient's minimum angle of resolution. The major feature of all of them is that a given pattern is enlarged bodily or reduced to find the threshold size at which the judgment can be made correctly.

The most familiar of these tests is the Snellen chart. In a normal observer in best focus the resolution limit is between 30 seconds of arc and 1 minute of arc. The standard testing procedure is to enlarge the pattern until resolution can be achieved. Commonly the overall size of the letter is five times the width of each limb (Fig. 17-7). The easiest description is afforded by the Landolt C. The reference letter is a ring with an outer diameter subtending 5 minutes of arc at the observer's eye and an inner diameter subtending 3 minutes of arc. A gap 1 minute of arc wide is made in the ring, and the ring is presented with its opening in one of, say, four possible positions: up, down, right, or left. The subject has to indicate in which direction the C is pointing. At an observation distance of 6 m (20 feet), the overall size of the letter is 8.73 mm and the gap is 1.75 mm. If this is the subject's threshold, that is, if his minimum angle of resolution is 1 minute of arc, the visual acuity is identified as 6/6 or 20/20. However, suppose that he has a minimum angle of resolution of 0.75 minute of arc, that is, at 6 m he can resolve a letter with a feature that subtends 1.3 mm and whose overall size is 6.5 mm; such a letter has a gap that subtends 1 minute of arc at 4.5 m, or 15 feet, and would be resolvable by an observer with 1 minute of arc resolution at such a distance. The subject is then said to have visual acuity of 6/4.5 or 20/15.

Illiterate E and Landolt's C tests are based on the same principle as Snellen's charts. One may distinguish these from certain repetitive patterns such as gratings or checkerboards. In these the corresponding feature size must always be clearly understood; in a grating it is half the length of a period; in a checkerboard it is the side length of a square.

On the whole, single features such as individual-style letter charts are to be preferred, because under certain conditions of defocus, repetitive patterns may at times be spuriously resolved at a size for which a patient cannot consistently make correct judgments on letters.

All letters in the alphabet are not equally legible[37]; most charts do not use the whole alphabet. Test charts have been created with letters in other scripts.

Instruments occasionally have been designed that permit zooming of letters until they can be resolved, but the multiple-choice psychophysical technique of letter charts with several letters to the row has never been bettered in the practical situation.

The procedure of requiring a patient to read a letter chart rests on facilities for verbal communication that may not always be satisfied. A patient may not be able to understand the request or to indicate to the examiner what his performance actually is. For this reason, several so-called "objective" techniques of measuring visual acuity have been devised. They use a nonverbal response mode, but it cannot always be guaranteed that the results will be equivalent, because they may be channeled through different neural circuits. This has been made clear particularly by the case of one patient[3] who was manifestly blind by all observable criteria, but whose grating "resolution" measured by evoked potentials was normal.

The two most prominent objective measuring techniques for the minimum angle of resolution

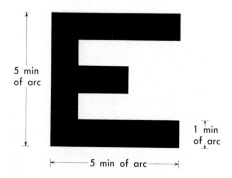

FIG. 17-7   20/20 Snellen's letter.

involve neural electrical potentials and oculomotor responses.

The evoked potential technique[30] is based on the presentation of a differentiated spatial pattern to the subject and measuring the changes in the electroencephalogram (EEG) that accompany the presentation. In the most sophisticated modern versions of this test the stimulus consists of a change merely in the internal light distribution in the pattern without any overall changes in total light reaching the eye. Examples are the instantaneous exchange of light and dark squares in a checkerboard or the replacement of a uniform field with a grating of the same average luminance. Whenever the pattern dimension is too small to be resolved, no changes are expected in the evoked potential on stimulus presentation. Use of temporal repetition and a signal averager can allow good measurements of resolution.

Pursuit and optokinetic eye movements are released by target movements, usually with little or no "voluntary" components. Here again targets with spatial differentiations too small to be resolved would not be expected to lead to associated smooth eye movements, and we clearly have a good principle for acuity measurement.[15] A variant of the eye movement method, observation of the relative frequency of voluntary fixations, recently has been the primary vehicle for accumulating information about the developments of visual acuity in infants.[12] In one of two equivalent but separated patches of the infant's visual field a grating is shown, and an observer notes the relative frequency of voluntary fixations on the two; the expectation is that a field with a differentiated pattern will be favored for fixation. However, one needs to remember that this technique presupposes access to and integrity of the oculomotor pathways.

When there is a lack of concordance of results with the various measuring techniques, the origin obviously has to be sought in difference in the pathways used in them.[9] Evoked potential recordings with electrode placements favoring the visual cortex would probe the most elementary pathways, but letter recognition and verbalization involve many other cortical areas. Whatever technique is applied, attention has to be given to the method of identifying a threshold. Even when there is no resolution, an EEG blip occasionally may occur synchronously with a stimulus, a randomly occurring saccade (although a smooth movement is unlikely) land on the target, or a subject may guess correctly the letter presented or the target's direction if it is an illiterate E or a grating. Special procedures have

been devised to ensure that objective techniques separate "signal" from "noise." Threshold determination is, of course, one of the time-honored problems of psychophysics. The method of constant stimuli with forced choice has been applied effectively as has the method of staircases. In either case, the usual value of thresholds is the target size at which the subject responds correctly on 75% of occasions. In clinical practice it works well to indicate the number of letters a patient misses in a line of Snellen's letters or can read beyond it (e.g., 20/15 − 1 or 20/20 + 2).

Thresholds obtained with a rigorous psychophysical method give not only a mean value of, say, the minimum angle of resolution, but also a standard error of this mean. Such a number has the virtue of permitting conclusions about whether the threshold is significantly different statistically in one situation as compared with another. It has been found that the standard error of the minimum angle of resolution, in common with that of other sensory limits, remains an approximately constant proportion of the mean (Weber's law).[44]

This finding suggests that a logarithmic scale be applied to the minimum angle of resolution, for example, the size of the letters in a visual acuity chart increase in geometric proportion as follows: 20/16, 20/20, 20/31, 20/39, 20/48, 20/61, 20/76, 20/95, 20/120, 20/149, 20/186, and 20/232. In practice, variations of such a scheme have been followed for nearly 100 years.[35] There is medicolegal significance in the identification of the percentage loss of visual acuity as a consequence of disease or injury. An earlier attempt by Snell and Sterling[38] led to a system of measurement in which any increase by 1 minute of arc in the minimum angle of resolution was regarded as reducing the visual efficiency to 86% of its previous value. Table 17-2 indicates several ways for specifying visual acuity levels: minimum angle of resolution, Snellen's acuity, Snell-Sterling's efficiency rating, Snellen's fraction (that is, the reciprocal of the minimum angle of resolution), and the logarithm of Snellen's fraction.

Identical numbers can give considerably different impressions, depending on the mode of presentation. As mentioned before, because the ratio

$$\frac{\Delta \text{ MAR}}{\text{mean MAR}}$$

is approximately constant, the logarithmic scale is the most appropriate. In it all reductions of acuity by a given factor constitute equivalent decrements. For example, the step from 20/10

TABLE 17-2 Visual Acuity Equivalents in Different Notations

MAR (minutes of arc)	Snellen's visual acuity		Snell-Sterling's visual efficiency (%)	Snellen's fraction	Log visual acuity relative to 20/20
	Feet	Meters			
0.5	20/10	6/3	109	2.0	0.3
0.75	20/15	6/4.5	104	1.33	0.1
1.00	20/20	6/6	100	1.0	0
1.25	20/25	6/7.5	96	0.8	−0.1
1.5	20/30	6/9	91	0.67	−0.18
2.0	20/40	6/12	84	0.5	−0.3
2.5	20/50	6/15	76	0.4	−0.4
3.0	20/60	6/18	70	0.33	−0.5
4.0	20/80	6/24	58	0.25	−0.6
5.0	20/100	6/30	49	0.2	−0.7
6.0	20/120	6/36	41	0.17	−0.78
7.5	20/150	6/45	31	0.133	−0.88
10.0	20/200	6/60	20	0.10	−1.0
20.0	20/400	6/120	3	0.05	−1.3

to 20/20 is equivalent to the steps from 20/20 to 20/40, or from 20/200 to 20/400.

FACTORS INFLUENCING VISUAL ACUITY

Because all optical, anatomic, and physiologic elements are at or near their peak performance when a subject exhibits what we call normal visual acuity, a diminution of function in any of these constituent elements will manifest itself in a reduction in visual acuity. The list of factors influencing visual acuity is legion,[42] and no attempt will be made to give an exhaustive account of them here. However, there are some stimulus variables whose effects are of more universal interest and have been well documented.

Refractive error

As soon as the optics of the eye are defocused, the point-spread function widens, and two stars, to be identified as separate, need to be farther apart than in the fully focused state. The width of the defocused point-spread function depends directly on the amount of defocus and inversely on the pupil size. For normal observation of a Snellen chart, the data in Figure 17-8 are typical. However, there are some complications. Because of optical peculiarities, some repetitive patterns, for example, gratings or checkerboards, occasionally can be resolved with a defocused optical system when letters of a similar size cannot. Another important variable is pupil size. Depth of focus increases with

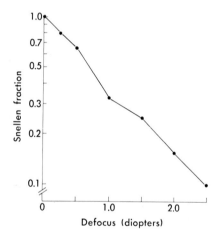

FIG. 17-8 Visual acuity (Snellen's fraction) as a function of defocus for a typical eye. The ordinates are plotted on logarithmic coordinates. (Data from Laurance.[23])

reduction in pupil size; thus the curve in Figure 17-8 will be less steep in a patient with a 2 mm pupil than shown. That a young hyperope can compensate for the refractive error by accommodation and hence may have no deficit in unaided acuity needs no special mention. However, it also must be remembered that retention of the state of zero accommodation is an active process. Thus blurring a young emmetropic eye with a +2 D lens may not make it exactly 2 D myopic—with good anchor points missing accommodation may be active and the defocus could be more than 2 D and, more important, quite unstable. In astigmatic imagery, the point-spread function will have different dimensions in the various directions. There will be meridional variation in acuity leading to a choppy performance on letter charts.

Retinal eccentricity

Only in the center of the fovea are the conditions appropriate for maximum acuity. Even 1 degree away from it there is a reduction to about 60% of maximum[52]; the function of visual acuity with eccentricity is shown in Figure 17-9. Data on the fall-off of cone[7] and ganglion cell[6] density with eccentricty in the human retina have recently become available. It is true that cones are farther apart as distance from the fovea increases, but rods remain closely packed and could, in theory, have been connected to carry good spatial information. The reduction in image quality in the retinal periphery is certainly nowhere near as severe as the reduction in acuity. The immediate cause is an increase in retinal summation areas, that is, the area from which excitatory signals converge on a ganglion cell. Because the visual cortex appears to be organized in processing modules,[20] each presumably with a constant number of input lines, one seeks concordance with the cortical magnification ratio (that is, the number of degrees of visual

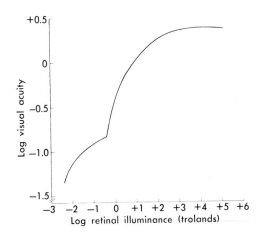

FIG. 17-10 Visual acuity (Snellen's fraction) as a function of luminance. (Data from Shlaer.[34])

field represented in a millimeter of visual cortex).

Visual acuity and hyperacuity seem to fall off at different rates with eccentricity,[46] but both exhibit better values for a given angle of eccentricity in the temporal than in the nasal visual field.[11]

Luminance

Data from Shlaer's definitive study[34] of the effect of luminance on visual acuity are shown in Figure 17-10. The evidence points to a separate rod and cone branch of the curve. Rods asymptote at a value of about 8 minutes of arc, and this is the acuity usually found in the absence or complete dysfunction of cones.[36] Visual acuity remains constant over a wide range of photopic luminances, extending from the level of full moonlight to that of a bright sky on a sunny day. Very high luminances cause an unexplained reduction in acuity,[54] even in adjoining zones of moderate luminance.

Contrast

When contrast is reduced there is a reduction in resolution. This occurs over a large range of retinal illumination levels, particularly in the range below 90 trolands.[39] Although stereoscopic acuity also suffers seriously when contrast is reduced, vernier alignment acuity is less severely affected.[50]

Pupil size

With pupil size below about 2.5 mm, the eye's point spread function in good focus becomes progressively wider, and a reciprocal relation-

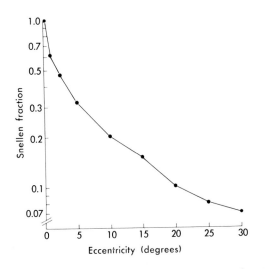

FIG. 17-9 Visual acuity (Snellen's fraction) as a function of retinal eccentricity. (Data from Wertheim.[40])

ship is expected between minimum angle of resolution and pupil size. Depending on the quality of the optics of the peripheral zones of the pupil, visual acuity remains approximately constant,[24] in the range of 2.5 to 6 mm, beyond which the aberrations begin to widen the point-spread function again.

Exposure duration

Although there is progressive reduction of visual acuity with decreasing exposure duration in the millisecond range, this can be offset by increasing illumination[16] to ensure constancy of the number of absorbed quanta. However, visual acuity in most observers is not as good for target exposures in the range of 100 to 500 msec as for longer durations, even though retinal summation is no longer a factor.[2] Vernier acuity seems relatively immune to reduction in exposure duration, but this is not the case for stereoscopic acuity.[50]

Target and eye movements

There is a decrement in certain visual functions during saccades and also in the general case in which there is significant movement of the retinal image. A target moving at moderate velocities, a few tens of degrees per second for at least half a second, can induce good enough pursuit eye movement to ensure acuity not far from normal. However, small movements of the image do not detract from acuity[22,49]—strict stability of the retinal image is not a requirement for optimum resolution.

Meridional variations in acuity

Differences in acuity in the various retinal meridians have been reported widely. They require grating or similar targets that permit the selective evaluation of the function one meridian at a time. The usual finding is that horizontal and vertical meridians are favored, although this is not universally so. The differences rarely exceed 15%, and there are claims for an etiologic influence connected with uncorrected astigmatism.[10]

Interaction effects

Visual acuity suffers when targets are too close together. Thresholds rise and occasionally may even double when a competing target is presented within a few minutes of arc. That this is not purely optical in origin is demonstrated by the nonmonotonic relationship between threshold and intertarget distance; the diminution of performance is maximal at a distance of 2 to 5 minutes of arc and disappears for larger and

smaller distances. The effect can be observed with ordinary visual acuity[14] and also vernier[48] and stereoscopic acuity.[4]

Developmental aspects

The difficulties of assessing the resolving capacity of the infant had, for a long time, left the time course of visual acuity development unclear. By the time ordinary methods—illiterate E's, for example—can be used, visual acuity is normal. It takes several months after birth for the full development of pursuit eye movement, and therefore it is not easy to differentiate between inability to resolve a pattern and inability to execute the movement that would betray resolution. Preferential-looking methods, using the frequency of intersaccadic fixation in regions containing a pattern as compared with those not containing a pattern, have yielded fairly consistent results in the hands of dedicated experimentalists. Reasonable indication of the state of development of visual acuity with infant age is given in Fig. 17-11. The subject has been reviewed thoroughly by Dobson and Teller.[9] When evoked potential is used as the measure, the data routinely come up with thresholds that are lower. This may be because evoked potentials tap off at an earlier state of elaboration of the visual acuity signal than do eye movements or verbal responses; however, it must not be for-

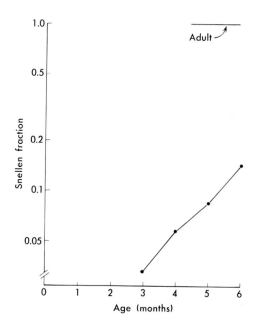

FIG. 17-11 Visual acuity as a function of age in the infant. (Data from Dobson and Teller.[9])

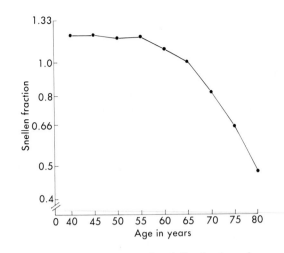

FIG. 17-12 Fiftieth percentile of distribution of measured visual acuity in the population, graphed as a function of age. (Data from Weymouth.[51])

gotten that evoked responses are based on an averaging procedure often effectively summing many hundreds of stimuli. Active research is in progress on the possible interference with normal development (for example, by patching one eye or failing to correct the optical defects engendered by aphakia or aniridia). The interest was sparked by Wiesel and Hubel's observation[53] in 1963 that cats whose eyes were kept artificially closed in their first few weeks of life had visual behavior and single-cell responses in the visual cortex that differed from the norm. There appears to be a clear need for the visual system to be exposed to appropriate optical stimuli during a critical period of development, but it is as yet too early to identify the exact period and the nature of the needed stimuli in the human infant. See the discussion of amblyopia below.

Hyperacuity development in infants proceeds at a rate different than that of visual acuity.[33] In early infancy vernier acuity can in fact be poorer than visual acuity, but this reverses as development proceeds.

Aging

Because good visual acuity depends on the integrity of a variety of structures in the eye and visual pathways, it is natural to expect its maintenance into old age to be an exception rather than the rule. Figure 17-12, showing the 50th percentile of the measured visual acuity of a population as a function of age above 40 years, may be used as a guide.

SINUSOIDAL GRATING TARGETS

We saw earlier in this chapter that the optical spread in the eye constitutes one possible limit to resolution. It would be advantageous to have a test that probes the retinal and neural stages of the visual acuity processing alone, bypassing, so to speak, the eye's optics. As it happens, there is one mode of illuminating the retina that creates a pattern largely independent of the optical quality of the eye: Young's interference fringes (Fig. 17-13). When two monochromatic coherent point sources are imaged in the pupil, light diverging from them into the vitreous will form a system of interference fringes whose angular spacing in object space is given by the formula λ/a, in which λ is the wavelength and a is the separation of the sources in the plane of the pupil. When laser light of wavelength 623 nm is used, fringe spacing of 1 minute of arc occurs with a source separation of 2.14 mm in the pupil, fringe spacing of 2 minutes of arc (minimum angle of resolution = 1 minute of arc) with a source separation of 1.07 mm, and so on. The retinal image is a sinusoidal grating, that is, a grating whose intensity profile is sinusoidal. Its major viture is that it retains very high contrast and constant fringe spacing regardless of the state of refraction or aberrations. The procedure has been used to find the resolution limit of the visual system when the optical factors have been eliminated,[5,41] disclosing that retinal resolution matches that of good optics with a 2 to 2.5 mm pupil. Gratings with finer fringes, created by separating the source images beyond 2.5 mm, are not resolved.

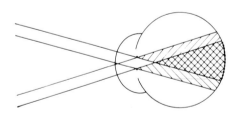

FIG. 17-13 Basis for the interference fringe method of measuring resolution of retinal and central stages of the visual system, bypassing refractive stage. A pair of coherent point sources is imaged in the plane of the pupil. Wherever the two bundles overlap in the image space, a system of interference fringes is formed. Spacing of the fringes in angular measure in the eye's object space is given by λ/a radians, where λ = wavelength of light and a = separation of the two point sources. When λ = 623 nm and a = 1.0 mm, fringe peaks are 2.14 minutes of arc apart.

However, the clinical utility of the test is still an open matter. Careful ophthalmoscopic and retinoscopic examination will give an excellent indication of the optics of an eye, making it unnecessary to bypass the eye's optics just to ascertain whether they caused an acuity deficit. A much more important question concerns the capacity for resolution of the retinal and central stages when they cannot be reached via the standard optical imaging route because of opacities in the media. If it were possible to smuggle a system of interference fringes into the vitreous, one could in principle reach a conclusion as to the integrity of the neural stages prior to instituting surgical relief for the opacities of the media. The difficulty in the way of this approach is apparent from Figure 17-13. Fringes of a given spacing arise from the interference of coherent beams from two points in the pupil a fixed distance apart. For maximum contrast, the intensity of the two beams must be equal. When the effective intensity of one beam is reduced to k times the other $(1 > k > 0)$, the interference fringe contrast is reduced to $2\sqrt{k}/(1 + k)$. The essential precondition for the application of a sinusoidal grating interference fringe test that bypasses the optics of the eye is that pairs of locations can be found in the media that allow the admission of twin coherent beams whose image-sided intensities are not excessively different. The psychophysical safeguards when using a grating ("Do you now see a set of stripes?") are somewhat more cumbersome than when using letters ("Please read the letters on this line of the chart"), but do not constitute a crippling disadvantage for such a test.

There has been a great deal of interest in sinusoidal grating targets used via the ordinary optics of the eye. In 1956 Schade[32] found that sinosoidal gratings with fringe spacing of 5 to 8 minutes of arc can be seen when they have a remarkably low contrast, often much less than 1%, while fringes with finer spacing (that is, higher spatial frequency) and also with coarser spacing (that is, lower spatial frequency) have to have higher contrast to be visible. The basic element of the test is a grating target of given spatial frequency, expressed in cycles/degree of visual angle. Its contrast is changed by keeping the mean luminance constant and varying the difference between the luminance at the peaks (L_{max}) and troughs (L_{min}) of the sinusoidal luminance profile of the grating target until the observer's threshold is reached. The modulation M is given by the expression

$$M = \frac{L_{max} - L_{min}}{L_{max} + L_{min}}$$

This formula originally was proposed by Michelson[27] for the visibility of interference fringes and gives what should be called the "Michelson" contrast, which is applicable to repetitive patterns. For a single target with peak luminance L_{max} seen against a uniform background of luminance L, the Weber fraction $(L_{max} - L)/L = \Delta L/L$ has become the standard.

Modulation sensitivity measurements are made in the spatial frequency range of 0.5 cycles/degree (where each sinusoidal fringe covers 2 degress of visual angle) and 20 or 30 cycles/degree (where it covers 3 or 2 minutes of arc). Thresholds usually are plotted as the reciprocal of the Michelson contrast on logarithmic coordinates. Thus the situation where $L_{max} = 101$, $L_{min} = 99$ and $M = 2/200 = 0.01$ would be represented by a modulation sensitivity of 100. Similarly, when $L_{max} = 110$ and $L_{min} = 90$, $M = 20/200 = 0.1$ would mean a modulation sensitivity of 10. Modulation sensitivity curves, which combine the effect of optical, neural, and behavioral stages of vision, can be obtained under a variety of conditions; a typical one for central fixation and photopic luminance is shown in Figure 17-14. The curve exemplifies the band-pass characteristics of the human visual system, which also is apparent in the temporal domain (see Chapter 18). Its origin is largely in the center-surround organization of neural elements in the retina and visual projection. An excitatory center flanked by inhibitory surrounds is a characteristic of retinal ganglion cells and also of cortical neurons, and these are well matched by light patterns such as gratings that can deliver the appropriate stimulus to the various components of the receptive field at the same time. Unless only a few cycles are shown at a time, gratings are not localized sufficiently to probe, say, the fovea that has a diameter of 30 minutes of arc.

In one application of the modulation sensitivity approach, the target modulation is set at 1 (that is, $L_{min} = 0$) and a threshold is obtained by varying the spatial frequency until the field is no longer seen as striped. The test then is a determination of visual acuity for a grating target. On the other hand, when the spatial frequency is set at values below this cut-off spatial frequency and the modulation varied until the field begins to appear uniform and no longer striped, thresholds map the contrast detection for coarser-than-resolution targets, in this case sinusoidal

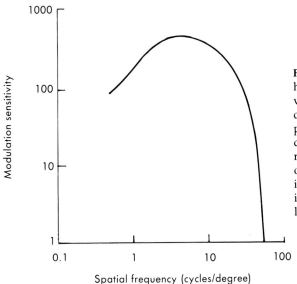

FIG. 17-14 Modulation sensitivity curve for normal human observer at high photopic luminance and foveal vision. Axis of abscissae refers to spatial frequency of grating targets with sinusoidal luminance profile, i.e., number of complete grating cycles in each degree of visual angle. Modulation sensitivity is reciprocal measure of grating contrast needed for threshold. The curve shows the spatial bandpass characteristics of visual system: contrast sensitivity is higher in intermediate range and falls off for both higher and lower spatial frequencies.

gratings. A great deal of work is in progress to determine whether such stimulus manipulation in the domain of contrast can aid in the diagnosis of ophthalmic disorders, but the results are not yet definite.[1]

AMBLYOPIA

Amblyopia is a condition in which there is reduced visual acuity in the eye that does not exhibit any explicit abnormality on detailed examination. It is usually unilateral, and specific etiologic factors have been identified, including the presence, at an early formative stage of visual development, of an uncorrected difference in refractive state between the two eyes (anisometropic amblyopia) or a sustained lack of binocular fixation (strabismic amblyopia). Other factors such as congenital cataract or oculomotor instability (e.g., nystagmus) may also be involved.

Animal models of amblyopia exist. They have their basis in the pioneering work of Wiesel and Hubel,[53] who raised kittens with one eye sutured and observed changes in the organization of the visual cortex. This had led to many studies concerning the so-called critical period, i.e., the time span during which visual functional integrity is needed for subsequent development of normal adult vision (see Mitchell and Timney[29] for review). More recently a thorough study[18] was conducted on monkeys, who were raised from infancy with one eye optically blurred, induced by atropinization. Resolution

and contrast sensitivity, measured behaviorally, were reduced, but the retina and all other eye tissues were histologically normal. In the lateral geniculate nuclei, however, cells belonging to the parvocellular stream from the affected eye were smaller and in the visual cortex anatomic and physiologic changes were found in structures associated with the processing of fine spatial detail originating in the blurred eye.

As we have seen earlier in this chapter, one can differentiate between simple resolving capacity, localizing ability, and letter or feature recognition. Grating resolution, vernier acuity, and Snellen acuity, respectively, are individual tests for these capabilities. Ordinarily, the diagnosis of amblyopia would be based on simple Snellen acuity alone. It is, therefore, of interest to inquire about the extent to which reductions in this measure are mirrored also by reductions in the others. It turns out that there is a fundamental difference between anisometropic and strabismic amblyopia.

Insofar as it has been measured, contrast discrimination for small fields[28] or high spatial frequency gratings is reduced in all kind of amblyopia.[19] Vernier alignment and bisection of spatial intervals, which fall into the category of hyperacuity, are also poorer in all kinds of amblyopia than in the normal. In anisometropic amblyopes the ratio between hyperacuity and ordinary visual acuity is the same as in a normal eye.[26] In strabismic amblyopia, hyperacuity and grating resolution also are down in proportion, but there is in addition a more severe reduction in letter acuity. This extra loss in strabismic amblyopia emphasizes the point made earlier about the need to invoke a further mechanism, specifically, form vision, to distinguish between pure resolution and Snellen letter performance.

In reviewing the etiology of the amblyopias, Levi[25] comes to the conclusion that the origin of the difference between anisometropic and strabismic amblyopia lies in the ontology of visual acuity and hyperacuity. Visual acuity develops more slowly than hyperacuity in infancy.[33] Strabismic amblyopia becomes manifest at an earlier age than anisometropic amblyopia, at a time when the ratio between hyperacuity and visual acuity is still rather low. Anisometropic amblyopes, on the other hand, have a little longer span of normal development before their pathology emerges. Therefore they have a chance to achieve a stage where the ratio between the two acuities has already reached a normal level, though their development is arrested before either of these two functions has gained the full adult capability, which may be at age 6 or even later.

REFERENCES

1. Arden GB: Recent developments in clinical contrast sensitivity testing, in Breinin GM, Siegel IM, eds: Advances in diagnostic visual optics, Berlin, Springer-Verlag, 1983.
2. Baron WS, Westheimer G: Visual acuity as a function of exposure duration, J Opt Soc Am 63:212, 1973.
3. Bodis-Wollner I, et al: Visual association cortex and vision in man: pattern evoked occipital potentials in a blind boy, Science 198:629, 1977.
4. Butler T, Westheimer G: Interference with stereoscopic acuity: spatial, temporal and disparity tuning, Vision Res 18:1387, 1978.
5. Campbell FW, Green DG: Optical and retinal factors affecting visual resolution, J Physiol (Lond) 181:576, 1965.
6. Curcio CA, Allen KA: Topography of ganglion cells in the human retina, J Comp Neurol 300:5, 1990.
7. Curcio CA, Sloan KR, Kalina RE, et al: Human photoreceptor topography, J Comp Neurol 292:497, 1990.
8. Curcio CA, Sloan KR, Packer O, et al: Distribution of cones in human and monkey retina: individual variability and radial symmetry, Science 236:579, 1987.
9. Dobson V, Teller D: Visual acuity in human infants: a review and comparison of behavioral and electrophysiological studies, Vision Res 18:1469, 1978.
10. Emsley HH: Irregular astigmatism of the eye, effect of correcting lenses, Trans Opt Soc Lond 27:28, 1925.
11. Fahle M: Zum Einfluss von Gesichtsfeldort und Reizorientieurung auf verschiedene Wahrnehmungsleistungen, in Herzau W, ed: Pathophysiologie des Sehens, Stuttgart, Ferdinand Enke, 1984.
12. Fantz RL: Pattern vision in young infants, Psychol Record 8:43, 1958.
13. Fechner GT: Elemente der Psychophysik, Leipzig, Breitkopf & Härtel, 1860.
14. Flom MC, Weymouth FW, Kahneman D: Visual resolution and contour interaction, J Opt Soc Am 53:1026, 1963.
15. Goldmann H: Objektive Sehschärfenbestimmung, Ophthalmologica 105:240, 1942.
16. Graham CH, Cook C: Visual acuity as a function of intensity and exposure time, Am J Psychol 49:654, 1937.
17. Hecht S, Mintz EU: The visibility of single lines at various illuminations and the retinal basis of visual resolution, J Gen Physiol 22:593, 1939.
18. Hendrickson AE, Movshon JA, Eggers HM, et al: Effects of early unilateral blur on the macaque's visual system, II, Anatomical observations, J Neuroscience 7:1327, 1987.
19. Hess RF, Howell ER: The threshold contrast sensitivity function in strabismic amblyopia: evidence for a two-type classification, Vision Res 17:1049, 1977.
20. Hubel H, Wiesel TN: Functional architecture of macaque monkey visual cortex, Proc R Soc Lond B 198:1, 1977.
21. Jennings JAM, Charman WN: Off-axis image quality in the human eye, Vision Res, 21:445, 1981.
22. Keesey UT: Effects of involuntary eye movements on visual acuity, J Opt Soc Am 50:769, 1960.
23. Laurance L: Visual optics and sight testing, 3rd ed, London, School of Optics, 1926.
24. Leibowitz H: The effect of pupil size on visual acuity for photometrically equated test fields at various levels of luminance, J Opt Soc Am 42:416, 1952.
25. Levi DM: Visual acuity in strabismic and anisometropic amblyopia, Pediatric Ophthalmology 3:289, 1990.
26. Levi DM, Klein SA: Hyperacuity and amblyopia, Nature 298:268, 1982.
27. Michelson AA: On the application of interference methods to spectroscopic measurements, Phil Mag Series V 27:484, 1891.
28. Miller EF II: The nature and cause of impaired vision in the amblyopic eye of a squinter, Am J Optom Arch Am Acad Optom 32:10, 1955.
29. Mitchell DE, Timney B: Postnatal development of function in the mammalian visual system, in Darian-Smith I, Ed: American Physiological Society Handbook of Physiology—vol III, part I, The nervous system, 1984.
30. Regan D: Evoked potentials in psychology, sensory physiology and clinical medicine, London, Chapman & Hall, 1972.
31. Rolls ET, Cowey A: Topography of the retina and striate cortex and its relationship to visual acuity in rhesus and squirrel monkeys, Exp Brain Res 10:298, 1970.
32. Schade OH Sr: Optical and photoelectric analog of the eye, J Opt Soc Am 46:721, 1956.
33. Shimoyo S, Held R: Vernier acuity is less than grating acuity in 2- and 3-month-olds, Vision Res 17:77, 1977.
34. Shlaer S: The relation between visual acuity and illumination, J Gen Physiol 21:165, 1937.
35. Sloan LL: Measurement of visual acuity, Arch Ophthalmol 45:704, 1951.

36. Sloan LL: Congenital achromatopsia: a report of 19 cases, J Opt Soc Am 44:117, 1954.

37. Sloan LL, Rowland WM, Altman A: Comparison of three types of test target for the measurement of visual acuity, Q Rev Ophthalmol 8:4, 1952.

38. Snell AC, Sterling S: Percentage evaluation of macular vision, Arch Ophthalmol 54:443, 1925.

39. Van Nes FL, Bouman MA: Spatial modulation transfer in the human eye, J Opt Soc Am 57:401, 1967.

40. Wertheim T: Uber die indirekte Sehschärfe, Z Psychol 7:172, 1894.

41. Westheimer G: Modulation thresholds for sinusoidal light distributions on the retina, J Physiol 152:67, 1960.

42. Westheimer G: Visual acuity, Ann Rev Psychol 16:359, 1965.

43. Westheimer G: Optical properties of vertebrate eyes, in Fuortes M, ed: Handbook of sensory physiology, vol 7/2, Physiology of photoreceptor organs, Berlin, Springer-Verlag, 1972, p 449.

44. Westheimer G: The scaling of visual acuity measurements, Arch Ophthalmol 97:327, 1979.

45. Westheimer G: The spatial sense of the eye, Proctor Lecture, Invest Ophthalmol Vis Sci 18:893, 1979.

46. Westheimer G: The spatial grain of the perifoveal retina, Vision Res 22:157, 1982.

47. Westheimer G: The Prentice Lecture, Visual acuity and hyperacuity: resolution, localization, form, Amer J Optom and Physiol Optics 64:567, 1987.

48. Westheimer G, Hauske G: Temporal and spatial interference with vernier acuity, Vision Res 15:1137, 1975.

49. Westheimer G, McKee SP: Visual acuity in the presence of retinal-image motion, J Opt Soc Am 65:847, 1975.

50. Westheimer G, Pettet MW: Contrast and duration of exposure differentially affect vernier and stereoscopic acuity, Proc Roy Soc London B241:42, 1990.

51. Weymouth FW: The effect of age on visual acuity, in Hirsch MJ, Wick RE, eds: Vision of the aging patient, Radnor, Chilton, 1960.

52. Weymouth FW, et al: Visual acuity within the area centralis and its relation to eye movements and fixation, Am J Ophthalmol 11:947, 1928.

53. Wiesel TN, Hubel DH: Single-cell responses in striate cortex of kittens deprived of vision in one eye, J Neurophysiol 26:1003, 1963.

54. Wilcox WW: The basis of the dependence of visual acuity on illumination, Proc Natl Acad Sci USA 18:47, 1932.

55. Wülfing EA: Über den kleinsten Gesichtswinkel, Z Biol 29:199, 1892.

CHAPTER
18

The Temporal Responsiveness of Vision

WILLIAM M. HART, Jr., M.D., Ph.D.

The vertebrate visual system has evolved in such a way as to allow a practical interpretation of the external physical world, with which it has only indirect contact, through sensations initiated by radiant energy (see Chapter 13). This energy covers an extremely broad dynamic range, a fact that has required that the visual system also be able to adapt to the available light, whether at very high or very low levels of luminance (see Chapter 16). Another class of specialized visual properties deals with both rapid and slow changes of radiant energy as a function of time. The visual system responds to such changes in a manner that allows nearly instantaneous interpretation of a rapidly changing environment. Through a built-in editorial capacity, it avoids being overwhelmed by an excessive amount of information. Subjectively, visual images appear to be stable, and objects appear to move smoothly in time and space. Yet most of what we see are only selected portions of a potentially infinite variety of images taken from our surroundings. The visual system periodically samples the images cast on the retina. It then stores, integrates, differentiates, erases, and performs other operations, resulting in the perception of apparently stable scenes. Because the radiant energy arriving at the eye differs continuously from moment to moment and place to place, interpretations of these variations must take place in a nearly synchronous fashion. The temporal responsiveness of the visual system is necessarily limited; a finite amount of time is required to collect and process the information in any image. This chapter describes some of the physiologic phenomena that determine these limits.

Although visual experiences generally tend to conform well to the spatiotemporal order of the external physical world, they are never a perfect representation of reality. This is a result of the limited responsiveness of physiologic mechanisms in the visual system. These mechanisms edit all visual information, condensing or discarding redundant or irrelevant features, while enhancing and retaining relevant information. Functionally useful visual information consists of variations of radiant energy in either time or space. That which is visually significant is the presence of "something different": a change in an image. Contrasting boundaries of

ACKNOWLEDGEMENT

This chapter is an adaptation and extension of the work of Gerard M. Schickman, who in prior editions of this text developed the major concepts covered herein. The importance of his contributions lay in his ability to define critical issues and to clarify difficult concepts. Our understanding of the temporal properties of the visual response has thereby been enriched.

W.M.H.

This work was supported in part by Research Grant EY 06582 from the National Eye Institute, National Institutes of Health.

light in the retinal image and changes in their location or magnitude are all that is relevant. The visual system responds appropriately by emphasizing borders and by detecting temporal changes in their locations. It acts as a differentiator and as an integrator, separating disparate image features from one another and grouping similar sensations together. It integrates energy across time and space to enhance sensitivity, and it functions as a comparator and an extrapolator to fill in apparent voids in visual content. It serves to interpret a constantly changing pattern of stimulation, using a time-based, continuous search for invariances and orderly relations within retinal images.

SHORT- AND LONG-TERM EVENTS IN VISION

While the eye must be capable of distinguishing among many different levels of luminance, it also must cope with many different rates of change in luminance. The photochemical events that initiate vision are quite rapid.[3,92] Absorption of light energy by photopigments and the initiation of pigment bleaching take place within microseconds. Subsequent electrical events within photoreceptors can be recorded within milliseconds after exposure to a flash of light.[19,27,103] Although the initial stages of the bleaching process are rapid, subsequent thermal events are slower. Complete dissociation of rhodopsin into all-*trans*-retinal and opsin requires minutes of continuous light exposure. The bleaching process continues to a certain extent even in total darkness, following a very short flash exposure; thus radiant excitation of a visual receptor may be essentially complete before the subsequent molecular changes have run their course.[135]

At low levels of illumination the visual task of detection is facilitated by temporal summation (see below). At high levels of illumination the eye no longer faces a detection task. Here the problem is one of differentiation. So much visual information is available that it must be broken down into its most important components. Under such conditions, the eye acts as an intermittent sampling device, making fixatory pauses of brief duration during which it takes in task-related information. While reading, such fixatory pauses may last 200 to 300 msec.[130] Saccadic refixation movements from one point to another require approximately 10 to 80 msec, depending on the angular distance between the two points. Such movements may be repeated as often as three to five times per second, as the viewer scans a scene of high visual content.[144]

While the extraction of detailed information from individual glimpses is a form of differentiation, the illusion of image continuity and stability is the result of storage and comparison operations that are performed between successively captured samples of the surrounding scene.

Short-term changes in an image require a high speed of responsiveness by the visual system; speed of storage is important for image continuity and stability. The upper limiting time for visual storage and temporal integration varies from 10 msec to 1 second depending on the nature of the task. On the other hand, such processes work at cross purposes with the need to replace old information with new, a process termed "erasure."[6] Pathologic failures of this function can result in the superposition of temporally sequential images. This type of visual disturbance, called "palinopsia," is occasionally seen in patients with extensive damage to the visual cortex.[30] Troxler's phenomenon (see Chapter 16) is another example of a temporally dependent visual process. An image cast on a fixed retinal location tends to fade from view after a few seconds. It can be restored to view by slight movement over the retinal surface. This phenomenon demonstrates the reliance of the visual system on temporal, as well as spatial, changes, to capture visual information.

Long-term changes in image features invoke a different class of visual response. An example is the visual system's ability to adapt to changes in the apparent spatial distribution of objects in the field of view. Although a spectacle lens may improve a patient's acuity by providing an optimal image at the fovea, its curvatures produce a variable prismatic effect, depending on the distance from its optical center. This accounts for the distortion frequently reported by patients with new glasses. Shifts of fixation from the center to the periphery of the lens cause a deflection of the line of sight through an angle that changes with eccentricity. Thus movements by either the eye or the head seem to alter the relative position of objects seen through the lens. After a few days, however, these disturbing distortions disappear as the patient's visual response patterns adapt. When this long-term adjustment is complete, the patient can remove and replace the glasses, encountering no difficulty in spatial perception as the appropriate set of responses occurs automatically. This ability of the visual system to compensate for spatial distortion is one of its most remarkable and useful capacities.[57,104]

VISUAL PHYCHOPHYSICS OF TEMPORAL PHENOMENA

The temporal responsiveness of the visual system has been most exhaustively studied with the techniques of psychophysics. Only recently have conventional neurophysiologic methods begun to yield explanations at a cellular level for the phenomena that have been so well described at a behavioral level. The first half of this chapter reviews some of the central features of the psychophysics of temporal phenomena in vision. The second half of the chapter summarizes the findings of neurophysiologic and anatomic studies that illustrate some of the physiologic mechanisms underlying the behavioral phenomena.

TEMPORAL SUMMATION

Although photoreceptor absorption of a single quantum of light can trigger a neural event,[55] several quanta must be absorbed in the completely dark-adapted eye to elicit a sensation.[59] A group of quantal absorptions must occur within a restricted retinal area (spatial summation) and during a limited period of time (temporal summation) to constitute an adequate stimulus. During this period of temporal integration, up to about 0.1 second, the retina sums the effects of individual quantal absorptions. The maximum time over which this temporal summation can occur is termed the "critical duration of vision." The simplest experimental method of demonstrating temporal summation uses single test lights projected on a dark background in the visual field of a dark-adapted eye. Even this relatively simple test design involves multiple variables, such as the luminance and size of the projected spot of light, its spectral composition, its location in the visual field, its shape, luminance gradients at its borders, and its internal uniformity. Temporal variables include the speed of onset of the test light, its duration, and the speed of its extinction. Despite these many complications fairly simple general rules seem to govern the visual response to isolated lights.

CRITICAL DURATION

The period of time during which a light stimulus can be summed by the retina is called the "critical duration." By convention, critical duration is represented by the symbol Tc. Determining how long a light must shine to be seen against a dark background depends primarily on the luminance of the test spot of light. To reach the threshold of visibility an intense light need not remain on as long as a weak one. To measure threshold perception in a dark-adapted eye, one can begin with a relatively intense light and then adjust the duration of exposure on repeated trials until a sufficiently short interval is reached so that an observer can detect only 50% of its presentations. Under these conditions only a very short flash will be needed. If the luminance of the test flash is then reduced further, the observer will detect fewer than 50% of the flash presentations. To restore performance to the 50% detection level the duration of the flash must be increased in proportion to its reduction in luminance. A twofold reduction in luminance requires a doubling of the duration, and a threefold reduction in luminance requires a tripling of the duration to remain at threshold. Such reciprocity holds for flashes shorter than the critical duration. Within this interval a constant product of luminance (B) and duration (t) achieves a constant effect by maintaining the stimulus at the threshold level. Since the product (Bt) is proportional to the total luminous energy of the test flash, it is said that flashes of equal energy produce equal threshold effects. The relationship

$$Bt = K$$

(where K is a constant value) is Bloch's law of vision. This relationship states that, within the period of the critical duration, a given amount of luminous energy will have the same effect regardless of its distribution in time.

The Bunsen-Roscoe law of photochemistry is an analog of Bloch's law of vision. It describes the physical phenomenon of temporal summation of light energy by chemical reactions that are driven by light. Over a wide range of luminance, photochemical reactions have rates that are proportional to the total luminous energy driving the reaction, and not to the flux level or rate at which light energy is introduced into the reaction. Identical photochemical effects can be achieved by low levels of illumination introduced over long periods of time and by higher levels of illumination applied over shorter intervals. This reciprocal property is of value to photographers, who use balanced variations in diaphragm aperture sizes and exposure duration to achieve equivalent degrees of film exposure with greater or less motion blur and depth of field. The total effect of exposure is determined by the number of quanta absorbed by the photosensitive emulsion on the film surface. Within certain limits the same reciprocal relationship between quantal absorptions and duration of exposure is found in the retina's sensitivity for light detection. In a manner analogous to photochemical reactions, the retina accumulates the results of sufficiently rapid energy input until a criterion of performance is met, such as threshold detection.

Beyond the critical duration, temporal summation by the visual system ceases. The effect of a test light then becomes dependent on its luminance alone rather than on the product of its luminance and duration. Thus it is necessary to specify, when thresholds are being measured, whether the threshold is being determined with the minimum amount of energy or with the minimum level of luminance. Measurement of threshold energy requires flashes shorter than the critical duration,[126] whereas measurement of threshold luminance (probably more useful for the practical assessment of visual function) requires test flashes longer than the critical duration. Clinical examination of the visual field, so-called perimetry, employs test spots of light that are longer than the critical duration of vision. This constitutes a tactical device for eliminating time as a variable for perception of the test light. Spots of light presented for longer time periods than the critical duration are visible solely as a function of their luminance, relative to the surrounding or adapting level of luminance (that is, contrast).

The visual system's capacity for temporal summation is not a constant but varies complexly according to a variety of test variables, such as stimulus size and background luminance.[126] Temporal summation also is critically dependent on whether the task required of the observer is one of simple detection of light or of correct identification of image content. Figure 18-1, a plot of energy vs. duration for various test stimuli, illustrates some of these determinants. Each curve represents a set of conditions that are equivalent in that they produce a particular level of visual performance, for example, detection of a flash against a background (A and B), matching of test brightness to a criterion (C, open circles), or 50% correct identifications of binary digits presented in triads (C, filled circles). Note that for short presentations of the test stimuli the curves have horizontal segments, indicating that a constant luminance-duration product is needed to reach the criterion level of performance. The break in each curve defines the critical duration. This is seen to be longer for small than for large test areas[116] and longer for dark than for lighter backgrounds.[115] The critical duration also is longer for complex perceptual tasks than for the relatively simple task of light

detection.[67,68] A positive slope of unity above the break in each curve indicates that stimulus luminance values for threshold task performance are constant, and the product Bt increases linearly with time. In other words, for durations that exceed the critical period, the stimulus luminance needed for a threshold effect becomes independent of time.

Temporal summation interacts with acuity-related tasks in a manner analogous to that for luminance detection. Figure 18-2 illustrates results obtained when test stimuli were Landoldt C optotypes of various sizes.[67] Background luminances were adjusted until observers could just barely detect the critical detail (opening of the C) with a probability of about 80%. Exposure duration of the background was 10 msec. Luminances and exposure times were reciprocally varied to maintain a constant product. Six target sizes were used, allowing determinations for six different energy levels, for each of which the probability of detection was plotted as a function of duration. As in Figure 18-1 the data fit curves having a horizontal segment and a sloping segment. The break between the two segments defines the critical duration. For short exposures constant energy is associated with a constant level of detection. Detectability drops, however, as exposures longer than the critical duration increasingly fail to compensate for decreases in luminance (remember that the product of luminance and time is being kept constant). Notice that the critical durations for luminance detection shown in Figure 18-1 have upper limits of approximately 0.1 second while those for the acuity-related tasks in Figure 18-2 are longer, having maximum values of approximately 0.4 second. The critical duration tends to vary as a function of the level of acuity required for the task: it is relatively short for the detection of coarse spatial detail and relatively long for finer detail. Exposure duration of the structured image, and not the total energy, appears to be the determining variable for detection of the gap in the Landoldt ring. The detection task improves with time up to a maximum of 400 msec at phototopic luminances.[9] These findings suggest the participation of a central nervous mechanism in determining the critical duration for an acuity-dependent task.

TEMPORAL SUMMATION OF SPECTRALLY DIFFERENT LIGHT STIMULI

The temporal responsiveness of the visual system to colored light stimuli varies in a complex manner. Measurements of critical durations for

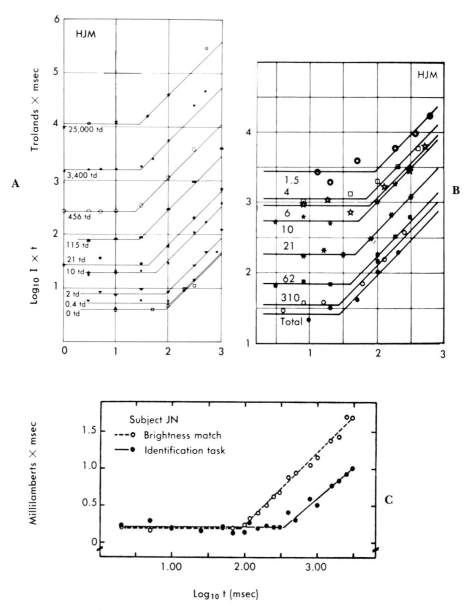

FIG. 18-1 Luminance-duration reciprocity and its breakdown above stimulus-dependent and task-dependent critical duration. **A**, Variation of threshold energy (retinal illuminance × duration) with duration of 1-degree foveal test field on different backgrounds. (Data of Roufs.[115]) **B**, Variation of threshold energy with duration for foveal test fields having different diameters in minutes of arc, and for whole-eye stimulation (total). (Data of Roufs and Meulenbrugge.[116]) **C**, Open circles indicate test field energy (luminance × duration) required to match brightness of 10-degree test flashes of different durations to that of standard 10 msec flash. Filled circles indicate background energy required for 50% contrast reading of binary digits (black on white) as function of background duration. (Data of Kahnemann and Norman.[68])

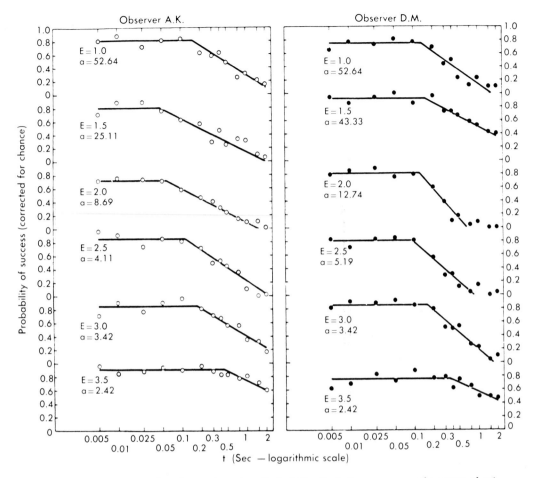

FIG. 18-2 Luminance-duration reciprocity. Probability that observer correctly reported orientation of gap in black Landolt C, as related to duration of its white 8-degree background. For each curve, product (background luminance × duration) was held constant at value E; a is width of gap in minutes of arc for C presented on each background. (Data of Kahneman.[67])

different colors have indicated that short wavelength lights are integrated over longer intervals than are long wavelength lights.[131] This apparent separation of color channels indicates that temporal summative properties are at least partially differentiated at an early stage of visual perception.[82] Measurements of critical durations for threshold changes in luminance or wavelength of monochromatic lights are compared in Table 18-1. Threshold detection of changes in wavelength requires a constant product of wavelength change times duration, up to a critical duration.[108,109] Beyond this period threshold detection of wavelength change depends on the magnitude of wavelength change alone. Of course this rule also applies to increments of luminance. However, critical durations for hue shifts are found to vary according to the spectral region being studied. These periods of temporal summation are markedly longer than for luminance changes, and they are inversely related to wavelength. The critical duration for blue light (short wavelength) is greater than that for red light (long wavelength). The critical duration for detection of wavelength change at the red end of the spectrum at photopic levels of luminance is about 0.1 second, which is similar to that for integration of luminance stimuli in the dark-adapted eye. For lights at the blue end of the spectrum critical durations for wavelength change are up to two and one-half times as long, or .25 second.

TABLE 18-1   Critical Duration for Wavelength Pulses and Luminance Pulses[109]

Retinal illuminance (td)	Wavelength (nm)	Critical duration (milliseconds)	
		for $\Delta\lambda$	for ΔL
0.1	527	—	96
	600	—	90
10.0	600	110	64
	580	160	62
	527	250	68
	480	250	56
110.0	527	94	40

The temporal responsiveness of the visual system is related to the length of the critical duration; the visual system can be expected to respond more rapidly to changes in luminance than to changes in spectral composition and, in general, to respond more rapidly to changes in spectral composition at the red end of the spectrum than at the blue end of the spectrum. This property of the visual system is used to advantage in the experimental method called "heterochromatic flicker photometry" (see Chapter 13). This process employs rapid alternation of two light stimuli that differ in color but that are alternated at a frequency exceeding that of the responsiveness of the visual system to change in wavelength. The test subject varies the luminance of one of the two stimuli to achieve a perception of minimal flicker. This eliminates luminance differences between the two test lights, since the temporal responsiveness of the visual system is adequate to detect luminance change at the frequency chosen. The end point of the method produces two spectrally different lights of equivalent luminance. When stationary (not flickering), these two lights may not subjectively appear to be equal in brightness, although their luminances are identical.

THE BROCA-SULZER EFFECT

When a light is first turned on, it is not seen instantly but requires a certain amount of time to reach threshold. It requires still longer to attain its full subjective brightness, because its excitatory effects undergo temporal summation in the visual system. Since temporal summation is limited by the critical duration, however, brightness levels off to a plateau as the duration of the light stimulus increases. Figure 18-3 shows the time course of subjective brightness following the onset of light stimuli of various strengths. For relatively bright stimuli, a transient peak of brightness occurs before the plateau is reached. This is called the Broca-Sulzer effect.[18] This effect can produce the seeming paradox of a short flash appearing brighter than a longer flash of the same luminance. The luminance of a short flash adjusted to match the apparent brightness of a continuous light reaches a minimum at flash durations of 50 to 100 msec. Further increases of flash duration require higher levels of luminance for matching to the same brightness standard, again rising to a plateau.

A similar experimental technique employs measurement of luminance of a long flash varied to match the apparent brightness of a very short flash of fixed luminance. If plotted as a function of the duration of the short flash, this luminance is seen to peak when the short flashes are 50 to 100 msec long. These experiments show that a duration of 50 to 100 msec is optimal for subjective flash brightness. Since the Broca-Sulzer effect occurs under a broad range of conditions, including both light and dark adaptation in virtually all areas of the retina without regard to the spectral composition of the light,[69] it must be determined by a rather uniform underlying neural mechanism.

At very long durations of flash stimulus, visual efficiency declines. This is another manifestation of Troxler's phenomenon (see Chapter 16). When a small stationary spot of light is projected onto the retina, it will, if held in position, fade away within several seconds. The lower the luminance of the spot, the sooner it will disappear. It has been established that such targets fade away from view long before they have bleached an appreciable fraction of the retinal photopigment[105]; thus Troxler's phenomenon depends mainly on neural rather than photochemical processes.[20] Since the disappearance time is longer with increasing target sizes at a given eccentricity from the fovea, it appears to be related to the receptive field sizes of retinal ganglion cells. (See Chapters 19, 22, and 23 for complete discussions of neural receptive fields and their properties.) If the target is relatively small compared to the size of the receptive fields, it more rapidly fades from view when fixed in position. There is a receptive field gradient of small to large when moving from the central retina to the peripheral retina[64]; smaller stationary targets fade more rapidly from view in the central visual field than do larger targets. As a spatially fixed image disappears, its back-

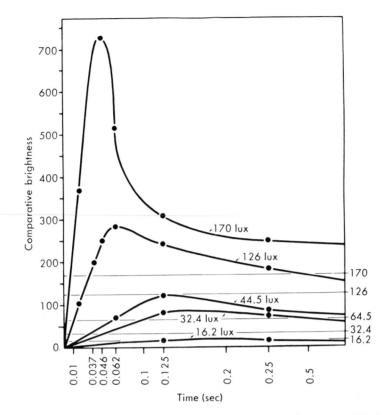

FIG. 18-3 Brightness of flashes having various luminances, as functions of flash duration. (Data of Broca and Sulzer.[18])

ground fills in the area it once occupied. The visual system seems to extrapolate conditions across the image boundary, creating a perceptual continuity. This phenomenon also seems to be related to the fact that the physiologic blind spot and some pathologic defects in the visual field cannot be detected under casual gaze.[49,136]

CONTROL OF FIXATION

Eye movements are organized into a series of specialized patterns that allow the visual system to take maximal advantage of the information contained in images. The principal patterns are those of the fixation maintenance system, the saccadic system, and the smooth pursuit or tracking system (see Chapter 5). The fixation maintenance system serves to sustain an object of interest in a relatively stable position on the foveal receptors of the retina, so that the object can be examined with the retinal area having the higher visual acuity. Fixation must at the same time avoid stabilization of the image on the retina for too long a period, lest the contrast-

ing contours of the image be lost from view.[1,112] (See Troxler's phenomenon, Chapter 16). In fact, the fixation maintenace system has an inherent and regular instability of position that is quite small but constant. A series of residual, small-angle drifts, microsaccades, and tremor movements of the eye are constantly present.[124,133] The drifts are monocular, independent between the two eyes,[28] and they have amplitudes of up to 6 minutes of arc, whereas the microsaccades or "flicks" are binocularly correlated. The flicks tend to be corrective, returning the image detail of interest toward the optimal fixation point at the center of the fovea. The microsaccades have amplitudes of 1 to 20 minutes of arc and take approximately 25 msec. Superimposed upon the slow drifts of the eye are tremors with frequencies of 30 to 80 Hz and amplitudes of 10 to 30 seconds of arc.[35,36] These movements are very small and cannot be detected without suitable optical magnification of the eye.[111] Data extracted by the foveal photoreceptors about the location of contours and other details within a retinal image constitute a constantly changing stream of visual information.

SACCADIC MOVEMENTS

Saccades are rapid, volitionally initiated movements of the eye. As saccades move the eye's line of sight from one visual detail to another, there is little or no subjective impression of blur or illusory movement of the external visual scene.[90,91] This absence of illusory movement during image motion across the retina is associated with an elevated visual threshold during the period of the saccade. It is as if vision were temporarily "turned off" during movement of the eye. This avoids confusion by rapidly changing and essentially unusable information during the saccadic movement. The elevation of visual threshold during saccades can be measured experimentally by using test flashes that are synchronized with movements of the eye[145,146] (Fig. 18-4).

One hypothesis explaining this reduced sensitivity during movements is that displacement of the test area on the retina during the course of the movement causes a "retinal smear," which effectively spreads the test flash over a larger retinal area and at a reduced average lu-minance at any one point. This explanation is inadequate, since bright flashes of extremely brief periods, having no significant smear at all, show the same effect.[134] In addition, the suppression effect actually begins before the movement of the eye.[84,144] This anticipatory phenomenon rules out the possibility that the geometry of the movements or that shifts to less sensitive areas of peripheral retina can explain the reduced sensitivity. It further suggests that saccadic suppression may act to facilitate or initiate the saccadic movement rather than result from it. It has been said that "it is not the proprioceptors of the eye muscles, that cause the visual system to be 'blind' during eye movements, but rather that the 'blind mind' allows the eye to start its movement."[84]

OSCILLOPSIA

Although visual suppression is an integral feature of saccadic movements, it does not occur during movements caused by nonsaccadic mechanisms. If the movement is not initiated volitionally, illusory movement of the environment will be perceived. Motion of an image across the retina, which is not "anticipated" by the brain, will result in the perception of movement. When caused by disease of the vestibular

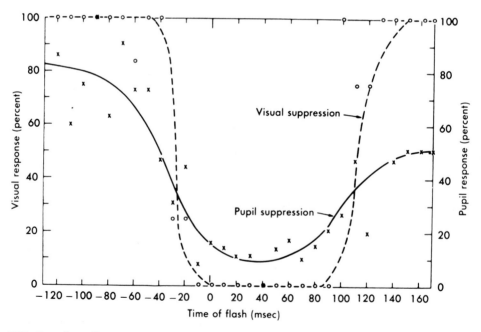

FIG. 18-4 Saccadic suppression. Time course of visual and pupillary responsiveness to test flashes presented before, during, or after 8-degree saccadic eye movements that start at time 0. (Data of Zuber, Stark, and Lorber.[146])

system, the phenomenon of illusory movement of the environment is called "oscillopsia." Vestibular disorders that cause nystagmus are associated with spinning or oscillating movements of the external visual scene, a sensation familiar to all children who have experienced postrotatory vertigo.

Diseases that interfere with vestibulo-ocular reflexes or with the fixation maintenance system often produce symptoms of illusory movement of the environment. Brainstem damage can produce an impairment of such reflexes, resulting in illusory movement of the environment during such tasks as walking on a level surface. During the act of walking, movements of the body are transmitted to the eyes. If uncorrected by the vestibulo-ocular and fixation maintenance systems, these movements result in apparent bobbing up and down of the horizon. This symptom was first emphasized by Dandy, who encountered it in patients he had treated for Ménière's disease with bilateral sectioning of the vestibular nerves.[31] Oscillopsia is sometimes termed "Dandy's symptom."

PURSUIT MOVEMENTS

Although tracking of small objects is in part a voluntary function,[123] such movements are almost unsuppressible when involved in pursuit of very large images in the visual field. At least two different populations of cortical neurons respond to moving objects in the visual field. One group of cells is excited by relative movements of elements within adjacent areas of the retinal image, whereas another is excited by movements of the entire image across the retina.[17] Involuntary tracking seems to compensate for general image movement, maintaining the image position on the retina. Such reflexive tracking of movement of extended objects in the visual field is the basis for several useful clinical tests. The optokinetic drum is a rotating cylinder that may be several inches in diameter or large enough to surround the head of an observer at a viewing distance of several feet. Vertical contrasting stripes cover the surface of the drum. As the stripes of the drum move past the observer, the eyes will exhibit a series of smooth tracking movements, followed by corrective saccadic (jerk) movements. The alternating slow pursuit and rapid saccadic movements are termed "optokinetic nystagmus (OKN)." This sort of test has been useful in estimating visual function in illiterate patients and in infants.[7,86,87,110,120] It also is helpful in establishing the intactness of the afferent visual system in patients who falsely claim or believe they have suffered visual loss. In addition, the OKN test can be used to test the intactness of the subcortical association pathways that link the visual cortex with the cortical areas involved in oculomotor function. Disruption of these pathways is frequently the result of large hemispheric lesions of the brain, such as neoplasms or infarctions. When these association pathways are interrupted, smooth pursuit movements are not accompanied by the normal corrective saccadic movements.[86] This defect is found when deep hemispheric lesions are located ipsilateral to the direction of horizontally moving OKN stimuli.

MASKING

In addition to saccadic suppression there are other masking mechanisms that serve to cancel the perception of current image detail, preparing the retina to receive new information. Four categories of masking have been studied: the masking of light by light, the masking of pattern by light, the masking of pattern by structurally related pattern, and the masking of pattern by structurally unrelated pattern. The first of these phenomena will be discussed.

Masking of light by light

The masking of light by light is similar to saccadic suppression, having nearly the same speed of response. When two spots of light overlap or coincide, an interaction between them can be observed: one alters the visibility or detectability of the other.[29,122] (See also Crawford's experiment, Chapter 16). One of the lights, called the "masking" or "conditioning stimulus," causes a change in the visual threshold for perception of the other light, called the "test stimulus." Similar to masking is the phenomenon of metacontrast, in which the conditioning and test stimuli are presented to adjacent but nonoverlapping locations.[2,4,54,118] The usual procedure for masking experiments is to present the two stimuli repeatedly but with varying intervals of time between them. The luminance of the conditioning stimulus is held constant, while that of the test stimulus is adjusted to measure the threshold of perception.

Figure 18-5 illustrates a typical masking curve. The masking stimulus had a duration of 250 msec and was repeated with a frequency of 1 per second. The masking curve plots the threshold intensity of the test stimulus as a function of the time difference between onset of the masking stimulus and onset of the test stimulus. With onset of the masking stimulus there was a

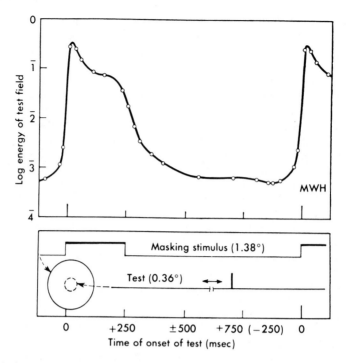

FIG. 18-5 Masking. Time course of threshold variation due to 50 footlambert, 250 msec masking flash, measured with "impulse" test flash. Lower panel shows flash diameters and field configuration. Last seven data points are same as first seven. (Data of Sperling.[122])

2.5 log unit rise in threshold for the test flash. Note that threshold began to rise almost 100 msec before the onset of the masking flash and that the maximum point on the threshold curve was nearly coincident with the onset of the masking stimulus. Threshold then dropped within 150 msec to a plateau. It then began to drop again, just before the time when the masking light was extinguished. Threshold returned to its dark value after a few hundred msec.

The rise in the test flash threshold that occurs before the onset of a masking stimulus has been termed "backward masking." This phenomenon has been attributed to the differing latencies for afferent conduction of high and low luminances of visual stimuli. Response latencies vary reciprocally with the intensity of stimulation. Thus a weak stimulus must precede a strong one to arrive coincidentally at the cerebral cortical areas that mediate conscious visual perception. There is also a lateral inhibitory effect that results in a decrease in the masking effect of a stimulus as it increases in size. The converse, an increase in masking effect with decreasing size of the masking stimulus, is apparently due to a combination of reduced lateral inhibition and to the increasing proximity of the borders of the

masking and test stimuli. While the presence of light per se has a masking effect on the detectability of light, the presence of a pattern (contrasting border of the adapting stimulus) similarly has an additional masking effect for detection of a test light. A possible basis for masking and metacontrast may be interactions between sustained and transiently responding neural elements.[15,16]

PHI MOVEMENT

Stimulus combinations similar to those used for masking and metacontrast experiments can produce the appearance of movement, as if one stimulus had crossed the space between the two and become the other. This kind of apparent motion, called "phi movement," has been studied extensively.[81] If two light stimuli are used to produce the effect, the brighter they are or the longer the interval between them, the more distant they must be from one another to give optimal subjective phi movement.

The fact that smoothly continuous displacement of a retinal image is not required for the sensation of movement has been the foundation of the television and motion picture industries. Successive displacements of stationary details in a frame-by-frame sequence gives rise to a perceptual continuity. This effect is similar to but different from the sense of continuity constructed by the visual system during a series of refixation saccades. Despite the fact that movement in a motion picture image may appear to be smooth and continuous, the temporal discontinuity of the light still can be detected as a flicker, especially in the peripheral visual field. The visual system seems to have the capacity to abstract spatiotemporal discontinuities from purely temporal changes, processing the two forms of information in separate ways.[70]

The masking of a test flash by a conditioning flash is a complex interaction. The degree of masking varies with the time interval between the two flashes, and the masking of one flash by another can be counteracted by a third flash presented shortly thereafter. This effect is called "disinhibition."[113] Similar interactions may be studied with multiple flashes presented sequentially over long intervals. When flashes are separated from one another by about 1 second or more, their subjective brightness and other characteristics appear to be independent of one another, like isolated flashes. If, however, the frequency of recurrence of the flashes is increased, perceptible interactions begin to occur between successive flashes. What appears at low frequency rates as a discrete succession of separate flashes will take on a flickering appearance as the frequency rises. At higher frequencies the flicker becomes too rapid to be seen, and the light appears to be continuous.

CRITICAL FLICKER FREQUENCY AND TALBOT'S LAW

The transition point from a flickering appearance to one of a continuous light is termed the "critical flicker frequency" (CFF). The change-over with increasing frequencies from flicker to fusion is not an abrupt one but takes place over a transitional range. Within this range one frequency may be designated as the boundary between the two modes of appearance. This frequency, customarily the one with a 50% probability of being seen as flickering, is called the CFF. It is a simple measure of the temporal resolving power of the visual system. Above the CFF, brightness conforms to the Talbot plateau law, which holds that subjectively fused intermittent light and objectively steady light of the same color and brightness have exactly the same time-averaged luminance per unit time.[83] The so-called Talbot brightness of a flash train equals that of a steady light created by spreading the luminous energy of each flash uniformly throughout the interval of time from its onset to the onset of the next flash.

Brücke brightness enhancement

A phenomenon related to the Broca-Sulzer effect (the transient peaking of brightness when a light is turned on) is called the Brücke brightness enhancement effect.[107] When a light is flickered on and off, its apparent brightness varies according to the frequency of flicker, reaching a maximum over a narrow range of frequencies at approximately 5 to 20 Hz, depending on the luminance of the flickering light. The apparent brightness of the flickering light can be adjusted to match that of a steadily illuminated standard.[10] As the flicker frequency is increased above the range of brightness enhancement, the apparent luminance of the flickering light drops, gradually approaching a plateau. For a flickering light with a 50% duty cycle, the luminance of each flash will be exactly twice that of the steady standard being used for comparison. This is the time-averaged luminance of the flickering light, as predicted by the Talbot plateau law.

Determinants of CFF

Many variables of the intermittent stimulus interact to determine the value of the CFF. Some of these variables include the luminance of the test field, its spectral composition, retinal position, size, temporal waveform, duty cycle, duration, and the number of stimuli in a multiflash train. The effects of some of these variables on the CFF are discussed next.

The Ferry-Porter law

CFF increases with the luminance of the intermittent stimulus, rising in direct linear proportion to the logarithm of flash luminance. This rise in CFF occurs over a wide range of luminance and is termed the "Ferry-Porter law."[42,106] Figure 18-6 shows data that verify this property for a foveal test field over a range of retinal illuminance of 10,000 to 1.[60] The linearity of this relationship tends to break down at very high luminances.

Spectral composition

Equal energy spectral lights have different luminances (see Chapter 13). Thus, according to the Ferry-Porter law, spectrally different lights of equal energy should have different CFF values. If the energies of the different wavelengths of flashing stimuli are adjusted to match them

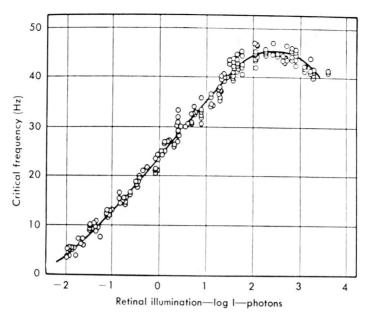

FIG. 18-6   Critical flicker frequency at rod-free fovea as influenced by retinal illuminance (photons = trolands) of test field, showing conformity to the Ferry-Porter law over range of four logarithmic units. (From Hecht S, Verrijp CD: J Gen Physiol 17:251, 1933.)

for brightness under photopic conditions, their respective CFFs should then be identical and should follow the Ferry-Porter logarithmic function as brightness increases. This prediction has been tested,[58] as shown in the data of Figure 18-7. Except for minor variations, the upper (cone) branch of the flicker function was the same for all of the seven different wavelengths of light that had photopically matched luminances. At low levels of retinal illumination (the rod branch) the results were different for differing wavelengths, because photopically equated brightnesses are not equal in the scotopic range. Wavelengths for which rod sensitivity greatly exceeded cone sensitivity (for instance at the blue end of the spectrum) determined CFF over wider ranges of retinal illumination at the lower end of the scale than did wavelengths for which rod and cone sensitivities are more nearly the same (at the red end of the spectrum). This explains the horsetail shape of the graph in Figure 18-7.

Retinal position

Since the CFF function for rods differs from that for cones, the CFF for a test stimulus that is confined to a limited area of the retina will depend on the relative proportion of rods and cones in the stimulated area. Population densities of the two types of photoreceptor vary from one part of the retina to another,[102] and the extent to which each population is activated by light is a function of retinal illuminance. If the test light is confined to the fovea, it will activate only cones, and the CFF function will rise according to the Ferry-Porter law as luminance changes. However, if the same test light is presented to an extrafoveal area of retina, it will stimulate rods at low luminances and cones at higher luminances, giving rise to a bipartite CFF function. (Fig. 18-8).[60]

The lower maximum CFF values found with increasing retinal eccentricity result from the relative decrease in cone populations, leaving predominantly rods to determine the flicker function. Below the retinal illuminance indicated by log I = −1, rods alone determine the flicker function for the 2-degree test field. The range over which the Ferry-Porter law is applicable decreases with a reduction in the number of cones in the tested area and finds its maximum expression in the fovea, which contains a pure cone mosaic.

The Granit-Harper law

CFF also increases linearly with the logarithm of the stimulus area. This relationship, called the "Granit-Harper law," holds true for stimuli

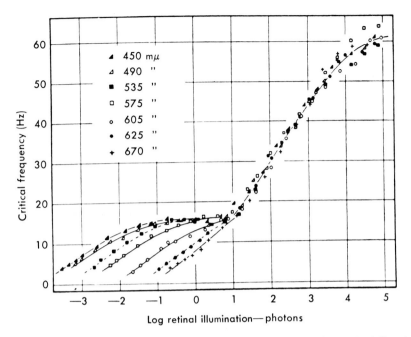

FIG. 18-7   Critical flicker frequency of 19-degree test field as related to retinal illuminance (photons = trolands), for monochromatic lights of different wavelengths having equal photopic brightness. (From Hecht S, Shlaer S: J Gen Physiol 19:965, 1936.)

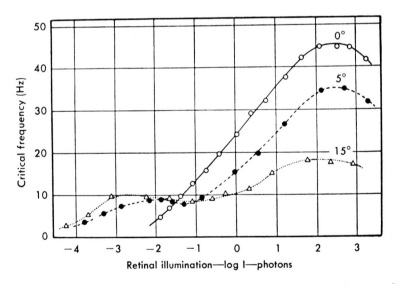

FIG. 18-8   Critical flicker frequency of a 2-degree white test field as related to retinal illuminance (photons = trolands), measured at fovea, 5 degrees above fovea, and 15 degrees above fovea. (From Hecht S, Verrijp CD: J Gen Physiol 17:251, 1933.)

within a 1000 to 1 range of luminances and with retinal eccentricities up to 10 degrees.[52] For foveally centered stimuli it remains true for all sizes up to approximately 50 degrees in diameter.[44,114] CFF, however, depends on the proportion of rods and cones within the stimulated area at photopic luminances. When the stimulus intensity and level of adaptations are such that both rods and cones are being stimulated, the CFF vs. area curve will have two branches, of which only the cone branch conforms to the Granit-Harper law.

As the curves in Figure 18-8 indicate, the CFF for small targets is greatest at the fovea at any level of photopic illuminance. However, larger targets in the periphery may have higher values of CFF than those closer to or surrounding the fovea. This may explain why a television screen seems to flicker less when viewed in the central visual field than it does when seen in the peripheral visual field. Differential retinal sensitivities and spatial summations by rod and cone subsystems, as well as receptive field sizes and densities, may be responsible for this complex interaction of field size and retinal eccentricity. In addition, receptive fields in the peripheral retina are predominantly transient in character, whereas the more densely concentrated receptive fields of the foveal retina are predominantly sustained in their responses.[47]

Background luminance

If the flickering test field is surrounded by darkness, the CFF is found to depend not only on the luminance and other characteristics of the test field but also on stray light scattered within the ocular media or reflected from the illuminated area onto other portions of the retina. An observer may respond to flicker in the scattered halo of stray light even when the test field appears to be steady. To avoid this phenomenon test fields commonly are presented against a lighted background, which can be used to control the adaptation level of the eye, to mask stray light, and also to vary the contrast at the border of the test field. In general, the highest CFF is obtained with a surround that is matched to the Talbot brightness of the test area, a condition that minimizes border contrast.[11]

Adaptation

The level of retinal adaptation determines CFF, largely because it governs the relative sensitivity of rod and cone mechanisms. Increasing levels of light adaptation reduce the size and change the organization of retinal receptive fields in a manner that enhances the mechanisms of inhibitory interaction.[8] In general, the higher the level of light adaptation, the higher will be the CFF for a given stimulus.

Clinical use of CFF

A number of attempts have been made to use measures of the CFF for the diagnosis of disease. Electroretinographic recordings and evoked cortical potentials in response to flickering stimuli have been used to test the integrity of the retinocortical pathway[132] (see Chapter 21). The detection of flicker at various locations within the visual field has been used as a form of clinical perimetry.[65,96] However, this type of perimetry is rather cumbersome and is not known to yield diagnostic information that is not available by more conventional types of perimeteric examination.

FLICKER PERCEPTION AND LINEAR FILTER THEORY

Through the use of theoretic models of the behavior of the visual system in response to flickering stimuli, orderly rules have been devised that predict the value of CFF from properties of the flickering stimuli.[32–34,85,121] If the visual system is viewed as a "black box" (an electrical circuit of unknown components), its properties can be characterized by analyzing the way in which its inputs (visual stimuli) are altered to produce an output (visual sensation). Operations performed on the input "signal" include differentiation, integration, and filtering, among others. This approach to studying the temporal responsiveness of vision was taken by DeLange.[32–34] The temporal fluctuations of a continuous variable (such as a visual stimulus) make up its waveform. It is possible to express any repetitive waveform, such as flicker, as a sum of elementary sinusoidal components (sine waves, cosine waves, or both). One of these components is called the "fundamental" and is equal in frequency to the repetition rate of the original waveform. All other components, called "harmonics," are integral multiples of the fundamental frequency. Any complex waveform that is repetitive can be reduced to a particular mixture of these components. The property of any one sinusoidal component that expresses how much of it is used is its amplitude, which in turn is the maximum extent to which the sinusoid deviates above or below its average value.

Mathematically, all sinusoids have average values of zero. A sum of sinusoids that reconstitutes a complex waveform will also have an average value of zero, unless a steady nonzero component called the "DC component" is included in the mixture. The DC component expresses the average value by which the integral of a complex waveform differs from zero. This provision is particularly necessary for the theoretic treatment of light, which cannot have negative values. In linear filter theory the DC component is analogous to the Talbot brightness (the average level of luminance of a time-varying light stimulus). The general method by which a repetitive waveform is reduced to its sinusoidal and DC components is called "Fourier analysis," and the components thus obtained are often called "Fourier components."[129]

The process by which Fourier components are added together to produce a complex waveform is called "summation." Summation is a linear process, and signal processing systems that sum their inputs to produce an output are said to be linear. When the input to such a linear system is a sinusoid, the output will be a sinusoid of the same frequency. When the input is a complex waveform equivalent to a weighted sum of sinusoids of differing frequencies, the output will also be a sum of sinusoids having those same frequencies.

Two properties of a signal processing system may cause variations in content of its output: (1) system gain (ratio of output amplitude to input amplitude) may not be the same for sinusoids of all frequencies; and (2) the system may introduce a varying degree of time lag or "phase shift" between the input and output components, depending on their frequencies. A linear system with frequency-dependent gain and phase shift is called a "linear filter" and can be described completely by plots of its gain and phase shift, measured as a function of the frequencies of its sinusoidal inputs. A plot of gain vs. frequency defines what is called the "attenuation characteristic" of a linear filter. DeLange's approach to the visual system was to attempt to determine the attentuation characteristic of the visual system as if it were a linear filter. He used a range of frequencies of sinusoidally changing light stimuli, while measuring the "output" of vision: the subjective perception of flicker. Unlike observations that can be made on electrical circuits, he was studying a physiologic sensory system. The output "signal" was not physically accessible but only detectable in the psychophysical behavior of human observers.

A nonlinear signal processing system is one that, when given a sinusoidal input, will produce either a nonsinusoidal output or a sinusoid of a different frequency. However, such a system may act sufficiently linearly with low amplitude inputs to allow its analysis to proceed as if it were actually linear. DeLange made the essential assumption that small signal linearity would hold for the visual system. He argued that the visual system is not truly linear but that it is possible to treat it as a combination of linear and nonlinear parts. For example, the validity of Talbot's law establishes that for stimuli near the CFF, the system behaves linearly for the perception of brightness. This is true because the subjective brightness of a flickering stimulus at the CFF matches the brightness of a continuous light source, the luminance of which has been set to the time-averaged value of the flickering light. If the signal delivered to the visual system's brightness evaluator were proportional to some nonlinear transformation of the input, for example its logarithm, a steady light would produce a brightness that would be different from that of the fluctuating light with equal time-averaged luminance.

Since Talbot's law can be experimentally verified, DeLange accepted the assumption that temporal averaging of light stimuli took place before brightness was evaluated by the visual system and before any nonlinear transformation took place. Thus linearity was assumed for the visual system when the inputs were small (close to threshold). For this reason DeLange decided to measure the amplitudes of sinusoidally varying light stimuli, necessary to reach flicker threshold at different frequencies. This allowed determination of the frequency-dependent attenuation characteristics of the visual system as if it were a linear filter.

Results of this kind of experiment, done at several different levels of luminance, are shown in Figure 18-9.[71] Sensitivity and threshold values are reciprocally related. The attentuation characteristics have been plotted with threshold values increasing downward and sensitivity values increasing upward along the logarithmic ordinate. The ordinate values are expressed as a "threshold modulation ratio." This ratio is the extent to which the sinusoidally modulated light deviates from its average or DC luminance level. Although the amplitude of sinusoidally modulated light cannot be larger than its DC value (negative values of luminance are physically impossible), it is possible for the amplitude to take on any smaller value, which in turn may be calculated as a fraction of the DC level. This fraction, the "modulation ratio," is defined as 100

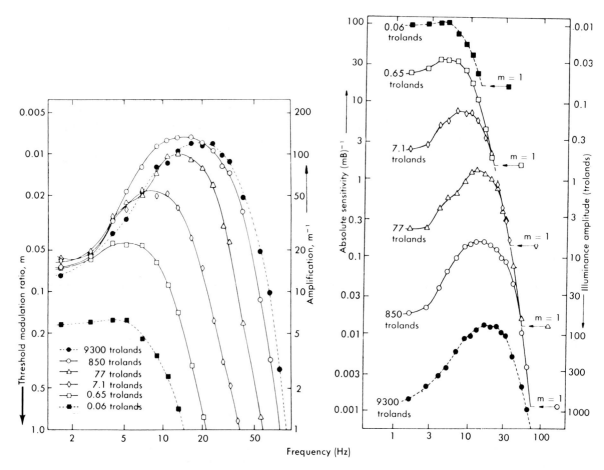

FIG. 18-9 Flicker sensitivity. Visual attenuation characteristics measured with sinusoidal variation about different average values of retinal illuminance. Left panel shows modulation ratios, m, increasing downward, that correspond to just detectable flicker at each of frequencies tested. Right panel shows absolute amplitudes, increasing downward, of retinal illuminance variation required for just noticeable flicker at various frequencies. Absolute sensitivity, increasing upward, is reciprocal of threshold absolute amplitude at each frequency. (Data of Kelly.[71])

times the ratio of the amplitude of the sinusoidal change to the DC level. Since both parts of this fraction are in the same units, the modulation ratio is itself a dimensionless number. It is a means of expressing amplitude as a percentage deviation of the fluctuating stimulus from its average value.

In the left half of Figure 18-9, the threshold modulation ratio is shown as a function of flicker frequency. Each curve was obtained by adjusting the amplitude of the sinusoidally modulated light to attain threshold at various frequencies, while the average retinal luminance was being held constant. Since the average luminance controls the level of adaptation, each of the curves represents the visual atten-

tuation characteristics for a single level of adaptation, and each expresses the flicker fusion boundary for that condition. Depending on the level of adaptation, any combination of stimulus frequency and modulation amplitude below a given curve is seen as flickering, whereas any combination lying above the curve is seen as a steady light. Notice that increasing the level of adaptation enlarges the areas seen as flicker, a finding consistent with the higher values of CFF at higher luminances predicted by the Ferry-Porter law. These attenuation characteristics, however, far transcend the Ferry-Porter law in generality. Note that the curves in the left half of Figure 18-9 are widely separated at high frequencies, but they come together at low frequencies. This indicates that low-frequency flicker reaches its threshold at a nearly constant value of modulation ratio for all levels of adaptation in the photopic range, whereas higher frequency flicker perception shows threshold values that change both with frequency and with the level of adaptation.

DeLange found that these response properties were the same for waveforms that were not sinusoids, as long as their fundamental frequencies were the same. One curve expressed the response for all wave shapes for a given level of adaptation, and only the fundamental frequency of the waveform was of importance for flicker detection. The highest frequency components of a stimulus waveform seem to be erased or ignored by the visual system. A square waveform gave the same result as a sinusoid. At high levels of luminance the sensitivity for flicker detection peaked at a frequency of approximately 15 to 20 Hz. This is the Brücke brightness enhancement effect, sometimes called resonance.[33] It is as if the visual system were "tuned" to this frequency at high luminances. At lower luminances the modulation ratio curves decline smoothly and do not show this tuning phenomenon.

The right half of Figure 18-9 shows that the modulation ratio may not be the most appropriate measure for expressing attenuation characteristics. These curves were plotted on an absolute, rather than a relative, scale. At the higher frequencies of sinusoidal flicker, the absolute sensitivity for flicker detection drops. Flicker at each frequency in this high range has a unique threshold amplitude, as shown on the right-hand side of the series of curves. The continuity of the frequency-amplitude relation throughout this range (referred to by Kelly as a master curve[73]) reveals that flicker sensitivity is independent of the level of adaptation, and it is determined solely by the absolute amplitude of luminance modulation above and below the DC level. This is a necessary characteristic for a system that is truly linear.

In the low-frequency range, however, any of several input amplitudes may be just detectable as flicker for a given frequency. This means that system gain changes with adaptation level at low frequencies, a condition that is not consistent with linearity. Kelly has proposed a theoretic model that fits the experimental data and that assumes operation by two different stages.[74] The first stage, which accounts for the linear high frequency behavior of flicker thresholds, is thought to involve neural processes at or near the receptor level. The second stage, accounting for the nonlinear low frequency behavior, is possibly the result of lateral inhibition in the neural network of the retina.

FLICKER SENSITIVITY IN RELATION TO STIMULUS COLOR AND SIZE

The attenuation characteristics of the visual system vary systematically with the color of the flickering stimulus.[33,34,53,72] For example, a flickering blue light requires a much higher modulation or lower frequency to be detected as flickering, whereas green or red lights have CFF values that are much higher. Low-frequency behavior, being affected by lateral inhibition, is also highly dependent on the field size of the flickering stimulus. The curves shown in the right half of Figure 18-9 were all obtained with a white 68-degree test field that was uniformly illuminated throughout the central area of 50 degrees. Beyond this limit luminance dropped smoothly to zero at the margin of the field. In the frequency range below 10-20 Hz the threshold values for flicker lie below DeLange's, which were obtained with a small, white 2-degree test field at the center of a 60-degree adapting surround.

A comparison of DeLange's high-frqeuency data with Kelly's (for similar levels of adaptation) confirms the expectation from the Granit-Harper law that increased field sizes should raise the CFF for otherwise equivalent test fields. Whereas increasing field sizes result in increasing flicker sensitivity for a given frequency, the opposite effect is demonstrated at lower frequencies. This in part is why Kelly assumed that lateral inhibitory interactions at the retinal level serve to reduce flicker sensitivity at lower frequencies for increasing stimulus sizes.[74]

ELECTROPHYSIOLOGY OF TEMPORAL RESPONSIVENESS

The temporal and spatial sensitivities of the visual system are precisely organized by excitatory and inhibitory interactions among neural elements of the afferent visual system. Although the earliest electrophysiologic studies of these cells were chiefly concerned with the spatial organization of receptive fields, subsequent studies also have revealed some of the mechanisms that characterize their temporal properties. Many of these physiologic properties can be linked to the behavioral measures of temporal responsiveness demonstrated in psychophysical experiments. The bulk of experimental work on the neural circuitry of the vertebrate visual system has been done in amphibians and small mammals such as the cat,* although much information also has been obtained from nonhuman primates.[39]

PHOTORECEPTORS

Variations of temporal responsiveness have particular significance in the organization of the afferent pathways that originate in rod and cone photoreceptors. Aside from the differences in rates of dark adaptation between rods and cones (see Chapter 16), rod responses have a greater average latency and duration than those of cones. The latency of ganglion cell responses to rod activity is uniformly greater than that for cone-initiated events.[50] Since there is convergence of both rod and cone signals on the same ganglion cells in the retina, neural signals in optic nerve fibers can contain information originating in either type of photoreceptor. At photopic levels of retinal adaptation only cone-initiated signals are transmitted in the optic nerve. This appears to be more the result of the differing temporal responses of the rod and cone systems than only saturation of the rod system by high light levels. Cone-initiated responses, by virtue of their greater rapidity, appear to preempt the attention of the ganglion cell, rendering it refractory to the more sluggishly initiated signals arising from rods. Thus the functional independence of rod and cone systems is, at least in part, due to differences of timing within the neural circuitry of the retina. This is a general property of the afferent visual system. As reviewed by Hess,[61] individual neurons within the retino-geniculo-cortical pathways have the properties of neural filters along the dimensions of size, time, orientation, and contrast. These filtering properties are spread across the entire retinotopic map of the visual field, and can be found in the individual elements of the neural circuitry from the retina through and beyond the primary visual cortex.

Photoreceptor potentials in vertebrate retinas were first studied by extracellular techniques. The use of small extracellular electrodes to record mass electrical responses from localized regions of the retina (a local electroretinogram or ERG) has allowed study of receptor potentials arising from cells within a restricted area of the retina.[143] Rod and cone receptor potentials of the cynomolgus monkey (Fig. 18-10) demonstrate that their responses differ markedly in timing.

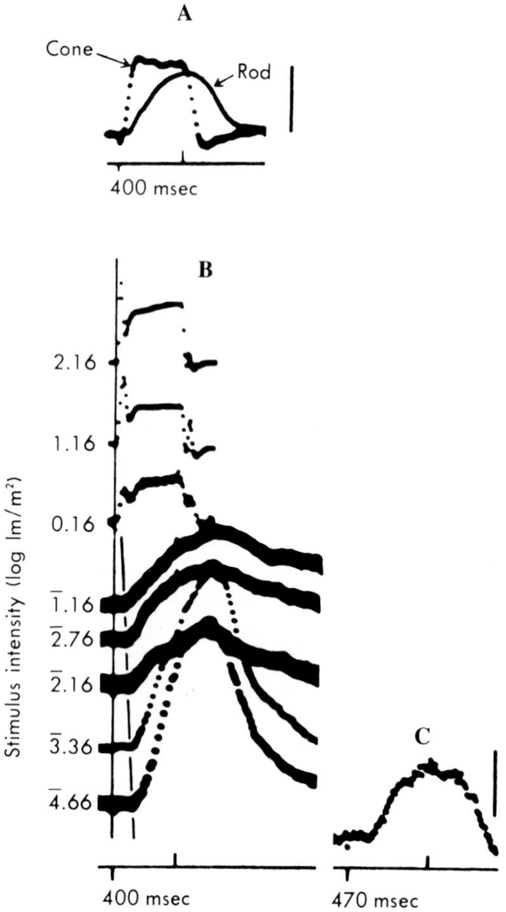

*References 37, 38, 40, 79, 119, 125, 140

FIG. 18-10   Cone and rod late receptor potentials compared. **A,** Potentials elicited by stimuli equalized for number of quanta per unit retinal area, wavelength 560 nm (cone) and 508 nm (rod). **B,** Relative latencies of cone late receptor potentials (top three records) and rod late receptor potentials (lower five records) as functions of stimulus intensity. Latency of rod late receptor potential decreases approximately linearly with increase of log stimulus intensity. **C,** Pure rod late receptor potential, peripheral retina, low stimulus intensity. (Data of Whitten and Brown.[142])

Scotopic rod receptor potentials have a greater latency and duration than those of cone potentials and cannot be made to resemble the latter by any variation of stimulus intensity. Under mesopic conditions of adaptation the two types of receptor potential can be reliably distinguished from one another by their decay rates, the rod receptor potential being more prolonged. At photopic levels of adaptation the rod component disappears entirely, suggesting that its response is completely lost rather than simply saturated, as cones, in turn, become increasingly more active.[142]

While rod and cone activities vary markedly with differing levels of light adaptation, the neural circuitry through which their signals are processed makes maximal use of the available information about contrast and temporal variation in image components. Thus rod-and-cone-mediated vision can show remarkably similar performance for tasks of spatial and temporal discrimination, if the levels of light adaptation are properly defined and performance is measured relative to the differing threshold for the two systems.[62]

Microelectrode techniques have allowed intracellular recordings to be obtained from photoreceptors in the cat.[101] After electrophysiologic characterization of the cell's responses, it can be stained by iontophoretic application of a dye so that the cell's morphology may be studied after histologic sectioning of the retina. Intracellular recordings from cones of the cat (Fig. 18-11) show slow hyperpolarizations. At low levels of intensity these consist of two components. One, due to the cone signal alone, increases in amplitude with increasing light intensity. The other, due to rod intrusion, becomes progressively more prolonged with brighter stimuli. The peak amplitude of response as a function of stimulus intensity is plotted for two different wavelengths of stimuli. The response curve for the 441 nm (blue) stimulus has a biphasic shape,

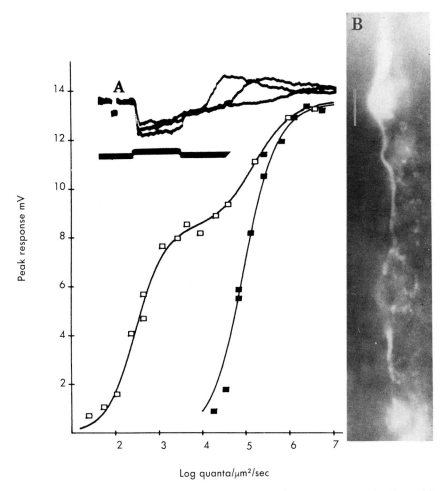

FIG. 18-11   **A,** Microelectrode recordings of responses of cat cone to varying intensities of light stimuli.—□—, 441 nm stimuli; —■—, 647 nm stimuli. Three tracings at top left superimposed for three intensities of stimulus: 4.0, 4.6, and 5.2 log quanta/μm²/sec. Calibration pulse 4.1 mV; flash length 540 msec. **B,** Procion-stained cone that produced the electrical responses recorded at left. Calibration bar 10 μm. (From Nelson R, et al.[101])

the result of mixing of rod and cone signals. The slow hyperpolarization in the intracellular response is known to have the spectral characteristics of rods. The response curve on the right, for the 647 nm (red) light, has a single S-shaped curve in the higher intensity ranges, and it is a pure cone response. The fact that cones in the cat retina show physiologic response properties like those of rods has been accounted for by the demonstration of direct synaptic connections between rod spherules and cone pedicles[76] (see Chapter 19).

BIPOLAR CELLS AND HORIZONTAL CELLS

The temporal differences of response timing found for rods and cones are partially preserved in subsequent neural elements of the retina, including horizontal cells and bipolar cells. Like photoreceptors, these cells respond with slow electrical potentials, although these may be either hyperpolarizations or depolarizations. In addition, the responses of bipolar cells show some degree of spatial organization, as reflected in their receptive field properties. The receptive field of a visual neuron is the locus of all points within the visual field at which light stimuli are effective in eliciting a response from the cell. A response may be a change in potential or firing rate (see Chapter 19). Bipolar cells receiving cone input can be divided into those with on-center and off-center receptive field properties

(responding to the onset or offset of a light respectively). This functional organization of bipolar cells has been found in all vertebrate retinas that have been studied with intracellular recordings.[93,97,141]

In many species bipolar cell receptive fields also have a concentric organization: a surrounding area of response that is opposite in polarity from that of the center. The basis for this response pattern is thought to be provided by the circuitry of the horizontal cells, which have broad dendritic distributions and large receptive fields receiving input from many photoreceptors. They in turn synapse directly with bipolar cells.

The horizontal cells of the cat retina are of two morphologic types (Fig. 18-12). The A type horizontal cell is a large stellate neuron having no axon. The B type horizontal cells (Bhc) is smaller, and it has more numerous dendrites and a very long axon extending some 300 μm from its cell body to end in a large axon terminal (Bat).[13,43,48,75,100] The axon terminal has numerous branches extending over a broad area of the outer plexiform layer. The axon terminal of the B type horizontal cells is thought to be electrically independent from the cell's dendritic system and appears to function in an isolated fashion.[101] One B type axon terminal with its many branches receives and integrates input from as many as 3000 rods.[138] The dendritic trees of both

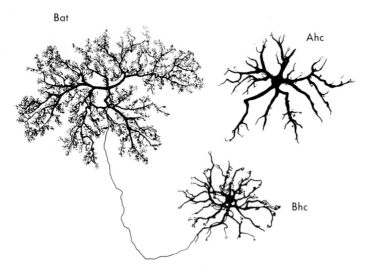

FIG. 18-12 Drawings of Golgi-stained horizontal cells of the cat retina. Ahc, A type of horizontal cell (note absence of axon). Bhc, B type horizontal cell. Note long axon of B type cell separating dendritic plexus at one end of cell (Bhc) from extensive ramifications of axon terminal at other end (Bat). Dendrites of both A and B type cells contact only cones, whereas axon terminal of B type cell contacts only rods. (From Nelson R, et al.[101])

the A and B type horizontal cell bodies possess numerous clusters of small terminals that contact cone pedicles, ending as the lateral elements of synaptic triads at ribbon synapses.[75] (See Chapter 19 for a description of photoreceptor synapses.) By contrast, the axon terminal of the B type horizontal cell has terminals that contact only rod spherules, similarly occupying the lateral positions of synaptic triads at photoreceptor ribbon synapses.

Intracellular recordings from the various elements of the horizontal cell system of the cat retina have been followed by iontophoresis of fluorescent dyes to allow anatomic identification after physiologic characterization of these cells.[101] Recordings obtained from horizontal cells of the cat are shown in Figure 18-13. Responses of the somas of both A and B type cells are shown, as well as the responses of an axon terminal of a B type horizontal cell.

All three cells responded to light stimuli with slow hyperpolarization. The differences in their waveforms were due to the relative contributions of rod and cone input to their responses. Responses were recorded to rod-saturating 400 nm (blue) light stimuli of increasing intensity. The highest intensity stimuli were followed by the largest (downward) peak deflections and the longer slow potentials. The dendritic systems (somas) of the A and B type horizontal cells had

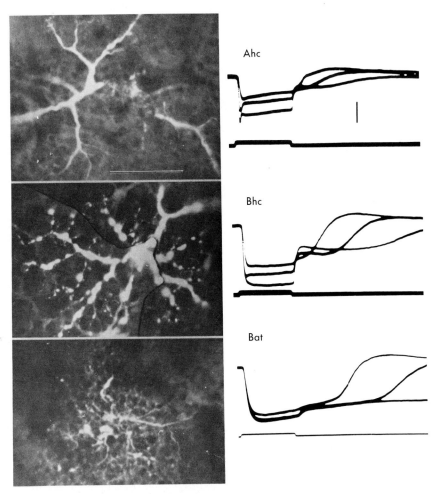

FIG. 18-13   Intracellular recordings of horizontal cell responses to rod-saturating 400 nm blue light stimuli *(right)*, and Procion-stained preparations of same cells *(left.)* Calibration bar in micrograph 50 μm. Three responses to increasing photopic stimulus intensities superimposed for each group of recordings. Greatest peak deflections and longest-lasting slow potentials ("rod aftereffects") correspond to highest intensities of stimuli. Stimulus duration 520 msec, calibration deflection 10 mV. (From Nelson, R, et al.[101])

conelike responses that were brisk and increased in amplitude with increasing stimulus intensities in the photoptic range of luminance. By contrast, the axon terminal response of the B type cell was less brisk and was essentially satured at all stimuli, characteristics of a pure rod response. Note that the rodlike response had a somewhat greater latency of peak effect and much longer duration of activity than did the conelike response. The responses recorded from the cell bodies of both A and B type horizontal cells showed a mixture of rod and cone activity. This is to be expected, since we know that scotopic and mesopic stimuli will elicit a significant rod component in recordings of cone responses in the dark-adapted cat retina (Fig. 18-11).

BIPOLAR PATHWAYS TO GANGLION CELLS

In the cat retina there is an anatomic and a functional separation of rod and cone pathways through bipolar cells to ganglion cells. The rod pathway is at least a four-neuron chain from photoreceptor to ganglion cell. Rods form direct synapses with rod bipolar cells. The receptive field sizes of rod bipolars are far greater than their dendritic field sizes. The axon terminals of the B type horizontal cells probably account for this large area of spatial integration for rod signals. Rod bipolars, which respond with slow potentials, are found in both on- and off-center varieties.[12] These bipolar cells then synapse with amacrine cells located in the inner plexiform layer. In the cat retina the general rule appears to be that rod bipolars uniformly contact amacrine cells, which, in turn, synapse with ganglion cells.[77,78]

The cone pathway to ganglion cells has a smaller number of synaptic elements. Cones, which also receive inputs directly from adjacent rods, form synaptic connections with the cell bodies of both A and B type horizontal cells (although not with the axon terminal of the B type). Cones also form direct synaptic connections with cone bipolar cells. In addition, cone bipolars, similar to their rod counterparts, have receptive fields organized into on- and off-center varieties. Cone bipolars in the cat retina are known to form direct synaptic connections with both on and off types of ganglion cells. A major difference between rod and cone pathways to the ganglion cell is illustrated by the shortest series of synaptic connections for rods: photoreceptor to bipolar to amacrine to ganglion cell, whereas the shortest afferent chain for cone input is cone to bipolar cell to ganglion cell.

GANGLION CELL RESPONSES

Ganglion cells have been classified both anatomically and functionally. One anatomic classification is based on ganglion cell body size and dendritic morphology.[14] The alpha cell is a large-bodied ganglion cell with a broadly ramifying dendritic tree and a large axon. Similarly, the beta cell has a relatively large cell body, but it has a more restricted and bushy dendritic arborization.[80] Gamma cells are those with small cell bodies and small axons. This anatomic classification has been found to correlate well with the three basic physiologic classes, X, Y, and W.[24,25,41,128] (See the following discussion and Chapters 19 and 23.)

Intracellular recordings followed by dye injections of cat ganglion cells have shown a strict correlation between the strata of dendritic branching of ganglion cells and their receptive field response characteristics. Ganglion cells of all morphologic types with off-center responses have dendritic trees that arborize in the outer one third of the inner plexiform layer (called "sublamina a"). Ganglion cells with on-center responses, no matter what their cell body sizes, have dendritic trees that branch in the inner two-thirds of the inner plexiform layer (called "sublamina b"), closer to the ganglion cell bodies.[99]

Figure 18-14 illustrates some of the morphologic and functional characteristics of alpha, beta, and gamma cells. The drawings of Procion-stained ganglion cells include three gamma cells (in the top portion of the figure), one alpha cell in the bottom left of the figure, and one beta cell in the bottom right. Both of the cells (alpha and beta) drawn at the bottom of the figure had on-center responses and dendritic trees that arborized in strata confined to sublamina b. The three gamma cells at the top of the figure had off-center responses and dendritic trees arborizing in strata confined to sublamina a. Both alpha and beta ganglion cells in the cat retina receive the majority of their synaptic input from cone bipolar cells. Those cells with the smallest dendritic field sizes are clustered most densely in the area centralis (the functional equivalent of the primate fovea). With increasing degrees of eccentricity from the area centralis, ganglion cell dendritic trees and receptive field sizes increase, whereas the density of ganglion cell bodies decrease.[137,139]

Every point on the cat retina appears to be covered by at least one off-center and one on-center cell of each of the alpha and beta types. Each of these two types of ganglion cell (alpha

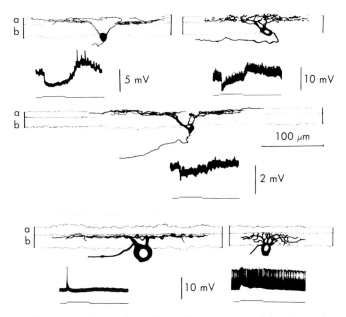

FIG. 18-14   Intracellular recordings of ganglion cell responses and drawings of same cells after staining with Procion. Cells with dendritic strata confined to sublamina a of inner plexiform layer *(top three cells)* all had off-center responses to light flashes. These three cells had small cell bodies and small axons (gamma cells). Lower two ganglion cells had dendritic strata confined to sublamina b of inner plexiform layer and had on-center responses. Cell at bottom left was of alpha morphologic type and had brisk, phasic (transient) response. Cell at bottom right was of beta morphologic type and had brisk response with both phasic (transient) and tonic (sustained) components. (From Nelson, R, et al.[99])

and beta) appears to be arranged in a regular mosaic pattern that spreads across the entire retina.

It is estimated that between 50% and 60% of all ganglion cells in the cat retina are other than alpha or beta types.[46] There are at least 21 different morphologic types of ganglion cells in addition to the alpha and beta varieties.[77] Examples of the gamma cell variety are shown in Figure 18-14 (the top three cells). Some gamma cells have been found to be driven solely by rod input. This subtype of gamma cell appears to branch exclusively in sublamina a of the inner plexiform layer; it has an off-center response, and it is thought to have receptive field input primarily through the amacrine cells of the rod system.[99]

There are numerous functional classifications of ganglion cells in vertebrate retina.[21,41,45,51,117] A widely used nomenclature[41] classifies cells, according to their physiologic responses, as X or Y. X cells, which exhibit linear spatial summation, are usually sustained or tonic in their responses. Y cells, which have nonlinear spatial summation, are usually transient or phasic in their re-

sponses. Generally, both X and Y cell types respond briskly, although the latency of the X (sustained) type is significantly shorter than that of the Y (transient) type.[23] W cells[117] have large receptive fields; they respond sluggishly, and they have slow axon conduction velocities. Distinctions between transient and sustained response types[26,66] and brisk and sluggish response types[24,25] also have been studied. Whereas transient cells always show phasic responses, sustained response patterns can have both transient and sustained components.[66]

A number of studies have linked the physiologic classes with the morphologic characteristics of ganglion cells in the cat retina. The best correlation is that between the alpha morphologic class and the Y physiologic class. These are large-bodied ganglion cells with large axons and very broad dendritic trees. They respond briskly and transiently. Such a cell is illustrated in the bottom left of Figure 18-14. Beta cells correlate with the X type of physiologic response. These ganglion cells also have large cell bodies, but they differ in having smaller axons and compact, bushy dendritic trees. They respond briskly with sustained or tonic rates of spike generation. Such a cell is illustrated in the bottom right of Figure 18-14. Notice that the response of this cell (its rate of spike generation) showed both transient and sustained components. The three cells illustrated in the top half of the figure are from the gamma morphologic class. Gamma cells frequently have physiologic responses matching those of the W cell. They have small cell bodies and small axons, more sluggish responses to light, and slow axon conduction velocities. The three cells at the top of the figure had dendrites branching in sublamina a of the inner plexiform layer, as well as off-center receptive fields. The cell at the top left showed a slow, sustained hyperpolarization to light and a discharge of spikes occurring after the offset of the light stimulus. The sluggish and transient response of this cell was similar to that reported for rod-dominated gamma cells.[99]

The functional contribution to vision by differing classes of ganglion cell has been studied in the *Macaque* with selective destruction of beta ganglion cells by exposure to the neurotoxicant acrylamide monomer.[95] This poison evidently spares other neurons within the visual system. Behavioral testing of these monkeys found normal sensitivity for stimuli of high temporal and low spatial frequencies, but large reductions of contrast sensitivity at low temporal and high spatial frequencies. This evidence suggests that slower conducting beta cells carry information weighted toward high visual (spatial) acuity, but do not carry information about rapid temporal changes in visual stimuli. The larger, more rapidly conducting ganglion cells, on the other hand, are primarily tuned to the transmission of rapidly changing visual information and are sensitive only to the lower spatial frequencies, *i.e.* are of poor spatial acuity.

The relative contribution of rod and cone input to ganglion cells has been estimated by measuring sensitivities at various wavelengths. Rod-dominated ganglion cells are very sensitive in the dark-adapted state to low energies of blue light, but they require up to 3 log units greater flux of red light to respond under similar conditions. Ganglion cells that receive a strong input from cones as well as rods tend to have brisk responses, whether they are phasic (transient) or tonic (sustained).

There are a greater number of synaptic connections in the rod pathway to ganglion cells than there are for the cone pathway, and there is physiologic evidence to show that the latency of responses of cone input to ganglion cells is very much shorter than that of rod input. This is illustrated by the responses of the cells in Figure 18-14. The two cells at the bottom are an alpha and a beta cell with on-center responses (of the sort found to have Y and X physiologic properties, respectively). The latency of peak response of these cells after the onset of the light stimulus was less than 100 msec. The cell at the top left, however, being of the gamma morphologic class (the cell type often found to be of the W physiologic type), had a latency of peak off-response that occurred several hundred msec after the offset of the light stimulus. Thus we know that both transient and sustained types of ganglion cells, receiving inputs from both rods and cones, have brisk responses, large cell bodies, and large axons.

When both rods and cones are active, cone signals tend to dominate in the transient component and rod signals in the sustained component of the ganglion cell response. Those cells that are believed to have predominately or exclusively rod input have small cell bodies, sluggish responses, and small axons. It is apparent that throughout the neural circuitry of the retina there is a marked difference in the temporal responsiveness to rod and cone input.

THE RESPONSIVENESS OF RETINAL NEURONS TO FLICKER

As the frequency of a flickering light increases, flicker sensitivity rises to a peak whose height and center frequency increase with adaptation level (see Fig. 18-9). This peak is located in the range of frequencies between 5 and 20 Hz. This phenomenon is the Brücke brightness enhancement effect, which has approximately the same frequency response as the Broca-Sulzer effect for single flashes (see Fig. 18-3). When wavelength rather than luminance is the modulated variable, this peak response no longer is demonstrable.[109] This finding is consistent with other evidence for a functional separation of color and luminance channels between retina and cortex.

There is evidence that the Brücke brightness enhancement effect is at least in part retinal in origin. Figure 18-15 shows data obtained by recording from single ganglion cells of a cat's retina, whose receptive fields were being stimulated by small spots of sinusoidally modulated light.[22] In *A*, the maximum spike response frequency of the ganglion cell discharge is plotted (on a relative scale) as a function of stimulating frequency with a constant modulation ratio of 50%. A peak response occurred near 10 Hz for both on-center and off-center ganglion cells. *B* shows that the mean number of impulses per second recorded from the same two ganglion

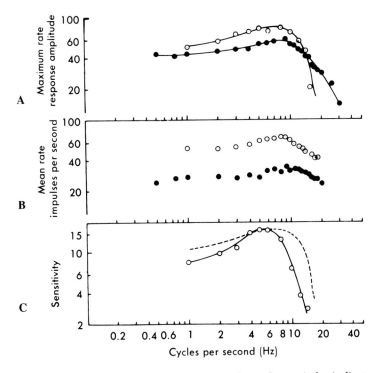

FIG. 18-15 Flicker response of retinal ganglion cells of cat. Open circles indicate on-center cell; filled circles indicate off-center cell. **A,** Maximum rate of cell discharge for different frequencies of sinusoidally modulated light having constant modulation ratio of 0.5. **B,** Mean rate of cell discharge (conditions same as in **A**). **C,** Sensitivity function (attenuation characteristic). Sensitivity is reciprocal of modulation ratio, m, needed to produce just noticeable fluctuation of ganglion-cell discharge rate at each frequency of sinusoidal stimulation tested. Dashed line is maximum-response function of on-center cell in **A**. (Data of Cleland and Enroth-Cugell.[22])

cells also reached a maximum when stimulus frequency was about 10 Hz, although the discharge of the on-center cell was more rapid than that of the off-center cell. *C* shows the attenuation characteristics recorded for the on-center cell of *A* and *B*, with a peak of about 6 Hz. Thus it seems that the frequency responses of cat retinal ganglion cells mimic some features of human flicker sensitivity.

FAST AND SLOW OPTIC NERVE AND OPTIC TRACT FIBERS

Corresponding to the two brisk classes of retinal ganglion cells (X and Y) are two populations of optic nerve fibers distinguished by their conduction velocities—fast for transient cells and slower for sustained cells.[21,45] (Fig. 18-16.) These axon groups couple transient retinal ganglion cells to transiently firing cells in the lateral geniculate nucleus, and sustained retinal cells to sustained geniculate cells.[21]

Conduction velocity differences among monkey geniculostriate neurons appear to be important for color coding.[94] Signal transmission times for successive stages of the retinocortical pathway are related to conduction velocities and path lengths, as summarized in Table 18-2.[66] When both rods and cones are active, the cone signals tend to dominate in the transient component and the rod signals in the sustained component of ganglion cell responses.[56] The responses of sustained cells have shorter latencies than those of transient cells, but they take longer to reach the visual cortex. Thus the cortical arrival times for the two types of signals differ by less than their retinal latencies.

The generalization in which afferent neurons of the retino-geniculo-cortical pathways are distinguished by their conduction velocities has been carried over by visual psychophysicists into a dichotomy based on the sizes of cells in the lateral geniculate body.[88,89] The larger cells in the two ventral layers comprise the magnocellular groups, while the smaller cells of the four dorsal layers are the parvocellular group. This distinction has been abbreviated as the "M-cell"

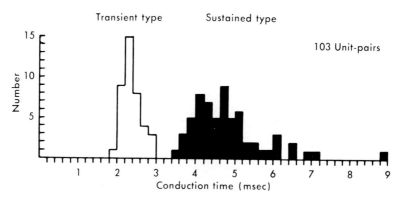

FIG. 18-16   Frequency histogram of retinogeniculate conduction times. Note that all transient retinal ganglion cells (white bars) fell into group with short conduction times: all sustained cells (black bars) made up group with longer conduction times. (Data of Cleland, Dubin, and Levick.[21])

TABLE 18-2   Calculation of Retinogeniculate and Retinocortical Conduction Times

	Transient	Sustained
Latency of ganglion cell response to photic stimulation (present results, standard spot)	38 to 56 msec	19 to 24 msec
Intraretinal axon lengths for these cells (present results)	5.6 to 8.0 mm	3.5 to 4.0 mm
Intraretinal conduction velocity[127]	3.5 to 4.9 meters/sec	1.5 to 1.8 meters/sec
Estimated intraretinal conduction time for these cells (present results)	1.1 to 2.3 msec	1.7 to 2.6 msec
Extraretinal axon lengths for these cells (present results)	34.0 to 35.5 mm	33.0 to 34.5 mm
Extraretinal conduction velocity[127]	29 to 39 meters/sec	9 to 14 meters/sec
Estimated extraretinal conduction time for these cells (present results)	0.9 to 1.2 msec	2.3 to 3.8 msec
Total estimated retinogeniculate conduction time (present results)	2.0 to 3.5 msec	4.0 to 6.4 msec
Measured retinogeniculate conduction time[21]	1.8 to 3.0 msec	3.4 to 8.6 msec
Impulse initiation in LGN[63]	0.3 msec	0.3 msec
Time for LGN (optic radiation) to cortex[63]	1.0 to 1.8 msec (complex cell)	1.6 to 3.6 (simple and hypercomplex cells)
Total estimated retinocortical conduction time for these cells (present results)	3.0 to 5.3 msec	5.6 to 10.0 msec
Total estimated latency to photic stimulation at cortex (assuming a cortical response) i.e., ganglion cell latency + retinocortical conduction time (present results)	41.0 to 61.3 msec	24.6 to 34.0 msec
Measured latency of the cortical cells to photic stimulation	Not available (complex cell)	Not available (simple and hypercomplex cells)

From Ikeda H, Wright MJ: J Physiol (Lond) **227**:769, 1972.[66]

and "P-cell" pathways of the afferent visual system. There is both physiologic and psychophysic evidence for a partial segregation of various visual functions (e.g., perception of form, color, movement, stereopsis, etc.) into either the M-cell or P-cell pathways, and this parallel segregation is maintained well into the circuitry of the visual cortex (see Chapter 23). The M-cell pathway is characterized as mediating high contrast sensitivity and fast temporal resolution, but having low spatial resolution and no color sensitivity. The P-cell channel on the other hand is seen as carrying information about color discrimination and high spatial resolution, but having poor temporal responsiveness and low contrast sensitivity.

CORTICAL INFORMATION PROCESSING

Studies of spatial and temporal contrast sensitivity in the cat cortex demonstrate parallel processing of pattern and motion information in visual areas 17 and 18.[98] Cells in the visual cortex have a predominance of Y cells (transient type, longer response latency) and X cells (sustained type, short response latency). The relatively high spatial frequencies to which X cells respond, coupled with a response predominately to low and intermediate temporal frequencies, make them ideally suited to pattern discrimination. The Y cells, with a preference for relatively low spatial frequencies, and intermediate to high temporal frequencies, are best suited for response to motion detection within the visual field. Unlike area 17 (striate cortex), which receives axons with a broad spectrum of conduction velocities from X, Y, and W cells, area 18 (part of extrastriate visual cortex) lacks input from X cells. The Y cell input to area 18 permits a response to movement information entering this area more or less simultaneously with pattern information processing in area 17. The physiology of the visual cortex is covered more completely in Chapter 23. Developmental defects in the neural circuitry of the visual cortex, such as in strabismic amblyopia (see Chapter 24), have been found associated with a deficit in the temporal integration of sequenced stimuli. Altmann[5] attributed this to a marked reduction of the duration of visual persistence in the amblyopic visual system, suggesting that the effect is due to a shortening of normally sustained neuronal responses. This could presumably result from a loss of dentritic ramifications in neural elements of the visual cortex receiving input from the P-cell pathway.

REFERENCES

1. Adler FH, Fliegelman M: Influence of fixation on the visual acuity, Arch Ophthalmol 12:475, 1934.
2. Alpern M: Metacontrast, J Opt Soc Am 43:648, 1953.
3. Alpern M, Maaseidvaag F, Ohba N: The kinetics of cone visual pigments in man, Vision Res 11:539, 1971.
4. Alpern M, Rushton WAH: The nature of rise in threshold produced by contrast flashes, J Physiol (Lond) 189:519, 1967.
5. Altmann L, Singer W: Temporal integration in amblyopic vision, Vision Res 26:1959, 1986.
6. Averbach E, Coriell AS: Short-term memory in vision, Bell System Tech J 40:309, 1961.
7. Barany R: The clinical aspects and theory of train nystagmus, Arch Augenheilkd 88:139, 1921.
8. Barlow HB, Fitzhugh R, Kuffler SW: Change of organization in the receptive fields of the cat's retina during dark adaptation, J Physiol (Lond) 137:338, 1957.
9. Baron WS, Westheimer G: Visual acuity as a function of exposure duration, J Opt Soc Am 63:212, 1973.
10. Bartley SH: Brightness comparisons when one eye is stimulated intermittently and the other eye steadily, J Psychol 34:165, 1952.
11. Berger C: Illumination of surrounding field and flicker fusion frequency with foveal images of different sizes, Acta Physiol Scand 30:161, 1954.
12. Boycott BB, Kolb H: The connections between the bipolar cells and photoreceptors in the retina of the domestic cat, J Comp Neurol 148:91, 1973.
13. Boycott BB, Peichl L, Wässle H: Morphological types of horizontal cell in the retina of the domestic cat, Proc R Soc Lond (Biol) 203:229, 1978.
14. Boycott BB, Wässle H: The morphological types of ganglion cells of the domestic cat's retina, J Physiol (Lond) 240:397, 1974.
15. Breitmeyer BG: Metacontrast with black and white stimuli: evidence for inhibition of on- and off-sustained activity for either on- or off-transient activity, Vision Res 18:1443, 1978.
16. Breitmeyer BG, Ganz L: Implications of sustained and transient channels for theories of visual pattern masking, saccadic suppression, and information processing, Psychol Rev 83:1, 1976.
17. Bridgeman B: Visual receptive fields sensitive to absolute and relative motion during tracking, Science 178:1106, 1972.
18. Broca A, Sulzer D: La sensation lumineuse en fonction du temps, J Physiol Path Gen 4:632, 1902.
19. Brown KT, Watanabe K, Murakami M: The early and late receptor potentials of monkey cones and rods, Symp Quant Biol 30:457, 1965.
20. Clarke FJJ, Belcher SJ: On the localization of Troxler's effect in the visual pathway, Vision Res 2:53, 1962.
21. Cleland BG, Dubin MW, Levick WR: Sustained and transient neurones in the cat's retina and lateral geniculate nucleus, J Physiol (Lond) 217:473, 1971.
22. Cleland BG, Enroth-Cugell C: Cat retinal ganglion cell responses to changing light intensities: sinusoidal modulation in the time domain, Acta Physiol Scand 68:365, 1966.
23. Cleland BG, Enroth-Cugell C: Quantitative aspects of gain and latency in the cat retina, J Physiol (Lond) 206:73, 1970.
24. Cleland BG, Levick WR: Brisk and sluggish concentrically organized ganglion cells in the cat's retina, J Physiol (Lond) 240:421, 1974.
25. Cleland BG, Levick WR: Properties of rarely encountered types of ganglion cells in the cat's retina and an overall classification, J Physiol (Lond) 240:457, 1974.
26. Cleland BG, Levick WR, Sanderson KJ: Properties of sustained and transient ganglion cells in the cat retina, J Physiol (Lond) 228:649, 1973.
27. Cone RA: The early receptor potential of the vertebrate eye, Symp Quant Biol 30:483, 1965.
28. Cornsweet TN: Determination of the stimuli for invol-

untary drifts and saccadic eye movements, J Opt Soc Am 46:987, 1956.

29. Crawford BH: Visual adaptation in relation to brief conditioning stimuli, Proc R Soc Lond (Biol) 134:283, 1947.

30. Critchley M: Visual perseveration, Trans Ophthalmol Soc UK 71:91, 1951.

31. Dandy WE: Meniere's disease: its diagnosis and treatment, South Med J 30:621, 1937.

32. DeLange H: Relationship between critical flicker frequency and a set of low-frequency characteristics of the eye, J Opt Soc Am 44:380, 1954.

33. DeLange H: Research into the dynamic nature of the human fovea-cortex systems with intermittent and modulated light, I, Attenuation characteristics with white and colored light, J Opt Soc Am 48:777, 1958.

34. DeLange H: Research into the dynamic nature of the human fovea-cortex systems with intermittent and modulated light, II, Phase shift in brightness and delay in color perception, J Opt Soc Am 48:784, 1958.

35. Ditchburn RW, Foley-Fisher JA: Assembled data in eye movements, Opt Acta 14:113, 1967.

36. Ditchburn RW, Ginsborg BL: Involuntary eye movements during fixation, J Physiol (Lond) 119:1, 1953.

37. Dowling JE: Synaptic organization of the frog retina: an electron microscopic analysis comparing the retinas of frogs and primates, Proc R Soc Lond (Biol) 170:205, 1968.

38. Dowling JE, Boycott BB: Neural connections of the retina: fine structure of the inner plexiform layer, Symp Quant Biol 30:393, 1965.

39. Dowling JE, Boycott BB: Organization of the primate retina: electron microscopy, Proc R Soc Lond (Biol) 166:80, 1966.

40. Dowling JE, Werblin F: Organization of retina of the mudpuppy, Necturus maculosus, I, Synaptic structure, J Neurophysiol 32:315, 1969.

41. Enroth-Cugell C, Robson JG: The contrast sensitivity of retinal ganglion cells of the cat, J Physiol (Lond) 187:517, 1966.

42. Ferry ES: Persistence of vision, Am J Sci 44:192, 1892.

43. Fisher SK, Boycott BB: Synaptic connexions made by horizontal cells within the outer plexiform layer of the retina of the cat and the rabbit, Proc Roy Soc Lond (Biol) 186:317, 1974.

44. Foley PJ: Interrelationships of background area, target area and target luminance in their effect on the critical flicker frequency of the human fovea, J Opt Soc Am 51:737, 1961.

45. Fukuda Y: Receptive field organization of cat optic nerve fibers with special reference to conduction velocity, Vision Res 11:209, 1971.

46. Fukuda Y, Stone J: Retinal distribution and central projections of Y-, X-, and W-cells of the cat's retina, J Neurophysiol 37:749, 1974.

47. Fukuda Y, et al: Functional significance of conduction velocity in the transfer of flicker information in the optic nerve of the cat, J Neurophysiol 29:698, 1966.

48. Gallego A: Horizontal and amacrine cells in the mammal's retina, Vision Res 11(Suppl 3): 35, 1971.

49. Gassel MM, Williams D: Visual function in patients with homonymous hemianopia, III, The completion phenomenon, Brain 86:229, 1963.

50. Gouras P: The effects of light-adaptation on rod and cone receptive field organization of monkey ganglion cells, J Physiol (Lond) 192:747, 1967.

51. Gouras P: Identification of cone mechanisms in monkey ganglion cells, J Physiol (Lond) 199:533, 1968.

52. Granit R, Harper P: Comparative studies on the peripheral and central retina, II, Synaptic reactions in the eye, Am J Physiol 95:211, 1930.

53. Green DG: Sinusoidal flicker characteristics of color sensitive mechanisms of the eye, Vision Res 9:591, 1969.

54. Growney R, Weisstein N: Spatial characteristics of metacontrast, J Opt Soc Am 62:690, 1972.

55. Hallett PE: Quantum efficiency and false positive rate, J Physiol (Lond) 202:421, 1969.

56. Hammond P: Chromatic sensitivity and spatial organization of LGN neurone receptive fields in cat: cone-rod interaction, J Physiol (Lond) 225:391, 1972.

57. Harris, CS: Perceptual adaptation to inverted, reversed and displaced vision, Psychol Rev 72:419, 1965.

58. Hecht S, Shlaer S: Intermittent stimulation by light, V, The relation between intensity and critical frequency for different parts of the spectrum, J Gen Physiol 19:965, 1936.

59. Hecht S, Shlaer S, Pirenne MH: Energy, quanta, and vision, J Gen Physiol 25:819, 1942.

60. Hecht S, Verrijp CD: Intermittent stimulation by light, III, The relation between intensity and critical fusion frequency for different retinal locations, J Gen Physiol 17:251, 1933.

61. Hess RF: The Eldrige-Green lecture, Vision at low light levels: role of spatial, temporal and contrast filters, Ophthal Physiol Opt 10:351, 1990.

62. Hess RF, Norby K: Spatial and temporal properties of human rod vision in the achromat, J Physiol (Lond) 371:387, 1986.

63. Hoffmann KP, Stone J: Conduction velocity of afferents to cat visual cortex: a correlation with cortical receptive field properties, Brain Res 32:460, 1971.

64. Hubel DH, Wiesel TN: Receptive fields of optic nerve fibers in the spider monkey, J Physiol (Lond) 154:572, 1960.

65. Hylkema BS: Examination of the visual field by determining the fusion frequency, Acta Ophthamol 20:181, 1942.

66. Ikeda H, Wright MJ: Receptive field organization of "sustained" and "transient" retinal ganglion cells which subserve different functional roles, J Physiol (Lond) 227:769, 1972.

67. Kahneman D: Temporal summation in an acuity task at different energy levels—a study of the determinations of summation, Vision Res 4:557, 1964.

68. Kahneman D, Norman J: The time-intensity relation in visual perception as a function of the observer's task, J Exp Psychol 68:215, 1964.

69. Katz MS: Brief flash brightness, Vision Res 4:361, 1964.

70. Keesey UT: Flicker and pattern detection: a comparison of thresholds, J Opt Soc Am 62:446, 1972.

71. Kelly DH: Visual responses to time-dependent stimuli, I, Amplitude sensitivity measurements, J Opt Soc Am 51:422, 1961.

72. Kelly DH: Visual responses to time-dependent stimuli, IV, Effects of chromatic adaptation, J Opt Soc Am 52:940, 1962.

73. Kelly DH: Sine waves and flicker fusion, Doc Ophthalmol 18:16, 1964.

74. Kelly DH: Theory of flicker and transient responses, I, Uniform fields, J Opt Soc Am 61:537, 1971.

75. Kolb H: The connections between horizontal cells and photoreceptors in the retina of the cat: electron microscopy of Golgi preparations, J Comp Neurol 155:1, 1974.

76. Kolb H: The organization of the outer plexiform layer in the retina of the cat: electron microscopic observations, J Neurocytol 6:131, 1977.

77. Kolb H: The inner plexiform layer in the retina of the cat: electron microscopic observations, J Neurocytol 8:295, 1979.

78. Kolb H, Famiglietti EV: Rod and cone bipolar connections in the inner plexiform layer of the cat retina, Science 186:47, 1974.

79. Kolb H, Nelson R: Neural architecture of the cat retina, in Osborne N, Chader G, eds: Progress in retinal research, Oxford, Pergamon Press, 1984, p 21.

80. Kolb H, Nelson R, Mariani A: Amacrine cells, bipolar cells and ganglion cells of the cat retina: a Golgi study, Vision Res 21:1081, 1981.

81. Korte A: Kinematoskopische Untersuchungen Z Psychol 72:193, 1915.

82. Krauskopf J, Mollon JD: The independence of the temporal integration properties of individual chromatic mechanisms in the human eye, J Physiol (Lond) 219:611, 1971.

83. Landis C: An annotated bibliography of flicker fusion phenomena covering the period 1740-1952, Washington, DC, Armed Forces, National Research Council, 1953.

84. Latour PL: Visual thresholds during eye movements, Vision Res 2:261, 1962.

85. Levinson JZ: Flicker fusion phenomena, Science 160:21, 1968.

86. Ling W, Gay AJ: Optokinetic nystagmus: a proposed pathway and its clinical application, in Smith JL, ed: Neuro-ophthalmology, vol 4, St Louis, CV Mosby, 1968.

87. Linksz A: Visual acuity in the newborn with notes on some objective methods to determine visual acuity, Doc Ophthalmol 34:259, 1973.

88. Livingstone M, Hubel D: Psychophysical evidence for separate channels for the perception of form, color, movement, and depth, J Neurosci 7:3416, 1987.

89. Livingstone M, Hubel D: Segregation of form, color, movement, and depth: anatomy, physiology, and perception, Science 240:740, 1988.

90. MacKay DM: Visual stability, Invest Ophthalmol 11:518, 1972.

91. MacKay DM: Visual stability and voluntary eye movements, in Jung R, ed: Handbook of sensory physiology, Central processing of visual information: integrative functions and comparative data, vol 7/3A, Berlin, Springer-Verlag, 1973, pp 307-331.

92. Mainster MA, White TJ, Stevens CC: Mathematical analysis of rhodopsin kinetics, Vision Res 11:435, 1971.

93. Marchiafava PL, Weiler R: Intracellular analysis and structural correlates of the organization of inputs to ganglion cells in the retina of the turtle, Proc R Soc Lond B 208:103, 1980.

94. Marrocco RT, Brown JB: Correlation of receptive field properties of monkey LGN cells with the conduction velocity of retinal afferent input, Brain Res 92:137, 1975.

95. Merigan WH, Eskin TA: Spatio-temporal vision of macaques with severe loss of P beta retinal ganglion cells, Vis Res 26:1751, 1986.

96. Miles PW: Flicker fusion fields, Arch Ophthalmol 43:661, 1950.

97. Miller RF, Dacheux RF: Synaptic organization and ionic basis of on and off channels in mudpuppy retina, I, Intracellular analysis of chloride-sensitive electogenic properties of receptors, horizontal cells and amacrine cells, J Gen Physiol 67:639, 1976.

98. Movshon JA, Thompson ID, Tolhurst DJ: Spatial and temporal contrast sensitivity of neurones in areas 17 and 18 of the cat's visual cortex, J Physiol (Lond) 283:101, 1978.

99. Nelson R, Famiglietti EV, Kolb H: Intracellular staining reveals different levels of stratification for on-center and off-center ganglion cells in the cat retina, J Neurophysiol 41:472, 1978.

100. Nelson R, et al: Horizontal cells in cat retina with independent dendritic systems, Science 189:137, 1975.

101. Nelson R, et al: Neural responses in rod and cone systems of the cat retina: intracellular records and Procion stains, Invest Ophthalmol 15:935, 1976.

102. Østerberg GA: Topography of the layer of rods and cones in the human retina, Acta Ophthalmol Suppl 6, 1935.

103. Pak WL: Rapid photoresponses in the retina and their relevance in vision research, Photochem Photobiol 8:495, 1968.

104. Pick HL Jr, Hay JC: Gaze-contingent adaptation to prismatic spectacles, Am J Psychol 79:443, 1966.

105. Pirenne MH, Marriott FHC: Visual functions in man, in Davson H, ed: The eye, vol 2, New York, Academic Press, 1962.

106. Porter TC: Contributions to the study of flicker, Proc R Soc Lond A 70:313, 1902.

107. Rabelo C, Grusser OJ: Die Abhängigkeit der subjektiven Helligkeit intermittierenden Lichtreize von der Flimmerfrequenz: Untersuchungen bei verschiedenen Leuchtdichte und Feldgrosse, Psychol Forsch 26:299, 1961.

108. Regan D, Tyler CW: Some dynamic features of color vision, Vision Res 11:1307, 1971.

109. Regan D, Tyler CW: Temporal summation and its limit for wavelength changes: an analog of Bloch's law for color vision, J Opt Soc Am 61:1414, 1971.

110. Reinecke RD: Review of optokinetic nystagmus from 1954-1960, Arch Ophthalmol 65:609, 1961.

111. Riggs LA, Armington JC, Ratliff F: Motions of the retinal image fixation, J Opt Soc Am 44:315, 1954.

112. Riggs LA, et al: The disappearance of steadily fixated visual test objects, J Opt Soc Am 43:495, 1953.

113. Robinson DN: Disinhibition of visually masked stimuli, Science 154:157, 1966.

114. Roehrig WC: The influence of area on the critical flicker-fusion threshold, J Psychol 47:317, 1959.

115. Roufs, JAJ: On the relation between the threshold of short flashes, the flicker-fusion frequency and the visual latency, Institute for Perception Research, Eind-

hoven, The Netherlands, Annual Progress Report no 1, 1966, pp 69-77.

116. Roufs JAJ, Meulenbrugge HJ: The quantitative relation between flash threshold and the flicker fusion boundary for centrally fixated fields, Institute for Perception Research, Eindhoven, The Netherlands, Annual Progress Report no 2, 1967, pp 133-139.

117. Rowe MH, Stone J: Naming of neurones: classification and naming of cat retinal ganglion cells, Brain Behav Evol 14:185, 1977.

118. Schiller PH, Smith MC: Detection in metacontrast, J Exp Psychol 71:32, 1966.

119. Sjostrand FS: Ultrastructure of retinal rod synapses of the guinea pig eye as revealed by three dimensional reconstructions from serial sections, J Ultrastruct Res 2:122, 1958.

120. Smith JL: Optokinetic nystagmus, Springfield, IL, Charles C Thomas, Publisher, 1963.

121. Sperling G: Linear theory and the psychophysics of flicker, Doc Ophthalmol 18:3, 1964.

122. Sperling G: Temporal and spatial visual masking, I, Masking by impulse flashes, J Opt Soc Am 55:541, 1965.

123. Stark L: Neurological control systems: studies in bioengineering, New York, Plenum, 1968.

124. St-Cyr GJ: Signal and noise in the human oculomotor system, Vision Res 13:1979, 1973.

125. Sterling P: Microcircuitry of the cat retina, Ann Rev Neurosci 6:149, 1983.

126. Stewart BR: Temporal summation during dark adaptation, J Opt Soc Am 62:449, 1972.

127. Stone J, Freeman RB Jr: Conduction velocity groups in the cat's optic nerve classified according to their retinal origin, Exp Brain Res 13:489, 1971.

128. Stone J, Fukuda Y: Properties of cat retinal ganglion cells: a comparison of W-cells with X- and Y-cells, J Neurophysiol 37:722, 1974.

129. Stuart RD: An introduction to Fourier analysis, New York, John Wiley, 1961.

130. Taylor EA: The spans: perception, apprehension and recognition as related to reading and speed reading, Am J Ophthalmol 44:501, 1957.

131. Uetsuki T, Ikeda M: Adaptation and critical duration for Stiles mechanisms, J Opt Soc Am 61:821, 1971.

132. Van der Tweel LH: Relation between psychophysics and electrophysiology of flicker, Doc Opththamol 18:287, 1964.

133. Verheijen FJ: A simple after-image method demonstrating the involuntary multidirectional eye movements during fixation, Opt Acta 8:309, 1961.

134. Volkmann FC: Vision during voluntary saccadic eye movements, J Opt Soc Am 52:571, 1962.

135. Wald G, Brown PK: The molar extinction of rhodopsin, J Gen Physiol 37:189, 1953.

136. Walls GL: The filling-in process. Am J Optom 31:329, 1954.

137. Wässle H, Boycott BB, and Illing RB: Morphology and mosaic of on- and off-beta cells in the cat retina and some functional considerations, Proc Roy Soc Lond B 212:177, 1981.

138. Wässle H, Peichl L, Boycott BB: Topography of horizontal cells in the retina of the domestic cat, Proc Roy Soc Lond B 203:269, 1978.

139. Wässle H, Peichl L, Boycott BB: Morphology and topography of on- and off-alpha cells in the cat retina, Proc Roy Soc Lond B 212:157, 1981.

140. Werblin FS: Functional organization of a vertebrate retina: sharpening up in space and intensity, Ann NY Acad Sci 193:75, 1972.

141. Werblin FS, Dowling JE: Organization of the retina of the mudpuppy, Necturus maculosus, II, Intracellular recordings, J Neurophysiol 32:339, 1969.

142. Whitten DN, Brown KT: Photopic suppression of monkey's rod receptor potential, apparently by a cone-initiated lateral inhibition, Vision Res 13:1629, 1973.

143. Whitten DN, Brown KT: The time courses of late receptor potentials from monkey cones and rods, Vision Res 13:107, 1973.

144. Yarbus AL: Eye movements and vision, Haigh B, trans, New York, Plenum, 1967.

145. Zuber BL, Stark L: Saccadic suppression: elevation of visual threshold associated with saccadic eye movements, Exp Neurol 16:65, 1966.

146. Zuber BL, Stark L, Lorber M: Saccadic suppression of the pupillary light reflex, Exp Neurol 14:351, 1966.

GENERAL REFERENCES

Bartley SH: Temporal features of input as crucial factors in vision, in Neff WD, ed: Contributions to sensory physiology, vol 3, New York, Academic Press, 1968, pp 82-135.

Grusser OJ, Grusser-Cornehls U: Neuronal mechanisms of visual movement perception and some psychophysical and behavioral correlations, in Jung R, ed: Handbook of sensory physiology, Central processing of visual information: integrative functions and comparative data, vol 7/3A, Berlin, Springer-Verlag, 1973, pp 333-429.

Jameson D, Hurvich LM, eds: Handbook of sensory physiology; Visual psychophysics, vol 7/4, Berlin, Springer-Verlag, 1972.

Kelly DH: Flicker, in Jameson D, Hurvich LM, eds: Handbook of sensory physiology, vol 7/4, Berlin, Springer-Verlag, 1972, pp 273-302.

Levick WR: Receptive fields of retinal ganglion cells, in Fuortes MGF, ed: Handbook of sensory physiology; physiology of photoreceptor organs, vol 7/2, Berlin, Springer-Verlag, 1972, pp 531-566.

MacLeod DIA: Visual sensitivity, Annu Rev Psychol 29:613, 1978.

Ronchi L: An annotated bibliography of variability and periodicities of visual responsiveness, Florence, Italy, Fond G Ronchi, 1972.

Van de Grind WA, Grusser OJ, Lunkenheimer HU: Temporal transfer properties of the afferent visual system: psychophysical, neurophysiological and theoretical investigations, in Jung R, ed: Handbook of sensory physiology; central processing of visual information: integrative functions and comparative data, vol 7/3A, Berlin, Springer-Verlag, 1973, pp 431-573.

CHAPTER
19

The Retina

ADOLPH I. COHEN, Ph.D.

DEVELOPMENT OF THE RETINA

The eye is an externalized portion of the brain. The neural retina is, in fact, a derivative of and an extension of the diencephalon. The optic nerve, which connects the retina with higher visual centers, is structurally and functionally a tract of the central nervous system, rather than a peripheral nerve. The layers of collagen bundles in the cornea and sclera are continuous with those of the dural investment of the optic nerve and, via that connection, with that of the brain. The clear fluid in the eye most closely resembles the cerebrospinal fluid of the brain, rather than any other body fluid. The blood vessels of the retina are structurally identical with those of the brain proper.

In the human, formation of the eye[75] begins with lateral outpouchings of the prosencephalon (the precursor of the telencephalon and diencephalon) during the third week of development (2.6 mm stage). These enlarge to form primary optic vesicles whose lateral aspects invaginate during the fourth week of development to form double-walled optic cups. These continue to enlarge, primarily on their dorsal and lateral aspects, to form more mature double-walled optic cups whose concavities are directed lateroventrally. Because the optic vesicles

are outpouchings of the hollow neural tube, the cavity in each optic vesicle is initially continuous with that of the neural tube. The neural tube's system of connected cavities develops into the hollow, fluid-filled ventricular system of the brain. Each optic vesicle's lumen becomes cut off from the lumen of the neural tube because of total obliteration of the lumen in the optic stalk that connects the optic vesicle to the neural tube. However, an important residuum of this cavity persists between the two walls of the optic cup in the adult vertebrate, between the retina and the pigment epithelium. Clinicians refer to this space in the human eye as the subretinal space, and it is this space that enlarges in detachment of the retina, but it is, in fact, the ocular ventricle.

The fates of the two walls of the embryonic optic cup in the vertebrate eye are as follows: the outer wall, closest to the brain proper, remains as a sheet of cells, one cell thick, and becomes the pigment epithelium. The invaginated inner wall, facing the future vitreous chamber of the eye, becomes several structures. Over most of its central extent it becomes the neural retina, a relatively thick multicellular tissue, but the peripheral extent of this layer remains one cell thick. This peripheral, one-cell-thick extension from the retina becomes physically attached to the corresponding peripheral portion of the pigment epithelium, also one cell thick, and this double epithelium forms a peripheral extension of the double-walled optic cup. This persists in the adult eye as the two-layered epithelium of

This work was supported in part by Research Grant EY 00258-28 from the National Eye Institute, National Institutes of Health.

the ciliary body and iris. Between these adherent layers of pigment epithelium and nonneural epithelium, the ventricular space is essentially obliterated.

Because of the invagination process during development and the spherical organization of the eye, the retinal surface facing the vitreous chamber is its inner surface; that facing the ocular ventricle and pigment epithelium is its outer surface. Had the invagination not occurred, the inner or vitreous surface of the retina would have faced the outside of a sphere. This reveals its homology to the outer or pial surface of the brain. Similarly, in the absence of invagination the outer surface of the retina would have faced the cavity of a hollow sphere. Thus its homology is to the inner or ventricular surface of the brain. In an anterior facing eye, as in the human, the inner layer of the optic cup is sometimes designated the anterior layer; the outer layer is the posterior layer.

Paralleling the situation at the pial surface of the brain, all the cell membrane at the inner surface of the retina belongs to a mosaic of processes of glial cells, and the surface is covered by a basal lamina. This surface with its covering (Fig. 19-1) constitutes the vaguely defined "inner limiting membrane" (ILM) of the retina.[52]

The outer surface of the retina and the inner surface of the pigment epithelium face the ocular ventricle. The margins of all cells facing *brain* ventricles are joined by presumptively adhesive structures that were once called terminal bars but are now called zonulae adherens, that is, adherent girdles. These form a sort of collar around each cell at the surface, and the proteins of these attachment specializations stain intensely with certain procedures. The same cytologic description holds true for the cells facing the ocular ventricle, that is, the photoreceptors and intervening Müller cells. These cells are joined by zonulae adherens. In thick sections of retina this line of intense stain at the outer or ventricular surface of the retina was originally interpreted as representing a membrane, hence the term "external limiting membrane" (ELM) of the retina (Fig. 19-2). It forms a useful marker for the retinal surface at the ventricle.[20,21] In

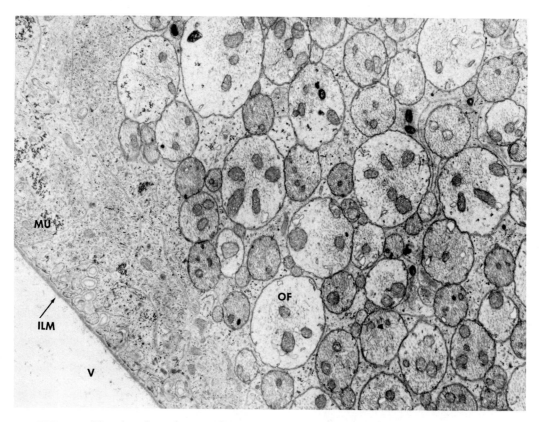

FIG. 19-1   Vitreal surface of retina of rhesus monkey. Note vitreous, V; inner limiting membrane, ILM; foot processes of glial cells of Müller, MU; optic fibers, OF. (Magnification × 14,000.)

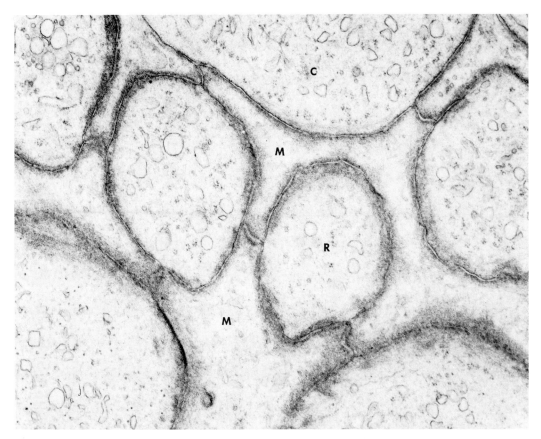

FIG. 19-2 Tangenital section of human retina at level of external limiting membrane. Note glial cells of Müller, M; separating rods, R; cones, C. (Magnification × 26,400.)

many epithelia of the body, each cell junction contains a junctional complex, consisting of a zonula adherens, a zonula occludens (tight junction), and gap junctions, but each cell's junctional specialization at the external limiting membrane consists solely of a zonula adherens.

PIGMENT EPITHELIUM

The outer layer of the optic cup or pigment epithelium (PE) is the homolog of the epithelium of choroid plexus of the brain. In regions of the brain in which choroid plexus forms, the wall of the neural tube remains one cell thick, and this sheet of cells is invaginated into a brain ventricle before ingrowing tufts of capillaries. The epithelium remains intact and persistently intervenes between the capillaries and the ventricular volume. The capillaries of choroid plexus exhibit fenestrated endothelial cells, and various molecules introduced into the blood readily leak out of the capillaries, apparently through these fenestrae. However, the choroid plexus epithelium forms an effective barrier for these sub-stances. Included in the junctional complex on the ventricular side of plexus epithelium, joining these epithelial cells to one another, is a tight or occluded intercellular zone that largely restricts the ability of material to enter or leave the ventricle by passage *between* these cells. Thus to enter or leave a ventrical via choroid plexus, material must pass largely through the cells of the epithelium itself, suggesting that this is a site for control and selectivity.

Similarly, although the pigment epithelium (Fig. 19-3) has some specialized functions, which are described in connection with the photoreceptors, these are superimposed on some persistent choroid plexus functions. The pigment epithelium is backed by fenestrated (Fig. 19-4) choroid capillaries.[84] Included in the junctional complex system girdling the inner aspect of the cells facing the ocular ventricle is an occluded zone (Fig. 19-5) that resists intercellular movements of molecules across the epithelium thus facilitating control of transport by the epithelial cells. The layer of cells of the pigment ep-

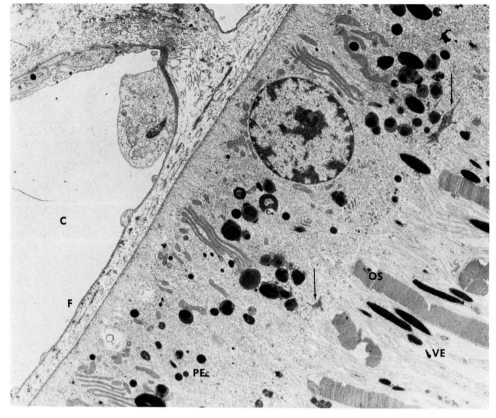

FIG. 19-3 Pigment epithelium, PE, of rhesus monkey. Note ventricle, VE; outer segments, OS; choroid capillary, C, with its fenestrated inner wall, F. Arrows indicate terminal bars. (Magnification × 4250.)

FIG. 19-4 Inner wall of human choroid capillary. C, showing tight junction, T, between endothelial cells and fenestrations, F, in endothelial cell wall. (Magnification × 50,000.) (From Moyer FH, in Straatsma BR, et al, eds: The retina: morphology, function, and clinical characteristics, UCLA Forum Med Sci no 8, Los Angeles, University of California Press, 1969. Reprinted by permission of the Regents of the University of California.)

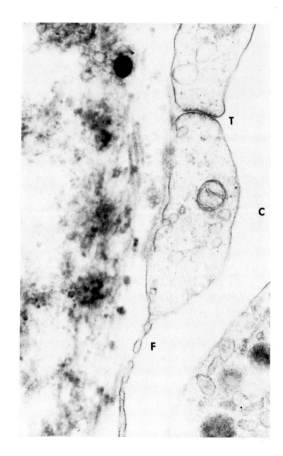

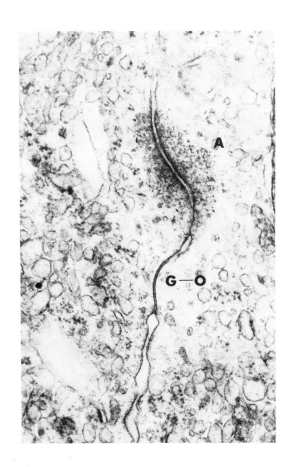

FIG. 19-5 Terminal bar of human pigment epithelium showing an adherent junction. A, and a zone, G-O, facing the retina where freeze-fracturing reveals gap junctions between strands of a zonula occludens (tight junction). (Magnification × 48,000.)

ithelium, thus joined by occluded junctions, forms a barrier of considerable electrical resistance known as the "R" membrane.[14] In addition to occluded junctions, the junctional complexes between pigment epithelial cells include gap junctions that probably electrically couple the epithelial cells to one another. The functional significance of the arrangement is still unclear.

CELLULAR ORGANIZATION OF THE RETINA

The retina develops from a primitive, pseudostratified neuroepithelium, whose tall, thin cells run the full retinal thickness, reaching both inner and outer surfaces. Within the cells of this epithelium, nuclei migrate toward the ventricle, and nuclear and cell division occurs at this level. Before or after these events, the cells' nuclei are located away from the ventricle, where they form a single thick band. Eventually certain cells cease dividing and differentiate into one of the varieties of nerve or glial cells of the mature retina. These lose their connections with the retinal surfaces. The first mature cells to be recognizable are the ganglion cells of the retina, which form the nerve cell layer closest to the vitreous chamber. The sequence of appearance of other cell varieties is less precise. However, the sequence of appearance of recognizable synapses does not necessarily correspond with the sequence of appearance of cell types, because synapses involving the photoreceptors are the first to appear and reach their mature organization and numbers.

Eventually the retina reaches its well-known layered appearance (Fig. 19-6). The layers of cell nuclei are as follows:

1. The outer nuclear layer (ONL), which contains the cell bodies of the photoreceptors.
2. The inner nuclear layer (INL), which contains the cell bodies of horizontal neurons, bipolar neurons, amacrine neurons, interplexiform neurons, displaced ganglion cells, and those of the glial cells of Müller.
3. The ganglion cell layer, which contains the cell bodies of most of the ganglion cells, displaced amacrine cells and those of some astroglial cells.

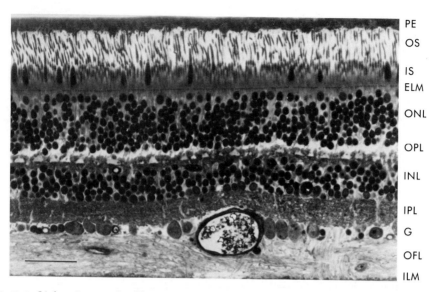

PE
OS
IS
ELM
ONL
OPL
INL
IPL
G
OFL
ILM

FIG. 19-6 Light micrograph of human retina illustrates its layered structure. PE, Pigment epithelium; OS, outer segments of photoreceptors; IS, inner segments of photoreceptors; ELM, external limiting membrane; ONL, outer nuclear layer (photoreceptor cell bodies); OPL, outer plexiform or synaptic layer; INL, inner nuclear layer; IPL, inner plexiform or synaptic layers; G, ganglion cell layer; OFL, optic fiber layer; and ILM, inner limiting membrane. Bar indicates 50 μm.

Between the ONL and INL is the outer synaptic layer (OSL), also called the outer plexiform layer (OPL). Here take place synaptic interactions of photoreceptors, horizontal cells, and bipolar neurons. Between the INL and the ganglion cell layer is the inner synaptic layer (ISL), also called the inner plexiform layer (IPL). Here take place synaptic interactions involving bipolar neurons, amacrine cells, ganglion cells, and in certain retinas, such as those of birds, interactions with terminals of centrifugal fibers to the retina from extraretinal sources.

Recently, interplexiform neurons have been identified in a number of species, including the goldfish, cat, cebus monkey, and human retinas. These neurons have their cell bodies in the INL and processes in both synaptic layers. Cytologic examination suggests that they convey information from the IPL to the OPL, and histochemical analyses suggest that in different species these cells may use different transmitter molecules.[34] In the human retina, Linberg and Fisher[74] have serially reconstructed portions of interplexiform neurons. They are both presynaptic and postsynaptic to amacrine processes and can make synapses on amacrine cell bodies. In the OPL they synapse on bipolar processes and unidentified processes entering photoreceptor terminals. Mariani[76] also has reported that macaque retinas contain biplexiform cells

that resemble ganglion cells in receiving input from amacrine and bipolar neurons but, in addition, have processes in the outer plexiform layer that receive an input from rods. Like ganglion cells, they contribute an axon to the optic fiber layer.

The expanded processes of glial cells of Müller fully occupy the retinal face on the vitreous chamber. Between this face and the ganglion cells lies the layer of optic fibers. The optic fibers consist of the axons of the ganglion cells and, in most species, including humans, are unmyelinated while within the retina. In most species these course across the retina to a central point, the optic nerve head or optic papilla, where they turn and leave the globe as the optic nerve. In some species the exit of the axons of ganglion cells is via a band or stripe, and the collection of axons into an optic nerve occurs just outside the eye.

The glial cells of Müller fall into a class of cells termed "ependymoglia." They retain the primitive condition in extending in their height, the full thickness of the retina, and the dual name indicates that they are glial cells and also are fulfilling a role corresponding to that of the ependymal cells that line other ventricular cavities of the brain. As already noted, at the inner retinal surface their expanded "feet" form a complete mosaic occupying the vitreous face of the retina.

At the outer surface of the retina, where the Müller cells reach the surface, they separate the individual photoreceptors from one another, and microvillous processes of the Müller cells form so-called "fiber baskets" about the bases of the portions of the photoreceptors protruding into the ventricle. In the retina Müller cell processes fill in almost all volumes not occupied by nerve cells, relatively rare astroglia, or blood vessels. Most retinas, including primate retinas, lack oligodendroglial cells.

There appears to be no physical barrier to the diffusion of molecules of moderate size from the vitreous through the retina into the ocular ventricle. Proteins with a Stokes radius of 3 nm diffuse freely past the ELM while those with a radius of 3.6 nm or greater are blocked. There is no hindrance to electric current.[17] The cell junctions linking the photoreceptors and Müller cells at the level of the external limiting membrane lack occluded zones, although small gap junctions are sometimes seen between adjacent Müller cells at this level. This again parallels the situation in the brain in that, apart from the epithelium of the choroid plexus, the cells facing the ventricles seem to lack complete circumferentially occluding junctions. Substances injected into brain ventricles readily enter the tissue of the brain.

BLOOD SUPPLY OF THE RETINA

During the development of the optic cup, a cleft forms in the ventral aspect of the cup and optic stalk. In the retina this extends dorsally to the site of the future nerve head.[75] Along this groove run blood vessels that gain access to the inner surface of the developing retina. Branches of these vessels eventually come to supply the inner retina. The cleft through which they reach the retinal inner surface progressively heals, uniting the divisions of retina it formerly separated, and the penetrating main blood vessels become restricted to a residue of the cleft in the center of the optic nerve head. In most animals the capillaries derived from the branches of arteries originating at the nerve head tunnel into and supply the inner two thirds of the retina, the choroidal circulation apparently sufficing to supply the remaining outer retina via regulated transport across the PE. This is the situation in humans. However, in some animals, such as the rabbit, blood vessels are both superficial (that is, on the vitreous surface) and confined to rather limited regions of the retina, whereas in others, such as the flying squirrel, capillaries penetrate the full thickness of all retinal regions, even lying just below the outer retinal margin denoted by the external limiting membrane. The junctions of endothelial cells in retinal vessels are tight or occluded. Thus to enter or leave the retina, most substances require active transport across the endothelial cells. The capillaries are surrounded by a basal lamina and by intermittent pericytes (mural cells),[53] which are also covered by a basal lamina.

RETINAL NEUROANATOMY AND ITS PHYSIOLOGIC SIGNIFICANCE

What does the retina do and how is it organized to accomplish its functions? The input to the retina is a time-varying two-dimensional display of an image in its focal plane. The image consists of patches of illumination varying in shape, intensity, and spectral content. The information input is received by the photoreceptors. The output of the photoreceptors is processed by a variety of subsequent retinal neurons and finally by the retinal ganglion cells whose axons leave the retina for higher brain centers. If we consider the information in the encoded output of the latter cells, we can then return to address how the retina produced this encodement from the information it received.

The information leaving the retina via axons of the ganglion cells represents a small number of information processing streams[30] parceling certain types of information contained in the visual input to axons with particular routing. The axons of the ganglion cells have several principal as well as minor destinations, and the cells are sometimes classified by their axonal targets. Thus, in primates, those ganglion cells that, via the optic nerve, synapse on cells of the parvocellular (small cell) layers of the dorsal lateral geniculate nucleus (DLGN) are sometimes called "P" cells (also B cells or $P\beta$ cells), while those connecting to the cells of the magnocellular (large cell) layers of the DLGN are sometimes called "M" cells (also A cells or $P\alpha$ cells). Both systems are responsive to dark versus light and can indicate brightness. However, the information to the parvocellular DLGN contains sustained responses with good resolution of wavelengths, shape, fine stereopsis, and moderate resolution of contrast, whereas that to the magnocellular DLGN has good temporal resolution and excellent spatial contrast sensitivity, as required for discerning movements and flickering light, but poor wavelength sensitivity and a cruder ability than the P systems for responding to textures and subtle patterns.[104,105] An earlier view of spatial and chromatic interactions in the DLGN is that of Wiesel and Hubel.[126] The retina also has outputs to the outermost layers of the superior colliculus, where the information directly or indirectly interacts with motor pathways influencing the extraocular muscles, visually concerned cerebellar pathways, such as those dealing with head and neck movements, and with vestibular and auditory centers. Rostral to the colliculus is the pretectal region, which indirectly receives retinal information important for the parasympathetic and sympathetic regulation of the pupil and ciliary muscle. Indications of optic nerve input are also found in the nucleus of the accessory optic tract. In addition, some ganglion cell information passes directly to the suprachiasmatic nucleus of the hypothalamus, which is a center that influences circadian rhythms and pineal activity.

One important role for the retina is to maintain the perception of contrast over the 12 log unit range of illumination in which vision is possible. This requires mechanisms not only within the photoreceptors, but also within the neuronal networks of the postreceptoral retina.

PHOTORECEPTORS

The photoreceptors of the retina[21] are cells whose structure has suggested to many that they are evolutionarily related to the ciliated ependymal cells that line brain ventricles. The cells are bipolar (see Fig. 19-6). Their cell bodies lie in the ONL, with those of cones tending to be larger and lying closer to the outer retinal surface than those of rods. Their synaptic terminals lie at the outer aspect of the OPL. From the cell body, an elongated portion of the cell protrudes into the ventricular space. This is structurally divided into two portions, linked by a ciliary derivative. There is an outer segment, whose apex reaches the inner aspect of the pigment epithelium, and an inner segment, which connects to the cell body within the retina (Fig. 19-7).

Slightly below the apex of the inner segment, and lying eccentrically, is a basal body from which arises a ciliary stalk. This stalk links the inner to the outer segment, and the nine pairs of microtubules in the stalk (which lacks the central pair of microtubules seen in motile cilia) continue as a sort of backbone, eccentrically in the outer segment.

At the apex of the inner segment is a large collection of mitochondria, and this region of the cell is sometimes known as the ellipsoid. The remainder of the inner segment has more usual cell organelles, including ribosomes and a Golgi region. In certain species the apical portion of the inner segment may have a colored oil drop-

let or other specialized organelles. In some species, but not in mammals, the ventricular portions of the cell may extend or contract in the radial direction in response to light. In these species the name myoid is sometimes applied to the portion of the inner segment closest to the retinal surface at the external limiting membrane, because this is where the active process responsible for the translational movement is thought likely to occur.

Before turning to the outer segments, the apparent site of initiation of visual signals, one must remark on the two varieties of photoreceptors, the rods and cones. As the names imply, these are morphologic terms. Originally the morphologic distinction was that in rods the inner and outer segments were both cylindrical and of similar diameter, whereas in cones the outer segment was conical and the inner segment of clearly greater diameter than the outer. In current usage photoreceptors are often called cones on morphologic grounds if the inner segment is of considerably greater diameter than a short outer segment, whether the latter is clearly conical or not.

The importance of the distinction in shapes was first recognized by Schultze, who in 1866 pointed to the correlation that rods tended to be the numerically dominant photoreceptor variety in animals whose activity extended into the range of twilight and night, whereas strictly diurnal animals tended to be very rich in cones. This correlation of the period of animal activity and shape of the dominant variety of photoreceptor hints at something related to the optical properties of the photoreceptors. Photoreceptor diameters are of the same order of magnitude as the wavelengths of light in water. Photoreceptors can act as wave guides and, particularly in cones, the shape of the inner segment may act to concentrate light on the outer segment. However, much remains to be understood about the function of photoreceptor shapes. The evidence is rather overwhelming that the identification of a receptor as a rod or cone is a very useful probabilistic indicator for the presence of other photoreceptor and visual properties—the general spectral area of the absorption maxima of visual pigments, ability to follow flickering light, certain ultrastructural details of the photoreceptors, frequency of certain retinal neuronal classes, and so on. Presumably these all relate to a heightened efficiency for the visual tasks of the animal. However, the shape of the cells is by no means a certain indicator for the presence of any particular property, and in a relatively few spe-

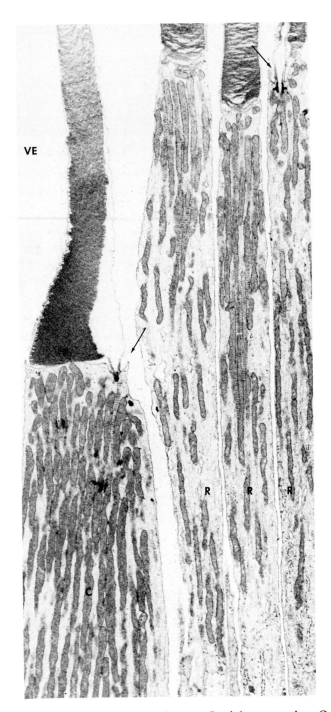

FIG. 19-7 Ventricular portions of rods, R, and cones, C, of rhesus monkey. Outer segments (*above*) are linked to inner segments (*below*) by ciliary connective *(arrows)*, and these portions of photoreceptors are surrounded by ventricular space, VE. (Magnification × 7700.)

cies the decision as to whether a given receptor should be called a rod or cone on morphologic grounds is not readily made.

The outer segments of both rods and cones contain many double-membrane discs or flattened saccules (Fig. 19-8). At the inner or vitread end of the outer segments of rods, membranes from adjacent pairs of evaginations of the plasma membrane combine to form hollow discs whose lumina are continuous with extracellular space. However, in rods, apart from this small zone, one observes that most of the discs apparently have become isolated from the cell membrane (Figs. 19-8, A and B, and 19-9, A) and from each other, and the disc lumina thus are isolated from extracellular space. The individual discs are seen completely and uniformly separated from each other, but some special techniques have demonstrated fine filaments linking rims of adjacent discs and rims to the plasma membrane. On the other hand, in cones one observes in inframammalian species that virtually all the discs in the outer segments retain their connection with the cell membrane, and therefore the disc lumina retain their continuity with extracellular space. However, in mammalian cones, while the discs in the inner third of the outer segment have their membranes confluent with the cell membrane (Figs. 19-8, C and D, and 19-9, B), in the outer two thirds the cone discs seem isolated. Occasionally special techniques reveal persistent connections of distal mammalian discs of cones to the plasma membrane.

The discs are of great importance because the visual pigments, which capture the photons to begin the visual process, appear to be built into the discs. Although visual pigment molecules also are present in the plasma membrane of the outer segment, they constitute a small fraction of those in disc membranes and are not optimally oriented for interaction with light. The visual pigments are insoluble and detergents must be employed to bring them into solution. This demonstrates that they are intrinsic membrane proteins. Also supporting this view are studies with polarized light that indicate that the light-capturing or chromophore portions of the visual pigment molecules lie in planes essentially parallel to the planes of the discs. Visual pigment molecules may constitute in excess of 50% of the protein of the outer segments. The pigments are combinations of the aldehyde of vitamin A and various proteins. Their chemistry is discussed in Chapter 14.

Outer segments are capable of regeneration. If outer segments of rods or cones are destroyed via experimental retinal detachments, they may regenerate on reattaching the retina. Similarly, rod outer segments may break down because of vitamin A deficiency, but if vitamin A refeeding is initiated before the whole cell deteriorates, the outer segments may reform.

The volume surrounding the photoreceptor inner and outer segments contains a gel, now termed the interphotoreceptor matrix (IPM), which stains for acid mucopolysaccharides.[42] This proves to be rich in chondroitin-6-sulfate. The portion surrounding the photoreceptors is organized as a sheath. That surounding the cones is distinctive in that it binds peanut lectin (PL)[47,57] and that surrounding rods binds the lectin, wheat germ agglutinin (WGA). When the lectins are conjugated to fluorescent dyes such as FITC or rhodamine,[54] the organized gels can be visualized (Figs. 19-10 and 19-11). Thus distinctive acid mucopolysaccharides relate to the two receptor classes. In rats apparent gel redistribution and/or changes in staining properties are triggered by light-dark transitions.[120]

In 1961 Droz noted that radiolabeled protein from the inner segment was moving into the outer segment. Putting this observation together with observations of possibly forming saccules at the base of rod outer segments and observations of fragments of outer segments in cells of the PE, it was suggested[4,20] that rod saccules might be in continuous formation. That this was indeed the case was proved by the elegant work of Young.[129] By supplying a pulse of a radioactive amino acid, he was able to show that amino acids were incorporated into rod discs and into rhodopsin, the rod pigment, and the pulse could be followed as a band of radioactivity, detected in autoradiographs, at both the levels of light and electron microscopy. With time this band of radioactive protein was located at increasingly sclerad levels of outer segments and eventually in fragments of outer segments ingested (phagosomes) by the cells of the PE[136] (Fig. 19-12).

However, in cones of both frogs[130] and monkeys,[131] no banding was seen, only a diffuse labeling of the outer segments. This appears to be due to the confluence of the membrane of cone discs with the plasma membrane, which permits the mixing and randomization of newly added molecules of photopigment by diffusion. Cone discs also are shed,[52,111] and an interesting distinction from rods has been observed. The shedding of rod discs largely occurs shortly after morning, as when lights come on in an animal room,[6,71] but the time of peak shedding of cone discs varies in different species, sometimes occurring at the end of the day,[95,133,134,135] but some-

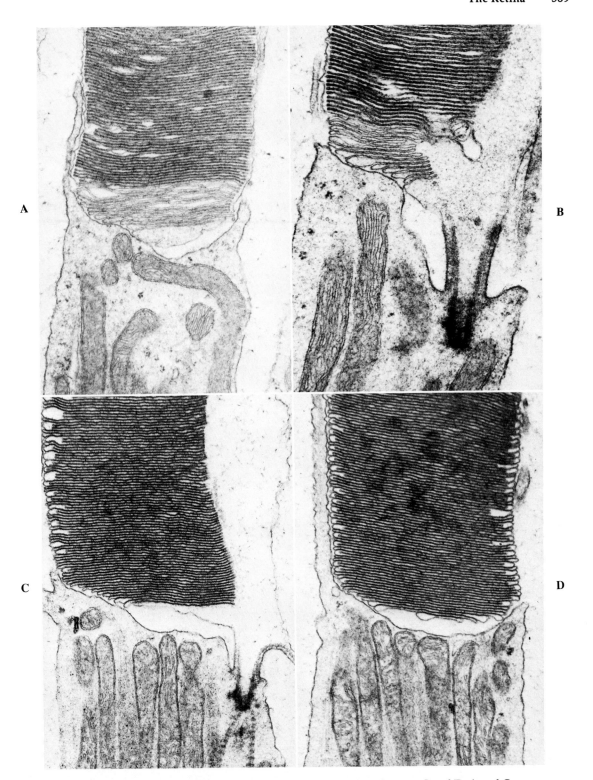

FIG. 19-8   Bases of outer segments of rhesus rods, **A** and **B**, and cones, **C** and **D**. **A** and **C** are cut at right angles to **B** and **D**. Note plasma membrane infolding to form saccules in **A** (magnification × 37,000) and total separation of outer and inner segments in **B** (magnification × 30,000). Similar phenomena are observed in **C** (magnification × 22,500) and **D** (magnification × 25,000) except that almost all saccules are seen to connect with the plasma membrane.

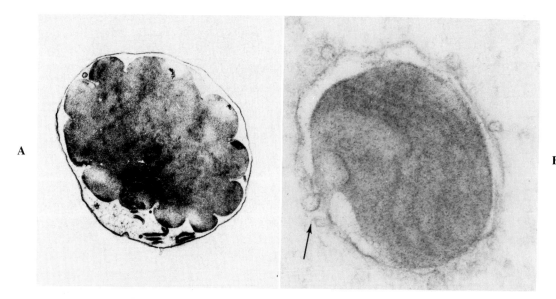

FIG. 19-9   A, Cross section of human rod outer segment. (Magnification × 40,000). **B,** Cross section of distal portion of outer segment of rhesus cone. Note plasma membrane infolding at arrow to form disc. (Magnification × 54,500.) (**A** from Cohen AI: Anat Rec 152:63, 1965.)

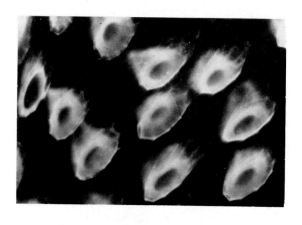

FIG. 19-10   Single fluorescent exposure with FITC filter set. Cone matrix domains prominent; rod matrix domains barely discernible. (Courtesy of J. G. Hollyfield, Ph.D.)

FIG. 19-11   Double exposure with FITC filters followed by rhodamine filter sets. Both rod and cone matrix domains are prominent. (Courtesy of J.G. Hollyfield, Ph.D.)

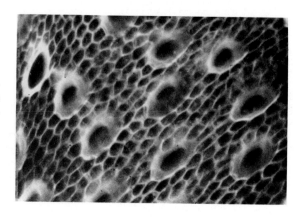

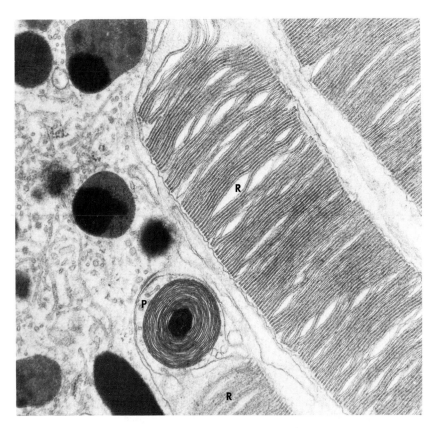

FIG. 19-12 Rod outer segments, R, abutting on pigmented epithelium of rhesus monkey. Note phagosome, P, forming at rod tip. (Magnification × 29,000.)

times occurring in the morning as with rods.[43] These studies point to disc shedding as a normal photoreceptor phenomenon. These results require that some rod and cone discs are replaced each day and further suggest that certain pathologic conditions may be explained by an imbalance in the production and destruction of discs. For example, in the RCS strain of rats in which an inherited receptor dystrophy occurs, Dowling and Sidman[35] observed accumulating discs and rhodopsin in the ocular ventricle during the onset of the pathologic process. However, this is by no means the typical inherited receptor dystrophy. In another receptor dystrophy, which occurs in mice, no membranes accumulate in this area. Both inherited lesions somewhat resemble the human disease called retinitis pigmentosa.

The functional significance of disc renewal and of the temporal differences in phagosome formation in rods and cones is unclear. There is a possibility that in the course of a normal exposure to light the radiation irreversibly denatures a certain fraction of the photopigment.

Possibly it is unsaturated lipid of the discs that is broken down. It has been shown in certain species that rods are surprisingly sensitive to damage by a prolonged exposure to light.[67,91]

Another interesting fact about photoreceptors in all species studied thus far is their high content of the free amino acid taurine. This seems to be concentrated at the level of their inner segments and cell bodies.[97] In a cat a diet deficient in taurine results in a loss of the photoreceptors, with cones succumbing first.[49] Moreover, it has been shown that when infant monkeys were raised on a commercial human milk formula (which in the past lacked taurine despite its high level of human milk) retinal cones deteriorated.[117] In some neurons taurine may have an osmoregulatory role. However, the actual role of taurine in photoreceptors is unknown.

Receptor outer segment
Pigment epithelium relations

Pigment epithelial cells are implicated in the ocular transport of vitamin A and its derivatives, and in most species the close approximation of the photoreceptor outer segments to the pigment epithelial cells of their processes is important for the most efficient regeneration of visual pigment. The regeneration of visual pigment is one factor in dark adaptation after the significant bleaching of such pigment. However, when substantial levels of visual pigment are bleached in isolated retinas free of PE, dark adaption produces not only a fairly rapid return of cone-initiated electrophysiologic response, but also a much slower (tens of minutes) return of rod response.

Where the apices of receptor outer segments approach the PE, they are well draped by long microvillous or sleevelike processes extending from these cells. In the inner aspect of the cells of the PE, and in their processes, are found numerous melanosomes. In some species, but not noticeably in mammals, these cytoplasmic granules move into and out of these processes in response to the intensity of light. In a state of light adaptation, when these particles are in pigment cell processes between outer segments, they obviously minimize the scattering of light from one receptor to another. However, it should be noted that by far the greatest amount of melanin pigment in the eye lies in numerous melanophores in the uveal coat. The bulk of absorption of stray light in the eye thus occurs in the latter, but some light is backscattered out of the eye. This is what permits the use of the ophthalmoscope and certain sophisticated photometric devices used in studying the dynamics of photopigment bleaching in the living eye.

The phenomenon of detachment of the retina consists of the physical separation of the retina from its close approximation to the PE. However, there is no convincing evidence for specialized membrane junctions between the photoreceptors and the latter cells. All the parameters that contribute to attachment are probably not known and many are not well understood, and the importance of different parameters may vary in different species. These parameters include the following:

1. Factors regulating the volume of the fluid in the ocular ventricle.
2. Acid mucopolysaccharides, known to be present in the fluid of the ocular ventricle, which could contribute to its viscosity or to the cohesion of neighboring membranes.
3. A barb action of the elongated melanosomes in the long microvilli from the PE.

It is well known that retinas are easily removed from some eyes (elderly human) but that others resist with such force that outer segments are torn from the photoreceptors and left behind adherent to the PE (many squirrels). An hour's dark adaptation facilitates the removal of some retinas (frog). Punctate retinal perforations in monkeys cause a rapidly spreading detachment in a retina otherwise removed with difficulty. When photoreceptors vanish in mice with inherited receptor dystrophy, after a time the remaining retina is detached with more difficulty than before.

The PE also has phagocytic functions. As noted earlier, portions of the tips of outer segments are ingested and digested in the PE.[52,134,136] The membrane of the outer segment heals over. It is not yet clear how this terminal fragmentation is accomplished. The morphologic evidence in one study[108] pointed to the active participation of the epithelial cells, because processes of the PE gave the appearance of pinching off the tips of the outer segments. However, in another study,[132] the morphologic evidence pointed to an independent mechanism in the receptor outer segments, because fragments seemed to be forming without the participation of the PE.

Another interesting relation of the PE to the outer segments has recently come to light. Laties et al.[70] noted that the relationship of the axis formed by the aligned inner and outer segments to the plane of the retina at the external limiting membrane was often not perpendicular. Indeed, this proved to vary progressively from the perpendicular as one examined retina farther and farther from that lying on the optic axis of the eye. An analysis of the optical aspects of the phenomenon by Laties and Enoch[69] revealed that the receptor axes are so tipped as to orient them to the exit pupil of the eye rather than to the center of the ocular sphere. This maximizes the ability of any one photoreceptor to capture light.

There is good evidence that during the act of accommodation, the contraction of the ciliary muscle drags the choroid and PE forward (see Chapter 11) and the retina likewise to some extent. This shifting is unequal because of the "tacking down" of the retina at the nerve head and possibly through the resistance of uveal vessels. However, this shearing could alter the orientation of receptor outer segments.

Finally, it has been known since the last century that the regeneration of bleached photopigment was facilitated by and often required the presence of the PE in close proximity to the outer segments. It is now clear that after bleaching of photopigment, the 11-*cis*-retinaldehyde has been converted to all-*trans*-retinaldehyde. There is then a conversion to all-*trans*-retinol by a dehydrogenase. The PE is the site where reoxidation of retinol to retinal occurs, as well as reisomerization of the all-*trans*-isomer to the 11-*cis*-isomer. Important carrier proteins are involved in moving these vitamin A derivatives between the photoreceptors and PE in both directions.[16,18]

Distribution of photoreceptors and other neurons within the retina
Central regions and foveas

Almost all retinas contain more than one variety of photoreceptor. While all-rod or all-cone retinas *may* exist, claims of the existence of such retinas must be taken with caution. In any event, the existence of photoreceptors with differing visual pigments within the class of rods or among cones[21] in some retinas raises questions as to how different types of photoreceptors are distributed in retinas.

Retinal regions usually are functionally specialized. This specialization may be inferred from the differences in the local relative concentrations of the varieties of receptors and other cells. One functional subdivision commonly considered is a distinction between regions with an organizational bias for detecting gross form and movements versus regions organizationally biased for inspecting detail. Regions biased for inspecting detail are richer in cones by virtue of containing thinner cones and more of them per unit area than elsewhere and more ganglion

cells per unit area as well. Such a region is termed a "central" region and usually is a circular patch of retina, as in the human, cat, and bird, but in some animals, such as ground squirrels, there is a central band running horizontally across the retina. This is sometimes called a visual streak. A more precise definition of "central" region, which makes the remainder of the retina "peripheral," includes physiologic and psychophysical, as well as neuroanatomic, distinctions. It is important to note that in terms of area, "central" regions may occupy a rather small portion of the total area of retinas. Thus in a conventional, nonphysiologic sense, much of the functional periphery of the retina is still physically rather central in the fundus. Physiologically, central regions tend to be free of major blood vessels and in certain retinas even capillaries. In the human the extent of the cone-rich area is about 5.5 mm in diameter, and it tends to be variably demarked by the presence of yellow, nonphotolabile carotenoids in photoreceptor axons and some inner retina cells.[106,107] The pigment is largely zeaxanthin.[48] These pigments give the region the name, *macula lutea*. It therefore is referred to as the macular region. The intensity of the yellow pigment, which has some effect on color perception, varies considerably from individual to individual.

In some species, including humans, the center of the cone-rich region contains a pit or fovea. In the human the full depression occupies about 5 degrees of arc or about 1.5 mm on the retina (Fig. 19-13). In the center of the fovea is a region of 54 minutes of arc or about 260 μm in extent on the retina, and in this region the

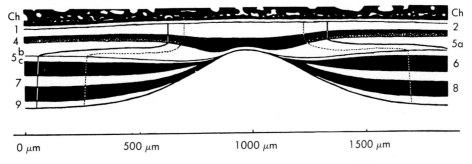

FIG. 19-13 Semidiagrammatic representation of changes in relative thickness and position of retinal layers brought about by foveal excavation in adult human eye; peculiar topical functional relationship of photoreceptor layer, 2, and deeper layers, 4 to 9, caused by latter's displacement owing to formation of fovea. Broken lines indicate rodless territory; white dots, rod cell nuclei; solid lines, region of high photoreceptor (rods plus cones) density. (From Polyak S: The retina, Chicago, University of Chicago Press, 1941.)

only photoreceptor type present, in terms of form, are cones. This region is sometimes called the central fovea or foveola. Although a general definition of "central" fitting all vertebrates would make the macula the central region of the human retina, most physiologists confine "central" to the fixation center or foveola in the human and other foveate primates. Cones in this region have the finest diameters of the retinal cones (1.5 μm), and this is the region of the highest concentration of cones in the retina. Foveas occur in other primates and in certain fish and birds. Certain predatory birds may have a fovea in each of two well-separated central retinal regions. Functionally the fovea is the position of the retina to which, by turning the eyeball, a person brings the image of whatever is of greatest psychologic interest in the visual field. To perform an inspection of a static object, the eye, by small movements (saccades), moves successively to the foveal position the elements in the image of the visual field essential to discrimination and evaluation, such as borders of contrast. Anatomically, the retina in the central fovea consists entirely of the outer and inner segments of the photoreceptors, the photoreceptor cell bodies, and the intervening glial cell processes. The axons of the photoreceptors, the so-called Henle fibers, are swept horizontally and leave the foveal area. The terminals of foveal cones, the horizontal neurons and bipolar neurons with which they interact, and those amacrine cells and ganglion cells that receive information from the foveal cones are centrifugally and laterally displaced so that, in the foveolar region, all these elements are missing, and they are minimized elsewhere in the fovea. Although qualitatively it is easy to imagine that this arrangement minimizes possible disturbing effects in the light path for this critical area, no satisfactory quantitative statement of this advantage has been forthcoming, probably because the extent to which tissue in front of the fovea would scatter light is hard to estimate. The foveola is surrounded by a parafoveal region, and this by a perifoveal region. The circle defined by the limits of the parafovea has a diameter of 2500 μm and that defined by the limits of the perifovea, a diameter of 5500 μm.

If one imagines a vertical line passing through the central fovea, thus separating nasal retina from temporal retina, axons from ganglion cells of the temporal retina will project to the DLGN and superior colliculus on the same side of the brain as the eye, whereas ganglion cells from the nasal half of the retina will cross in the optic chiasm and terminate in the DLGN and superior colliculus of the contralateral brain. A recent finding that is important in understanding retinal pathology is that the expected ipsilateral projecting cells in and around the fovea can generate 2° to 3° of bilateral representation in the geniculocortical pathways, because they are intermingled with contralaterally projecting cells on the nasal side of the foveal pit. This helps explain the phenomenon of macular sparing in unilateral damage to the visual pathway.[73]

In the human retina most of our early knowledge of the quantitative distribution of rods and cones was based on a horizontal section across the retina (Fig. 19-14) from Østerberg.[98] However, recent studies by Farber et al.[40] and Curcio et al.,[25] while confirming the general distribution drawn from Østerberg's report, supply more precise information for all retinal regions. The main points to note are as follows. The adult human retina has about 80 to 110 million rods and 4 to 5 million cones. Cone numerical density peaks in the fovea at about 199,000 cones/mm^2 (but with much higher or lower values in particular individuals) and then falls off sharply in all directions, although there is some concentration of cones along the horizontal meridian, particularly in the nasal retina. Cones continue to be present even in the most peripheral retina, although color perception in this region is very poor. The area for useful color vision in humans has a diameter of 9 mm centered on the fovea. Three types of primate cones with pigments showing peak absorption in the yellow, green, or blue have been identified by spectrophotometry (Chapter 22) and the genes for the human cone pigments have been identified.[87] Good evidence suggests that the rod-free center of the fovea (foveola) may be deficient in cones with a peak absorption in the blue.[1] The human rod numerical density peaks in a somewhat elliptical ring whose long axis parallels the horizontal meridian with the nerve head as one focus of the ellipse and the macula as the other. The highest rod concentration (ca. 160,000/mm^2) along this configuration occurs in the superior retina. It is important to realize that when light levels are in the photopic range of cone function, their activity tends to command all retinal output, even in animals where cones total but a few percent of rods. Color vision may differ in lower primates and other diurnal mammals but it both occurs and may be of high quality in birds, reptiles, amphibians, and fish. The region of the optic nerve head has no retina or photoreceptors and therefore produces a blind spot in the subject's visual field. Many retinas exhibit cones in animals in

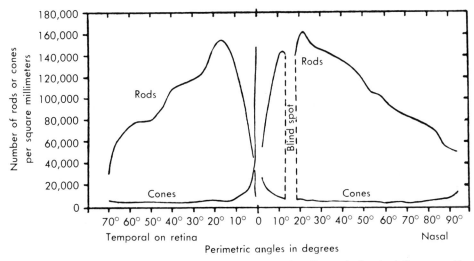

FIG. 19-14   Distribution of rods and cones in human retina. Instead of retinal distances, Østerberg's values for corresponding perimetric angles are given. Although approximate only,
especially at higher angles, such values are more useful in practice than distances on the retina. Note distribution of rods and cones on nasal side in and near fovea, not given on this
graph, would be approximately the same as distribution on temporal side of retina, which is
seen on left of vertical passing through 0 degree on angle scale. (After Østerberg; from Pirenne M: Vision and the eye, London, Pilot Press, 1948.)

which there is little or no evidence of color vision. Thus the more general function of cones
probably relates to vision at higher levels of
light.

In the interpretation of analyses of the INL in
the literature, one may be misled by an unhappy
tendency to refer to this layer as "the bipolar
layer." Although it certainly contains the somal
regions of these neurons, it also contains those
of horizontal and amacrine neurons, interplexiform neurons, rare "displaced" ganglion cells,
and the somal regions of the glial cells of Müller.
If cell counts were to be made of this layer by
measuring the concentrations of cell nuclei
across the retina, they would lump these cell varieties together on an unwarranted assumption
that their relative concentrations are the same
across the retina. Not only would one like to
have individual data for the frequency of these
individual cell varieties, but as there are different types of horizontal, bipolar, and amacrine
cells, one ultimately would want to have figures
for their individual distributions. Although
technical problems at the moment make it difficult to obtain such data, it is important to recognize the existence of the problem.

The situation for the distribution of ganglion
cells is somewhat better, because, apart from
some astroglial nuclei, the neuronal nuclei in
this region belong only to ganglion cells and
"displaced" amacrines. However, there are several varieties of ganglion cells in terms of size
and distribution of processes. Some information
does exist as to their distribution; thus it is fair to
state that the macula region in the human retina
is rich in small ganglion cells and that, by comparison to the concentration of cones in this region, it seems likely that there are enough small
ganglion cells to permit the consideration that
each could receive information via intermediate
cells from a rather small population of cones. A
chain of information transmission in which the
ratio of receptors connected via intermediates to
ganglion cells approaches 1:1 is what one might
idealize for a region of high-detail discrimination. In contrast to low information convergence
in such regions, in other retinal regions there is
a high ratio of rods to ganglion cells and, as expected, a high sensitivity to detecting light but
poor form discrimination.

SYNAPTIC CONNECTIONS OF THE RETINA

Receptor terminals fall into two morphologic
categories,[21] spherules and pedicles. As these
terms imply, spherules are small and round and
pedicles are large and have flat bases facing the
rest of the OPL. In humans and in those other
mammals having clearly defined rods and
cones, rods end in spherules and cones in pedicles, but in many nonmammalian species both
rods and cones may terminate in pedicles, with
those of rods usually being smaller. In some

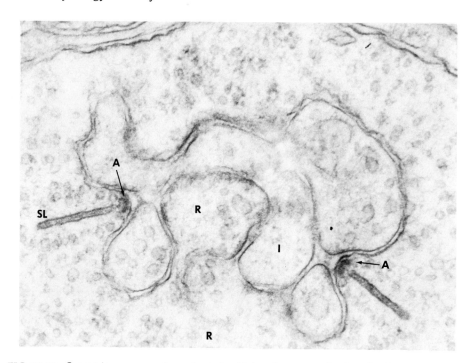

FIG. 19-15 Synaptic processes invaginated within a human rod spherule, R. Note synaptic lamella, SL; arciform densities beneath lamellae, A *(arrows);* invaginated neurites, I. (Magnification × 74,500.)

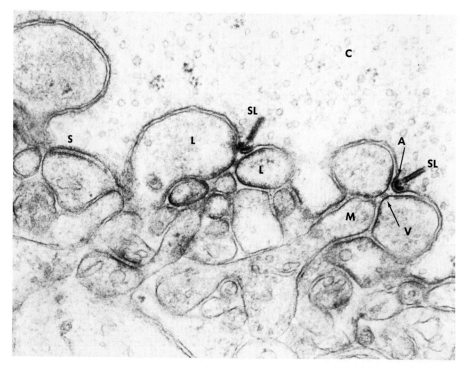

FIG. 19-16 Synaptic region of pedicle of cone, C, of rhesus monkey. Note synaptic lamellae, SL, and underlying arciform density, A. Synapses may be partially invaginated triads that involve two lateral, L, and one medial, M, component, probably of horizontal cell and bipolar cell origin, respectively, or superficial synapses, S, probably from another type of bipolar neuron. Also note small circular profiles in synaptic cleft, V *(arrow).* (Magnification × 60,000.)

mammals, such as gray squirrels, all the terminals seem to be pedicles, and in others, for example, mice, in which almost all receptors seem rodlike, some receptors ending in pedicles are found among those ending in spherules.

Processes of horizontal cells and bipolar neurons are deeply invaginated in rod spherules (Fig. 19-15), but only superficially invaginated into the bases of pedicles (Fig. 19-16). The typical appearance of invaginated synaptic processes has a pair of horizontal cell processes flanking a bipolar dendrite lying between but slightly vitread to them (triads). Lying within the receptor terminal, in a plane that passes between the contacting horizontal processes, is a membranous lunate plate, or synaptic lamella. This is often called a synaptic ribbon because of its appearance in sections. Underlying the lunate plate, paralleling its concavity, is the so-called arciform density. The receptor terminal is full of synaptic vesicles, and a halo of these surrounds the lamella, whose function is unknown. Cone terminals also have superficial, noninvaginated synaptic contacts on their base and, in addition, send out processes ending on nearby cone pedicles and spherules. Recent evidence suggests that these interreceptor contacts[100] contain a so-called "gap" junction, which in some neuronal junctions permit the electrotonic spread of current between the cells they join. In addition, just sclerad to the external limiting membrane (ELM), short processes from foveolar cone inner segments contact some neighboring cones, and elsewhere in the macular region cone-to-rod contacts are seen, as well as some rod-rod contacts. It is not yet clear whether these, like the interterminal contacts, contain gap junctions.

A recent summary of retinal neuronal connections is that of Stell,[112] and a generalized diagram of synaptic connections in the vertebrate retina is given in Figure 19-17.[32] However, the diagram omits the interplexiform neuron whose cell body is in the INL. This cell type receives inputs in the IPL and to project to the OPL. Horizontal cells occur in the outer portion of the INL and are neurons whose processes are disposed in a manner suggesting a role in the horizontal integration of retinal activity. Their activity has been studied in very few species. In fish there may be three layers of these cells, and these are further distinguished by their large size and the presence of putative electrotonic junctions that join cells in the same layer to one another and may permit the spread of current from one cell to another. Some physiologic evidence in turtles also suggests such linkage of horizontal cells. In most species there seem to be at least two varieties of these cells. Sometimes only one type has a well-defined axon, but this may be a technical problem. Mammalian horizontal cells are conventionally neuronal in appearance, and there is no anatomic evidence suggesting that they are electronically linked. It is now well established[11] that primate retinas have two types of horizontal cells (H1 and H2), which have dendrites forming paired or triadic contacts with cones. The H1 horizontal cell contacts both rods and cones. In rod spherules the synapse made by the bipolar dendrite tends to be flanked by processes originating in horizontal cells.

Turning to bipolars, there is considerable variation in different species as to form and connectivity. In primates cone pedicles may be in synaptic contact with four varieties of cone bipolars. One of these, the invaginating, midget bipolar, has its dendrites enter the triads, where it forms the central elements. There also are flat midget bipolars, so called because their contacts on the pedicle base are not invaginated, and diffuse bipolars, both flat and invaginating.[62]

All primate cones are contacted by at least one invaginating and one flat midget bipolar and commonly by other cone bipolars, but the contacts of one midget bipolar seem confined to one cone. The terminals of the invaginating cone bipolars, midget or diffuse, are located in the vitread half of the IPL, whereas those of the flat bipolars, midget or diffuse, are located in the sclerad half of the IPL. In addition, there are rod bipolars whose dendrites synapse in the triads of a group of spherules. Moreover, there is an overlap of synaptic fields of adjacent rod bipolars. All rod bipolars have their synaptic terminals in the vitread half of the IPL. In other species, certain fish, for example, single bipolars contacting both rods and cones have been reported. In certain fish, central processes of some triads have proved to originate in a particular class of horizontal cells; thus central triad processes are not invariably of bipolar origin.

Despite the fact that in higher primates rods outnumber cones by about 16 or 17 to 1, there is a greater convergence of rods than of cones onto bipolar neurons, and this, combined with the saturation of rod signaling in these species at modest light levels, means that under many situations, cone-initiated activity can dominate neuronal signaling even where rods locally outnumber cones in the retina. Although the light levels at which rod signaling saturates may vary among species, cone signaling sometimes can

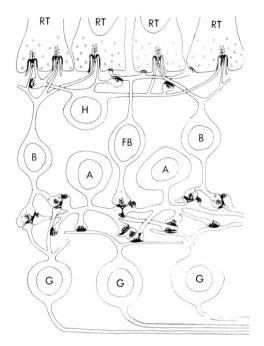

FIG. 19-17 Summary diagram of arrangements of synaptic contacts found in vertebrate retinas. In outer synaptic layer, processes from bipolar, B, and horizontal cells, H, penetrate into invaginations in receptor terminals, RT, and terminate near synaptic ribbons, lamellae, of receptor. Processes of flat bipolar cells, FB, make superficial contacts on bases of some receptor terminals. Horizontal cells make conventional synaptic contacts onto bipolar dendrites and other horizontal cell processes (not shown). Since horizontal cells usually extend farther laterally in outer synaptic layer than do bipolar dendrites, distant receptors can presumably influence bipolar cells via horizontal cells. In inner synaptic layer, two basic synaptic pathways are suggested. Bipolar terminals may contact one ganglion cell dendrite and one amacrine process at ribbon synapses (left side of diagram) or two amacrine cell, A, processes (right side of diagram). When latter arrangement predominates in a retina, numerous conventional synapses between amacrine processes (serial synapses) are observed, and ganglion cells, G, are contacted mainly by amacrine processes (right side of diagram). Amacrine processes in all retinas make synapses of conventional type back onto bipolar terminals (reciprocal synapses). (From Dowling JE: Invest Ophthalmol 9:655, 1970.[32])

dominate retinal activity even where cones are but 2% to 3% of the photoreceptors.

Before considering the terminations of these bipolar varieties in the IPL, since both amacrine cell processes and dendrites of ganglion cells are involved in these junctions, one must consider the disposition of the two latter cell varieties. An amacrine cell is a neuron with no morphologically definable axon. In most cases the somal regions of these cells lie at the inner aspect of the INL. From the soma of the cell, an inwardly directed process arises that simply branches and rebranches into finer processes. If these occur at a fairly precise horizontal level, the cell is said to show a stratified disposition of processes and may be unistratified or bistratified, depending on whether the processes spread on one or two levels. Stratified amacrine cells tend to be moderately branched. Amacrine cells also may exhibit a diffuse or nonstratified but highly branched dispersion of their processes with the horizontal extent of the volume of spreading being wide or narrow. Another variety is "displaced" in the sense that its soma occurs in the layer of ganglion cells rather than in the inner aspect of the INL, and its principal process is then directed outward. Some amacrine cells possess large, dense core vesicles in their cytoplasm and processes, and these probably correspond to cells that histochemical studies reveal to contain dopamine. Some of the recently described interplexiform neurons of the fish and cebus monkey (a new-world monkey) have OPL terminals containing dopamine.[34]

The ganglion cells, large or small, also may be classified by how their dendritic expanses are distributed—unistratified, bistratified, multistratified, or diffuse—and like the amacrine cells, some ganglion cells are "displaced" by having their somas occur near amacrine somas in the INL. In one species the axons of these "displaced" ganglion cells have been reported to terminate in a distinctive region of the optic tectum. Ganglion cells may be small cells of the midget variety, which sometimes contact but one midget bipolar. Thus a color-coded path could exist from a single cone to this midget ganglion cell via a midget bipolar. Of the larger ganglion cells, there is something of a spectrum, in that from one or more levels of fairly precise stratifications of dendrites, one can go to a single, thicker stratification of dendrites (diffusely stratified) and to a partly globular disposition of dendrites (diffuse).

In birds it is quite certain that centrifugal fibers from the isthmooptic nucleus of the midbrain enter the retina via the optic nerve and synapse on certain amacrine cells.[24,33] Less secure evidence for centrifugal fibers exist for some amphibians and fish, but evidence for the existence of such a system in mammals is exceedingly thin.

The analysis of synaptic connections in the inner plexiform layer is facilitated by the fact that cells depolarizing to light "off" appear to have their connections in the outer (sclerad) half of the IPL, while those depolarizing to light "on" appear to have their connections in the inner (vitread) half. Cells responding both at on and off have terminals in both regions. Anatomically, the analysis is additionally facilitated by the fact that the terminals of bipolar neurons are distinctive at the electron microscope level. The bipolar axon branches to some extent, and the branches end in large "bags" filled with synaptic vesicles. A number of synaptic ribbons, strongly resembling those in photoreceptors, occur at various points in each bipolar terminal perpendicular to and against the cell membrane. In a given section the plane of each lamella or ribbon in the terminal passes between two, closely opposed, contacting processes on the adjacent outer surface of the terminal. Such an arrangement is termed a dyad; however, serial reconstructions of a retinal *volume* may suggest more than two postsynaptic elements in the area. The two contacting processes in a dyad may contain synaptic vesicles and therefore may originate in amacrine cells, or one may contain vesicles but the other may be free of them and be identifiable as a dendrite originating in a ganglion cell (Fig. 19-18). Often a single vesicle-filled process is seen to make contact with a bipolar terminal, and the synaptic structure suggests that, in this case, the bipolar is postsynaptic. Since this presynaptic amacrine process may sometimes branch off a process about to terminate in a dyad, or a presynaptic contact may even be seen *within* a postsynaptic amacrine element of a dyad, the possibility of inhibitory feedback of stimulation via a reciprocal synapse arrangement is suggested. Amacrine-to-amacrine synapses frequently are seen in the IPL, and in certain species serial chains of inter-amacrine synapses are seen. Four or five processes may be involved in such a chain, but it is not clear how many cells are involved. Short serial chains sometimes may be seen in the periph-

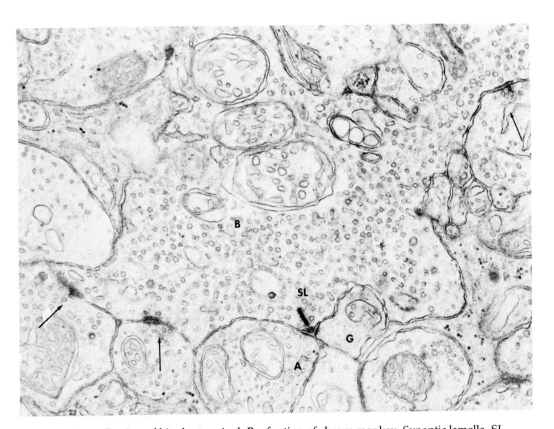

FIG. 19-18 Portion of bipolar terminal, B, of retina of rhesus monkey. Synaptic lamella, SL, indicates "dyad" synapse with adjacent postsynaptic processes from an amacrine, A, and ganglion, G, cell. Amacrine cell contacts *(arrows)* that are presynaptic to the bipolar are also evident. (Magnification × 26,000.)

eral retina of primates. Finally, processes of amacrine cells often are seen to terminate on the outer aspects of the somas of ganglion cells and on their principal dendrites.

A statistical analysis of the frequency of amacrine-amacrine versus amacrine-ganglion dyads and other amacrine synapses per given area of the IPL in sections supports the impression obtained from Golgi and methylene blue studies that retinas proportionally richer in amacrine cells (pigeons and rabbits) have a proportionally greater extent of the IPL volume that is devoted to amacrine cell processes and their synapses. This seems to correlate with the presence of more complex data-processing operations in these retinas. An impression also coming from such studies is that in some species there may exist a class of ganglion cells whose synaptic contacts are largely or even exclusively with amacrine cells. There is no evidence that the primate retina falls into such a group, although it is likely that different varieties of primate ganglion cells differ both as to the kinds of amacrine and bipolar cells with which they interact and in the frequency of contacts they make with such cells.

Some ganglion cells in the bovine, rabbit, and dolphin retinas have been reported to possess collaterals making intraretinal synapses.[28] More recently collateral and other synapses on nerve fibers and cell bodies in the ganglion cell and nerve fiber layer have been reported in the rabbit.[56] A similar picture seems to be emerging for primate retinas.[63] In primates many of the fibers involved are immunoreactive to antibodies for γ-aminobutyric acid (GABA). This additional synaptic zone remains to be fully evaluated both as to the generality of its occurrence and functional significance.

Retinal synaptic mechanisms and putative chemical neurotransmitters

Before entering into a discussion of the information obtained from studying the electrical activity of retinal cells, it is worth summarizing what is known of synaptic mechanisms in the retina. The photoreceptors have terminals rich in synaptic vesicles and evidence strongly indicates that the transmitter of the photoreceptor is glutamate, an excitatory (depolarizing) amino acid. Interphotoreceptor contacts between cones, or rods and cones, have frequently been noted[21] and appear to include gap junctions,[100] indicating the possibility of electrotonic interactions between these cells. Evidence for such coupling between cones in the retina of the

turtle has been presented.[7] The evidence is quite strong that horizontal, bipolar, and ganglion cells possess receptors for glutamate.[83] Thus glutamate may be the basic molecule involved in the most direct vertical path of communication in the retina.[82] There appear to be subtypes of glutamate receptors as defined by their differential reactivity to various glutamate analogs. For some of these subtypes the responsivity of a cell to glutamate may be strongly influenced by the presence of certain cofactors (e.g., glycine) and the cell's state of polarization. Particular groups of neurons of normally positioned or "displaced" amacrine cells may contain one or more putative transmitters or neuromodulators[36] such as acetylcholine (acting at nicotinic or muscarinic receptors on target cells), glycine, taurine, dopamine, serotonin, or γ-aminobutyric acid (GABA).[77] These presumably function in modulating the photoreceptor, bipolar, ganglion cell information stream. Depending on the species, interplexiform neurons[34,77] whose cell bodies lie in the IPL but which have targets in the OPL may contain dopamine, glycine, or GABA. They appear to modulate horizontal cell activity and possibly photoreceptor output in the OPL as a function of events in the IPL. In addition, various neuroactive peptides may occur in amacrine cells, varying somewhat with species.[12,60] These include substance P, neurotensin, enkephalin, glucagon, and cholecystokinin. Enzymes for the synthesis of the indoleamine, melatonin, have been located in the photoreceptors and cone bipolars of the human and other retinas.[125] Melatonin and dopamine may have diurnally regulated interactions in the retina and with cells of the pigment epithelium. In addition to possible synaptic involvement, these agents may have paracrine roles, such as influencing the disposition of melanosomes in the processes of pigment epithelial cells, the length of cones in certain fish, as well as a possible influence on disc shedding from photoreceptor outer segments. Another molecule of recent interest as a neuromodulator is adenosine. Receptors for adenosine have been located on certain neurons in both the inner and outer retina, including displaced amacrine cells containing acetylcholine or GABA.[9]

The action of a neurotransmitter or neuromodulator, promoting excitation or inhibition, is both a parameter of the nature of the agent and of the membrane mechanisms determining the response of a particular cell to the agent. For example, the action of acetylcholine on skeletal muscle is excitatory, but its action on cardiac muscle is inhibitory.

Finally, when transmitter or neuromodulatory substances are released, it is obviously desirable to terminate their presence by enzyme action or other mechanisms after they have carried out their signaling function. Thus the glial cells of Müller appear to take up and metabolize glutamate. Light can cause the release of dopamine.[64] Excess released dopamine is recaptured at specialized reuptake sites on dopaminergic cells.

Electrical activity and information processing by retinal neurons

To attempt to discern how the retina processes visual information,[14] one ideally studies the activity of specific cells of different types in specific retinal areas and relates their responses to specific spatial and temporal stimulus patterns in the visual field of the animal. A recent summary of this approach is given by Dowling.[32] The electrical activity of individual cells can be recorded by intracellular electrodes and sometimes by extracellular electrodes while an animal is held in a frame with its eyes immobilized and with the stimuli projected onto a screen whose surface includes the visual field of the animal. Any portion of the receptor mosaic where appropriate stimuli from the visual field evoke or modify responses from a visual system neuron under investigation is referred to as part of the "receptive field" of that cell. This is a physiologic concept. The cell in question may be at any level in the chain of nerve cells processing visual information. It also is important to realize that there is considerable overlapping of receptive fields of cells near each other in the retina.

Within a cell's receptive field, one sometimes distinguishes physiologically distinct regions, such as a "center" and a "surround." When a small spot of light, at an intensity above background, is first positioned on the center and then on the surround, opposite responses are often elicited, with a diminished or absent response if the spot of light is expanded to stimulate simultaneously both center and surround. One also can see center-surround effects with spots of "darkness," the illumination of the dark spot being well below that of the background. The spatial dimensions of receptive field centers are one determinant of spatial resolution—the smaller the center the smaller the possible spatial resolution.

Depending on the parameters being studied, the stimuli presented in receptive field analysis may have to be specified with reference to size, shape and orientation, intensity, contrast with background, hue, level and hue of background illumination, whether the stimulus is steady or in motion, and, if in notion, the direction and speed of motion.

Of course, one can obtain valuable information from the gross electrical responses of the retina. Electrodes across the eye "see" a summation of the various individual cell responses as attenuated by various geometries of the cells in the retina and by variations in the resistances in the extracellular pathways in the eye. The techniques can be refined by presenting stimuli to specific regions of the retina while supplying a steady background illumination to minimize responses from scattered light and by refining the data through computer averaging techniques. It also is possible to project gratings or other patterns directly on the retina, sometimes bypassing the optics of the eye. The results of such studies have provided much of the background for the advances in the study of information processing, and since they do not usually involve entering the eye, they can be carried out on intact animals or human subjects. These methods also have yielded valuable clinical information. Such gross electrical studies of the eye are described in Chapter 21. In addition, a duplex retina with its population of rods and cones modifies the signals reaching ganglion cells as a function of its adaptational state, that is to say, when it is dark adapted to a lower level of illumination or when it is light adapted to a more intense illumination. Altering the adaptational level involves both photochemical and electrochemical changes in the receptors and probably at subsequent retinal processing levels. These are treated in Chapter 16.

The most elegant methods for studying information processing involve intracellular recordings because of the certainty that information is being derived from single cells and because it is often possible to mark the cell from which the record was obtained by injecting dyes into the cell and then processing the tissue for histology. In the case of the fluorescent dye Procion yellow, the dye diffuses throughout the entire cell, and when processed tissue is observed by fluorescence microscopy, the form of the entire cell may be observed with a clarity matching that given by the Golgi method (Fig. 19-19). Cells also may be marked by injecting the enzyme horseradish peroxidase through the recording electrode. Much of the activity of this enzyme survives fixation, and an electron-dense

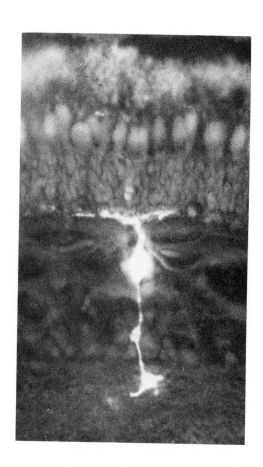

FIG. 19-19   Fluorescent bipolar cell in section of goldfish retina fixed after injection of Procion yellow subsequent to electrical recording. No magnification given. (From Kaneko A: J Physiol [Lond] 207:623, 1970.)

product can be generated to permit locating the cell and its processes in the electron microscope. Thus the electrical record may be associated with a particular cell type.

However, intracellular recording is greatly facilitated by having large cells available for penetration, and for this reason most of the intracellular data come from amphibians or fish.

Extracellular records of the activity of single cells are most easily obtained from large ganglion cells at the retinal face. It proves to be relatively difficult to obtain records from small ganglion cells. Thus it is important to remember in evaluating schemes of retinal data processing that they may be based on an unrepresentative sampling. Certain types or sizes of cells may less frequently or even never have been successfully observed by either the intracellular or extracellular methods.

The electrical activity of most retinal cells does not include "spikes," that is, propagated all-or-none discharges. The cell dimensions are such that disturbances spreading electrotonically from an active locus of the cell apparently are adequate for activating synaptic mecha-

nisms elsewhere in the same cell. However, some amacrine cells show some spiking discharges riding on depolarizations, and the ganglion cells, whose axons travel considerable distances, have conventional all-or-none behavior with propagated discharges.

It cannot be emphasized too strongly, in considering the following brief summation of the electrical activity of retinal cell types and retinal information processing, that the intracellular data are derived from a few species and from a field in which rapidly appearing reports of research sometimes bring rapid remodelings of working hypotheses. The description of electrical activity will begin with the receptors and follow the visual pathways, but it should be appreciated that, historically, the earliest cells studied were the ganglion cells of the retina and that much of the basic concept of receptive fields and their functional organization originated with studies of ganglion cell activity.

Before turning to what is known of the electrical responses of various retinal neurons, there are two important statements that can be made about the visual process. First, all evidence points to a functional organization in the retina and higher visual system that is relativistic and directed at discerning local contrasts that establish borders between areal elements in the complex image of the visual field, rather than mechanisms for assaying the absolute levels of light in local areas. Indeed, it is the case that a retinal locus receiving an image of an area perceived as "black" at a high level of illumination may actually be receiving a greater absolute quantity of light than a retinal locus receiving an image of an area perceived as "white" at a dim illumination if, in the former instance, the "black" area is receiving *relatively* much *less* light than its general surround and in the latter instance, if the "white" area is receiving *relatively* much *more* light than its surround. Moreover, the color perceived to be present in a patch will depend on the nature of the perceived color in its surround. The second important point is that the neural networks of the visual apparatus are more keyed to detecting fluctuations in the retinal image caused by changes in local relative intensity than for detecting steady displays. One source of this fluctuation is movement of the image of the visual field on the retina. The latter fact raises an important point regarding movements of the eye. In their normal function eyes cannot hold their positions for more than 1 or 2 seconds, and in the case of humans, when objects in the visual field are intentionally fixed on the fovea, they drift off, and continual corrections of eye position must be made to restore the intended positioning. Moreover, if by elaborate optical means the image of the visual field is made to hold its position on the retina despite eye movements, the image fades and is no longer seen by the observer. This explains why the shadows of the blood vessels of the retina are not in constant view in superimposition on the field of vision, because by having a fixed relation to the retina and the pathway of light, they are "adapted" out of the perceived image. The important point therefore is that a normal fine instability of the eye contributes to the normal visual process.

One of the major surprises in the field of retinal physiology was the discovery by a number of investigators[10,59,118] that vertebrate photoreceptors hyperpolarize when exposed to flashes of light. Not only was this the reverse of the well-known behavior of invertebrate photoreceptors, but it also seemed contrary to the conventional wisdom that nerve cells excite other nerve cells by releasing an appropriate quantity of transmitter agent when their terminals are depolarized, and it is certainly the case that pho-

toreceptors signal second-order cells. One may consider that the vertebrate photoreceptors normally are neither in absolute darkness nor in intense light. They signal shifts toward darkness by depolarizing and proportionally increasing their liberations of a chemical transmitter (neurohumor) and shifts toward light by hyperpolarizing and proportionally reducing the release of neurohumor.

It has been known by deduction from the findings of Hecht et al.[51] that single rods may be excited by a single quantum of light. What these workers actually found is that at the absolute threshold for vision, a flash bringing small numbers of quanta to the photoreceptors had some of these quanta captured by a group of rods of such a number that made it unlikely that any individual rod in the group caught more than one. Direct studies on individual rods by Baylor et al.[8] confirm this sensitivity to a single photon. One must concede that for a single rod to be excited by the capture of a single photon represents an exquisite sensitivity. If photoreceptors are exquisitely sensitive near their absolute threshold in total darkness, yet maximally releasing transmitter in this state, second-order cells are detecting a reduction in the amount of transmitter released against the largest possible background.

Is there evidence pointing to whether photoreceptors are diminishing or increasing their putative release of a putatively excitatory neurohumor in response to light? Such evidence has been sought in the electrical behavior of the second-order cells, the horizontal and bipolar cells, and seems to support the maximum release of transmitter in the dark. Another indication that photoreceptor transmitters are turning over maximally in the dark has been seen when comparing their terminals after exposure to the enzyme horseradish peroxidase in either the light or dark. The enzyme is taken up passively in vesicles that are known to be forming from terminal plasma membrane during synaptic activity. The retinas are fixed for electron microscopy. Some enzyme activity survives fixation and can be used to generate an electron-dense product that appears in recently formed terminal vesicles. Since peroxidase-containing vesicles prove to be much more numerous in photoreceptor terminals of dark retinas, this indicates a more vigorous synaptic activity in the dark.[101,102] There also is an interesting morphologic consequence of the enhanced release of synaptic vesicles in the dark. When such vesicles discharge by exocytosis, their membrane fuses with the synaptic membrane, which tends to increase its area because the process for recycling this membrane by endocytosis usually is slower than exocytosis. Thus the synaptic terminals of dark-adapted cones have a more complex morphology, that is deeper invaginations and larger surface area than in light-adapted cones.[103]

Studies with extracellular electrodes on retinal slices showed that in the dark a current is flowing into the outer segment from the rest of the photoreceptor. The effect of a flash of light is to diminish this dark current,[99] and a number of studies indicate that this diminution is achieved largely by decreasing the conductance for sodium ion across the plasma membrane of the outer segment. The extent of reduction of the dark current by light quanta seems adequate to explain the required modulation of transmitter output for receptor signaling. The light effect can be mimicked to a large extent by manipulating the concentration of external calcium ions, leading to the suggestion that calcium ions normally may be involved in the control of sodium current in the outer segment. By this hypothesis, light causes an increase in calcium activity in outer segments and calcium blocks the sodium channels. Recently, however, studies by Yau and Nakatani[127] and Matthews et al.[78] have made it evident that light causes a decrease rather than an increase in calcium activity in outer segments. It now seems evident that in the dark a low level of calcium ions enters outer segments along with sodium ions. This entry of calcium ions is countered by the activity of a counterporting mechanism that exchanges intracellular calcium and potassium for external sodium. Since, in the dark, calcium enters the cell along with sodium via the light-modulated channels, and as the exchange mechanism is not regulated by light, when the light-sensitive channel is closed, the continuing operation of the exchange mechanism decreases intracellular calcium.

The main agent in regulating the channels for the entry of sodium is cyclic guanosine monophosphate (cGMP). Photoreceptors are extraordinarily rich in cyclic GMP. Light causes losses of cyclic GMP by a complex mechanism called the cyclic GMP cascade, wherein bleached rhodopsin activates a nucleotide-binding protein, and this intermediate activates a cyclic GMP phosphodiesterase that hydrolyzes cyclic GMP to GMP. Patch clamp studies by Fesenko et al.[41] and by Nakatani and Yau[86] have shown that cyclic GMP can act on the inner face of the plasma membrane of the rod outer segment to open conductances. Yau and Nakatani[128] also have

shown that this effect is suppressed by light. It is therefore clear that a channel involved in transduction in rods, and also in cones,[19,50] is light-sensitive, because appropriate levels of cGMP keep it open in the dark, while the loss of cGMP through the activation of cGMP phosphodiesterase via the light-initiated cGMP cascade allows the channel to close. To complete the story, cGMP is regenerated from GTP by the activity of guanylate cyclase. Early studies showed that chelating calcium rapidly and massively increased cGMP levels in photoreceptors,[22] suggesting that this enzyme is inhibited by calcium. This proves to be the case and, in addition, the enzyme requires the presence of a protein cofactor.[61] The significance of the light-insensitive mechanism exchanging calcium and potassium for sodium is thus seen as a way to promote the resynthesis of cGMP by reducing the calcium level after light has caused a loss of this cyclic nucleotide.

Recording from single rods of a salamander, Bader et al.[3] found a dark membrane potential of about −45 mV, which could be driven to −75 mV by a bright flash. At bright flash intensities, a sharp transient hyperpolarization was seen initially, which then fell to a plateau of lesser hyperpolarization. Control of the membrane potential by injecting current showed that the reversal or blocking potential for the light response was about 0 mV.

Although the alteration by light of a membrane conductance to sodium in outer segment largely explains potential changes in receptors, certain complexities seem to require the existence of voltage-controlled conductances, possibly to potassium and calcium, in as yet unknown locations in the cell, and Fain et al.[37,38] have presented evidence to support this view. Werblin[123] has presented evidence for a voltage-induced regenerative hyperpolarization in rods. If present in cones, such a property could help explain how adequate signals reach the distant terminals of foveal cones.

Intracellular recordings from amphibian rods and cones by Norman and Werblin[92] have revealed differences that to a first approximation are likely to be reflected in the differential behavior of mammalian rods and cones, in which such recordings are not yet feasible. Both rods and cones hyperpolarize to light flashes, but rods recover more slowly than do cones from bright flashes presented against a dark background, and rods have a lower absolute threshold to flashes presented against a dark background. The magnitude of the response of both rods and cones is graded over 3 log units of intensity of light flashes presented against a dark background. With brighter flashes, both show amplitude saturation (although the rise times to reach these amplitude maxima continue to decrease with increasing flash intensities). However, when light flashes are presented against illuminated backgrounds, the threshold for the response of cones is raised in relation to the background intensity, but they continue to respond over 3 log units of intensity above background; that is, their response curve is simply shifted. On the other hand, the response of rods to flashes against illuminated backgrounds also is elevated in threshold but is very poorly responsive to increasing flash intensity; that is, their response is essentially saturated. Attwell[2] has recently reviewed factors regulating the synaptic output of photoreceptors. Isolated whole individual rods of the tiger salamander show time constants of voltage response to injected current that are 170 times those of intact rods in this retina. This appears to relate to the existence of extensive gap junctions between the rod inner segments in this retina, which allows the diffusion of current actively developed in a single rod. In primate retinas gap junctions between photoreceptors involve rod-and-cone terminals, as well as cone-to-cone terminals, but no rod-to-rod contacts. Although small junctions via processes occasionally are seen at the bases of inner segments that involve rods, or rods with cones, or cones, it is not established that these are gap junctions.

Nunn et al.[93] used glass suction electrodes to record responses of individual cones in the isolated retina of the monkey, *Macaca fascicularis*. The cones responded in one half to one third the time for rod responses in the same retina. This property may contribute to cone-initiated vision having a faster response time than rod-initiated vision, while the latter can integrate more discrete events over time before responding, a feature perhaps useful in dim light vision. These receptor properties may be based, in part, on the fact that most discs in rod outer segments appear to be isolated from the plasma membrane, whereas most cone discs are connected to this membrane.

The more rapid recovery of cones than rods to light flashes often has been held to account partly for the ability of cone-initiated vision to more readily follow higher flicker frequencies of bright (photopic) light than can rod vision in the dim (scotopic) light range. However, under certain circumstances it has been shown that the rods of the skate,[46] and possibly those of humans,[23] can adapt and begin to follow fast flicker.

A further aspect of receptor physiology has been discerned by potassium-sensitive electrodes. These reveal that the onset of light causes a decrease in extracellular potassium in the ventricular space about the outer and inner limbs of the photoreceptors. This produces a greater hyperpolarization of the apical (ventricle-facing) aspect of the pigment epithelial cells than of their basal aspect and creates a transepithelial potential, which in rod-dominated retinas persists beyond the termination of the flash. The effect is of short duration and hard to detect in cone-dominated retinas, probably because of temporal differences in the recovery processes of rods and cones. This potential, variably attenuated by some opposing retinal potentials in different species, largely accounts for the c wave of the electroretinogram (ERG). The use of current source-density analysis and potassium electrodes has also revealed that in amphibians approximately 95% of the total membrane conductance of Müller cells is located in their end feet, which form the retinal face on the vitreous.[21,89,90] These cells appear to be potent spatial buffers for potassium resulting from light-induced neuronal activity. The action of potassium on the Müller cells appears related to the origin of the b-wave of the electroretinogram.[122] Almost all the potassium ion entering these glial cells would be shunted out of the cell onto the face of the retina.[90]

The earliest records of potentials from what we now know to be horizontal cells were obtained from fish and were termed "S" (slow) potentials. These fell into two groupings—one sensitive to color ("C" type) in that the cell's membrane potential shifted in the hyperpolarizing or depolarizing direction as a function of wavelength and another ("L" type) whose membrane potential when disturbed by luminosity of any wavelength always was displaced in the hyperpolarizing direction. In the mudpuppy, an amphibian with small eyes but with extraordinarily large retinal cells, Werblin and Dowling[124] were able to record from all principal types of retinal neurons and then mark the cells (Fig. 19-20). All horizontal cells hyperpolarized to light. However, from later studies in other species it is now clear that while horizontal cells with a sole input from rods or a single type of cone will hyperpolarize to white light, others subserving cone vision may depolarize to some wavelengths and hyperpolarize to others; thus their inputs come from more than one type of cone. Horizontal cells only sensitive to light intensity or luminosity are called "L" type. These have been well studied in the cat.[109,110] Those

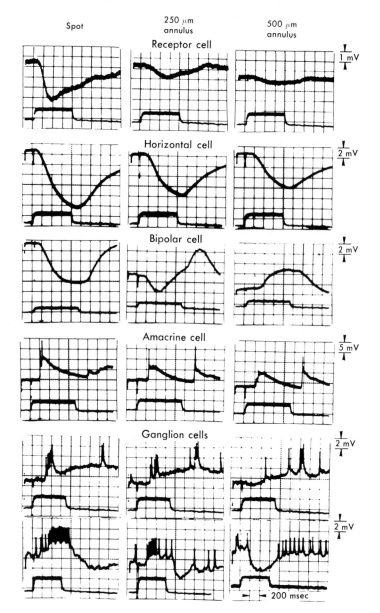

FIG. 19-20 Recordings show major response types in *Necturus* retina and difference in response of a given cell type to a spot and to anuli of 250 and 500 μm radii. Receptors have relatively narrow receptive fields, so that annular stimulation evokes very little response. Small potentials recorded on annular stimulation were probably due to scattered light. Horizontal cell response over broader region of retina, so that annular stimulation with same energy as that of the spot (left column) does not reduce response significantly (right columns). Bipolar cell responds by hyperpolarization when center of its receptive field is illuminated (left column). With central illumination maintained (right trace; note lowered baseline of recording and elevated baseline of stimulus trace in records) annular illumination antagonizes sustained polarization elicited by central illumination, and response of opposite polarity is observed. In middle column, anulus was so small that it stimulated center and periphery of field simultaneously. Amacrine cell was stimulated under same conditions as was bipolar cell and gave transient responses at both onset and cessation of illumination. Its receptive field was somewhat concentrically organized, given a larger on response to spot illumination and a larger off response to annular illumination of 500 μm radius. When an anulus of 250 μm radius, cell responded with large responses at both on and off. Ganglion cell shown in upper row was of transient type and gave bursts at both on and off. Its receptive field organization was similar to that of amacrine cell illustrated. Ganglion cell shown in lower row was of sustained type. It gave a maintained discharge of impulses with spot illumination. With central illumination maintained, large annular illumination (right column) inhibited impulse firing for duration of stimulus. Smaller anulus (middle column) elicited brief depolarization and discharge of impulses at on, and brief hyperpolarization and inhibition of impulses at off. (From Werblin FS, Dowling JE: J Neurophysiol 32:339, 1969.)

whose polarity is color sensitive are called "C" type and have been studied in animals with good color vision like fish.[58,113] Horizontal cells are often coupled by electrotonic "gap" junctions, and their effects often feed back on to cones, possibly to rods, and perhaps feed forward on to bipolars. However, to return to *Necturus*, bipolar cells exhibited a behavior that was influenced by the spatial distribution of light in their receptive field. This field could be subdivided into a central and peripheral region. When a spot of light fell solely in the central region of their receptive field, the membrane potentials of many of the bipolar cells shifted in the depolarizing direction, the remainder in the hyperpolarizing direction.

These cells have come to be defined as depolarizing and hyperpolarizing bipolars on the basis of this response to light on their centers. These same bipolar classes can be viewed in another way. In one class, light on their centers causes depolarization, where in the other, darkness on their centers causes depolarization. When a test spot of light (or darkness) is enlarged to include the surround of the receptive field, the previous center response is antagonized, thus contrast between a center and its surround enhances the center response in either class. Thus bipolar neurons are responding to contrast, not simply light intensity, and these center versus surround phenomena are also evident at the ganglion cell level. In the photopic range spatial detail is best detected by brightness contrast rather than color contrast. The best detectors of brightness contrast are red or green cones, the relatively sparce blue cones less so. Brightness contrast is poorly detected by rods operating in the scotopic range. In recognizing temporal detail, i.e., to see whether a light is flickering, luminance contrast is also better than color contrast. The two bipolar classes, depolarizing and hyperpolarizing, may function as part of the system discriminating relatively bright centers in dark surrounds and the converse, dark centers in bright surrounds.

The likely anatomic basis for the center of this receptive field is the population of photoreceptors with which these bipolars are in direct synaptic contact, whereas the surround may represent another population of photoreceptors by which the bipolars are indirectly influenced, via horizontal neurons. In *Necturus* an anulus of light falling solely on the periphery exerted an effect on the center only when the latter was also illuminated, but in most retinas an effect of an anulus of light on a center is seen without center illumination and gives the opposite effect to center illumination.

The dichotomy of neurons represented by those that either depolarize or hyperpolarize to light has given rise to the description that the visual system contains "on" and "off" pathways as well as a terminology for indicating whether two linked neurons in an information chain both shift their polarity in the same or opposite directions in response to light. Neurons that depolarize in response to an increase in the intensity of light above background in their receptive field are termed "on" cells, whereas those that depolarize in response to the offset or diminution of light compared to background are termed "off" cells. Since light diminishes the sodium current entering photoreceptors, all photoreceptors hyperpolarize in response to increasing light and depolarize to diminishing light and are therefore "off" cells. Bipolars that depolarize to light are "on" cells, whereas those that hyperpolarize to light are "off" cells. As the latter mimic the polarization responses of photoreceptors, the synapse between them is said to be "sign conserving." Conversely, the synapse between photoreceptors and those bipolars that depolarize to light is termed "sign inverting." Because some types of bipolars possess dendrites that end exclusively within triads of cones (invaginating bipolars) and the dendrites of others end superficially on cones (flat bipolars), a suggestion has been advanced that these classes may be respectively identical with depolarizing and hyperpolarizing bipolars. However, some studies by Lasansky[68] in the salamander do not support this view. While cone-initiated "on" or "off" pathways contain several morphologic types of cone-driven bipolars and ganglion cells addressed by the latter,[114] the rod pathway is more complex. In the rabbit,[26,27] cat,[85] and primate[31] all rods connect with rod bipolars with a sign inverting synapse, i.e., these bipolars are depolarized in the light. This corrects an earlier view.[88] The rod-driven bipolar synapses with a particular amacrine cell, the AII amacrine, in a sign-conserving synapse. This specialized amacrine cell makes two types of output connections, one utilizing electrotonic gap junctions, the other chemical synapses. When this amacrine is depolarized at light "on," via its extensive gap junctions, it depolarizes "on" cone bipolars whose release of excitatory transmitter leads to "on" cone ganglion cells being depolarized. At the same time the depolarization of the AII amacrine activates inhibitory chemical synapses (apparently using glycine as a transmitter), which it makes with dendrites of cone ganglion cells of the "off" pathway. These cells thus hyperpolarize to light. When the rod bipolar is hyperpolarized in the dark, the AII amacrine is hyperpolarized. This produces a disinhibition (therefore depolarization) of the "off" cone ganglion cell plus the canceling of electrotonic depolarization of the "on" cone bipolar and therefore a canceling of the depolarizing input to the "on" cone ganglion cell. Thus cone information and rod information can feed through some of the same ganglion cells.

The two bipolar classes (depolarizing versus hyperpolarizing) likely differ in responsiveness to the same photoreceptor neurohumor, a possibility favored by the observation that only depolarizing bipolars lose their responsiveness in chloride-free media[79] or in the presence of the glutamate analogue 2-amino-4-phosphonobutyric acid (APB).[80] Hyperpolarizing bipolars lose their antagonistic surround only under these circumstances. However, the possibility of two different neurohumors has not been eliminated. The two bipolar classes may function in detecting relatively bright centers in darker surrounds, or the converse.

Intracellular recordings from cells identified as amacrine cells have been accomplished in the salamander *Necturus*, some fish, turtles, and in the cat and rabbit. Although the major morphologic and electrophysiologic subtypes occur across different species, there appears to be a considerable variety in minor populations of these cells. One of a variety of neuroactive substances may be possessed by particular amacrine cells and a single type of amacrine cell sometimes possesses more than one such substance. Among other tasks, particular amacrine cells probably serve in abstracting particular environmental features to permit ganglion cells to respond to such things as movements in particular directions or to objects of particular sizes, orientations, shapes, or patterns. Successful living in aquatic, aerial, arborial, and different ground-dwelling environments all require these visual mechanisms. Many amacrine cells respond with slow electrotonic changes in potential, while others show transient responses, such as a few spikes both at light on and light off. In *Necturus*[124] some cells exhibited a center-surround organization, as did half the amacrine cells studied by Toyoda et al.[119] in the carp. In *Necturus* some amacrine effects on bipolar neurons could be evoked by stimuli at distances, suggesting a chain of amacrine cells bringing this influence, possibly via the serial synapses sometimes seen involving groups of these cells.

The release of amacrine cell transmitter or modulatory substances can be complex. For example, the starburst amacrine cell of rabbits,[39] so named for the disposition of its processes, possesses both acetylcholine and GABA. Acetylcholine in the retina is typically an excitatory transmitter inducing depolarization in target cells, whereas GABA is typically inhibitory. O'Malley and Masland[96] have shown that a flashing light caused the release of acetylcholine but not GABA. High potassium levels caused both to be released, but if calcium ion is absent, high potassium only induced GABA release. Their interpretation is that acetylcholine release is likely based on the release of synaptic vesicles but that GABA release is likely to be carrier mediated.

Some amacrine cells, and some ganglion cells as well (discussed later), exhibit transient depolarizing responses at "light on," as well as at "light off." Such "on-off" cells are believed to receive direct or indirect input from both depolarizing and hyperpolarizing bipolars. On the other hand, cells exhibiting sustained or transient depolarization only at "light on" or only at "light off" are thought to receive input only from depolarizing and hyperpolarizing bipolars, respectively.

Turning to ganglion cells, recordings from single ganglion cells can be obtained extracellularly at the retinal face, from single, surviving active optic nerve axons in small bundles teased from the nerve, or by intracellular recordings. It is possible to classify ganglion cells by a number of physiologic, as well as anatomic, criteria. Ganglion cells fire "all-or-none" spike discharges. In retinas of primates and certain mammals (for example, cat), many ganglion cells have a low, sustained firing rate in total darkness. In addition to naming ganglion cells by the destination of their axons, or by their shape, like bipolar cells they are often referred to by their discharge patterns, i.e. "on" cells, "off" cells, or "on-off" cells. These characteristics relate anatomically to their dendrites extending to the inner (vitread) half of the IPL for "on" inputs, to the outer (sclerad) half of the IPL for "off" inputs and to both IPL halves for "on-off" inputs. Apart from this generalization, it should be remembered that individual ganglion cells summate the effects of numerous impinging inputs of electrotonic or chemical synapses and the location of a synapse on a cell is also of possible significance. In mammals, an individual ganglion cell may be driven by a stimulus exciting cones, or either rods or cones, but not exclusively by rods.

Ganglion cells usually exhibit a center-surround response organization based on their bipolar input as modified by amacrine cell influences.

Ganglion cells largely fall into one of two major groups characterized by whether their discharge pattern is sustained or phasic. A ganglion cell exhibiting a sustained discharge is not responsive to the rearrangement of dark and bright elements in its receptive field provided that the net illumination is constant, whereas phasic ganglion cells would respond to each such change. Ganglion cell inputs to the magnocellular DLGN and to the superior colliculus are generally phasic. Physiologists also recognize discharge characteristics called "brisk" versus "sluggish". A ganglion cell type called the "w" cell type has also been described[115,116] in rabbits. These are quite small, numerous, have slow conductance rates, can be brisk or sluggish and may lack a surround influence. The more complex types may respond to non-uniformity in their receptive field.

The destinations of axons of ganglion cells of the rhesus monkey have been investigated anatomically with the horseradish peroxidase tracing technique by Bunt et al.[15] and electrophysiologically by Schiller and Malpeli.[104,105] The latter find that the fast-conducting axons from the retina tend to end in the magnocellular layers of the dorsolateral geniculate nucleus (DLGN), whereas axons of medium conduction velocity project to the parvocellular layers of the DLGN. The majority of cells projecting to the superior colliculus were phasic and not color opponent (discussed later). The conclusions from the peroxidase studies differed in that *all* rhesus ganglion cells projected to the parvocellular layers of the DLGN, but only the largest ganglion cells of the peripheral retina and about 25% of the ganglion cells of the parafovea also projected to the magnocellular layers. Scattered ganglion cells of a wide range of sizes also projected to the superior colliculus (SC). If peroxidase injected in the parvocellular DLGN can label *all* retinal neurons, it follows that the labeling of some retinal ganglion cells via peroxidase injected into the magnocellular layers or colliculus must be occurring via collaterals. This situation in the monkey appears to differ from that in the cat, in which the "W" cells tend to project to the superior colliculus and to some large cells of the DLGN, sustained discharging (tonic) cells appear to project only to the DLGN, and phasic discharging cells seem to project to both the DLGN and SC.

Early studies of the electrical discharges of ganglion cells were those on the eel by Adrian and Matthews, the frog by Hartline, and a variety of animals by Granit and various coworkers. Later studies were performed by Kuffler,[65] who reviewed the earlier work. Their findings led to some important generalizations. Kuffler had paid critical attention to the correlation of the behavior of these cells with the position and sizes of the spots of light and discerned that within the receptive field of a ganglion cell there was a central region whose response to light tended to be antagonized by light positioned in its surround. Thus some of the brevity of firing in a phasic cell could be attributed to an inhibitory effect of a surround. A later report by Barlow et al.[5] showed that adaptational effects played a role in defining these center-surround mechanisms, the antagonistic surround effect often being greatly diminished in the dark-adapted state. Kuffler[65] considered it likely that ganglion cells with sustained firing to light (tonic cells) had a fairly direct and uncomplicated input from bipolars, whereas those ganglion cells exhibiting transient responses to light (phasic cells) had a more complex input. This early view seems well supported by Werblin and Dowling's interpretations[124] based on their intracellular recordings of ganglion cell activity in *Necturus*. They found one type of ganglion cell with a receptive field organization quite similar to those of bipolars. Central illumination produced a sustained depolarization and sustained firing of this cell that could be inhibited in a sustained fashion by illumination of the surround. The second type of ganglion cell gave a phasic discharge, and many ganglion cells of this type fired phasically to moving stimuli passing through their receptive fields. Werblin and Dowling suggest that the important source of input to the phasic cells are amacrine cells, whereas bipolars are the important input to ganglion cells exhibiting tonic responses.

In mammalian retinas there is a distinct tendency for the mean size of the receptive fields of ganglion cells to increase with distance from a central area or fovea. However, in any given retinal region there is a wide spread of sizes of the receptive fields of ganglion cells.

In species with color vision the behavior of individual ganglion cells to spectral light consists of those responsive to a broad range of wavelengths (broad-band) or black versus white, and those excited or inhibited by relatively narrow portions of the spectrum (color opponent). Gouras[44,45] notes that the broad-band types receive signals from two cone varieties whose activation transiently (phasically) excites the receptive field center of the ganglion cell and inhibits in its surround. On the other hand, color opponent ganglion cells typically have sustained (tonic) responses. In one type, one wavelength on the receptive field center excites while another inhibits (red versus green or blue versus yellow). In another opponent type, one wavelength that has actions only on the receptive field center may be countered by another wavelength that acts only on the surround. Schiller and Malpeli[104,105] found that in the macaque "on" color-opponent ganglion cells projected to layers 5 and 6 of the DLGN, whereas "off" color-opponent cells projected to layers 3 and 4. The transient broad-band ganglion cells projected to layers 1 and 2, but some projected to the superior colliculus. In the visual cortex of primates (but in the retinas of many other vertebrates) one finds so-called double opponency, i.e., a situation fully combining spatial and color opponency. In this case one wavelength (e.g., red) has an excitatory tonic effect on a receptive field center but an inhibitory effect on the surround so that no effect is seen if both are illuminated by red. For the same cell some other wavelength (e.g., green) may have an inhibitory effect on the center but an excitatory effect on the surround so that, again, no effect is seen if green illuminates both. However, for the above cell, if simultaneously red illuminates the center and green the surround, a marked excitatory response is seen, whereas if green illuminates the center and red the surround a marked inhibition is observed. This physiology appears to play a role in discerning borders of color contrast.

DeValois[29] has pointed out that when the luminance of both center and surround are increased in color-opponent systems, antagonism persists, but if instead of a luminance increase there is a spectral shift, one can obtain synergy. For example, if a center is being stimulated by a long wavelength and the surround by a middle wavelength, a color shift to wavelengths in the shorter part of the spectrum can both undo the antagonism of the surround and enhance the activity of the center.

Hubel and Wiesel[55] had earlier observed ganglion cells in the retina of the spider monkey that were excited by certain wavelengths and inhibited by others, and DeValois et al.[29] had observed cells in the DLGN that were similarly excited or inhibited by different wavelengths. This had raised the question as to whether spatial and chromatic information sometimes might move to the lateral geniculate via the same channel as had been observed earlier in goldfish by Wagner et al.[121] The central processing of information is discussed in Chapter 23.

Confirming earlier studies on cats, Gouras and Link[45] also have noted that certain perifoveal ganglion cells responded to rod-initiated stimuli in dim light but switched to cone-initiated inputs when cone thresholds were exceeded. Signals above the threshold for cone-initiating firing of these ganglion cells took less time to reach the ganglion cells than did those from rods when tested just above rod threshold. Using different stimulating wavelengths, Gouras observed that in a moderate state of dark adaptation, the same cell could send either rod- or cone-initiated signals, but not simultaneously. Thus the receptive field of some perifoveal ganglion cells in the monkey appears to be organized into two superimposed fields. In recording from optic nerve inputs at the level of the monkey lateral geniculate nucleus, Wiesel and Hubel[126] confirmed the existence of these dual-function ganglion cells, but found ganglion cells with a sole cone input to be in the majority, even at 10 degrees off the fovea, and found no signs of ganglion cells with a sole-rod input.

One of the most seminal investigations in visual data processing was that of Lettvin et al.[72] This dealt with the presentation in the visual fields of frogs of complex stimuli rather than simple spots of light. Recording from axons of retinal ganglion cells near their termination in the optic tectum of the frog, they discovered cells that were preferentially activated by one of a variety of such complex stimuli as straight or curved, black and white borders, moving spots of light, and spots of light with changing intensity. The frog has some unmyelinated fibers in its optic nerve, and Lettvin et al. associated sustained activity in the presence of a static, contrasting border with such fibers. Other unmyelinated fibers were active when small spots were moving across a complex patterned background. Some myelinated fibers were active when moving edges passed through the receptive field of their ganglion cells, and still others responded to dimming spots.

Thus one line of investigation has become the search for the presence of nerve cells in the visual system that respond solely to stimuli of particular types, such as moving spots, borders, or bars of contrast (black on white or white on black), with attention paid to the size of spots, width of bars, and preferential responses to particular directions of movement, wavelength sensitivity, and the presence of surrounds with opponent mechanisms.

It was discerned that at the retinal level there were some species in which ganglion cells exhibited only a fairly simple, center-surround mechanism of circular configuration. In the same animals cells specifically responsive to more complex inputs were discerned only at such higher levels as the visual cortex and superior colliculus. Retinas in this group include those of the cat, monkey, and presumably humans. Other animals, such as rabbits, ground squirrels, and pigeons, had retinas in which additional categories of ganglion cells could be found that responded best to borders or bars and to motions in particular directions. It was apparent that the presence of ganglion cells with such properties correlated with the presence of a relatively greater proportion of amacrine cells in the inner retina. The percentage of ganglion cells that exhibit phasic behavior tends to be greater in the complex retinas. As noted earlier, the various classes of amacrine cells with their unique transmitters and connections play a role in creating the field properties of the ganglion cells.

One may imagine populations of specific, first-order cells connected to some second-order cells, populations of specific, second-order cells connected to some third-order cell, and so on to achieve a higher degree of specificity of response in some nth-order cell. Clearly some vertebrates carry out more stages of the data processing in the retina than do others, and operations may vary with retinal region, that is, a particular region of a retina may be more complex than another.

It should be clear from the preceding discussion that the retina is organized to permit the lateral interaction of nerve cell networks and that this often can take the form of lateral inhibition. Certain perceptive phenomena therefore may be explicable on the basis of processing at the retinal level.

To summarize the foregoing discussion, one can consider the retina (and higher visual system) to have parallel depolarizing (on-center) and hyperpolarizing (off-center) informational pathways, with a neuron assigned to a pathway by the polarity of its response to the onset of light on its receptive field. Opposite effects occur with light offset, and cells that exhibit "on-off" behavior are thought to connect to both information streams. Passing from a simplistic application of this scheme to the behavior of particular neurons, such as a type of amacrine cells or a specific "W" ganglion cell, requires understanding that cells can hyperpolarize not only as a result of the impingement of an inhibitory transmitter, but also in response to the withdrawal of an excitatory transmitter, and conversely, cells depolarize not only in response to the impingement of an excitatory transmitter, but also to the withdrawal of an inhibitory transmitter. Moreover, polarization shifts can be the product of complex summations inasmuch as individual neurons can be postsynaptic to a variety of cells with chemical and electrotonic inputs. These inputs can influence not only surround effects and the duration of responses, but whether the response occurs at all, as in some cells influenced by the size, movement, direction, or orientation of the stimulus at the level of the receptive field. In primates, many of the more complex behaviors are first evident in visual cortex.

ROLE OF GLIA

The retina normally contains three types of glia: fibrous astrocytes, the empendymoglial cell of Müller, and the phagocytic microglia that are of extraretinal origin. In most retinas the axons of the retinal ganglion cells are unmyelinated until they leave the eye and pass through the cribriform plate, at which point they encounter oligodendroglia and become myelinated. Only rarely are human retinas found with some intraretinal myelinated axons and oligodendroglia, although in some retinas this is normally evident in local regions, such as in the visual streak of the rabbit retina.

The electrical activities of retinal cells doubtlessly are accompanied by movements of ions across membranes. Kuffler et al.[66] having noted that astroglia in the optic nerve of the frog exhibited slow potential changes as potassium accumulated about them during optic nerve discharges, Miller and Dowling[81] were led to investigate potential changes in the principal glial cell of the retina, the Müller cell, during retinal activity. In *Necturus* they found that the responses of the retinal Müller cells were indeed highly simlilar to those observed by Kuffler et al. in the optic nerve. Miller and Dowling made the reasonable suggestion that the b wave of the ERG (Chapter 21) may largely reflect potential changes in the Müller cells. Based on further studies by a number of investigators, the current detailed hypothesis contains the following elements. The membrane potential of the Müller cell may reflect its behavior as a potassium electrode. After a light flash, the level of extracellular potassium falls near the receptors[94] and the apices of the Müller cells, a factor probably underlying a Müller cell contribution to PIII of the ERG, but then increases at the OPL level of the retina and more slowly at a deeper level. The source of this increased extracellular potassium appears to be the activity of depolarizing bipolars in the outer retina and depolarizing third-order neurons in the inner retina, and these effects of locally increased extracellular potassium on Müller cells seem responsible for the appearance of local current sinks in these cells. Elegant studies by Newman[87] and others[13] were carried out to determine the regional ion selective and membrane conductance properties of isolated retinal Müller cells. Pressure injection of potassium ion near the endfeet of these cells, the vitreous facing portion when in the retina, produced depolarizations 7 times those obtained with similar injections on the lateral cell surfaces and 24 to 50 times those obtained from the cell regions normally near the external limiting membrane. This non-uniform conductance suggests that K^+ ion liberated by the action of retinal neurons is taken up by the Müller cells and predominantly discharged at its endfoot surface on the vitreous. This helps explain the origins of the b wave of the retinal electroretinogram. Temporal and magnitude differences in these radial Müller cell currents are reflected in the changing transretinal potentials representing the initial and sustained portions of the b wave. Sustained increases in extracellular potassium in the inner retina consequent to backgrounds of light that do little bleaching also have been suggested as a source of "network adaptation."

Glia undoubtedly have phagocytic functions in pathologic states and certainly functions that are still unknown. Because of differences in the vegetative metabolism of retinas of different species, partly because of differences in vascularity, one is handicapped in finding animal retinas whose glia may be useful in predicting the spectrum of functions of glia in primate retinas.

REFERENCES

1. Ahnelt PK, Kolb H, Pflug R: Identification of a core photoreceptor, likely to be blue sensitive, in the human retina, J Comp Neurol 255:18, 1987.
2. Attwell D: The photoreceptor output synapse, in Osborn N, Chader G, eds: Progress in retinal research, vol 9, Oxford, Pergamon Press, 1990.
3. Bader CR, MacLeish PR, Schwartz EA: Responses to light of solitary rod photoreceptors isolated from tiger salamander retina, Proc Natl Acad Sci USA 75:3507, 1978.
4. Bairati A Jr, Orzalesi N: The ultrastructure of the pigment epithelium and of the photoreceptor-pigment epithelium junction in the human retina, J Ultrastruc Res 9:484, 1963.
5. Barlow HB, FitzHugh R, Kuffler SW: Change of organization in the receptive fields of the cat's retina during dark adaptation, J Physiol (Lond) 137:338, 1957.
6. Basinger S, Hoffman R, Matthews M: Photoreceptor shedding is initiated by light in the frog retina, Science 194:1074, 1978.
7. Baylor DA, Fuortes MGF, O'Bryan PM: Receptive fields of cones in the retina of the turtle, J Physiol (Lond) 214:265, 1971.
8. Baylor DA, Lamb TD, Yau K-W: Responses of rods to single photons, J Physiol 288:613, 1979.
9. Blazynski C: Discrete distributions of adenosine receptors in mammalian retina, J Neurochem 54:648, 1990.
10. Bortoff A: Localization of slow potential responses in the *Necturus* retina, Vision Res 4:627, 1964.
11. Boycott BB, Hopkins JM, Sperling HG: Cone connections of the horizontal cells of the rhesus monkey's retina, Proc R Soc Lond B 229:345, 1987.
12. Brecha NC, Karten HJ: Localization of neuropeptides in adult and developing retina, in Hilfer SR, Sheffield JB, eds: Molecular and cellular basis of visual acuity, New York, Springer-Verlag, 1984.
13. Brew H, Gray PTA, Mobbs P, et al: Endfeet of retinal glial cells have higher densities of ion channels that mediate K^+ buffering, Nature 324:466, 1986.
14. Brindley GS: Physiology of the retina and visual pathway, 2nd ed, Baltimore, Williams & Wilkins, 1970.
15. Bunt AH, et al: Monkey retinal ganglion cells: morphometric analysis and tracing of axonal projections, with a consideration of the peroxidase technique, J Comp Neurol 164:265, 1975.
16. Bunt-Milam AH, Saari JC: Immunocytochemical localization of two retinoid-binding proteins in vertebrate retina, J Cell Biol 97:703, 1983.
17. Bunt-Milam AH, Saari JC, Klock IB, et al: Zonulae adherentes pore size in the external limiting membrane of the rabbit retina, Invest Ophthalmol Vis Sci 26:1377, 1985.
18. Chader GJ: Retinoids in ocular tissues: binding proteins, transport, and mechanisms of action, in McDevitt DS, ed: Cell biology of the eye, New York, Academic Press, 1982.
19. Cobbs WH, Barkdoll AE III, and Pugh EN Jr: Cyclic GMP increases photocurrent and light sensitivity of retinal cones, Nature 317:64, 1985.
20. Cohen AI: Vertebrate retinal cells and their organization, Biol Rev 38:427, 1963.
21. Cohen AI: Rods and cones, in Fuortes MGF, ed: Handbook of sensory physiology, vol. 7/2, Berlin, Springer-Verlag, 1972.
22. Cohen AI, Hall IA, Ferrendelli JA: Calcium and cyclic nucleotide regulation in incubated mouse retinas, J Gen Physiol 71:595, 1978.
23. Conner JD, MacLeod DIA: Rod photoreceptors detect rapid flicker, Science 195:698, 1977.
24. Cowan WM, Powell TPS: Centrifugal fibres in the avian visual system, Proc R Soc Lond (Biol) 158:232, 1963.
25. Curcio CA, Sloan KR, Kalina RE, et al: Human photoreceptor topography, J Comp Neurol 292:497, 1990.
26. Dacheux RF, Raviola E: Physiology and anatomy of a rod bipolar and amacrine cell in the rabbit retina, Invest Ophthalmol Vis Sci 25(Suppl):203, 1984.

27. Dacheux RF, Raviola E: The rod pathway in the rabbit retina: a depolarizing bipolar and amacrine cell, J Neurosci 6:331, 1986.

28. Dawson WW, Lieberman H: Growing evidence for the ganglion cell of Marenghi, Invest Ophthalmol Vis Sci 18(Suppl):117, 1978.

29. DeValois RL, et al: Response of single cells in monkey lateral geniculate nucleus to monochromatic light, Science 127:238, 1958.

30. DeYoe A, Van Essen DC: Concurrent modeling streams in monkey visual cortex, TINS 11:219, 1988.

31. Dolan RP, Schiller PH: Evidence for only depolarizing rod bipolar cells in the primate retina, Visual Neuroscience 2:421, 1989.

32. Dowling JE: Organization of vertebrate retinas, Invest Ophthalmol 9:655, 1970.

33. Dowling JE, Cowan WM: An electron microscopic study of normal and degenerating centrifugal fiber terminals in the pigeon retina, Zeit Zellf 71:14, 1966.

34. Dowling JE, Ehinger B: Synaptic organization of the amine-containing interplexiform cells of the goldfish and cebus monkey retinas, Science 188:270, 1975.

35. Dowling JE, Sidman RL: Inherited retinal dystrophy in the rat, J Cell Biol 14:73, 1962.

36. Ehinger B: Cellular location of the uptake of some amino acids into the rabbit retina, Brain Res 46:293, 1972.

37. Fain GL, Quandt FN, Gershenfeld HM: Calcium-dependent regenerative responses in rods, Nature 269:707, 1977.

38. Fain GL, et al: Contribution of a caesium-sensitive conductance increase to the rod photoresponse, Nature 272:467, 1978.

39. Famiglietti EV Jr: "Starburst" amacrine cells and cholinergic neurons: mirror-symmetric ON and OFF amacrine cells of the rabbit retina, Brain Res 26:138, 1983.

40. Farber DB, Flannery JG, Lolley RN, et al: Distribution patterns of photoreceptors, protein, and cyclic nucleotides in the human retina, Invest Ophthalmol Vis Sci 26:1558, 1985.

41. Fesenko EE, Kolesnikov SS, Lyubarsky AL: Induction by cyclic GMP of cationic conductance in plasma membrane of retinal rod outer segment, Nature 313:310, 1985.

42. Fine BS, Zimmerman LE: Observations on the rod and cone layer of the retina, Invest Ophthalmol 2:446, 1963.

43. Fisher SK, Pfeffer BA, Anderson DH: Both rod and cone disc shedding are related to light onset in the cat, Invest Ophthalmol Vis Sci 24:844, 1983.

44. Gouras P: Identification of cone mechanisms in monkey ganglion cells, J Physiol (Lond) 199:533, 1968.

45. Gouras P, Link K: Rod and cone interaction in dark-adapted monkey ganglion cells, J Physiol (Lond) 184:499, 1966.

46. Green DG, Siegal IM: Double branched flicker fusion curves from the all-rod skate retina, Science 188:1120, 1975.

47. Hageman GS, Johnson LV: Chondroitin-6-sulfate glycosaminoglycan is a major constituent of primate cone photoreceptor matrix sheath, Curr Eye Res 6:639, 1987.

48. Handelman GJ, Dratz EA, Reay CC, et al: Carotenoids in the human macula and whole retina, Invest Ophthalmol Vis Sci 29:850, 1988.

49. Hayes KC, Carey RE, Schmidt SY: Retinal degeneration associated with taurine deficiency in the cat, Science 188:949, 1975.

50. Haynes L, Yau K-W: Cyclic GMP-sensitive conductance in outer segment membrane of catfish cones, Nature 317:61, 1985.

51. Hecht S, Shlaer S, Pirenne MH: Energy, quanta, and vision, J Gen Physiol 25:819, 1942.

52. Hogan MJ: Role of the retinal pigment epithelium in macular disease, Trans Am Acad Ophthalmol Otolaryngol 76:64, 1972.

53. Hogan MJ, Alvarado JA, Weddell JE: Histology of the human eye, Philadelphia, WB Saunders, 1971.

54. Hollyfield JG, Rayborn ME, Landers RA, et al: Insoluble interphotoreceptor matrix domains surround rod photoreceptors in the human retina, Exp Eye Res 51:107, 1990.

55. Hubel DH, Wiesel TN: Receptive fields of optic nerve fibers in the retina of the spider monkey, J Physiol (Lond) 154:572, 1960.

56. Hughes A: New perspectives in retinal organization, in Osborne N, Chader G, eds: Progress in retinal research, Oxford, Pergamon Press, 1985.

57. Johnson LV, Hageman GS, Blanks JC: Interphotoreceptor matrix domains ensheath vertebrate cone photoreceptor cells, Invest Ophthalmol Vis Sci 27:129, 1986.

58. Kaneko A: Physiological and morphological identification of horizontal, bipolar and amacrine cells in goldfish retina, J Physiol 207:623, 1970.

59. Kaneko A, Hashimoto H: Recording site of single cone response determined by an electrode marking technique, Vision Res 7:847, 1967.

60. Karten HJ, Brecha N: Neuropeptides in the vertebrate retina, in Bradford HF, ed: Neurotransmitter interaction and compartmentation, New York, Plenum, 1982, p 719.

61. Koch K-W, Stryer L: Highly cooperative feedback control of retinal rod guanylate cyclase by calcium ions, Nature 334:64, 1988.

62. Kolb H: Cone pathways in the mammalian retina, in Hilfer SR, Sheffield JB, eds: Molecular and cellular basis of visual acuity, New York, Springer-Verlag, 1984.

63. Koontz MA, Hendrickson AE, Ryan MK: GABA-immunoreactive synaptic plexus in the nerve fiber layer of primate retina, Visual Neuroscience 2:19, 1989.

64. Kramer SG: Dopamine: a retinal neurotransmitter, I, Retinal uptake, storage, and light-stimulated release of H3-dopamine in vivo, Invest Ophthalmol 10:438, 1971.

65. Kuffler SW: Discharge patterns and functional organization of mammalian retina, J Neurophysiol 16:37, 1953.

66. Kuffler SW, Nicholls JG, Orkand RK: Physiological properties of glial cells in the central nervous system of amphibia, J Neurophysiol 29:768, 1966.

67. Kuwabara T, Gorn RA: Retinal damage by visible light, Arch Ophthalmol 79:69, 1968.

68. Lasansky A: Organization of the outer synaptic layer

in the retina of larval tiger salamander, Philos Trans R Soc Lond (Biol) 265:471, 1976.

69. Laties A, Enoch J: An analysis of retinal receptor orientation, I, Angular relationship of neighboring photoreceptors, Invest Ophthalmol 10:69, 1971.

70. Laties A, Liebman P, Campbell C: Photoreceptor orientation in the primate eye, Nature 218:172, 1968.

71. LaVail MM: Rod outer segment disk shedding in rat retina, Science 194:1071, 1976.

72. Lettvin JY, et al: What the frog's eye tells the frog's brain, Proc Inst Radio Eng 47:1940, 1959.

73. Leventhal AG, Ault SJ, Vitek DJ: The nasotemporal division in primate retina: the neural bases of macular sparing and splitting, Science 240:66, 1988.

74. Linberg KA, Fisher SK: Ultrastructure of the interplexiform cell of the human retina, Invest Ophthalmol Vis Sci 24(Suppl):259, 1983.

75. Mann I: The development of the human eye, New York, Grune & Stratton, 1950.

76. Mariani AP: Biplexiform cells: ganglion cells of the primate retina that contact photoreceptors, Science 216:1134, 1982.

77. Massey SC, Redburn DA: Transmitter circuits in the vertebrate retina, Prog in Neurobiol 28:55, 1987.

78. Matthews HR, Torre V, Lamb TD: Effects on the photoresponse of calcium buffers and cyclic GMP incorporated into the cytoplasm of retinal rods, Nature 313:582, 1985.

79. Miller RF, Dacheux RF: Synaptic organization and ionic basis of on and off channels in mudpuppy retina, I, Intracellular analysis of chloride-sensitive electrogenic properties of receptors, horizontal cells, bipolar cells, and amacrine cells, J Gen Physiol 67:639, 1976.

80. Miller RF, Dacheux RF: Synaptic organization and ionic basis of on and off channels in mudpuppy retina, II, Chloride-dependent ganglion cell mechanisms, J Gen Physiol 67:661, 1976.

81. Miller RF, Dowling JE: Intracellular responses of the Müller (glial) cells of the mudpuppy retina: their relation to b-wave of the electroretinogram, J Neurophysiol 33:323, 1970.

82. Miller RF, Slaughter MM: Excitatory amino acid receptors in the vertebrate retina, in Morgan WW, ed: Retinal transmitters and modulators: models for the brain, vol II, Boca Raton, CRC Press, 1985, p 124.

83. Miller RF, Slaughter MM, Dick E: Excitatory, inhibitory, and peptidergic pathways in the mudpuppy retina, in Bradford HF, ed: Neurotransmitter action and compartmentation, New York, Plenum, 1982.

84. Moyer FH: Development, structure, and function of the retinal pigmented epithelium, in Straatsma BR, et al, eds: The retina: morphology, function and clinical characteristics, UCLA Forum Med Sci, no 8, 1969.

85. Muller F, Wassle H, Voigt T: Pharmacological modulation of the rod pathway in the cat retina, J Neurophysiol 59:1657, 1988.

86. Nakatani K, Yau K-W: cGMP opens the light-sensitive conductance in retinal rods, Biophys J 47:356a, 1985.

87. Nathans J, Thomas D, Hogness DS: Molecular genetics of human color vision: the genes encoding blue, green, and red pigments, Science 232:193, 1986.

88. Nelson R, et al: Neural responses in the rod and cone system of the cat retina: intracellular records and Procion stains, Invest Ophthalmol 15:946, 1976.

89. Newman EA: Membrane physiology of retina glial (Müller) cells, J Neurosci 5:2225, 1985.

90. Newman EA, Odette LL: Model of electroretinogram b-wave generation: a test of the K^+ hypothesis, J Neurophysiol 51:164, 1984.

91. Noell WK, et al: Retinal damage by light in rats, Invest Ophthalmol 5:450, 1966.

92. Norman RA, Werblin FS: Control of retinal sensitivity, I, Adaptation in rods and cones, J Gen Physiol 67:37, 1974.

93. Nunn BJ, Schnapf JL, Baylor DA: Spectral sensitivity of single cones in the retina of Macaca fascicularis, Nature 309:264, 1984.

94. Oakley B II, Green DG: Correlation of light-induced changes in retinal extracellular potassium concentration with c-wave of the electroretinogram, J Neurophysiol 39:1117, 1976.

95. O'Day WT, Young RW: Rhythmic daily shedding of outer segment membranes by visual cells in the goldfish, J Cell Biol 76:593, 1978.

96. O'Malley DM, Masland RH: Co-release of acetylcholine and γ-aminobutyric acid by a retinal neuron, Proc Natl Acad Sci USA 86:3414, 1989.

97. Orr HT, Cohen AI, Lowry OH: The distribution of taurine in the vertebrate retina, J Neurochem 26:609, 1976.

98. Østerberg G: Topography of the layer of rods and cones in the human retina, Acta Ophthalmol 6(Suppl):8, 1935.

99. Penn RD, Hagins WA: Signal transmission along retinal rods and the origin of the electroretinographic a-wave, Nature (Lond) 223:201, 1969.

100. Raviola E, Gilula NB: Intramembrane organization of specialized contacts in the outer plexiform layer of the retina: a freeze-fracture study in monkey and rabbits, J Cell Biol 65:192, 1975.

101. Ripps H, Shakib M, MacDonald ED: Peroxidase uptake by photoreceptor terminals of the skate retina, J Cell Biol 70:86, 1978.

102. Schacher SM, Holzman E, Hood DC: Uptake of horseradish peroxidase by frog photoreceptor synapses in the dark and the light, Nature 249:261, 1974.

103. Schaeffer SF, Raviola E: Ultrastructural analysis of functional changes in the synaptic endings of turtle cone cells, Symp Quant Biol 40:521, 1975.

104. Schiller PH, Malpeli JG: Properties and tectal projections of monkey retinal ganglion cells, J Neurophysiol 40:428, 1977.

105. Schiller PH, Malpeli JG: Functional specificity of lateral geniculate nucleus laminae in the rhesus monkey, J Neurophysiol 41:788, 1978.

106. Snodderly DM, Aurna JD, Delori FC: The macular pigment, II, Spatial distribution in primate retinas, Invest Ophthalmol Vis Sci 25:674, 1984.

107. Snodderly DM, Brown PK, Delori FC, et al: The macular pigment, I, Absorbance spectra, localization, and discrimination from other yellow pigments in primate retinas, Invest Ophthalmol Vis Sci 25:660, 1984.

108. Spitznas M, Hogan MJ: Outer segments of photorecep-

tors and the retinal pigment epithelium, Arch Ophthalmol 84:810, 1970.

109. Steinberg RH: Rod and cone contributions to S-potentials from the cat retina, Vision Res 9:1319, 1969.

110. Steinberg RH, Schmidt R: Identification of horizontal cells as S-potential generators in the cat retina by intracellular dye injection, Vision Res 10:817, 1970.

111. Steinberg RH, Wood I, Hogan MJ: Pigment epithelial ensheathment and phagocytosis of extrafoveal cones in human retina, Philos Trans R Soc Lond (Biol) 277:459, 1978.

112. Stell WK: The morphological organization of the vertebrate retina, in Fuortes MGF, ed: Handbook of sensory physiology, vol 7/2, Berlin, Springer-Verlag, 1972.

113. Stell WK, Lightfoot DO: Color-specific interconnections of cones and horizontal cells in the retina of the goldfish, J Comp Neurol 159:473, 1975.

114. Sterling P: Microcircuitry of the cat retina, Ann Rev Neurosci 6:149, 1983.

115. Stone J, Fukuda Y: The naso-temporal division of the cat's retina re-examined in terms of Y, X and W cells, J Comp Neurol 155:377, 1974.

116. Stone J, Hoffman K: Very slow-conducting ganglion cells in the cat's retina: a major new functional type? Brain Res 43:610, 1972.

117. Sturman JA, et al: Retinal degeneration in primates raised on a synthetic human milk formula, Int J Dev Neurosci 2:121, 1984.

118. Tomita T: Electrophysiological study of the mechanisms subserving color coding in the fish retina, Symp Quant Biol 30:559, 1965.

119. Toyoda JI, Hashimoto H, Ohtsu K: Bipolar-amacrine transmission in the carp retina, Vision Res 13:295, 1973.

120. Uehara F, Matthes MT, Yasumura D, et al: Light-evoked changes in the interphotoreceptor matrix, Science 248:1633, 1990.

121. Wagner HG, MacNichol EF Jr, Wolbarscht ML: The response properties of single ganglion cells in the goldfish retina (part 2), J Gen Physiol 43:45, 1960.

122. Wen R, Oakley B II: Electroretinogram b-wave and slow PIII components are produced by Müller cell responses to retinal potassium, Soc Neurosci (Abstract) 15:922, 1989.

123. Werblin FS: Regenerative hyperpolarization in rods, J Physiol 244:53, 1975.

124. Werblin FS, Dowling JE: Organization of the retina of the mudpuppy, *Necturus maculosis*, II, Intracellular recording, J Neurophysiol 32:315, 1969.

125. Wiechmann AF, Hollyfield J: HIOMT immunoreactivity in the vertebrate retina: a species comparison, Exp Eye Res 49:1079, 1989.

126. Wiesel TN, Hubel DH: Spatial and chromatic interactions in the lateral geniculate body of the rhesus monkey, J Neurophysiol 29:1115, 1966.

127. Yau K-W, Nakatani K: Light-induced reduction of cytoplasmic free calcium in retinal rod outer segment, Nature 313:579, 1985.

128. Yau K-W, Nakatani K: Light-suppressible, cyclic GMP-sensitive conductance in the plasma membrane of a truncated rod outer segment, Nature 317:252, 1985.

129. Young RW: The renewal of the photoreceptor cell outer segments, J Cell Biol 33:61, 1967.

130. Young RW: A difference between rods and cones in the renewal of outer segment protein, Invest Ophthalmol 8:222, 1969.

131. Young RW: The renewal of rod and cone outer segments in the rhesus monkey, J Cell Biol 49:303, 1971.

132. Young RW: Shedding of discs from rod outer segments in the rhesus monkey, J Ultrastruc Res 34:190, 1971.

133. Young RW: The daily rhythm of shedding and degradation of cone outer segment membranes in the lizard retina, J Ultrastruc Res 61:172, 1977.

134. Young RW: The daily rhythm of shedding and degradation of rod and cone outer segment membranes in the chick retina, Invest Ophthalmol Vis Sci 17:105, 1978.

135. Young RW: Visual cells, daily rhythms and vision research, Vision Res 18:573, 1978.

136. Young RW, Bok D: Participation of the retinal pigment epithelium in the rod outer segment process, J Cell Biol 42:392, 1969.

CHAPTER 20

The Optic Nerve

DOUGLAS R. ANDERSON, M.D.

HARRY A. QUIGLEY, M.D.

NORMAL PHYSIOLOGY
The axons

Functionally, the optic nerve begins at the ganglion cells in the retina. The axons arising from these cells course toward the exit of the optic nerve from the eye. From the nasal side the axons take the straight course toward the optic nerve head. The axons from the macular region around the fovea form the spindle-shaped *papillomacular bundle,* which enters the temporal sector of the optic nerve head. The fovea is normally situated below the midpoint of the nerve head; thus this papillomacular bundle enters the optic disc inferior to its equator. Axons from the remaining retinal regions take an arcuate course around the *papillomacular bundle* to enter the optic nerve head at the superior and inferior poles. The retinal nerve fiber layer is thickest in these arcuate bundles as they approach the upper and lower sectors of the optic disc.[159,176] When the nerve bundles are illuminated by green light, a brilliant back-scattering of light occurs against a dark background caused by the absorption of green light by the melanin of the retinal pigment epithelium and choroid. The brightness of the reflections from the nerve fiber layer is in direct proportion to the thickness of the layer (Fig. 20-1).

The optic nerve can be considered to have four portions: the intraocular portion (optic nerve head, optic disc, optic papilla); the intraorbital portion; a small intracanalicular portion (within the optic canal); and a small intracranial portion that merges into the optic chiasm and optic tract. From there the axons complete their course to their central nervous sytem terminals.

By this pathway the 1 million axons that pass from each eye into the optic nerve conduct partially processed visual information from the retinal ganglion cells to the lateral geniculate body, superior colliculus, hypothalamus, and certain midbrain centers. There are now considered to be two parallel pathways in the anterior visual pathways carrying different types of visual information.[196] The luminance pathway, also called M (for magnocellular), utilizes larger retinal ganglion cells with larger diameter axons that synapse in the magnocellular layers of the lateral geniculate body. They are most sensitive to changes in luminance at low light levels, subserve motion perception, and are relatively insensitive to color. Only a small proportion of all ganglion cells are part of the M pathway. The color or P (for parvocellular) pathway consists of smaller ganglion cells that project to the parvocellular lateral geniculate layers and preferentially carry information on color and fine detail. This group includes the majority of retinal ganglion cells, including the midget cells of the foveal area.

While coursing through the retinal nerve fiber layer and the optic nerve head, the nerve fibers are unmyelinated, keeping the retina sufficiently transparent for light to reach the photoreceptors in the outer retina. After passing through the lamina cribrosa to enter the intraorbital portion, the fibers gain a myelin sheath, which insulates the axons. From this point on-

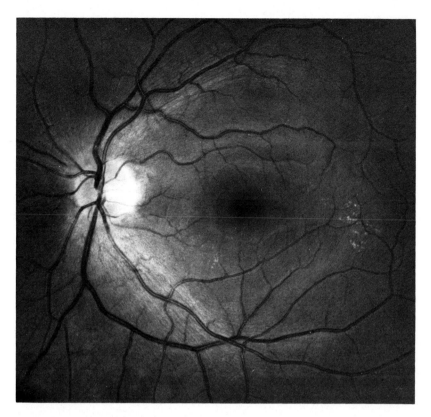

FIG. 20-1 Fundus photograph in which can be seen the course of axons in the retina toward the optic disc. (Courtesy P. Juhani Airaksinen, M.D.)

ward the impulse is carried by *saltatory conduction* typical of white matter tracts and myelinated peripheral nerves. Depolarization occurs only at the nodes of Ranvier, with the impulse jumping from node to node. With this saltatory conduction, the impulse passes along the axon more rapidly than it would by conduction of an action potential, such as in an unmyelinated fiber. Saltatory conduction also conserves metabolic energy, because only the exposed portion of the axon membrane at the node needs to be repolarized, not the entire length of the axon. With demyelinating disease, the naked axon segments presumably conduct the impulse by propagation of an action potential in the unmyelinated region; this slower conduction is the apparent explanation for a prolonged latency in the visually evoked response (VER) in demyelinating diseases.

In the monkey and human retrobulbar optic nerve all fibers are myelinated and conduct impulses toward the brain. Amphibian optic nerves contain a substantial number of nonmyelinated fibers. The optic nerve of birds contains fibers that originate from cell bodies in the brain and terminate in the retina. The function of such fibers is speculative, but they may modulate retinal responses.

The primate optic nerve has a narrower distribution of fiber diameter than is present even in other vertebrates (Fig. 20-2). While the cat optic nerve shows clear groups of large, medium, and small axons, the monkey and human nerve have a nearly unimodal distribution.[187,191]

The number of fibers in each monkey and human optic nerve is approximately 1 million, but there is considerable variation from person to person, and even between two fellow eyes.[187,191] The number of fibers appears to be related to the size of the optic disc as it is seen clinically (and to the area of the optic nerve just behind the eye).[165] The larger the optic disc, the more the number of fibers. This makes intuitive sense, as the ganglion cells send their axons through the future nerve head during the first trimester of embryological life.[72] At that gestational age there is no extracellular matrix in the sclera and no Bruch's membrane, each of which

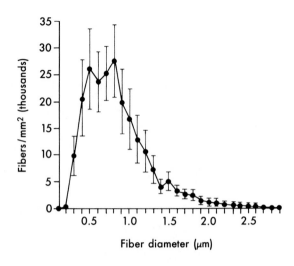

FIG. 20-2 The density of optic nerve fibers in the normal Macaque monkey is plotted against their diameter. The distribution is quite unimodal, though two potential groups make up the main peak and one further group is suggested near 1.5 μ diameter. (From Sanchez RM, Dunkelberger G, Quigley HA: Invest Ophthalmol Vis Sci 27:1342, 1986.[191])

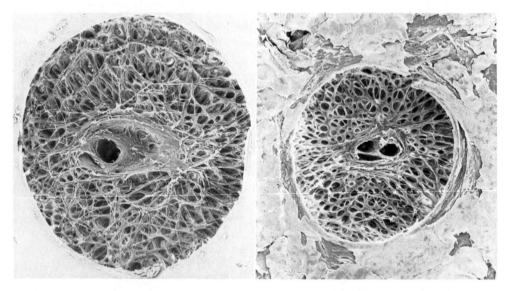

FIG. 20-3 Scanning electron micrographs of human optic nerve heads. All but the connective tissues have been digested away, showing the pore structure of the lamina cribrosa. While one disc is large and the other is small, both are from normal eyes. (From Quigley HA, Brown AE, Morrison JC, et al: Arch Ophthalmol 108:51, 1989.[165])

forms the delimiting features of the optic disc in the adult eye. Rather, these structural elements are laid down in response to the volume of nerve tissue present; hence, disc area is partly a result of fiber number.

There are more than twice the number of axons in a fetal primate eye than in the the adult eye.[184] It is believed that ganglion cells die if their axons do not successfully synapse with appropriate targets in the brain. After birth, this attrition of optic nerve fibers slows dramatically. During a 75-year human life, the further loss of ganglion cells, presumably from aging, encompasses only 25% of the total.[28,135,187]

The size of the opening for the optic nerve varies considerably among normal persons, more than is explained by variation in the number of nerve fibers (Fig. 20-3), and along with the variation in fiber number gives rise to a variety of disc appearances (cup-disc ratio). There are racial differences in disc diameter, with blacks having larger discs[31,165] and hence larger cups. Some disease states are more common in eyes with small disc size (e.g., optic disc drusen and ischemic optic neuropathy). In glaucoma, the most common optic neuropathy, disc size appears not to be a significant risk factor in damage.

Intracellular movement of molecules and organelles from one location to another occurs within the cytoplasm of every cell. Neurons are no exception. Indeed, intra-axonal movement is particularly striking and easily studied by virtue of its directional orientation along the length of axons that extend a distance many hundred times greater than the cell body width. The movement along axons seems to occur by at least two different processes: rapid axonal transport and slow axoplasmic flow.[10,193,225]

Rapid axonal transport is bidirectional, orthograde from the ganglion cell body to the axon terminal and retrograde from the terminal to the ganglion cell body. This active transport requires metabolic energy, which is obtained from adenosine 5'-triphosphate (ATP) produced locally within each axon segment along the way. Among the items transported, membrane-associated protein synthesized in the rough endoplasmic reticulum of the ganglion cell body is seemingly carried in membrane-bound vesicles of smooth endoplasmic reticulum along the surface of the microtubules, reaching the lateral geniculate body of small monkeys within 3 to 5 hours (200 to 400 mm/day) (Fig. 20-4). Pinocytotic vesicles containing samples of the extracellular space in the lateral geniculate body are carried back to the ganglion cell body at a similar or slightly slower speed. Transmitter substance made in the cell body is transported to the axon terminal. A variety of chemical messages, hormones, and foreign material such as toxins and viruses can be passengers in this system.

In contrast, *slow axonal flow* can be traced as the movement of soluble protein synthesized in the cell body toward the axon terminal at a rate of only 1 to 3 mm *per day*. It may be visualized as a glacierlike movement of the entire cytoplasmic column (including the cytoskeletal structure, in part composed of microtubules[90]) into and along the axon, replacing the material catabolized downstream.

The glia

The predominant glial element in the optic nerve head is the astrocyte. The astrocytes weave together to form a dense structure in which there are tunnels coordinated with astrocyte-lined openings in the lamina cribrosa.[6,7,18,19] Through these tunnels pass the bundles of axons. Their organization and their many intracellular filaments are in keeping with their func-

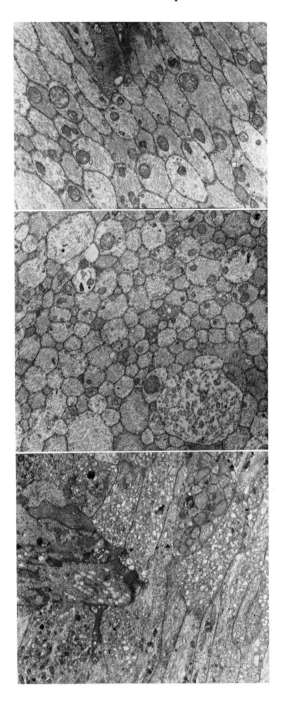

FIG. 20-4 The normal appearance of unmyelinated axons of the optic nerve head above changes as they enter the lamina cribrosa area in the human glaucomatous eye. The normal axons *(top)* have microtubules, neurofilaments, and occasional mitochondria. With obstruction of their axonal transport induced by elevated intraocular pressure, axons are swollen with vesicles adjacent to a laminar beam *(bottom)*. (From Quigley HA, Addicks EM, Green WR, et al: Arch Ophthalmol 99:635, 1981.[160])

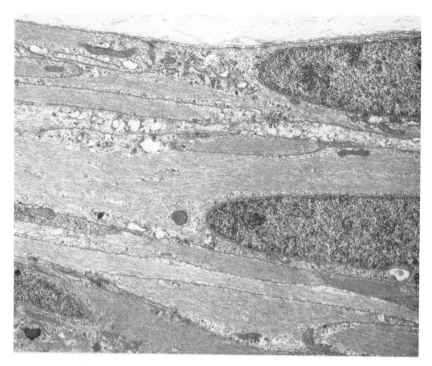

FIG. 20-5   Astrocytes of the optic nerve head in a monkey eye with substantial optic atrophy (transmission electron micrograph). Dense intracellular filaments and extensive interdigitation characterize these glial cells that have many gap junctions between each other (not shown). (From Quigley HA, Hohman RM, Addicks EM: Am J Ophthalmol 93:689, 1982.[171])

tion to support the bundles of nerve fibers as they turn to enter the optic nerve from the retina (Fig. 20-5). Astrocytes also provide a cohesiveness to the neural compartment by arranging themselves to form an interface (demarcated by a basal lamina) with all mesodermal structures, for example, with the vitreous at the disc surface, with the surrounding choroid and sclera, with the collagenous bundles of the lamina cribrosa, and with blood vessels. Apart from their obvious support function, astroglia in the nerve head presumably also serve to moderate conditions for neuronal function, for example, by absorbing excess extracellular potassium ions released by depolarizing axons and by storing glycogen for use during transient oligemia. They function in the nerve head like the Müller cells of the retina (see Chapter 19).

Behind the lamina cribrosa fibrous astrocyte processes mingle among the axons and line the pial septa. Intrafascicular oligodendrocytes are aligned in columns next to the fibrous septa along with astrocyte nuclei. The oligodendrocytes form and maintain the myelin sheaths, as they do elsewhere in the central nervous system (CNS).

The blood vessels

The central retinal artery enters the optic nerve midway in its orbital course and courses anteriorly in the center of the nerve (Fig. 20-6). It provides some branches to the intraorbital portion of the nerve (but not the optic nerve head), but its main function is to supply the retina (Fig. 20-7). The main arterial supply to optic nerve itself is from various orbital branches that penetrate the dura mater, spread over the pia mater, and send branches into the septa of the optic nerve. Anteriorly, the posterior ciliary arteries penetrate the sclera, sending branches both to the choroid and to the optic nerve. These branches to the optic nerve supply the optic nerve head, the lamina cribrosa, and the optic nerve immediately behind the globe. The details of the arterial supply[15,80,119] command considerable interest because of the presumed relevance to the pathophysiology of glaucomatous optic neuropathy. There has been debate about some of the anatomic details, in part because of apparent individual variations in anatomy, as well as differing interpretations of the physiologic implications of the anatomic features.

Branches of the posterior ciliary artery that

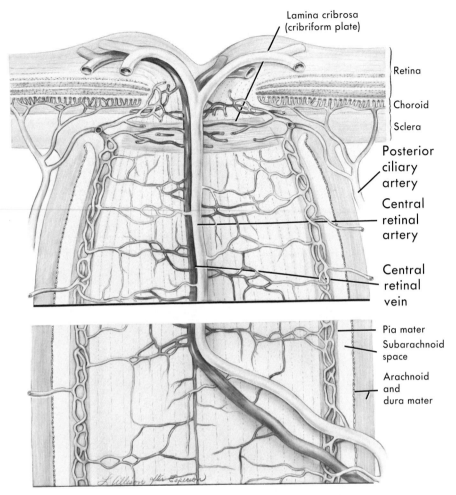

FIG. 20-6 Vascular supply and drainage of the optic nerve.

enter the choroid break up into the capillary network of the choriocapillaris, with its fenestrated endothelium. However, the branches that enter the optic nerve have all the features of CNS vessels. Pericytes (mural cells) engulf the capillaries, and the nonfenestrated endothelium has tight junctions. Because of these fundamental anatomic differences, the physiology of the microvasculature in the optic nerve head differs from that of the choroidal vessels. The optic nerve microvascular bed resembles anatomically the retinal and CNS vessels. The optic nerve vessels share with those of the retina (and of the CNS in general) the physiologic properties of autoregulation[63,201,220,221] and the presence of the blood-brain barrier.

Because of autoregulation, the rate of blood flow in the optic nerve is not much affected by intraocular pressure (IOP), whereas the blood flow in the choroid falls as IOP is elevated.[3,4] In

principle, if there were no change in the vascular resistance produced by a regulatory mechanism, then raising the blood pressure would increase the flow through the vessels. However, in the retina and optic nerve, as in the brain, the vascular tone is increased by autoregulation when blood pressure rises, increasing the resistance to flow, so that the flow level is not affected by the elevated blood pressure. This retinal autoregulation is witnessed clinically by the well-known narrowing of retinal arteries in cases of arterial hypertension. Elevated IOP compresses the vein, increasing the total resistance to flow through the arteriovenous circuit, which—were it not for autoregulation—would reduce the blood flow for a given level of arterial blood pressure. However, autoregulation compensates for venous compression by reducing the vascular tone in other parts of the circuit as IOP rises, so that blood flow is maintained despite

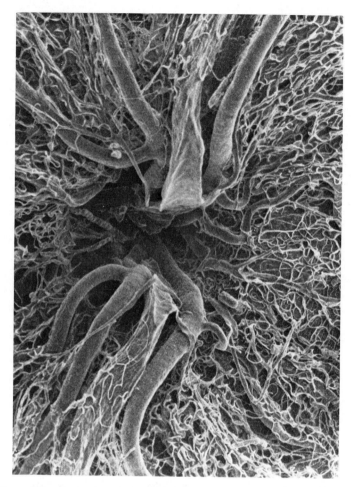

FIG. 20-7   Cast of blood vessels of the optic nerve head in a monkey eye. Large retinal blood vessels emanate from the central disc, while the dense plexus of capillaries supplying the anterior nerve head branch out from them. (From Quigley HA, Hohman RM, Addicks EM, et al: Invest Ophthalmol Vis Sci 25:918, 1984.[173])

the venous compression caused by intraocular pressure.

Such autoregulation of blood flow seems to be accomplished in part as a response to the degree of arterial stretching (when blood pressure rises or falls) and in part as metabolic autoregulation. The latter is a response of the vascular tone to local conditions such as carbon dioxide (CO_2) concentration, pH, or oxygen level. CO_2 is a particularly powerful vasodilator. Whenever CO_2 accumulates because of inadequate blood flow, the vessels dilate and blood flow increases. Autonomic influence may affect the central retinal artery in the orbit, but there is no autonomic innervation to the blood vessels anterior to the lamina cribrosa,[113,91] and local control in the nerve head and retina seems to be mainly by autoregulation.

Because of the blood-brain barrier, intravascular protein and fluorescein cannot cross the vascular endothelium to enter the retina or optic nerve. However, both protein and fluorescein (and presumably many other substances) leak from choroidal vessels rather freely. The choroid is not separated from the optic nerve head by a cellular layer that has tight junctions. Hence, extracellular materials may diffuse into the extracellular space of the optic nerve head and lamina cribrosa (Figs. 20-8 and 20-9).[33,41,56,61,66,67,96,140,141,217] In clinical angiograms fluorescein diffuses toward the center of the optic disc from its boundary with the choroid.

The extracellular space of the nerve head may also permit bulk flow from the vitreous cavity through the anterior portion of the nerve substance to the subarachnoid space.[82] This flow

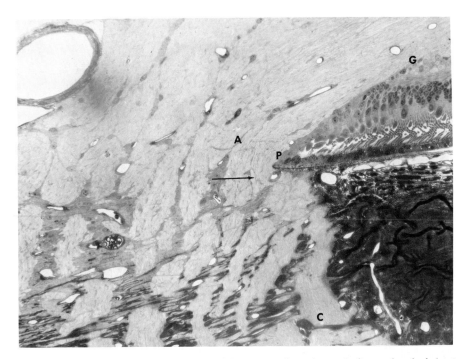

FIG. 20-8 Optic fibers exiting from retina of rhesus monkey. Arrow indicates level of chorio-capillaris. There is no impermeable barrier between axons of optic nerve and these vessels. Locations of retinal ganglion cells, G, their axons, A, and pigmented epithelium, P, are indicated. Note collagen bundles of lamina cribrosa, C, are confluent with those of scleral region. (Magnification × 270.) (Courtesy Adolph I. Cohen, Ph.D.)

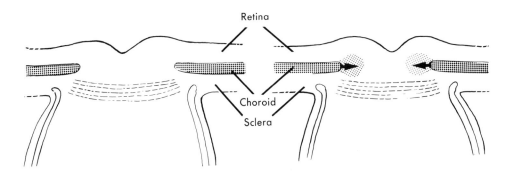

FIG. 20-9 Diffusion of extracellular material from choroid into optic nerve head.

probably increases with the greater pressure gradient caused by increased IOP. The amount of such flow must be small compared to the rate of aqueous humor formation, because it is not enough to handle the load when the trabecular meshwork is obstructed. Moreover, the reverse flow that would be produced by elevated sub-arachnoid pressure has not been recognized to produce a change in IOP.

PAPILLEDEMA (OPTIC NERVE-HEAD SWELLING)

A variety of intracranial conditions may result in papilledema. The apparent basis of the nerve-head swelling is some obstruction of cerebro-spinal fluid exit, which results in an elevated intracranial (hydrostatic) pressure. In some instances this may be confined to certain intracranial compartments. Because the sub-

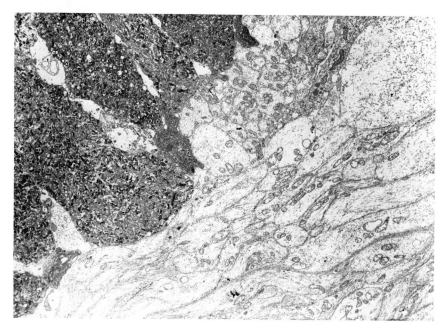

FIG. 20-10   Electron micrograph showing axonal swelling in papilledema from a patient who had orbital neoplasm. Some of the axons *(center)* are of normal size. Others, to the upper right, are grossly swollen with watery cytoplasm and disrupted neural filaments. On the left, some axons are packed with mitochondria and laminate dense bodies. Here and there the extracellular space is slightly enlarged. Magnification × 7600. (Courtesy Mark O. M. Tso, M.D. From Topics in neuro-ophthalmology, Thompson S, ed, Baltimore, Williams & Wilkins, 1979, p 171.[213])

arachnoid space extends through the optic canal into the vaginal sheaths of the optic nerve, its hydrostatic pressure can be transmitted as far forward as the junction of the dura mater and lamina cribrosa with the sclera. In cases of increased intracranial pressure, distension of the sheaths of the optic nerve can be appreciated by ultrasonic echography[36,37,142] and by computed tomography. The pressure can be relieved surgically.[211]

The central retinal vein, as it crosses the optic nerve sheaths in the mid-orbit (see Fig. 20-6), is subject to external compression by the subarachnoid pressure. When the subarachnoid pressure exceeds venous pressure, compression of the vein increases resistance to flow at that point and elevates slightly the venous pressure upstream.[188] If spontaneous venous pulsations are present in the optic disc, as happens in many normal individuals, they disappear when the elevated central retinal venous pressure exceeds the normal IOP. Therefore, spontaneous venous pulsations seen ophthalmoscopically at the disc suggest that subarachnoid pressure in the optic nerve sheaths is not elevated, at least at the moment of observation, unless the IOP is also elevated.

It is now thought that the main pathophysiologic event is an impairment of slow axoplasmic flow.[12,129,133,213,216] The tissue pressure of the axons within the eye is equal to IOP, whereas in the orbit the intra-axonal tissue pressure is governed by the subarachnoid pressure. The lamina cribrosa is the partition that separates the two pressure compartments,[57] where axons are subjected to this pressure gradient. Under normal conditions the IOP is greater than the subarachnoid pressure and the gradient may be thought of as augmenting the movement of axoplasm out of the eye. However, when intracranial pressure equals or exceeds IOP, the forces of slow axoplasmic flow encounter a diminished or reverse pressure gradient. The axons in the optic nerve head become distended.[212,214,215] Unlike other types of central nervous system edema, there is no primary glial swelling or expansion of the extracellular space, but such changes may occur secondarily.

Although slow axoplasmic flow is impaired, the axon often continues to function. Visual function may be quite normal in chronic papilledema for a long time, except that the physiologic blind spot is enlarged when the swollen disc displaces the inner retina next to the optic nerve head. In experimental papilledema it has been shown that fast axonal transport is also affected,[129,214] but seemingly only after the axonal swelling is established.[12,17,180] The blockage of rapid axonal transport may be the secondary result of a disruption of intra-axonal anatomy or a vascular embarrassment produced by the swelling. Because blockage of rapid transport can be a lethal injury to the axon, this stage of experimental papilledema may correspond to the advanced clinical cases in which visual obscuration and frank visual loss occur.[68] Experimental evidence suggests that the usual translucent swelling of papilledema (made pink by the accompanying hyperemia) may represent obstruction of slow axonal flow, while superimposed cotton-wool patches seen in advanced cases may represent impaired rapid axonal transport.[70,125,126,127,128]

Not all swellings of the optic nerve head are papilledema due to increased subarachnoid pressure. For example, anterior ischemic optic neuropathy in which the nerve head swells is most likely an infarction of the anterior optic nerve. With cytoplasmic death, alterations in pH and osmotic pressure result in a pale swelling of axons and of other tissue elements, along with accumulation of extracellular fluid.[108,181] "Cotton-wool spots" appear at the boundary of the ischemic and the nonischemic regions. They represent accumulations of smooth endoplasmic reticulum and other membranous structures that are carried by either orthograde or retrograde axonal transport.[129,181,195] These structures pass through nonischemic segments of the axon but accumulate wherever an ischemic segment of the axon is encountered. Other swellings may occur as a result of neoplastic infiltration, inflammation, acute glaucoma, and hereditary neuropathy.

OPTIC ATROPHY

Nonglaucomatous optic atrophy is characterized by a loss of axons (and their retinal ganglion cells) in response to a lethal insult to the cell. With loss of its substance, the optic disc flattens and turns pale. Some causes of optic atrophy include acute ischemic episodes, trauma, demyelinating diseases, and compression of the optic nerve by tumor.

The nature and location of the lesion determine which axons are affected. Localized insults, which occur most often in the anterior optic nerve and retina, injure bundles of axons and in the visual field produce scotomas and other visual field defects that are shaped like the course of nerve fiber bundles. Although lesions of the posterior optic nerve also can rarely injure bundles of axons and produce nerve fiber bundle defects,[77,93,94,95] the usual compressive lesion in this location almost always has a diffuse effect or affects preferentially the small diameter macular fibers, resulting in a central scotoma.

Whichever the underlying etiology of optic atrophy, the integrity of the axon is interrupted anatomically or physiologically at some point in its course. This can be experimentally modeled by crushing or cutting the nerve fibers.[65] The proximal segment of the axon, being disconnected from its ganglion cell, promptly degenerates (Wallerian). It is no longer part of the cell body and no longer receives support through the orthograde axonal transport mechanism.[8,166,178]

There remains the ganglion cell and the attached fragment of axon that extends from the ganglion cell to the site of injury. In some cold-blooded species the retinal ganglion cells undergo chromatolysis (hypertrophy of the rough endoplasmic reticulum), increasing the synthesis of cytoplasmic components and producing regeneration of the axon until it connnects with its proper receptor. Until recently it was believed that mammalian retinal ganglion cells did not retain the ability to regenerate.[64] It is now clear that the milieu at the site of injury determines the capacity for neural regeneration. Aguayo and coworkers[1] have shown that mammalian optic nerve fibers can not only regenerate, but reestablish connections with their target sites in the central nervous system if provided with a segment of peripheral nerve tissue as a bridge within which to grow. While only a small proportion of rodent optic nerve fibers will regenerate in these experimental conditions, the possibility of inducing regeneration in the human visual pathway is intriguing.

However, without a peripheral nerve graft, an experimentally injured monkey optic nerve degenerates beginning about 4 to 6 weeks after the insult. The degeneration of the axon is not progressively retrograde; seemingly the ganglion cell and axon die simultaneously.[8,166,178] The degeneration of the ganglion cell (and its attached axon fragment) follows the principle that central neurons degenerate after an injury if they fail to reestablish contact with an end organ within some inherent time limit.[65,148,205,219]

When atrophy occurs, the astroglia migrate into the spaces vacated by the degenerated axons (Fig. 20-11).[166] Blood vessels are reduced in number but remain in proportion to the glial and neuronal tissue that persists and requires nutrition. When optic atrophy occurs, the typically red color of the optic disc rim becomes pale. The normal redness results from extensive

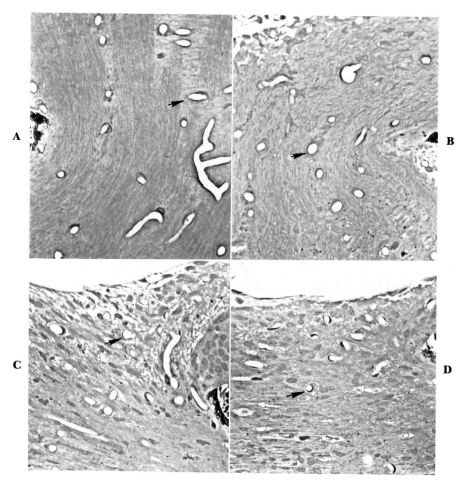

FIG. 20-11   The histologic changes in experimental optic atrophy at the optic disc in a monkey eye. In **A**, *upper left*, the normal nerve bundles course past capillaries *(open areas)*. As the bundles atrophy in **B** and **C**, and are totally absent in **D** *(lower right)*, the remaining tissue consists only of astrocytes and capillaries. (From Quigley HA, Hohman RM, Addicks EM: Am J Ophthalmol 93:689, 1982.[171])

light scattering within the disc with absorption of shorter visible wavelengths by the red blood cells in the disc capillaries.[44] Presumably the axon bundles of the disc rim are transparent and conduct light into the deeper tissues where perhaps glia scatter the light and the blood imparts a red color. With atrophy, the pallor hypothetically results from three factors: (1) there are fewer axon bundles to conduct light into the deeper tissue; (2) the astrocytes now occupy a larger proportion of the tissue and they are more reflective of white light; and (3) the total thickness of rim tissue is thinner, which allows more white light to reflect directly from the collagen of the lamina cribrosa beneath.[164,171,179]

GLAUCOMA
Role of IOP

IOP has been consistently found to be one of the most important risk factors in glaucomatous injury (Fig. 20-12).[21,22,79,103] A graph of the rate of initial visual field loss versus IOP level shows no IOP at which there is a sudden rise in relative risk.[198] At every level of IOP there is a risk of glaucomatous damage, though it increases exponentially with increasing pressure. The effect is such that the risk of damage is 40 times higher at an IOP of 40 mm Hg than at 15 mm Hg. We observe a substantial number of eyes with glaucomatous excavation and field loss with a normal IOP simply because a small percentage of a large number of persons with normal pressure is a large number.

RISK OF SUBSEQUENT GLAUCOMATOUS FIELD LOSS

BASELINE INTRAOCULAR PRESSURE (MM HG)	PERCENT DEVELOPING FIELD DEFECT*	RELATIVE RISK
< 16	0.8	1.0
16–19	1.4	1.7
20–23	3.1	4.0
≥ 24	8.4	10.5

*Over a one- to 13-year follow-up period. Modified from Armaly and associates.

FIG. 20-12 This table shows that the risk of developing visual field loss in glaucoma eyes increases by a factor of 10 when intraocular pressure is above 24 mm Hg compared to below 16 mm Hg. (From Sommer A: Am J Ophthalmol 107:186, 1989.[198])

Additional evidence that IOP produces damage is that unilateral IOP elevation produces unilateral nerve damage[139] and that experimentally produced pressure elevation in animals results in glaucomatous nerve damage (Figs. 20-13 and 20-14).[62,157] If the IOP level is associated with glaucoma injury, it is logical that therapeutic lowering of IOP would be protective. Until recently, there was only retrospective data to support this concept.[107,111,223] Two reports now indicate that medical lowering of IOP decreases the rate of initial glaucoma damage in those with untreated IOP between 20 and 30 mm Hg.[54,102] Additionally, the lower the pressure achieved surgically, the less the incidence of further visual field loss.[69a,139a,190a,223]

Though IOP is clearly involved, there must be other relevant pathogenic factors that ac-

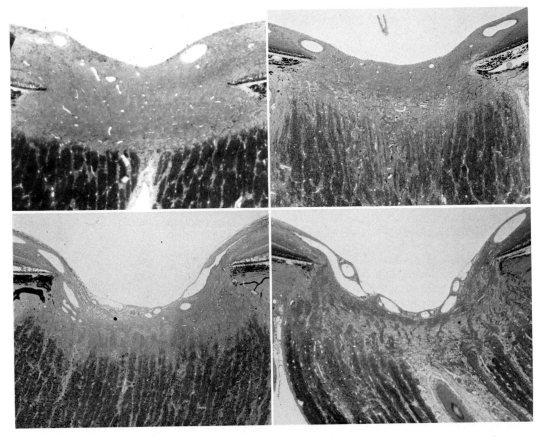

FIG. 20-13 Changes in the optic nerve head in experimental monkey glaucoma showing the development of changes identical to human glaucomatous damage. From normal appearance *(upper left)*, loss of neural tissue and compression of lamina cribrosa leads to excavation of disc surface *(bottom right)*. (From Quigley HA, Hohman RM, Addicks EM, et al: Invest Ophthalmol Vis Sci 25:918, 1984.[173])

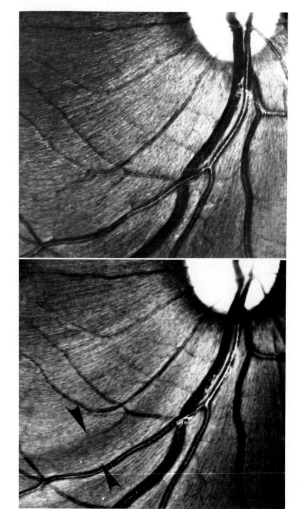

FIG. 20-14 Nerve fiber layer photograph of monkey eye prior to development of wedge-shaped defect *(above)* and with defect (between arrows *below*). This finding is identical in position and appearance to those seen in human eyes that develop early glaucoma damage. (From Quigley HA, Hohman RM, Addicks EM, et al: Invest Ophthalmol Vis Sci 25:918, 1984.[173])

count for wide individual variation in the level of pressure that is required to produce damage, or for wide variation in the degree of damage from a given pressure. Among the factors that correlate with susceptibility to glaucoma damage are increasing age,[21,22] myopia,[40,147,150] and vascular disease.[79,114,115] It is not known whether these factors relate to neuronal resistance to injury, to differences in the viscoelastic properties of the lamina cribrosa connective tissue, to abnormal regulation of blood flow and nutrition to

axons, or to other mechanisms. In face of this ignorance about other elements in the pathogenic process, all studies of pathogenesis revolve around effects of IOP.

Mechanical considerations

The eye is a closed structure whose internal fluid pressure is normally higher than atmospheric pressure. The IOP generates forces in the eyewall that are relevant to optic nerve function and disease. The IOP exerts a force from the inside of the eye outward on the whole scleral coat. The sclera is thereby stretched, producing a tension parallel to the scleral circumference, which increases with increasing IOP.

In the infant eye, when IOP is chronically elevated, the eye stretches considerably and stays larger,[156,189] even after the pressure is relieved. This expresses the fact that the sclera and cornea have not yet cross-linked their extracellular matrix components, chiefly collagens, into a rigid structure,[20] but can be remolded by prevailing forces and later become cross-linked in an expanded size. When IOP is successfully lowered, there may be some degree of reversibility of any cup enlargement,[39,86,87,104,120,138,145,149,155,156,194,204,209] a reflection of some tissue elasticity. However, because collagen deposition and cross-linking is ongoing while the eye is under stretch, much of the ocular and scleral canal enlargement of the infant eye remain permanent.

In the adult eye the eyewall stretches elastically (or viscoelastically) as the IOP increases, but the stretch of the sclera is slight and completely reversible with no permanent ocular enlargement. A possible exception is the permanent disturbance of the plates in the lamina cribrosa. (It should be noted that the intraocular pressure-volume relationship, or ocular rigidity, may result in large part from alterations in choroidal blood volume in addition to the small reversible elastic changes in globe size. (See Chapter 8.)

The optic nerve head is a weak spot in the sclera by virtue of having 300 to 500 openings for the passage of axon bundles.[43] It is well-known that a hole in a continuous structure would be a location where the stress of IOP would generate the greatest strain.[165] The resistance to viscoelastic elongation is much less at the optic nerve head than in the remainder of the sclera. This has been shown in enucleated eyes and recently in live monkey eyes.[116,117,226] Perhaps it is no surprise that the site of axon injury in glaucoma is the nerve head at the level of the sclera.[14,160]

The most characteristic feature of glaucomatous optic neuropathy is excavation of the optic disc (see Fig. 20-13). This is visible clinically as a deepening of the disc floor, narrowing of its rim of tissue, and an undermining of the rim.[53,157,160] Histologically, the process involves two major elements: compression of 10 or so perforated plates of the lamina cribrosa and posterior rotation of the lamina on its insertion into the sclera (Figs. 20-15 and 20-16). This process can be duplicated in its clinical and histologic appearance in the normal monkey eye if chronic IOP elevation is experimentally produced,[144,173] and in otherwise normal human eyes that suffer increase in IOP from injury, in-

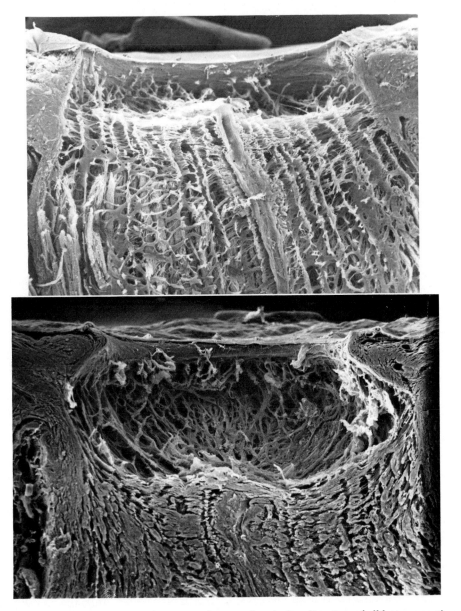

FIG. 20-15 Preparations of the human optic nerve head after digestion of all but connective tissues (scanning electron microscopy). The optic nerve head is cut in half with optic nerve below and vitreous cavity above. In the normal eye *(above)* the lamina cribrosa passes from one side of the opening to the other with a gentle backward curve. In the glaucoma-damaged eye, the lamina is compressed and its insertion into the sclera is rotated posteriorly.

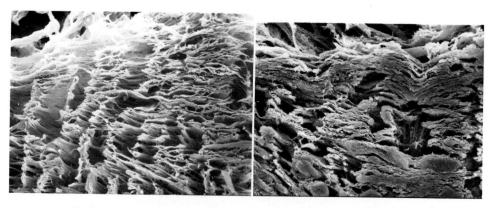

FIG. 20-16 Higher power view of lamina cribrosa as in Figure 20-15. The successive plates of the lamina through which axon bundles pass in the normal eye *(left)* are compressed together in the glaucoma damaged example *(right)*.

flammation, or outflow obstruction. A suggestion from nearly a century ago that astrocytes are preferentially killed in glaucoma has not been confirmed by modern studies.[169] Loss of axons alone (from transection of the optic nerve) results only in a pale disc without excavation, but excavation occurs rapidly if subsequent pressure elevation is induced.[146]

Glaucomatous axon damage accompanies the stretching and rearrangement of the lamina cribrosa,[172] and occurs at IOP above the statistically normal level in many human eyes, as in the experimental monkey or secondary glaucoma. Such excavation with accompanying nerve fiber loss also occurs with a normal IOP found commonly in the population.[92] There are minimal, if any, differences between the clinical appearance and functional loss from glaucoma related to the IOP level prevailing during damage. It has been common to think separately about the pathogenesis of glaucomatous eyes whose IOP is "normal" (so-called low-tension glaucoma). The incorrect assumption has been that if IOP is normal, the physical effects of IOP must play no role in the damage. Yet, as soon as IOP exceeds atmospheric pressure there are physical forces generated at the nerve head by it. There are forces exerted upon the nerve head at IOP between 10 and 20 mm Hg. Conceivably, if the individual eye has a lower resistance to laminar deformation, it may undergo excavation in this pressure range. Recent reports show that even among eyes with glaucoma but IOP in the normal range, the greater damage tends to occur in the eye with the higher IOP.[38,42]

The relationship between deformation of nerve head structure and glaucoma injury is made clearer by comparing the connective tis-

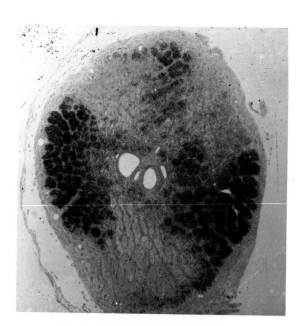

FIG. 20-17 A cross-section of an optic nerve from a human eye with moderate glaucoma damage. Black areas are remaining myelinated axons, while lighter areas are atrophic. Note the major loss of upper and lower nerve areas in an hourglass-shaped pattern. These zones are most susceptible to axon loss and correspond to areas of the lamina cribrosa that have the lowest density of connective tissue support.

sue of the lamina cribrosa[157,158,177] to the nerve fiber injury pattern in glaucoma (Fig. 20-17).[167] The structural support of the laminar tissues is less dense in the upper and lower poles of the nerve head,[43] just as these areas lose nerve fibers most rapidly in glaucoma.[167] The backward movement of laminar plates in the upper and lower nerve head is more pronounced than that through the mid-nerve head.[160] The upper and lower nerve head areas contain fibers of the mid-peripheral visual field that is known to lose function earliest in glaucoma.

The above facts suggest that IOP may alter the physical configuration of the nerve head, and that such alterations may be an important step in initiating glaucoma injury. The axons passing through this area might quite simply be compressed by or against the supportive tissue, leading to their dysfunction and the death of their cell bodies. To explain why some individuals are more susceptible than others, it might be supposed that the pressure-induced distortion in one eye may be greater than in another. Mechanical compression of nerve fibers can serve to injure them terminally. The modern exposition of this concept originates from the clinical observations by Maumenee.[123,124]

Vascular considerations

The influence of IOP on blood flow to the eye is another potentially important factor. The extraluminal tissue pressure (the IOP) tends to collapse blood vessels with flaccid walls when the force of IOP on the vascular wall exceeds the force of intraluminal pressure. Because normal IOP exceeds the orbital venous pressure, the central retinal vein and vortex veins, for example, are constricted at their exits from the eye. The retinal and choroidal arteries are also subject to compressive forces, but the effect is presumably less because, in arterioles, a mild elevation of IOP reduces the transmural pressure difference only slightly.

The resistance to blood flow at the point of venous collapse, added to the resistance that already exists in the arteriovenous pathway, works toward impairing the volume of blood flow through the circuit. Upstream from the constriction the intravascular pressure is raised. In particular, the venous pressure at the inlet to the constricted segment is the same as the IOP. For this reason the *perfusion pressure* (the arteriovenous pressure difference) for intraocular blood flow up to the point of venous constriction is in essence the arterial pressure minus the IOP.

In addition to direct external compression, the vessels may be distorted or kinked as the lamina cribrosa is distorted by the pressure. The capillaries of the lamina cribrosa at the level of the slcera are contained within the very connective tissue beams that distort, stretch, break, and reheal in the excavation process,[85,136,157] and this may result in small vessel compression or tearing.

Despite the resistance caused by either vascular kinking or by direct compression, blood flow in the retina and optic nerve of experimental animals is little affected by elevation of IOP,[63,174,201] up to a certain limit. This is evidence that autoregulatory relaxation of muscle tone exists at some other point along the arteriovenous pathway to compensate for the pressure-induced constriction. This coincides with the clinical experience that in many people modest elevation of IOP for short periods does not produce a detectable functional loss. Marked IOP elevation in angle closure glaucoma and glaucomatocyclitic crisis may persist for a week or more without producing detectable damage to the optic nerve.[45,46,182] Many patients with chronic ocular hypertension suffer no measurable optic nerve damage.[11] Neuronal tissue would not be expected to survive if the IOP in these clinical situations had produced ischemia.

Nonetheless, there are a number of clinical observations that suggest that poor vascular function may contribute to glaucomatous damage. For example, carotid artery occlusion, acute hypotension, and drastic therapeutic alteration in blood pressure seem to have exacerbated the course of glaucomatous optic nerve damage in some eyes.[48,49,51,59,74,75,99,106,186] Such examples are sometimes striking. However, obvious vascular influences are not recognized in the majority of glaucoma eyes, and only a minority of those with acute vascular insufficiency suffer optic nerve damage.

To explain the fact that the eyes of some people suffer more from pressure than others, anatomic variation that produces more compression, distortion, or kinking of vessels in one eye than another might be postulated. Alternatively, those eyes with increased susceptibility to glaucoma damage may have impaired autoregulatory reserve in the optic disc[55,71,152,153,218] leading to poor nutrition at an IOP that would not impair vascular function in the presence of normal autoregulatory responsiveness. For example, vascular sclerosis in the larger vessels that supply the disc capillaries may reduce their ability to dilate when needed for autoregulation.

As another explanation, autoregulatory capacity of the nerve head might be adversely affected by circulating vasoconstrictors, the amount of which may vary from one person to another. These vasoconstrictors may escape from the choriocapillaris and diffuse into the optic disc.[200] There they could alter vascular tone and limit the autoregulatory response of the microvasculature to the forces generated by the IOP.

As described above, the preferential loss of nerve fibers at the vertical poles of the nerve head suggests that study of regional function or anatomy might provide clues to pathogenesis. Since the lamina cribrosa has a lower density of connective tissue beams in the upper and lower nerve head, and since the capillaries supplying the lamina are within the beams, the intercapillary distance for nerve bundles in these susceptible regions is greater. If vascular function decreases with positional shifts in laminar beams, these regions might suffer preferentially because of their larger capillary spacing

Alternatively, Hayreh[81,83] proposed that there may be a "watershed zone" between sectors supplied by separate branches of the posterior ciliary arteries. The postulate is that the boundary zone between sectors supplied by separate branches would be most vulnerable to ischemia. This theory is based upon fluorescein angiographic observations of choroidal vascular filling. Experimental measurements in monkeys do not show significant regional differences in blood flow across the nerve head in normal or glaucomatous monkey eyes.[174] More accurate methods to measure regional optic nerve head blood flow and its autoregulation in human eyes are needed.

In optic atrophy, whether from orbital trauma or experimental glaucoma, the number of capillaries in the nerve head decreases in proportion to the loss of neural tissue. This accounts for the absolute fluorescein filling defect that corresponds to the region of tissue loss in glaucomatous cups in clinical fluorescein angiograms.[60,192,202,207,208] There is no difference between experimental glaucoma and primary optic atrophy in this readjustment in the volume of tissue occupied by capillaries.[173] While there were reports from blind human eyes with glaucoma suggesting a preferential loss of capillaries, this has not been true in material studied by light and electron microscopy.

Other considerations

Several other aspects of anatomy and physiology may be relevant to our understanding of the pathogenesis of glaucomatous optic neuropathy.

There are individual variations in the angle at which the optic nerve leaves the eye. This may lead to an associated misalignment or atrophy of the several layers of peripapillary tissues (pigment epithelium, choriocapillaris, deeper choroid, and sclera). This congenital misalignment and acquired atrophy of peripapillary tissue accounts for zones of tissue disarray around the disc in the form of crescents or halos, which are common in glaucoma (Fig. 20-18).* This obliqueness of nerve exit and the associated

_____

*References 13,35,58,100,101,139,190

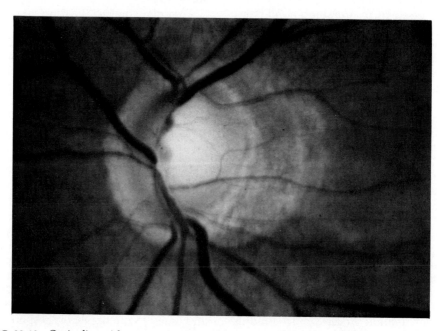

FIG. 20-18   Optic disc with crescentic peripapillary zone of retinal pigment epithelial depigmentation on the left optic nerve head on the temporal side.

crescents or halos may relate to the presence of glaucoma damage.[13,84] In many discs the nerve exits in an upper nasal direction. There is a flattened lower temporal lip of peripapillary tissue with a crescent-shaped area of exposed choroid. Perhaps this regional difference in anatomy leads in some way to the increased susceptibility to injury of the inferior temporal sector of the disc. Conceivably, regional vascular supply may correspond to the tilt of a particular disc, as does the makeup of the connective tissue beams of the lamina cribrosa.[165] The latter may affect the mechanical forces transmitted to axons or to blood vessels by the IOP. The area of contact between the optic nerve tissue and the adjacent layers of choroid and sclera is also related to the peripapillary configuration. The area of contact may be relevant, if the susceptibility factor in glaucoma is a limitation of autoregulation by diffusion of vasoactive substances from the general circulation through the choroid to the optic nerve head.[200]

One documented pathophysiologic effect of elevated IOP on the axons is blockage of retrograde and orthograde rapid axonal transport. Barany (cited by Lampert[112]) first suggested that blockage of axonal transport might occur as the axon passes from the compartment governed by the IOP to the lower pressure compartment of the intraorbital portion of the optic nerve.[29,30,57] In monkeys, cats, and dogs increasing IOP does block retrograde and orthograde rapid axonal transport at the lamina cribrosa.[16,62,130,131,133,157,162,163,168,170,200] There is also evidence of blockage of axonal transport in subacute and chronic glaucoma of both monkeys[62,132] and humans.[160] Such blockage, if maintained, is a lethal injury to the neuron.

It would intuitively seem that the pressure gradient should impair mainly retrograde transport but serve to assist orthograde movement. Yet both are blocked by elevated IOP. Moreover, it can be questioned whether the pressure gradient would directly influence these active transport processes as much as it would affect passive movement (see earlier discussion on papilledema). Therefore recent speculation has been that the demonstrated blockages are caused either by pinching of the axons[73] (by the distorted laminar beams) or by regional ischemia.

Artificial increases in IOP can affect the electrical activity of retinal ganglion cell axons. In some experiments it is clear that this occurs only at extreme levels of IOP, and results from decreases in blood flow in the retina.[69] There has been conflicting evidence as to whether certain types of retinal ganglion cells preferentially become dysfunctional or recover fastest from such severe experimental conditions in animal eyes.[2,69] Clinical recordings of ganglion cell activity are possible with the pattern-evoked electroretinogram (pERG)[121] and indirectly via the visually evoked response recorded over the occipital cortex. Both in experimental monkeys[98,122] and in humans with glaucoma[210] there is a reduction in pERG response proportional to the extent of glaucoma injury. Unfortunately, the low signal-to-noise ratio and variability of pERG testing may ultimately limit its clinical usefulness.

Thus, although much has been learned in the last two decades about glaucomatous neuropathy, the factors that account for vulnerability to damage have not been definitively demonstrated. When we understand the pathophysiologic mechanism that determines the degree of damage produced by a given level of IOP, we may be able to predict the degree of risk represented by each individual's prevailing IOP. We may also be able to attack these susceptibility factors therapeutically. Meanwhile, the clinician can judge whether the individual is susceptible to IOP damage only by observing if damage has begun or is continuing. At present the IOP is the only component of the damage mechanism toward which we can aim therapy.

Results of glaucomatous damage

By whatever mechanism, the axons may be damaged in bundles or diffusely throughout the optic nerve cross section.[14] Perhaps most typical is a preferential loss in the vertical sectors of the disc[9,32,89,97,105,109,149,183,185,203,204] accompanied by some degree of loss diffusely.[97,143,160,161,197]

Loss of axons in bundles is seen distinctly by ophthalmoscopy or in fundus photographs as defects in the normal nerve fiber layer appearance.[175,199] Visual function in each retinal region declines in relation to the loss of nerve fibers serving that region. Scotomas and other defects in the mid-peripheral visual field occur as large numbers of axons die.[26,34,47,50,76,78,134,222] In these visual field defects visual sensation in the affected region is less than in surrounding regions. In most cases the excavation of the disc and nerve fiber layer defects can be appreciated to be locally worse in the sector corresponding to the diminished field sensitivity.

With diffuse loss of axons, the physiologic cup enlarges concentrically[97,143,197] and may be difficult to distinguish from a physiologic cup of the same size, unless comparison can be made to the previously documented status of the disc or is made to the contralateral, less affected eye.[5,14,23] In these eyes loss of the nerve fiber layer pattern diffusely at the upper or lower disc pole may provide additional evidence of damage. With diffuse axon loss, the visual sensation is reduced diffusely throughout the visual field.[5,21,118,137,143] Since a general decline in visual sensation is also produced by opacity of the ocular media, this finding is nonspecific. In addition, by standard visual field testing, there may be a diffuse or localized change in contrast sensitivity,[24,25,137,206] color sensitivity,[27,52,137,154] and acuity[151] in affected retinal regions, including the fovea.[5] There is accumulating evidence that chronic glaucoma leads to a selectively greater loss of larger retinal ganglion cells (Fig. 20-19), especially the M-pathway group.[167] This suggests that functions subserved by these cells should be tested in improving the sensitivity of detection of early glaucoma.

The disc excavation, nerve fiber layer defects, and field loss develop over a period of years. At times the progression appears to be a succession of acute events. In other cases a gradual worsening occurs.

After acute glaucoma, even though the pressure may have been severely elevated for several hours or days, the optic nerve may not be recognizably affected at all.[45,46,182] When it is affected, the clinical manifestations differ from those of chronic glaucoma. Only scattered anecdotal observations of the optic nerve during

acute glaucoma exist. Swelling of the optic nerve head has been observed during an acute attack,[110,227,228] and in acute experimental glaucoma.[112] After the swelling resolves, the disc may be pale, with or without corresponding defects in the visual field. After an acute attack, there is no evacuation such as in chronic glaucoma. However, excavation will occur subsequently if there is a residual chronic pressure elevation.

REFERENCES

1. Aguayo AJ, Vidal-Sanz M, Villegas-Perex MP, et al: Axonal regrowth and connectivity from neurons in the adult rat retina, in Agardh E, Ehinger B, eds: Retinal signal systems, degenerations and transplants. Amsterdam, Elsevier, 1986, pp 257-270.

2. Alder VA, Constable IJ: Effect of hypoxia on the maintained firing rate of retinal ganglion cells, Invest Ophthalmol Vis Sci 21:450, 1981.

3. Alm A, Bill A: The oxygen supply to the retina, II, Effects of high intraocular pressure and of increased arterial carbon dioxide tension on uveal and retinal blood flow in cats: a study with radioactively labelled microspheres including flow determinations in brain and some other tissues, Acta Physiol Scand 84:306, 1972.

4. Alm A, Bill A: Ocular and optic nerve blood flow at normal and increased intraocular pressures in monkeys *(Macaca irus):* a study with radioactively labelled microspheres including flow determinations in brain and some other tissues, Exp Eye Res 15:15, 1973.

5. Anctil JL, Anderson DR: Early foveal involvement and generalized depression of the visual field in glaucoma, Arch Ophthalmol 102:363, 1984.

6. Anderson DR: Ultrastructure of human and monkey lamina cribrosa and optic nerve head, Arch Ophthalmol 82:800, 1969.

7. Anderson DR: Ultrastructure of the optic nerve head, Arch Ophthalmol 83:63, 1970.

8. Anderson DR: Ascending and descending optic atrophy produced experimentally in squirrel monkeys, Am J Ophthalmol 76:693, 1973.

9. Anderson DR: Clinical evaluation of the glaucomatous fundus, in symposium on glaucoma, transactions of the New Orleans Academy of Ophthalmology, St Louis, CV Mosby, 1975, p 95.

10. Anderson DR: Axonal transport in the retina and optic nerve, in Glaser JS, ed: Neuro-ophthalmology: symposium of the University of Miami and the Bascom Palmer Eye Institute, vol IX, St Louis, CV Mosby, 1977, p 140.

11. Anderson DR: The management of elevated intraocular pressure with normal optic disks and visual fields, I, Therapeutic approach based on high risk factors, Surv Ophthalmol 21:479, 1977.

12. Anderson DR: Papilledema and axonal transport, in Thompson HS, Daroff R, Frisén L, et al, eds: Topics in neuro-ophthalmology, Baltimore, Williams and Wilkins, 1979, p 184.

13. Anderson DR: Correlation of the peripapillary anatomy with the disc damage and field abnormalities in glaucoma, Doc Ophthalmol Proc Ser 35:1, 1983.

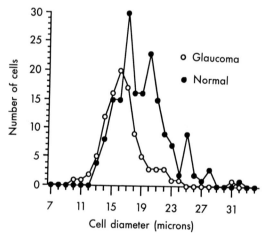

FIG. 20-19 Glaucoma injury to retinal ganglion cells selectively targets larger cells first. In this graph of number of cells against their size the glaucoma eye (open circles) has a substantial reduction in the cells larger than 17 microns in size relative to normal eyes at this location in the human retina. (From Quigley HA, Dunkelberger GR, Green WR: Am J Ophthalmol 107:453, 1989.)

14. Anderson DR: What happens to the optic disc and retina in glaucoma? Ophthalmol 90:766, 1983.

15. Anderson DR, Braverman S: Reevaluation of the optic disk vasculature, Am J Ophthalmol 82:165, 1976.

16. Anderson DR, Hendrickson AE: Effect of intraocular pressure on rapid axoplasmic transport in monkey optic nerve, Invest Ophthalmol 13:771, 1974.

17. Anderson DR, Hendrickson AE: Failure of increased intracranial pressure to affect rapid axonal transport at the optic nerve head, Invest Ophthalmol 16:423, 1977.

18. Anderson DR, Hoyt WF: Ultrastructure of the intraorbital portion of human and monkey optic nerve, Arch Ophthalmol 82:506, 1969.

19. Anderson DR, Hoyt WF, Hogan MJ: The fine structure of the astroglia in the human optic nerve and optic nerve head, Trans Am Ophthalmol Soc 65:275, 1967.

20. Arciniegas A: Vitrectomy: approach for progressive myopic diseases, J Ocular Ther Surg 3:71, 1984.

21. Armaly MF: Ocular pressure and visual fields: a ten-year follow-up study, Arch Ophthalmol 81:25, 1969.

22. Armaly MF: Lessons to be learned from the collaborative glaucoma study, Surv Ophthalmol 25:139, 1980.

23. Armaly MF, et al: Biostatistical analysis of the collaborative glaucoma study, I, Summary report of the risk factors for glaucomatous visual-field defects, Arch Ophthalmol 98:2163, 1980.

24. Atkin A, et al: Abnormalities of central contrast sensitivity in glaucoma, Am J Ophthalmol 88:205, 1979.

25. Atkin A, et al: Interocular comparison of contrast sensitivities in glaucoma patients and suspects, Br J Ophthalmol 64:858, 1980.

26. Aulhorn E, Harms H: Early visual field defects in glaucoma, in Leydhecker W, ed: Glaucoma: Tutzing Symposium (1966), Basel, S Karger, 1967, p 151.

27. Austin D: Acquired colour vision defects in patients suffering from chronic simple glaucoma, Trans Ophthalmol Soc UK 94:880, 1974.

28. Balazsi AG, Rootman J, Drance SM, et al: The effect of age on the nerve fiber population of the human optic nerve, Am J Ophthalmol 97:760, 1984.

29. Barany E: Experiments on axoplasmic flow, in Etienne R, Paterson GD, eds: International glaucoma symposium (Albi 1974), Marseille, Diffusion Générale de Librairie, 1975, p 83.

30. Barany E: Ability of retrograde axoplasmic flow to overcome pressure gradients: preliminary communication, Doc Ophthalmol Proc Ser 16:215, 1978.

31. Beck RW, Messner DK, Musch DC, et al: Is there a racial difference in physiologic cup size? Ophthalmol 92:873, 1985.

32. Begg IS, Drance SM, Goldman H: Fluorescein angiography in the evaluation of focal circulatory ischaemia of the optic nervehead in relation to the arcuate scotoma in glaucoma, Can J Ophthalmol 7:68, 1972.

33. Ben-Sira I, Riva CE: Fluroescein diffusion in the human optic disc, Invest Ophthalmol 14:205, 1975.

34. Brais P, Drance SM: The temporal field in chronic simple glaucoma, Arch Ophthalmol 88:518, 1972.

35. Buus, DR, Anderson DR: Peripapillary crescents and halos in normal-tension glaucoma and ocular hypertension, Ophthalmol 96:16, 1989.

36. Byrne SF: Evaluation of the optic nerve with standardized echography, in Smith JL, ed: Neuro-opthalmology now! Field, Rich, and Associates, 1986, pp 45–66.

37. Byrne SF, Glaser JS: Orbital tissue differentiation with standardized echography, Opthalmol 90:1071, 1983.

38. Cartwright MJ, Anderson DR: Correlation of asymmetric damage with asymmetric intraocular pressure in normal tension glaucoma, Arch Ophthalmol 106:898, 1988.

39. Chandler PA, Grant WM: Lectures on glaucoma, Philadelphia, Lea & Febiger, 1965, p 327.

40. Chisholm IA, et al: Prognostic indicators in ocular hypertension, Can J Ophthalmol 15:4, 1980.

41. Cohen AI: Is there a potential defect in the blood-retinal barrier at the choroidal level of the optic nerve canal? Invest Ophthalmol 12:513, 1973.

42. Crichton A, et al: Unequal intraocular pressure and its relation to asymmetric visual field defects in low tension glaucoma. Ophthalmol 96:1312, 1989.

43. Dandona L, Quigley HA, Brown AE, et al: Quantitative regional structure of the normal human lamina cribrosa, Arch Ophthalmol 108:393, 1990.

44. Delori FC, Pflibsen KP: Reflectance properties of the optic disc, in Non-invasive assessment of the visual system, 1989 Technical Digest Series, vol 7, Washington, DC, Optical Society of America, 1989, pp 154–157.

45. Douglas GR, Drance SM, Schulzer M: The visual field and nerve head following acute angle closure glaucoma, Can J Ophthalmol 9:404, 1974.

46. Douglas GR, Drance SM, Schulzer M: The visual field and nerve head in angle-closure glaucoma: a comparison of the effects of acute and chronic angle closure, Arch Ophthalmol 93:409, 1975.

47. Drance SM: The glaucomatous visual field, Br J Ophthalmol 56:186, 1972.

48. Drance SM: Some factors in the production of low tension glaucoma, Br J Ophthalmol 56:229, 1972.

49. Drance, SM: The visual field of low tension glaucoma and shock-induced optic neuropathy, Arch Ophthalmol 95:1359, 1977.

50. Drance SM, Fairclough M, Thomas B, et al: The early visual field defect in glaucoma and the significance of nasal steps, Doc Ophthalmol Proc Ser 19:119, 1979.

51. Drance SM, Morgan, RW, Sweeney VP: Shock-induced optic neuropathy: a cause of nonprogressive glaucoma, N Engl J Med 288:392, 1973.

52. Drance SM, et al: Acquired color vision changes in glaucoma: use of a 100-hue test and Pickford anomaloscope as predictors of glaucomatous field change, Arch Ophthalmol 99:829, 1981.

53. Emery JM, et al: The lamina cribrosa in normal and glaucomatous human eyes, Trans Am Acad Ophthalmol Otolaryngol 78:OP-290, 1974.

54. Epstein DL, Drug JH, Hertzmark, E, et al: A long term clinical trial of timolol therapy versus no treatment in the management of glaucoma suspects, Ophthalmol 96:1460, 1989.

55. Ernest JT: Pathogenesis of glaucomatous optic nerve disease, Trans Am Ophthalmol Soc 73:366, 1975.

56. Ernest JT, Archer D: Fluroescein angiography of the optic disc, Am J Ophthalmol 75:973, 1973.

57. Ernest JT, Potts AM: Pathophysiology of the distal portion of the optic nerve, I, Tissue pressure relationships, Am J Ophthalmol 66:373, 1968.

58. Fantes FE, Anderson DR: Clinical histologic correlation of human peripapillary anatomy, Ophthalmol 96:20, 1989.

59. Feldman F, Sweeney VP, Drance SM: Cerebrovascular studies in chronic simple glaucoma, Can J Ophthalmol 4:358, 1969.

60. Fishbein SL, Schwartz B: Optic disc in glaucoma: topography and extent of fluorescein filling defects, Arch Ophthalmol 95:1975, 1977.

61. Flage T: Permeability properties of the tissues in the optic nerve head region in the rabbit and monkey: an ultra-structural study, Acta Ophthalmol 55:652, 1977.

62. Gaasterland D, Tanishima T, Kuwabara T: Axoplasmic flow during chronic experimental glaucoma, I, Light and electron microscope studies of the monkey optic nervehead during development of glaucomatous cupping, Invest Ophthalmol Vis Sci 17:838, 1978.

63. Geijer C, Bill A: Effects of raised intraocular pressure on retinal, prelaminar, laminar, and retrolaminar optic nerve blood flow in monkeys, Invest Ophthalmol Vis Sci 18:1030, 1979.

64. Goldberg S, Frank B: Will central nervous systems in the adult mammal regenerate after bypassing a lesion? A study in the mouse and chick visual systems, Exp Neurol 70:675, 1980.

65. Grafstein G: The nerve cell body response to axotomy, Exp Neurol 48:32, 1975

66. Grayson M, Laties AM: Ocular localization of sodium fluorescein: effects of administration in rabbit and monkey, Arch Ophthalmol 85:600, 1971.

67. Grayson M, Tsukahara S, Laties AM: Tissue localization in rabbit and monkey eye of intravenously-administered fluorescein, in Shimizu K, ed: Fluorescein angiography: Proceedings of the International Symposium on Fluorescein Angiography, Tokyo, 1972, Tokyo, Igaku Shoin, 1974, p 235.

68. Grehn F, Knorr-Held S, Kommerell G: Glaucomatous-like visual field defects in chronic papilledema, Arch Klin Exp Ophthalmol 217:99, 1981.

69. Grehn F, Prost M: Function of retinal nerve fibers depends on perfusion pressure: neurophysiologic investigations during acute intraocular pressure elevation, Invest Ophthalmol Vis Sci 24:347, 1983.

69a. Greve EL, Dake CL: Four-year follow-up of a glaucoma operation, Internat Ophthalmol 1:139, 1979.

70. Griffin JW, et al: The pathogenesis of reactive axonal swellings: role of axonal transport, J Neuropathol Exp Neurol 36:214, 1977.

71. Grunwald GB, et al: Retinal autoregulation in open-angle glaucoma, Ophthalmol 91:1690, 1984.

72. Haden HC: The development of the ectodermal framework of the optic nerve, with especial reference to the glial lamina cribrosa, Am J Ophthalmol 30:1205, 1947.

73. Hahnenberger RW: Effects of pressure on fast axoplasmic flow: an in vitro study in the vagus nerve of rabbits, Acta Physiol Scand 104:299, 1978.

74. Harrington DO: The pathogenesis of the glaucoma field: clinical evidence that circulating insufficiency in the optic nerve is the primary cause of visual field loss in glaucoma, Am J Ophthalmol 47:177, 1959.

75. Harrington DO: Pathogenesis of the glaucomatous visual field defects: individual variations in pressure sensitivity, in Newell FW, ed: Glaucoma: transactions of the fifth conference, Princeton, NJ, 1960, New York, Josiah Macy, Jr Foundation, 1961, p 259.

76. Harrington DO: The Bjerrum scotoma, Am J Ophthalmol 59:646, 1965.

77. Harrington DO: Differential diagnosis of the arcuate scotoma, Invest Ophthalmol 8:96, 1969.

78. Hart WM Jr, et al: Quantitative visual field and optic disc correlates early in glaucoma, Arch Ophthalmol 96:2206, 1978.

79. Hart WM Jr, et al: Multivariate analysis of the risk of glaucomatous visual field loss, Arch Ophthalmol 97:1455, 1979.

80. Hayreh SS: Blood supply of the optic nerve head and its role in optic atrophy, glaucoma, and oedema of the optic disc, Br J Ophthalmol 53:721, 1969.

81. Hayreh SS: Pathogenesis of visual field defects: role of the ciliary circulation, Br J Ophthalmol 54:289, 1970.

82. Hayreh SS: Fluids in the anterior part of the optic nerve in health and disease, Surv Ophthalmol 23:1, 1978.

83. Hayreh SS: Interindividual variation in the blood supply of the optic nerve head, Doc Ophthalmol 59:217, 1985.

84. Heijl A, Samander C: Peripapillary atrophy and glaucomatous visual field defects, Docum Ophthalmol Proc Ser 42:403, 1985.

85. Hernandez MR, Andrzejewska WM, and Neufeld AH: Changes in the extracellular matrix of the human optic nerve head in primary open angle glaucoma, Am J Ophthalmol 109:180, 1990.

86. Hetherington J: Discussion of paper by Richardson, Invest Ophthalmol 7:140, 1968.

87. Hetherington J Jr, Shaffer RN, Hoskins HD Jr: The disc in congenital glaucoma, in Etienne R, Paterson GD, eds: International glaucoma symposium (Alibi, France, 1974), Marseille, Diffusion Générale de Librarie, 1975, p 127.

88. Hiller R, Kahn HA: Blindness from glaucoma, Am J Ophthalmol 80:62, 1975.

89. Hitchings RA, Spaeth GL: The optic disc in glaucoma, I, Classification, Br J Ophthalmol 60:778, 1976.

90. Hoffman PN, Lasek RJ: The slow component of axonal transport: identification of major structural polypeptides of the axon and their generality among mammalian neurons, J Cell Biol 66:351, 1975.

91. Hogan MJ, Feeney L: The ultrastructure of retinal blood vessels, I, The large vessels, J Ultrastruct Res 9:10, 1963.

92. Hollows FC, Graham PS: Intraocular pressure, glaucoma, and glaucoma suspects in a defined population, Br J Ophthalmol 50:570, 1966.

93. Hoyt WF: Anatomic considerations of arcuate scotomas associated with lesions of the optic nerve and chiasm: a Nauta axon degeneration study in the monkey, Bull Johns Hopkins Hosp 111:57, 1962.

94. Hoyt WF, Luis O: Visual fiber anatomy in the infrageniculate pathway of the primate, Arch Ophthalmol 70:69, 1962.

95. Hoyt WF, Luis O: The primate chiasm, Arch Ophthalmol 70:69, 1963.

96. Isukahara I, Yamashita H: An electron microscopic study on blood-optic nerve and fluid-optic nerve barrier, Arch Klin Exp Ophthalmol 196:239, 1975.

97. Iwata K: Retinal nerve fiber layer, optic cupping, and visual field changes in glaucoma, in Bellows JG, ed: Glaucoma: contemporary international concepts, New York, Masson, 1979, p 139.

98. Johnson MA, Drum B, Quigley HA, et al: Pattern-evoked potentials and optic nerve fiber loss in monocular laser-induced glaucoma, Invest Ophthalmol Vis Sci 30:897, 1989.

99. Jonasson F: Dangerous antihypertensive treatment, Br Med J 2:1218, 1979.

100. Jonas JB, Naumann GOH: Parapapillary chorioretinal atrophy in normal and glaucoma eyes, II, Correlations, Invest Ophthalmol Vis Sci 30:919, 1989.

101. Kasner O, Feuer WJ, Anderson DR: Possibly reduced prevalence of peripapillary crescents in ocular hypertension, Can J Ophthalmol 24(5):211, 1989.

102. Kass MA, Gordon MO, Hoff MR, et al: Topical timolol administration reduces the incidence of glaucomatous damage in ocular hypertensive individuals, Arch Ophthalmol 107:1590, 1989.

103. Kass MA, et al: Risk factors favoring the development of glaucomatous visual field loss in ocular hypertension, Surv Ophthalmol 25:155, 1980.

104. Kessing SV, Gregersen E: The distended disc in early stages of congenital glaucoma, Acta Ophthalmol 55:431, 1977.

105. Kirsch RE, Anderson DR: Clinical recognition of glaucomatous cupping, Am J Ophthalmol 75:442, 1973.

106. Klewin KM, Appen RE, Kaufman PL: Amaurosis and blood loss, Am J Ophthalmol 86:669, 1978.

107. Kolker AE: Visual prognosis in advanced glaucoma: a comparison of medical and surgical therapy for retention of vision in 101 eyes with advanced glaucoma, Trans Am Ophthalmol Soc 75:539, 1977.

108. Kroll AJ: Experimental central retinal artery occlusion, Arch Ophthalmol 79:453, 1968.

109. Kronfeld PC: The optic nerve, In Symposium on Glaucoma, Transactions of the New Orleans Academy of Ophthalmology, St Louis, CV Mosby, 1967, p 62.

110. Kronfeld PC: Glaucoma and the optic nerve: a historical review, Surv Ophthalmol 19:154, 1974.

111. Kronfeld PC, McGarry HI: Five year follow-up of glaucomas, JAMA 136:957, 1948.

112. Lampert PW, Vogel MH, Zimmerman LE: Pathology of the optic nerve in experimental acute glaucoma; electron microscopic studies, Invest Ophthalmol 7:199, 1968.

113. Laties AM: Central retinal artery innervation: absence of adrenergic innervation to the intraocular branches, Arch Ophthalmol 77:405, 1967.

114. Leske MC: The epidemiology of open-angle glaucoma: a review, Am J Epidemiol 118:166, 1983.

115. Leske MC, Podgor MJ: Intraocular pressure, cardiovascular risk variables, and visual field defects, Am J Epidemiol 118:280, 1983.

116. Levy NS, Crapps EE: Displacement of optic nerve head in response to short-term intraocular pressure elevation in human eyes, Arch Ophthalmol 102:782, 1984.

117. Levy NS, Crapps EE, Bonney RC: Displacement of the optic nerve head: response to acute intraocular pressure elevation in primate eyes, Arch Ophthalmol 99:2166, 1981.

118. Lichter PR, Standardi CL: Early glaucomatous visual field defects and their significance to clinical ophthalmology, Doc Ophthalmol Proc Ser 19:111, 1979.

119. Lieberman MF, Maumenee AE, Green WR: Histologic studies of the vasculature of the anterior optic nerve, Am J Ophthalmol 82:405, 1976.

120. Lister A: The prognosis in congenital glaucoma, Trans Ophthalmol Soc UK 86:5, 1966.

121. Maffei L, Fiorentini A, Bisti S, et al: Pattern ERG in the monkey after section of the optic nerve, Exp Brain Res 59:423, 1985.

122. Marx MD, Podos SM, Bodis-Wollner I, et al: Flash and pattern electroretinograms in normal and laser-induced glaucomatous primate eyes, Invest Ophthalmol Vis Sci 27:378, 1986.

123. Maumenee AE: The pathogenesis of visual field loss in glaucoma, in Brockhurst RJ, Boruchoff SA, Hutchinson BT, et al, eds: Controversy in ophthalmology, Philadelphia, WB Saunders, 1977, p 301.

124. Maumenee AE: Visual field loss in glaucoma, in Symposium on glaucoma, Transactions of the New Orleans Academy of Ophthalmology, St Louis, CV Mosby, 1981, p 160.

125. McLeod D: Clinical sign of obstructed axoplasmic transport, Lancet 2:954, 1975.

126. McLeod D: Ophthalmoscopic signs of obstructed axoplasmic transport after ocular vascular occlusions, Br J Ophthalmol 60:551, 1976.

127. McLeod D, et al: The role of axoplasmic transport in the pathogenesis of retinal cotton-wool spots, Br J Ophthalmol 61:177, 1977.

128. McLeod D, et al: Fundus signs in temporal arteritis, Br J Ophthalmol 62:591, 1978.

129. Minckler DS, Bunt AH: Axoplasmic transport in ocular hypotony and papilledema in the monkey, Arch Ophthalmol 95:1430, 1977.

130. Minckler DS, Bunt AH, Johanson GW: Orthograde and retrograde axoplasmic transport during acute ocular hypertension in the monkey, Invest Ophthalmol Vis Sci 16:426, 1977.

131. Minckler DS, Bunt AH, Klock IB: Radioautographic and cytochemical ultrastructural studies of axoplasmic transport in the monkey optic nerve head, Invest Ophthalmol Vis Sci 17:33, 1978.

132. Minckler DS, Sapeth GL: Optic nerve damage in glaucoma, Surv Ophthalmol 26:128, 1981.

133. Minckler DS, Tso MOM, Zimmerman LE: A light microscopic, autoradiographic study of axoplasmic transport in the optic nerve head during ocular hypotony, increased intraocular pressure, and papilledema, Am J Ophthalmol 82:741, 1976.

134. Morin JD: Changes in the visual fields in glaucoma: static and kinetic perimetry in 2,000 patients, Trans Am Ophthalmol Soc 77:622, 1979.

135. Morrison JC, Brown AE, Quigley HA: Aging changes in the rhesus monkey optic nerve, Invest Ophthalmol Vis Sci 31:1623, 1990.

136. Morrison JC, Dorman-Pease ME, Dunkelberger GR, et al: Optic nerve head extracellular matrix in primary optic atrophy and experimental glaucoma, Arch Ophthalmol 108:1020, 1990.

137. Motolko M, Drance SM, Douglas GR: The early psychophysical disturbances in chronic open-angle glau-

coma: a study of visual functions with asymmetric disc cupping, Arch Ophthalmol 100:1632, 1982.

138. Neumann E, Hyams SW: Intermittent glaucomatous excavation, Arch Ophthalmol 90:64, 1973.

139. Nevarez J, Rockwood EJ, Anderson DR: The configuration of peripapillary tissue in unilateral glaucoma, Arch Ophthalmol 106:901, 1988.

139a. Odberg T: Visual field prognosis in advanced glaucoma, Acta Ophthalmol Scand 182 (Suppl): 27, 1987.

140. Okinami S, Ohkuma M, Tsukahara I: Kuhnt intermediatry tissue as a barrier between the optic nerve and retina, Arch Klin Exp Ophthalmol 201:57, 1976.

141. Olsson Y, Kristensson K: Permeability of blood vessels and connective tissue sheaths in retina and optic nerve, Acta Neuropathol 26:147, 1973.

142. Ossoinig KC, Cennamo G, Byrne SF: Echographic differential diagnosis of optic-nerve lesions, Doc Ophthalmol Proc Ser 29:327, 1981.

143. Pederson JE, Anderson DR: The mode of progressive disc cupping in ocular hypertension and glaucoma, Arch Ophthalmol 98:490, 1980.

144. Pederson JE, Gaasterland DE: Laser-induced primate glaucoma, I, Progression of cupping, Arch Ophthalmol 102:1689, 1984.

145. Pederson JE, Herschler J: Reversal of glaucomatous cupping in adults, Arch Ophthalmol 100:426, 1982.

146. Pederson JE, Radius R: Personal communication, 1985.

147. Perkins ES, Phelps CD: Open angle glaucoma, ocular hypertension, low-tension glaucoma, and refraction, Arch Ophthalmol 100:464, 1982.

148. Perry GW, Wilson DL: Protein synthesis and axonal transport during nerve degeneration, J Neurochem 37:1203, 1981.

149. Phelps CD: Recognition of glaucomatous cupping, in Blodi FC, ed: Current concepts in ophthalmology, vol 4, St Louis, CV Mosby, 1974, p 72.

150. Phelps CD: Effect of myopia on prognosis in treated primary open-angle glaucoma, Am J Ophthalmol 93:622, 1982.

151. Phelps CD, Remijan PW, Blondeau P: Acuity perimetry, Doc Ophthalmol Proc Ser 26:111, 1981.

152. Pillunat LE, Stodtmeister R, Wilmanns I, et al: Autoregulation of ocular blood flow during changes in intraocular pressure, Graefe's Arch Clin Exp Ophthalmol 223:219, 1985.

153. Pillunat LE, Stodtmeister R, Wilmanns I: Pressure compliance of the optic nerve head in low tension glaucoma, Br J Ophthalmol 71:181, 1987.

154. Poinoosawmy D, Nagasubramanian S, Gloster J: Colour vision in patients with chronic simple glaucoma and ocular hypertension, Br J Ophthalmol 64:852, 1980.

155. Quigley HA: The pathogenesis of reversible cupping in congenital glaucoma, Am J Ophthalmol 84:358, 1977.

156. Quigley HA: Childhood glaucoma: results with trabeculotomy and study of reversible cupping, Ophthalmol 89:219, 1982.

157. Quigley HA, Addicks EM: Chronic experimental glaucoma in primates, II, Effect of extended intraocular pressure elevation on optic nerve head and axonal transport, Invest Ophthalmol Vis Sci 19:137, 1980.

158. Quigley HA, Addicks EM: Regional differences in the structure of the lamina cribrosa and their relation to glaucomatous optic nerve damage, Arch Ophthalmol 99:137, 1981.

159. Quigley HA, Addicks EM: Quantitative studies of retinal nerve fiber layer defects, Arch Ophthalmol 100:807, 1982.

160. Quigley HA, Addicks EM, Green WR, et al: Optic nerve damage in human glaucoma, II, The site of injury and susceptibility to damage, Arch Ophthalmol 99:635, 1981.

161. Quigley HA, Addicks EM, Green WR: Optic nerve damage in human glaucoma, III, Quantitative correlation of nerve fiber loss and visual field defect in glaucoma, ischemic neuropathy, papilledema, and toxic neuropathy, Arch Ophthalmol 100:135, 1982.

162. Quigley HA, Anderson DR: The dynamics and location of axonal transport blockade by acute intraocular pressure elevation in primate optic nerve, Invest Ophthalmol 15:606, 1976.

163. Quigley HA, Anderson DR: Distribution of axonal transport blockade by acute intraocular pressure elevation in the primate optic nerve head, Invest Ophthalmol Vis Sci 16:640, 1977.

164. Quigley HA, Anderson DR: The histologic basis of optic disc pallor in experimental optic atrophy, Am J Ophthalmol 83:709, 1977.

165. Quigley HA, Brown AE, Morrison JC, et al: The size and shape of the optic disc in normal human eyes, Arch Ophthalmol 108:51, 1989.

166. Quigley HA, Davis EG, Anderson DR: Descending optic nerve degeneration in primates, Invest Ophthalmol Vis Sci 16:814, 1977.

167. Quigley HA, Dunkelberger GR, Baginski TA, et al: Chronic human glaucoma causes selectively greater loss of large optic nerve fibers. Ophthalmol 95:357, 1988.

168. Quigley HA, Flower RW, Addicks EM et al: The mechanism of optic nerve damage in experimental acute intraocular pressure elevation, Invest Ophthalmol Vis Sci 19:505, 1980.

169. Quigley HA, Green WR: The histology of human glaucoma cupping and optic nerve damage: clinicopathologic correlation in 21 eyes, Ophthalmol 86:1803, 1979.

170. Quigley HA, Guy J, Anderson DR: Blockade of rapid axonal transport: effect of intraocular pressure elevation in primate optic nerve, Arch Ophthalmol 97:525, 1979.

171. Quigley HA, Hohman RM Addicks EM: Quantitative study of optic nerve head capillaries in experimental optic disc pallor, Am J Ophthalmol 93:689, 1982.

172. Quigley HA, Hohman RM, Addicks EM, et al: Morphologic changes in the lamina cribrosa correlated with neural loss in open-angle glaucoma, Am J Ophthalmol 95:673, 1983.

173. Quigley HA Hohman RA, Addicks EM, et al: Blood vessels of the glaucomatous optic disc in experimental primate and human eyes, Invest Ophthalmol Vis Sci 25:918, 1984.

174. Quigley HA, Hohman RM, Sanchez RM, et al: Optic nerve head blood flow in chronic experimental glaucoma, Arch Ophthalmol 103:956, 1985.

175. Quigley HA, Miller NR, George T: Clinical evaluation

of nerve fiber layer atrophy as an indicator of glaucomatous optic nerve damage, Arch Ophthalmol 98:1564, 1980.

176. Radius RL: Thickness of the retinal nerve fiber layer in primate eyes, Arch Ophthalmol 98:1626, 1980.

177. Radius RL: Regional specificity in anatomy at the lamina cribrosa, Arch Ophthalmol 99:478, 1981.

178. Radius RL, Anderson DR: Retinal ganglion cell degeneration in experimental optic atrophy, Am J Ophthalmol 86:673, 1978.

179. Radius RL, Anderson DR: The mechanism of disc pallor in experimental optic atrophy: a fluorescein angiographic study, Arch Ophthalmol 97:532, 1979.

180. Radius RL, Anderson DR: Fast axonal transport in early experimental disc edema, Invest Ophthalmol Vis Sci 19:158, 1980.

181. Radius RL, Anderson DR: Morphology of axonal transport abnormalities in primate eyes, Br J Ophthalmol 65:767, 1981.

182. Radius RL, Maumenee AE: Visual field changes following acute elevation of intraocular pressure, Trans Am Acad Ophthalmol Otolaryngol 83:OP-61, 1977.

183. Radius RL, Maumenee AE, Green WR: Pit-like changes of the optic nerve head in open-angle glaucoma, Br J Ophthalmol 62:389, 1978.

184. Rakic P, Riley KP: Overproduction and elimination of retinal axons in the fetal monkey, Science 219:1441, 1983.

185. Read RM, Spaeth GL: The practical clinical appraisal of the optic disc in glaucoma: the natural history of cup progression and some specific disc-field correlations, Trans Am Acad Ophthalmol Otolaryngol 78:OP-225, 1974.

186. Reese AB, McGavic JS: Relation of field contraction to blood pressure in chronic primary glaucoma, Arch Ophthalmol 27:845, 1942.

187. Repka MX, Quigley HA: The effect of age on normal human optic nerve fiber number and diameter, Ophthalmol 96:26, 1989.

188. Rios-Montenegro EN, Anderson DR, David NJ: Intracranial pressure and ocular hemodynamics, Arch Ophthalmol 89:52, 1973.

189. Robin AL, Quigley HA, Pollack IP, et al: An analysis of visual acuity, visual fields, and disk cupping in childhood glaucoma, Am J Ophthalmol 88:847, 1979.

190. Rockwood EJ, Anderson DR: Acquired peripapillary changes and progression in glaucoma, Graefe's Arch Ophthalmol 226:510, 1988.

190a. Roth SM, et al: The effects of postoperative corticosteroids on trabeculectomy and the clinical course of glaucoma: 5-year follow-up study, Ophthalmic Surgery, in press, Dec 1991.

191. Sanchez RM, Dunkelberger G, Quigley HA: The number and diameter distribution of axons in the monkey optic nerve, Invest Ophthalmol Vis Sci 27:1342, 1986.

192. Schwartz B, Rieser JC, Fishbein SL: Fluorescein angiographic defects of the optic disc in glaucoma, Arch Ophthalmol 95:1961, 1977.

193. Schwartz JH: Axonal transport: components, mechanisms, and specificity, Annu Rev Neurosci 2:467, 1979.

194. Shaffer RN, Hetherington J Jr: The glaucomatous disc in infants: a suggested hypothesis for disc cupping,

Trans Am Acad Ophthalmol Otolaryngol 73:929, 1969.

195. Shakib M, Ashton N: Ultrastructural changes in focal retinal ischaemia, Br J Ophthalmol 50:325, 1966.

196. Shapley R: Visual sensitivity and parallel retinocortical channels, Annu Rev Psychol 41:635, 1990.

197. Shiose Y, Ohmi Y, Kawase Y, et al: Glaucoma and the optic disc, I, Studies on cup and pallor in the optic disc, Jpn J Clin Ophthalmol 32:51, 1978.

198. Sommer A: Intraocular pressure and glaucoma, Am J Ophthalmol 107:186, 1989.

199. Sommer A, Quigley HA, Robin AL, et al: Evaluation of nerve fiber layer assessment, Arch Ophthalmol 102:1766, 1984.

200. Sossi N, Anderson DR: Blockage of axonal transport in optic nerve induced by elevation of intraocular pressure: effect of arterial hypertension induced by angiotensin I, Arch Ophthalmol 101:94, 1983.

201. Sossi N, Anderson DR: Effect of elevated intraocular pressure on blood flow: occurrence in cat optic nerve head studied with iodoantipyrine I^{125}, Arch Ophthalmol 101:98, 1983.

202. Spaeth GL: Fluorescein angiography: its contributions towards understanding the mechanisms of visual loss in glaucoma, Tr Am Ophthalmol Soc 73:491, 1975.

203. Spaeth GL: Morphological damage of the optic nerve, in Heilmann K, Richardson KT, ed: Glaucoma: concepts of a disease; pathogenesis, diagnosis, therapy, Philadelphia, WB Saunders, 1978, p 138.

204. Spaeth GL: Appearances of the optic disc in glaucoma: a pathogenetic classification, in Symposium on glaucoma, Transactions of the New Orleans Academy of Ophthalmology, St Louis, CV Mosby, 1981, p 114.

205. Spencer PS, Schaumburg HH: Ultrastructural studies of the dying-back process, IV, Differential vulnerability of PNS and CNS fibers in experimental central-peripheral distal axonopathies, J Neuropathol Exp Neurol 36:300, 1977.

206. Stamper RL, Hsu-Winges C, Sopher M: Arden contrast sensitivity testing in glaucoma, Arch Ophthalmol 100:947, 1982.

207. Talusan E, Schwartz B: Specificity of fluorescein angiographic defects of the optic disc in glaucoma, Arch Ophthalmol 95:2166, 1977.

208. Talusan ED, Schwartz B, Wilcox LM Jr: Fluorescein angiography of the optic disc; a longitudinal follow-up study, Arch Ophthalmol 98:1579, 1980.

209. Thompson AH: Physiological and glaucoma cups, Trans Ophthalmol Soc UK 40:334, 1920.

210. Trick GL: Retinal potentials in patients with primary open-angle glaucoma: physiological evidence for temporal frequency tuning deficits, Invest Ophthalmol Vis Sci 26:1750, 1985.

211. Tse D, et al: Optic nerve sheath fenestration in pseudotumor cerebri; a lateral orbitotomy approach, Arch Ophthalmol 106:1458, 1988.

212. Tso MOM: Axoplasmic transport in papilledema and glaucoma, Trans Am Acad Ophthalmol 83:OP-771, 1977.

213. Tso MOM: Pathology and pathogenesis of papilledema, in Thompson HS, Daroof R, Frisén L, et al, eds: Topics in neuro-ophthalmology, Baltimore Williams & Wilkins, 1979, p 171.

214. Tso MOM, Fine BS: Electron microscopic study of human papilledema, Am J Ophthalmol 82:424, 1976.

215. Tso MOM, Hayreh SS: Optic disc edema in raised intracranial pressure, III, A pathological study of experimental papilledema, Arch Ophthalmol 95:1448, 1977.

216. Tso MOM, Hayreh SS: Optic disc edema in raised intracranial pressure, IV, Axoplasmic transport in experimental papilledema, Arch Ophthalmol 95:1458, 1977.

217. Tso MOM, Shih C-Y, McLean IW: Is there a blood-brain barrier at the optic nerve head? Arch Ophthalmol 93:815, 1975.

218. Ulrich WD, Ulrich C, Bohne B-D: Deficient autoregulation and lengthening of diffusion distance in anterior optic nerve circulation in glaucoma: electro-encephalo-dynamographic investigation, Ophthalmol Rees 18:253, 1986.

219. Veraa RP, Grafstein B: Cellular mechanisms for recovery from nervous system injury: a conference report, Exp Neurol 71:6, 1981.

220. Weinstein JM, et al: Optic nerve blood flow and its regulation, Invest Ophthalmol Vis Sci 23:640, 1982.

221. Weinstein JM, et al: Regional optic nerve blood flow and its autoregulation, Invest Ophthalmol Vis Sci 24:1559, 1983.

222. Werner EB, Beraskow J: Temporal visual field defects in glaucoma, Can J Ophthalmol 15:13, 1980.

223. Werner EB, Drance SM, Schulzer M: Trabeculectomy and the progression of glauocmatous visual field loss, Arch Ophthalmol 95:1374, 1977.

224. Williams LW, Gelatt KN, Gunn GG, et al: Orthograde rapid axoplasmic transport and ultrastructural changes of the optic nerve, I, Normotensive and acute ocular hypertensive beagles, Glaucoma 5:117, 1983.

225. Wilson DL, Stone GC: Axoplasmic transport of proteins, Annu Rev Biophys Bioeng 8:27, 1979.

226. Zeimer RC, Ogura Y: The relation between glaucomatous damage and optic nerve head mechanical compliance, Arch Ophthalmol 107:1232, 1989.

227. Zimmerman LE: Discussion, in Symposium on glaucoma: Transactions of the New Orleans Academy of Ophthalmology, St Louis, CV Mosby, 1967, p 192.

228. Zimmerman LE, deVenecia G, Hamasaki DI: Pathology of the optic nerve in experimental acute glaucoma, Invest Ophthalmol 6:109, 1967.

CHAPTER 21

Electrical Phenomena in the Retina

ELIOT L. BERSON, M.D.

The continued growth of knowledge about electrical phenomena in the retina both in normal subjects and in patients with retinal disease precludes a comprehensive review in a single chapter. Nevertheless, ophthalmologists have expressed a need for a summary of this subject to gain a better understanding of retinal degenerations in humans and to have a basis for further research. This chapter has been written in an effort to fulfill this need; the text, modified and expanded from the previous edition, presents some recent advances.

THE ELECTRORETINOGRAM
Origin of components

In 1865 Holmgren[184] showed that an alteration in electrical potential occurred when light fell on the retina. Dewar[100] recorded this light-evoked electrical response or electroretinogram (ERG) from humans for the first time in 1877. The response of the dark-adapted eye to white light was separated by Einthoven and Jolly[123] into an early cornea-negative a-wave, then a cornea-positive b-wave, a slower, usually cornea-positive c-wave, and in some mammals a small

d-wave or off effect coincident with cessation of illumination (Fig. 21-1). Granit[167,168] identified three components or processes (P-I, P-II, and P-III) that disappeared successively from the ERG of a cat during deepening anesthesia and considered the ERG as a summation of these processes; his analysis (Fig. 21-2) has provided a frame of reference for more recent studies.

Tomita[335,336] showed that ERG components could be localized by depth recording with microelectrodes within the frog retina. Components of the ERG, recorded from within the retina, also could be recorded at the cornea with similar waveform. From a series of depth recordings in the cat retina Brown and Wiesel[76] found a correlation between amplitude maxima and retinal layers respectively for the a-, b-, and c-wave; they clearly demonstrated that at least part of the a-wave is generated in a layer distal or external to that responsible for the b-wave. Brown and Watanabe[74] found that a large a-wave could be recorded in the local foveal ERG of the monkey where photoreceptors are in abundance and the remaining neuropile is scant, whereas the a-wave was much smaller and the b-wave relatively larger in the peripheral retina, where the inner nuclear layer is more prominent. In retinas of cold-blooded vertebrates Murakami and Kaneko[245] divided P-III into distal and proximal components; distal P-III was recorded in the receptor layer and proximal P-III in the inner nuclear layer. Distal P-III has been correlated with the onset of the a-wave of

From the Berman-Gund Laboratory for the Study of Retinal Degenerations, Harvard Medical School, Massachusetts Eye and Ear Infirmary, Boston, Massachusetts. This work was supported in part by the Retinitis Pigmentosa Foundation Fighting Blindness, Baltimore, Maryland.

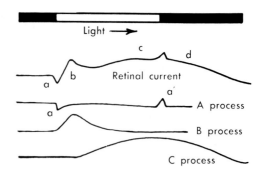

FIG. 21-1   Diagram of Einthoven and Jolly's analysis of retinal response (top tracing) into three components or processes, A, B, and C. (From Adrian ED, Matthews, R: J Physiol (Lond) 63:378, 1927.)

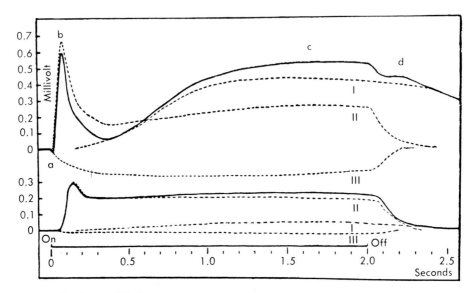

FIG. 21-2   Analysis of ERG at two stimulus intensities. Upper tracing, 14 mL. Lower tracing, 0.14 mL. The a-wave has been broadened slightly out of proportion to demonstrate its derivation more clearly. Duration of stimulus was 2 seconds. (From Granit R: Sensory mechanisms of the retina, London, 1947, Oxford University Press.)

the ERG in the monkey.[75] Witkovsky, Dudek, and Ripps[359] subdivided distal P-III in the carp into a faster component (fast P-III), which is generated by photoreceptors, and a slower component (slow P-III), which appears to be generated by the distal portions of the Müller cells.

Armington, Johnson, and Riggs[15] (Fig. 21-3) observed that the a-wave recorded at the cornea from the human eye under dark-adapted or scotopic conditions consists of two components; the earlier cornea-negative component (a_p) has the spectral sensitivity of the cone system and is little affected by light adaptation, whereas the later cornea-negative component (a_s) is much depressed by light adaptation and has the spectral sensitivity of the rod system.[15]

The cellular origin of the b-wave (P-II) of the ERG has also been clarified. Following central

retinal artery occlusion in monkeys[161] and humans,[178] cells in the inner nuclear layer are destroyed whereas photoreceptors appear intact, and the b-wave is eliminated while the a-wave is preserved. Large responses similar in waveform to the b-wave have been observed when the tips of microelectrodes are on opposite sides of the inner nuclear layer.[174] Microelectrode studies in the mud puppy (Necturus) by Miller and Dowling[237] (Fig. 21-4) and in the frog by Newman[255,256] provide evidence for the Müller cell as the site of generation of the b-wave. The waveforms of the intracellularly recorded Müller cell potential and the extracellularly recorded b-wave of the ERG are similar, particularly at low stimulus intensities. The Müller cell does not generate an a-wave. Furthermore, the latency of the Müller cell response and the b-wave

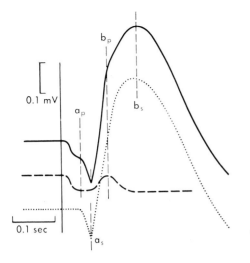

FIG. 21-3 Analysis of ERG in dark-adapted human eye as the resultant of photopic *(dashed line)* and scotopic *(dotted line)* components. The a-wave is composed of photopic (a_p) and scotopic (a_s) components, and the b-wave is similarly composed of photopic (b_p) and scotopic (b_s) components. (From Armington JC, Johnson EP, Riggs LA: J Physiol (Lond) 118:289, 1952.)

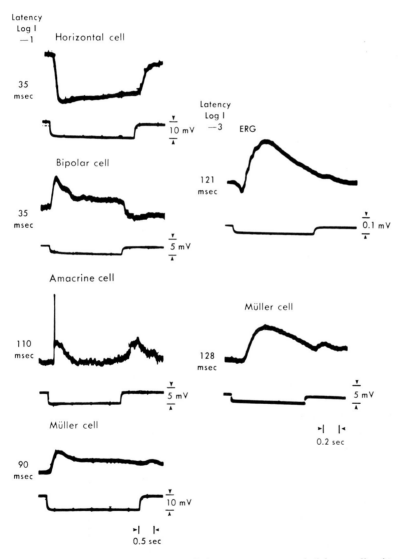

FIG. 21-4 Comparison of ERG with intracellular responses recorded from cells of inner nuclear layer of mud puppy. All responses were evoked by light flashes that illuminated entire retina evenly. Müller (glial) cell response closely matches b-wave in latency and waveform, especially at relatively low intensities *(right)*. Latencies and waveforms of neuronal and Müller cell responses are compared on left. (From Miller RF, Dowling JE: J Neurophysiol 33:323, 1970.)

correspond closely over a wide range of stimulus intensities, and stimulus intensity–response amplitude relations agree over a stimulus range of 5 to 6 log units. Intracellular responses from other cells in the inner nuclear layer of the mud puppy do not match the ERG b-wave (Fig. 21-4).[107,237]

Although the b-wave is generated proximal to the photoreceptors, rhodopsin content of the retina after exposure to bright light is linearly related to the log threshold of the b-wave in the normal rat. Furthermore, rats fed a vitamin A–free diet show a decline in rhodopsin levels in the retina and a parallel rise of the log threshold of the ERG b-wave.[106]

Adrian[1,2] recognized the separate contributions of the rod and cone systems in the generation of ERG responses. Stimulus conditions that favored cones (photopic) resulted in small b-wave responses of short latency, whereas stimulation of the rod receptor system under scotopic conditions produced relatively large cornea-positive b-wave responses of longer latency. Under conditions of complete dark adaptation the peak sensitivity of the major cornea-positive ERG b-wave in response to single flashes of light (presented at 2-second intervals) was near 504 nm, and the ERG spectral sensitivity curve approximated the absorption spectrum of rhodopsin. Under conditions of steady white light adaptation sufficient to eliminate the rod contribution to the ERG, the peak sensitivity of the ERG b-wave in response to single flashes shifted from 504 nm to about 555 nm (the so-called Purkinje shift).[192]

Psychophysical studies on humans by Stiles[325] and Wald[354] have shown that at least three cone mechanisms, defined by their spectral sensitivity curves, can be revealed by measurement of thresholds to narrow band light stimuli presented in the presence of intense chromatic backgrounds. Three cone mechanisms (Fig. 21-5), defined by their spectral sensitivity curves, also can be separated in the ERG b-wave recorded at the cornea of the cynomolgus monkey by a similar approach.[236,268,344] ERG b-waves recorded in response to narrow band stimuli superimposed on an intense yellow background reveal the short wavelength (blue) mechanism with its maximum sensitivity near 440 nm. Narrow band stimuli presented on a purple background reveal a middle wavelength (green) mechanism, with maximum sensitivity near 540 nm. When the background is blue-green, narrow band stimuli elicit a long wavelength (red) mechanism, with maximum sensitivity near 580 nm. In each case the chromatic

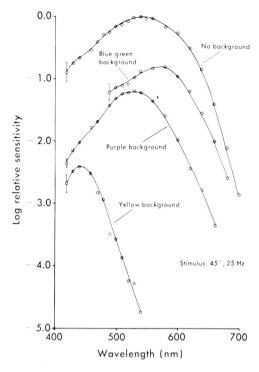

FIG. 21-5 Spectral sensitivity curves describing response of monkey cone mechanisms to 25 Hz stimulus under conditions of dark adaptation or in presence of intense chromatic backgrounds. Sector disc (50% duty cycle) was used to present flickering stimuli (25 Hz). Stimulus subtended visual angle of 45 degrees and was centrally superimposed on 68-degree background. Spectral sensitivity data were based on log relative quantum flux at retina necessary to elicit criterion amplitude in ERG. Red cone mechanism showed best separation on blue-green (Wratten 47) adapting field of 6.2 log troland intensity, green cone mechanism on purple (Wratten 35) adapting field of 5.8 log troland intensity, and blue cone mechanism on yellow (Corning 3482) adapting field of 7.2 log troland intensity. Data points (o) are an average from three animals. Vertical lines equal ±1 SD (average). (From Mehaffey L III, Berson EL: Invest Ophthalmol 13:266, 1974.)

background eliminated the rod contribution and most, if not all, of the contributions from two cone mechanisms. The spectral sensitivity curves of these three mechanisms, derived from measurement of ERG b-waves, approximate cone pigment absorption data from individual cones obtained with microspectrophotometric measurements by Marks, Dobelle, and MacNichol[229] and by Brown and Wald.[73] Therefore it is important to recognize that ERG b-waves can provide a measure of cone and rod system activity in monkeys and in humans, even though evidence from the mud puppy indicates that the b-wave reflects activity of the glial cells (Müller cells) and is not generated directly by retinal neurons.

Microelectrode studies, complemented by observations on the effects of various retinotoxic agents, have helped to define the cellular origin of the c-wave (P-I). Steinberg, Schmidt, and Brown[324] recorded a c-wave intracellularly from the pigment epithelium of the cat. Noell[258] showed that intravenously administered sodium iodate, which severely injured the pigment epithelium, selectively reduced the c-wave in the rabbit. Dowling and Ripps[115] found that application of sodium aspartate to the all-rod retina of the skate (Fig. 21-6, middle tracings) suppresses the responses of proximal elements but leaves relatively unaffected the electrical activity of the photoreceptors (a-wave) and pigment epithelium (c-wave). Removal of the aspartate-treated retina from the eyecup, which contains the pigment epithelium, eliminated the c-wave (Fig. 21-6, bottom tracings). Although the pigment epithelium must be present to generate a c-wave, the rods certainly contribute to or lead to the response, because the spectral sensitivity of the dark-adapted c-wave response corresponds with the absorption spectrum of rhodopsin in the rods and not that of melanin in the pigment epithelium.[104,169]

Clinical usefulness of ERG testing in establishing the site of visual loss derives in part from the fact that the a-, b-, and c-waves are generated by cells distal to the ganglion cells. Electroretinographic testing can help to distinguish abnormalities in the pigment epithelium and outer and inner nuclear layers from abnormalities in the ganglion cell layer or optic nerve.[150,151,191] For example, the ERG in response to flashes of light is very small or nondetectable in patients with advanced retinitis pigmentosa[196] and congenital amaurosis of Leber[179] (diseases that involve the photoreceptors or pigment epithelium or both) but is normal in patients with Tay-Sachs disease,[92] glaucoma, or neuromyelitis optica (diseases that involve ganglion cells or the optic nerve).

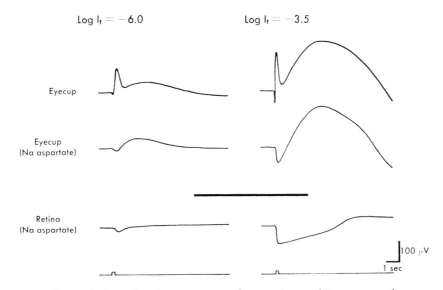

FIG. 21-6 Effects of Na (sodium) aspartate on electroretinographic responses from eyecup and isolated retina of skate. Responses were elicited by 0.2-second stimuli at two intensities (log I_t = −6.0 and −3.5). Upper traces were recorded from untreated eyecup preparation and show a-, b-, and c-waves of normal ERG. After immersion for 3 minutes in Ringer's solution containing 50 mmol L-sodium aspartate (middle tracings), b-wave was suppressed, but a- and c-waves were essentially unaltered. Removing aspartate-treated retina from eyecup eliminated c-wave. Log I_t values give filter density attenuating test beam (log $I_t \sim -D$), where log I_t = 0 corresponds to 1.1 mW cm^{-2}. (From Dowling JE, Ripps H: J Gen Physiol 60:698, 1972, copyright © 1972, Rockefeller University Press.)

Physiologic basis

In 1896 von Helmholtz[348] recognized that current flowing from vitreous to sclera, which should hyperpolarize the synaptic terminals of rods and cones, caused light to appear brighter, whereas current flowing from sclera to vitreous, which should depolarize the terminals, caused light to look dimmer. Intracellular recordings from the inner segments of the carp and *Necturus* receptors revealed a resting potential of -30 to -40 mV and a hyperpolarizing response of the photoreceptors to light. Toyoda and coworkers[337] made the interesting observation in *Necturus* cone inner segments and *Gekko* rod outer segments that during the response to light the resistance of the cell membrane rose substantially, whereas passive hyperpolarization of the cell by passing current into it does not routinely affect membrane resistance. The dark current (steady flow of radial current that causes a standing voltage gradient in the interstices between rods of the rat retina) is reduced by the action of light, thus increasing the cell membrane potential.[170] Toyoda and associates[337] suggested that the action of light on receptors was to make their membranes less permeable to ions such as sodium whose passive entry tends to depolarize the membranes. Externally applied calcium has been shown to reduce the dark current of lizard cones.[367]

Visual excitation in rods begins with the absorption of a photon of light by the photopigment rhodopsin (Fig. 21-7). The resulting change in conformation of rhodopsin (Rh) facilitates binding of rhodopsin to the G-protein transducin (T). This interaction results in a replacement of GTP for GDP in the alpha subunit of many molecules of transducin that in turn causes the alpha unit to split off from the beta-gamma part of the enzyme. $T\alpha$-GTP binds to and causes the release of an inhibitory γ-subunit of cyclic GMP phosphodiesterase (PDE). Removal of γ-subunits leads to activation of PDE and activated PDE then hydrolyzes a large number of molecules of cyclic guanosine monophosphate (cGMP).[286] This light-dependent decrease in cGMP leads to hyperpolarization of vertebrate photoreceptors through closure of cation channels. Resynthesis of cGMP by the enzyme guanylate cyclase restores the cGMP concentration to the dark level.[21,329,361]

The ionic conductance that generates the electrical response to light has been referred to as the cGMP-activated conductance; light modulates the conductance by changing the intracellular concentration of cGMP.[130,361] In darkness Na^+, Ca^{2+}, and Mg^{2+} enter the rod outer

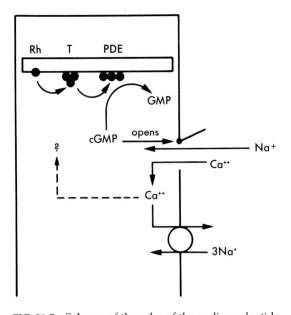

FIG. 21-7   Scheme of the roles of the cyclic nucleotide cascade and Ca^{2+} in phototransduction. The upper portion of the diagram shows how cyclic guanosine monophosphate (cGMP) regulates the light-sensitive channel in the surface membrane of the outer segment. In darkness the internal level of free cGMP is relatively high. cGMP binds to the channels, increasing their conductance (channel door open) and allowing Na ions to enter. Light closes the channel by activating the nucleotide cascade: (1) illumination of the outer segment photoisomerizes rhodopsin (Rh), (2) activated rhodopsin catalytically activates the GTP-binding protein transducin (T), (3) active T removes inhibition from the cGMP phosphodiesterase (PDE), and (4) activated PDE hydrolyzes cGMP to GMP. This product cannot open the channel, and the channel closes. The role of Ca^{2+} is diagrammed in the lower part of the figure. Ca ions enter the rod through open light-sensitive channels and are extruded by a $Na^+ - Ca^{2+}$ exchanger. The exchanger transports three Na ions inward for each Ca ion that moves outward. On illumination, entry of Ca^{2+} is blocked and continued extrusion by the exchange lowers the internal free Ca^{2+}. Internal Ca^{2+} has little direct effect on the light-sensitive channel, but controls it indirectly by modulating the nucleotide cascade. The sites and mechanism of action of the Ca^{2+} effects need to be worked out (dotted line). Ca^{2+} seems to inhibit the cyclase, which synthesizes cGMP and probably prolongs the activation of PDE by excited rhodopsin. Ca^{2+} appears to participate in a negative feedback loop, which accelerates recovery of the flash response and mediates light adaptation. (From Baylor DA: Invest Ophthalmol Vis Sci 28:34, 1987.)

segment through the cGMP conductance; Ca^{2+} is pumped out by the $Na^+ - Ca^{2+}$ exchange carrier in the outer segment while Na^+ is pumped out by a $Na^+ - K^+$ pump in the inner segment. The exit pathway for Mg^{2+} is not known nor is the possible modulation by Ca^{2+} of the cGMP phosphodiesterase well understood. In the light, closure of the cGMP-regulated conductance, together with continued Ca^{2+} efflux through the exchange, causes the free Ca^{2+} concentration to fall. A negative feedback exists such that a fall in Ca^{2+} in the outer segment is associated with a rise in cGMP levels while a rise in Ca^{2+} is associated with a fall in cGMP levels. Therefore, Ca^{2+} appears to serve an important role as an internal messenger for sensitivity modulation whereby rod photoreceptors can light adapt, i.e., adjust their sensitivity according to the intensity of the ambient illumination.[128,232,361]

The cGMP-gated channel from bovine retina consists of a single type of polypeptide of relative molecular mass of 63,000 (63K).[199] Channel activation occurs by the cooperative binding of at least 3 molecules of cGMP,[175,369] raising the possibility that the functional channel is composed either of several 63K polypeptides with 1 or 2 cGMP binding sites or of only a single polypeptide with 3 or more cGMP binding sites.

Cone conductance is also gated by cGMP with involvement of a G-protein and a cGMP phosphodiesterase.[362] There also appears to be a negative feedback on light sensitivity mediated by changes in internal Ca^{2+} resulting from Ca^{2+} fluxes through the light-regulated cGMP-activated conductance and a $Na^+ - Ca^{2+}$ exchange.[87,362] Cones do not show signs of light adaptation in the absence of this Ca^{2+} feedback.[232,250] Details of the light-activated cGMP cascade in cones await further study.[361]

Faber first suggested that the b-wave of the ERG reflected the activity of the Müller cells, the glial cells of the retina.[127] Other studies tend to support this idea, since it appears that the b-wave depends on current flow along the Müller cell in response to increases in extracellular potassium ion concentrations $[K^+]_o$, Kuffler and Nicholls[212] noted that glial cells in the optic nerve showed slow potential changes as potassium accumulated about them during optic nerve discharge and that the glial cell behaved like a potassium electrode. More recently, Dick and Miller[102] in the mud puppy and Kline, Ripps, and Dowling[201] in the skate, using potassium-sensitive electrodes, observed two sites of potassium ion efflux in response to light, one in the distal retina in the region of the outer plexi-

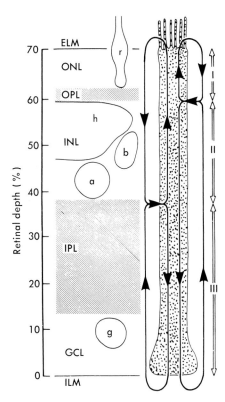

FIG. 21-8 Drawing of the skate retina. Relative retinal thickness is based on the dimensions observed in O_sO_4-fixed sections (70% retinal depth corresponds to about 105 μm). The Müller cell (stippled) extends from the internal limiting membrane (ILM) at the vitreal surface of the retina to the external limiting membrane (ELM) in the outer nuclear layer (ONL). Proposed current flow set up around the Müller cell is indicated by arrows. There is a distal current sink at the interface regions I and II and a proximal current sink at the interface of regions II and III. Cell types: g, ganglion; a, amacrine; b, bipolar; h, horizontal; r, receptor; GCL, ganglion cell layer; IPL, inner plexiform layer; INL, inner nuclear layer; OPL, outer plexiform layer. (From Kline R, Ripps H, Dowling JE: Proc Natl Acad Sci USA 75:5727, 1978.)

form layer and the second more proximally in the vicinity of the amacrine cells. The $[K^+]_o$ accumulation in the distal retina was faster and more transient in nature than that in the proximal retina.[198,201]

Kline, Ripps, and Dowling[201] proposed a model that attempts to explain how current flow in the extracellular space along the Müller cell generates the b-wave voltage (Fig. 21-8). Sites at which potassium is released by active neurons are at the interface of regions I and II and II and

III respectively; at these sites, called current sinks, current flows into the Müller cell, producing the various current paths shown in Figure 21-8. Considering the b-wave as it is clinically recorded at the cornea as a transretinal potential, the contribution to the b-wave voltage from the proximal sink is relatively negligible (that is, because of the location of the proximal sink midway along the Müller cell, there are two opposite currents of approximately the same magnitude). On the other hand, the distal current sink is asymmetrically placed along the Müller cell and therefore gives rise to the large cornea-positive potential recorded as the b-wave. The distal $[K^+]_0$ source is critical for the generation of the b-wave, and Dick and Miller[102] and Kline and coworkers[201] have suggested that the $[K^+]_0$ in the distal retina derives from the activity of the depolarizing bipolar cells. This model continues to be studied with current source density analysis[255,256,347] and selective glial-toxic agents[331] to determine whether other retinal cells also are contributing to the b-wave response.

The physiologic basis of the c-wave, a very slow response relative to the a- and b-waves, depends on depletion of potassium ions in the extracellular space between the photoreceptors and pigment epithelium distal to the external limiting membrane; following a flash of light, potassium ions presumably move into photoreceptor cells and the distal Müller cell processes, thereby creating an ionic imbalance across the apical surface of the pigment epithelium. This change results in the large, slow cornea-positive potential, which is referred to as the c-wave of the ERG.[261,262] It should be noted that the c-wave as recorded at the cornea represents the summation of a cornea-positive component generated by the apical membranes of the pigment epithelial cells and a cornea-negative component generated by the distal portions of the Müller cells (that is, slow P-III).

Separation of rod and cone components

Review of the spectral sensitivity functions of the rod and cone systems reveals (Fig. 21-9) that the rods *(solid curve)* are more sensitive than the cones *(dashed curve)* across almost the entire visible spectrum; this difference diminishes in the long wavelength portion of the spectrum, and with very long wavelength (deep red) stimuli (λ > 680 nm), cone function may be isolated. The rod contribution to the ERG can be separated by recording from the dark-adapted subject and stimulating with a relatively *dim* short wavelength (blue) or *dim* long wavelength (orange-red) light stimulus. One would anticipate that the cones could be isolated simply by presenting

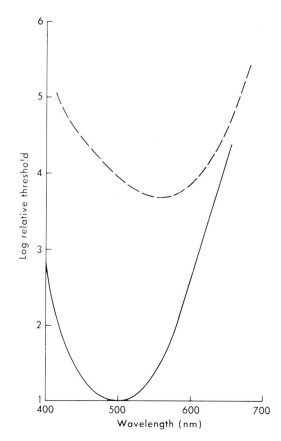

FIG. 21-9 Continuous line is CIE (Commission International de l'Eclairage) scotopic luminosity curve (rod spectral sensitivity function) derived from psychophysical measurements and placed at level for normal human subjects; dashed line is Wald's photopic luminosity curve (spectral sensitivity function for the cone mechanisms under photopic conditions) derived from psychophysical measurements of peripheral retinal function. ERG spectral sensitivity curves for normal rod and cone systems also respectively approximate solid line and dashed line curves.

single flashes of deep red light, but in fact, with the Grass photostimulator as the light source, single flashes of this deep red light are too dim to elicit an easily detectable cone ERG at the cornea from a normal subject, much less an ERG from a patient with retinal degeneration. In clinical testing, stimuli bright enough to elicit a cone response not only from normal subjects but also from patients with retinal disease can be achieved, without signal averaging, only with broad-band filters (for example, Wratten 26, λ > 600 nm). Such a stimulus, presented well above threshold, elicits not only an early cornea-positive b-wave (photopic x-wave)[243] from the cones but also a later cornea-positive b-wave from the rods. If the stimulus is well above rod threshold, as is the usual white light stimulus used for testing patients with suspected retinal disease, the ERG a- and b-waves are generated by both the rod and cone systems.

The cone response can be seen in relative isolation by stimulating the eye in the presence of a background light sufficient to eliminate the rod contribution to the ERG.[153] White light flickering stimuli presented at 25 to 30 flashes/sec (25 to 30 Hz) separate the red and green cone responses from the rod response; rod responses fuse to a repetitive white light stimulus above 20 Hz, and this results in a nondetectable rod ERG.[103,105,149,176] Therefore the peak sensitivity of the dark-adapted ERG to a 25 Hz stimulus (a response from the cone system) is near 555 nm (see Fig. 21-5). Flicker fusion frequency for red and green cones is 50 to 60 Hz.

The cone and rod contributions to the human ERG are respectively represented in recordings from a patient with dominant stationary night blindness (Fig. 21-10, *top*) and a patient with congenital rod monochromatism (Fig. 21-10, *bottom*). Responses (columns 1 and 2) were obtained to scotopically balanced light stimuli (long wavelength and short wavelength lights matched in brightness under conditions of complete dark adaptation to elicit equal-amplitude rod ERG b-waves near threshold from a normal subject).[44,46] These scotopically balanced stimuli,

when presented well above threshold, elicit equal ERG responses from the rod monochromat (*bottom*, columns 1 and 2), but they elicit unequal responses both from the patient with only cone function (*top*, columns 1 and 2) and the normal subject with cone and rod function (*middle*, columns 1 and 2). Figure 21-10 (extreme right column) illustrates that the rod monochromat (*bottom*) has no detectable response to white flickering (30 Hz) stimuli in contrast to the response of the normal subject (*middle*) and the patient with dominant stationary night blindness (*top*). Long wavelength and short wavelength light stimuli also can be photopically balanced, that is, matched in brightness to elicit equal-amplitude 30 Hz responses from a normal subject near threshold. Single flashes of these photopically balanced lights, presented in the presence of a full-field background light sufficient to eliminate the rod contribution to the ERG (Fig. 21-10, columns 3 and 4, *bottom row*), will elicit matched responses from the normal subject (*middle row*) and the patient with night blindness and only cone function (*top row*). Lights matched in brightness for subjects with normal cone pigments will elicit mismatched responses from a protanope or deuteranope.[157]

ERGs often are described as photopic or scotopic responses; this usually refers to the fact that the responses were recorded under phot-

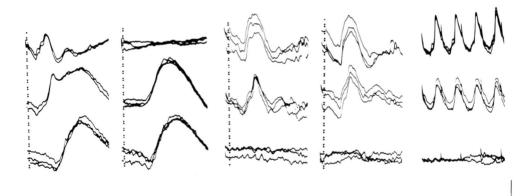

FIG. 21-10   ERG responses to scotopically balanced red ($\lambda > 600$ nm, column 1) and blue ($\lambda < 470$ nm, column 2) light stimuli, to photopically balanced orange ($\lambda > 550$ nm, column 3) and blue-green ($\lambda < 550$ nm, column 4) stimuli in presence of 5 to 10 ft-L background light, and to flickering (30 Hz) white stimuli (column 5) are shown successively from top to bottom for patient with night blindness (Nougaret type), normal subject, and congenital rod monochromat. Two or three responses to same stimulus are superimposed; calibration symbol signifies 60 milliseconds horizontally and 50 μV vertically for columns 1 and 2, 30 milliseconds horizontally and 50 μV vertically for columns 3 and 4, and 60 milliseconds horizontally and 100 μV vertically for column 5; corneal positivity is an upward deflection; stimulus onset, vertical hatched line for columns 1 to 4, and shock artifacts for column 5. (From Berson EL, Gouras P, Hoff M: Arch Ophthalmol 81:207, 1969.)

opic (light-adapted) or scotopic (dark-adapted) conditions. This description does not necessarily define which receptor system(s) has generated the response, particularly in patients with retinal disease. Scotopic ERGs to relatively intense white light stimuli usually represent contributions from both the rod and cone systems; scotopic ERGs to relatively dim white light can be generated by the rods alone. Photopic ERGs may represent either responses from the light-adapted or dark-adapted cone[159] system, and the temporal aspects of the light-adapted and dark-adapted cone ERG responses are different from each other. In patients with retinal disease, dark-adapted cone thresholds can approximate dark-adapted rod thresholds,[228] and then the minimal white light stimulus required to elicit a near threshold ERG b-wave response will be almost the same for both receptor systems. Therefore stimulus wavelength, stimulus brightness, state of retinal adaptation, stimulus frequency, and application of the concept of balanced or matched light stimuli are all important in separating the rod and cone system contributions to abnormal ERG responses.[42,157]

Summation of rod and cone electroretinogram components

The human ERG recorded at the cornea in response to a full-field (Ganzfeld) stimulus is a mass response generated by cells across the entire retina; loss of half the photoreceptors across the retina is associated with approximately a 50% reduction in ERG amplitude.[16] An ERG ob-

tained in response to a constant test stimulus is proportional in size to the area of the image of the test field on the retina, and there appears to be no interaction between one area of the retina and another in generating response amplitudes even when regions illuminated are small and near to each other.[66,68,70]

Gouras recorded ERGs intraretinally (note that the polarity is reversed) in the perifovea of the rhesus monkey (Fig. 21-11) and found that responses (left column) to a dim, short wavelength light (that is, responses only from the rod system) and responses (middle column) to a narrow band, deep, long wavelength light (that is, responses in this experiment only from the cone system) algebraically summate when both light stimuli (right column) are presented together at varying time intervals. Because the responses were generated independently, they appear in any position relative to each other, depending on the time interval of the stimulus flashes, and algebraically summate under all conditions.[152]

ERGs recorded at the cornea in humans in response to stimuli bright enough to stimulate the cone and rod systems also represent an algebraic summation of cone and rod contributions. For example, Figure 21-10 (left column) illustrates responses to long wavelength light (λ > 600 nm); the response from the normal dark-adapted subject (*middle*) represents the algebraic summation of the response from a dominant stationary night-blind patient (*top*) with only cone function and that from a rod monochromat (*bottom*) with only rod function.[42]

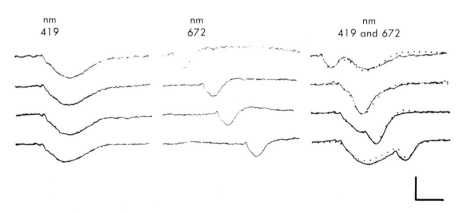

nm
419

nm
672

nm
419 and 672

FIG. 21-11 ERG recorded from within perifoveal retina to 10-millisecond pulses of monochromatic light (419 and 672 nm) covering 24.6 mm^2 of retina. Each trace is sum of 10 responses. Traces on left are responses to 419 nm, alone, and begin with stimulus. Those in middle are responses to 672 nm, alone, and only upper trace begins with stimulus, the stimulus being delayed progressively in lower traces. Traces on right are responses to both stimuli together. Dotted lines show algebraic sum of separate responses to 672 and 419 nm. Calibration signifies 0.1 mV vertically and 0.1 second horizontally. (From Gouras P: J Physiol (Lond) 187:455, 1966.)

The peak-to-peak ERG amplitude recorded from a patient with dominant stationary night blindness (normal or near-normal cone function and no detectable rod function) and a rod monochromat or patient with advanced cone degeneration (normal rod function and no detectable cone function) are respectively about 100 μV and 300 μV in response to white light stimuli, whereas the ERG to the same white light stimuli, recorded from a normal dark-adapted young adult, would be approximately 400 μV in amplitude. The ERG of a young adult with ocular albinism (reduced pigmentation with increased internal reflection of the stimuli within the eye) is usually well above 400 μV.[206] The amplitude of a child's ERG gradually increases during the first year of life and approaches that of a normal adult around age 1; rod and cone components were not separated in this study.[368] The ERG amplitude of a normal young child sedated with a barbiturate such as thiopental (Pentothal) can be reduced as much as 50% below that of a normal adult whereas Ketamine appears to have no significant effect on amplitudes.

Although the rods outnumber the cones 13 to 1 in the normal human retina,[267,360] the cone system pathway accounts for 20% to 25% of the ERG response amplitude. In response to single flashes of light on chromatic backgrounds, the blue cone mechanism contributes maximally a few microvolts to the total cone ERG response (to white light) of 75 to 100 μV in the normal subject, whereas the red and green cone mechanisms contribute the rest in approximately equal amounts.[236] Although the red and green cone contributions, as well as the rod contribution, can be detected in response to single flashes, present recording techniques require signal averaging to identify the small contribution from the blue cone mechanism. Therefore the ERG responses to single flashes of white light in the dark-adapted state from the rod monochromat (normal rod function, no detectable cone function) and the blue (π_1) cone monochromat (apparently normal blue cone and normal rod function, no red or green cone function) are approximately the same. Differences in ERG spectral sensitivity of the dark-adapted monkey eye obtained respectively in responses to 25 and 50 Hz flickering stimuli (Fig. 21-12) can be explained by a summation of the

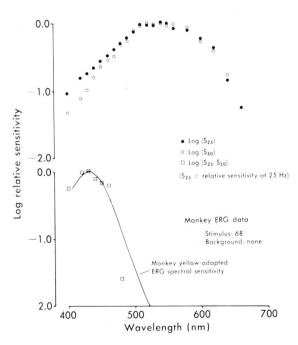

FIG. 21-12 ERG spectral sensitivity data describing monkey dark-adapted cone responses to 25 Hz (●) and 50 Hz (○) narrow-band stimuli subtending visual angle of 68 degrees. Subtraction, on linear basis, of the two sets of data yields difference points (□), shown here normalized on log plot. Curve drawn through points is spectral sensitivity curve of blue cone mechanism isolated with flickering (25 Hz) stimuli in presence of intense yellow adapting field (see Fig. 21-5). (From Mehaffey L III, Berson EL: Invest Ophthalmol 13:266, 1974.)

blue, green, and red cone mechanisms at the lower frequency and by the fact that only the green and red cone mechanisms contribute to responses at the higher frequency.[236]

Temporal aspects of electroretinogram

The temporal aspects of the cone and rod ERG responses depend on stimulus intensity and state of retinal adaptation. Figure 21-13 illustrates that relatively dim short wavelength light elicits slow, small responses from the rod system, and more intense light stimuli result in faster and larger responses.[44,60] Figure 21-14 (columns 1 and 2) shows cone ERG responses from a normal subject and a patient with dominant (Nougaret-type) stationary night blindness (no detectable rod function) to demonstrate that the cornea-positive b-waves are slower in response to dim light stimuli than comparable oscillations (designated 0) recorded from the same subjects in response to more intense light stimuli. Marked delays in cone responses are seen in two children with early retinitis pigmentosa (columns 3 and 4). With regard to the state of retinal adaptation, the light-adapted rod ERG b-waves in response to long (left column) and short (right column) wavelength stimuli (Fig. 21-15) are faster than the dark-adapted responses with stimulus intensity held constant. Similarly, for the cone system, ERG b-waves

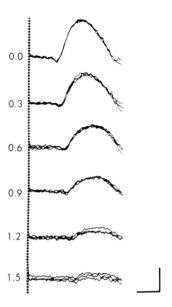

FIG. 21-13   Rod ERGs for normal subject in response to dim, short-wavelength (λ < 470 nm) light stimuli. Stimulus intensity has been successively diminished with neutral density filters (0.0 to 1.5 log units) to obtain responses. Cornea positivity is upward deflection. Two or three consecutive responses to same stimulus are superimposed. Stimulus onset is vertical hatched line. Calibration symbol (*lower right*) signifies 50 milliseconds horizontally and 100 μV vertically. Amplitudes and latencies of response depend on stimulus intensity (see text).

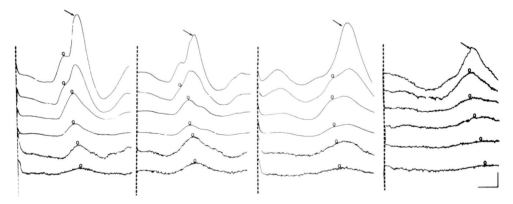

FIG. 21-14   ERG responses successively from left to right for normal subject, patient with Nougaret nyctalopia, young patient with dominant retinitis pigmentosa with reduced penetrance, and older patient with same condition. In each column stimulus intensity has been successively diminished from top to bottom with neutral density filters (0.0, 0.3, 0.6, 1.0, 1.3, and 1.6 log units). Each trace is computer summation of 150 responses to flashes of yellow light (Wratten 15) in presence of background light of 5 to 10 ft-L. Stimulus onset, vertical hatched line; corneal positivity is upward deflection, and calibration symbol, lower right corner, is 10 milliseconds horizontally and 20 μV vertically for top four responses in columns 1 to 3, and 4 μV vertically for lower two responses in columns 1 to 3 and all responses in column 4. Stimulus onset to peak of responses (*arrow*) is cone implicit time. The peak may be h-wave off effect of Nagata.[247] Circles (o) indicate comparable peaks in responses for each patient and illustrate gradually prolonged timing of response with decreasing stimulus intensity. (From Berson EL, Gouras P, Hoff M: Arch Ophthalmol 81:207, 1969).

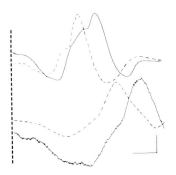

FIG. 21-16 ERG cone responses summed by computer for Nougaret nyctalope (*top*) and patient with dominant retinitis pigmentosa with reduced penetrance (*bottom*). Dashed line for each patient is response to maximum yellow-light stimulation (noted in Fig. 21-14) in presence of 10 ft-L white background light; solid line represents cone response to this same yellow light under dark-adapted conditions; stimulus onset, vertical hatched line; corneal positivity is upward deflection, and calibration symbol (lower right corner) is 10 msec horizontally for both patients, 20 μV vertically for Nougaret nyctalope, and 4 μV vertically for patient with retinitis pigmentosa. (From Berson EL, Gouras P, Hoff M: Arch Ophthalmol 81:207, 1969.)

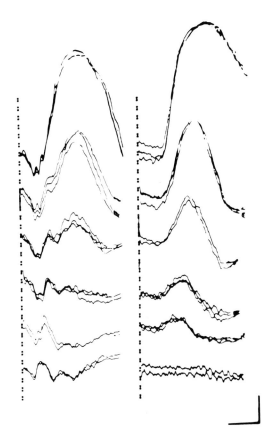

FIG. 21-15 ERG responses from normal subject elicited by scotopically matched long-wavelength (left column, $\lambda > 550$ nm) and short-wavelength (right column, $\lambda < 550$ nm) light stimuli. Top row of traces recorded in dark-adapted state. Responses to same two stimuli (i.e., stimulus intensity held constant) in presence of increasing white full-field steady background are shown successively from top to bottom—dark, 0.06, 0.16, 0.5, 0.8, and 5.0 ft-L. With increasing intensity of adapting lights, rod responses to scotopically balanced stimuli become diminished in amplitude, and implicit times become shorter. Early cone component is clearly visible only in response to long-wavelength stimulus in presence of background light. Stimulus onset is noted by vertical hatched line. Calibration symbol, lower right, signifies 60 milliseconds horizontally and 50 μV vertically. Cornea positivity is an upward deflection. (From Berson EL, Gouras P, Gunkel RD: Arch Ophthalmol 80:58, 1968.)

from the dark-adapted cone system are slower than the ERGs from the light-adapted cone system, again with stimulus intensity held constant (Fig. 21-16).[42]

Boynton and Riggs,[63] Asher,[17] and Fry and Bartley[139] have emphasized the importance of stray light in interpreting ERG responses. Light is scattered by small heterogeneities of the transparent media and by the choroid; for example, it is estimated that the minimum scatter outside a focal image on the retina is about 10% of the incident light flux at the plane of the pupil.[220] The importance of stray light was demonstrated in experiments in which a stimulus flash subtending a small angle at the eye produced a slightly larger ERG when it fell on the disc than when it fell on the retina.[17,63] With a focal light source the ERG recorded at the cornea would be expected to be a summation of responses of different amplitudes and latencies; the part of the retina stimulated with direct (more intense) light would generate faster, larger responses, and the part of the retina stimulated with stray light (less intense) would generate slower, smaller responses. Similarly, ERGs recorded in the presence of an overhead room light or focal background illumination could be expected to result in a similar phenomenon; that is, part of the retina would be exposed to bright focal background illumination and part of the retina would be exposed to relatively dim stray background light. Under these conditions some of the photoreceptors would respond more quickly in the presence of the more intense background, and some would respond more slowly in the presence of a less intense background.

With the above considerations in mind, a full-field (Ganzfeld) system has been used to record the human ERG[41,78,157,274]; this system incorporates a full-field stimulus[260] and a full-field background (Fig. 21-17). All the receptors are stimulated in a relatively homogeneous manner. Under conditions of dark adaptation or in the presence of a full-field background, recordings become remarkably reproducible with respect to amplitudes and latencies, even in children with variable fixation.[41,78,274] Possible differences in retinal illumination due to the size

of the pupil are minimized by dilating all patients' pupils with 10% phenylephrine hydrochloride and 1% cyclopentolate hydrochloride prior to testing.

Technique for recording the human electroretinogram

Electroretinographic testing became feasible clinically in 1941 when Riggs[281] discovered that a stable electrical connection with the cornea could be achieved for more than an hour with a silver disc electrode mounted in a scleral contact lens. When the lens was placed on the eye, the silver made contact with a physiologic saline solution between it and the cornea. A reference or

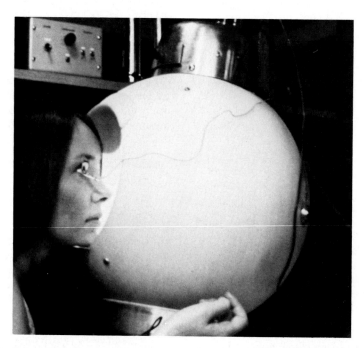

FIG. 21-17   Ganzfeld system. Stroboscope light (Grass PS 2) enclosed in case and attached to top of diffusing sphere illuminates inner white surface of this dome (40 cm in diameter), providing a full-field stimulus. Lights are recessed in top of dome so that patient can be tested in presence of steady full-field background light. During the test the patient, with contact lens electrode in place, sits with her head supported by chin rest. This dome can be mounted on a wall with the opening toward the floor so that an adult or young child can be tested in a reclining position. Wavelength of test flash can be modified by filters interposed between light source and dome. The original prototype[42,131] of this dome was constructed by Gunkel. Electrode attached to patient's forearm is grounded to amplifier common ground terminal through junction box located in case on top of dome. For routine testing, responses are differentially amplified at a gain of 1000 (3 db down at 2 Hz and 300 Hz) and d.c. coupled with 220 uF in series with an oscilloscope. If responses are to be photographed in superposition, a rapid decay phosphor in the oscilloscope is recommended. Waveforms obtained with this system are equivalent to those obtained with a battery-powered amplification system previously described.[274] Signal averaging is used for responses with amplitudes less than 10 μV; responses are differentially amplified at a gain of 10,000 (3 db down at 2 Hz and 300 Hz), attenuated at 60 Hz by a notch filter (Q = 30), amplified at a gain of 1 to 20 by a bandpass filter (Q = 16) for 30 Hz flicker and summed by a computer with bipolar artifact reject buffer.[54]

neutral electrode was placed on the skin over the cheekbone. Some electrical noise could be eliminated by placing the recording electrode and reference electrode close together, that is, a double-electrode contact lens with the recording electrode as part of a corneal contact lens and the reference electrode as part of the lid speculum (Fig. 21-18).[219]

A patient with the contact-lens electrode on the topically anesthetized cornea sits in front of the ganzfeld dome during the test (Fig. 21-17). Sedation or anesthesia usually is required to perform this test in children under age 6. Ambient electrical noise is minimized by surrounding the patient and the dome with a grounded copper enclosure. Recording equipment is placed outside the enclosure. With appropriate shielding of the patient and the dome, and with appropriate preamplifiers, signal averaging is not necessary for routine testing.

The rate of presentation and duration of the stimuli used to elicit the ERG can affect the amplitudes and latencies of responses to successive flashes of light. This problem can be obviated by using a brief flash (10 microseconds in duration) presented at 2-second intervals to evaluate rod

or cone function. Furthermore, stimulation of the dark-adapted patient with suprathreshold white flicker will light adapt the patient so that the rods cannot be tested immediately thereafter. Sequential testing of first the rods and then the cones with reliable measurements of amplitudes and latencies can be accomplished by dark adapting the patient for 30 to 45 minutes and then presenting first single flashes of dim short and long wavelength stimuli, then single flashes of dim white light, then white flicker (30 Hz), and finally single flashes of short wavelength, long wavelength, and white light stimuli in the presence of a steady white background light sufficient to eliminate the rod contribution to the ERG.

Once the patient is dark adapted, the lens is placed on the topically anesthetized eye; the actual testing time with this protocol for a cooperative patient can be as little as 10 to 15 minutes per eye. Although published values can be used as a guideline,[47,50] it is recommended that normal ranges for amplitude and b-wave implicit times (time interval between stimulus onset and the peak of the major cornea-positive component of the rod or cone b-wave response) be obtained for each ganzfeld system by testing normal subjects of different ages prior to evaluating patients with retinal disease or suspected retinal disease.

Full-field electroretinogram responses in retinal degenerations

The conventional ophthalmoscopic evaluation of the patient with retinal degeneration to determine how much of the macula and how much of the periphery appear visibly involved[135] can be complemented, extended, and often redefined by an ERG evaluation of how much the cones are involved (both macular and peripheral cones) and how much the rods are involved (both macular and peripheral rods).[29] Cone and rod system responses algebraically summate in ERGs from normal subjects and appear to algebraically summate in ERGs from patients with retinal disease. Separation of the rod and cone components in ERGs from normal subjects has provided a basis for separation of these components in the ERGs from patients with retinal disease (Figs. 21-19 to 21-22).

When ERGs are obtained in response to a full-field test stimulus, generalized involvement of a photoreceptor system has been associated not only with a reduction in ERG amplitude but also with a delay in ERG b-wave implicit time. These reductions in amplitude and delays in implicit time have been demonstrated for the rod

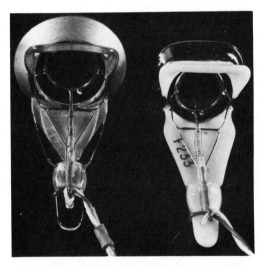

FIG. 21-18 Double-electrode (Burian-Allen) contact lenses used to obtain ERG responses. Although adult-sized lens (*left*) has been used successfully in most patients over age 6, small speculum (*right*) should be available to evaluate young children with small interpalpebral fissures. The two leads from lens are connected to differential inputs of an amplifier via junction box located in case on top of dome (Fig. 21-17) and are current limited by 2 mA fuses. (From Rabin AR, Berson EL: Arch Ophthalmol 92:59, 1974.)

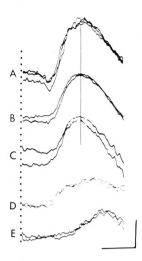

FIG. 21-19 Rod ERGs to blue light successively from top to bottom for normal subject, A; patient with central chorioretinal scar, B; patient with peripheral chorioretinal scar, C; patient with early stage of sex-linked retinitis pigmentosa, D; patient with early stage of dominant retinitis pigmentosa, E. Two or three consecutive responses to same stimulus are superimposed. Calibration symbol (lower right corner) signifies 60 milliseconds horizontally and 50 μV vertically; cornea positivity is upward deflection; stimulus onset is vertical hatched line. Vertical line has been extended from peak of normal rod b-wave response through b-waves of patients with focal chorioretinal scars, B and C, to show that these rod implicit times are within normal range in contrast to delayed rod implicit times in patients with widespread hereditary retinitis pigmentosa, D and E. (From Berson EL, Gouras P, Hoff M: Arch Ophthalmol 81:207, 1969.)

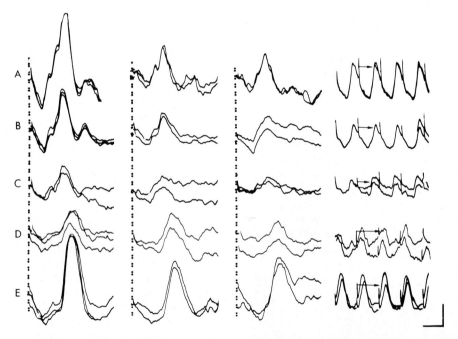

FIG. 21-20 Cone ERGs from top to bottom for normal subject, A; patient with central chorioretinal scar, B; patient with large peripheral chorioretinal scar, C; patient with moderately advanced sex-linked retinitis pigmentosa, D; patient with early stage of dominant retinitis pigmentosa with reduced penetrance, E. Left column of responses was obtained with single flashes of white light stimuli (32 $\times$ 10^3 ft-L) in presence of adapting field of 10 ft-L; second and third columns represent responses of long-wavelength ($\lambda > 550$ nm) and short-wavelength ($\lambda < 550$ nm) photopically matched lights in presence of same background light; fourth column illustrates responses to flickering white light stimuli (30 Hz) without background light. Two or three responses to same stimulus are usually superimposed; calibration symbol (lower right corner) signifies 30 milliseconds horizontally and 50 μV vertically for columns 1 to 3 and 60 milliseconds horizontally and 100 μV vertically for column 4. Cornea positivity is upward deflection. Stimulus onsets are vertical hatched lines for columns 1 to 3 and vertical shock artifacts in column 4. Cone implicit times are shown with arrows in column 4. (From Berson EL, Gouras P, Hoff M: Arch Ophthalmol 81:207, 1969.)

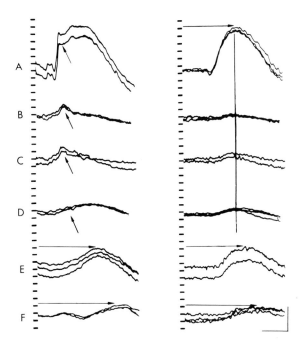

FIG. 21-21 ERGs to scotopically balanced light stimuli successively from top to bottom for normal subject, A; three patients with sector retinitis pigmentosa, B, C, and D; two children with recessively inherited retinitis pigmentosa, E and F. Responses on left are obtained with red light stimuli (Wratten 26, $\lambda > 600$ nm) and on right with scotopically matched blue light stimuli (Wratten 47, Wratten 47A, and Wratten 47B, with 0.6 neutral density filter. $\lambda < 470$ nm). Two to three responses to same stimulus are superimposed; calibration symbol (lower right corner) signifies 50 milliseconds horizontally and 100 μV vertically; cornea positivity is upward deflection; stimulus onset is vertical hatched line. Solid vertical line is extended from positive peak of normal rod ERG b-wave through b-waves of patients with localized retinitis pigmentosa; horizontal arrows designate rod b-wave implicit times. Oblique arrows (left column) designate splitting of early cornea-positive oscillation from cone system and later cornea-positive component from rod system. (From Berson EL, Howard J: Arch Ophthalmol 86:653, 1971.)

system in ERG b-wave responses from rats depleted of vitamin A[259] and for the cone system in ERG b-wave responses recorded from cats fed a taurine-free diet, with casein as the source of protein.[275,296,297] These reductions in amplitude and delays in b-wave implicit time occur in the early stages of these degenerations at a time when nearly all the rod (rat) and cone (cat) photoreceptors are partially affected. In contrast to the widespread but apparently partial involvement of the photoreceptor systems in the early stages of diet-induced retinal degenerations,[106,259,296] focal but complete destruction of photoreceptors (following photocoagulation) either in the periphery or in the macula of humans has been associated with reductions in ERG b-wave amplitudes without delays in ERG b-wave implicit times.[136]

Studies of the temporal aspects of the human ERG have provided criteria that allow separa-tion of localized retinal diseases (localized chorioretinal scars or localized macular degenerations) from the early stages of widespread pigmentary retinal degenerations (degenerations that involve all or nearly all the photoreceptors across the entire retina). For example, patients with delimited chorioretinal scars secondary to old toxoplasmosis that are either localized in the macula or in the peripheral retina show reduced amplitudes of the rod (Fig. 21-19) and cone (Fig. 21-20) components in the ERG but have normal ERG b-wave implicit times.[46] In contrast, patients with widespread pigmentary retinal degenerations[41,42,51,52] have delayed rod (Fig. 21-19) or cone system (Fig. 21-20) b-wave implicit times or both.

Patients with dominantly inherited sector retinitis pigmentosa have bone spicule pigmentation and retinal arteriolar narrowing in one or more quadrants of the fundus, and they have

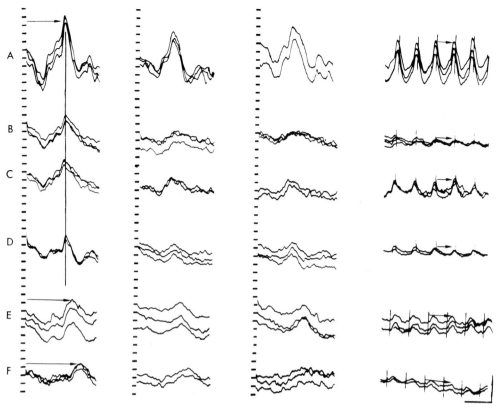

FIG. 21-22 Cone ERGs successively from top to bottom for normal subject, A; three patients with sector retinitis pigmentosa, B, C, and D; two children with widespread recessively inherited retinitis pigmentosa, E and F. Left column was obtained with single flashes of white light (32×10^3 ft-L) in presence of steady background light of 10 ft-L; second and third columns represent respectively responses to photopically matched long-wavelength (Cinnemoid 5, $\lambda > 550$ nm) and short-wavelength (Cinnemoid 16, $\lambda > 550$ nm) lights in presence of same adapting light; fourth column illustrates responses to flickering white light stimuli (30 Hz) without background light. Two or three responses to same stimulus are superimposed. Calibration symbol (lower right corner) signifies horizontally 25 milliseconds for columns 1 to 3 and 50 milliseconds for column 4; calibration signifies vertically 40 µV for columns 1 to 3 and 100 µV for column 4. Cornea positivity is upward deflection; stimulus onset is vertical hatched lines for columns 1 to 3 and vertical shock artifacts in column 4. Cone implicit times are shown with arrows in columns 1 and 4 for some patients. Solid line has been extended vertically from major positive peak of normal cone b-wave through b-waves of three patients with sector retinitis pigmentosa. (From Berson EL, Howard J: Arch Ophthalmol 86:653, 1971.)

normal psychophysical dark-adaptation rod thresholds in part of the retina and abnormal thresholds in other parts of the retina.[43,135,207] Studies of the ERG in dominant sector retinitis pigmentosa, which is minimally, if at all, progressive, have shown that this type of retinitis pigmentosa can be distinguished from widespread autosomal recessive retinitis pigmentosa, which is clearly progressive, on the basis of the temporal aspects of the ERG.[43,44] In sector retinitis pigmentosa, rod (Fig. 21-21) and cone (Fig. 21-22) ERG b-wave implicit times are normal (patients B, C, and D), whereas in widespread

recessive retinitis pigmentosa the rod (Fig. 21-21) and cone (Fig. 21-22) ERG implicit times are markedly delayed (patients E and F), even at a stage when the amplitudes of the ERG in the sector and widespread types are comparably reduced.

Some observations on ERG amplitudes and implicit times in patients with retinal disease are summarized in Tables 21-1 and 21-2. Conclusions[28] based on these data are as follows:

1. Cone and rod ERG b-wave implicit times are normal in the ganzfeld ERG in sector

TABLE 21-1 ERG* in Sector or Stationary Retinal Disease

Type	Cases	Cone ERG (b wave)		Rod ERG (b wave)	
		Amplitude	Implicit time	Amplitude	Implicit time
Sector retinitis pigmentosa	11	Reduced	Normal	Reduced	Normal
Stationary night blindness	20	Normal or reduced	Normal	Absent or normal for one flash	Normal if present
Macular degenerations	40	Reduced	Normal	Reduced	Normal
Chorioretinal scars	50	Reduced	Normal	Reduced	Normal

*Ganzfeld, clear media, dilated pupil.

TABLE 21-2 ERG* in Widespread, Progressive, Pigmentary Retinal Degenerations

Type	Cases	Cone ERG (b wave)		Rod ERG (b wave)	
		Amplitude	Implicit time	Amplitude	Implicit time
Dominant retinitis pigmentosa with reduced penetrance	8	Normal or reduced	Delayed	Reduced	Delayed
Dominant retinitis pigmentosa with complete penetrance	11	Normal or reduced	Normal	Reduced	Delayed
Autosomal recessive retinitis pigmentosa	75	Reduced	Delayed	Reduced	Delayed or normal
Sex-linked retinitis pigmentosa	7	Reduced	Delayed	Reduced	Delayed

*Ganzfeld, clear media, dilated pupil; large enough responses to separate into rod and cone components.

retinitis pigmentosa or localized retinal disease.

2. Cone or rod ERG implicit times or both are markedly delayed in the early stages of widespread progressive retinitis pigmentosa.

3. Substantially delayed cone ERG b-wave implicit times can be used to separate practically all patients with night blindness (that is, those patients with elevated rod psychophysical thresholds to an 11-degree white test light in the Goldmann-Weekers dark adaptometer in all areas of the remaining visual field) and progressive forms of widespread retinal degenerations from the patients with stationary night blindness or localized retinal degenerations (Fig. 21-23).

4. A normal cone implicit time with delayed rod implicit time can be seen in progressive retinitis pigmentosa of the dominant type (Fig. 21-24).

Individual patients have been followed over a decade from the stage of normal-appearing fundi and abnormal full-field ERGs to the stage of visible fundus abnormalities of retinitis pigmentosa and further reduction in ERG amplitudes.[50] In every family with retinitis pigmentosa in which an older affected relative has become nearly blind, the younger affected relatives have shown not only reduced ERGs but also delays in ERG b-wave implicit times.[28,29] Delayed cone b-wave implicit times have been observed not only in retinitis pigmentosa but also in other progressive widespread retinal degenerations with night blindness, including choroideremia,[305] generalized choroidal sclerosis,[28] and progressive albipunctate dystrophy.

It is important to note that the delays in cone b-wave implicit times seen in the early stages of most types of retinitis pigmentosa are observed under conditions of light adaptation (that is, in the presence of steady-state white 30 Hz flickering stimuli or single flashes of white light in

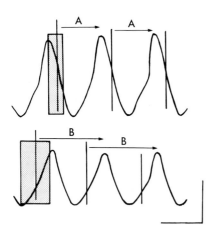

FIG. 21-23 Diagrammatic tracing to illustrate temporal aspects of cone ERG in response to 30 Hz white stimulus in normal subjects and patients with retinal disease. Stippled bar represents normal range (mean ± 2 SD) for time of onset of stimulus flash in top tracing and abnormal range (mean ± 2 SD) for time of onset in lower tracing. Vertical lines are representative for time of onset of each stimulus flash. Upper horizontal arrows, A, represent cone implicit time for patient with sector retinitis pigmentosa or localized retinal disease; and lower horizontal arrows, B, represent cone implicit time for patient with widespread recessively inherited retinitis pigmentosa. Note phase shift in relationship of stimulus artifact and response peak for B compared with A. For upper tracing, calibration symbol (lower right corner) signifies horizontally 25 milliseconds for all patients; calibration symbol signifies vertically 50 μV for normal patients and less than 50 μV vertically for patients with sector retinitis pigmentosa, chorioretinal scars, or retinal degenerations confined to macula. For lower tracing, calibration symbol (lower right corner) signifies horizontally 25 milliseconds and vertically 50 μV or less for patients with widespread recessively inherited retinitis pigmentosa.

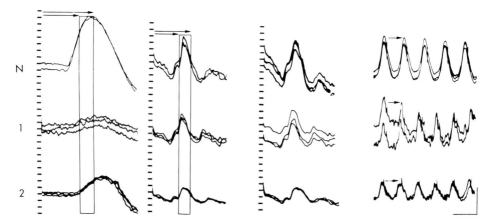

FIG. 21-24 ERGs for normal subject, N, and two children, 1 and 2, with early stages of dominant retinitis pigmentosa with complete penetrance. Left column illustrates rod responses to dim, short-wavelength (λ < 470 nm) light. Second and third columns are cone responses to photopically matched long-wavelength (λ > 550 nm) and short-wavelength (λ < 550 nm) light flashes respectively in presence of 10 ft-L white background light. Fourth column illustrates cone responses to 30 Hz white flickering light. Horizontal arrows designate range for normal rod b-wave implicit times (left column) and cone b-wave implicit times (second column). Vertical bar defining this range (mean ± 2 SD) in normal response has been extended through responses of these patients. Patients 1 and 2 have reduced rod and cone amplitudes, but implicit times of rod b-waves are delayed and cone b-waves are normal. Two or three consecutive responses to same stimulus are superimposed. Calibration symbol (lower right corner) signifies horizontally 50 milliseconds for columns 1 and 4 and 25 milliseconds for columns 2 and 3. Calibration symbol signifies vertically 100 μV for columns 1 and 4 and 40 μV for columns 2 and 3. Stimulus onset is vertical hatched line for columns 1 to 3 and vertical shock artifact in column 4.

the presence of a steady white background sufficient to eliminate the rod contribution to the ERG). However, these same patients under dark-adapted conditions may have normal cone b-wave implicit times (Fig. 21-25). Under dark-adapted conditions, in response to blue and red test stimuli, matched in brightness for the rods, patients can have no clearly detectable rod function to blue or red light (Fig. 21-25, columns 1 and 2) but can have an easily detectable cone response to a red light stimulus that is usually normal in b-wave implicit time (Fig. 21-25, column 2). With light adaptation afforded by steady-state white 30 Hz stimulus conditions, cone b-wave implicit times are substantially shorter for normal subjects and minimally shorter for patients; representative responses are illustrated in Figure 21-25, column 3. Similar differences between normal subjects and patients have been observed in cone b-wave implicit times recorded to single flashes of the same red light stimulus

under dark-adapted and light-adapted conditions. These full-field ERGs would suggest that the patients have a defect in light adaptation of their cone system or, stated in another way, the cone system of these patients functions as if it were relatively dark-adapted even in the light.[30,32,288]

More recently it has been shown in normal subjects that among stimuli matched in brightness for the cone system, the light stimulus that was brightest for the rods elicited the fastest cone b-wave implicit time.[289] Responses from patients with retinitis pigmentosa with detectable rod ERGs and different cone b-wave implicit times have demonstrated that cone b-wave implicit time to white flicker is inversely proportional to the log amplitude of the dark-adapted rod b-wave to blue light; a tenfold reduction in rod amplitude was associated with about a 5.5 msec slowing in cone b-wave implicit time.[57] These results would suggest that it

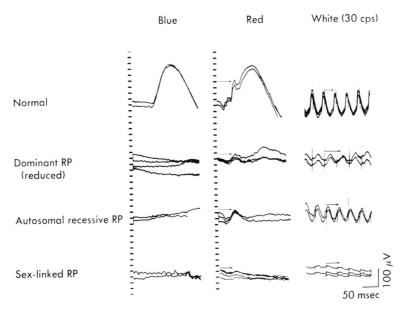

FIG. 21-25   ERGs in early retinitis pigmentosa (RP). Full-field ERG responses to blue ($\lambda < 470$ nm) and red ($\lambda > 600$ nm) light stimuli matched in brightness for the rods and white (30 Hz) light for a normal subject and representative young patients having dominant with reduced penetrance, autosomal recessive, and sex-linked retinitis pigmentosa. Responses in columns 1 and 2 were obtained after 45 minutes of dark adaptation. Cone b-wave implicit times (column 2) in normal subjects were confirmed by computer subtraction of the rod isolated response to blue light from the combined cone and rod response to red light with the residual component to red light being due to cone function. Stimulus onset is designated by vertical hatched lines in columns 1 and 2 and vertical shock artifacts in column 3. Arrows designate cone b-wave implicit times under dark-adapted (column 2) and light-adapted (column 3) conditions. Responses to 30 Hz flicker were considered delayed if greater than 32 milliseconds. Calibration symbol, lower right, designates 50 milliseconds horizontally and 100 μV vertically. (From Berson EL: Light deprivation and retinitis pigmentosa, Vision Res 20:1179, 1980.)

is the loss of rod photoreceptors among remaining cones that apparently leads to abnormal rod-cone interaction and that can account in large part for the delays in cone b-wave implicit times seen in widespread progressive forms of retinitis pigmentosa.[34,57,289]

In the case of affected males with no affected female relatives the question often arises as to whether they have sex-linked or autosomal recessive retinitis pigmentosa. In most cases males with sex-linked disease are virtually blind by age 30 to 40, whereas males and females with autosomal recessive disease usually retain vision until age 45 to 60. A study of obligate female carriers of sex-linked retinitis pigmentosa, who were in most cases asymptomatic, has revealed that 22 out of 23 tested, or 96%, could be detected on the basis of abnormal full-field ERGs.[47] Obligate carriers (age 9 to 55 with 6 or less diopters of myopia) had ERGs that were either reduced in amplitude to single flashes of white light under dark-adapted conditions (that is, $<350 \mu V$), or delayed in cone b-wave implicit time (that is, >32 msec), or both (Fig. 21-26, A) in one or both eyes. Rod-isolated responses to blue light proved less sensitive in detecting carriers than combined cone and rod responses to single flashes of white light under dark-adapted conditions. Some obligate carriers were detected on the basis of delays in cone ERG b-wave implicit times to 30 Hz flicker as the only abnormality. A few older obligate carriers with symptoms had very small or even nondetectable full-field ERGs.[47]

Among obligate carriers of childbearing age, a patch of bone spicule pigmentation or an abnormal tapetal-like reflex in the macula was observed in the fundus with the ophthalmoscope in less than half of those who could be detected with the ERG. Daughters of obligate carriers had either normal ERGs (Fig. 21-26, B, patient 3) or abnormal ERGs (Fig. 21-26, B, patients 2 and 7) similar to those recorded from obligate carriers. The abnormal ERGs of carriers of sex-linked retinitis pigmentosa contrasted with the normal full-field ERGs and normal fundi observed in 20 obligate female carriers of autosomal recessive disease.[47]

Once carrier females of sex-linked disease are identified, affected male relatives would know

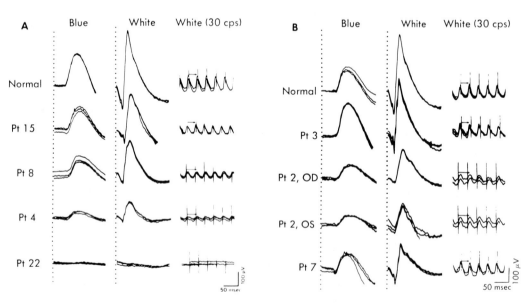

FIG. 21-26   **A,** ERG responses from a normal subject and four obligate female carriers of sex-linked retinitis pigmentosa. Pt (patient) 15, age 39; Pt 8, age 41; Pt 4, age 51; Pt 22, age 70. **B,** ERG responses for a normal subject and three daughters of obligate carriers of sex-linked retinitis pigmentosa, Pt 3, age 23; Pt 2, age 21; Pt 7, age 20. Pt 2 had bone spicule pigmentation only in OS. Pt 3 and Pt 7 had normal fundus examination results OU. For both **A** and **B** stimulus onset is designated by the vertical hatched lines for columns 1 and 2, and vertical shock artifacts for column 3. Cornea positivity is an upward deflection. Arrows in column 3 designate cone b-wave implicit times. (From Berson EL, Rosen JB, Simonoff EA: Am J Ophthalmol 87:460, 1979.)

they have sex-linked disease with a relatively poor visual prognosis and that all their daughters would be carriers and all their sons would be normal. Female relatives identified as carriers of sex-linked retinitis pigmentosa would know they have a 50% chance of having an affected son and a 50% chance of having a carrier daughter with each childbirth.

In families with autosomal dominant and autosomal recessive retinitis pigmentosa, younger siblings of clearly affected individuals have been evaluated with the full-field ERG at a stage when these siblings (age range 6 to 20 years) had minimal or no changes visible with the ophthalmoscope. The numbers of siblings with abnormal ERGs (reduced and delayed responses) expressed as percentages of the total number of siblings tested in families with the dominant and recessive types of retinitis pigmentosa agreed respectively with the percentages predicted from the mendelian laws that define dominant and recessive patterns of inheritance (Table 21-3). The mendelian patterns described previously for families in which some members had advanced stages of retinitis pigmentosa[23] have been confirmed in a study of families in which some members have the early stages.[26] Available data indicate that patients age 6 or over with normal full-field cone and rod amplitudes and normal cone and rod b-wave implicit times will not develop hereditary retinitis pigmentosa at a later time. Therefore the ERG, separated into rod and cone components, can be used in families with retinitis pigmentosa to establish the diagnosis of normality or abnormality relatively early in life and thus can help to

determine visual prognosis in younger siblings of clearly affected individuals.[26,28,29,31]

Although retinitis pigmentosa is usually a slowly progressive disease and the long-term prognosis can be estimated in early life based on genetic type,[32] the course of this disease on a year-to-year basis has only recently been defined with the ERG. Whereas the original report[196] suggested that the majority of adults had nondetectable (<10 μV) responses, more recent studies with more sensitive recording techniques have shown that the majority of patients under age 50 have large enough responses to quantitate and follow. With band-pass filtering and signal-averaging with a bipolar artifact reject buffer, it has been possible to record ERGs as low as 1 μV to single flashes of white light and with band-pass filtering to record responses as low as 0.05 μV to 30 Hz flicker.[10,54] Among 94 patients, ages 6 to 49 years, with the common forms of retinitis pigmentosa, full-field ERGs declined significantly over a 3-year interval in 66 of 86 patients (77%) with detectable responses at baseline.[54] Patients lost, on average, 16% of remaining full-field ERG amplitude per year to single flashes of white light (95% confidence limits, 13.1 to 18.6%) and 18.5% of remaining amplitude per year to 30 Hz white flicker (95% confidence limits, 15.1 to 21.5%).[54] Caution must be exercised in applying these population ERG results to predict longitudinal patterns in individual patients, since standard deviations derived from standard errors indicated considerable variation around the mean for these patients. However, these results should prove useful in planning interventions in

TABLE 21-3   Retinitis Pigmentosa, the Electroretinogram, and Mendel's Laws*

Type	Families with at least one affected patient†	Siblings‡ with subnormal ERGs	Siblings§ with normal ERGs	Siblings affected with subnormal ERGs	Prediction of affected siblings ‖
A (Dominant retinitis pigmentosa with complete penetrance)	6	5	6	$\frac{5}{11} = 45.5\%$ ←——→	50%
B (Autosomal recessive retinitis pigmentosa)	18	10	29	$\frac{10}{39} = 25.6\%$ ←——→	25%

*Age range of affected patients and their siblings was 6 to 20 years.
†Fundus examination showed visible changes of retinitis pigmentosa.
‡Fundus examination showed no visible abnormalities or minimal pigmentary changes.
§Fundus examination showed no visible abnormalities.
‖Percentages were predicted from laws of mendelian inheritance.

a similar population to alter the course of retinitis pigmentosa, particularly if monitored by full-field electroretinographic testing.[54]

Molecular genetic techniques have provided a new approach to defining hereditary retinal diseases. Analyses of leukocyte DNA have revealed specific gene defects in forms of autosomal dominant retinitis pigmentosa[119,120] as well as in autosomal recessive gyrate atrophy of the choroid and retina,[187,233,240,241,276] sex-linked cone degeneration-protan type,[279] sex-linked blue cone monochromacy,[252] and sex-linked choroideremia.[93] The rhodopsin gene mutations so far found in some forms of dominant retinitis pigmentosa (Proline-23-Histidine, Proline-347-Leucine, Proline-347-Serine, and Threonine-58-Arginine) have segregated perfectly with the disease in families so far studied and only one mutation has been found in a given family. In these families all patients so far studied with these rhodopsin gene mutations have had abnormal full-field rod ERGs.[55,119,120]

A wide range of ERG amplitudes has been observed among patients of comparable age with rhodopsin, Proline-23-Histidine, suggesting that some factor(s) other than this gene defect itself is involved in the expression of this form of dominant retinitis pigmentosa. Functional assessment of patients with this gene defect over years may help to reveal risk factors that are associated with a faster or slower course, with possible implications for therapy.[55]

Electroretinograms in stationary forms of night blindness

Although the majority of patients with severe night blindness in all quadrants of the fundus have progressive retinal degenerations, some patients with night blindness due to retinal malfunction have stationary diseases. It is the normality or near normality of the cone system in full-field ERGs that allows separation of stationary forms of night blindness from practically all forms of night blindness associated with early stages of retinitis pigmentosa.[182]

One type of stationary night blindness is dominantly inherited nyctalopia (Nougaret type). These patients (Fig. 21-10, top row) have a normal fundus appearance and have normal or nearly normal cone ERGs, but they show no evidence of a rod ERG a-wave or b-wave. Fundus reflectometry studies have indicated that even though these patients are night blind, rhodopsin kinetics are normal[83] and cone pigment kinetics are also normal or nearly normal.[7] The absence of the rod a-wave and the electrooculogram (EOG) light rise suggest that this condition affects the proximal part of the rod photoreceptor or possibly the synaptic site between the rod photoreceptor and more proximal retinal cells.[80,83,155]

Another type of stationary night blindness is congenital nyctalopia with myopia (-3.5 to -14.5 D). This form of night blindness, sometimes designated as the Schubert-Bornschein type, is inherited by either a sex-linked or autosomal recessive mode. These patients cannot attain normal dark-adapted rod thresholds and have fundus findings of myopia. They show no rod ERG b-wave in response to dim blue-light stimuli, and they have a characteristic cornea-negative response to white light in the dark-adapted state and a smaller cornea-negative response and a cornea-positive component in the light-adapted state (Fig. 21-27).[182,298] The waveforms in congenital nyctalopia with myopia can be explained by retention of the a-wave and b-wave from the cone system and the a-wave from the rod system with an absence of the b-wave from the rod system; the ERG is a summation of all three components in the dark-adapted state and only the cone a- and b-wave in the light-adapted state.[81,83] The defect appears to be some abnormality in intraretinal transmission of the response from the rod photoreceptors to the proximal retinal cells. Application of a high concentration of magnesium (which tends to inhibit the release of transmitter at nerve terminals) to the skate retina results in a selective loss of the b-wave and a waveform similar to that observed in patients with congenital nyctalopia with myopia.[116,285] Rhodopsin kinetics measured by fundus reflectometry are normal, and the light rise of the EOG is preserved, so that this condition is thought to involve a defect that is more proximal in the retina than is the defect in the Nougaret nyctalope. ERG amplitudes are reduced (Fig. 21-27) in recessive nyctalopia with myopia compared with those from normal emmetropes; this probably occurs because of the known reduction of ERG amplitudes seen in patients with moderate axial myopia as the only finding.[59,101,271]

The ERG abnormality in congenital nyctalopia with myopia has been reported as an acquired defect in a patient with malignant melanoma who developed retinal toxicity presumably secondary to intake of vincristine. Vincristine exerts its effect by binding to tubulin subunits, thereby inhibiting the assembly of microtubules. Ripps has hypothesized that a defect in assembly of microtubules with consequent impairment of transport of cytoplasmic components could explain the impairment of synaptic

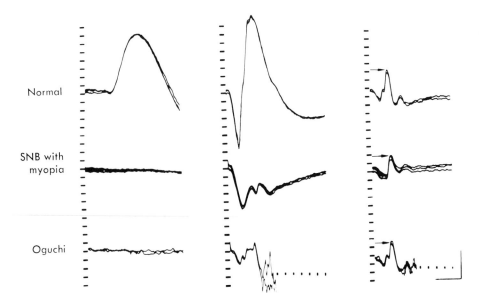

FIG. 21-27 ERGs from normal emmetropic subject (*top row*), patient with congenital stationary night blindness (SNB) with moderate myopia (*middle row*), and emmetropic patient with Oguchi's disease (*bottom row*). Responses were obtained to dim blue ($\lambda < 470$ nm) light (*left*) and white (16×10^3 ft-L) flashes (*middle*) after 1 hour of dark adaptation. Responses to white (16×10^3 ft-L) flashes in presence of steady 10 ft-L white background sufficient to eliminate rod contribution are illustrated in right column. Stimulus onset is vertical hatched line. Cornea positivity is upward deflection. Two or three successive responses are illustrated. Horizontal arrows (*right column*) designate cone b-wave implicit times. Responses from this patient with Oguchi's disease are often interrupted by reflex blinking, so latter part of some responses cannot be illustrated. Calibration symbol (lower right corner) designates 50 milliseconds horizontally and 100 μV vertically for all tracings. Stimulus flash duration was 10 microseconds.

transmission in this condition.[285] Similar ERGs have also been observed in an elderly patient with a cutaneous malignant melanoma who developed sudden onset of night blindness prior to administration of any anti-metabolite therapy. This suggests that this type of ERG abnormality can represent a paraneoplastic effect of the melanoma itself.[45]

Recessively inherited stationary night blindness can occur without myopia. In this form, sometimes designated as the Riggs type, the patient retains only a cone ERG, has a normal appearance to the fundus, and after prolonged dark adaptation attains only normal dark-adapted cone threshold on psychophysical testing. In another type, called Oguchi's disease, the patients usually require 2 to 12 hours to attain normal dark-adapted rod thresholds and show a characteristic change from a golden brown fundus in the light-adapted state to a normal color fundus in the dark-adapted state (the Mizuo phenomenon). Following 1 hour of dark adaptation (Fig. 21-27), patients with Oguchi's disease have no rod b-wave in response to dim

blue light, a cornea-negative response to white light, and a normal cone response (Fig. 21-27, right column) to white light in the presence of a background light sufficient to eliminate the rod contribution to the ERG. Following complete dark adaptation (after 12 hours) some patients have a normal rod b-wave amplitude and normal rod b-wave implicit time, but only in response to one or two flashes of light.[157] The test flash used to elicit the ERG, although relatively dim, can be intense enough to light adapt the rod system. Rhodopsin kinetics are normal, and the light rise of the EOG is preserved; therefore the defect in Oguchi's disease, as well as in congenital nyctalopia with myopia, appears to be located more proximal in the retina than is the defect in the Nougaret nyctalope.

Another type of autosomal recessively inherited stationary night blindness is fundus albipunctatus. Patients have many yellow-white deposits in the deep retina, with greatest density in the posterior pole outside the macula.[80,230] Results of fundus reflectometry in one adult patient showed that both rod visual pigment and foveal cone pigment regenerate slowly. This patient had half-times of recovery for rod and cone pigment of about 60 and 20 minutes respectively, values approximately 20 and 16 times greater than those found in normal subjects. These changes in visual pigment levels paralleled the prolonged cone and rod limbs of his dark-adaptation curve. This patient's ERG and light rise of the EOG, abnormal after short-term dark adaptation, reached normal values within 3 hours of dark adaptation.[80] Other patients studied with the full-field ERG showed normal cone and rod amplitudes and normal b-wave implicit times after full dark adaptation.[230] The findings in fundus albipunctatus point to an abnormality in visual pigment regeneration and suggest an abnormality in the relationship between the photoreceptors and pigment epithelium.[80] The composition of the yellow-white lesions and their relationship to the abnormality of visual pigment regeneration are not known.

The defect in adaptation in Oguchi's disease differs from that in fundus albipunctatus in several respects. First, in Oguchi's disease the rod mechanism is selectively affected while the cone limb of the dark-adaptation curve as measured by psychophysical testing proceeds at a normal rate. Second, the rate of rhodopsin regeneration in Oguchi's disease as measured by fundus reflectometry appears normal because the defect presumably occurs proximal to the photoreceptors. Third, relatively weak illumination will delay the appearance of the rod branch of the dark-adaptation curve as measured by psychophysical testing by more than 30 minutes in Oguchi's disease, whereas exposure to a similar light produces a smaller effect in fundus albipunctatus.[284]

Miyake and coworkers[242] have subdivided the Schubert-Bornschein type of stationary night blindness into a complete and an incomplete form, based in part on ERG testing. The complete form showed no detectable rod response to dim blue light while the incomplete form had reduced but measurable rod responses to blue light and reduced cone function as well. Patients with the incomplete form were slightly myopic or mildly hyperopic. The long-term course of patients with the incomplete form remains to be documented.

For all types of stationary night blindness, correlation of the electrophysiologic findings with electron-microscopic studies remains to be done. It is interesting that these diseases, involving either the rod photoreceptor or cells proximal to the rod photoreceptor, are not associated with pigment migration or attenuation of the retinal vessels, whereas these latter findings are characteristically seen in patients with rod photoreceptor cell degeneration and retinitis pigmentosa.

Advances in electro-optical technology have resulted in night-vision devices that allow patients with stationary night blindness, as well as patients with moderately advanced retinitis pigmentosa, to use their cones to function under scotopic (starlight or moonlight) conditions or, if necessary, under dim photopic conditions (dusk). These light-amplifying devices have been incorporated into a monocular pocketscope or binocular goggle, which can be used as an aid to alleviate the symptom of night blindness.[27,46]

Hereditary diseases affecting the retina—some therapeutic considerations

Electroretinographic testing has allowed early detection of abnormal retinal function in some hereditary diseases affecting the retina and thereby has provided an opportunity for assessing the efficacy of therapeutic trials. The importance of early diagnosis was emphasized when the abnormal ERG (abnormal cone and rod function) in a patient with hereditary abetalipoproteinemia (Bassen-Kornzweig's disease) and night blindness was reversed to normal within hours with large doses of orally administered vitamin A. An older affected patient with a more advanced stage of this disease did not respond to this treatment.[163] Vitamin E also has been reported as necessary to preserve retinal function in these patients over the long term.[58]

Another potentially treatable hereditary disease associated with night blindness and retinal degeneration is gyrate atrophy of the choroid and retina. Patients with this autosomal recessive disorder have myopia, constricted visual fields, elevated dark adaptation thresholds, small or nondetectable full-field ERGs, and chorioretinal atrophy distributed around the peripheral fundus and sometimes near the optic disc. The chorioretinal atrophy differs in extent among young patients of comparable age.[49] Patients develop cataracts and usually become virtually blind between ages 40 to 50 due to extensive chorioretinal atrophy. Biochemical abnormalities include 10- to 20-fold elevations of plasma ornithine,[48,49,234,309,333] hypolysinemia,[48,234] hyperornithinuria,[49,333] and virtual absence of ornithine ketoacid transaminase (OKT) in extracts of cultured skin fibroblasts[49,263,300,324,339] and in cultured lymphocytes.[194,341] Genetic heterogeneity appears to exist, since some patients have shown a 30% to 50% fall in plasma ornithine levels within a week when given orally administered vitamin B_6 (300 to 500 mg/day), whereas other patients have not responded.[49,356] All patients so far studied have shown a decline in plasma ornithine levels of 50% or more when placed on a low-protein (15 g/day), low-arginine diet.[299,342] Some have shown increased areas of atrophy despite lowering of plasma ornithine.[53] It remains to be established whether any degree of biochemical responsiveness to diet, vitamin B_6, or both in patients with gyrate atrophy of the choroid and retina will alter ERG function or the course of this degeneration over the long term. Many years will be required to show whether or not stabilization has occurred in young patients, if one takes into account the natural history of the ocular disease.[49]

The retinal degeneration observed in Refsum's disease (heredopathia atactica polyneuritiformis) also may be amenable to treatment. Patients with this autosomal recessively inherited disease characteristically have a peripheral neuropathy, ataxia, and an elevated cerebrospinal fluid protein level with a normal cell count.[277] Ocular findings include an atypical retinitis pigmentosa–like appearance in the peripheral fundus and reduced or nondetectable ERGs.[278] Some have anosmia, deafness, pupillary abnormalities, lens opacities, electrocardiographic malfunction, skeletal abnormalities, and skin changes resembling ichthyosis. A diagnosis depends ultimately on the demonstration of an elevated serum phytanic acid.[277] Patients have shown a defect in alpha-hydroxylation of phytanic acid, and this enzyme defect can be detected in extracts of cultured skin fibroblasts.[318] Pathogenesis of this disease appears to involve a replacement of the long-chain fatty acids in phospholipids and triglycerides with phytanic acid derived from dietary sources. Accumulation of phytanic acid in many tissues then leads to consequent malfunction. Treatment with a low-phytol, low-phytanic acid diet (that is, excluding green leafy vegetables, animal fats, and milk products), while maintaining body weight, has led to lowered serum phytanic acid levels, improved nerve conduction times, and lowered cerebrospinal fluid protein levels.[125,277,278,319] Two patients, one followed for many years and the other for more than 10 years, have shown stabilization of their retinitis pigmentosa and hearing impairment.[278] A third patient with a mild form followed for 4 years on a low-phytol, low-phytanic acid diet has shown

stable full-field ERGs over this interval.[34] The long-term effects on retinal function continue to be studied.

At the time of detection most patients so far studied with gyrate atrophy or Refsum's disease have shown full-field ERGs that have been very small or nondetectable. Gyrate atrophy and Refsum's disease have been detected in the early stages in two patients; these patients had large enough responses to separate into rod and cone components (Fig. 21-28). Interestingly, the full-field rod and cone responses from these patients, although reduced in amplitude, were within normal range with respect to b-wave implicit times. Similarly, a patient with the early stages of hereditary abetalipoproteinemia was not reported to show marked delays in cone or rod b-wave implicit times.[163] The normal temporal aspects of these ERGs contrast with the substantially delayed cone or rod b-wave implicit times, or both, recorded from patients with early stages of the more common forms of progressive widespread hereditary retinitis pigmentosa.

Focal electroretinograms

The total cone population in the human retina is approximately 6.8×10^6; the number of cones in the central macula (central 10 degrees) is maximally 4.4×10^5; therefore the central macula contains maximally 7% of the total retinal cone population.[267,360] The foveola (1 degree 40 min) contains about 30,000 cones compared with 130 million receptors across the entire retina. This could explain the inability of the full-field ERG system to detect abnormalities confined to the foveola, to the fovea (5 degrees), or to the central macula; a patient can lose foveal photoreceptor function and have 20/200 vision with a normal full-field ERG. Conversely, a patient with advanced retinitis pigmentosa and less than 10-degree central fields can still retain 20/20 vision and have a reduced full-field ERG.

One difficulty in recording the small foveal or macular cone ERG at the cornea is that scattered light from a focal test stimulus can evoke a response from many receptors outside the macula, and therefore the foveal or macular ERG cannot be seen in isolation. Furthermore, the macula (18.4 degrees) contains as many rods as cones, and the macular rod ERG can thereby obscure the contribution from the macular or foveal cones. Biersdorf and Diller[56] used computer averaging with a small test stimulus (flickering red stimulus, <4-degree visual angle) superimposed on a large (50-degree) background sufficient to eliminate the rod contribution and ob-

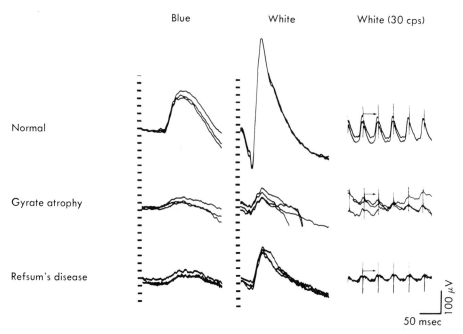

FIG. 21-28   Full-field ERGs to single flashes of dim blue ($\lambda < 470$ nm) light, single flashes of white light under dark-adapted conditions, and white 30 Hz flickering light for a normal subject, a 12-year-old female with gyrate atrophy of the choroid and retina, and a 30-year-old male with Refsum's disease. Stimulus onset is designated by the vertical hatched lines in columns 1 and 2 and the vertical shock artifacts in column 3. Arrows (column 3) designate cone b-wave implicit times. The responses of these patients, although reduced in amplitude, fall within the normal range with respect to b-wave implicit time for the rod isolated response to blue light (normal range, 71 to 108 milliseconds in this test system) and for the cone isolated response to 30 Hz flicker (normal range, 25 to 32 milliseconds).

tained a focal ERG at the cornea from the macular area. They compared the ratio of the ERG response produced by stimulation of the macula to that obtained by light flashed on the optic disc to try to account for the problem of stray light; they reported that this technique could be used to detect macular degenerations in patients when their visual acuity decreased to the 20/40 to 20/80 range.

Riggs, Johnson, and Schick[193,282] have isolated photopic (cone) responses by stimulating the eye with a barred stimulus pattern; each time the bars shift position, the stripes that are dark become light and vice versa. With phase alternation of this stimulus pattern, the overall amount of light on the retina is always the same and the amount of stray light outside the stimulus area proper also remains relatively constant. The response from the cone system to a stimulus (19-degree visual angle) presented at 8 to 10 alternations/sec is a sinusoidal waveform with amplitudes up to 7 to 8 μV. When the visual angle of the stimulus was <2 degrees and centrally placed on the fovea, this response was barely detectable even with signal averaging.

Foveal and parafoveal cone ERGs also have been elicited with a hand-held, two-channel stimulator ophthalmoscope (Fig. 21-29). This instrument has one light source for both stimulus and surround in the base of the instrument.[287] The stimulus light channel, contained within the body of the instrument, can be focused on the fundus by a focusing knob. The surround light channel is conducted from the base to the head of the instrument by a fiber-optic and prism housing. The optics in the head of the instrument are arranged so that lights from the stimulus and surround channels are reflected by a mirror to enter the patient's pupil coaxially and in maxwellian view. The stimulus centered within the surround is viewed on the fundus by the examiner through the lens assembly in the head of the instrument. With this instrument the levels of stimulus retinal illuminance and surround retinal illuminance can be precisely adjusted. The surround light is used not only to minimize the effect of stray light from the stimulus but also to provide sufficient retinal illumination to visualize retinal landmarks.

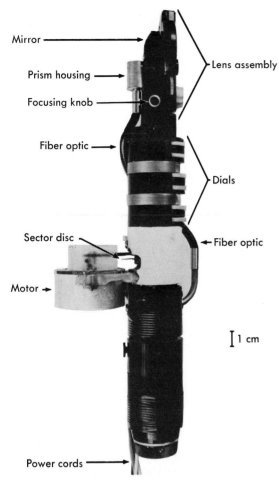

Mirror

Prism housing

Focusing knob

Fiber optic

Sector disc

Motor

Power cords

Lens assembly

Dials

Fiber optic

1 cm

FIG. 21-29 Two-channel stimulator ophthalmoscope. Stimulus channel internal to instrument; surround (or background) channel conducted in fiber optic bundle as shown. A motor-driven sector disc is used to regulate frequency of stimulus. Dials can be used to modify size, wavelength, and intensity of stimulus. Instrument weighs little more than a standard direct ophthalmoscope. (From Sandberg MA, Berson EL, Ariel M: Arch Ophthalmol 95:1805, 1977.)

The eye to be tested is dilated with a mydriatic to facilitate visualization of the fundus. A double-electrode contact lens is placed on the topically anesthetized cornea and a ground electrode on the forehead; the stimulus on the fundus can be visualized through the contact lens without difficulty. Responses are differentially amplified, tuned by a bandpass filter, and computer averaged. The computer is triggered by a photocell in the stimulator ophthalmoscope. The signal-averaging computer contains a bipolar artifact reject buffer so that voltages >5

μV, presumably due to eye movements, are eliminated from the averaged response. The examiner can compensate for small eye movements by adjusting this hand-held instrument. If eye movements occur that are so large that the examiner cannot keep the stimulus on the area of interest, the examiner interrupts the computer averaging by releasing a foot pedal switch. For a given retinal area at least three consecutive computer summations are performed; this typically requires about 3 minutes of recording time.[292]

Representative focal cone ERGs to a 4-degree white (4.8 log troland) flickering stimulus centered within a 10-degree white (5.5 log troland) steady annular surround are illustrated (Fig. 21-30) for a normal subject (*top row*), a patient with a one-disc diameter central macular scar (*second row*), and a patient with strabismic amblyopia (*bottom row*) with the stimulus centered on the fovea or centered 5 degrees nasal to the foveola. Recordings done at two stimulus frequencies (42 Hz, illustrated, as well as 28 Hz, not illustrated) established the relationship of stimulus onset to the corresponding (that is, next plus one) response peak. Normal subjects showed smaller responses in the parafovea than the fovea consistent with the known fall in cone density with increasing eccentricity from the foveola. The patient with a macular scar showed responses indistinguishable from noise when the stimulus was centered within the scar but normal responses when the stimulus was centered outside of the scar in a parafoveal area that appeared normal on ophthalmoscopic examination. For the patient with strabismic amblyopia the stimulus could be maintained on the fovea or parafovea despite variations in eye position, and a normal ERG was recorded in both areas. A congenital rod monochromat showed responses (not illustrated) that were indistinguishable from noise. These findings helped to establish that these ERGs were focal responses generated by the cone system under these test conditions.[292]

Foveal cone ERGs are illustrated (Fig. 21-31) for a normal subject (normal range: 0.18–0.56 μV) and three patients with juvenile hereditary macular degeneration with visual acuities ranging from 20/60 to 20/200. These patients had normal full-field flicker cone ERGs, but foveal responses were reduced in amplitude (that is, < 0.18 μV) without (patient 1) or with (patient 2) delays (that is, >38 milliseconds) in b-wave implicit time or indistinguishable from noise (patient 3). Focal cone ERGs elicited with the stimulator ophthalmoscope have proved useful for detecting and quantitating macular malfunction

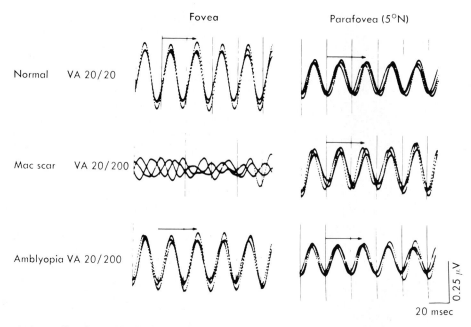

FIG. 21-30   Focal cone ERGs from a normal subject, a patient with a 1-disc diameter central macular scar, and a patient with strabismic amblyopia elicited with a 4-degree, 42 Hz white flickering stimulus centered on the fovea (left column) or centered 5 degrees nasal to the foveola (right column). Responses represent computer summation of 128 sweeps; three consecutive runs are illustrated. Arrows designate b-wave implicit times for detectable responses. (From Sandberg MA, Jacobson SG, Berson EL: Am J Ophthalmol 88:702, 1979.)

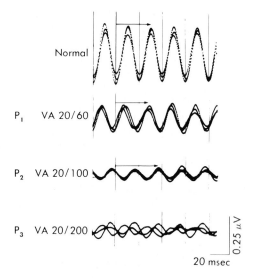

FIG. 21-31   Foveal cone ERGs for a normal subject and three patients (P$_1$, P$_2$, and P$_3$), ages 11, 13, and 23 respectively, with juvenile hereditary macular degeneration (Stargardt's disease). Responses represent computer summation of 128 sweeps; three consecutive runs are illustrated. Arrows designate b-wave implicit times for detectable responses. (From Sandberg MA, Jacobson SG, Berson EL: Am J Ophthalmol 88:702, 1979.)

in all patients tested with early stages of juvenile hereditary macular degeneration with visual acuity reduced to 20/50 or below. Patients with visual acuity less than 20/100 had smaller and slower foveal cone ERGs than those with better visual acuity.[291] Similar testing has been performed on patients with hereditary retinitis pigmentosa with reduced and delayed full-field cone ERGs, and all of those tested with 20/40 or below have shown foveal cone ERGs that are reduced in amplitude with normal b-wave implicit times[292] (Fig. 21-32).

Foveal cone ERGs elicited with a spot stimulus have been compared to midperipheral cone ERGs elicited by an annular stimulus concentric with the fovea in three young patients with dominant retinitis pigmentosa with reduced penetrance positioned on a bite bar before a maxwellian view optical system. Focal cone ERGs were recorded from the green and red cone systems in combination by a method of rod silent substitution. With this method two alternating lights of different wavelength, matched in brightness for the rods, were presented to the same retinal area; the brighter light for the green and red cones was designated as the stimulus increment (I_s) and the dimmer light as the back-

Foveal cone ERGs

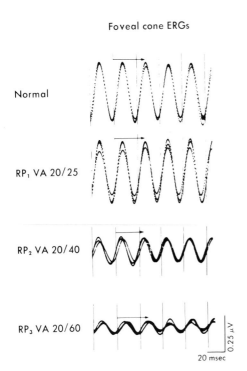

Normal

RP₁ VA 20/25

RP₂ VA 20/40

RP₃ VA 20/60

0.25 μV

20 msec

FIG. 21-32 Foveal cone ERGs from a normal subject, a 17-year-old patient with dominant retinitis pigmentosa with reduced penetrance (RP₁), a 32-year-old patient with autosomal recessive retinitis pigmentosa (RP₂), and a 24-year-old patient with sex-linked retinitis pigmentosa (RP₃). Three consecutive computer summations ($n = 256$) are shown. Arrows designate b-wave implicit times. (From Sandberg MA, Jacobson SG, Berson EL: Am J Ophthalmol 88:702, 1979.)

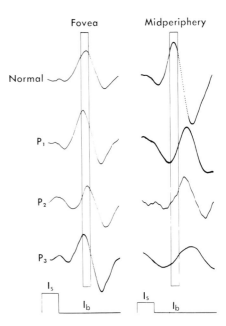

FIG. 21-33 Focal ERGs from the green and red cone systems in combination for a normal subject and three young patients (P₁, P₂, and P₃) with dominant retinitis pigmentosa with reduced penetrance in response to a 3.75-degree diameter spot centered on the foveola (left column) and a 38 to 44 degree diameter annulus concentric with the foveola (right column). I_s at 556 nm (1700 photopic trolands) is alternated at 5 Hz with I_b at 500 nm (120 photopic trolands). Vertical bars designate normal limits for b-wave implicit time. Calibration markers signify onset and duration of 20 milliseconds I_b horizontally and 0.25 μV vertically. (From Sandberg MA, Effron MH, Berson EL: Invest Ophthalmol Vis Sci 17:1096, 1978.)

ground (I_b). This method was chosen so that cone ERGs unmodified by any rod contribution could be measured at low levels of cone adaptation; testing could be done at a low frequency to separate the b-wave of one response from the a-wave of the next response. In these three patients with full-field cone ERGs that were normal or nearly normal in amplitude but substantially delayed in b-wave implicit time, foveal cone ERGs elicited with rod silent substitution were normal in amplitude and b-wave implicit time, whereas midperipheral cone ERGs were minimally reduced but substantially delayed (Fig. 21-33). These findings support the idea that the abnormal full-field cone ERGs seen in these patients are due to an abnormal extrafoveal cone contribution to their full-field responses.[290]

Efforts have been made to simulate in normal subjects the abnormal midperipheral cone ERGs seen in these patients. Minimal reductions in

amplitude with substantial delays in b-wave implicit time could be recorded from normal subjects in the midperiphery when the brightness of I_b was reduced more than the brightness of I_s while still maintaining rod silent substitution. This was not observed in normal subjects when the brightnesses of I_b and I_s were proportionately diminished (that is, neutral density effect or simulation of decreased visual pigment in the photoreceptors) or when the area of I_b and I_s was decreased (that is, reduced width of annulus or simulation of decreased numbers of photoreceptors). These findings support the idea that the abnormal midperipheral cone ERGs observed in young patients with dominant retinitis pigmentosa with reduced penetrance are due in part to a lower than normal state of light adaptation of the cone system and that reduced amount of visual pigment in the photoreceptors or reduced numbers of photoreceptors cannot be solely responsible for their abnormal cone ERGs.[290] These findings, in addition to those obtained with full-field ERG testing (Fig. 21-25), suggest that many patients with retinitis pigmentosa have a defect in the mechanism by which their cone system adapts to light.

THE PATTERN ELECTRORETINOGRAM

The pattern electroretinogram (PERG) is the retinal response to a phase reversing patterned stimulus, usually a grating or checkerboard, displayed on a television screen.[193] The pattern elements (checks or bars) periodically reverse position so that the bright bars become dim and vice versa (that is, they reverse in phase), although the sum of all bars has a constant brightness at all times. Thus the stimulus is fully described as a phase-reversing pattern with constant overall mean luminance. Four parameters specify the main characteristics of a pattern stimulus; namely, overall screen brightness

(mean luminance, cd/m²), brightness contrast of neighboring bars or checks (percent of contrast), rate of pattern reversal (temporal frequency, Hz), and bar or check size (spatial frequency, cycles per degree). Responses can be reliably assessed only when the stimulus is known to be focused on the retina and to be stable on the fovea during testing.

Maffei and Fiorentini[225,226] identified a significant difference between the PERG and the flash ERG. The PERG amplitude decreased several weeks after the optic nerve was cut in the cat, but the flash-elicited ERG b-wave remained large (Fig. 21-34). Since the progressive reduction of PERG amplitude correlated with ganglion cell degeneration following optic nerve section, the PERG was thought to originate in the inner retina of the cat proximal to the origins of the b-wave.

Speckreijse, Estevez, and van der Tweel[316] have emphasized that the PERG may result from changes in local luminance conditions within the retina and need not require a spa-

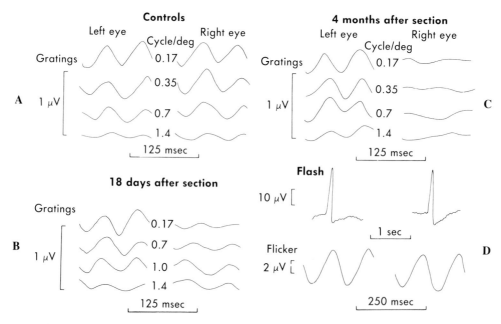

FIG. 21-34   Examples of pattern-reversal ERGs recorded from one cat before and after the section of the right optic nerve. **A,** Control records obtained from the two eyes before the section of the optic nerve. **B** and **C,** Records obtained 18 days and 4 months after the optic nerve section. Each record is the average of 500 responses. Stimulus: vertical sinusoidal grating reversed in contrast 16 times per second; contrast, 30%; mean luminance, 10 cd/m². The spatial frequency is indicated next to each record. **D,** ERG in response to 50-msec light flashes (250 trolands) and to light flickering at 8 Hz (mean luminance, 10 cd/m²; amplitude of square-wave modulation, 40%) recorded from the two eyes 4 months after section of the right optic nerve. (From Maffei L, Fiorentini A: Science, 211:953, February, 1981.)

tially sensitive generator. Since photoreceptors at any retinal location of the stimulus are periodically subjected to local pattern changes (that is, from a dim to bright bar condition and vice versa), they may respond as though stimulated by a flash of light. These researchers propose that differences between responses to dim and bright grating bars may add up to the PERG at the cornea.

Although linear components dominant in flash ERGs are present with a phase reversal pattern stimulus within the retina,[307] these linear components are thought by others to cancel each other from the different parts of the pattern and leave only nonlinear, even harmonic components in the PERG at the cornea. Baker and Hess[18] found that linear components of the human ERG were independent of spatial frequency, whereas the nonlinear even harmonics showed bandpass spatial characteristics (that is, their components were largest for a given pattern bar size and were smaller for wider or narrower bars). Hess and Baker[181] applied this analysis to human PERGs and found that they exhibited spatial bandpass characteristics. Sieving and Steinberg[307] used microelectrodes to record the PERG within the cat retina and identified significant PERG currents in the proximal retina. These generators depended on the pattern temporal frequency (that is, the rate of phase reversals) and showed spatial bandpass characteristics, suggesting that they were spatially organized. Baker et al.[19] recorded in the monkey retina and found a proximal retinal origin for the PERG under some conditions. However, when the PERG is recorded at the cornea, it represents a complex summation of activity from many retinal layers, and reports that designate a site of retinal origin for the PERG must be considered in terms of the specific stimulus conditions that were used.

The PERG may have clinical value in monitoring inner retinal disease in patients with known preservation of the outer retina as monitored by the focal flash ERG.[14] Abnormal PERG responses have been found in glaucoma, temporary occlusion of the central retinal artery, optic nerve trauma, and in some types of amblyopia. However, PERG responses can be interpreted as reflecting inner retinal disease only in areas in which the outer retina is functionally intact, since the PERG has been reported to be abnormal in macular degenerations involving the photoreceptors.[217] The PERG could provide a new dimension in the functional assessment of the inner retina, although more research is needed on the cellular origin of this response.[218]

Foveal function in the electroretinogram and the visually evoked cortical potential

Whereas the fovea contributes a small percentage (estimated <2%) of the response amplitude of the full-field ERG from all the cones across the entire retina, the visually evoked cortical potential (VECP) recorded at the occiput is dominated by the foveal cones.[272,283] This is undoubtedly due in part to the fact that the ratio of foveal to extrafoveal representation is increased by a factor of about 1000 in the area striata[283] compared with that in the retina. In addition, the foveal projection in the area striata is located superficially at the occipital pole, whereas the peripheral retinal projection is located deeper (more anteriorly) in the occipital lobe; therefore the foveal projection is relatively close to the scalp electrodes placed over the occipital pole to record the VECP.

The waveform of the VECP (also called the VER, or visually evoked response) is variable and complex; a typical waveform (Fig. 21-35) to a slowly repetitive stimulus contains the primary response (waves 1, 2, and 3), the secondary response (4 and 5), and the after discharge (rhythmic waves beginning with wave 6).[24,144] Rietveld, Tordoir, and Duyff[280] found that a unit retinal area, 25 minutes of arc from the foveal center, contributed to the VECP only 0.1 as much as the fovea itself. It has been estimated that the central 2-degree area generates 65% of the response. The implicit times are related within limits to stimulus intensity, but they are not much shortened by stimuli with field size greater than 1 degree.[345]

The effects of image blur of the test stimulus, attention of the subject, binocular rivalry, and other variables on the VECP are well described in other texts.[206,272,273,315] The problem of stray

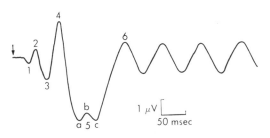

FIG. 21-35 Representative VECP recorded with monopolar electrode (inion-ear) in response to white light stimulus. Cumulation of 50 sweeps of computer. (From Bergamini L, Bergamasco B: Cortical evoked potentials in man, Springfield, IL, Charles C Thomas, Publisher, 1967.)

light has been minimized by use of pattern-reversal stimulation to elicit the VECP, and with this technique, abnormalities have been detected in patients with strabismic amblyopia.[315] The VECP is also abnormal in optic atrophy,[189] although no data exist to quantitate the degree of damage necessary to produce a significant alteration of the VECP. It has had limited, if any, value in assessing macular function behind a lens opacity because a smaller than normal response can result from the reduction of stimulus intensity and image blur on the retina produced by the opacity.[206]

Variable fixation of the eyes presents a technical problem in placing the stimulus on the fovea, and this problem has limited application of VECP testing in evaluation of central foveal (<2 degrees) function in patients with suspected disease. This problem of variable fixation has been minimized by viewing the stimulus on the central fovea during testing.[124,183,188,190,287,301] As an example, the two-channel stimulator ophthalmoscope (Fig. 21-29) has been used to elicit focal cone visually evoked cortical responses.[287] For this testing a 5 Hz stimulus, 1.5 degrees or smaller, is centrally superimposed on a steady 10-degree background. Bipolar re-

sponses are recorded between the inion and vertex with a ground electrode attached to the patient's ear lobe. The sensitivity of this technique is illustrated in the detection of abnormal foveolar function in a patient with a foveolar cyst that subtended 30 minutes of arc and visual acuity reduced to only 20/25 (Fig. 21-36). When a stimulus larger than the cyst was centered on the cyst (area A), the patient could see the flickering stimulus, and focal cone VECPs were within the normal range. When a stimulus that subtended 10 minutes of arc was centered on the cyst, the patient could not see the flickering stimulus, and the focal cone VECP was indistinguishable from noise. When the 10-minute stimulus was positioned just nasal to the cyst in a portion of the foveola that appeared normal on ophthalmoscopic examination (area B), the patient could see the flickering stimulus and the VECP was clearly detectable. With a weak stimulus increment and a 1.5-degree flickering stimulus centrally superimposed on a steady 10-degree background, all patients who have been tested with visual acuity of 20/25 or below and juvenile hereditary macular degeneration have shown abnormal focal cone VECPs. Abnormal VECPs have been either shifted in phase with or

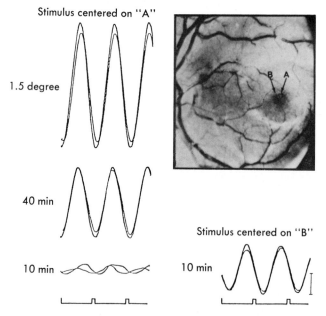

FIG. 21-36 Focal cone VECPs from left eye of patient with bilateral foveolar cysts; responses were obtained to 7.0 log troland white stimuli of varying diameter flickering at 5 Hz. Stimuli were centrally superimposed on steady 5.0 log troland white background. Fundus photograph of left eye from this patient illustrates foveolar cyst. The stimulus was centered on cyst (area A) or just nasal to cyst (area B). Two runs to same stimulus condition are superimposed; calibration (*lower right*) is 1 μV and vertical deflections (*lower row*) indicate onset and duration of each stimulus. (From Sandberg MA, Berson EL, Ariel M: Arch Ophthalmol 95:1805, 1977.)

without reductions in amplitude or so reduced in amplitude as to be indistinguishable from noise (Fig. 21-37).[287]

Although the VECP can be a sensitive index of central visual malfunction, it has not been helpful in separating visual loss on a retinal basis from visual loss due to disease in the optic nerve or cerebral cortex. The VECP has been abnormal in macular degeneration, optic atrophy, and strabismic amblyopia. In contrast, the foveal cone flash ERG, if abnormal, helps to localize the site of visual loss to the preganglion cell retina; the foveal cone ERG has been abnormal in patients with hereditary macular degeneration[191,292] (visual acuity of 20/50 or less), but it has been normal in patients with optic atrophy[191] or strabismic amblyopia.

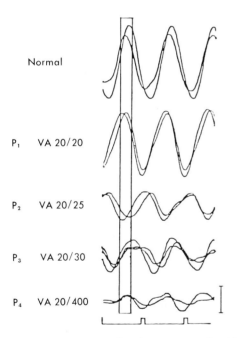

EARLY RECEPTOR POTENTIAL
Origin of components

The early receptor potential (ERP) is a rapid response (Fig. 21-38) that can be detected when the retina is stimulated with an intense flash of light.[72,89] The stimulus intensity required to generate the ERP is approximately 10^6 times brighter than that required to elicit the ERG (Fig. 21-39).[89] The human ERP is completed within 1.5 msec and is followed by the leading edge of the a-wave of the ERG.[35,82,143,365] The human ERP recorded at the cornea has a waveform similar to that recorded at the cornea or intraretinally from other animals. The initial cornea-positive phase, R1, has been associated with the conversion of lumirhodopsin to metarhodopsin I,[269] and the later cornea-negative phase, R2, with the conversion of metarhodopsin I to metarhodopsin II in the rat retina.[90] In the rat the action spectrum of the ERP corresponds with the absorption spectrum of rhodopsin.[89] ERP amplitude is linearly proportional to the amount of unbleached rhodopsin in the rat retina. Although rhodopsin is the predominant visual pigment in frog, monkey, and human retinas, the ERP in these species is generated primarily by cone visual pigments.[145-147] In humans, Goldstein and Berson[148] found that 60% to 80% of the total amplitude of the ERP is generated by the cones and 20% to 40% by the rods, and Carr and Siegel[82] confirmed the cone dominance of the human ERP by showing that the ERP action spectrum of the dark-adapted eye matched the human photopic luminosity curve (with peak sensitivity near 555 nm).

The ERP response consists of a photostable component (probably about 5% of the response)

FIG. 21-37 Focal cone VECPs from a normal subject and members of a family with juvenile hereditary macular degeneration (i.e., Stargardt's disease); responses were elicited to a 1.5-degree, 5 Hz, 5.6 log troland white stimulus centered on 10-degree, 5.0 log troland steady white background. Stimulus was centered on foveola during testing. P_1 through P_4 were 14, 11, 13, and 17 years of age, respectively. P_1 has normal fundus and normal VECP; P_2, P_3, P_4 had fundus abnormalities and abnormal VECPs. Vertical bar defines normal range of peak latencies. At least two runs to same stimulus condition are superimposed; calibration (*lower right*) is 1 μV and vertical deflection (*lower row*) indicate onset and duration of stimulus. (From Sandberg MA, Berson EL, Ariel M: Arch Ophthalmol 95:1805, 1977.)

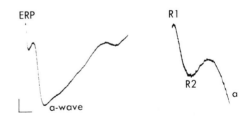

FIG. 21-38 Normal human ERP followed by a-wave of ERG (left tracing); cornea-positive peak, R1, and later cornea-negative, R2, of ERP are designated (right tracing). Stimulus onset is at beginning of each trace, and upward deflection from beginning represents cornea positivity. Calibration symbol signifies 2 milliseconds horizontally and 100 μV vertically for left tracing, and 0.5 milliseconds horizontally and 50 μV vertically for right tracing. (From Berson EL, Goldstein EB: Arch Ophthalmol 83:412, 1970.)

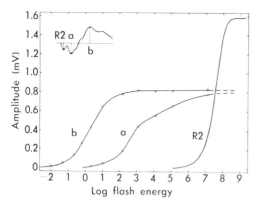

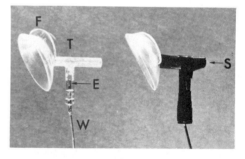

FIG. 21-39 Amplitudes of R2, a-wave, and b-wave in ERG of dark-adapted albino rat as functions of log of stimulus flash energy. On this semilog plot a response such as R2, which is proportional to flash energy, becomes a rapidly upward curving line. Data for a- and b-wave amplitudes were obtained from single rat, leaving sufficient time between flashes to allow eye to dark adapt. Data similar to these have been obtained from more than 10 animals. Uniform illumination of entire retina was obtained by placing small, uniformly illuminated section of Ping-Pong ball over eye. Pentobarbital, 50 mg/kg was used for anesthesia; homatropine (1%), to dilate pupil. Flash duration 0.7 millisecond; white light. Log (flash energy) = 0 corresponds to 1 quantum/rod. Amplitudes were measured from baseline as shown in diagram. (From Cone RA: Cold Spring Harbor Symp Quant Biol 30:483, 1965.)

and a photolabile component (about 95% of the response).[71] The photostable component can be recorded from the eyecup (without retina) preparation in the frog and is presumably generated by light stimulation of melanin granules in the pigment epithelium. The photolabile component is generated in the receptor outer segments, and regeneration of this component can be correlated with the regeneration rate of photoreceptor visual pigments.

Physiologic basis

The lack of a measurable latency, as well as the correlation of components of the ERP with the accumulation of specific photoproducts of bleaching, supports the idea that this response is generated in the receptor outer segments. ERP amplitude depends not only on the concentration of unbleached visual pigment in the receptor but also on the orientation of the visual pigments within the outer segments,[69,91] the orientation of the outer segment membrane,[13]

and the chemical environment of the receptors.[69,270] When the retina is heated, the ERP disappears at just the temperature at which the visual pigment molecules lose their regular orientation.[91] The ERP is thought to depend on charge displacement in the outer segments during photochemical reactions. One possible reason for the cone dominance of the human ERP, even though rhodopsin is the predominant visual pigment, is that many cone disc lumina are continuous with the extracellular space (the vitreous and therefore the cornea), whereas the majority of rod outer segment discs are isolated from and surrounded by a plasma membrane and therefore are "shielded" from the vitreous and cornea. Charge displacement in the "unshielded" cone discs could explain the cone dominance of the human and monkey ERP recorded at the cornea.

Technique for recording the human early receptor potential

In contrast to the double-electrode contact lens used for recording the ERG, a special scleral lens with the electrode in a side arm (Fig. 21-40) is required to record the ERP.[35] This lens was designed to eliminate the photovoltaic artifact that occurs within the first millisecond after light strikes a metallic electrode. The lens and side

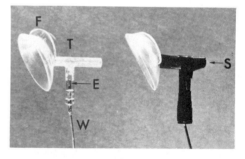

FIG. 21-40 Lenses for recording human ERP. Black tape has been removed from T-tube of left lens to show electrode, E. Letters designate silver recording electrode, E, mounted in plastic T-tube, T. T-tube is attached to inferior corneal curvature of lens. Electrode is shielded from light with black tape (right lens) to prevent photovoltaic artifacts. Contact between electrode and cornea is through saline bridge. Saline solution is introduced at S through polyethylene tube attached to T-tube. Movement of upper and lower lids was limited by lid flange, F, and T-tube. Wire lead, W, from electrode is plugged into junction box, which is in turn connected to preamplifier. Electrical resistance between front of cornea and electrode was less than 32,000 Ω. (From Berson EL, Goldstein EB: Arch Ophthalmol 83:412, 1970.)

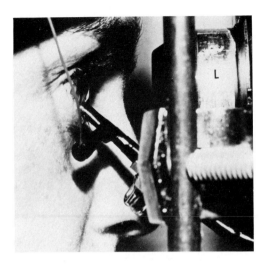

FIG. 21-41 Side view of subject with scleral contact lens electrode for recording ERP on topically anesthetized right eye. Stimulus from electronic flash gun is focused into eye through condensing lens, L. T-tube attached to lens, covered with black tape during testing, shields silver recording electrode from stimulus. (From Berson EL, Goldstein EB: Arch Ophthalmol 83:412, 1970.)

arm are filled with saline solution to ensure a saline bridge between the cornea and the recording electrode, and the side arm is covered with black tape to protect the recording electrode from exposure to the stimulus flash, as well as reflected light from the eye. The response is conducted to the electrode in the side arm. The reference electrode is taped to the forehead, and the ground is attached behind the ear. The routine ganzfeld, used to record the ERG, cannot be used to record the ERP because the light stimulus is too dim. The patient therefore sits in front of a flash gun (shielded), and the stimulus flash is presented in maxwellian view to maximize stimulus intensity (Fig. 21-41).

Early receptor potential responses in retinal disease

The ERP obtained under conditions of dark adaptation has been found to be subnormal in amplitude in young patients with dominant forms of retinitis pigmentosa (Fig. 21-42),[35] as well as sex-linked[36] and autosomal recessive retinitis pigmentosa.[334] The temporal aspects of R2 have not been delayed in patients with delays in ERG implicit times[35] (Fig. 21-43). The abnormal ERP amplitudes localized a defect in the receptor outer segments even at a time when affected children had 20/20 visual acuity, full fields with

conventional perimetric testing, and minimal or absent changes on ophthalmoscopic examination. In many retinitis pigmentosa patients it has not been determined whether the photoreceptors are altered primarily or become altered secondary to some change in the pigment epithelium. Possible explanations[35] for the decrease in ERP amplitude could be a decrease in the concentration of unbleached visual pigment in the diseased receptors, a change in the orientation of the outer segment membrane, a change in the orientation of visual pigment molecules within the outer segments, a change in the chemical environment of the receptors, or possibly a decrease in the number of photoreceptors, or any combination of these.

In addition to the reduction in ERP amplitude, patients with early retinitis pigmentosa have shown faster than normal ERP recovery rates during dark adaptation after a bleaching flash. These abnormal ERP recovery rates could be described by exponential functions, and the half-times of regeneration in children with dominant disease were about twice as fast as the half-times of regeneration recorded from normal subjects tested under the same bleaching conditions.[37] The half-times of regeneration have appeared to be characteristic for a given family. Although loss of rod function may contribute to the acceleration of ERP recovery rates in patients with retinitis pigmentosa, it is difficult to explain the faster than normal recovery rates of patients with retinitis pigmentosa on the basis of loss of rod function alone.[38] Since the human ERP has been shown to be generated primarily by the cones and since ERP recovery rates have been correlated with regeneration rates of visual pigments, the faster than normal ERP recovery rate in patients with early retinitis pigmentosa suggested as one possibility that some abnormality in the cone pigment regeneration process had occurred in these diseased retinas. Faster than normal recovery rates were measured in both dominant and sex-linked retinitis pigmentosa.[35-38] The precise mechanism responsible for these abnormal recovery rates under these test conditions remains to be defined.

Although no complications have been reported in recording the human ERP, the response is technically more difficult to obtain than the ERG, because it involves careful positioning of the patient in maxwellian view and isolation of the recording electrode from the stimulus flash. Although the ERP has provided a valuable dimension for clinical research, the ERG remains at this time the preferred electro-

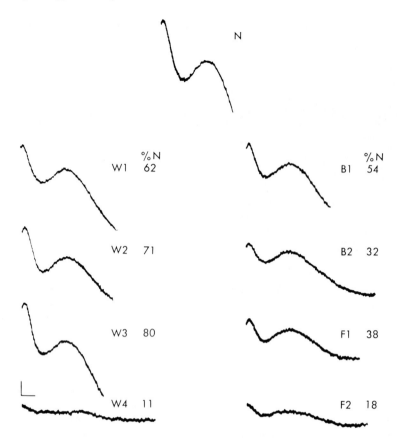

FIG. 21-42 Representative ERPs for normal subject, N, and eight patients with dominantly inherited retinitis pigmentosa, families W, B, and F. Responses to single flashes of white light recorded after patient had been dark adapted for a minimum of 1 hour. Amplitudes (from cornea-positive peak, R1, to cornea-negative peak, R2) for each patient are expressed as percentage of average normal response of 191 μV. Averages are based on 10 to 20 responses for each patient, except F1 and F2, which are based on two or three responses. Stimulus onset is at beginning of trace. Calibration symbol (lower left corner) is 50 μV vertically and 0.5 millisecond horizontally. (From Berson EL, Goldstein EB: Arch Ophthalmol 83:412, 1970.)

physiologic test for routine diagnostic evaluation of retinal function.

Clinical pathologic correlations

Postmortem examination of a donor eye from a 24-year-old male with sex-linked retinitis pigmentosa provided an unusual opportunity to correlate the ultrastructural abnormalities observed in remaining cones and rods with findings obtained, 3 weeks prior to death, with psychophysical and electroretinographic testing.[332] This patient noted a slight decrease in visual acuity and night blindness but did not report a deficiency in his visual field. Because of his poor general health, only limited testing could be done prior to death. Bone spicule pigmentation was distributed 45 to 60 degrees anterior to the fovea in all quadrants.

This patient had a 50% reduction in cone density in the foveola and a gradual diminution in cone density out to about 60 degrees, where the cone density increased; cone density appeared normal in the far periphery. Cone outer segments were considerably shortened in length in the foveola, and the inner segments appeared slightly increased in diameter (Fig. 21-44). In the parafovea cone inner segments were directly apposed to the pigment epithelium, and no organized cone outer segments could be seen (Fig. 21-45). In the far periphery cones appeared

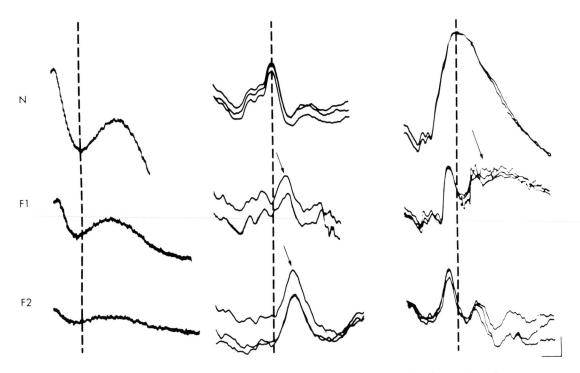

N

F1

F2

FIG. 21-43 ERPs (column 1) and ERGs (columns 2 and 3) for normal subject, N, and two children with dominant retinitis pigmentosa with reduced penetrance. Responses in column 2 are cone responses to 32×10^3 ft-L white light flash in presence of steady white background light of 10 ft-L. Responses in column 3 are dark-adapted ERGs to single flashes of long-wavelength light ($\lambda > 550$ nm) of sufficient intensity to elicit both cone and rod components in response. Arrows point to delayed cone (column 2) and rod (column 3) b-waves. Rod component in column 3 is so delayed in F1 compared with normal that clear splitting of rod and cone components can be seen. Stimulus onset is at beginning of each trace. Two or three consecutive responses are superimposed for responses in columns 2 and 3. Dashed line has been vertically extended from peak of R2 of normal subject through responses of F1 and F2 (see text). Calibration symbol (lower right corner) is 50 μV vertically and 0.5 millisecond horizontally for column 1, 12.5 milliseconds horizontally and 50 μV vertically for column 2, and 25 milliseconds horizontally and 30 μV vertically for column 3. (From Berson EL, Goldstein EB: Arch Ophthalmol 83:412, 1970.)

slightly shortened with respect to outer segment length. Rods were first seen 60 degrees anterior to the fovea at the anterior edge of the bone spicule pigmentation and were slightly reduced in length in the far periphery. Although shortened about 25% in length, remaining peripheral rods had well ordered discs (Fig. 21-46) and intact cell bodies.

Visual acuity reduction to 20/80 was consistent with the reduced cone density and reduced outer segment length in the central fovea. Psychophysical dark-adaptation threshold in the fovea was elevated 4 log units above normal rod threshold and 1.4 log units above normal cone threshold, and this was consistent with absence of rods in this region and reduced length of remaining cone outer segments. In the periphery

dark-adaptation thresholds were minimally elevated and the rods were only slightly shortened in length. The patient had constricted visual fields with I-4 and III-4 white test lights and retained full kinetic visual fields only with a V-4 white test light in the Goldmann perimeter (even though no detectable organized cone outer segments were seen in the midperiphery at the time of death); this constriction of his visual field was consistent with the decreased cone density from the fovea through the midperiphery. ERG amplitudes were reduced more than 90% below normal, and this was compatible with widespread photoreceptor loss and structural abnormalities in the remaining photoreceptors. This correlation of premortem findings obtained with psychophysical and

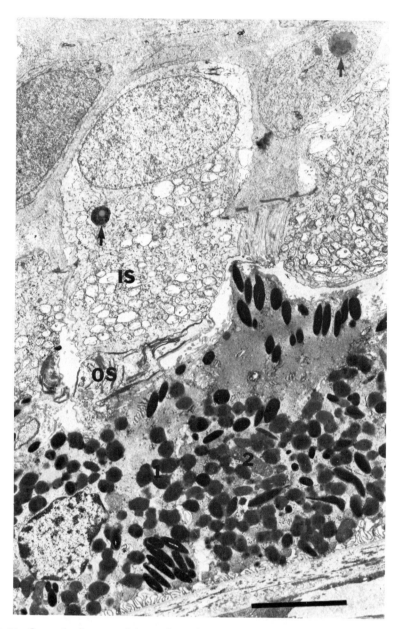

FIG. 21-44   Cones in the central fovea from donor eye with sex-linked retinitis pigmentosa have enlarged inner segments (IS) and distorted remnants of outer segments (OS). Autophagic vacuoles *(arrows)* are seen in the perinuclear cytoplasm. Pigment epithelial cells contain large numbers of melanolysosomes (1), lysosomes (2), and few free melanin granules. Apical protrusions of these cells extend between cone inner segments. Horizontal bar (*lower right*) is 5 µm. (From Szamier RB, et al: Invest Ophthalmol Vis Sci 18:145, 1979.)

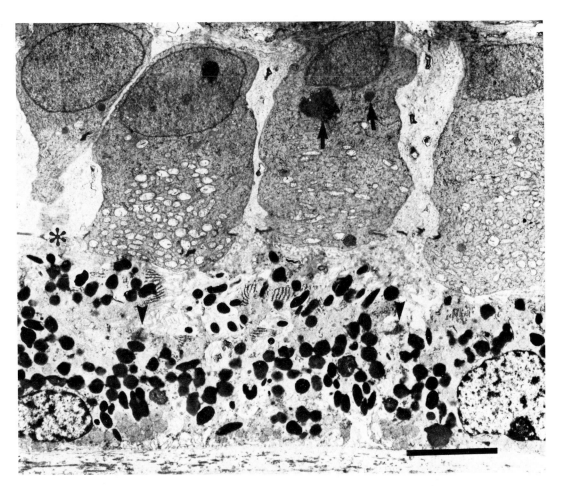

FIG. 21-45 Same case as Figure 21-44. Parafoveal cones have no organized outer segments and small portions of their inner segments extend beyond the external limiting membrane *(asterisk)*. Autophagic vacuoles *(arrows)* are present in cone cell bodies. Protrusions of the pigment epithelial cells extend proximal to their apical tight junctions *(arrowheads)*. Horizontal bar, lower right, represents 5 μm. (From Szamier RB, et al: Invest Ophthalmol Vis Sci 18:145, 1979.)

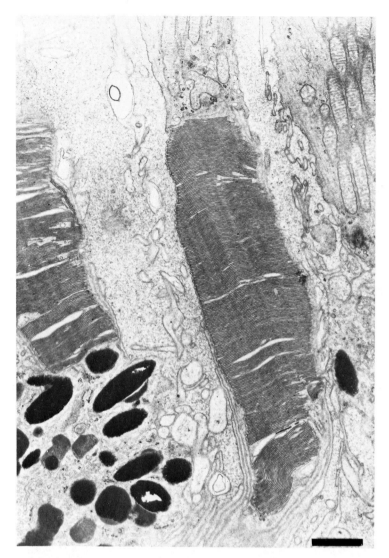

FIG. 21-46   Representative rods in the far periphery of donor eye with sex-linked retinitis pigmentosa have outer segments shortened in length with well-ordered discs. Outer segments are surrounded by microvillous processes of the pigment epithelium. Some processes extend up to the inner segments and are distended. Free melanin granules are prominent in the apical portion of the pigment epithelium. Horizontal bar (lower right) is 1 μm. (From Szamier RB, et al: Invest Ophthalmol Vis Sci 18:145, 1979.)

electroretinographic testing with postmortem ultrastructural observations supports the idea that these tests provide an index of the extent and type of photoreceptor involvement in a patient with hereditary retinitis pigmentosa.[31,332]

THE ELECTRO-OCULOGRAM

As early as 1848 Du Bois-Reymond reported that a difference in electrical potential of about 6 mV existed between the cornea and the back of the eye. The human eye behaves like a dipole, oriented along its anteroposterior axis with the cornea positive to the posterior pole. Movement of the eye will cause changes of the potential in one electrode placed near the inner canthus relative to another placed near the outer canthus of the eye. The record of eye movement obtained by this means is called the electro-oculogram, or the EOG. For eye excursions up to 30 degrees, a linear relationship with an accuracy of about 1.3 degrees exists between the EOG potential and the excursion of the eye. EOGs should not be confused with electromyograms, which are recordings of changes in potentials of individual contracting muscle fibers.

The EOG consists of at least two separate potentials, one that is insensitive and the other that is sensitive to light. Under usual recording conditions the subject with electrodes near the inner and outer canthus alternately observes fixation lights spaced 30 degrees apart, and the potential is measured under conditions of dark adaptation after prior exposure to room illumination.[12] The light-insensitive potential (or standing potential) per 30 degrees of eye excursion decreases slightly over a period of 8 or 9 minutes, at which time the so-called dark trough or lowest potential recorded in the dark-adapted state can be measured (Fig. 21-47). After exposure to light, the potential per 30 degrees of eye excursion gradually increases and reaches a peak in 10 to 15 minutes (light rise of the EOG), at which time the response under conditions of light adaptation may be more than twice that of the potential recorded under conditions of dark adaptation. The standing potential recorded from electrodes placed near the canthi can vary from 20 μV/degree to 5 μV/degree in normal subjects,[11] due in part to the placement of the electrodes. Therefore the EOG has been most

reliably interpreted as a ratio of peak voltage obtained in the light-rise potential over the minimum voltage obtained in the dark-trough or standing potential without changing the placement of the electrodes during the test.[12] This ratio is usually greater than 1.8 in normal human subjects under age 50. After the light-rise peak, the cornea-positive oscillations vary in voltage in a damped sinusoidal manner.

Origin of the components of the electro-oculogram

Microelectrode studies have located a large direct current (DC) component just distal to the outer margin of the outer nuclear layer of the retina,[76] and clinical studies suggest that the pigment epithelium is responsible for this standing potential. Lasansky and DeFisch[214] measured a transmembrane potential of 20 to 30 mV in the isolated pigment epithelium and choroid of the toad with the pigment epithelium surface positive with respect to the choroidal surface.

The apical membranes of the retinal pigment epithelial cells (RPE), facing the photoreceptors across the subretinal space, are electrically isolated to some extent from the basal (basolateral) membranes facing the choroid by the apical tight junctions of the RPE cells. Microelectrode recordings from the anesthetized or decerebrate cat (Fig. 21-48) have shown two light-evoked basal membrane responses that follow the apical-K^+ response (that is, RPE component of the ERG c-wave). The first basal membrane response, called the delayed basal hyperpolarization, is dependent on the decrease in subretinal $[K^+]_0$. The second basal membrane response, called the light peak depolarization, is not clearly associated with K^+ changes. The two basal membrane potentials are thought to be the origins, respectively, of the fast oscillation (sometimes seen as the slight decline in voltage in the EOG after light onset) and the light peak or slow oscillation (seen as the slow rise in voltage in the EOG after light onset).[322,323]

Initially the light rise of the EOG was thought to be initiated by rod activity, but it has since become clear that the cones also contribute to the response.[162] This latter conclusion is based not only on studies of the action spectrum of this response in the dark-adapted and light-adapted state, but it also is consistent with the observation that human subjects without rod function can have a light-rise response.

The light rise of the EOG has been reported to be eliminated experimentally by central retinal artery occlusion,[155,161] and this remains to be reconciled precisely with the findings with mi-

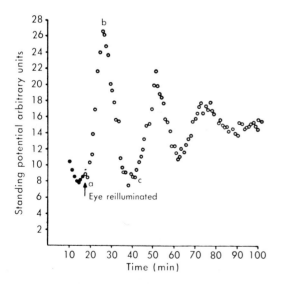

FIG. 21-47 Normal human EOG. Open circles are data describing oscillations of potential after reillumination of dark-adapted eye. Solid circles imply reading taken in darkness. Note initial transient fall in potential, a, first light peak, b, and first light trough, c. (From Arden GB, Barrada A, Kelsey JH: Br J Ophthalmol 46:449, 1962.)

FIG. 21-48 Diagrammatic summary of the three light-evoked responses showing their relative time-courses and amplitudes. The initial 6 min. of the response to maintained illumination are shown. The first response (*top*) is a hyperpolarization of the apical membrane that reaches its maximum at 4 sec. This is followed by two responses of the basal membrane: the delayed basal hyperpolarization, peaking at 20 sec and the light-peak depolarization reaching its peak at 300 sec. The offset of illumination produces a similar sequence of responses but of the opposite polarity (not shown). (From Steinberg RH, Linsenmeier RA, Griff ER: Vision Res 23:1321, 1983.)

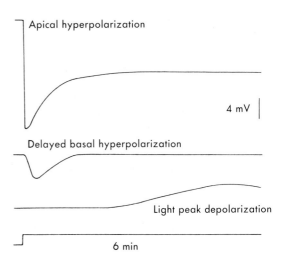

croelectrode studies in the cat, as described earlier. More work is needed to understand the physiologic basis of the EOG.

Electro-oculogram responses in retinal disease

The light-insensitive potential of the electro-oculogram provides a means of measuring the function of the pigment epithelium without having to stimulate the photoreceptors.[205] It is also a method for quantitating ocular movements. The test must be interpreted with caution if the patient has macular degeneration and poor fixation. In the early stages of retinitis pigmentosa the light rise of the EOG is reduced, but the standing potential is normal even at a time when the ERG is markedly abnormal or even nondetectable. In advanced stages the standing potential of the EOG becomes reduced. In advanced choroideremia, when only sclera is visible in large areas, both the light rise and the standing potential are absent. In patients with progressive cone-rod degeneration,[39] in whom both photoreceptor systems are abnormal, the light rise is affected early in the condition, but the standing potential is relatively preserved (Fig. 21-49). In contrast, in progressive cone degeneration[40] the light-rise to dark-trough ratio appears to be relatively preserved even though the patient has a widespread abnormality in the cone system. Patients with dominant, Nougaret-type, stationary night blindness with normal cone function and no detectable rod function have a markedly diminished light-rise response, whereas in recessive congenital stationary night blindness (both Oguchi's disease and recessive nyctalopia with myopia) the cornea-positive response of the EOG is normal.

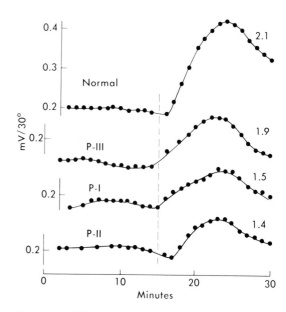

FIG. 21-49 EOG responses for normal subject and three patients, P-I, P-II, and P-III, with progressive cone-rod degeneration. Vertical hatched line indicates time of onset of 5 ft-L background light during test; ratio of light peak to dark trough shown on right above each response; scale (*left*) indicates amplitude of EOG response in mV/30 degrees of visual angle. (From Berson EL, Gouras P, Gunkel RD: Arch Ophthalmol 80:68, 1968.)

Therefore the EOG (as well as ERGs) can help to distinguish the dominant type of stationary night blindness from the recessive types. In chloroquine retinopathy[266] the EOG is abnormal in the advanced stages when large areas of the retinal pigment epithelium are abnormal, but in the very early stage, the EOG is normal.[164]

The ERG is usually abnormal in conditions in which the EOG is abnormal, but four exceptions have been observed clinically in which the patient has a normal or nearly normal ERG with an abnormal EOG light-rise to dark-trough ratio. These conditions are butterfly-shaped pigment dystrophy of the fovea,[99] fundus flavimaculatus,[99] advanced drusen,[208] and vitelliform dystrophy or Best's disease.[98,137] More recent studies of patients with fundus flavimaculatus have shown that most patients have normal EOGs[132,257] particularly when the light rise is evaluated with a ganzfeld dome rather than with a small diameter x-ray viewing box.[134] Patients with dominant drusen also have been reported to have normal EOGs.[133] Vitelliform macular dystrophy deserves special attention because the EOG is abnormal even in asymptomatic "carriers" of this condition who have no abnormalities visible with the ophthalmoscope.[94,98] Therefore the EOG can serve as a genetic marker to identify this autosomal dominant disease in families in which a "skipped" generation is suggested by history or routine ocular examination. The EOG also has been considered as an aid in distinguishing true dysgenesis neuroepithelialis of Waardenburg from congenital amaurosis of Leber; in both types of retinal degenerations the ERG is absent, but the former has a normal or nearly normal EOG and the latter has a nondetectable EOG.[179]

When the EOG is expressed as a ratio, it should be remembered that the ratio depends not only on the function of the pigment epithelium but also on the photoreceptors. Therefore when EOG ratios are found to be abnormal, it does not necessarily follow that the pigment epithelial cells alone are abnormal; the contribution of the pigment epithelium is separated in the light-insensitive component or dark trough of the EOG but not in the ratio of the light rise to the dark trough.

MICROELECTRODE STUDIES OF THE VERTEBRATE RETINA

Electrophysiologic measurements have provided a noninvasive method to monitor and to try to understand retinal function in normal human subjects and patients with retinal disease. Interpretations derived from these data are limited by the fact that large numbers of cells generate responses recorded at the cornea and that the physiologic bases for many abnormalities in these responses are not known. More detailed understanding of the organization of the retina at the cellular level is needed in normal vertebrates. Studies of animals with hereditary retinal degenerations (for example, *rd* and *rds* mice,[61,84,88,215,216,223,293,338,343] Royal College of Surgeons[117,244] and Wag Rij rats,[213] Irish setters,[4,5,222] miniature French poodles,[4,5,358] Norwegian elkhounds,[4] baboons,[340] Alaskan malamutes[286] and the Abyssinian cat[251]) and research on animals with nutritionally induced retinal degenerations (for example, vitamin A-deficient rats,[106,259] vitamin A-deficient ground squirrels,[25] and taurine-deficient cats[295-297]) should also help to provide a basis for further understanding of human retinal degenerations. Findings in animal models of hereditary degenerations[295] and nutritionally induced retinal degenerations[33] have been reviewed. This section focuses on microelectrode studies of the normal vertebrate retina that have increased our understanding of its organization at the cellular level. Some clinical implications will also be considered.

Recordings from mud puppy retina

The ability to record from single cells with microelectrodes and to identify with stains the cell from which the recording is taken represents a significant advance in the past 20 years that undoubtedly will help in understanding the organization of the vertebrate retina. The mud puppy has been studied in great detail by Werblin and Dowling[357] because this amphibian has cells with large perikarya that facilitate intracellular recording. Responses (Fig. 21-50) have been obtained to a spot of light about 100 μm in diameter focused on the electrode or centered on annuli 250 or 500 μm in diameter.

The photoreceptors (Fig. 21-50) increase their membrane potential; they hyperpolarize for the duration of illumination. The photoreceptors respond poorly to both small and large annuli. Spot and annulus presented together show no differences compared with a spot stimulus alone. The photoreceptor cells appear to have a small field and respond relatively autonomously. In contrast, horizontal cells respond with large hyperpolarizing responses (L-type of S-potential, see subsequent discussion) over large retinal areas. When spot and annulus are presented simultaneously, summation is observed, and this is consistent with anatomic observations that horizontal cells have input from

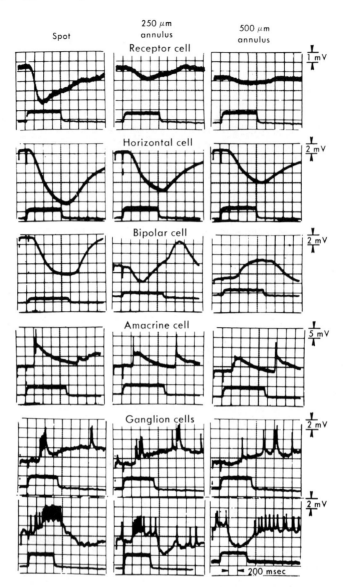

FIG. 21-50 Intracellular recordings from neurons of mud puppy retina. Responses were elicited with spot of light focused on electrode (left column) and with small and large annulus (center and right columns). Distal retinal neurons respond with slow, graded, mostly hyperpolarizing potentials: proximal neurons respond with depolarizing, mostly transient potentials. (From Werblin FS, Dowling JE: J Neurophysiol 32:339, 1969.)

receptors over a wide field. Two types of bipolar cells have been demonstrated in the mud puppy retina. In one type, spot illumination elicits a sustained hyperpolarizing potential (Fig. 21-51, left). For the other type, spot illumination results in a sustained depolarizing potential. Depolarizing bipolar cells have been called on-bipolar cells and hyperpolarizing bipolars have been termed off-bipolar cells.[239] For either bipolar cell

type, when the central region is stimulated, addition of annular illumination antagonizes or reduces the sustained potential produced by the central spot (Fig. 21-51, *right*). Therefore, at the bipolar layer, an antagonistic center-surround organization can be observed with appropriate stimulus conditions.[107]

In contrast to the slow graded potentials seen in the distal retina (receptors, horizontal cells,

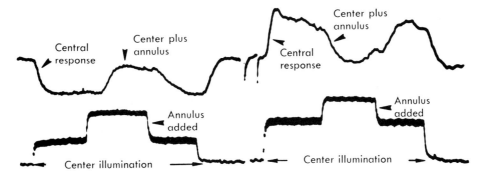

FIG. 21-51 Antagonistic effect of annular illumination on response of hyperpolarizing (*left*) and depolarizing (*right*) types of bipolar cells. In each case, central illumination was maintained steadily while annulus was flashed. (From Werblin FS, Dowling JE: J Neurophysiol 32:339, 1969.)

and bipolar cells), the neurons in the proximal retina of the mud puppy respond mostly with depolarizing and transient potentials. Amacrine cells respond transiently to static retinal illumination with on and off responses to illumination anywhere in their receptive field (Fig. 21-50). Only a few spikes are seen riding on the transient depolarizations; thus it is not clear whether the slow potentials or the spikes are the important component of signal transmission of the amacrine cell. Reciprocal synapses of amacrine cell processes back onto bipolar terminals, just adjacent to bipolar ribbon synapses, raise the possibility of some feedback mechanisms; the transient depolarizing response of the amacrine cell therefore could represent some negative feedback mechanism of amacrine cells on bipolar cells. Amacrine cells respond similarly to a bright spot on a dark background or a dark spot on a light background, a feature of many motion-sensitive and directionally sensitive cells. Amacrine cell responses may account for the directionally sensitive responses of on- and off-type ganglion cells (Fig. 21-50).

On the basis of microelectrode recordings from single cells, the outer plexiform layer of the mud puppy appears concerned with static or spatial aspects of illumination, whereas the inner plexiform layer is concerned more with dynamic or temporal aspects of illumination. Two physiologic types of ganglion cells may be related to the primary input into each type. One type receives direct input from bipolar cells and has a receptive field organization similar to bipolar cells; central illumination depolarizes the cell, whereas surround illumination inhibits this type in a sustained fashion (Fig. 21-50, lower-most responses). This type predominates in mammalian retinas. The second type of ganglion cell receives its major input from the amacrine cell and responds transiently to retinal illumination similar to the responses of amacrine cells (Fig. 21-50, fifth row). Therefore each type of ganglion cell may be carrying to the brain information processed in the two plexiform layers.[107,110]

Recordings from horizontal cells

When microelectrodes are inserted into certain regions of the inner nuclear layer of the fish retina, a response (Fig. 21-52) of large amplitude (10 to 50 mV) can be recorded superimposed on a negative resting potential (10 to 50 mV). This response, usually negative, is maintained for the duration of light stimulation. This response was named S-potential by Motokawa to acknowledge the discoverer, Svaetichin[330]; the cellular origin for this potential was not clear in 1959. Using intracellular marking techniques of Stretton and Kravitz,[328] Kaneko[195] showed in 1970 that these S-potentials are produced by horizontal cells. S-potentials have subsequently been recorded from many vertebrate horizontal cells, including the cat and monkey. One unusual characteristic of S-potentials is their large receptive field. Watanabe and Tosaka[355] showed that stimuli several millimeters away from the recording microelectrode influenced the size of S-potentials in the fish. The S-potential could be reduced by cutting the retina between the light stimulus and the recording electrode; this supported the idea that current and not scattered light was spreading from one region of the retina to the other. The receptive fields appeared

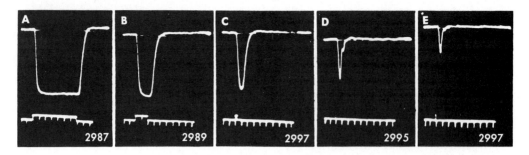

FIG. 21-52 Recordings of S-potentials from fish elicited at different millisecond durations (A, 500; B, 150; C, 20; D, 5; E, 0.5) of light stimuli (constant intensity and amplification). Time marks, 70 milliseconds. Light stimulus marked on time scale. (From Svaetichin G: Acta Physiol Scand 29 (Suppl 106):565, 1953.)

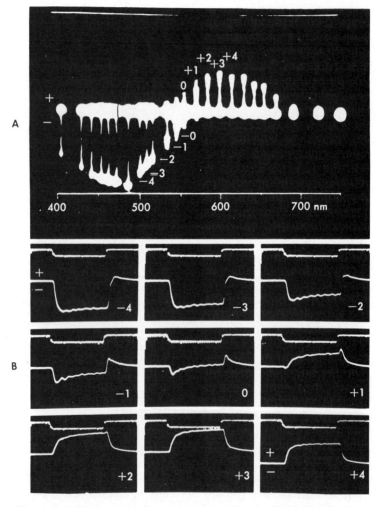

FIG. 21-53 Changes in time course of responses from C-unit of Mugil's retina as function of wavelength. **A,** Recording of response amplitude as function of wavelength. **B,** Responses recorded as function of time. Each numbered record was taken simultaneously with response peak bearing same number as in **A.** In **B,** top tracing in each record indicates time in tenths and hundredths of a second. Deflection of top tracing is due to output of photocell circuit used to monitor light flash (duration 0.3 second). Records taken at approximately 3-second intervals. (From MacNichol EF Jr, Svaetichin G: Am J Ophthalmol 46:26, 1958.)

larger than single horizontal cells, and this has raised the possibility that horizontal cells are electrically coupled to one another[249] or that perhaps horizontal cells synapsing on cones could in turn relay signals to other horizontal cells.

S-potentials can be separated into two distinct classes: one class produces a negative or hyperpolarizing response to all wavelengths (so-called luminosity or L-units)[248]; the other (Fig. 21-53) produces a hyperpolarizing response to long wavelength stimuli and a depolarizing response to short wavelength stimuli (so-called chromaticity or C-units).[224] The L-units have been thought to play a role in brightness perception, and the C-units have been thought to play a role in color vision. A red-adapting light not only depressed the contribution of a red-sensitive mechanism but also enhanced the contribution of a green-sensitive mechanism to the same L-unit[227] (Fig. 21-54). Specific cone mechanisms in C-units have been studied by determining action spectra in the presence of selective chromatic adaptation in fish; a green-sensitive and possibly a red-sensitive mechanism have been isolated in this way.[248] Rods also contribute to S-potentials in the mammalian retina, but it appears that rod and cone signals add their effects independently to this response.[320,321]

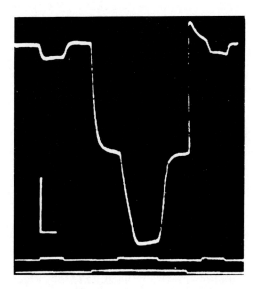

FIG. 21-54 Amplification of response to short-wavelength stimulation by red background light in L-unit of pike. Middle record shows duration of short-wavelength stimulus; lower one shows duration of red-adapting light. (From Maksimova EM, Maksimov VV, Orlov OY: Biofizika 11:472, 1966.)

Microelectrode studies in the turtle by Baylor, Fuortes, and O'Bryan[22] showed that a depolarizing potential in a cone could be detected whenever a neighboring horizontal cell was hyperpolarized by current passed through a second microelectrode. This finding suggested that horizontal cell terminals continuously release a hyperpolarizing transmitter on cones that can be reduced by hyperpolarizing the horizontal cell.

Recordings from horizontal cells in the perfused retina of the turtle also have shown that low levels of calcium, high levels of magnesium, and cobalt hyperpolarize the horizontal cell membrane and suppress the response to light but only partially affect the response of receptor cells. These results are interpreted as consistent with the idea that a depolarizing transmitter is released by photoreceptors in darkness. The hyperpolarizing response to light of the horizontal cells then would result from a reduction in the amount of transmitter released.[85]

The following arrangement is possible on the basis of available data. In the dark, cones may release a depolarizing transmitter on horizontal cells,[79] and horizontal cells may release a hyperpolarizing transmitter on cones.[22] One class of horizontal cells receives a direct input from one class of cones (C-unit), and another class receives an input from more than one class of cones and possibly rods (L-units). In this circuit the horizontal cells can provide a negative feedback mechanism. When a photoreceptor is stimulated by light, the photoreceptor membrane hyperpolarizes and the concentration of the depolarizing transmitter released by the photoreceptors becomes reduced. This leads to hyperpolarization of the horizontal cells and a resultant decrease in the release of hyperpolarizing transmitter back onto the photoreceptor cell. Therefore horizontal cells could increase the dynamic range over which cones function, could increase spatial contrast, and could even mediate color opponent properties to individual cones.[160]

Retinal neurotransmitters

Available evidence supports the idea that in darkness vertebrate photoreceptors are partially depolarized and release neurotransmitter onto second-order neurons (the horizontal and bipolar cells). Light hyperpolarizes the photoreceptors and depresses the release of transmitter; the light response of second-order neurons is therefore thought to occur secondary to a decrease of neurotransmitter secretion from the receptor terminal.

The vertebrate retina has more than 20 different neuroactive agents that are thought to be released from retinal neurons.[122] Fast excitatory and inhibitory retinal pathways appear to be mediated by 4 or 5 agents while the rest serve a regulatory or modulatory role.[109] The main excitatory pathway appears to be mediated primarily by L-glutamate (photoreceptors and bipolar cells) and by acetylcholine (cholinergic amacrine cells); whereas inhibitory pathways are subserved mainly by gamma aminobutyric acid (GABA) in horizontal cells and amacrine cells and by glycine in amacrine cells.[108] The glutamate analogue, 2-amino-4 phosphorobutyric acid, can block all of the "on" activity in the retina, suggesting that L-glutamate mediates transmission of this information from receptors to depolarizing bipolar cells.[294,312] The excitatory amino acid antagonist, ($\pm$) cis-2, 3 piperidine dicarboxylic acid blocks on-center ganglion cell responses in the mud puppy retina,[313] suggesting that a single transmitter substance from bipolar terminals is signaling "on" activity in the inner plexiform layer.

In the inner plexiform layer several neurotransmitters (GABA, glycine, dopamine, acetylcholine, and an indoleamine) have been identified by histochemical and other methods and associated with amacrine cells.[121,166,231,253,346] Certain amacrine cells appear to accumulate one or another of these substances, and it appears likely that different pharmacologic types of amacrine cells make different connections and perform different functions. For example, dopaminergic amacrine cells of the rabbit retina, called interamacrine cells, make synaptic contacts only with other amacrine cells, suggesting that they may play a modulating role in the retina.[113,121]

Interplexiform cell

In teleost fish and new-world monkeys, fluorescence microscopy has revealed dopamine-containing retinal neurons whose perikarya are found in the inner portion of the inner nuclear layer among amacrine cells and whose processes extend not only in the inner plexiform layer but also to the outer plexiform layer.[121] These neurons, called interplexiform cells, have been found in a variety of species,[62,114] but only in the teleost fish and new-world monkeys have these cells shown dopamine fluorescence. The input to the interplexiform cells is from the amacrine cells, whereas the output is in both plexiform layers and is particularly noticeable in the outer plexiform layer with respect to synapses onto horizontal cells and some bipolar cell dendrites.[111,112,114] These cells do not contact gan-

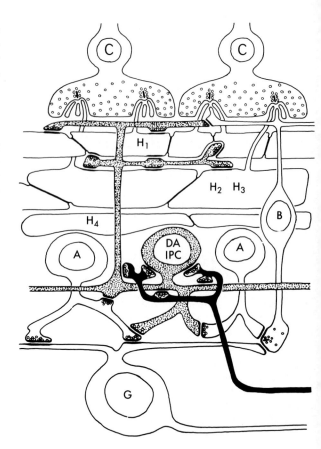

FIG. 21-55 Schematic diagram of the synaptic connections of the dopaminergic interplexiform cells (DA/IPC) in the white perch retina. The input to these neurons is in the inner plexiform layer from amacrine cells (A) and centrifugal fibers (filled processes). The interplexiform cell processes make synapses onto amacrine cell processes in the inner plexiform layer but do not contact the ganglion cells (G) or their dendrites. In the outer plexiform layer the processes of the interplexiform cells make synapses mainly onto the cone horizontal cells (H_1, H_2, and H_3) and occasionally onto bipolar cell dendrites. No synapses have been seen between interplexiform cell processes and photoreceptors or rod horizontal cells (H_4). C, cone photoreceptor. (From Dowling JE: Sem Neurosci 1:35, 1989.)

glion cells or photoreceptor terminals. These interplexiform cells are of particular interest because they appear to provide a pathway for information flow from the inner to the outer retina (Fig. 21-55).

The effects of dopamine on cells in the outer plexiform layer have been studied to consider the possible role of the interplexiform cell.[177] Dopamine depolarizes horizontal cells and depresses their responsiveness to light. Dopamine slightly hyperpolarizes a depolarizing bipolar cell, increases the amplitudes of responses to central spot illumination, and decreases the amplitudes of responses to annular illumination. These observations have led to the proposal that one role of the interplexiform cells is to regulate center-surround antagonism in the outer plexiform layer; activation of interplexiform cells could enhance bipolar cell center responsiveness while depressing lateral inhibitory effects initiated by horizontal cells. In the light and in short-term darkness the interplexiform cells are turned off and horizontal cells function maximally; in prolonged darkness the interplexiform cells become active, releasing dopamine and reducing lateral inhibition, thereby making the retina a better photodetector.[108,109]

Oscillatory potentials

The vertebrate ERG elicited with high-intensity light stimuli shows not only a large a-wave but also a series of rhythmic oscillations superimposed on the b-wave (that is, the b-wave is here defined as beginning at the trough of the cornea-negative a-wave). These rhythmic oscilla-

tions are called oscillatory potentials, and representative responses from a normal human subject recorded at the cornea are shown in Figure 21-56.[366] The oscillatory potentials are most easily detected in the mesopic state, and recordings from humans have revealed that the threshold and spectral sensitivity, as well as temporal and adaptational characteristics, differ from those of the b-wave.[349–352] Depth profile studies in the frog by Brindley[67] and others[364] have shown that the maximum amplitude of oscillatory potentials was in the inner nuclear layer. Ogden[264] and Ogden and Wylie[265] found that the maximum amplitude of the first three oscillatory potentials of the pigeon, chicken, and monkey ERG were at the level of the inner plexiform layer and suggested that axon terminals of bipolar cells, amacrine cell processes, and dendrites of ganglion cells could be involved in generation of these responses. Korol and coworkers[204] showed that intravitreal injection of glycine led to damage to amacrine cells and disappearance of oscillatory potentials in the ERG of the rabbit. In the mud puppy Wachtmeister and Dowling[352] found that the oscilla-

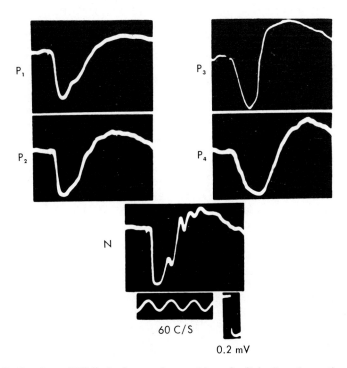

FIG. 21-56 Dark-adapted ERGs in four patients with early diabetic retinopathy visible with the ophthalmoscope. These four patients lacked the oscillatory potentials that are seen in the normal (N) dark-adapted ERG. Flash intensity was 37.5 J. (From Yonemura D, Aoki T, Tsuzuki K: Arch Ophthalmol 68:49, 1962.)

tory potentials reversed in polarity as a function of depth of their electrodes, thereby reflecting a radial flow of current in the retina; they also found that these potentials were selectively depressed by GABA, glycine, glutamate, and dopamine but not by acetylcholine. They suggested that the oscillatory potentials are generated by inhibitory feedback synaptic circuits within the retina. Heynen and coworkers[180] studied current source and sink profiles of the oscillatory potentials of the primate (macaque) ERG; they concluded that the oscillatory potentials are generated more proximal than the a- and b-waves, most probably by the bipolar cells, although the interplexiform cell cannot be excluded as a generator.

Oscillatory potentials have been considered of clinical importance because they have been shown to disappear in patients with diabetic retinopathy[6,77,202,366] (Fig. 21-56), as well as in other diseases with known inner retinal ischemia, including central retinal vein occlusion and sickle cell retinopathy. Changes in retinitis pigmentosa, central retinal artery occlusion, Behcet's disease, and siderosis have also been described.[317] In prediabetic eyes with no visible abnormalities on ophthalmoscopic examination, the oscillatory potentials have been reported to be normal in amplitude,[363,366] subnormal in amplitude,[363,366] supernormal,[310] or delayed in peak latency with or without reductions in amplitude.[366] Yonemura and Kawasaki[366] have claimed, based on a retrospective study, that a rapid decline in the amplitude of the oscillatory potential would predict an impending progression of retinopathy into the proliferative stage. More recently the oscillatory potential amplitudes have been considered useful in predicting progression of retinopathy to the more severe proliferative stages.[65,311] Bresnick et al.[65] have reported that eyes with reduced oscillatory potential amplitudes have at least a tenfold increased risk of developing Diabetic Retinopathy Study high-risk characteristics than do eyes with normal potentials. The ERG appears, in this respect, to be providing more information than ophthalmoscopy alone.[65] Comparison of the relative sensitivity of the oscillatory potentials, fluorescein angiography, and vitreous fluorophotometry in the same prediabetic eyes, to determine the earliest changes in diabetic retinopathy, remains to be done.

Scotopic threshold response

The scotopic threshold response (STR) is a small, slow, cornea-negative wave from a fully dark-adapted eye elicited by the dimmest flash that results in recordable ERG activity (Fig. 21-57). The response was named by Sieving, Frishman, and Steinberg[303] because the STR is recorded with flashes very near psychophysical absolute threshold.[131] An STR has now been identified specifically in the ERG of human,[9,306] monkey,[308,353] cat,[303] and dog.[64]

The STR is driven primarily by the onset of the light flash, and very little or no separate activity is noted at stimulus cessation. The STR is elicited best with large or diffuse stimuli. Signal averaging techniques are helpful in studying the fine details of the STR,[306] and the STR can also be recorded from normal human subjects (Fig. 21-57). Stimuli used to elicit the STR are so dim that the b-wave is not recorded, and the STR can be observed without other ERG components.

Because the STR is a negative wave in the ERG, one might be misled to think that it derives from the photoreceptors, like the a-wave. However, microelectrode recordings in the cat retina showed that the STR was maximum in the proximal retina, when the electrode was positioned between the inner plexiform and inner nuclear layers.[303] Further, intravitreal injections of aspartate abolished the STR but not the a-wave, indicating that the STR originates postsynaptic to the photoreceptors.[353] The STR is selectively abolished by GABA and glycine, which are neuroactive substances accumulated and used by amacrine cells.[246] The STR does not originate from ganglion cells, since eliminating these cells did not abolish the STR.[302]

The physiologic importance of understanding the STR lies in several areas. First, the STR allows the ERG to be used to probe quantal light sensitivities of the retina within 0.7 log units above absolute human visual threshold.[306] Second, the hypothesis that the STR derives from proximal retinal release of potassium, to which the Müller cells respond,[138] allows the refinement of Müller cell models of retinal current flow. Third, the STR may reflect activity of a specific neural pathway through the inner retina in starlight, in which the signal passes from rod bipolars, to A-II amacrine cells and only afterwards exits the retina through ganglion cells.[314]

The STR may provide clinical information about proximal retinal malfunction, particularly involving the rod pathway. In males with juvenile X-linked retinoschisis (Fig. 21-58), the STR is reduced or absent, whereas the a-wave remains normal.[304] The STR has also been found to be reduced in preproliferative diabetic retinopathy,[8,9] similar to the finding of reduced oscillatory potentials.[65]

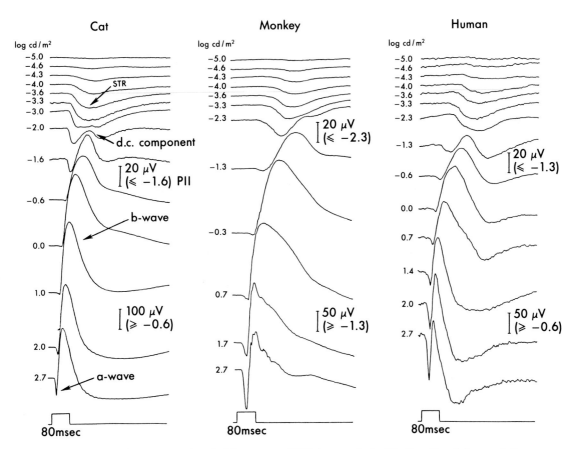

FIG. 21-57 The scotopic threshold response (STR) is recorded with dim stimuli from a fully dark-adapted eye. These ERG intensity series for the cat, monkey, and human all show similar ERG components at comparable stimulus intensities. The single difference is the faster latency of the STR and b-wave for the cat compared with monkey and human. Since 80 msec Ganzfeld stimuli were used for all recordings after full pupillary dilation, the effective retinal illuminances were similar across species. Human psychophysical threshold was near −5.0 log cd/m² for this subject, and an STR is identified with intensity only 0.4 to 0.7 log units higher. Since the d.c. component and b-wave (both part of PII) require brighter stimuli, the STR is recorded with minimal interference from other components. (From Sieving PA, Wakabayashi K: Clin Vis Sci, 6:171, 1991.)

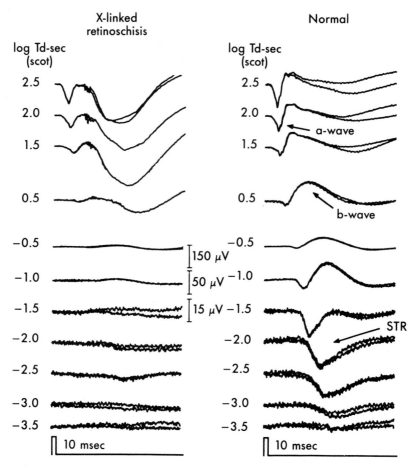

FIG. 21-58   Clinical ERGs recorded from a patient with juvenile X-linked retinoschisis and from a normal subject. Despite the small amplitude of the STR, it is reproducible, as shown by two successive traces at each intensity (averaging 10 responses for each trace). The STR is greatly reduced in juvenile retinoschisis, whereas the amplitude and shape of the photoreceptor a-wave remains normal. (From Murayama K, Kuo C-Y, Sieving PA: Clin Vis Sci 6:317, 1991.)

Recordings from ganglion cells and optic nerve fibers

In 1938 Hartline[171] observed three distinct types of responses from three separate fibers in records of action potentials recorded with microelectrodes from the optic nerve fibers of the frog eye (Fig. 21-59). In *A* the fiber responds with a rapid burst of impulses when the light is turned on. Although the light is kept constant, this soon dies down to a steady, slower discharge. No response to cessation of illumination can be recorded from this fiber. In *B* a different fiber responds as the previous one, but the impulses stop completely, although the light is kept on. In *C* another fiber gives no response when the light is turned on or throughout the entire duration of illumination, but when the light is turned off, there is a rapid burst of impulses. These fibers have been respectively termed "on," "on-off," and "off" units. In the frog each of these responses is peculiar to a particular fiber, which never gives any other type of response regardless of the conditions of stimulation or adaptation of the retina. An increase in illumination produces an increase in the frequency of discharge, and the sensitivity of the retina is diminished by light adaptation and increased by dark adaptation. The B fibers are extremely sensitive to any movement of the retinal image, whether it be a spot of light or a small shadow on the uniformly illuminated retina. The response in the C fibers to cessation of light stimulation usually

FIG. 21-59   Oscillographic records of action potentials in three single intraocular optic nerve fibers of frog's eye, showing three characteristic response types. **A,** Response to illumination of retina consisting of initial burst of impulses followed by maintained discharge lasting throughout illumination. No response to cessation of illumination in this fiber (off response in this record is partly due to retinal potential and partly to another fiber which discharged several small impulses). **B,** Response only to onset and cessation of light. **C,** Response only to cessation of illumination. In this record, time is marked in fifths of seconds, and signal marking period of illumination fills white line immediately above time marker. (From Hartline H: Am J Physiol 121:400, 1938.)

subsides in a few seconds, and the discharge in these fibers can be abruptly suppressed at any time merely by reillumination of the retina.

Hartline[172] explored the retinal surface with a small spot of light and could map an area from which responses could be recorded in a single fiber when the spot was turned on or off. He termed this region the receptive field of the fiber. In the frog many fields were of the order of 1 mm in diameter—much larger than the diameter of rods (6 μm), although it roughly agreed with the spread of the dendritic tree of some ganglion cells. Hartline observed that the response type (on, on-off, or off) remained unchanged in all points of the receptive field of a particular fiber. The sensitivity of the receptive field was greatest in the central region and diminished in the peripheral region of the field. Over the central portion Hartline was able to show that threshold intensity was inversely proportional to area of illumination. Furthermore, summation could be observed in one receptive field; a ganglion cell could show activity in response to two subthreshold stimuli presented in separate areas of its receptive field in which either stimulus presented alone elicited no activity from the ganglion cell.[173]

The concept of a receptive field as described by Hartline has been modified on the basis of observations in the mammalian retina. Recordings from ganglion cells in the cat showed that different response types could be obtained in the same ganglion cell by moving the same test spot to different positions. The receptive field could be subdivided into concentric zones (Fig. 21-60); a circular central zone of high sensitivity yielded either on or off responses, and outside this central zone was a concentric annular zone of lower sensitivity that yielded the opponent type of response (off responses if the center had on responses, on responses if the center had off responses).[185,210] Kuffler[211] showed interactions if the central zone and surround were stimulated simultaneously; the center and surround were functionally antagonistic (Fig. 21-61).

These antagonistic surrounds described by Kuffler are to be distinguished from silent surrounds described by Barlow[20] in the frog. Silent inhibitory surrounds do not themselves generate an impulse from a given ganglion cell, although light-on in a silent surround can reduce the response to light-on in the center of the receptive field of that ganglion cell. The concept of a receptive field is further complicated by such observations as the fact that some ganglion cells in the cat can be excited by a stimulus as distant as 45 degrees from the center of a conventional receptive field.[235] Therefore the definition of a receptive field of a ganglion cell must include some statement of the specificity of effects on that ganglion cell.[221]

The light-induced responses of the monkey retina show separate and independent contributions from both the rod and cone receptor systems, and the ERG (Fig. 21-11) represents a summation of these contributions.[152] In contrast, the output of the ganglion cell represents activity usually from one or the other photoreceptor,

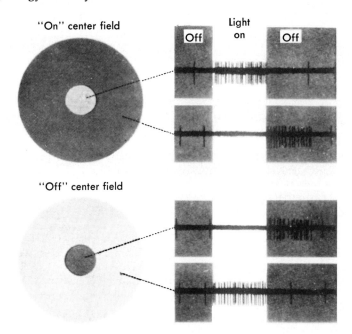

FIG. 21-60   Concentric fields are characteristic of retinal ganglion cells. *Top,* oscilloscope recording shows strong firing by on-center type of cell when spot of light strikes field center. If spot hits an off area, firing is suppressed until light goes off. *Bottom,* responses of another cell of off-center type. (From The visual cortex of the brain by D. Hubel, Copyright © 1963 by Scientific American, Inc. All rights reserved.)

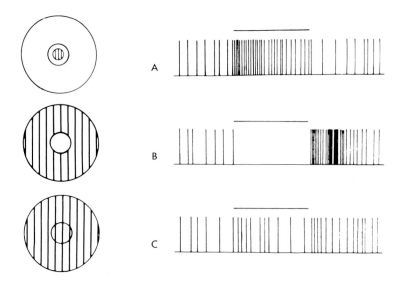

FIG. 21-61   On-center receptive field in the cat. **A,** Spot of light directed into center causes vigorous discharges. **B,** Surround illuminated by ring of light inhibits background discharge and causes responses when light is turned off. **C,** Light covering entire receptive field has relatively small effect when turned on and off because in this example antagonistic actions in center and surround almost cancel each other. Illumination, indicated by dark line, lasts 0.5 second. (From Kuffler SW: Invest Ophthalmol 12:794, 1973; drawn from unpublished records, Kuffler, 1953.)

and the ganglion cell becomes refractory to input from the other (Fig. 21-62). Interestingly, cone bipolar cells appear to synapse directly onto ganglion cells in the cat and probably in the monkey, whereas rod bipolar cells appear to synapse on an amacrine cell called the A-II amacrine cell; this amacrine cell, which receives almost exclusive input from the rod system, in turn synapses on ganglion cells to form a major pathway for rod signals leaving the retina.[129,203,254] The A-II, or rod, amacrine cell, between rod bipolar and ganglion cells, could possibly account for the observation[165] that threshold signals from the rods reach ganglion cells later than those from the cones in the monkey perifovea.

Hubel and Wiesel found the receptive fields of the spider monkey had sharply demarcated on centers with antagonistic off surrounds or the reverse.[186] Those centers nearest the fovea had a diameter as small as 4 minutes of arc (20 μm) on the retina, and some in the periphery had a diameter of about 2 degrees. Responses were rarely color specific. In contrast, in the rhesus monkey color opponency could be easily demonstrated, especially in the fovea and foveola.[158] Gouras showed that many on-center ganglion cells received excitatory signals from only one cone mechanism and contributions from another cone mechanism in the surround. One type of cell discharged transiently to maintained stimuli of any wavelength (so-called phasic); this type received signals from both green- and red-sensitive cone mechanisms, both of which excite in the center and inhibit in the periphery of the cell's receptive field. The second type discharged continuously to maintained stimuli of appropriate wavelength (so-called tonic); this type received excitatory signals from only one cone mechanism, either blue-, green-, or red-sensitive in the center, and inhibition from another cone mechanism in the periphery of its receptive field.

Whereas most tonic cells showed color opponency, phasic cells did not show this phenomenon. Gouras[156] found that the tonic cells had slower conduction velocities than the phasic cells. Tonic cells tended to show linear summation and phasic cells nonlinear summation over their receptive fields.[97] Tonic cells were more common near the fovea where small ganglion cells predominate, and phasic ganglion cells were more common toward the retinal periphery where ganglion cells are generally larger; however, both cell types were found adjacent to one another across the retina.[154] A small fraction of ganglion cells in the monkey

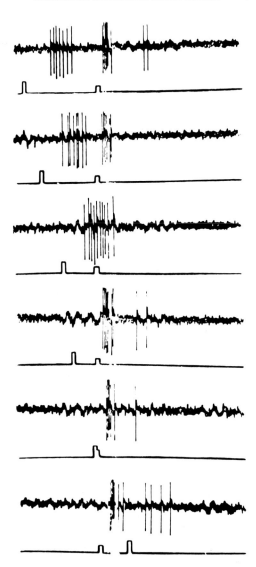

FIG. 21-62 Responses of dark-adapted perifoveal ganglion cell stimulated with two light pulses, one that affects rods (460 nm, larger photocell response) and one that affects cones (672 nm, smaller photocell response). Rod stimulus is delivered at different times relative to cone stimulus. Stimuli cover 24.6 mm² of retina, including center of cell's receptive field. Oscillograph of photocell's response is below each of cell's responses. Duration of each oscillograph is 0.5 second. Positivity is upward. (From Gouras P, Link K: J Physiol (Lond) 184:499, 1966.)

retina did not have properties of tonic or phasic cells; these cells lacked center-surround organization.[95,96]

Monkey tonic and phasic retinal ganglion cells have several similarities respectively with cat X (sustained) and Y (transient) ganglion cells described by Cleland, Dubin, and Levick,[86] Enroth-Cugell and Robson,[126] and Fukada.[140] Both tonic and X cells predominate in the central retina and have slower conducting axons than phasic and Y cells. An important difference is that monkey tonic ganglion cells show color opponency, whereas cat X cells do not. Cats also have another ganglion cell system (called the W system) with conduction latencies longer than the X and Y systems[326,327]; no exact counterpart in the monkey retina has yet been described.

The major subdivision of ganglion cells into tonic or X-like and phasic or Y-like cells is particularly important, since Dreher, Fukada, and Rodieck[118] and Kruger[209] have found that lateral geniculate cells with X-like properties (strong, sustained responses to stationary stimuli, unresponsiveness to fast-moving stimuli, and relatively long response latency) receive excitatory input from retinal cells with relatively slow-conducting axons, whereas lateral geniculate nucleus cells with Y-like properties (transient, weak responses to stationary stimuli, responsiveness to fast-moving stimuli, relatively short response latency) receive excitatory input from retinal cells with relatively fast-conducting axons. Moreover, these cells appear anatomically segregated within the monkey lateral geniculate nucleus with X-like cells in the parvocellular layers and Y-like cells in the magnocellular layers.[118,209]

The X-Y (tonic-phasic) separation appears to be an advance in understanding two parallel systems that leave the retina and carry different aspects of the physical image of light on the photoreceptors to the central nervous system. It will be of interest to see if the X and Y systems are differentially affected in various diseases such as amblyopia, glaucoma, and toxic optic neuropathies.

Single cell approach

Although investigations of the retina are concerned with over 100 million cells, relatively few neuronal types are present, and repeating units are evident. Information derived from microelectrode recordings from single cells have begun to reveal arrangements within the retina and its projection through the optic nerve to the lateral geniculate nucleus and visual cortex.[211] Receptive fields become more complex as one ascends through successive cell layers. For example, within the monkey cortex some cells respond only to light oriented in a particular way on the retina, others respond to particular configurations, dimensions, or directions of movement, and others respond only to certain wavelength bands. One problem now is to understand further not only the patterns of connections within the retina and between the retina and cortex but also the integrative mechanisms of these connections at synaptic sites. Another clinically relevant problem is the further definition of the relationship of the cone and rod photoreceptors to the pigment epithelium. Electrophysiologic and psychophysical studies combined with collaborative molecular genetic, immunocytochemical, and biochemical investigations would seem to have the best chance for clarifying these problems. Such research could provide some of the new dimensions needed to help patients with diseases involving the neuronal units responsible for vision.

ACKNOWLEDGMENT

The author thanks Dr. Paul A. Sieving for his contribution to the sections on the pattern electroretinogram and the scotopic threshold response.

REFERENCES

1. Adrian ED: Electric responses of the human eye, J Physiol (Lond) 104:84, 1945.
2. Adrian ED: Rod and cone components in the electric response of the eye, J Physiol (Lond) 105:24, 1946.
3. Adrian ED, Matthews R: Action of light on the eye; discharge of impulses in the optic nerve and its relation to electrical changes in the retina, J Physiol (Lond) 63:378, 1927.
4. Aguirre GD: Inherited retinal degenerations in the dog, Trans Am Acad Ophthalmol Otolaryngol 81:667, 1976.
5. Aguirre GD, et al: Pathogenesis of progressive rod-cone degeneration in miniature poodles, Invest Ophthalmol Vis Sci 23:610, 1982.
6. Algvere P, Gjotterberg M: The diagnostic value of the oscillatory potentials of the ERG and fluorescein angiography in diabetic proliferative retinopathy, Ophthalmologica 168:97, 1974.
7. Alpern M, Holland MG, Ohba N: Rhodopsin bleaching signals in essential night blindness, J Physiol (Lond) 225:457, 1972.
8. Alward GW: The scotopic threshold response in diabetic retinopathy, Eye 3:626, 1989.
9. Alward GW, Vaegan, Billson FA: The scotopic threshold response in man, Clin Vis Sci 4:373, 1989.
10. Andréasson SOL, Sandberg MA, Berson EL: Narrowband filtering for monitoring low-amplitude cone elec-

troretinograms in retinitis pigmentosa, Am J Ophthalmol 105:500, 1988.

11. Arden GB, Barrada A: Analysis of the electrooculograms of a series of normal subjects, Br J Ophthalmol 46:468, 1962.

12. Arden GB, Barrada A, Kelsey JH: New clinical test of retinal function based upon the standing potential of the eye, Br J Ophthalmol 46:449, 1962.

13. Arden GB, Ikeda H: Effects of hereditary degeneration of the retina on the early receptor potential and the corneofundal potential of the rat eye, Vision Res 6:171, 1966.

14. Arden GB, Vaegan, Hogg HC: Clinical and experimental evidence that the pattern electroretinogram (PERG) is generated in more proximal retinal layers than the focal electroretinogram (FERG), Ann NY Acad Sci 338:580, 1982.

15. Armington JC, Johnson EP, Riggs LA: The scotopic a-wave in the electrical response of the human retina, J Physiol (Lond) 118:289, 1952.

16. Armington JC, et al: Summation of retinal potentials, J Opt Soc Am 51:877, 1961.

17. Asher H: The electroretinogram of the blind spot, J Physiol (Lond) 112:40P, 1951.

18. Baker CL, Hess RF: Linear and non-linear components of human electroretinograms, J Neurophysiol 51:952, 1984.

19. Baker CL, et al: Current source density analysis of linear and nonlinear components of the primate electroretinogram, J Physiol 407:155, 1988.

20. Barlow HB: Summation and inhibition in the frog's retina, J Physiol (Lond) 119:69, 1953.

21. Baylor DA: Photoreceptor cells and vision, Invest Ophthalmol Vis Sci 28:34, 1987.

22. Baylor DA, Fuortes MGF, O'Bryan P: Receptive fields of cones in the retina of the turtle, J Physiol (Lond) 214:265, 1971.

23. Bell J: Retinitis pigmentosa and allied diseases of the eye, in Pearson K, ed: Treasury of human inheritance, vol 2, London, Cambridge University Press, 1922.

24. Bergamini L, Bergamasco B: Cortical evoked potentials in man, Springfield, IL, Charles C Thomas, Publisher, 1967.

25. Berson EL: Experimental and therapeutic aspects of photic damage to the retina, Invest Ophthalmol 12:35, 1973.

26. Berson EL: Retinitis pigmentosa, the electroretinogram, and Mendel's laws, Trans Pa Acad Ophthalmol Otolaryngol 26:109, 1973.

27. Berson EL: Night blindness: some aspects of management, in Faye E, ed: Clinical low vision, Boston, Little, Brown, 1976, pp 301-306.

28. Berson EL: Retinitis pigmentosa and allied retinal diseases: electrophysiologic findings, Trans Am Acad Ophthalmol Otolaryngol 81:659, 1976.

29. Berson EL: Hereditary retinal diseases: classification with the full-field electroretinogram, in Lawwill T, ed: Documenta Ophthalmologica Proceedings Series, no 13, Fourteenth ISCERG Symposium, Louisville, KY, May 10 to 14, 1976, The Hague, Dr W Junk BV, 1977, pp 149-171.

30. Berson EL: Light deprivation and retinitis pigmentosa, in Symposium: Intense light hazards in ophthalmic diagnosis and treatment, 1979, Houston, Vision Res 20:1179, 1980.

31. Berson EL: Hereditary retinal diseases: applications of electrophysiological and psychological testing, in Proenza LM, Enoch JM, Jampolsky A, ed: Clinical applications of psychophysics, Cambridge, England, Cambridge University Press, 1981, pp 170-197.

32. Berson EL: Retinitis pigmentosa and allied diseases: applications of electroretinographic testing, Int Ophthalmol 4:7, 1981.

33. Berson EL: Nutrition and retinal degenerations: vitamin A, taurine, ornithine, phytanic acid, Retina 2:236, 1982.

34. Berson EL: Electroretinographic findings in retinitis pigmentosa, Jpn J Ophthalmol 31:327, 1987.

35. Berson EL, Goldstein EB: The early receptor potential in dominantly inherited retinitis pigmentosa, Arch Ophthalmol 83:412, 1970.

36. Berson EL, Goldstein EB: The early receptor potential in sex-linked retinitis pigmentosa, Invest Ophthalmol 9:58, 1970.

37. Berson EL, Goldstein EB: Recovery of the human early receptor potential during dark adaptation in hereditary retinal disease, Vision Res 10:219, 1970.

38. Berson EL, Goldstein EB: Cone pigment regeneration, retinitis pigmentosa, and light deprivation, Vision Res 12:749, 1972.

39. Berson EL, Gouras P, Gunkel RD: Progressive cone rod degeneration, Arch Ophthalmol 80:68, 1968.

40. Berson EL, Gouras P, Gunkel RD: Progressive cone degeneration, dominantly inherited, Arch Ophthalmol 80:77, 1968.

41. Berson EL, Gouras P, Gunkel RD: Rod responses in retinitis pigmentosa, dominantly inherited, Arch Ophthalmol 80:58, 1968.

42. Berson EL, Gouras P, Hoff M: Temporal aspects of the electroretinogram, Arch Ophthalmol 81:207, 1969.

43. Berson EL, Howard J: Temporal aspects of the electroretinogram in sector retinitis pigmentosa, Arch Ophthalmol 86:653, 1971.

44. Berson EL, Kanters L: Cone and rod responses in a family with recessively inherited retinitis pigmentosa, Arch Ophthalmol 84:288, 1970.

45. Berson EL, Lessell S: Paraneoplastic night blindness with malignant melanoma, Am J Ophthalmol 106:307, 1988.

46. Berson EL, Rabin AR, Mehaffey L: Advances in night vision technology: a pocketscope for patients with retinitis pigmentosa, Arch Ophthalmol 90:427, 1973.

47. Berson EL, Rosen JB, Simonoff EA: Electroretinographic testing as an aid in detection of carriers of x-chromosome-linked retinitis pigmentosa, Am J Ophthalmol 87:460, 1979.

48. Berson EL, Schmidt SY, Rabin AR: Plasma amino acids in hereditary retinal disease: ornithine, lysine and taurine, Br J Ophthalmol 60:142, 1976.

49. Berson EL, Schmidt SY, Shih VE: Ocular and biochemical abnormalities in gyrate atrophy of the choroid and retina, Ophthalmol 85:1018, 1978.

50. Berson EL, Simonoff EA: Dominant retinitis pigmentosa with reduced penetrance; further studies of the electroretinogram, Arch Ophthalmol 97:1286, 1979.

51. Berson EL, et al: Rod and cone responses in sex-linked retinitis pigmentosa, Arch Ophthalmol 81:215, 1969.

52. Berson EL, et al: Dominant retinitis pigmentosa with reduced penetrance, Arch Ophthalmol 81:226, 1969.

53. Berson EL, et al: A two year trial of low protein, low arginine diets or vitamin B$_6$ for patients with gyrate atrophy, in Cotlier E, Maumenee I, Berman E, eds: Birth defects: original article series, vol 18, New York, Alan R Liss, 1982, pp 209-218.

54. Berson EL, et al: Natural course of retinitis pigmentosa over a three-year interval, Am J Ophthalmol 99:240, 1985.

55. Berson EL, et al: Ocular findings in patients with autosomal dominant retinitis pigmentosa and a rhodopsin gene defect (Pro-23-His), Arch Ophthalmol 109:92, 1991.

56. Biersdorf WR, Diller DA: Local electroretinogram in macular degeneration, Am J Ophthalmol 68:296, 1969.

57. Birch DG, Sandberg MA: Dependence of cone b-wave implicit time on rod amplitude in retinitis pigmentosa, Vision Res 27:1105, 1987.

58. Bishara S, et al: Combined vitamin A and E therapy prevents retinal electrophysiological deterioration in abetalipoproteinemia, Br J Ophthalmol 66:767, 1982.

59. Black RK, Jay B, Kolb H: Electrical activity in the eye in high myopia, Br J Ophthalmol 50:629, 1966.

60. Bornschein H, Goodman G, Gunkel RD: Temporal aspects of the human electroretinogram, Arch Ophthalmol 57:386, 1957.

61. Bowes C, et al: Retinal degeneration in the *rd* mouse is caused by a defect in the β subunit of rod cGMP-phosphodiesterase, Nature 347:677, 1990.

62. Boycott BB, et al: Interplexiform cells of the mammalian retina and their comparison with catecholamine-containing retinal cells, Proc R Soc Lond (Biol) 191:353, 1975.

63. Boynton RM, Riggs LA: The effect of stimulus area and intensity upon the human retinal response, J Exp Psychol 42:217, 1951.

64. Brabander B, Zrenner E: The scotopic threshold response (STR) in the electroretinogram of dog, Doc Ophthalmol, 1991 (in press).

65. Bresnick GH, et al: Electroretinographic oscillatory potentials predict progression of diabetic retinopathy, Arch Ophthalmol 102:1307, 1984.

66. Brindley GS: The effect on the frog's electroretinogram of varying the amount of retina illuminated, J Physiol (Lond) 134:353, 1956.

67. Brindley GS: Responses to illumination recorded by microelectrodes from the frog's retina, J Physiol (Lond) 134:360, 1956.

68. Brindley GS: Additivity in the electroretinogram, J Physiol (Lond) 137:51, 1957.

69. Brindley GS, Gardner-Medwin AR: The origin of the early receptor potential of the retina, J Physiol (Lond) 182:185, 1966.

70. Brindley GS, Westheimer G: The spatial properties of the human electroretinogram, J Physiol (Lond) 179:518, 1965.

71. Brown KT: The electroretinogram: its components and their origin, Vision Res 8:633, 1968.

72. Brown KT, Murakami M: A new receptor potential of the monkey retina with no detectable latency, Nature 201:626, 1964.

73. Brown PK, Wald G: Visual pigments in single rods and cones of the human retina, Science 144:45, 1964.

74. Brown KT, Watanabe K: Isolation and identification of a receptor potential from the pure cone fovea of the monkey retina, Nature 193:958, 1962.

75. Brown KT, Watanabe K, Murakami M: The early and late receptor potentials of monkey cones and rods, Cold Spring Harbor Symp Quant Biol 30:457, 1965.

76. Brown KT, Wiesel TN: Localization of origins of electroretinogram components by intraretinal recording in the intact cat eye, J Physiol (Lond) 158:257, 1961.

77. Brunette JR: Oscillatory potentials; a clinical study in diabetics, Can J Ophthalmol 5:373, 1970.

78. Brunette JR: A standardizable method for separating rod and cone responses in clinical electroretinography, Am J Ophthalmol 75:833, 1973.

79. Byzov AL, Trifonov YA: The response to electric stimulation of horizontal cells in the carp retina, Vision Res 8:817, 1968.

80. Carr RE, Ripps H, Siegel IM: Visual pigment kinetics and adaptation in fundus albipunctatus, in Documenta Ophthalmologica proceedings series, Eleventh IS-CERG Symposium, Bad Nauheim, West Germany, The Hague, Dr W Junk BV, 1974, pp 193-204.

81. Carr RE, Siegel IM: Electrophysiologic aspects of several retinal diseases, Am J Ophthalmol 58:95, 1964.

82. Carr RE, Siegel IM: Action spectrum of the early human receptor potential, Nature 225:88, 1970.

83. Carr RE, et al: Rhodopsin and the electrical activity of the retina in congenital night blindness, Invest Ophthalmol 5:497, 1966.

84. Carter-Dawson LD, LaVail MM, Sidman RL: Differential effect of the rd mutation on rods and cones in the mouse retina, Invest Ophthalmol Vis Sci 17:489, 1978.

85. Cervetto L, Piccolino M: Synaptic transmission between photoreceptors and horizontal cells in the turtle retina, Science 183:417, 1974.

86. Cleland BG, Dubin MW, Levick WR: Sustained and transient neurones in the cat's retina and lateral geniculate nucleus, J Physiol 217:473, 1971.

87. Cobbs WH, Pugh EN Jr: Two components of outer segment membrane current in salamander rods and cones, Biophys J 49:280a, 1986.

88. Cohen AI: Some contributions to the cell biology of photoreceptors, Proctor lecture, Invest Ophthalmol Vis Sci 25:1354, 1984.

89. Cone RA: The early receptor potential of the vertebrate eye, Cold Spring Harbor Symp Quant Biol 30:483, 1965.

90. Cone RA: Early receptor potential: photoreversible charge displacement in rhodopsin, Science 155:1128, 1967.

91. Cone RA, Brown PK: Dependence of the early receptor potential on the orientation of rhodopsin, Science 156:536, 1967.

92. Copenhaver RM, Goodman G: The electroretinogram in infantile, late infantile, and juvenile amaurotic family idiocy, Arch Ophthalmol 63:559, 1960.

93. Cremers FPM, et al: Cloning of a gene that is rear-

ranged in patients with choroideraemia, Nature 347:674, 1990.

94. Cross HE, Barr L: Electro-oculography in Best's macular dystrophy, Am J Ophthalmol 77:46, 1974.

95. DeMonasterio FM: Properties of ganglion cells with atypical receptive-field organization in retina of macaques, J Neurophysiol 41:1435, 1978.

96. DeMonasterio FM, Gouras P: Functional properties of ganglion cells of the rhesus monkey retina, J Physiol 251:167, 1975.

97. DeMonasterio FM, Gouras P, Tolhurst DJ: Concealed colour opponency in ganglion cells of the rhesus monkey retina, J Physiol 251:217, 1975.

98. Deutman AF: Electro-oculography in families with dystrophy of the fovea, Arch Ophthalmol 81:305, 1969.

99. Deutman AF, et al: Butterfly-shaped pigment dystrophy of the fovea, Arch Ophthalmol 83:558, 1970.

100. Dewar J: The physiological action of light, Nature 15:433, 1877.

101. Dhanda RP: ERG in myopic retinal degenerations, in Nakajima A, ed: Jpn J Ophthalmol 10(Suppl):325, 1966.

102. Dick E, Miller RF: Light-evoked potassium activity in mudpuppy retina: its relationship to the b-wave of the electroretinogram, Brain Res 154:388, 1978.

103. Dodt E: Cone electroretinogram by flicker, Nature 168:783, 1957.

104. Dodt E: Ein Doppelinterferenzfilter-Monochromator besonders hoher Leuchtdichte, Bibl Ophthalmol 48:32, 1957.

105. Dodt E, Wadenstein L: The use of flicker electroretinography in the human eye, Acta Ophthalmol 32:165, 1954.

106. Dowling JE: Nutritional and inherited blindness in the rat, Exp Res 3:348, 1964.

107. Dowling JE: Organization of vertebrate retinas, Invest Ophthalmol 9:655, 1970.

108. Dowling JE: The retina: an approachable part of the brain, Cambridge, MA, Harvard University Press, 1987.

109. Dowling, JE: Neuromodulation in the retina: the role of dopamine, Sem Neurosci 1:35, 1989.

110. Dowling JE, Dubin MW: The vertebrate retina, in Darien-Smith I, ed: Handbook of sensory physiology, section I, vol III, part I, Bethesda, MD, American Physiological Society, 1984, pp 317-339.

111. Dowling JE, Ehinger B: Synaptic organization of the interplexiform cells of the goldfish retina, Science 188:270, 1975.

112. Dowling JE, Ehinger B: The interplexiform cell system, I, Synapses of the dopaminergic neurons of the goldfish retina, Proc R Soc Lond (Biol) 201:7, 1978.

113. Dowling JE, Ehinger B: Synaptic organization of the dopaminergic neurons in the rabbit retina, J Comp Neur 180:203, 1978.

114. Dowling JE, Ehinger B, Heddon WL: The interplexiform cell: a new type of retinal neuron, Invest Ophthalmol Vis Sci 15:916, 1976.

115. Dowling JE, Ripps H: Adaptation in skate photoreceptors, J Gen Physiol 60:698, 1972.

116. Dowling JE, Ripps H: Neurotransmission in the distal retina: the effect of magnesium on horizontal cell activity, Nature 242:101, 1973.

117. Dowling JE, Sidman RL: Inherited retinal dystrophy in rats, J Cell Biol 14:73, 1962.

118. Dreher B, Fukada Y, Rodieck RW: Identification, classification and anatomical segregation of cells with X-like and Y-like properties in the lateral geniculate nucleus of old-world primates, J Physiol 258:433, 1976.

119. Dryja TP, et al: Mutations within the rhodopsin gene in patients with autosomal dominant retinitis pigmentosa, N Engl J Med 323:1302, 1990.

120. Dryja TP, et al: A point mutation in the rhodopsin gene in one form of retinitis pigmentosa, Nature 343:364, 1990.

121. Ehinger B: Connections between retinal neurons with identified neurotransmitters, Vision Res 23:1281, 1983.

122. Ehinger B, Dowling JE: Retinal neurocircuitry and transmission, in Bjorklund A, Hokfelt T, Swanson LW, eds: Handbook of chemical neuroanatomy, vol 5, Amsterdam, Elsevier, 1987, pp 389-446.

123. Einthoven W, Jolly WA: The form and magnitude of the electrical response of the eye to stimulation by light at various intensities, Q J Exp Physiol 1:373, 1908.

124. Eisenberg MF, Copenhaver RM: A fiber optic ophthalmoscope for focal retinal stimulation, Med Res Eng 6:23, 1967.

125. Eldjarn L, et al: Dietary effects on serum phytanic acid levels and on clinical manifestation in heredopathia atactica polyneuritiformis, Lancet 1:691, 1966.

126. Enroth-Cugell C, Robson JG: The contrast sensitivity of retinal ganglion cells of the cat, J Physiol 187:517, 1966.

127. Faber DL: Dissertation, Buffalo, NY, 1969, State University of New York.

128. Fain GL, Matthews HR: Calcium and the mechanism of light adaptation in vertebrate photoreceptors, TINS 13:378, 1990.

129. Famiglietti EV, Kolb H: A bistratified amacrine cell and synaptic circuitry in the inner plexiform layer of the retina, Brain Res 84:293, 1975.

130. Fesenko EE, Kolesnikov SS, Lyubarsky AL: Induction by cyclic GMP of cationic conductance in plasma membrane of retinal rod outer segment, Nature 313:310, 1985.

131. Finkelstein D, Gouras P, Hoff M: Human electroretinogram near the absolute threshold of vision, Invest Ophthalmol 7:214, 1968.

132. Fishman GA: Fundus flavimaculatus: a clinical classification, Arch Ophthalmol 94:2061, 1978.

133. Fishman GA, Carrasco C, Fishman M: The EOG in familial drusen, Arch Ophthalmol 94:231, 1976.

134. Fishman GA, et al: Electrooculogram testing in fundus flavimaculatus, Arch Ophthalmol 97:1896, 1979.

135. Franceschetti A, François J, Babel J: Les hérédodégénérescences chorio-rétiniennes, vol 1, Paris, Masson, 1963, pp 325-338, 351-369.

136. François J, de Rouck A: Behavior of ERG and EOG in localized retinal destruction by photocoagulation, in Burian HM, Jacobson JH, eds: Clinical electroretinography, Proceedings of the Third International Sym-

posium, Highland Park, IL, 1964, Oxford, Pergamon Press, 1966, pp 191-202.

137. François J, de Rouck A, Férnandez-Sasso D: Electro-oculography in vitelliform degeneration of the macula, Arch Ophthalmol 77:726, 1967.

138. Frishman L, Steinberg RH: Intraretinal analysis of the threshold dark-adapted ERG of cat retina, J Neurophysiol 61:1221, 1989.

139. Fry GA, Bartley SH: The relation of stray light in the eye to the retinal action potential, Am J Physiol 111:335, 1935.

140. Fukada Y: Receptive field organization of cat optic nerve fibers with reference to conduction velocity, Vision Res 11:209, 1971.

141. Furukawa T, Hanawa I: Effects of some common cations on electroretinogram of the toad, Jpn J Physiol 5:280, 1955.

142. Gallego A: Horizontal and amacrine cells in the mammal's retina, Vision Res 3(Suppl):33, 1971.

143. Galloway NR: Early receptor potential in the human eye, Br J Ophthalmol 51:261, 1967.

144. Gastant H, Régis H: Visually evoked potentials recorded transcranially in man, in Symposium: the analysis of central nervous system and cardiovascular data using computer methods, SP72, Washington, DC, NASA, 1964.

145. Goldstein EB: Visual pigments and the early receptor potential of the isolated frog retina, Vision Res 8:953, 1968.

146. Goldstein EB: Contributions of cones to the early receptor potential in the rhesus monkey, Nature 222:1273, 1969.

147. Goldstein EB, Berson EL: Cone dominance of the human early receptor potential, Nature 222:1272, 1969.

148. Goldstein EB, Berson EL: Rod and cone contributions to the human early receptor potential, Vision Res 10:207, 1970.

149. Goodman G, Bornschein H: Comparative electroretinographic studies in congenital night blindness and total color blindness, Arch Ophthalmol 58:174, 1957.

150. Goodman G, Ripps H: Electroretinography in the differential diagnosis of visual loss in children, Arch Ophthalmol 64:221, 1960.

151. Goodman G, Ripps H, Siegel IM: Cone dysfunction syndromes, Arch Ophthalmol 70:214, 1963.

152. Gouras P: Rod and cone independence in the electroretinogram of the dark-adapted monkey's perifovea, J Physiol (Lond) 187:455, 1966.

153. Gouras P: visual adaptation: its mechanism, Science 157:583, 1967.

154. Gouras P: Identification of cone mechanisms in monkey ganglion cells, J Physiol (Lond) 199:533, 1968.

155. Gouras P: Relationships of the electro-oculogram to the electro-retinogram, in The clinical value of electroretinography, ISCERG Symposium, Ghent, Belgium, 1966, Basel, Switzerland, S Karger, 1968, pp 66-73.

156. Gouras P: Antidromic responses of orthodromically identified ganglion cells in monkey retina, J Physiol 204:407, 1969.

157. Gouras P: Electroretinography: some basic principles, Invest Ophthalmol 9:557, 1970.

158. Gouras P: Color opponency from fovea to striate cortex, Invest Ophthalmol 11:427, 1972.

159. Gouras P: Light and dark adaptation, in Fuortes MGF, ed: Handbook of sensory physiology, vol 7/2, New York, Springer-Verlag, 1972, pp 609-634.

160. Gouras P: S-potentials, in Fuortes MGF, ed: Handbook of sensory physiology, vol 7/2, New York, Springer-Verlag, 1972, pp 513-529.

161. Gouras P, Carr RE: Light-induced DC responses of monkey retina before and after central retinal artery interruption, Invest Ophthalmol 4:310, 1965.

162. Gouras P, Carr RE: Cone activity in the light-induced DC response of monkey retina, Invest Ophthalmol 4:318, 1965.

163. Gouras P, Carr RE, Gunkel RD: Retinitis pigmentosa in abetalipoproteinemia: effects of vitamin A, Invest Ophthalmol 10:784, 1971.

164. Gouras P, Gunkel RD: The EOG in chloroquine and other retinopathies, Arch Ophthalmol 70:629, 1973.

165. Gouras P, Link K: Rod and cone interaction in dark adapted monkey ganglion cells, J Physiol (Lond) 184:499, 1966.

166. Graham LT Jr: Comparative aspects of neurotransmitters in the retina, in Davson H, Graham LT Jr, eds: The eye, vol 6, New York, Academic Press, 1974, pp 283-342.

167. Granit R: The components of the retinal action potential in mammals and their relation to the discharge in the optic nerve, J Physiol (Lond) 77:207, 1933.

168. Granit R: Sensory mechanisms of the retina, London, Oxford University Press, 1947.

169. Granit R, Munsterhjelm A: The electrical response of dark-adapted frog's eyes to monochromatic stimuli, J Physiol (Lond) 88:436, 1937.

170. Hagins WA, Penn RD, Yoshikami S: Dark current and photocurrent in retinal rods, Biophys J 10:380, 1970.

171. Hartline H: The response of single optic nerve fibers of the vertebrate eye to illumination of the retina, Am J Physiol 121:400, 1938.

172. Hartline H: The receptive fields of optic nerve fibers, Am J Physiol 130:690, 1940.

173. Hartline H: The effects of spatial summation in the retina on the excitation of the fibers of the optic nerve, Am J Physiol 130:700, 1940.

174. Hashimoto Y, Murakami M, Tomita T: Localization of the ERG by aid of histological method, Jpn J Physiol 11:62, 1961.

175. Haynes LW, Kay AR, Yau K-W: Single cyclic GMP-activated channel activity in excised patches of rod outer segment membrane, Nature 321:66, 1986.

176. Hecht S: Rods, cones and the chemical basis of vision, Physiol Rev 17:239, 1937.

177. Hedden WL Jr, Dowling JE: The interplexiform cell system, II, Effects of dopamine on goldfish retinal neurones, Proc R Soc Lond (Biol) 201:27, 1978.

178. Henkel HE: Electroretinography in circulatory disturbances of the retina, Arch Ophthalmol 51:42, 1954.

179. Henkes HE, Verduin PC: Dysgenesis or abiotrophy? A differentiation with the help of the electro-retinogram (ERG) and electro-oculogram (EOG) in Leber's congenital amaurosis, Ophthalmologica 145:144, 1963.

180. Heynen H, Wachtmeister L, van Norren D: Origin of

the oscillatory potentials in the primate retina, Vision Res 25:1365, 1985.

181. Hess RF, Baker CL: Human pattern-evoked electroretinogram, J Neurophysiol 51:939, 1984.

182. Hill DA, Arbel K, Berson EL: Cone electroretinograms in congenital nyctalopia with myopia, Am J Ophthalmol 78:127, 1974.

183. Hirose T, Miyake Y, Hara A: Simultaneous recording of electroretinogram and visual evoked response, Arch Ophthalmol 95:1205, 1977.

184. Holmgren F: Method att objectivera effecten av ljusintryck på retina, Ups Läkaref Förh 1:177, 1865-1866.

185. Hubel D: The visual cortex of the brain, Sci Am 209(5):57, 1963.

186. Hubel D, Wiesel T: Receptive fields of optic nerve fibers in the spider monkey, J Physiol (Lond) 154:572, 1960.

187. Inana G, et al: Point mutation affecting processing of the ornithine aminotransferase precursor protein in gyrate atrophy, J Biol Chem 264:17432, 1989.

188. Inoue J, Takeo K, Akiba T: The visual evoked potentials to focal illumination of the retina by direct view ophthalmoscopy, Acta Soc Jpn Ophthalmol 77:1149, 1973.

189. Jacobson JH, Hirose T, Suguki TA: Simultaneous ERG and VER in lesions of the optic pathway, Invest Ophthalmol 6:279, 1968.

190. Jacobson SG, Sandberg MA: Nasal-temporal asymmetry of visual thresholds from known retinal areas in strabismic amblyopia, Invest Ophthalmol Vis Sci 19(Suppl):271, 1980.

191. Jacobson SR, et al: Foveal cone electroretinograms in strabismic amblyopia; comparison with macular scars, juvenile macular degeneration, and optic atrophy, Trans Ophthalmol Soc UK 99:353, 1980.

192. Johnson EP, Cornsweet TN: Electroretinal photopic sensitivity curves, Nature 174:614, 1954.

193. Johnson EP, Riggs LA, Schick AML: Photopic retinal potentials evoked by phase alternation of a barred pattern, in Burian HM, Jacobson JH, eds: Clinical electroretinography, Proceedings of the Third International Symposium, Highland Park, IL, 1964, Oxford, Pergamon Press, 1966, pp 75-91.

194. Kaiser-Kupfer MI, Valle D, Del Valle LA: A specific enzyme defect in gyrate atrophy, Am J Ophthalmol 85:200, 1978.

195. Kaneko A: Physiological and morphological identification of horizontal, bipolar and amacrine cells in goldfish retina, J Physiol (Lond) 207:623, 1970.

196. Karpe G: Basis of clinical electroretinography, Acta Ophthalmol 24(Suppl):84, 1945.

197. Karwoski CJ, Lu HK, Newman EA: Spatial buffering of light evoked potassium increases by retinal Müller (glial) cells, Science 244:578, 1989.

198. Karwoski CJ, Proenza LM: Light evoked changes in extracellular potassium concentrations in mudpuppy retina, Brain Res 145:515, 1978.

199. Kaupp UB, et al: Primary structure and functional expression from complementary DNA of the rod photoreceptor cyclic GMP-gated channel, Nature 342:762, 1989.

200. Kennaway NG, Weleber RG, Buist NRM: Gyrate atrophy of choroid and retina: deficient activity of ornithine ketoacid aminotransferase in cultured skin fibroblasts, N Engl J Med 297:1180, 1977.

201. Kline RP, Ripps H, Dowling JE: Generation of b-wave currents in the skate retina, Proc Natl Acad Sci USA 75:5727, 1978.

202. Kojima K, et al: ERGs in diabetes, in Nakajima A, ed: Retinal degenerations, ERGs and optic pathways, Fourth ISCERG Symposium, Hakone, Japan, 1965, Tokyo, Maruzen, 1966, pp 120-125; Jpn J Ophthalmol vol 10 (Suppl), 1966.

203. Kolb H, Famiglietti EV: Rod and cone pathways in the inner plexiform of cat retina, Science 186:47, 1974.

204. Korol S, et al: In vivo effects of glycine on retinal ultrastructure and averaged electroretinograms, Brain Res 97:235, 1978.

205. Krill AE: The electroretinogram and electrooculogram: clinical application, Invest Ophthalmol 9:600, 1970.

206. Krill AE: Hereditary retinal and choroidal diseases, New York, Harper & Row, 1972, pp 248-249.

207. Krill AE, Archer D, Martin D: Sector retinitis pigmentosa, Am J Ophthalmol 69:977, 1970.

208. Krill AE, Klien BA: Flecked retina syndrome, Arch Ophthalmol 74:496, 1965.

209. Kruger J: Stimulus dependent color specificity of monkey lateral geniculate neurons, Exp Brain Res 30:297, 1977.

210. Kuffler S: Discharge patterns and functional organization of mammalian retina, J Neurophysiol 16:62, 1953.

211. Kuffler S: The single-cell approach in the visual system and the study of receptive fields, Invest Ophthalmol 12:794, 1973.

212. Kuffler S, Nicholls JG: The physiology of neuroglial cells, Ergeb Physiol 57:1, 1966.

213. Lai YL, Jonas AM: Rat model for hereditary retinal degeneration, in Landers MB, III, et al, eds: Retinitis pigmentosa, New York, Plenum, 1976, pp 115-136.

214. Lasansky A, DeFisch FW: Potential, current, and ionic fluxes across the isolated retinal pigment epithelium and choroid, J Gen Physiol 49:913, 1966.

215. LaVail MM: Analysis of neurological mutants with inherited retinal degeneration, Friedenwald lecture, Invest Ophthalmol Vis Sci 21:638, 1981.

216. LaVail MM, Mullen RJ: Role of the pigment epithelium in inherited retinal degeneration analyzed with experimental mouse chimeras, Exp Eye Res 23:227, 1976.

217. Lawwill T: The bar-pattern electroretinogram for clinical evaluation of the central retina, Am J Ophthalmol 78:121, 1974.

218. Lawwill T: The bar pattern electroretinogram, in van Lith GHM, Lawwill T, eds: Documenta Ophthalmologica Proceedings Series 40, Twenty-first ISCEV Symposium, Budapest, 1983, Dordrecht, Dr W Junk, 1984, pp 1-10.

219. Lawwill T, Burian HM: A modification of the Burian-Allen contact lens electrode for human electroretinography, Am J Ophthalmol 61:1506, 1966.

220. Le Grand Y: Form and space vision, Bloomington, IN, Indiana University Press, 1967.

221. Levick WR: Receptive fields of retinal ganglion cells, in Fuortes MGF, ed: Handbook of sensory physiology,

Vol 7/2, New York, Springer-Verlag, 1974, pp 531-566.

222. Liu YP, et al: Involvement of cyclic GMP phosphodiesterase activator in an hereditary retinal degeneration, Nature 280:62, 1979.

223. Lolley RN, Farber DB: Abnormal guanosine 3′,5′-monophosphate during photoreceptor degeneration in the inherited retinal disorder of C3H/HeJ mice, Ann Ophthalmol 8:496, 1976.

224. MacNichol EF Jr, Svaetichin G: Electric responses from the isolated retinas of fishes, Am J Ophthalmol 46:26, 1958.

225. Maffei L, Fiorentini A: Electroretinographic responses to alternating gratings before and after section of the optic nerve, Science 211:953, 1981.

226. Maffei L, Fiorentini A: Electroretinographic response to alternating gratings in the cat, Exp Brain Res 48:327-334, 1982.

227. Maksimova EM, Maksimov VV, Orlov OY: Intensified interaction between signals of receptors in cells that are sources of S-potentials, Biofizika 11:472, 1966.

228. Mandelbaum J: Dark adaptation, some physiological and clinical considerations, Arch Ophthalmol 26:203, 1941.

229. Marks WB, Dobelle WH, MacNichol EF Jr: Visual pigments of single primate cones, Science 143:1181, 1964.

230. Marmor MF: Defining fundus albipunctatus, in Lawwill T, ed: Documenta Ophthalmologia proceeding series, no 13, Fourteenth ISCERG Symposium, Louisville, KY, May 10-14, 1976, The Hague, Dr W Junk, 1977, pp 227-234.

231. Masland RH, Livingstone CJ: Effect of stimulation with light on synthesis and release of acetylcholine by an isolated mammalian retina, J Neurophysiol 39:1210, 1976.

232. Matthews HR, et al: Photoreceptor light adaptation is mediated by cytoplasmic calcium concentration, Nature 334:67, 1988.

233. McClatchey AI, et al: Splicing defect at the ornithine aminotransferase (OAT) locus in gyrate atrophy, Am J Hum Genet 47:790, 1990.

234. McCulloch JC, et al: Hyperornithinemia and gyrate atrophy of the choroid and retina, Ophthalmol 85:918, 1978.

235. McIlwain JT: Some evidence concerning the physiological basis of the periphery effect in the cat's retina, Exp Brain Res 1:267, 1966.

236. Mehaffey L III, Berson EL: Cone mechanisms in the electroretinogram of the cynomolgus monkey, Invest Ophthalmol 13:266, 1974.

237. Miller RF, Dowling JE: Intracellular responses of the Müller (glial) cells of the mudpuppy retina: their relation to b-wave of the electroretinogram, J Neurophysiol 33:323, 1970.

238. Miller WH, Nicol GD: Evidence that cyclic GMP regulates membrane potential in rod photoreceptors, Nature 280:64, 1979.

239. Miller RF, Slaughter MM: Excitatory amino acid receptors of the retina: diversity of subtypes and conductance mechanisms, Trends in Neurosci, Amsterdam, Elsevier, 9:211, 1986.

240. Mitchell G, et al: An initiator codon mutation in ornithine delta aminotransferase causing gyrate atrophy of choroid and retina, J Clin Invest 81:630, 1988.

241. Mitchell GA, et al: At least two mutant alleles of ornithine and aminotransferase cause gyrate atrophy of the choroid and retina in Finns, Proc Natl Acad Sci USA 86:197, 1989.

242. Miyake Y, et al: Congenital stationary night blindness with negative electroretinogram: a new classification, Arch Ophthalmol 104:1013, 1986.

243. Motokawa K, Mita T: Uber eine einfachere Untersuchungs Methode und Eigenschaften der Aktionsstrome der Netzhaut des Menschen, Tohoku J Exp Med 42:114, 1942.

244. Mullen RJ, LaVail MM: Inherited retinal dystrophy: primary defect in pigment epithelium determined with experimental rat chimeras, Science 192:799, 1976.

245. Murakami M, Kaneko A: Subcomponents of PIII in cold-blooded vertebrate retinae, Nature 210:103, 1966.

246. Naarendorp F, Sieving PA: The scotopic threshold response of the cat ERG is suppressed selectively by GABA and glycine, Vis Sci 1991. (In press.)

247. Nagata M: Photopic flicker ERG in cases of congenital night blindness and total color blindness, in Henkes HE, van der Tweel LH, eds: Flicker, Proceedings of the symposium on physiology of flicker and flicker electroretinography, Amsterdam, Sept, 1963, The Hague, Dr W Junk, 1964, pp 352-366.

248. Naka K, Rushton WAH: S-potentials from luminosity units in the retina of fish (Cyprinidae), J Physiol (Lond) 185:587, 1966.

249. Naka K, Rushton WAH: The generation and spread of S-potentials in fish (Cyprinidae), J Physiol (Lond) 192:437, 1967.

250. Nakatani K, Yau K-W: Calcium and light adaptation in retinal rods and cones, Nature 334:69, 1988.

251. Narfstrom K: Progressive retinal atrophy in the Abyssinian cat, Invest Ophthalmol Vis Sci 26:193, 1985.

252. Nathans J, et al: Molecular genetics of human blue cone monochromacy, Science 245:831, 1989.

253. Neal MJ: Acetylcholine as a retina transmitter substance, in Bonting SL, ed: Transmitters in the visual process, Elmsford, NY, Pergamon Press, 1976, pp 127-143.

254. Nelson R, et al: Neural responses in the rod and cone systems of the cat retina: intracellular records and Procion stains, Invest Ophthalmol Vis Sci 15:946, 1976.

255. Newman EA: B-wave currents in the frog retina, Vision Res 19:227, 1979.

256. Newman EA: Current source density analysis of the b-wave of the frog retina, Am J Neurophysiol 43:1335, 1980.

257. Noble KG, Carr RE: Stargardt's disease and fundus flavimaculatus, Arch Ophthalmol 97:1281, 1979.

258. Noell WK: The origin of the electroretinogram, Am J Ophthalmol 38:78, 1954.

259. Noell WK, Delmelle MC, Albrecht R: Vitamin A deficiency effect on the retina: dependency on light, Science 172:72, 1971.

260. Norden LC, Leach ME: Calibration of the ERG stimulus, in Lawwill T, ed: Documenta Ophthalmologica Proceeding series, no 13. Fourteenth ISCERG Sympo-

sium, Louisville, KY, May 10-14, 1976, The Hague, Dr W Junk, 1977, pp 393-403.

261. Oakley B II: Potassium and the photoreceptor-dependent pigment epithelial hyperpolarization, J Gen Physiol 70:405, 1977.

262. Oakley B II, Green DG: Correlation of light-induced changes in retinal extracellular potassium concentration with c-wave of the electroretinogram, J Neurophys 39:1117, 1976.

263. O'Donnell JJ, Sandman RP, Martin SR: Gyrate atrophy of the retina: inborn error of L-ornithine; 2-ornithine; 2-oxoacid aminotransferase, Science 200:200, 1978.

264. Ogden T: The oscillatory waves of the primate electroretinogram, Vision Res 13:1059, 1973.

265. Ogden T, Wylie R: Avian retina, I, Microelectrode depth and marking studies of local ERG, J Neurophysiol 34:357, 1971.

266. Okun E, et al: Chloroquine retinopathy, a report of eight cases with ERG and dark-adaptation findings, Arch Ophthalmol 69:59, 1963.

267. Østerberg G: Topography of the layer of rods and cones in the human retina, Acta Ophthalmol 6(Suppl):1, 1935.

268. Padmos P, van Norren D: Cone spectral sensitivity and chromatic adaptation as revealed by human flicker electroretinography, Vision Res 11:27, 1971.

269. Pak WL: Some properties of the early electrical response in the vertebrate retina, Cold Spring Harbor Symp Quant Biol 30:493, 1965.

270. Pak WL, Rozzi VP, Ebrey TG: Effect of changes in the chemical environment of the retina on the two components of the early receptor potential, Nature 214:109, 1967.

271. Pallin O: The influence of the axial length of the eye on the size of the recorded b-potential in the clinical single-flash electroretinogram, Acta Ophthalmol (Suppl) Vol 101, 1969.

272. Perry NW, Childers DG: The human visual evoked response, Springfield, IL, Charles C Thomas, Publisher, 1969.

273. Potts AM, Nagaya T: Studies on the visual evoked response, II, The effect of special cortical activity, Invest Ophthalmol 6:657, 1967.

274. Rabin AR, Berson EL: A full-field system for clinical electroretinography, Arch Ophthalmol 92:59, 1974.

275. Rabin AR, Hayes KC, Berson EL: Cone and rod responses in nutritionally induced retinal degeneration in the cat, Invest Ophthalmol 12:694, 1973.

276. Ramesh V, et al: Molecular basis of ornithine aminotransferase deficiency in B-6-responsive and -nonresponsive forms of gyrate atrophy, Proc Natl Acad Sci USA 85:3777, 1988.

277. Refsum S: Heredopathia atactica polyneuritiformis: phytanic acid storage disease (Refsum's disease) with particular reference to therapeutic and pathogenetic aspects, in Tower DB, ed: The nervous system, vol 2, New York, Raven Press, 1975, pp 229-234.

278. Refsum S: Heredopathia atactica polyneuritiformis phytanic-acid storage disease, Refsum's disease: a biochemically well-defined disease with a specific dietary treatment, Arch Neurol 38:605, 1981.

279. Reichel E, et al: An electroretinographic and molecular genetic study of X-linked cone degeneration, Am J Ophthalmol 108:540, 1989.

280. Rietveld WJ, Tordoir WEH, Duyff JW: Contribution of the fovea and parafovea to the visual evoked response, Acta Physiol Pharmacol Neerl 13:300, 1965.

281. Riggs LA: Continuous and reproducible records of the electrical activity of the human retina, Proc Soc Exp Biol Med 48:204, 1941.

282. Riggs LA, Johnson EP, Schick AML: Electrical responses of the human eye to moving stimulus patterns, Science 144:567, 1964.

283. Riggs LA, Wooten BR: Electrical measures and psychophysical data on human vision, in Jameson D, Hurvich LM, eds: Handbook of sensory physiology, vol 7/4, New York, Springer-Verlag, 1972, pp 690-731.

284. Ripps H: Night blindness and the retinal mechanisms of visual adaptation, Ann R Coll Surg Engl 58:2, 1976.

285. Ripps H: Night blindness revisited: from man to molecules, Invest Ophthalmol Vis Sci 23:588, 1982.

286. Rubin LF: Hemeralopia in dogs, Trans Am Acad Ophthalmol Otolaryngol 81:667, 1976.

287. Sandberg MA, Berson EL, Ariel M: Visually evoked response testing with a stimulator-ophthalmoscope: macular scars, hereditary macular degeneration, and retinitis pigmentosa, Arch Ophthalmol 95:1805, 1977.

288. Sandberg MA, Berson EL, Effron MH: A defect in light adaptation in retinitis pigmentosa, Invest Ophthalmol Vis Sci 19(Suppl):259, 1980.

289. Sandberg MA, Berson EL, Effron MH: Rod-cone interaction in the distal human retina, Science 212:829-831, 1981.

290. Sandberg MA, Effron MH, Berson EL: Focal cone electroretinograms in dominant retinitis pigmentosa with reduced penetrance, Invest Ophthalmol Vis Sci 17:1096, 1978.

291. Sandberg MA, Hansen AH, Berson EL: Focal and parafoveal cone electroretinograms in juvenile macular degeneration, Ophthal Ped & Gen 3:83, 1983.

292. Sandberg MA, Jacobson SG, Berson EL: Focal cone electroretinograms in retinitis pigmentosa and juvenile macular degenerations, Am J Ophthalmol 88:702, 1979.

293. Sanyal S, Chader G, Aguirre G: Expression of retinal degeneration slow (rds) gene in the retina of the mouse, in La Vail M, Hollyfield JG, Anderson RE, eds: Retinal degeneration: experimental and clinical studies, New York, Alan R Liss, 1985, pp 235-256.

294. Schiller PH: The connections of the retinal on and off pathways to the lateral geniculate nucleus of the monkey, Vision Res 24:923, 1984.

295. Schmidt SY: Retinal degenerations, in Lajtha A: Handbook of neurochemistry, vol 10, New York, Plenum, 1985, pp 461-507.

296. Schmidt SY, Berson EL, Hayes KC: Retinal degeneration in cats fed casein, I, Taurine deficiency, Invest Ophthalmol 15:47, 1976.

297. Schmidt SY, et al: Retinal degeneration in cats fed casein, III, Taurine deficiency and ERG amplitudes, Invest Ophthalmol Vis Sci 16:673, 1977.

298. Schubert G, Bornschein H: Beitrag zur Analyse des Menschlichen Elektroretinogramms, Ophthalmologica 123:396, 1952.

299. Shih VE, Berson EL, Gargiulo M: Reduction of hyperornithinemia with a low protein, low arginine diet and pyridoxine in patients with a deficiency of ornithine-ketoacid transaminase (OKT) activity and gyrate atrophy of the choroid and retina, Clin Chim Acta 113:243, 1981.

300. Shih VE, et al: Ornithine ketoacid transaminase deficiency in gyrate atrophy of the choroid and retina, Am J Hum Genet 30:174, 1978.

301. Shipley T: The visually evoked occipitogram in strabismic amblyopia under direct-view ophthalmoscopy, J Pediatr Ophthalmol 6:97, 1969.

302. Sieving PA: Retinal ganglion cell loss does not abolish the scotopic threshold response (STR) of the cat and human ERG, Clin Vis Sci 6:149, 1991.

303. Sieving PA, Frishman LJ, Steinberg RH: Scotopic threshold response of proximal retina in cat, J Neurophysiol 56:1049, 1986.

304. Murayama K, Kuo C-Y, Sieving PA: Abnormal threshold ERG response in X-linked juvenile retinoschisis: evidence for a proximal retinal origin of the human STR, Clin Vis Sci 6:317, 1991.

305. Sieving PA, Niffenegger JH, Berson EL: Electroretinographic findings in selected pedigrees with choroideremia, Am J Ophthalmol 101:361, 1986.

306. Sieving PA, Nino C: Scotopic threshold response (STR) of the human electroretinogram, Invest Ophthalmol Vis Sci 29:1608, 1988.

307. Sieving PA, Steinberg RH: Proximal retinal contribution to the intraretinal 8 Hz pattern ERG of cats, J Neurophysiol 57:104, 1987.

308. Sieving PA, Wakabayashi K: Comparison of rod threshold ERG from monkey, cat and human, Clin Vis Sci 6:171, 1991.

309. Simell O, Takki K: Raised plasma ornithine and gyrate atrophy of the choroid and retina, Lancet 1:1031, 1973.

310. Simonsen S: ERG in diabetics, Sixth ISCERG Symposium, Ghent, Belgium, 1966, Basel, Switzerland, S Karger, 1968, p 403.

311. Simonsen S: Prognostic value of ERG (oscillatory potential) in selecting juvenile diabetics at risk of developing proliferative retinopathy, Metab Ped Ophthalmol 5:55, 1981.

312. Slaughter MM, Miller RF: 2-amino-4-phosphonobutyric acid: a new pharmacological tool for retina research, Science 211:182, 1981.

313. Slaughter MM, Miller RF: Bipolar cells in the mudpuppy retina use an excitatory amino acid neurotransmitter, Nature 303:537, 1983.

314. Smith RG, Freed MA, Sterling P: Microcircuitry of the dark-adapted cat retina: functional architecture of the rod-cone network, J Neurosci 6:3505, 1986.

315. Sokol S: The visually evoked cortical potential in optic nerve and visual pathway disorders, in Fishman GA, Sokol S, eds: Electrophysiologic testing in disorders of the retina, optic nerve, and visual pathway, San Francisco, American Academy of Ophthalmology, 1990, pp 105-141.

316. Spekreijse H, Estevez O, van der Tweel LH: Luminance responses to pattern reversal, in Pearlman JT, ed: Documenta Ophthalmologica Proceedings Series, no 2, Tenth ISCERG Symposium, Los Angeles, August 20-23, 1972, The Hague, Dr W Junk, 1973, pp 205-211.

317. Speros P, Price J: Oscillatory potentials: history, techniques, and potential use in the evaluation of disturbances of retinal circulation, Survey of Ophthalmol 25:237, 1981.

318. Steinberg D, et al: Studies on the metabolic error in Refsum's disease, J Clin Invest 46:313, 1967.

319. Steinberg D, et al: Phytanic acid in patients with Refsum's syndrome and responses to dietary treatment, Arch Intern Med 125:75, 1970.

320. Steinberg RH: Rod and cone contributions to S-potentials from the cat retina, Vision Res 9:1319, 1969.

321. Steinberg RH: Rod-cone interaction in S-potentials from the cat retina, Vision Res 9:1331, 1969.

322. Steinberg RH, Griff ER, Linsenmeier RA: The cellular origin of the light peak, in Kolder HEJW, ed: Documenta Ophthalmologica Proceedings Series 37, Slow potentials, and microprocessor applications, Proceedings of the twentieth ISCEV Symposium, The Hague, Dr W Junk, 1983, pp 1-11.

323. Steinberg RH, Linsenmeier RA, Griff ER: Three light-evoked responses of the retinal pigment epithelium, Vision Res 23:1315, 1983.

324. Steinberg, RH, Schmidt R, Brown KT: Intracellular responses to light from cat pigment epithelium: origin of the electroretinogram c-wave, Nature 227:728, 1970.

325. Stiles WS: Colour vision: the approach through the increment threshold sensitivity, Proc Natl Acad Sci USA 45:100, 1959.

326. Stone J, Fukuda Y: Properties of cat retinal ganglion cells: a comparison of W-cells with X- and Y-cells, J Neurophysiol 37:722, 1974.

327. Stone J, Hoffman K-P: Very slow-conducting ganglion cells in the cat's retina: a major, new functional type? Brain Res 43:610, 1972.

328. Stretton AOW, Kravitz EA: Neuronal geometry: determination with a technique of intracellular dye injection, Science 162:132, 1968.

329. Stryer L: Cyclic GMP cascade of vision, Ann Rev Neurosci 9:87, 1986.

330. Svaetichin G: The cone action potential, Acta Physiol Scand 29(Suppl 106):565, 1953.

331. Szamier RB, Ripps H, Chappell RL: On the glial-cell origin of the ERG b-wave, Invest Ophthalmol Vis Sci 19(Suppl):39, 1980.

332. Szamier RB, et al: Sex-linked retinitis pigmentosa: ultrastructure of the photoreceptors and pigment epithelium, Invest Ophthalmol Vis Sci 18:145, 1979.

333. Takki K, Simell O: Gyrate atrophy of the choroid and retina with hyperornithinemia (HOGA), Birth Defects XII:373, 1976.

334. Tamai A: Studies on the early receptor potential in the human eye, III, ERP in primary retinitis pigmentosa, Yonago Acta Med 18:18, 1974.

335. Tomita T: Studies on the intraretinal action potential, I, Relation between the localization of micropipette in the retina and the shape of the intraretinal action potential, Jpn J Physiol 1:110, 1950.

336. Tomita T: Electrophysiological study of the mechanisms subserving color coding in the fish retina, Cold Spring Harbor Symp Quant Biol 30:559, 1965.

337. Toyoda J, Nosaki H, Tomita T: Light-induced resist-

ance changes in single photoreceptors of *Necturus* and *Gekko,* Vision Res 9:453, 1969.

338. Travis GH, et al: Identification of a photoreceptor-specific mRNA encoded by the gene responsible for retinal degeneration slow *(rds),* Nature 338:70, 1989.

339. Trijbels JMF, et al: L-ornithine-ketoacid-transaminase deficiency in cultured fibroblasts of a patient with hyperornithinemia and gyrate atrophy of the choroid and retina, Clin Chim Acta 79:371, 1977.

340. Vainisi SJ, Beck BB, Apple DJ: Retinal degeneration in a baboon, Am J Ophthalmol 78:279, 1974.

341. Valle D, Kaiser-Kupfer MI, Del Valle LA: Gyrate atrophy of the choroid and retina: deficiency of ornithine aminotransferase in transformed lymphocytes, Proc Natl Acad Sci USA 74:5159, 1977.

342. Valle D, et al: Gyrate atrophy: amino acids and correction of hyperornithinemia with low arginine containing diet, J Clin Invest 65:371, 1980.

343. Van Nie R, Ivanyi D, Demant P: A new H-2-linked mutation, rds, causing retinal degeneration in the mouse, Tissue Antigens 12:106, 1978.

344. Van Norren D, Padmos P: Spectral sensitivity of macaque cones determined with an ERG method, report no IZF 1971-10, Amsterdam, Institute for Perception RVO-TNO, 1971.

345. Vaughn HG: The perceptual and physiologic significance of visual evoked responses recorded from the scalp in man, in Burian HM, Jacobson JH, eds: Clinical electroretinography, Proceedings of the Third International Symposium, Highland Park, IL, 1964, New York, Pergamon Press, 1966, pp 203-223.

346. Voaden MJ: Gamma-aminobutyric acid and glycine as retinal neurotransmitters, in Bonting SL, Transmitters in the visual process, Elmsford, NY, Pergamon Press, 1976, pp 107-125.

347. Vogel DA, Green DG: Potassium release and b-wave generation: a test of the Müller cell hypothesis, Invest Ophthalmol Vis Sci 19(Suppl):39, 1980.

348. von Helmholtz H: Handbuch der physiologischen Optik, 2nd ed, Leipzig, Voss, 1896.

349. Wachtmeister L: Luminosity functions of the oscillatory potentials of the human electroretinogram, Acta Ophthalmol 52:353, 1971.

350. Wachtmeister L: Stimulus duration and the oscillatory potentials of the human electroretinogram, Acta Ophthalmol 52:729, 1971.

351. Wachtmeister L: On the oscillatory potentials of the human electroretinogram in light and dark adaptation, Acta Ophthalmol 116(Suppl):1, 1972.

352. Wachtmeister L, Dowling JE: The oscillatory potentials of the mudpuppy retina, Invest Ophthalmol 17:1176, 1978.

353. Wakabayashi K, Gieser J, Sieving PA: Aspartate separation of the scotopic threshold response (STR) from the photoreceptor a-wave of the cat and monkey ERG, Invest Ophthalmol Vis Sci 29:1615, 1988.

354. Wald G: The receptors of human color vision, Science 145:1007, 1964.

355. Watanabe K, Tosaka T: Functional organization of the Cyprinid fish retina as revealed by discriminative responses to spectral illumination, Jpn J Physiol 9:84, 1959.

356. Weleber RG, Kennaway NG, Buist NRR: Vitamin B$_6$ in management of gyrate atrophy of choroid and retina, Lancet 2(8101):1213, 1978.

357. Werblin FS, Dowling JE: Organization of the retina of the mudpuppy, *Necturus maculosus,* II, Intra-cellular recording, J Neurophysiol 32:339, 1969.

358. Wetzel MG, et al: Fatty acid metabolism in normal miniature poodles and those affected with progressive rod-cone degeneration (prcd), in La Vail MM, Anderson RE, Hollyfield JG, eds: Inherited and environmentally induced retinal degenerations, New York, Alan R Liss, 1989, pp 427-439.

359. Witkovsky P, Dudek FE, Ripps H: Slow PIII component of the carp electroretinogram, J Gen Physiol 65:119, 1975.

360. Wyszechi G, Stiles WS: Color science, New York, John Wiley, 1967, p 206.

361. Yau K-W, Baylor DA: Cyclic GMP-activated conductance of retinal photoreceptor cells, Ann Rev Neurosci 12:289, 1989.

362. Yau K-W, Nakatani K: Sodium-dependent calcium efflux at the outer segment of the retinal cone, Biophys J, 53:473a, 1988.

363. Yonemura D, Aoki T, Tsuzuki K: Electroretinogram in diabetic retinopathy, Arch Ophthalmol 68:49, 1962.

364. Yonemura D, Hatta M: Studies of the minor components of the frog's electroretinogram, Jpn J Physiol 16:11, 1966.

365. Yonemura D, Kawasaki K: The early receptor potential in the human electroretinogram, Jpn J Physiol 17:235, 1967.

366. Yonemura D, Kawasaki K: New approaches to ophthalmic electrodiagnosis by retinal oscillatory potentials, drug-induced responses from retinal pigment epithelium, and cone potential, Doc Ophthalmol 48:163, 1974.

367. Yoshikami S, Hagins WA: Light, calcium and the photocurrent of rods and cones, Biophys Soc Ann Meeting Abstr 11:47a, 1971.

368. Zetterstrom B: Clinical electroretinogram in children during first year of life, Acta Ophthalmol 29:295, 1951.

369. Zimmerman AL, Baylor DA: Cyclic GMP-sensitive conductance of retinal rods consists of aqueous pores, Nature 321:70, 1986.

CHAPTER
22

Color Vision

WILLIAM M. HART, Jr., M.D., Ph.D.

Color is purely a sensory phenomenon and not a physical attribute. Human awareness of color arises out of subjective visual experiences in which given sensations are ascribed names. Agreement between individuals in color naming derives from a tacit acceptance that given sensations can be reliably described with color names. Indeed, the color names that individuals use for describing objects have a remarkable constancy, and even linguistic studies of highly diverse cultures show that, left to their own devices, people will codify their color sensations with fairly predictable language patterns. While this is true for a majority (approximately 85%) of the population, there is a great deal of heterogeneity of color perception among normal individuals. This is particularly true for distinguishing between red and green hues in the middle and long wavelength portions of the light spectrum. Affected individuals are described as being color deficient, and these variations in color vision have now been traced to a genetic polymorphism in the DNA sequences encoding for the pigmented apoproteins of cone photopigments.

The perception of color varies complexly as a function of multiple parameters, including the spectral composition of light coming from the object, the spectral composition of light emanating from surrounding objects, and the state of light adaptation in the subject just prior to viewing any given object. A remarkable and as yet incompletely understood phenomenon that is characteristic of color vision is that of color constancy. Color constancy refers to the phenomenon in which the apparent color of an object does not seem to vary appreciably when the wavelengths and intensity of light illuminating the object are altered. Thus an orange may appear to be orange in color when viewed in full sunlight on an open field on a cloudless day, and will likewise appear to be orange when viewed in the darkened confines of a home at night where the only illumination may be from an incandescent bulb that illuminates the object with a much different spectral composition than that found in sunlight. Color constancy appears to be related to a phenomenon in which: (1) colors acquire their appearance primarily by relative comparisons to other objects in their immediate vicinity and (2) these comparisons change only minimally with broad changes in spectral mixtures of light falling on scenes.

Since color is a perceptual phenomenon and not a physical property, it can more readily be studied by behavioral methods such as those used by psychologists and psychophysicists. Physiologists, however, have been attempting to unravel the cell biology of color perception using the techniques of neurophysiology and molecular biology.

COLOR AND THE VISIBLE SPECTRUM

Color sensations do not correspond directly to the visible spectrum, but are nonetheless fundamentally affected by the wavelength or spec-

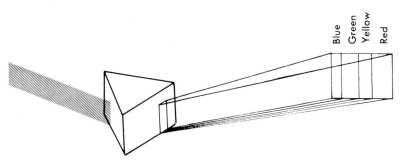

FIG. 22-1 Sunlight is bent from its straight path by prism. Short wavelength light is bent through greater angle than is long wavelength light.

tral composition of light. Isolated visible wavelengths, called monochromatic lights, are commonly named by the color sensations they evoke when seen in isolation. The rainbow of hues visible in the solar spectrum was first reported by Sir Issac Newton, who correctly supposed that individual components of the spectral mixture were in some way related to differential stimulation of photoreceptor units in the eye, providing the basis for the physical stimulus evoking color sensation.

If a prism is placed in the path of a narrow beam of sunlight, the path of the light beam will be refracted or bent toward the base of the prism (Fig. 22-1). The extent to which each wavelength component of the sunlight mixture is refracted depends upon the type of glass and the angle between the surfaces of the prism. The angle of refraction is also dependent upon wavelength, with the extent of refraction being roughly inversely proportional to the wavelength of light. In this manner short wavelengths are bent to a greater extent than are long wavelengths.

Snell's law describes the relationship between the refractive index of the prism and the angle of incidence of light on its surface:

$$n_m = \frac{\text{sine } i}{\text{sine } r}$$

where n_m is the refractive index, i is the angle between the incident beam of light and the normal or perpendicular to the glass surface, and r is the angle between the refracted ray and the normal.

As mentioned above, the extent of refraction by an optical surface varies with the wavelength of light, from which it follows that the index of refraction for an optical medium differs according to wavelength. Thus the index of refraction for each wavelength must be individually specified, such as by the symbol $n_{m\lambda}$. This variable

extent of refraction spreads a polychromatic white beam of light into its component wavelengths, a phenomenon referred to as spectral dispersion. The array of individual wavelengths thus exposed is referred to as the visible spectrum. The sensations that these individual wavelengths evoke are called the spectral colors.

The readily recognizable spectral colors include violet light at a wavelength of 430 nm, blue light of 460 nm, green light of 520 nm, yellow light of approximately 575 nm, orange light of 600 nm, and red light of 650 nm. Wavelengths falling between these values produce color sensations that are often given compound names, such as blue-green or yellow-green. Remember, though, that such stimuli remain monochromatic, and the sensations they evoke depend on much more than just wavelength and intensity. As implied above in the mention of color constancy, the color a given stimulus evokes depends critically on the context within which it is seen, a phenomenon called simultaneous color contrast. As will be outlined below, color is neurally encoded in the afferent visual system by cells whose receptive fields are tuned to the detection of simultaneous color contrasts.

Wavelength discrimination

Figure 22-2 shows a threshold curve for wavelength discrimination by the human eye. For each wavelength on the abscissa, the ordinate shows the threshold of wavelength change in nanometers that is required for a just noticeable difference. At wavelengths of approximately 500 nm, a normal observer is capable of detecting wavelength shifts as small as 1 nm. Toward the ends of the wavelength discrimination function, much larger shifts are required to be detectable, rising above 6 nm at the short wavelength end of the visible spectrum.

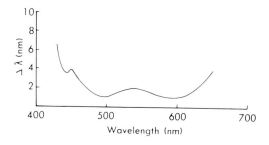

FIG. 22-2 Discrimination of wavelength by human eye. Change in wavelength, which can be just detected, $\Delta\lambda$, is plotted as a function of wavelength. (From Wright WD, Pitt FHG: Proc Physiol Soc 46:459, 1934.)

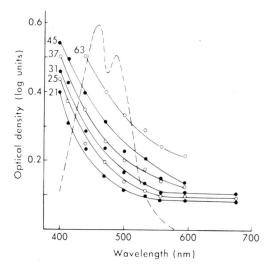

FIG. 22-3 Optical density of living human crystalline lenses plotted as function of wavelength (*solid lines*). Numbers refer to ages of observers. Broken line gives optical density of macular pigment as function of wavelength. (Modified from Said FS, Weale RA: Gerontologia [Basel] 3:213, 1959, and Ruddock KH: Vision Res 3:417, 1963.)

Spectral filtering by the ocular media

Optical transmission by the ocular media varies by tissue as well as by age. There is, for instance, a progressive yellowing of the lens with age (see Chapter 9), which can cause a detectable spectral shift in the sensitivity of the eye, manifest as a reduction in the relative sensitivity for blue light. Due to the phenomenon of color constancy, however, this shift is not noticeable to the casual observer.

Figure 22-3 shows the optical density of the human crystalline lens as a function of wavelength (solid lines). Superimposed on these curves is a line expressing optical density of the macular pigment as a function of wavelength. The lens of the eye preferentially absorbs shorter wavelengths, hence the perceptible yellowish cast to the adult crystalline lens. In the very young, short wavelength absorption is significant mostly for wavelengths of less than 450 nm, producing little or no visible spectral color shift. For people in the sixth or seventh decade of life, the optical absorption for wavelengths up to 550 nanometers becomes significant, producing a distinctly yellowish appearance. There is a great deal of interindividual variation in the extent of this phenomenon, so that in some elderly people the lens may appear pale yellow, while in others it may acquire a darker yellow or even brownish cast.

The trichromatic theory of human color vision

During the nineteenth century, two major theories to explain the properties of human color vision were developed by investigators studying the physical properties of light and the psychophysical properties of human color perception. These two principal theories are now referred to as the theory of trichromacy (or the Young-Helmholtz-Maxwell theory) and the opponent process theory. The development of these theories during the nineteenth century has been beautifully reviewed by Sherman,[44] who notes that contributions to the trichromatic hypothesis were dominated during the latter half of the nineteenth century by James Clerk Maxwell, the physicist. During the twentieth century, a heated debate concerning the correctness of these two hypotheses occurred, accompanied by the tacit supposition that they were mutually exclusive descriptions of the nature of color perception. However, over the past several decades, it has become apparent that human and nonhuman primate color vision is indeed mediated by an essentially trichromatic process at the receptor level, but is encoded for neural transmission in a physiologic paradigm of the color opponent process.

The earliest recorded outline of the trichromacy hypothesis is attributed to Thomas Young, who presented his ideas in the Bakerian lecture before the Royal Society in 1801, which was later published in the proceedings of that body in 1802.[55] In Young's words:

Now, as it is almost impossible to conceive each sensitive point of the retina to contain an infinite number of particles, each capable of vibrating in perfect unison with every possible undulation, it becomes necessary to suppose the number limited, for instance, to the three principal colors, red, yellow and blue.

Subsequent work by Helmholtz and Maxwell confirmed that the psychophysical responses of normal human observers could be best described by a theoretical system in which three primaries were necessary to account for the visual system's color categorization of visual stimuli. It was this seemingly irreducible need for at least three primaries in color observer behavior that was taken as evidence for a trichromatic process. It was not until the middle of the twentieth century that development of reflection densitometers and microspectrophotometers, followed by the use of microelectrophysiologic studies of individual photoreceptors, allowed the identification of three mutually exclusive classes of cones in the primate retina having differing, but overlapping, spectral sensitivities (Fig. 22-4).

One class of photoreceptors has a spectral sensitivity that peaks at approximately 440 to 450 nm. These receptors, which are most sensitive to the short wavelength end of the spectrum, are sometimes referred to as short wavelength sensitive (SWS) receptors, or blue cones.

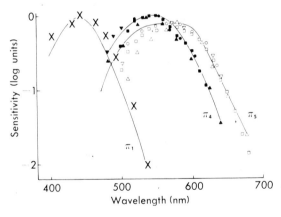

FIG. 22-4 Measurements of cone pigments and processes. Open symbols for red cones, closed symbols for green cones, crosses for blue cones. Measurements for red cones displaced downward 0.1 log unit for clarity. Curves from increment threshold measurements from Stiles.[46] ● and O, Selective bleaching measurements by reflection densitometry, from Rushton[42] and Baker and Rushton.[4] ▼ and ▽, Selective bleaching measurements by transmission through isolated retina, from Brown and Wald.[8] ■ and □, Increment threshold measurements against bright backgrounds (artificial monochromacy), from Brindley.[6] ▲, △, and X, increment thresholds against bright backgrounds, from Wald.[50]

A second class of middle wavelength sensitive (MWS) receptors has a spectral sensitivity that peaks at between 535 and 550 nm, sometimes referred to as green cones. The third class has a spectral sensitivity peaking at between 570 and 590 nm. These are referred to as long wavelength sensitive (LWS) photoreceptors or red cones.

The overlapping of the spectral sensitivities of these three clases of cones means that no individual class of cones can be stimulated in isolation by any one wavelength. There is one notable exception to this rule. Note from the curves in Figure 22-4 that although the spectral curves overlap broadly toward the short wavelength end of the spectrum, they diverge somewhat at longer wavelengths. At the extreme long wavelength end of the spectrum, the sensitivities for short and middle wavelength sensitive cones fall more rapidly than for long wavelength sensitive cones, so that for a narrow zone of optical frequencies in the vicinity of 650 nm long wavelength sensitive cones can be stimulated in near isolation.

The first direct confirmatory evidence for the presence of three classes of cones was derived from microspectrophotometry of individual photoreceptors teased from vertebrate retinal preparations. By aligning a single photoreceptor under a narrow beam of light, its spectral absorption could be determined before and after bleaching its visual pigment, yielding a so-called difference spectrum. While this difference spectrum does not accurately represent the spectral sensitivity of the receptor, it does give some idea of the wavelength of peak sensitivity. This type of measurement confirmed the presence of three peak sensitivities occurring at 414 to 424 nm, 522 to 539 nm, and 549 to 570 nm.[9,12,35]

In studies of cone outer segments taken from the central macular region of primate retinal preparations, only red and green cone photoreceptors are found. A clinical analog of this technique has been developed, called reflection densitometry.[4,42,51] Bleaching methods for studying isolated whole mount retinal preparations have also been used to determine difference spectra by measuring the extent to which monochromatic light can bleach photoreceptor pigments.[4,42] The various bleaching techniques, including reflection densitometry, have yielded data that agree fairly well with those for microspectrophotometry (Fig. 22-4).

Stiles[46] popularized and developed the psychophysical techniques that seem to best demonstrate the presence of individual cone "mechanisms." These increment threshold techniques are designed to select a monochromatic background that most effectively adapts two of the three cone types such that the third type of cone can be stimulated in relative isolation, allowing relatively independent determination of the threshold for one cone mechanism. The use of the term "relative" is important here, since it is impossible for any one wavelength to bleach any two cone photoreceptor types in complete isolation.

However, the use of increment threshold techniques has produced results that agree reasonably well with the spectral absorption data obtained from selective bleaching of isolated cones (Fig. 22-4). This is particularly true at photopic levels of adaptation. At somewhat lower levels of adaptation, three basic mechanisms have been defined by the Stiles technique, and which have been designated as the π_1, π_4, and π_5 mechanisms.

The π_1 mechanism most closely matches the microspectrophotometric values obtained from short wavelength sensitive cones. The π_4 mechanism most closely matches the values obtained from middle wavelength sensitive cones; however, the π_5 mechanism has a somewhat less exact match to the spectrophotometric data obtained from long wavelength sensitive cones. It has been proposed that the π_5 mechanism is the result of a neural integration of cone input involving contributions by both long and middle wavelength sensitive cones.

The opponent color theory

The other principal nineteenth century theory of color vision was the opponent color theory first put forth by Ewald Hering.[25] This theory was based largely on empirical observations of color appearances. The trichromatic theory, by itself, was not adequate to explain how mixtures of lights of different colors could produce lights of yet another color or even to appear colorless. Certain select pairs of colors such as red versus green or yellow versus blue were found to be mutually exclusive. (Mixing lights of such colors did not yield composite sensations). For instance, red light and green light mixed together produced an appearance of yellow, while mixing blue light with yellow light produced an appearance of white. Thus some colors seem to be mutually exclusive or opponents of one another. Nowhere in human language can one find colors described as being reddish-green, for instance, or bluish-yellow. Hering proposed that color vision was mediated by "opponent color" processes that would account for this

dual exclusivity of certain color pairs. Following Hering's statement of these ideas, the opponent color theory remained largely dormant until it was revived by the work of Hurvich and Jameson.[32] As noted previously in this chapter, a physiologic substrate for color opponent encoding has been found in the neurophysiologic properties of cellular elements in the afferent visual system. Excellent historical reviews of this subject are available.[5,41,54]

COLOR MIXING, METAMERIC MATCHES, AND COMPLEMENTARY WAVELENGTHS

One of the earliest pieces of evidence in favor of the trichromatic theory of color vision was that developed by Helmholtz and then Maxwell. Helmholtz[23] found that any colored light one wished to use as a reference could be matched by a suitable mixture of three strategically chosen lights mixed together. While Helmholtz established the qualitative nature of this relationship, it was later put on a quantitative basis by Maxwell (see below). It was the need for a minimum of three lights to match any color that was the earliest experimental evidence in support of Young's original theory.

Mixtures of light that produce identical-appearing colors are called metameric matches. Mixtures that are physically identical to one another (have identical spectral compositions) are said to be isomeric matches. A normal human observer can find combinations of three suitably chosen spectral lights that will exactly match the appearance of any other colored light. In other words, normal observers can alway produce metameric matches, but only if at least three spectral lights are given. In fact, depending on the three spectral lights being mixed, a large number of such matches can be found for any one test light shown to a color normal individual. While such metameric matches can be physically very different from one another (in terms of their spectral distributions), they nonetheless appear to be identical in color and brightness. This appearance of sameness is linked to the relative extent to which each of the three retinal cone classes are excited. Light mixtures that cause the same proportional stimulation of the three receptors will result in the same sensations. In those special cases of metameric matches of light seen as "white," it is often possible to achieve a match by the proper mixing of only two appropriately chosen spectral lights. Such pairs of monochromatic light sources are said to have complementary wavelengths.

Color triangles and the CIE chromaticity diagram

The results of metameric matching experiments are usually plotted in a graphic form, using a center of gravity rule to produce a so-called color triangle. This was the technique originally used by Maxwell in his color mixing experiments. The use of a triangular diagram was determined by the need to plot three separate coordinates in space. An example of the triangular plotting technique will be given here. If we suppose the use of three different monochromatic lights for reference wavelengths, we might designate them as "B", 459 nm and appearing blue; "G", 529 nm and appearing green; and "R", 650 nm and appearing red. A mixture of these three reference standards found to provide a match with a light that appears white could be expressed as follows:

W = bB + gG + rR

where W represents the white light being matched by the mixture of the three reference wavelengths, and b, g, and r are the coefficients representing the relative energies of the three reference lights (B, G, and R) being mixed. If we draw a triangle with its apexes arbitrarily defining the loci of B, G, and R, as in Figure 22-5, the center of gravity method for plotting point W within the triangle, is as follows. The location of point X can be defined along the straight line connecting G and R by the relative weights g and r:

$$\frac{XR}{XG} = \frac{g}{r}$$

Then let point W be defined along the line connecting B and X by the relative weights b and (g + r):

$$\frac{XW}{BW} = \frac{b}{(g + r)}$$

All lights that can be matched by some mixture of the reference wavelengths B, G, and R can be uniquely located in an analogous fashion. Special cases arise, however, where one must allow for a mixture of one of the three reference wavelengths with the light that is being matched. For example, when attempting to match a spectral light of 500 nm, we find the result:

a(500 nm) + rR = gG + bB,

meaning that a mixture of G and B came close but did not provide an exact match until we mixed a small amount of R into the 500 nm light.

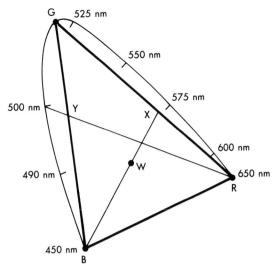

FIG. 22-5   Geometric derivation of a color triangle. (See text for explanation).

The location of 500 nm is then located relative to the BGR triangle as follows. Let the location for Y be defined along the line connecting B and G by the relative weights of b and g:

$$\frac{YB}{YG} = \frac{g}{b}$$

Then let the location for 500 nm be defined along the line connecting R and Y by the relative weights a and r:

$$\frac{YR}{Y500nm} = \frac{a}{r}$$

The location for 500 nm thus falls outside the triangle connecting B, G, and R. Similar results are found for matching other spectral lights, producing a curved line that passes directly through the points of the three reference wavelengths. This is called the spectrum locus curve.

The international commission on illumination (Commission Internationale de l'Éclairage or CIE) established an international standard in 1931 for plotting human trichromatic metameric matching data. Values obtained from a group of normal trichromats were averaged, yielding values for a hypothetical "standard observer." This standard, summarized in the CIE chromaticity diagram, is illustrated in Figure 22-6. Any straight line segment drawn in this diagram represents a series of colors that can be

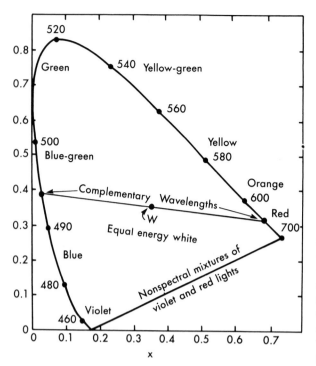

FIG. 22-6 The CIE chromaticity diagram. (See text for explanation.)

produced by mixing together various proportions of the two colors represented at the ends of the line. An example of this is the straight line drawn at the base of the triangular diagram in Figure 22-6, which connects the two extreme ends of the spectrum locus curve. This line represents a family of violets and purples that are multispectral mixtures of 400 nm (violet) and 700 nm (red) lights. Only points falling inside the perimeter of the spectrum locus curve and its closing straight line segment represent physiologically attainable color sensations. Points close to the center of the triangular diagram give the appearance of varying shades of white, while points close to the spectrum locus curve represent stimuli that have more intensely saturated color appearances. Points on the spectrum locus curve represent varying hues from red through orange, yellow, green, etc. A unique white denoted in the diagram by point W is the location of a mixture of equal energies of the three reference wavelengths in the mixture. A straight line drawn across the diagram through this point will intersect the spectrum locus curve at two points representing complementary wavelengths. That is to say that some mixed combination of the two spectral lights represented at each intersection of the straight line

with the spectrum locus curve can be found to provide metameric matches with the appearance of the light represented by the equal energy white. A line drawn from point W toward the spectrum locus curve represents a family of colors, all of the same hue but of varying saturation.

NEURAL ENCODING OF COLOR

Neural elements of the afferent visual system are characterized chiefly by their receptive field properties (see Chapters 19, 21, and 23). The receptive field of a visual cell encompasses all portions of the visual field in which a visually adequate stimulus can produce a neurophysiologic response. The receptive fields of neurons are classified as being colorcoded, if some aspect of the cells' responses are found to be specific for some color attribute. For instance, a cell may respond more vigorously to stimulation by light of one wavelength than of another, or the nature of the response may differ as a function of wavelength. The two broadest categories of such cells in the anterior visual system are opponent color cells and double opponent cells.

Opponent color cells

Tracing afferent visual pathways beyond the photo receptors, the first cells found to have specific color-related properties are the opponent color cells. Such cells have differing polarity of responses for differing portions of the visible spectrum. An example of an opponent color cell is shown in Figure 22-7. Stimulation by yellow light increases the tonic firing rate of such a cell, whereas stimulation by blue light inhibits or eliminates its rate of firing. Stimulation by similar-sized spots of white light produces no response. The latter phenomenon may be explained by presuming that simultaneous white light stimulation of both excitatory and inhibitory components of the cell's receptive field will result in a net zero response in firing rate. Opponency of such cells can be characteristically divided into two large groups: those having blue-yellow opponency, and those having red-green opponency. Red-green color opponent cells are tuned to detection of varying levels of stimulation of middle and long wavelength sensitive cones, and are best suited to the detection of red-green color contrasting borders. It is believed that there are also cells that sum the input of red and green cones to produce a yellow signal. Blue-yellow color opponent cells then detect levels of stimulation of blue cones as compared to the summed effect of stimulating both red and green cones.

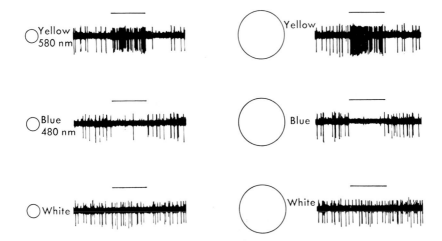

FIG. 22-7   Opponent color cell from the lateral geniculate nucleus of a rhesus monkey. Yellow light excites the cell, blue light inhibits it, and white light has little effect. Horizontal lines above the records indicate the duration of illumination. (From Wiesel TN, Hubel DH: J Neurophysiol 29:1115, 1966.)

Double opponent cells

Cells that have opponent receptive field properties for both color and space are said to be double opponent. Such cells have both centers and surrounds in their receptive fields, both of which are color coded.[36,37] The center of the receptive field may be stimulated by red light and inhibited by green light, while its surround has the opposite properties (Fig. 22-8). The uniform illumination of both center and surround will give little or no response without respect to wavelength. In most such cells white light mixtures will also not elicit a response when selectively stimulating either center or surround of the receptive field.

Double opponent cells are optimally organized for the detection of simultaneous color contrast. The phenomenon of simultaneous color contrast can be demonstrated by viewing restricted areas surrounded by contrasting color regions. For instance, a small field of gray surrounded by a field of red will appear to contain a greenish cast. Conversely, the same gray spot viewed in any region surrounded by green will acquire a reddish appearance. The general rule of simultaneous color contrast is that the color of

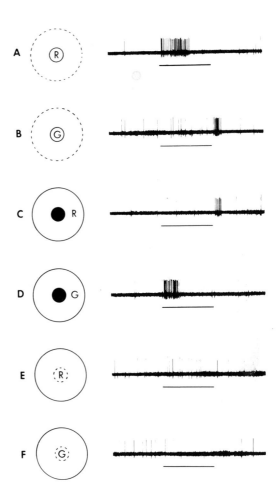

FIG. 22-8   Double opponent cell from striate cortex of rhesus monkey. Responses to **A**, red spot shone on the center of the receptive field; **B**, green spot; **C**, red anulus shone on the surround of the receptive field; **D**, green anulus; **E**, uniform red illumination of whole receptive field; **F**, uniform green illumination. (From Michael CR: J Neurophysiol 41:572, 1978.)

a restricted region will tend toward the complementary color of its surround.

Simultaneous color contrast is closely related to the phenomenon of color constancy referred to previously. The color that a given light will appear to have depends critically upon closely adjacent areas with which it is compared and contrasted. A localized area illuminated by monochromatic light of 585 nm wavelength can take on a variety of seemingly different colors, depending entirely on the areas surrounding it. For instance, a spot of 585 nm will acquire a green color when embedded in a surround of 650 nm but will appear to be red when surrounded by a field of 540 nm. When surrounded by a field of identical wavelength but 0.7 log unit brighter, it will acquire a gray appearance, whereas if the surround of the same wavelength is 2 log units brighter, the spot will appear to be black. Again, if the spot of 585 nm light is surrounded by a field of somewhat shorter wavelength, for instance 570 nm, but 1 log unit brighter, the spot will appear to be brown.

Cells in the retina having color opponent or double opponent neural properties belong to the general group of cells having tonic firing rates. Response gradations of these cells consist of temporal variations in rate of firing away from some resting value. Thus inhibition will produce a decrease in the rate of firing, while excitation will produce an increase. Such tonically firing cells generally belong to the class of ganglion cells having small somas and small axons, and are more slowly conducting. Additionally, they tend to synapse at the lateral geniculate body with cells having similar anatomic and physiologic properties. Thus color opponent and double opponent cells are also found in the lateral geniculate body. These are located in the four dorsal layers of the lateral geniculate body, making up the portion of that structure called the parvocellular division.

Retinal distribution of color-specific neurons

The trichromatic properties of human color vision are easily demonstrable out to between 20 and 30 degrees away from fixation. Beyond this limit color vision was once thought to be dichromatic or even monochromatic. However, recent work has established that, when suitable arrangements are made for spatial summation, all the essential properties of trichromatic color vision can be demonstrated well out into the periphery of the visual field.[33] Although large, contiguous areas are necessary to demonstrate these phenomena, one knows from subjective experience that a broad expanse like the sky, which has a uniform blue color, can be reliably identified as blue when viewed only by areas of the peripheral visual field.

The density of cones in the retina falls sharply outside the fovea, but cones of all three varieties are present, though in much smaller numbers, all the way to the ora serrata (see Chapter 19). The center of the fovea is unique both in having the highest spatial density of cones and in having a pure mosaic of red and green cones, with blue cones being eliminated from the photoreceptor population within the central ⅙ degree of the visual field. Although we are not consciously aware of it, all humans have a tiny area of blue blindness located at fixation. This can be demonstrated very easily by measuring spectral sensitivities with extremely small test objects. This psychophysical phenomenon is referred to as small field tritanopia[52], and it exactly matches the area of absent short wavelength sensitive cones in both human and nonhuman primate retina (see Figs. 22-12 and 22-13).[13,53]

Peculiarities of the blue cone system

Both visual acuity and contrast sensitivity are poorer in blue light than in red or green light.[7,19] This phenomenon is due not only to the absence of short wavelength sensitive cones in the foveal center but also to the relative scarcity of blue cones, which are much fewer in number in all retinal areas than are middle wavelength sensitive or long wavelength sensitive receptors. Blue cones are spread in a sparsely populated mosaic across the visual field. There is a much greater degree of neural convergence from short wavelength sensitive receptors on to their down stream neural components.[18] Blue light is color contrasted with yellow light and is encoded in the color opponent and double opponent cells that signal simultaneous contrast of blue and yellow in adjacent locations. The fact that this color contrast occurs in the absence of high levels of spatial acuity seems counterintuitive, since the greatest sensitivities for color discrimination and form discrimination are found at the center of the visual field. However, color contrast appears to provide the visual system with a means of "filling in" relatively large areas within a visual scene, enriching the image in a biologically useful way, but without participating in the high spatial discrimination typical of central (foveal) visual function. While foveal projections in the afferent visual system provide the neural basis for encoding fine spatial discrimination and shape recognition properties, color vision appears to amplify the available information within an image by providing a more varied means for discriminating between otherwise poorly contrasting subregions within a scene that would otherwise be difficult to distinguish from one another.

Color encoding in the cerebral cortex

The axons of color opponent and double opponent cells, arising from somas in the lateral geniculate nucleus, synapse with cells located in several layers of the striate cortex (see Chapter 23). The earliest studies of the electrophysiologic properties of striate cortical cells were concerned primarily with the spatial organization and the luminance, contrast, and temporal sensitivities of their receptive fields. Over the past several years physiologists have just begun to unravel the nature of color encoding in the striate and peristriate cortex. The first clue to color organization in the primary visual cortex was the finding of groups of cells that stain strongly for the presence of cytochrome oxidase.[26,28,31] These groups of cells are referred to as "blobs," since tangential sections of cortex tend to cut through parallel columns of such cells that are oriented perpendicular to the cortical layers and that stain strongly for cytochrome oxidase.[28] In the *macaque* the blobs form a repetitive polka-dot pattern of 200 micron-sized patches, spaced about 0.5 mm apart, covering the entire striate cortex. The blobs are arranged in parallel rows that meet the border between areas 17 and 18 at right angles. They are found in layers 2 and 3, and somewhat less prominently in layers 5 and 6, and are centered within ocular dominance columns[24,27] (see Chapter 23).

The receptive fields of striate cortical cells located between the blobs are characteristically tuned to specific spatial orientations, whereas cells within the blobs have no apparent orientation selectivity.[29] Blob cells also have relatively simple, concentric, center-surround receptive field properties, and are strongly associated with color differentiation. Color double opponency can be found in many of the blob cells of layers 2 and 3 in the *macaque*, and color sensitivity is also common in the blob cells of the lower cortical layers, 5 and 6.[47] Cells of the middle layers of striate cortex (the several sublaminae of layer 4) have properties that are determined by their positions relative to the locations of blob columns. Some cells of layer 4 that are in vertical register with the columns of blob cells (located above and below) lack spatial orientation and

have excitatory responses that are restricted to the two spectral extremes, red and blue. Layer 4 cells in register with interblob regions do not exhibit this property, but have instead excitatory responses to mid-spectral and broad-band stimuli, such as white, yellow, and green. White responders are clustered at interblob centers and are flanked to either side by yellow and green responders, separating them from the red and blue responsive cells of blob-registered locations.[15] It further appears that the cells of individual blob columns are devoted to one or the other major types of color opponency: red versus green or blue versus yellow. Blobs devoted to red/green opponency outnumber those of blue/yellow opponency by a ratio of about 3 to 1.[48]

In peristriate cortex (area 18 or V_2) rather than blobs, the pattern of cytochrome oxidase staining is one of parallel stripes of alternating widths, thick and thin. Cells within the thin stripe regions of area 18 are not orientation selective, show a high frequency of color-opponency, and probably receive their input directly from blob cells of area 17. Cells in the thick stripes and in the pale interstripe regions are orientation selective and are frequently sensitive to binocular disparity (probably concerned with stereo acuity). The thin stripes of area 18 appear to receive most of their input from the blobs of area 17, while the pale stripes receive the majority of their input from the interblob regions of area 17.[30] Thus an anatomic and functional segregation of form and color discrimination is maintained through the striate and into the peristriate visual cortex.

CONGENITAL DYSCHROMATOPSIAS

Inherited color vision deficits have been subdivided into groups according to the patterns in which colors are confused (Table 22-1). Two broad groups are represented, those in which reds and greens are confused with one another and those in which blues and yellows are confused. There are two principal varieties of red-green confusion, one called "protan" and the other "deutan," from the green for first and second. The third ("tritan") type of congenital defect is that in which blue and yellow confusions predominate. Congenital defects in color vision are further subdivided into anomalous trichromacy, dichromacy, and monochromacy. Anomalous trichromats are those who still require three primaries in order to match the full gamut of color but who do not accept the matches made by those with normal color vision. Dichro-

TABLE 22-1   Classification of Color-Deficient Observers

	Red deficient	Green deficient	Blue deficient
Anomalous trichromats	Protanomal	Deuteranomal	Tritanomal
Dichromats	Protanope	Deuteranope	Tritanope
Monochromats	Blue cone monochromats		
	Rod monochromats		

mats need only two primaries to match any colored light within their spectral range of vision, and will accept all matches made by normals. Monochromacy is a term used somewhat confusedly, having been applied to two different entities. Rod monochromats are those with a complete congenital absence of cone function, while blue cone monochromats have no red or green cone function but appear to have retinal pigments for both rods and blue cones. This latter disorder is rare and has features that mimic those of dichromacy, showing a need for two primaries to make some metameric matches at mesopic levels of retinal light adaptation.

Reflection densitometry[4,42] and heterochromatic increment threshold measures of Stile's π-mechanisms[46] have shown that one or more of the normal cone pigments are altered or missing altogether in individuals affected by congenital dyschromatopsia. Subjects with complete dichromacy have only two types of cones, each having normal spectral sensitivity characteristics, with the third type being absent. Protanopes are dichromats having normal green and blue cones, but an absence of cones containing long wavelength sensitive pigment. Conversely, deuteranopes have normal red and blue cones, but an absence of cones containing the middle wavelength sensitive pigment. While these subjects appear to have a normal numerical component of cones, those cones that should have contained a given variety of pigment, either red or green, have been genetically determined to contain the complementary variety. Anomalous trichromats have three classes of cones, containing three different pigments, but the pigment in one of the three has an abnormal spectral absorption. Protanomalous individuals, for instance, lack a normal red-sensitive pigment, but instead have cones containing pigment with a spectral absorption more nearly like that of the normal middle wavelength sensitive variety. As a consequence, the spectral absorption curves of

their red and green cones are more nearly alike.[43]

The molecular biology of the congenital dyschromatopsias

The inherited disorders of color vision are now reasonaby well understood. They are the result of a congenital absence or alteration in one or more of the cone photopigments.[1-3,32,45] Using the techniques of molecular genetics, Nathans et al. have isolated and sequenced human genomic complementary DNA clones that encode the apoproteins of the several cone pigments.[39] They have confirmed the hypothesis that congenital dyscromatopsias of the most common variety are caused by alterations in the genes encoding the red- and green-sensitive photopigments.[38] Color vision defects are produced by deletions of red or green pigment genes or by formation of hybrid genes comprised of portions of both red and green pigment genes, resulting from an unequal crossing over between genes that are located in tandem within the X chromosome. Differences in severity of the color vision defects are related to variations in the crossover sites. Even among color-normal trichromats, a certain degree of polymorphism has been found. Careful studies by Neitz et al. have shown that normal trichromats can be further subdivided by the patterns of the color matches that they make with the Rayleigh anomaloscope.[40] Thus even among color-normals there are detectable, discrete variations in capacities for discriminating between middle and long wavelength light. It is believed that most normal humans have, in fact, more than three different cone pigment types represented on the X chromosome.

The inherited dyschromatopsias are binocular, symmetrical, and do not change over time. They can generally be detected and characterized by the patterns created by mapping into the CIE chromaticity diagram those colors that the subjects find confusing. As shown in Figure 22-9,*A*, individuals with protan (red-deficient) congenital color defects will confuse colors represented by a family of straight lines that converge on a point in the diagram close to the red end of the spectrum locus curve. These lines are said to be isochromatic since they represent, for affected individuals, families of colors that are identical in appearance. The isochromatic lines for deutan and tritan congenital dyschromatopsias converge toward different loci. Those for tritan (blue-deficient) dyschromatopsia converge toward the short wavelength end of the spectrum locus curve, while those for deutan (green-deficient) dyschromatopsia converge toward a point located outside the perimeter of the CIE color triangle (Fig. 22-9).

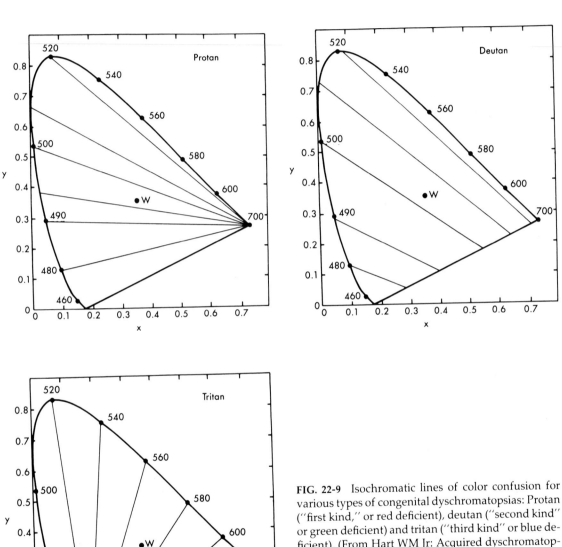

FIG. 22-9 Isochromatic lines of color confusion for various types of congenital dyschromatopsias: Protan ("first kind," or red deficient), deutan ("second kind" or green deficient) and tritan ("third kind" or blue deficient). (From Hart WM Jr: Acquired dyschromatopsias, Surv Ophthalmol 32:10, 1987.)

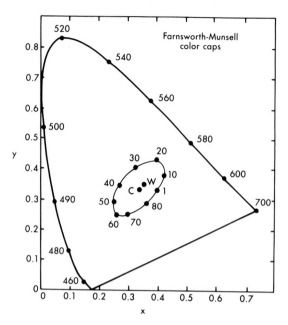

FIG. 22-10   CIE chromaticity coordinates for the color caps of the Farnsworth-Munsell 100-Hue test, C, standard illuminant used in clinical color vision testing. W, equal energy white. (From Hart WM Jr: Acquired dyschromatopsias, Surv Ophthalmol 32:10, 1987.)

Hue discrimination tests for characterizing abnormal color vision

The Farnsworth-Munsell 100 Hue Test[16] can be used to estimate both the nature and extent of defective color vision. It is largely a qualitative measure of color vision, however, which is unable to make subtle distinctions between similar types of color defects, such as extreme anomalous trichromacy versus pure dichromacy, but which nonetheless provides very useful information. The test consists of a series of 85 colored caps (15 colors in the original test design have since been eliminated). The colors of the caps correspond to an oval pattern of hues within the CIE chromaticity diagram, as diagramed in Figure 22-10. The 85 caps are divided into four approximately equal-sized groups that are stored in separate boxes. In the course of testing, a subject is asked to arrange the caps in a linear sequence between pairs of fixed referenced caps that are located at either end of each box. The order of the caps produced by the subject's arrangement is then plotted on a polar diagram such that correct ordering of caps will result in points close to the center of the circle, while in-

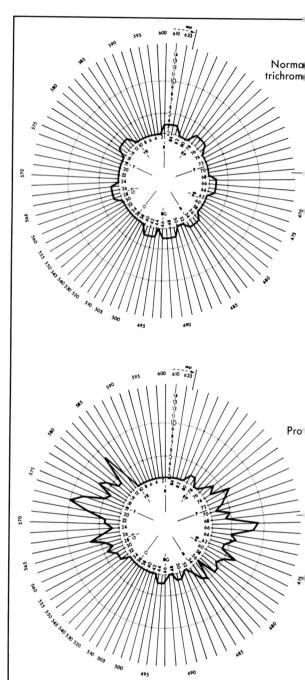

correct orderings or transpositions cause points to be plotted farther away from the center of the diagram[16] (Fig. 22-11).

Confusions between similar hues in patients with congenital color defects result in characteristic patterns in Farnsworth-Munsell polar plots. Transpositional errors are usually confined to

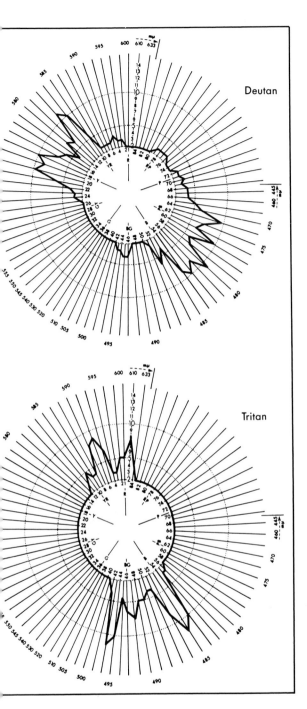

FIG. 22-11   Results of Farnsworth-Munsell 100-Hue test for a normal trichromat and for each of the three principal types of congenital dyschromatopsias. Compare patterns of isochromatic confusion lines in Figure 22-9 with positions of color caps in Figure 22-10. (From Hart WM Jr: Acquired dyschromatopsias, Surv Ophthalmol 32:10, 1987.)

ital dyschromatopsia will tend to confuse color caps from the hue circle that fall close to or nearly parallel the isochromatic lines associated with their particular type of congenital defect. A protanope will, for instance, confuse color caps in the regions of caps number 10 through 30 and from caps number 55-75. Likewise, an individual with a tritan defect will confuse caps 85-100 and caps 40-55. The presence of these two diametrically opposed zones of color confusion produces a pattern in the Farnsworth-Munsell diagram that defines an axis. Subjects with a tritan defect will have a polar pattern with a vertical axis while subjects with protan and deutan defects will show polar axes obliquely oriented from upper left to lower right. The differences in axial orientation for protan and deutan patterns are fairly small and are, therefore, relatively difficult to distinguish from one another by this test. This is because the orientations of isochromatic confusion lines for protan and deutan types, as plotted in the CIE chromaticity diagram, are very close to one another.

ACQUIRED DYSCHROMATOPSIAS

Acquired color vision defects, so called dyschromatopsias, are different from congenital color vision deficits in several respects. Most importantly, acquired defects in color vision are noticeable to the observer, whereas congenital defects usually are not. Additionally, acquired

restricted zones within the color circle that are located at directly opposite locations from one another. These patterns can be understood best by comparing the lines of isochromatic confusion shown in Figure 22-9 to the pattern of the Farnsworth-Munsell test caps plotted in the CIE diagram in Figure 22-10. Subjects with congen-

defects may be monocular or markedly asymmetric and may even vary from one part of the visual field to another. Acquired defects are commonly associated with reductions in visual acuity, changes in dark adaptation, and/or flicker discrimination. Acquired deficits are caused by a variety of diseases that damage the retina, the optic nerve, or the visual cortex. Toxic, vascular, inflammatory, neoplastic, demyelinating, and degenerative diseases are all well-recognized causes of acquired dyschromatopsias. The damage caused by these diseases is very nonselective, and the patterns of defect in hue discrimination caused by acquired disease are entirely different from those caused by the congenital, inherited abnormalities in photopigment composition. As a consequence of this, the color vision tests that were originally intended for the study of congenital dyschromatopsias produce somewhat confusing results when applied to patients with acquired diseases.

Classifications of acquired dyschromatopsias

In an attempt to bring order to the confusion caused by the highly variable findings found in patients with acquired color vision defects, Verriest proposed a classification based on extensive empirical observations on the nature of color vision disturbances found in ocular and neurologic disease.[17,49] His classification was based largely on the use of the Farnsworth-Munsell 100 hue test (see Table 22-2). Three major types of acquired dyschromatopsias called types I, II, and III are included in this classification. The first two varieties are associated with a major axis of defective hue discrimination in the red-green region of the Farnsworth-Munsell diagram, much like the patterns found for the protan and deutan varieties of congenital dyschromatopsias. Type I is protanlike, and is manifested as an acquired loss of discrimination between reds and greens with little or no loss of blue-yellow discrimination. This variety of dyschromatopsia is also associated with moderate to severe reductions in visual acuity. The type II dyschromatopsia is said to be deutanlike, and involves mild to severe confusion of reds and greens with a simultaneous but milder loss of discrimination between blues and yellows. Again, type II is usually associated with moderate to severe reductions in visual acuity. The third type of acquired color vision defect in the Verriest classification, type III, is said to be tritanlike, and is manifested by mild to moderate confusions of blue and yellow hues with a lesser or even absent impairment of red-green discrimination. In this third type of dyschromatopsia visual acuity may be normal or only mildly reduced.

Köllner's rule

In 1912 Köllner[34] published detailed findings on the study of color vision in patients with acquired ocular and neural disease. He made the observation that in patients with neural disorders there seemed to be a preponderance of damage to red-green discrimination with relative preservation of blue-yellow discrimination. On the other hand, patients with retinal or choroidal diseases more commonly showed evi-

TABLE 22-2   Verriest's Classification of Acquired Dyschromatopsias[49]

Name	Alternate names	Hue discrimination defect by Farnsworth-Munsell testing	Visual acuity
Type I	Acquired red/green, protan-like	Mild to severe confusion of red and green hues with little or no loss of blue/yellow discrimination	Moderate to severe reduction
Type II	Acquired red/green, deutan-like	Mild to severe confusion of red and green hues with a concomitant mild loss of blue/yellow discrimination	Moderate to severe reduction
Type III	Acquired blue/yellow, tritan-like	Mild to moderate confusion of blue and yellow hues with a lesser impairment of red/green discrimination (pseudoprotanomaly)	Normal to moderate reduction

From Hart WM Jr: Acquired dyschromatopsias, Surv Ophthalmol 32:10, 1987.[20]

dence of loss of blue-yellow discrimination with relative preservation of red-green discrimination. This phenomenon of predominant red-green loss in optic nerve disease and of blue-yellow discrimination loss in retinal and chroidal disease has since come to be known as Köllner's rule. However, there are numerous exceptions to Köllner's rule, and it would be false to assume that red-green discrimination is determined at a neural level while blue-yellow discrimination is determined at a retinal level. Rather there are anatomic peculiarities of the distribution of hue discrimination that produce the patterns of damage to color vision found in these various diseases. For instance, some primary diseases of the optic nerve, such as glaucoma, papilledema, or dominantly inherited optic atrophy, can result in a type III defect to color vision: a predominant loss of blue-yellow discrimination with preservation of visual acuity. On the other hand, other optic nerve diseases, such as demyelinating optic neuritis or neural compression by tumors, commonly produce profound reductions in acuity associated with relatively selective damage to red-green discrimination. There is no good evidence to support the idea that channels for one or another type of color discrimination are in any way selectively susceptible to damage by any particular class of optic nerve disease.

Spatial heterogeneity of color discrimination in the central visual field

It should be noted that the majority of color vision tests used for studying patients with acquired defects in color vision, especially the Farnsworth-Munsell 100 hue test, are actually tests of a very small portion of the central visual field. The colored caps used in this sorting test each subtend an angle of approximately 2° when held at a reading distance. (This size of visual stimulus was chosen for the Farnsworth-Munsell test in part because it subtends the same area of the visual field that was used in the original metameric matching experiments to produce the data for deriving the CIE chromaticity diagram.) Although consistent results can be obtained for large groups of normal trichomatic observers when using this area of the central visual field, it is important to understand that the distribution of color discrimination within this narrow region is not homogeneous. Variation in color discrimination within this area is most dramatically apparent as the presence of an absolute foveal defect for the perception of blue light. This phenomenon, referred to as small-field tritanopia or foveal tritanopia, is

most noticeable within the central 0.5°, and is attributable to two factors: the presence of macular xanthophyl pigment and the absence of short wavelength sensitive cones in the foveal cone mosaic.[10,52,53]

The foveal and perifoveal sensitivity for blue perception closely matches the anatomic distribution of blue cones in this region of the retina,[53] and the foveal defect for blue perception has been directly correlated with the reduced density of blue cones in this region (Fig. 22-12). Histochemical dyes have been used to selectively

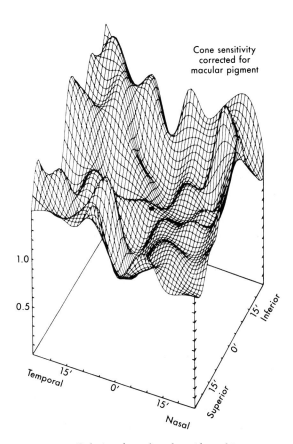

FIG. 22-12 Relative foveal and perifoveal increment sensitivity for blue cones, corrected for the absorption of blue light by the macular pigment. Area tested includes radius of 25 arc minutes within foveal center. Relative central scotoma (localized depression) for blue detection centered at fovea is demonstrated, as are local variations in sensitivity attributed to the low density of SWS (blue) cone receptors in foveal vicinity. (From Williams DR, et al: Punctate sensitivity of the blue sensitive mechanism, Vision Res 21:1357, 1981, with permission, copyright Pergamon Journals, Ltd.)

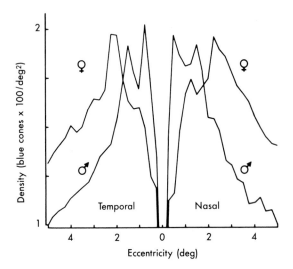

FIG. 22-13 Foveal and perifoveal density profiles for Procion-stained cones along the horizontal meridian of male and female *Macaque* retinas. (From de Monasterio FM, et al: Density profile of blue-sensitive cones along the horizontal meridian of *Macaque* retina. Invest Ophthalmol Vis Sci 26:289, 1985, used with permission of author and publisher.)

stain the short wavelength sensitive cones in retinal preparations.[14] An anatomic gap in the distribution of blue cones at the fovea has been convincingly demonstrated in the retinas of nonhuman primates that have trichromatic vision nearly identical to that of humans (Fig. 22-13).[13]

How acquired diseases produce their various patterns of color deficits

Because of the small blind spot for blue perception located at the center of the visual field, human observers making color judgments between the various caps of the Farnsworth-Munsell test must depend on comparisons between the more peripheral portions of the centrally viewed test objects in order to distinguish hues in the blue-yellow dimension of color space. Diseases of the retina and optic nerve produce characteristic patterns of damage in the central and pericentral portions of the visual field. For instance, the most common form of glaucoma notoriously damages the extracentral portions of the visual field, as evidenced by sparing of visual acuity until the latest stages of the disease. Apparently selective damage to blue-yellow discrimination with relative preservation of red-green discrimination and visual acuity (type III dyschromatopsia in the Verriest classification) is

common in chronic glaucoma.[22] This should be expected if damage to the extrafoveal visual field (outside the central half degree) exceeds that at the foveal center. In this situation the higher degree of red-green discrimination and visual acuity found in the foveal cone mosaic will be relatively preserved, but the perifoveal blue cone contribution to color discrimination will have been diminished.

Another common disease category for the type III acquired dyschromatopsias is toxic retinopathy. Antimalarial drugs, such as chloroquine or hydroxychloroquine, are often used in the treatment of autoimmune connective tissue disease, and are associated with a dose-dependent risk of retinal damage. In the early stages of antimalarial retinal toxicity, a ring-shaped region of damage to the pigment epithelium is characteristically found, and a corresponding ring of perifoveal depression of light sensitivity can be demonstrated by careful visual field testing.[21] At this stage of disease a type III acquired dyschromatopsia is found (Fig. 22-14), characterized by loss of discrimination between blues and yellows and with simultaneous relative preservation of visual acuity.

The converse interpretation can be made for diseases that preferentially damage the foveal cone representation in the center of the visual field. Toxic and nutritional damage to the optic nerve frequently results in small but deep areas of depressed visual function centered at "fixation," the foveal projection of the visual field. Such patients will often have sharply reduced visual acuity and red-green discrimination, but with relative preservation of blue-yellow discrimination (a type I or II dyschromatopsia in the Verriest classification)[11] (Fig. 22-15).

Although this visual field mechanism for determining the variety of acquired dyschromatopsia is not the only possible one, it is thoroughly consistent with all of the known patterns of color vision deficits in acquired diseases.[20]

REFERENCES

1. Alpern M, Moeller J: The red and green cone visual pigments of deuteranomalous trichromacy, J Physiol (Lond) 266:647, 1977.
2. Alpern M, Pugh EN Jr: Variation in the action spectra of erythrolabe among deuteranopes, J Physiol (Lond) 266:613, 1977.
3. Alpern M, Wake T: Cone pigment in human deutan colour vision defects, J Physiol (Lond) 266:595, 1977.
4. Baker HD, Rushton WAH: The red-sensitive pigment in normal cones, J Physiol (Lond) 176:56, 1965.
5. Boynton RM: Human color vision, New York, Holt Rinehart and Winston, 1979.

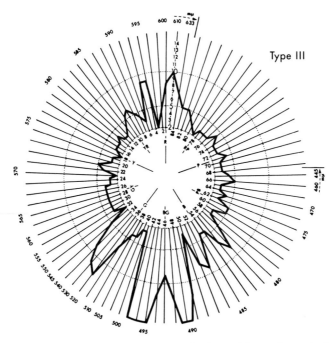

FIG. 22-14 Type III acquired dyschromatopsia in hydroxychloroquine retinal toxicity. Most transpositional errors are clustered at top and bottom of diagram, producing a nearly vertical axis typical for the tritan-like blue/yellow hue confusion of the type III color vision defect. This pattern is found in the earlier stages of toxicity, prior to the loss of central visual acuity. (Data redrawn from Pinckers et al: Acquired color vision defects, in Pokorny J, et al, eds: Congenital and acquired color vision defects, New York, Grune and Stratton, 1979, p 333.)

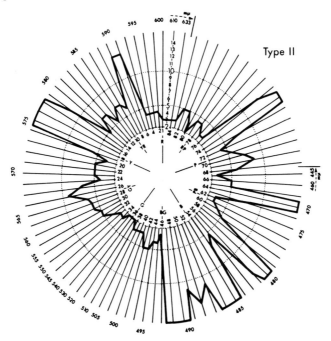

FIG. 22-15 Type II acquired dyschromatopsia in early stages of Leber's hereditary optic atrophy. Pattern of transpositional errors defines an oblique axis from upper left to lower right, indicating a protan- or deutanlike dyschromatopsia. (From Nikoskelainen E, et al: The early phase in Leber hereditary optic atrophy, Arch Ophthalmol 95:969, 1977, used with author's permission.)

6. Brindley GS: The effects on colour vision of adaptation to very bright lights, J Physiol (Lond) 122:332, 1953.

7. Brindley GS: The summation areas of human colour receptive mechanisms at increment threshold, J Physiol (Lond) 124:400, 1954.

8. Brown PK, Wald G: Visual pigments in human and monkey retinas, Nature 200:37, 1963.

9. Brown PK, Wald G: Visual pigments in single rods and cones of the human retina, Science 144:45, 1964.

10. Castano JA, Sperling HG: Sensitivity of the blue sensitive cones across the central retina, Vision Res 22:661, 1982.

11. Chisholm IA, Bronte-Stewart J, Awduche ED: Color vision in tobacco amblyopia, Acta Ophthalmol 48:1145, 1970.

12. Dartnall HJA, Bowmaker JK, Mollon, JD: Human visual pigments: microspectrophotometric results from the eyes of seven persons, Proc Roy Soc (Lond) 220(B):I15, 1983.

13. de Monasterio FM, McCrane EP, Newlander JK, et al: Density profile of blue-sensitive cones along the horizontal meridian of *Macaque* retina, Invest Ophthalmol Vis Sci 26:289, 1985.

14. de Monasterio FM, Schein SJ, McCrane EP: Staining of blue-sensitive cones of the macaque retina by a fluorescent dye, Science 213:1279, 1981.

15. Dow BM, Vautin RG: Horizontal segregation of color information in the middle layers of foveal striate cortex, J Neurophysiol 57:712, 1987.

16. Farnsworth D: The Farnsworth-Munsell 100 Hue Test Manual, Baltimore, Munsell Color Company, 1957.

17. Francois J, Verriest G: On acquired deficiency of color vision, Vision Res 1:201, 1961.

18. Gouras P: Identification of cone mechanism in monkey ganglion cells, J Physiol (Lond) 199:533, 1968.

19. Green DG: The contrast sensitivity of the colour mechanisms of the human eye, J Physiol (Lond) 196:415, 1968.

20. Hart WM Jr: Acquired dyschromatopsias, Survey Ophthalmol 32:10, 1987.

21. Hart WM Jr, Burde RM, Johnston GP, et al: Static perimetry in chloroquine retinopathy; perifoveal patterns of visual field depression, Arch Ophthalmol 102:377, 1984.

22. Hart WM Jr, Gordon MO: Color perimetry of glaucomatous visual field defects, Ophthalmol 91:338, 1984.

23. Helmholtz H: Physiological optics, in Southall JPC, ed: New York, Optical Society of America, 1924, vol 2, p 426.

24. Hendricksen AE, Hunt SP, Wu JY: Immunocytochemical localization of glutamic acid decarboxylase in monkey striate cortex, Nature 292:605, 1982.

25. Hering E: Outlines of a theory of the light sense (English translation), in Hurvich LM, Jameson D (eds): Cambridge, Harvard University Press, 1964.

26. Horton JC: Cytochrome oxidase patches: a new cytoarchitectonic feature of monkey visual cortex, Phil Trans R Soc Lond Ser B 304:199, 1984.

27. Horton JC, Hubel DG: Regular patchy distribution of cytochrome oxidase staining in primary visual cortex of Macaque monkey, Nature 292:762, 1981.

28. Hubel DH: Blobs and color vision, Cell Biophys 9:91, 1986.

29. Hubel DH, Livingston MS: Regions of poor orientation tuning selectivity coincide with patches of cytochrome oxidase staining in monkey striate cortex, Soc Neurosci Abst 7:118.12, 1981.

30. Hubel DH, Livingston MS: Segregation of form, color and stereopsis in primate area 18, J Neurosci 7:3378, 1987.

31. Humphrey AL, Hendrickson AE: Radial zones of high metabolic activity in squirrel monkey striate cortex, Soc Neurosci Abst 6:113.6, 1980.

32. Hurvich LM: Color vision deficiencies, in Jameson D, Hurvich LM, eds: Handbook of sensory physiology, vol V11/4: Visual psychophysics, Berlin, Springer Verlag, 1972, p 582.

33. Johnson MA: Color vision in the peripheral retina, Am J Optom Physiol Opt 63:97, 1986.

34. Köllner H: Die Störungen des Farbensinnes, Ihre klinische Bedeutung und ihre Diagnose, Berlin, S Karger, 1912.

35. Marks WB, Dobelle WH, MacNichol EF Jr: Visual pigments of single primate cones, Science 143:1181, 1964.

36. Michael CR: Color sensitive complex cells in monkey striate cortex, J Neurophysiol 41:1250, 1978.

37. Michael CR: Color vision mechanisms in monkey striate cortex: dual-opponent cells with concentric receptive fields, J Neurophysiol 41:572, 1978.

38. Nathans J, Piantanida TP, Eddy RL, et al: Molecular genetics of inherited variation in human color vision, Science 232:203, 1986.

39. Nathans J, Thomas D, Hogness DS: Molecular genetics of human color vision: the genes encoding blue, green and red pigments, Science 232:193, 1986.

40. Neitz J, Jacobs GH: Polymorphism in normal human color vision and its mechanism, Vision Res 30:621, 1990.

41. Pokorny J, Smith VC, Verriest G, et al, eds: Congenital and acquired color vision defects, New York, Grune and Stratton, 1979.

42. Rushton WAH: A cone pigment in the protanope, J Physiol (Lond) 168:345, 1963.

43. Rushton WAH, Powell DS, White KD: Pigments in anomalous trichromats, Vision Res 13:2017, 1973.

44. Sherman P: Colour vision in the 19th century; the Young-Helmholtz-Maxwell theory, Bristol, Adam Hilger, 1981.

45. Smith VC, Pokorny J: Spectral sensitivity of color-blind observers and the cone photopigments, Vision Res 12:2059, 1972.

46. Stiles WS: Color vision: the approach through increment-threshold sensitivity, Proc Natl Acad Sci USA 45:100, 1959.

47. Tootell RB, Silverman MS, Hamilton DL, et al: Functional anatomy of macaque striate cortex, III, Color J Neurosci 8:1569, 1988.

48. Tso DY, Gilbert CD: The organization of chromatic and spatial interactions in the primate striate cortex, J Neurosci 8:1712, 1988.

49. Verriest G: Further studies on acquired deficiency of color discrimination, J Opt Soc Am 53:185 195, 1963.

50. Wald G: The receptors of human color vision, Science 145:1007, 1964.

51. Weale RA: Photosensitive reactions in fovea of normal and cone-monochromatic observers, Opt Acta 6:158, 1959.

52. Williams DR, MacLeod DIA, Hayhoe MM: Foveal tritanopia, Vision Res 21:1341, 1981.

53. Williams DR, MacLeod DIA, Hayhoe MM: Punctate sensitivity of the blue-sensitive mechanism, Vision Res 21:1357, 1981.

54. Wyszecki G, Stiles WS: Color science, New York, Wiley, 1967.

55. Young, T: On the theory of light and colours, Philos Trans R Soc Lond (Biol) 92:12, 1802.

GENERAL REFERENCES

Boynton RM: Human color vision, New York, Holt Rinehart and Winston, 1979.

Boynton RM: Color vision, Ann Rev Psychol 39:69, 1988.

Dartnall HJA, ed: Photochemistry of vision, Handbook of sensory physiology, vol 7/1, New York, Springer Verlag, 1972.

Hurvich L: Color vision, Sunderland MA, Sinauer Associates, 1981.

Pokorny J, Smith VC, Verriest G, et al: Congenital and acquired color vision defects, New York, Grune & Stratton, 1979.

Sherman P: Colour vision in the 19th century, The Young-Helmholtz-Maxwell theory, Bristol, Adam Hilger, 1981.

CHAPTER 23

The Central Visual Pathways

JONATHAN C. HORTON, M.D., Ph.D.

The eye is a peripheral transducer responsible for converting patterns of light energy into neuronal signals that can be processed by the central nervous system. Vision begins with the capture of images focused by the optic media upon the photoreceptor matrix. Absorption of light by the photoreceptors activates a complex web of synaptic connections between horizontal cells, amacrine cells, and bipolar cells (see Chapter 19). Sensory information flowing through this retinal circuit ultimately converges upon a final common pathway: ganglion cells. These cells encode the visual image in a train of action potentials that is transmitted via the optic nerve to the brain.

The ganglion cells are the only cells in the retina that project from the eye to the brain. Their axons terminate in a thalamic relay nucleus called the lateral geniculate body. Postsynaptic neurons of the lateral geniculate body receiving retinal input project in turn to the primary visual cortex. The retino-geniculo-cortical pathway provides the neural substrate for visual perception. This chapter will concentrate upon the organization of this afferent sensory visual system, relying whenever possible upon evidence obtained directly from either clinical or pathological studies in humans. However, since most

ACKNOWLEDGMENT

This chapter is dedicated to Dr. William F. Hoyt: friend, mentor, and inspirational contributor to neuro-ophthalmology.

of our knowledge has been gained from laboratory work involving animals, frequent reference will be made to experimental studies in cats and monkeys.

Retinal ganglion cell targets

Although the lateral geniculate body is the main target of ganglion cells, at least nine other nuclei within the brain also receive retinal input (see Table 23–1). These projections were first identified by using silver impregnation stains that label degenerating axon terminals of ganglion cells after removal of one eye.[121] Results from these early anatomic studies have been confirmed in more recent years by employing modern axon tracing methods in primates.[57,145]

The superior colliculus receives a major input from a special class of retinal ganglion cells that projects only to the mesencephalon. Fibers comprising this projection leave the optic tract just before the lateral geniculate body and enter the brachium of the superior colliculus to reach the midbrain. Inputs from each eye segregate into a mosaic of alternating, irregular bands in the superficial gray layer of the optic tectum.[72,120] The superior colliculus contains a complete retinotopic map of the contralateral field of vision.[32] Application of an electrical pulse to any point on this retinotopic map evokes a saccade of appropriate direction and amplitude to shift fixation to the receptive field location of neurons at the stimulation site.[128,134] Lesions of the superior colliculus, combined with lesions of the cortical frontal eye fields, severely impair the ability of

TABLE 23-1 Retinal Ganglion Cell Projections

Target	Function
Lateral geniculate body	Visual perception
Pregeniculate nucleus	Visual perception
Superior colliculus	Visuomotor behavior; foveation
Pretectal nuclear complex	Pupillary responses
Suprachiasmatic nucleus	Circadian rhythms
Paraventricular nucleus	Neuroendocrine regulation
Supraoptic nucleus	Neuroendocrine regulation
Pulvinar	Unknown
Accessory optic system	Optokinetic reflexes
Nucleus of the optic tract	Optokinetic reflexes

monkeys to shift their gaze to targets of visual interest (Chapter 5). However, lesions of the superior colliculus do not produce a defect in the field of vision. Taken together these findings suggest that the superior colliculus is important for visual orienting and foveation but is not essential for analysis of sensory information leading to visual perception.

The pupillary light reflex is governed by a retinal projection that exits the optic tract before the lateral geniculate body to terminate bilaterally in a scattered, ill-defined cellular complex within the midbrain referred to as the "pretectal nuclei." Neurons of the pretectal nuclei send projections to the ipsilateral and contralateral Edinger-Westphal subdivisions of the oculomotor nuclei. Edinger-Westphal neurons provide parasympathetic input via an interneuron in the ciliary ganglion to control the sphincter pupillae of the iris (see Chapter 12).

Retinal ganglion cells also provide a small, mostly crossed input to the accessory optic system, a complex of three midbrain structures called the dorsal, lateral, and medial terminal nuclei.[28] These three subnuclei, and the nucleus of the optic tract, appear to supply sensory information about retinal image slip to the neuronal circuit mediating optokinetic reflexes (see Chapter 5).[62,132]

The pulvinar is the largest nuclear mass in the primate thalamus. It is comprised of at least two visual subnuclei called the inferior pulvinar and the lateral pulvinar. Each visual subnucleus contains a retinotopic map of the contralateral visual hemifield.[9] Only the inferior pulvinar appears to receive direct retinal input.[22] Both the inferior pulvinar and the lateral pulvinar send a projection to striate cortex and to extrastriate cortex.[11] The pulvinar thus provides a route from retina to visual cortex that bypasses the lateral geniculate body. However, this parallel pulvinar pathway is negligible compared with the main retino-geniculo-cortical projection. The role of the pulvinar in visual processing is unclear despite studies examining the effect of pulvinar lesions in behaving monkeys.[112] It is rather unsettling that the function of such a prominent visual nucleus should remain an enigma.

The suprachiasmatic nuclei receive a retinal projection that regulates circadian rhythms.[111] Recent human studies by Sadun suggest that the supraoptic and paraventricular nuclei also receive direct retinal input.[129,130] These additional retinohypothalamic pathways presumably contribute a light-mediated element to neuroendocrine regulation.

The issue of a reciprocal pathway from the brain to the retina arouses perpetual controversy among anatomists.[29] In birds a centrifugal projection connects the isthmo-optic nucleus with the retina. However, in mammals no reliable evidence is available to support the existence of a centrifugal pathway. The mammalian optic nerve should be regarded as a one-way pathway containing only ganglion cell axons bound from the retina to the brain.

THE RETINO-GENICULO-CORTICAL PATHWAY
Retina to lateral geniculate body

The superior visual field is focused upon the inferior retina and the temporal visual field is projected upon the nasal retina by virtue of the optical inversion produced by the media of the eye. The fixation point corresponds to the fovea, a small pit in the central retina specialized for best visual activity. The fovea defines the vertical meridian of the field of vision by splitting the retina into nasal and temporal halves. Ganglion cells located in temporal retina project ipsilaterally, while ganglion cells in the nasal retina project contralaterally by crossing at the optic chiasm. This pattern of central retinal terminations can be labeled in the monkey by injecting horseradish peroxidase, a retrograde axon tracer, directly into the optic tract (Fig. 23-1,A and B).[20,49,93,142] It can also be observed directly in patients who suffer a lesion that destroys one optic tract. Injury to the primary optic pathway occurring anywhere between the retina and the

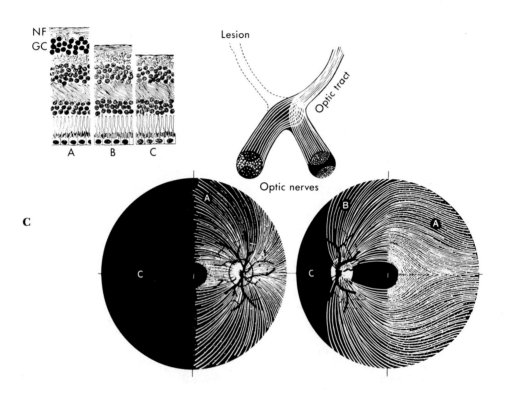

FIG. 23-1   **A,** Distribution of labeled cells in the right nasal retina and **B,** left temporal retina of the macaque monkey after injection of horseradish peroxidase tracer into the left optic tract. The vertical midline separating crossed and uncrossed ganglion cell projections passes through the fovea. Scale bar = 1 mm. (From Fukuda Y, et al: J Neurosci 9:2353, 1989.[49]) **C,** Schematic appearance of homonymous hemiretinal retrograde degeneration first observed by Hoyt in patients with a lesion of the optic tract. In this example the lesion is located in the right optic tract and remaining ganglion cells and fibers are sketched in white. The surviving ganglion cells and fibers correspond to the distribution of label shown above after horseradish peroxidase injection into the monkey's left optic tract. In zones A the retinae are normal. In zone B the retina contains no ganglion cells but is traversed by nerve fibers from the intact temporal retina. In zones C the retina contains neither ganglion cells nor nerve fibers. (From Hoyt WF, et al: Br J Ophthalmol 56:537, 1972.[71])

lateral geniculate body will produce degeneration of ganglion cells and fibers. This process of cellular degeneration requires several weeks, or even months, to become clinically apparent upon inspection of the ocular fundus. In normal individuals the ganglion cell axons are visible with an ophthalmoscope as they run across the inner surface of the retina in the nerve fiber layer. After injury to the optic tract, if sufficient time has elapsed, a characteristic pattern of homonymous hemiretinal atrophy develops in the ocular fundi, corresponding to the anatomic projections of nasal and temporal retinae (Fig. 23-1,C). The atrophic changes are most obvious in the eye contralateral to the lesion, where the nerve fibers that issue from the nasal and temporal aspects of the optic disc disappear and a horizontal, bowtie-shaped band of pallor appears on the optic disc.[71]

The superb visual acuity of humans is achieved at the fovea by thrusting aside all retinal elements except the photoreceptors, to minimize absorption and scattering of light. This unique primate specialization requires fibers from ganglion cells in temporal retina to follow a circuitous route to the optic disc to avoid passing over the fovea. The nerve fiber layer in temporal retina splits along a horizontal raphe, with axons originating from superior retina arching over the fovea and axons originating from inferior retina arching under the fovea (see Fig. 23-1,C).[157] This division of the nerve fiber layer, present only in temporal retina, defines the horizontal meridian of the visual field.

The horizontal raphe in the temporal nerve fiber layer results in a complex, discontinuous arrangement of ganglion cell axons at the optic disc. Cells in the temporal retina just above and below the horizontal meridian send their fibers via a roundabout route to enter the superior and inferior poles of the optic disc respectively. Although their cell bodies are situated close together in the retina, their fibers are widely sep-arated in the optic disc by other fibers that directly enter the nasal and temporal sides of the disc (see Fig. 23-1,C). Retinotopic organization is further complicated by intermingling between peripheral and central axons as they approach the optic disc.[109,115,123]

After leaving the eye at the optic disc, the ganglion cell fibers become invested with myelin to form the optic nerve. As they exit the globe the axons create an oval blind spot in the visual field that is easy to detect (Fig. 23-2). Close your right eye and hold the book at a distance of about 1 foot. By adjusting the book while staring at the cross hair the target within your blind spot will disappear. In humans the blind spot measures about 7.75° in vertical height by 5.0° in horizontal width.[161]

The retinotopic organization of ganglion cell fibers is generally preserved within the optic nerve.[70] Near the eye the ganglion cell fibers are precisely arrayed in a manner that duplicates their arrangement within the optic nerve head. Moving proximally toward the optic chiasm the fibers gradually scatter in position until the topography in the optic nerve becomes quite imprecise.[66,113] At least a third of the optic nerve is comprised of macular fibers. Near the globe the macular fibers are clustered into the central and temporal sectors of the optic nerve, but more proximally they intermingle with other fibers to distribute throughout all sectors of the optic nerve.[70] Fibers destined to decussate at the chiasm occupy a horizontal band through the optic nerve with a broad nasal base (Fig. 23-3).[152] Approaching the chiasm, these fibers shift position to occupy successively more nasal portions of the optic nerve, in anticipation of crossing.

At the optic chiasm the fibers originating from ganglion cells located nasal to the fovea cross into the contralateral optic tract (Fig. 23-4). Wilbrand observed that some ventral crossing fibers loop briefly into the opposite nerve before entering the optic tract (Wilbrand's knee).[165] At

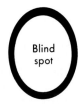

FIG. 23-2 Close the right eye and stare at the cross hair while holding the book at a distance of about one foot. When you succeed in projecting the blind spot target upon the optic disc of the left eye, the target will disappear.

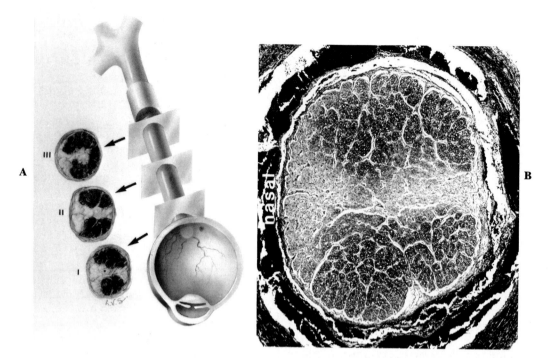

FIG. 23-3   **A**, Schematic diagram showing band atrophy of the left optic nerve due to a lesion destroying the crossed nasal retinal projection. **B**, Cross-section through the midorbital portion of the optic nerve (section II) stained with Luxol fast blue to reveal a pale horizontal band of atrophic nerve fascicles depleted of normal axons. (From Unsöld R, Hoyt WF: Arch Ophthalmol 98:1637, 1980.[152])

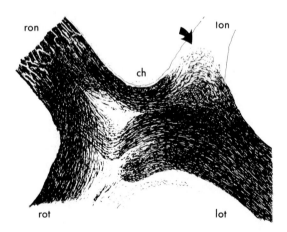

FIG. 23-4   Horizontal section stained by the Weigert method through the optic chiasm of a patient whose left eye was lost 24 years before death. The left optic nerve (lon) is completely atrophic. Note the course followed by fibers of the right optic nerve (ron) as they enter the right optic tract (rot) and left optic tract (lot). The arrow indicates the decussating fibers of Wilbrand's knee that detour into the fellow optic nerve. (From Polyak S: The vertebrate visual system, Chicago, University of Chicago Press, 1957.[121])

the chiasm the partial decussation of optic nerve fibers merges input from the two hemiretinas subserving the contralateral field of vision. Fibers from each eye representing common points in the visual field are aligned in approximate register, thereby maintaining a coarse retinotopic order in the optic tract. Fibers from the superior retinas occupy the dorsomedial portion of the optic tract, while those from the inferior retinas fill the ventrolateral optic tract.[70]

The lateral geniculate body

The lateral geniculate body is the principal thalamic visual nucleus linking the retina and the striate cortex. The majority of retinal ganglion cell fibers terminate in the lateral geniculate body. The nucleus consists of six principal cellular laminae separated by thin cell-free zones. The basic six laminae are often quite fragmented and irregular, making it difficult to recognize them clearly in some specimens.[60] Laminae 1, 4, and 6 receive axons from the contralateral nasal retina and laminae 2, 3, and 5 receive axons from the ipsilateral temporal retina.[110] This pattern of retinal input can be appreciated in Nissl-stained sections cut through the lateral geniculate body of a patient who died many years after loss of one eye (Fig. 23-5). Transneuronal atrophy is visible in laminae 2, 3, and 5 of the lateral geniculate body ipsilateral to the missing eye.

Each lamina of the lateral geniculate body contains a precise retinotopic map of the contralateral hemifield of vision. These maps are stacked in register so that a microelectrode passing along a dorsoventral projection line, like a toothpick through a club sandwich, would encounter cells sharing the same receptive field position in each lamina (Fig. 23-5).[158] The presence of multiple topographic maps, the variable laminar structure, and the folding of laminae around the hilum together result in an exceedingly complex internal three-dimensional retinotopic organization within the lateral geniculate body. Detailed maps have been compiled of the visual field representation in the macaque lateral geniculate body.[102] Comparable data are not available for the human. Central vision is thought to be represented in the caudal, 6-layered portion of the human lateral geniculate body. Rostrally, the lateral geniculate body is reduced to only 4 laminae by fusion of each pair of dorsal laminae. The periphery of the visual field is represented in this 4-layered region of the nucleus.

Draped over the dorsal convexity of the lateral geniculate body is a thin, crescent-shaped tier of cells called the pregeniculate or parageniculate nucleus. Little is known about the physiology or anatomy of this structure. It appears to receive innervation from the retina and from axon collaterals of principal cells of the lateral geniculate body. The pregeniculate nucleus may provide a recurrent inhibitory link to the lateral geniculate body.

The optic radiations

Neurons of the lateral geniculate body complete the relay of retinal input to the primary visual cortex by projecting to the ipsilateral occipital lobe. Their axons form a sheet of white matter called the optic radiations. Fibers representing the superior visual quadrant swing anteriorly around the temporal horn of the lateral ventricle before heading posteriorly toward the occipital lobe (see Fig. 23-9). This detour into the temporal lobe is known as Meyer's loop. Fibers representing the inferior visual quadrant reach the primary visual cortex by following a more direct posterior course within the white matter of the parietal lobe.

The primary visual cortex

The representation of vision in the cerebral cortex was explored early in this century by the clinical examination of soldiers wounded in battle.[63,86,141,144] Investigators constructed detailed retinotopic maps of primary visual cortex by matching visual field deficits with the trajectory of missiles penetrating the occiput. An updated version of these maps has been prepared recently with the aid of magnetic resonance, a high-resolution imaging technique that allows direct correlation of occipital lobe lesions with visual field defects in patients (Fig. 23-6).[68]

The upper and lower visual quadrants are represented in the lower and upper calcarine banks respectively, separated by the horizontal meridian along the base of the calcarine fissure. The fovea is represented at the occipital pole, where primary visual cortex usually extends about 1 cm onto the lateral convexity of the hemisphere. The vertical meridian corresponds to the perimeter of primary visual cortex located along the exposed medial surface of the occipital lobe (Fig. 23-6,A). Most of primary visual cortex is actually buried within the depth of the calcarine fissure (Fig. 23-6,B). The clearest view of the visual field map can be obtained by schematically unfolding and flattening visual cortex to

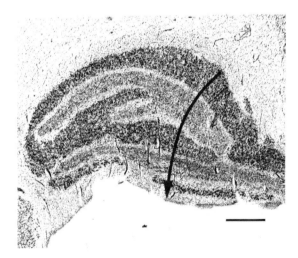

FIG. 23-5 Nissl stained section through the left lateral geniculate body from a 57-year-old man who died 23 years after enucleation of the left eye. Laminae 1,4, and 6 appear normal. Laminae 2 and 3 (fused) and 5 are pale due to transneuronal degeneration of their cells. The curved arrow marks a projection line through common retinotopic points in each laminae. Scale bar = 1 mm. (From Horton JC, Hedley-Whyte ET: Phil Trans R Soc Lond B 304:255, 1984.[67])

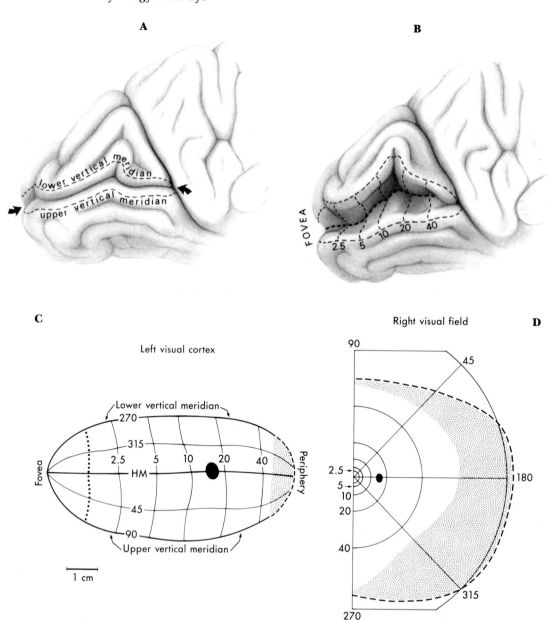

FIG. 23-6 **A,** Left occipital lobe showing location of striate cortex within the calcarine fissure (running between arrows). The boundary (*dashed line*) between striate cortex (V1) and extrastriate cortex (V2) contains the representation of the vertical meridian. **B,** View of striate cortex after opening the lips of the calcarine fissure. The dashed lines indicate the coordinates of the visual field map. The representation of the horizontal meridian runs approximately along the base of the calcarine fissure. The vertical dashed lines mark the isoeccentricity contours from 2.5° to 40°. Striate cortex wraps around the occipital pole to extend about 1 cm onto the lateral convexity where the fovea is represented. **C,** Schematic map showing the projection of the right visual hemifield upon the left visual cortex by transposing the map illustrated in **B** onto a flat surface. The row of dots indicates approximately where striate cortex folds around the occipital tip. The black oval marks the region of striate cortex corresponding to the contralateral eye's blind spot. It is important to note that considerable variation occurs among individuals in the exact dimensions and location of striate cortex. HM = horizontal meridian. **D,** Right visual hemifield plotted with a Goldmann perimeter. The stippled region corresponds to the monocular temporal crescent which is mapped within the most anterior 8 to 10% of striate cortex. (From Horton JC, Hoyt WF: Arch Ophthalmol 109:816, 1991.[68])

create an artificial planar surface (Fig. 23-6,C). The primary visual cortex contains a topographic but highly distorted representation of the contralateral hemifield of vision (Fig. 23-6,D).

The most striking feature of the visual field map is the enormous fraction of visual cortex assigned to the representation of central vision. Quantitative measurements in macaque monkey reveal that between 55 and 60% of the surface area of primary visual cortex is devoted to the representation of the central 10° of vision.[33,155] The linear cortical "magnification factor"—the millimeters of cortex representing one degree of visual field—has a ratio of more than 40:1 between the fovea (0° eccentricity) and the periphery (60° eccentricity).[33] The temporal crescent representation (shaded area, Fig. 23-6,D) constitutes less than 10% of the total surface area of primary visual cortex.[65,89] The representation of central vision is highly magnified compared with peripheral vision, so that the cortical area devoted to the central 1° of visual field roughly equals the cortical area allotted to the entire monocular temporal crescent.

The relatively magnified representation of the macula in primary visual cortex furnishes an important clue to how the cerebral cortex analyzes sensory information. The linear magnification factor of the retina is equal to about 250 μm of tissue per degree for all points in the visual field. The linear magnification factor of the retina must remain nearly constant, because the eye is engaged in processing an optical image of the visual environment. The steep gradient in visual acuity, from 20/20 centrally to 20/400 peripherally, is achieved by variation in the density of cells in the ganglion cell layer. In central retina the ganglion cells are stacked 6 to 8 cells deep, declining to a broken monolayer in peripheral retina. Free of any optical constraints, the cerebral cortex handles the richer flow of visual information emanating from the central retina in a different fashion. The cortical mantle maintains uniform thickness throughout primary visual cortex but allocates more tissue for the analysis of central vision. In the visual cortex the magnification factor, rather than the cell density, varies with eccentricity in the visual field representation. From the fovea to the periphery of the visual field a roughly parallel relationship exists between cortical magnification factor, ganglion cell density, and visual acuity. A similar strategy is employed by the somatosensory cortex to represent the most densely innervated regions of the body surface, as exemplified by the exaggerated size of the face, tongue, and hands of the homunculus.

The distorting effect of the cortical magnification factor can be appreciated at a glance by viewing the cerebral image of a visuscope target (Fig. 23-7).[147] In this experiment by Tootell and coworkers, a monkey was trained to view a flashing visuscope target while receiving an intravenous injection of ^{14}C-2-deoxyglucose, a radioactive tracer that accumulates preferentially in metabolically active brain regions. In an autoradiograph prepared from a section through the left visual cortex the cortical pattern of deoxyglucose uptake provides a direct view of the central portion of the retinotopic map. Note that

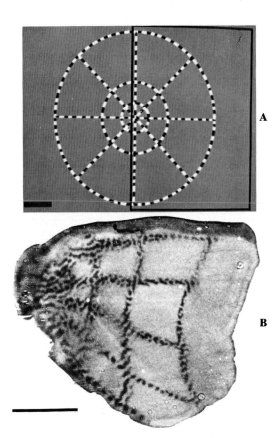

FIG. 23-7   A, Visuscope stimulus consisting of rings at 1°, 2.3°, and 5.4° viewed by monkey during a 2-deoxyglucose injection. The area enclosed by the solid black rectangle (not actually part of the original stimulus) indicates portion of visual field activating the animal's left occipital lobe. Scale bar = 2°. B, Corresponding 2-deoxyglucose autoradiograph of a tangential section through the left striate cortex showing pattern of activity generated by the stimulus in A. The fovea is represented at the far left, the periphery to the far right. Compare pattern of metabolic activity with the representation of the central 5° of visual field depicted in Figure 23-6,C. Scale bar = 1 cm. (From Tootell RBH, et al: J Neurosci, 8:1531, 1988.[147])

the rings and rays become thinner moving away from the center of the target because of the decline in cortical magnification factor with increasing eccentricity. The peripheral rings also appear more closely spaced in the cortical image than in the actual visual stimulus.

VISUAL FIELD EXAMINATION

Vision may be impaired by damage to the afferent visual pathway anywhere from the retina to the occipital lobe. The preservation of topographic order within the retino-geniculo-cortical pathway usually allows accurate localization of lesions causing a disturbance in vision by careful examination of the visual fields. The mapping and interpretation of the visual fields is a clinical art learned best by practice with patients. The goal of this section is merely to outline a few basic principles by correlating abnormalities in the visual fields with the anatomy of the sensory visual projection. A more extensive review of perimetry is available from other sources.[55,108,148]

Prechiasmal lesions

The crux of visual field analysis is to decide whether a lesion is located before, at, or behind the optic chiasm. A visual field deficit confined to one eye must be due to a lesion anterior to the chiasm involving either the optic nerve or the retina (Fig. 23-8, lesion 1). A visual field deficit in both eyes can result from either bilateral prechiasmal lesions or from a single lesion at or behind the chiasm. In attempting to distinguish between these two alternatives, the pattern of visual field loss can be helpful.

Certain patterns of visual field loss are characteristic of diseases that afflict the optic nerve. Glaucoma selectively injures axons that enter the superotemporal and inferotemporal poles of the optic disc. This pattern of nerve fiber loss produces arching, fan-shaped field defects that emanate from the blind spot and curve around fixation to terminate flat against the nasal horizontal meridian. This type of field defect, known as a Bjerrum scotoma, mirrors the arcuate course of fibers in the temporal retinal nerve fiber layer (see Fig. 23-1,C). Although nerve fiber layer defects are most commonly associated with glaucoma, they can occur from other diseases that attack the nerve fiber layer, optic disc, or distal optic nerve. Examples include optic disc drusen, pits, infarcts, or optic neuritis.

Certain diseases have a predilection for axons that serve the macula and the area of retina located between the macula and the optic disc. These fibers comprise the "papillomacular" bundle. When the papillomacular bundle is damaged, the patient develops a visual field defect that encompasses the blind spot and macula. This field defect is called a "cecocentral" scotoma. The papillomacular bundle emerges from the temporal aspect of the optic disc. Consequently, as the fibers of the papillomacular bundle degenerate, the temporal side of the optic disc develops marked pallor. The cecocentral scotoma is typical of the optic neuropathy caused by toxins like ethanol, tobacco, methanol, and ethambutol. It also occurs in patients with optic neuritis and Leber's optic neuropathy. The peculiar susceptibility of the papillomacular bundle to certain toxins, inflammatory processes, or hereditofamilial disorders, is a mystery.[119] We presume that the process— whatever it may be—must be acting fairly close to the optic nervehead, before the papillomacular bundle disperses throughout the optic nerve.

Inadequate blood supply to the optic disc results in ischemic optic neuropathy. This condition is frequently accompanied by an altitudinal pattern of visual field loss. Although the mechanism responsible for the altitudinal field loss is still under debate, the pattern is typical of optic disc ischemia, and therefore helps to localize the site of pathology.

Chiasmal lesions

The hallmark of chiasmal lesions is bitemporal hemianopia: the loss of vision in the temporal field of each eye (Fig. 23-8, lesion 2). For reasons that remain quite unclear, crossed fibers are more vulnerable than uncrossed fibers to compression of the optic chiasm by mass lesions. The most common culprit is a tumor arising from the pituitary gland within the sella turcica. Lesions situated at the junction of the optic nerve with the optic chiasm can produce an anterior chiasmal syndrome consisting of blindness in one eye and temporal hemianopia in the other eye (Fig. 23-8, lesion 3). The temporal hemianopia is usually most severe in the superior quadrant, a finding often attributed to injury of Wilbrand's knee of inferior crossed fibers (see Fig. 23-4).[165] Alternatively, the superior temporal hemianopia may be due simply to early compression of the optic chiasm. In rare cases a lesion just anterior to the chiasm will produce a temporal hemianopia in one eye only. This unusual visual field defect is caused by damage to crossing fibers that are segregated into the nasal portion of the optic nerve just before the chiasm.

Postchiasmal lesions

The decussation of fibers from the nasal hemiretinae at the chiasm aligns ganglion cells subserving the contralateral hemifield of vision in the postchiasmal segment of the visual pathway. Consequently, any lesion behind the chiasm will produce a homonymous hemianopia, namely a visual field defect involving matching portions of the overlapping temporal hemifield of the contralateral eye and the nasal hemifield of the ipsilateral eye (Fig. 23-8, lesions 5 and 8). It is important to realize that visual acuity will be entirely normal if the postchiasmal pathway in the other hemisphere is intact. Input from only half the fovea is sufficient for 20/20 Snellen visual acuity. A decrement in visual acuity should never be attributed to a unilateral postchiasmal lesion.

Frequently a homonymous hemianopia is incomplete and the visual field defects in each eye are incongruous (Fig. 23-8, lesions 4, 6, and 7). The degree of congruence depends upon how precisely inputs from each eye representing common retinotopic points are aligned at the site of the lesion in the visual pathway. As a general rule: the more congruent a visual field defect, the more posterior the lesion in the visual pathway.

Often it is difficult to ascertain whether a homonymous hemianopia is due to a lesion of the optic tract, lateral geniculate body, optic radiations, or visual cortex. A number of ancillary clues are available to guide the examiner. Usually a lesion of the optic tract produces a homonymous hemianopia with an afferent pupil defect in the contralateral eye (this localizing sign presupposes that both optic nerves and retinae are otherwise normal).[7] The afferent pupil defect in the contralateral eye occurs because ganglion cells in the nasal hemiretina outnumber those in the temporal hemiretina.[31] Consequently, a lesion of the optic tract damages more ganglion cell fibers driving the pupil reflex of the contralateral eye than the ipsilateral eye. This results in an afferent pupil defect in the contralateral eye. Small lesions of the brachium of the superior colliculus have been reported to produce an afferent pupil defect in the contralateral eye with no visual field defect in either eye.[40] The lesion causes selective injury to the asymmetric pupil fiber input to the pretectum from the two hemiretinae. No field defect occurs because retino-geniculate fibers are entirely spared.

Lesions of the lateral geniculate body are difficult to recognize with surety because they often occur in conjunction with lesions of the distal optic tract or proximal optic radiations. A homonymous hemioptic pattern of atrophy eventually appears in the ocular fundi after lesions that damage either the optic tract or the lateral geniculate body. Therefore, evidence of retrograde degeneration of ganglion cells and fibers (see Fig. 23-1,C) on fundus examination does not help one to differentiate between a lesion of the optic tract and a lesion of the lateral geniculate body. However, the presence or absence of an afferent pupil defect in the contralateral eye may be useful. An afferent pupil defect will develop after a lesion of the optic tract, but should not develop after a lesion of the lateral geniculate because axons governing the pupil reflex exit for the midbrain well before the lateral geniculate body.

Lesions involving the optic radiations or the visual cortex do not result in homonymous hemiretinal atrophy, because the primary projection from the retina to the lateral geniculate body remains completely intact. The only exceptions to this rule have been reported in patients suffering from congenital suprageniculate lesions. The fibers of the optic radiations spread out to form a broad fan of white matter after exiting from the lateral geniculate body. Injury to just a portion of the optic radiations occurs quite frequently and usually produces a partial homonymous hemianopia that appears roughly quadrantic.[42,154] For example, tumors of the temporal lobe may selectively injure Meyer's loop to cause a homonymous superior quadrantanopia (Fig. 23-8, lesion 6). Lesions of the white matter underlying the parietal lobe often result in a homonymous inferior quadrantanopia (Fig. 23-8, lesion 7).

Partial homonymous hemianopia also occurs from lesions that damage only a portion of the primary visual cortex. The conspicuous feature of an incomplete cortical hemianopia is the extreme degree of congruity. This congruity results because axons from right eye and left eye laminae of the lateral geniculate body terminate side-by-side in a finely dovetailed pattern of ocular dominance columns in visual cortex. Therefore, a cortical lesion produces equal damage to inputs corresponding to each eye for any given region of the visual field map. As a consequence, the visual field defects in each eye are virtually identical. By contrast, in the optic radiations the ocular inputs representing the same locus in the visual field are aligned less exactly so that lesions produce a more incongruous pattern of visual field loss. Occasionally, incongruous field loss is found in a patient with a cortical lesion: the incongruity reflects concomitant damage to the white matter underlying the cortex.

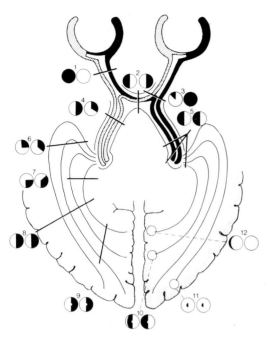

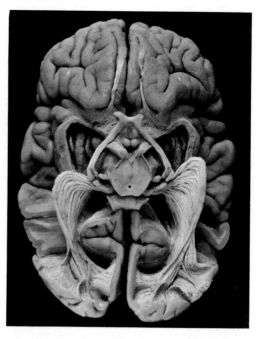

FIG. 23-8 Diagrammatic representation of the visual pathway showing abnormalities in visual fields produced by lesions at various levels. Visual fields are shown as viewed by patient, with black areas indicating areas of absent vision. Explanation for the field defect resulting from the lesion at each site is provided in the text. (Modified from Harrington DO, Drake MV: The visual fields: text and atlas of clinical perimetry, 6th ed, St Louis, CV Mosby, 1990.[55])

FIG. 23-9 Dissection showing the human retino-geniculo-cortical pathway viewed from the ventral aspect of the brain. The eyes and optic nerves have been severed at the optic chiasm. (From Gluhbegovic N, Williams TH: The human brain, Hagerstown, MD, Harper & Row, 1980.)

Macular sparing

Lesions in visual cortex sometimes produce a homonymous hemianopia with macular sparing (Fig. 23-8, lesion 9). In many patients macular sparing is nothing more than an artefact due to poor fixation during visual field testing. These factitious cases aside, macular sparing is a real cortical phenomenon that has perplexed clinicians for many years. In the past bilateral representation of the macula was invoked to explain macular sparing. According to this notion, macular vision is preserved after complete destruction of one occipital lobe because the macula is dually represented in the fellow occipital lobe. This explanation has become untenable in light of evidence from experiments in monkeys proving that the macula is not represented bilaterally in visual cortex.[37,147] In the representation of the fovea the receptive field centers of neurons do not stray more than $\frac{1}{12}$th of 1° into the ipsilateral visual field.[37]

A nasotemporal overlap across the vertical midline about 1° wide in central retina occurs in the decussation of ganglion cell axons at the chiasm.[20,49,93,142] This scatter in central projections has been offered as an explanation for macular sparing.[93] If correct, macular sparing would not be a special feature of lesions in visual cortex but would occur just as frequently after lesions of the optic chiasm or optic tract. Moreover, this theory could account at most for 1 to 2° of macular sparing. In practice, macular sparing usually extends beyond this eccentricity.

The extreme cortical magnification of the macula is the key to understanding the problem of macular sparing. In most individuals the vascular supply to primary visual cortex is provided by the posterior cerebral artery. After infarction of the territory of the posterior cerebral artery, a complete, macula-splitting homonymous hemianopia ensues. However, in some patients the occipital pole straddles the vascular territories of the posterior cerebral artery and the middle cerebral artery.[140] In these patients the occipital pole survives after posterior cerebral artery occlusion, due to perfusion by the middle cerebral artery. Because the representation of central vision is so magnified, the preservation of posterior visual cortex spares tissue devoted exclusively to macular vision. If only the occipital tip becomes infarcted, the converse is produced: a homonymous hemimacular field defect with peripheral sparing (Fig. 23-8, lesion 11).

The unpaired extreme nasal retina is represented along the anterior border of visual cortex near the confluence of the calcarine and parieto-occipital fissures (see Fig. 23-6). A lesion in this area causes a field defect limited to the temporal crescent of the contralateral eye (Fig. 23-8, lesion 12).[10] There is no other site behind the chiasm where a lesion can produce a visual field defect in one eye only. In practice such visual field defects are extremely rare, probably because few symptomatic lesions remain confined to such a small patch of visual cortex.

Complete bilateral injury or infarction of the occipital lobes results in total blindness. Lesions of both optic nerves, tracts, or the chiasm can also cause total blindness. These two situations can be differentiated by examination of the pupils. Pupillary responses to light will be absent in patients with total blindness of infrageniculate origin.

STRUCTURE AND FUNCTION OF THE LATERAL GENICULATE BODY

In the nervous system afferent information from every sensory system except olfaction passes through the thalamus before reaching the cerebral cortex. The lateral geniculate body is often called a thalamic "relay station," as if its function were merely to transmit a faithful copy of the retinal output to the visual cortex. Our intuition argues that the lateral geniculate body must do something more important than provide a simple conduit for information passing from the eye to the occipital lobe. The lateral geniculate body has been the subject of extensive investigation by researchers attempting to elucidate its role in visual perception. In this section we shall review current knowledge about the anatomy and physiology of the lateral geniculate body.

Receptive field organization

Cells in the visual system discharge action potentials spontaneously even in the absence of stimulation. For every cell this spontaneous activity can be influenced by stimulation with light in some region of the visual field. This special zone is called the "receptive field" of the cell.

Kuffler first described the receptive field properties of mammalian ganglion cells by recording extracellular potentials in the cat retina.[88] He made the landmark discovery that receptive fields of ganglion cells are organized in a remarkable concentric center-surround configuration. For on-center cells the field center is excited by light stimuli, whereas the surround is inhibited by light stimuli and excited by dark stimuli. For off-center cells the reverse holds true (see Chapter 19).

Neurons in the lateral geniculate body share with retinal ganglion cells the same basic center-surround arrangement of their receptive fields.[74,163] On-center cells respond with a burst of spikes when a small spot of light stimulates the field center (Fig. 23-10,A). The maximal response is obtained by choosing a spot size equal to the diameter of the receptive field center (Fig. 23-10,B). If the spot is larger than the field center the cell's response is attenuated, indicating antagonism between the center and the surround subfields (Fig. 23-10,C). A light annulus suppresses spontaneous activity and produces a brisk "off" response (Fig. 23-10,D). In the monkey on-center cells are slightly more numerous than off-center cells in the retina and in the lateral geniculate body.

Diffuse light is a mediocre stimulus for neurons with center-surround receptive field organization, because the field center and the surround have offsetting effects upon the cell's discharge rate. The center is slightly more effective than the surround in driving most retinal ganglion cells, so a weak "on" or "off" response occurs to diffuse light, depending on the cell type. The surround of geniculate cells is relatively more effective at canceling the center, making geniculate cells even less responsive to illumination of the entire receptive field. This enhancement of antagonism by the field surround is one putative function of the lateral geniculate body.[74]

The inputs of geniculate cells are wired together to generate the more elaborate receptive fields of cortical cells. Cells in visual cortex are virtually unresponsive to stimulation with diffuse light. Thus it appears that as receptive field requirements become more stringent in the hierarchy from retina to lateral geniculate body to visual cortex, diffuse light becomes progressively less effective as a stimulus.

Information about absolute light intensity is generally not important for the visual system, except perhaps for the small subclass of retinal ganglion cells that drives the pupil light reflex. Information about spatial discontinuities in pat-

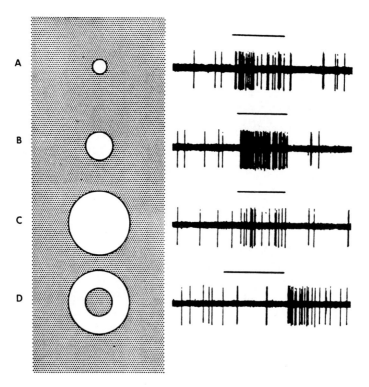

FIG. 23-10   Responses of an on-center neuron in the cat lateral geniculate body. Light stimuli are shown on left and the cell's action potentials, as recorded with an extracellular microelectrode, are shown on right. Straight horizontal lines above responses indicate when stimulus is on; stimulus duration is 1 second. Stimuli **A**, **B**, and **C** are spots 1°, 2°, and 14° in diameter centered in receptive field. Stimulus **D** is an annulus with inner diameter of 2° and outer diameter of 14°. (From Hubel DH, Wiesel TN: J Physiol (Lond) 155:385, 1961.[74])

terns of light energy is more useful for image analysis. Cells with center-surround receptive field organization are ideally suited for detecting such contrasts. Their best responses are elicited by contours illuminating just a portion of their receptive field. For example, a robust discharge would be elicited by a light stimulating the entire field center and only a portion of the field surround.

Synaptic inputs

The lateral geniculate body has always attracted the interest of anatomists because of its conspicuous, layered cellular architecture. Numerous theories have been devised to explain why the visual field representation in the lateral geniculate is stratified into multiple laminae. Le Gros Clark suggested that this arrangement serves color vision, with each pair of laminae assigned to one of the three cone systems: red, green, or blue.[23] Although his theory has long been refuted, it will become clear in the next few sections that his notion of functional specificity in the pattern of retinal connections to individual

laminae of the lateral geniculate body has been fully vindicated.

The axon terminals of single optic tract fibers can be labeled by anterograde filling with tracers like horseradish peroxidase (Fig. 23-11). In the cat individual optic tract fibers project to both the midbrain and the lateral geniculate body.[17] In the monkey, however, separate populations of optic tract fibers project to either the midbrain or the lateral geniculate body.[27,107] Moreover, any given optic tract fiber arborizes exclusively within a single geniculate lamina. Each axon terminal plexus makes about a 100 synaptic contacts over an area 50 to 100 μm wide. Although tract fibers end in a veritable spray of terminals, exquisite specificity is preserved in connections with geniculate cells. Serial reconstruction of synaptic circuits involving single retinogeniculate axons indicates that contact is made upon only a handful of the postsynaptic geniculate cells with dendrites available within the terminal field of a given optic tract fiber.[54] Each optic tract fiber may synapse with as few as 4 to 6 geniculate cells and each genic-

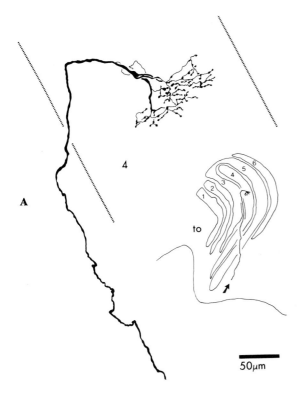

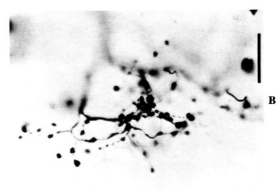

FIG. 23-11 **A**, Sketch of a single horseradish peroxidase labeled optic tract fiber terminating in parvocellular lamina 4 of the macaque lateral geniculate body. **B**, Higher power photomicrograph of the terminal plexus of the axon shown in **A**. Scale bar = 20 μm. (From Conley M, Fitzpatrick D: Vis Neurosci 2:287, 1989.[27])

ulate cell receives input from even fewer tract fibers. These anatomic studies of synaptic contacts made by individual optic tract fibers suggest that minimal divergence or convergence occurs in the processing of retinal information by the lateral geniculate body.

This conclusion is supported by physiologic evidence obtained in cats from simultaneous recording of the input and output of the lateral geniculate body. By placing one electrode in the retina and a second electrode in the lateral geniculate body, it is possible to correlate the firing patterns of cell pairs.[26] A single spike from a retinal ganglion cell fiber is sufficient to elicit a single spike from a geniculate cell. On-center ganglion cells trigger only on-center geniculate cells and off-center ganglion cells drive only off-center geniculate cells. Some geniculate neurons derive their excitatory input from only a single ganglion cell. For the majority of geniculate cells the excitatory input is provided by 2 or 3 ganglion cells.

The lateral geniculate body contains about 1,800,000 neurons.[24] The exact number of ganglion cells in the retina is a subject of endless debate, but 1 million is a reasonable estimate. Approximately 90% of the retinal ganglion cells terminate in the lateral geniculate body,[118] yielding a ratio of ganglion cell fibers to geniculate neurons of 1:2. This ratio is consistent with data suggesting that each geniculate cell receives input from 2 to 3 optic tract fibers and that each optic tract fiber contacts 4 to 6 geniculate cells. These average synaptic ratios probably vary with eccentricity and may differ slightly depending upon the geniculate lamina in question.

Magno versus parvo

Even upon casual inspection a striking difference is apparent in the morphology of neurons in the dorsal laminae and the ventral laminae of the primate lateral geniculate body. The two ventral laminae contain loosely packed cells with giant somas that exceed 30 μm in diameter. They are commonly referred to as the "magnocellular" laminae [Lat. *magnus*, great]. The four dorsal laminae are comprised of much smaller neurons and hence are known as the "parvocellular" laminae [Lat. *parvus*, small]. This anatomic dichotomy provides a powerful hint that neurons in dorsal and ventral laminae of the lateral geniculate body play different functional roles in the processing of visual information.

This view was bolstered by Enroth-Cugell and Robson,[41] who provided the first evidence that two distinct retinal ganglion cell populations project to the lateral geniculate body. Testing cat ganglion cells with stationary sinusoidal grating patterns, they found that some cells had a "null position" where contrast reversals gave no response. At the null position spatial summation of the receptor elements in the center and surround of the cell's receptive field canceled in a linear fashion. These units were termed "X" cells. Another class of retinal ganglion cells lacked a null position and hence demonstrated nonlinear spatial summation. These units were called "Y" cells. These two categories of cells differed in a number of other important respects.[41,48] In general, X cells had smaller receptive fields and gave more sustained, tonic responses to visual stimulation. Y cells had larger receptive fields and more transient, phasic responses. A few years after ganglion cells were classified as X or Y by physiologic criteria, two morphological cell types called "alpha" and "beta" were identified in the cat retina.[18] Correlative experiments later proved that α cells are the anatomic counterpart of Y cells, and β cells are equivalent to X cells.

In primate retina Polyak[121] used the Golgi method to identify at least five different types of ganglion cells. He called the two principal, most numerous varieties "midget" cells and "parasol" cells. Midget cells were named on the basis of their diminutive size, uniformity, and small dendritic trees. They are the most common ganglion cell type in the retina, especially in the macula. Parasol cells were identified by their larger cell bodies and more generous, umbrella-like dendritic arbors. Subsequent investigators have confirmed Polyak's classification scheme and drawn an analogy between primate parasol and midget cells and cat α and β cells respectively.[94,117,118,159] This parallel is supported by microelectrode recordings describing X and Y physiological cell types in monkey retina.[34] They resemble X(β) and Y(α) cells in the cat retina, except for their responses to colored stimuli. The cat has poor color vision and therefore only an occasional ganglion cell with color-selective responses. By contrast the macaque monkey shares with humans a highly developed trichromatic color system. Consequently, many cells in the monkey visual system are exquisitely sensitive to stimulus wavelength (see Chapters 19 and 22). Midget (or P(for **Primate**)β) cells in the primate retina have color-opponent receptive fields. The field center and the surround receive input from different cone types, for example: red on-center, green off-surround. Parasol (or Pα) cells have broad-band fields that share a

mixed cone input to the field center and surround. These differences in color responses are significant, for they are subsequently reflected in the properties of cells in the parvo and magno layers of the lateral geniculate body.

The Pα and Pβ, or more plainly, type A and type B, nomenclature is popular because it simplifies the problem of trying to categorize the diverse population of ganglion cells in the primate retina. However, it oversimplifies, inasmuch as a variety of subtypes are almost certain to exist among and in addition to Pα and Pβ cells. Moreover, the retina contains other morphological classes of ganglion cells with separate projections to other central targets (see the table on page 729).

Functional specificity of geniculate laminae

In the primate lateral geniculate body the parvocellular laminae receive input from the midget (Pβ, B) retinal ganglion cells, and the magnocellular laminae receive input from the parasol (Pα, A) cells.[94,107,118] This pattern of innervation implies that the color-opponent and broad-band retinal channels remain segregated at the level of the lateral geniculate body. Physiologic recordings comparing receptive field properties of cells in magno and parvo geniculate laminae have confirmed this supposition.

In the parvocellular laminae the majority of cells have color-selective responses. Wiesel and Hubel[163] described three principal types of parvocellular units. The most common cell (Type I) has a standard center-surround receptive field arrangement. The center and surround have different spectral sensitivities because they are fed by different cone systems. A typical cell might give an "on" response to a red spot and an "off" response to a green annulus. Type I cells account for about 80% of parvocellular units. A much less common cell class (Type II) lacks center-surround receptive field organization. Type II cells are comprised of only a field center that is supplied by input from antagonistic cone populations with different spectral sensitivity. Such cells have chromatically but not spatially opponent receptive fields. They give an "on" response to one color and an "off" response to another color anywhere in the receptive field. Finally, a small group of parvocellular units (Type III) has center-surround field organization but no color selectivity. The field center and surround receive undifferentiated input from all cone types. These cells account for less than 10% of parvocellular units.

The magnocellular laminae are populated with "color blind" broad-band cells that have center-surround receptive fields. The majority resemble the Type III cells found in the parvocellular laminae. Another variety of cell (Type IV), unique to magnocellular laminae, has a broad-band cone input to the field center and a tonic suppressive surround supplied by long wavelength cones. These cells respond with dramatic, prolonged silence to a large red spot.

Parvo cells and magno cells differ in other important receptive field parameters besides their color responses. At any given eccentricity the receptive fields of magno cells are several times larger than the fields of parvo cells. Magno axons conduct action potentials to striate cortex more rapidly than parvo axons. Magno cells have higher contrast sensitivity than parvo cells. To visual stimulation magno cells give rapid, phasic responses whereas parvo cells give slow, tonic responses. In these various respects a parallel can be drawn between X and Y cells in the cat and parvo and magno cells in the monkey.[39,133,138] Parvo cells show linear spatial summation when tested with sinusoidal gratings and therefore qualify as X cells. However, many magno cells also demonstrate linear spatial summation and hence should not be classified as Y cells.[136] Since the X and Y designation hinges upon the question of spatial summation, in the macaque monkey this classification system does not differentiate between parvo and magno cells. For this reason most investigators avoid the terms X and Y in the primate and refer instead to dorsal "color-opponent" and ventral "broad-band" cells. Strictly speaking these designations are also inaccurate because some cells in the dorsal laminae have broad-band color responses (Type III cells) and some cells in the ventral layers have red surrounds (Type IV cells). The original labels, "magno" and "parvo," probably are the most suitable, inasmuch as they are based upon an obvious and incontrovertible difference in cell size. The possible significance for visual function of the separate magno and parvo divisions of the lateral geniculate will become more evident in the next sections as their connections are traced through the visual cortex.

In parvocellular geniculate the on-center cells and off-center cells are segregated into separate laminae.[133] Laminae 5 and 6 receive input mostly from on-center retinal ganglion cells and consequently contain mostly on-center cells. Laminae 3 and 4 receive input largely from off-center ganglion cells and are more richly populated with off-center cells. This pattern of retinal innervation suggests that one major function of the primate lateral geniculate body is to sort retinal on-off channels into different laminae. However, on-center and off-center cells are intermingled throughout the magnocellular geniculate laminae with no loss of specificity in their inputs from on-center and off-center parasol retinal ganglion cells.

This paradox returns us to the puzzling issue of the function of the lateral geniculate body in visual processing. The response properties of geniculate cells are remarkably similar to those of their retinal inputs. A single excitatory postsynaptic potential from a ganglion cell is usually sufficient to evoke a discharge from a geniculate neuron. There is little divergence or convergence in the transmission of information through the lateral geniculate body. In all these respects the lateral geniculate body appears to behave as a relay nucleus.

The lateral geniculate body receives a massive projection from neurons in layer VI of the visual cortex.[52] This reciprocal corticogeniculate projection might be expected to influence profoundly the receptive fields of geniculate cells. It offers an anatomic substrate for potential modulation of retinal inputs at the geniculate level before transfer to visual cortex. However, reversible inactivation of the corticogeniculate input by cooling striate cortex produces only slight effects upon the response properties of cells in the lateral geniculate body.[6] This surprising result leaves us without a clear understanding of the role of the lateral geniculate body. Although the analogy of a "relay station" seems unsatisfactory, we have at present no better model for geniculate function.

THE PRIMARY VISUAL CORTEX

In 1782 a medical student named Francesco Gennari described a thin white stripe running through the gray matter of the occipital lobe (Fig. 23-12). This stria, visible to the naked eye in fresh or fixed specimens, prompted him to suggest that the cortex might contain anatomically distinct regions. Before Gennari's discovery anatomists had assumed that the cortex was a uniform sheet of tissue lacking any internal subdivisions. Today neurobiologists have partitioned the cerebral cortex into dozens of discrete areas serving various functions in the human repertoire. Ironically, in describing the first cortical area in the brain Gennari had no inkling that he had stumbled upon the primary visual cortex. More than a century elapsed before Henschen finally proved that the stria of Gennari is coextensive with the primary visual cortex.

The primary visual cortex is often called "stri-

FIG. 23-12   Coronal section through the human occipital lobe processed to reveal the distribution of myelin. The stria of Gennari is visible as a thin dark line running between the two arrows. In gross specimens it appears as a white band. It delineates the boundaries of primary visual cortex within the calcarine fissure.

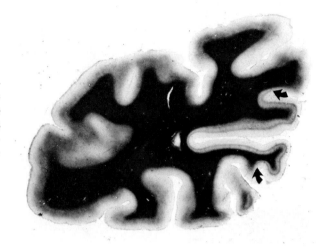

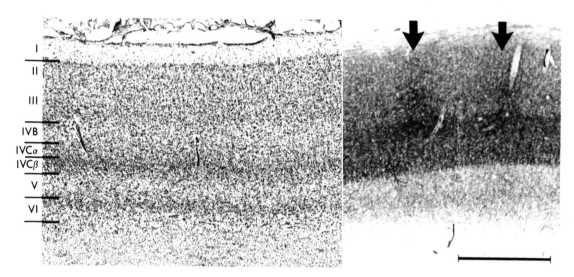

FIG. 23-13   Composite figure showing Nissl substance *(left)* and cytochrome oxidase *(right)* activity in a section of human striate cortex cut perpendicular to the pial surface *(top).* The Nissl stain for cell bodies reveals the cortical layers. The dark band of cytochrome oxidase activity in layer IV corresponds to the zone filled by geniculate afferents. Two cytochrome oxidase blobs are labeled with arrows. Scale = 1 mm.

ate cortex," referring to the prominent stria found by Gennari. Later Brodmann parceled the cerebral cortex into 47 different regions based upon subtle distinctions in cortical histology.[19] He assigned the arbitrary label of "area 17" to the primary visual cortex. In recent years other visual areas have been discovered in extrastriate cortex surrounding the primary visual cortex. The primary visual cortex has received the prosaic designation of "V1" [Visual area 1] and adjacent extrastriate visual areas are named V2, V3, V4, and so on. Primary visual cortex, striate

cortex, area 17, and V1 are all synonyms for the same piece of tissue.

Ocular dominance columns

In a tissue section of visual cortex stained for Nissl substance the most striking feature is the horizontal lamination of cell bodies (Fig. 23-13). There are six fundamental layers in the primate neocortex. In striate cortex some layers contain multiple sublayers, requiring neuroanatomists to append suffixes to laminar designations. Layer IVB includes the distinctive white myelin band that corresponds to the stria of Gennari. For many years this layer was thought to receive the projection from cells in the lateral geniculate body. This notion was debunked when the optic radiations were cut in a monkey and the stria of Gennari failed to degenerate.[25] The stria of Gennari is actually a dense, myelinated intracortical fiber plexus comprised of horizontally oriented pyramidal and stellate cell axons.[99]

Magno cells and parvo cells project to separate layers of striate cortex in the macaque monkey.[79] Magnocellular axons terminate in layer IVCα of striate cortex with minor branches entering the deeper portion of layer VI. Parvocellular axons innervate layer IVCβ and layer IVA, with small additional inputs to layer I and the upper portion of layer VI. Layer IVA is absent in humans, indicating that important differences exist among similar primate species in the cytoarchitecture of striate cortex.[67]

Axon terminals from right eye and left eye geniculate laminae are not randomly distributed in layer IVC of striate cortex, but rather, they are segregated into a system of alternating parallel stripes called ocular dominance columns.[79] These columns can be labeled by injecting a quantity of radioactive proline into one eye of a monkey.[82] After transport to the cortex via the geniculate body, the tracer is visible in autoradiographs of tissue sections cut through layer IVC. In humans the ocular dominance columns have been revealed in striate cortex by examining the distribution of cytochrome oxidase, a mitochrondrial enzyme.[67] This method exploits the fact that after monocular enucleation the levels of cytochrome oxidase diminish in columns formerly driven by the missing eye. In tangential sections from a patient who died many years after monocular enucleation, a mosaic of alternating light and dark stripes about 1 mm wide appears in layer IVC (Fig. 23-14). The light columns correspond to the ocular dominance columns of the enucleated eye.

LeVay[89] has reconstructed the complete pattern of the ocular dominance columns from serial autoradiographs in the macaque monkey (Fig. 23-15). In human striate cortex the ocular dominance columns are arranged in a very similar fashion.[65] They form a system of irregular parallel stripes oriented at right angles to the perimeter of striate cortex. As expected, ocular dominance columns are absent in the representation of the temporal monocular crescent. Near the monocular crescent representation the ocular dominance columns of the ipsilateral eye become relatively thin and fragmented. Presum-

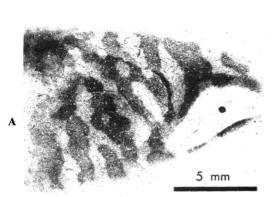

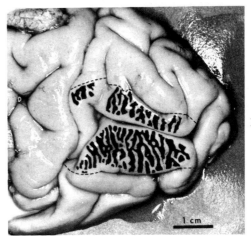

FIG. 23-14   **A,** Photomontage of serial tangential sections through layer IVC showing the ocular dominance columns in human striate cortex labeled by a histochemical stain for cytochrome oxidase in a patient who lost one eye many years before death. Metabolic activity is diminished in the pale columns corresponding to the missing eye. **B,** Partial reconstruction of the layout of the ocular dominance columns exposed on the medial surface of the right occipital lobe; the region illustrated in **A** is located at the lower right. The dotted line marks the V1-V2 border. (From Horton JC, Hedley-Whyte ET: Phil Trans R Soc Lond B 304:255, 1984.[67])

FIG. 23-15 The complete pattern of ocular dominance columns in striate cortex of the macaque monkey. The columns intersect the perimeter (vertical meridian; V1-V2 border) of striate cortex at right angles.
Ocular dominance columns are absent in the representation of the blind spot (solid oval) and the monocular crescent (far left). A few relieving cuts have
been made in the mosaic to reduce distortion. Note
that the ipsilateral eye columns (dark set) become fragmented and attenuated in the peripheral field representation. By flipping this figure left-to-right it can be
compared directly with Figure 23-6,C. (From LeVay et
al: J Neurosci 5:486, 1985.[89])

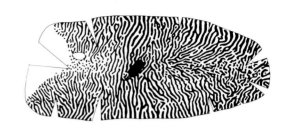

FIG. 23-16 Deoxyglucose autoradiograph of right
striate cortex in a monkey stimulated visually only
through the left eye. The pale oval corresponds to the
blind spot of the left eye. While viewing Figure 23-2
with both eyes open, the image of the blind spot target is processed within this zone. When the right eye
is closed, input to this zone is cut off and metabolic
activity drops. The blind spot target immediately becomes invisible. WM = white matter. Scale bar = 2
mm. (From Horton JC: Phil Trans R Soc Lond B
304:199, 1984.[64])

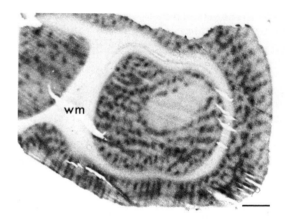

ably this appearance reflects the lower density
of ganglion cells beyond an eccentricity of 20°
in the ipsilateral temporal retina compared with
the contralateral nasal retina.[31]

Ocular dominance columns are also lacking
in the cortical representation of the blind spot.[89]
Their absence can be shown directly in the monkey by stimulating only the left eye with a random visual pattern during an injection of 2-
deoxyglucose.[64,87] In the right visual cortex a
pale oval is visible, corresponding to the blind
spot representation of the left eye (Fig. 23-16).
Of course, this area is not literally the blind spot
representation of the left eye, but rather a cortical region where cells are driven exclusively by
the right eye because the left eye contributes no
input. While viewing Figure 23-2 with both eyes
open, sensory information emanating from the
blind spot target is processed within this cortical
region. Upon closing the right eye the blind spot
"representation" falls silent and the blind spot
target fades from perception.

At the level of the lateral geniculate body no
binocular interaction occurs, because retinal afferents terminate in purely monocular laminae.
Convergence of afferents representing the right
eye and the left eye occurs only in striate cortex.
Binocular integration in the cortex is delayed beyond the initial tier of synaptic input by the segregation of geniculate afferents into ocular dominance columns. Microelectrode recordings in
macaque monkey confirm that neurons in layer
IVC are strictly monocular.[78] Cells that respond
to stimulation from either eye are found only
outside layer IV. Such cells owe their binocularity to convergence of inputs from monocular
cells in layer IV. The functional significance of
ocular dominance columns in humans and macaques is uncertain. In some species of primates
like the squirrel monkey the ocular dominance
columns are absent. In these animals the geniculate afferents representing right eye and left
eye synapse freely upon binocular cells in layer
IVC. This species difference in the organization
of the geniculostriate projection has no explanation.

Physiology of striate cortex

Hubel and Wiesel[75] were the first scientists to provide a coherent description of the receptive field properties of cells in striate cortex. Recording in anesthetized cats, they discovered new types of receptive fields never encountered at the level of the retina or lateral geniculate body. After cataloging the various cell types in striate cortex they proposed an ingenious model to explain how receptive fields are elaborated in the visual system.

Simple cells

The receptive fields of simple cells can be mapped into excitatory and inhibitory subdivisions with a small spot of light. They exhibit summation within their separate excitatory and inhibitory subfields and antagonism when both regions are stimulated simultaneously. In these respects simple cells are similar to the center-surround cells of the lateral geniculate body (Fig. 23-17,A and B). The critical distinction between geniculate cells and cortical simple cells lies with the spatial arrangement of their excitatory and inhibitory domains. For cortical simple cells these domains are not arrayed concentrically, but organized into parallel, flanking subfields separated by straight boundaries (Fig. 23-17). The geometry of the subfields varies considerably among simple cells. In the most common layout a narrow elongated region, either excitatory or inhibitory, is sandwiched between two symmetric subregions of the opposite type (Fig. 23-17,C and D). Some cells have subfields of unequal area (Fig. 23-17,E and F) and other cells have only two antagonistic subfields (Fig. 23-17,G). For all simple cells the best stationary stimulus is a slit or bar of light exactly the right dimensions to activate only an excitatory (on-response) or inhibitory (off-response) subfield. Diffuse light evokes a meager response, because excitatory areas and inhibitory areas cancel. Correct orientation of the light slit is crucial to obtain the maximum response. If the stimulating light bar is not parallel to the axis of the receptive field, it will stimulate part of the inhibitory subfield and fail to stimulate the entire excitatory subfield. Orientation selectivity is thus a cardinal feature of cortical simple cells. For the sake of illustration all the cells in Figure 23-17 are depicted with a preferred orientation of 45°. In fact, all orientations are represented equally in the visual cortex.

Simple cells also respond briskly to moving bars, slits, or edges, and sometimes the discharge pattern can be predicted from the arrangement of the excitatory and inhibitory subfields. Simple cells usually fire a burst of spikes just as a moving light slit enters an excitatory region. The most vigorous discharge is provoked by simultaneously leaving an inhibitory zone and entering an excitatory zone. Cells with symmetric subfield arrangements generally give an equal response to movement in either direction (see Fig. 23-17, C, D, and F). Cells with asymmetric subfields often give unequal responses to movement in opposite directions (see Fig. 23-17, E and G). The optimal speed of stimulus movement can also vary among simple cells.

Complex cells

The receptive fields of complex cells cannot be mapped with stationary stimuli into excitatory and inhibitory subregions. They give inconsistent on-off responses when tested with stationary slits or spots of light. However, when a light slit is swept across the receptive field, it elicits a sustained barrage of impulses (Fig. 23-18,D). A complex cell may respond to movement of the light stimulus anywhere within the receptive field, provided the stimulus is oriented correctly (Fig. 23-18). By contrast, a simple cell fires only

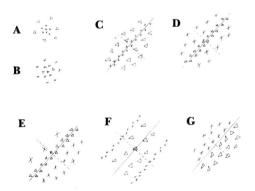

FIG. 23-17 Common arrangements of lateral geniculate and cortical receptive fields. **A**, "On" center geniculate receptive field. **B**, "Off" center geniculate receptive field. **C** to **G**, Various arrangements of simple cortical receptive fields. Crosses denote areas giving "on" responses, triangles denote areas giving "off" responses. Receptive-field axes are shown by continuous lines through field centers. (From Hubel DH, Wiesel TN: J Physiol (Lond) 160:106, 1962.[75])

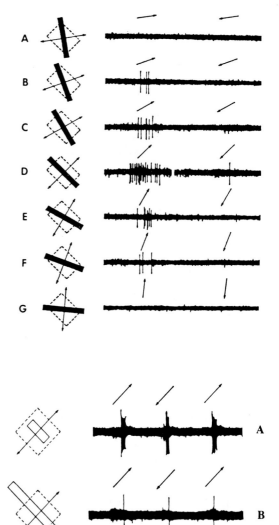

FIG. 23-18 Receptive field of a complex cell from monkey striate cortex. Outline of receptive field is given by dashed line. Orientations of bar stimuli are shown on left and responses to that particular orientation are shown on right. Arrows indicate direction of bar movement. (From Hubel DH, Wiesel TN: J Physiol (Lond) 195:215, 1968.[78])

FIG. 23-19 End-stopped complex cell recorded in monkey striate cortex. The activating region of the receptive field is outlined by the broken line on left. The moving slit of white light is represented by a solid rectangle and responses to movements are indicated by arrows over the oscilloscope tracings on right. *Top,* the stimulus is contained within activating region; *bottom,* it extends into antagonistic regions on either side and the cell's response is reduced. (From Hubel DH, Wiesel TN: J Physiol (Lond) 195:215, 1968.[78])

short bursts at the moment when the light slit crosses an interface between antagonistic subregions.

End-stopped cells

Ordinary complex cells show summation by responding more robustly as the length of a light stimulus is increased. The maximum response occurs when a slit or bar equals the full length of the cell's receptive field. Extending the stimulus beyond the length of the receptive field augments the response no further. A special subtype of complex cell behaves in a different fashion: the cell's response declines sharply as the stimulus exceeds the length of the activating portion of the receptive field (Fig. 23-19). The central activating region of these cells appears to be flanked by inhibitory subfields. Hubel and Wiesel[77] called these "hypercomplex" cells, assuming that they are higher-order complex cells constructed from standard complex cells. According to one model, excitatory input from a complex cell drives the activating region, while inhibitory input from neigboring complex cells accounts for the end-inhibition.

Years after Hubel and Wiesel invented the term "hypercomplex" cell, simple cells with end-inhibition were discovered in striate cortex.[38] The end-inhibition of these simple units may be generated by inhibitory input from geniculate cells or by inhibitory input from other simple cells flanking the end-stopped cell's activating region. Whatever the mechanism, this finding indicates that end-stopping is not a unique feature of complex cells and hence the term "hypercomplex" cell has been abandoned.

Receptive field hierarchy

Receptive fields undergo a remarkable transformation in the progression from lateral geniculate body to striate cortex. Cells in cortex respond best to suitably oriented bars or edges, rather than circular spots, and their responses depend critically upon the speed and direction of stimuli. How do geniculate cells generate the receptive fields of cortical cells?

Simple cells are concentrated in layer IV of striate cortex, the same cortical layer that receives the bulk of the projection from the lateral geniculate body.[51,75] Simple cells are also sprinkled throughout layer VI, another layer innervated by geniculate neurons. This finding is unlikely to be a coincidence: it suggests that simple cells receive their input directly from geniculate cells. The axons of simple cells ramify widely to synapse upon cells located in other cortical layers. Complex cells are common in all cortical layers except layer IV. The logical inference is that simple cells in layers IV and VI feed their input to complex cells situated outside layer IV.

Hubel and Wiesel[75] suggested that simple cell receptive fields are constructed from geniculate cell receptive fields. For example, the simple field in Figure 23-17,C might be generated by excitatory input from a row of geniculate cells with on-centers lined up as shown in Figure 23-20. In such a scheme a light stimulus falling within the narrow rectangular zone containing the geniculate on-centers will elicit a net response, despite partial stimulation of antagonistic field surrounds. The inhibitory subfields of the simple cell might derive from the off-surrounds of the geniculate cells, or perhaps from off-center geniculate cells placed in rows on either side of the on-center units. Alternatively, the flanking subfields might be due to inhibitory input from rows of on-center geniculate cells. With a little ingenuity all the receptive field types in Figure 23-17 can be generated by wiring together some combination of geniculate inputs.

The receptive fields of complex cells are probably built from simple cells that share the same orientation tuning. In one possible arrangement the receptive fields of simple cells are concatenated within the larger receptive field of a single complex cell (Fig. 23-21). A moving light slit will activate in succession each simple receptive field, eventually exciting a discharge from the complex cell. A stationary on-off stimulus elicits a feeble response because activation of only one

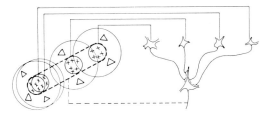

FIG. 23-20   Scheme proposed by Hubel and Wiesel to explain the organization of simple receptive fields. A large number of geniculate cells, four of which are illustrated in the upper right in the figure, have receptive fields with "on" centers arranged along a straight line in the retina. All of these project upon a single cortical cell and the synapses are supposed to be excitatory. The cortical cell receptive field will have an elongated "on" center indicated by the dotted lines in the receptive field diagram to the left. (From Hubel DH, Wiesel TN: J Physiol (Lond) 160:106, 1962.[75])

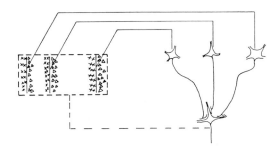

FIG. 23-21   Scheme proposed by Hubel and Wiesel to explain the organization of complex receptive fields. A number of cells with simple fields are imagined to project to a single complex cortical cell. In this example each simple cell has a receptive field arranged as shown to the left, composed of flanking excitatory and inhibitory zones (like those in Fig. 23-17,G) The boundaries of the field are staggered within an area outlined by the dotted lines. Sequential activation by a vertical edge stimulus moving across this rectangle, regardless of its position, will activate the simple cells and lead to excitation of the higher order cell. (From Hubel DH, Wiesel TN: J Physiol (Lond) 160:106, 1962.[75])

simple cell is not enough to drive the complex cell.

These circuit diagrams for receptive fields of simple cells and complex cells were published with a disclaimer that they "are obviously tentative and should not be interpreted literally."[75] Their stated purpose was simply to provide a conceptual framework for understanding the responses of cortical cells in terms of their inputs. To prove these models directly is difficult. For example, evidence that a given complex cell derives input from simple cells as shown in Figure 23-21 would require recording from the complex cell while searching with other microelectrodes to identify all the simple cells providing direct synaptic input. This sort of painstaking needle-in-a-haystack experiment is not feasible with current methods. One objection to the Hubel-Wiesel model stems from the observation that simple cells are actually quite scarce in striate cortex compared with complex cells. The circuit in Figure 23-21 would predict just the opposite. Data also suggest that cells with center-surround organization may synapse directly upon complex cells in macaque striate cortex. With new techniques and more experiments it will eventually be possible to unravel the neuronal circuits responsible for the receptive field properties of cells in visual cortex. The Hubel-Wiesel model will undoubtedly need amendment in the future. Whatever revision is ultimately required, the model has inspired a generation of scientists interested in the organization of the cerebral cortex.

The role of simple cells and complex cells in visual perception is unclear, although their receptive field properties are well defined. Simple cells and complex cells respond best to oriented contours, suggesting that they process information about borders or edges. If their function is to outline the boundaries comprising a visual scene, how are features like texture, shading, or perspective incorporated in the signals of cells in striate cortex? The preference of cortical cells for moving stimuli is also a puzzle. Are cortical cells specialized to handle the moving objects within our environment, and if so, which cells encode the stationary elements? Or do microsaccades provide enough movement to activate cortical cells while viewing stationary targets? Finally, if striate cortex contributes to perception by abstracting the line segments and contrasts from a visual image, do other cells at a higher stage in the hierarchy synthesize inputs from striate cells to enable us to appreciate the overall scene? These unanswered questions are testimony that our understanding of cortical visual processing is still quite incomplete.

Functional architecture

In a microelectrode penetration aimed perpendicular to the cortical surface, all cells selective for stimulus orientation respond best to the same orientation of a light slit or edge (Fig. 23-22).[75,78] This finding indicates that cells shar-ing the same orientation preference are grouped into columns. The aggregation into columns of cells sharing the same value for any given receptive field parameter is a commonly employed strategy in cortical processing. Orientation columns and ocular dominance columns are the two clearest examples in striate cortex. While the significance of columnar organization is not fully understood, it allows efficiency in patterns of intracortical projections. If the scheme in Figure 23-21 is correct, inputs from simple cells with any given orientation must converge upon complex cells in different layers sharing the same orientation. Presumably the most economical way of wiring the connections between these cells is to stack them into vertical columns spanning the cortex from pia to white matter.

In electrode penetrations tangential to the cortical layers the optimal stimulus orientation gradually shifts in either a clockwise or counterclockwise direction, with occasional reversals or abrupt shifts, indicating that orientation columns are arranged in a semi-orderly fashion. An advance of about 1 to 2 mm is usually sufficient to rotate 180° through a complete set of orientation columns.[80] The layout of the orientation columns has been visualized with the 2-deoxyglucose technique and with several new optical techniques that allow in vivo surface imaging of activity in striate cortex.[14,84,149] The orientation columns form a complicated latticework of stripes that intersect the ocular dominance columns randomly. The two columnar systems interweave so extensively that any given block of cortical tissue measuring a few mm² in surface area is endowed with a full complement of orientation columns (0° to 180°) and ocular dominance columns (right eye plus left eye). Such a module of cortical tissue contains cells responsive to all orientations presented in either eye (see Fig. 23-22).[82]

In an electrode penetration through the cortex the receptive fields of all cells cluster in the same part of the visual field (Fig. 23-23). There is some scatter in the exact position of each receptive field, so that any locus in the cortex corresponds to a region, rather than a single point in the visual field. This region, called the "aggregate receptive field," is defined as the product of scatter and field size of individual units. It is measured by circumscribing all the overlapping receptive fields plotted in a single vertical pass through the cortex.

Aggregate receptive field size varies in a parallel fashion with eccentricity.[81] Near the representation of the fovea the aggregate receptive fields are small. They become steadily larger as

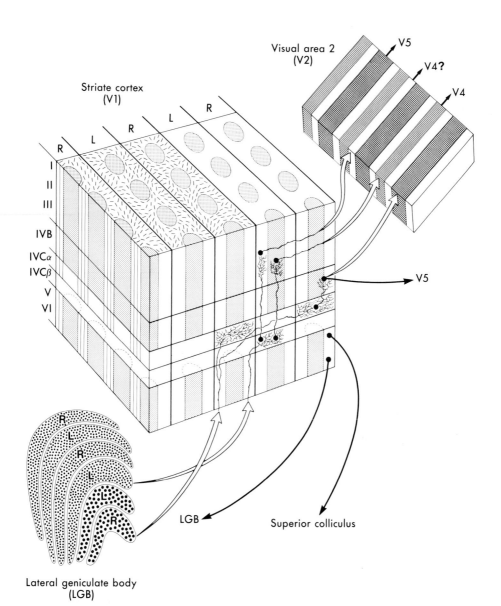

FIG. 23-22 Schematic diagram showing the magno and parvo pathways from the lateral geniculate body through V1 and V2 to areas V4 and V5. Each module of striate cortex contains a few complete sets of ocular dominance columns (R + L), orientation columns, and about a dozen cytochrome oxidase blobs (stippled cylinders, with a break in layer IVC). The orientation columns (depicted with hash marks on the cortical surface) extend through all layers except IVCβ. Their borders are not discrete; preferred orientation varies in a continuous, not stepwise, fashion with movement of a microelectrode parallel to the cortical layers. The magno stream courses through layer IVCα, layer IVB, thick stripes in V2, and V5. The parvo stream projects through layer IVCβ to layers II & III. A minor projection to layer IVA, found in the monkey but not the human, is omitted in this figure. Cells within the cytochrome oxidase blobs project to thin dark stripes in V2. Cells within the interblob regions project to pale thin stripes in V2. Both thin dark and thin pale stripes in V2 probably project to V4 and other targets. In striate cortex layers V and V1 send projections to the superior colliculus and the lateral geniculate body respectively.

FIG. 23-23 Drift in aggregate receptive field position determined by mapping fields during a 4 mm tangential electrode penetration through striate cortex. A few fields were mapped along each of four 100 μm segments spaced at 1 mm intervals. These four groups of fields are labeled 0, 1, 2, and 3. Each new set of fields was slightly above the previous set, consistent with the direction of movement of the electrode in the cortex. Roughly a 2 mm net movement through cortex was required to displace the aggregate receptive fields from one region (0 to 2, or 1 to 3) to a completely separately, non-overlapping region. lf 10° designates left fovea 10° away. (From Hubel DH, Wiesel TN: J Comp Neurol 158:295, 1974.[81])

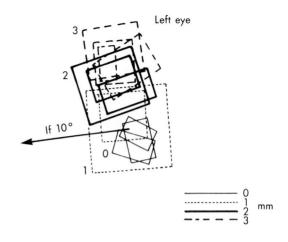

FIG. 23-24 Diagram showing how receptive field drift varies with eccentricity in the visual field. For the sake of illustration the right upper quadrant is shown in this figure. The circles represent aggregate receptive fields, namely, the collective territory occupied by all the receptive fields of cells encountered in a single microelectrode penetration perpendicular to the cortical surface. Each pair of circles represents the drift in aggregate receptive field position (*arrow*) accompanying a movement along the cortex of 1 to 2 mm. Both displacement and the aggregate field size vary with distance from the fovea, but they do so in a parallel fashion. Close to the fovea the fields are tiny, but so is the displacement accompanying 1 to 2 mm movement through the cortex. The greater the distance from the fovea, the greater the aggregate field displacement. (From Hubel DH, Wiesel TN: Proc R Soc Lond B 198:1, 1977.[82])

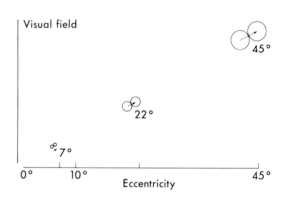

the recording microelectrode moves tangentially through the cortex towards the representation of the periphery of the visual field (Fig. 23-24). In macaque striate cortex a movement from one aggregate receptive field to an adjacent aggregate receptive field requires an electrode advance of about 2 mm. This value of 2 mm is a constant for all regions of striate cortex. It does not depend upon eccentricity, although of course the actual shift measured in degrees becomes greater the more peripherally the electrode moves in the visual field representation. A 2 mm electrode advance is also sufficient to traverse a full set of ocular dominance columns and orientation columns. This coincidence led Hubel and Wiesel[82] to hypothesize that striate cortex is diced into hundreds of modules, each containing a complete system of columns for analysis of visual information from any given portion of the visual field (see Fig. 23-22). More modules are allocated to central vision than peripheral vision, reflecting the higher cortical magnification of central vision. By the same token, modules representing central vision have much smaller aggregate receptive fields.

Cytochrome oxidase blobs

When Hubel and Wiesel suggested that striate cortex is subdivided into several hundred blocks of tissue, each containing a copy of the same basic visual processing unit, their module was a mere abstraction. It did not actually correspond to a real structure with defined boundaries that could be measured or photographed in a tissue section. A few years later strong anatomical support for their hypothesis was obtained from histochemical studies of striate cortex.[166] A stain for cytochrome oxidase revealed a spectacular array

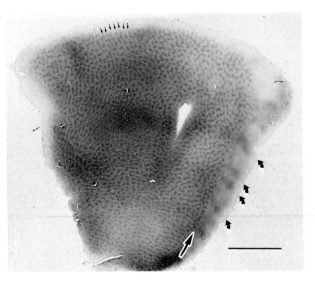

FIG. 23-25 The cytochrome oxidase stain reveals a regular array of blobs in layers II & III of a tangential section cut through striate cortex of the rhesus (macaque) monkey. The patches are arranged in long rows that are aligned with the ocular dominance columns in layer IVC. Refer to Figure 23-15 (right one-third of reconstruction) to view the layout of the ocular dominance columns in this particular region of cortex. The rows of cytochrome oxidase blobs intersect the V1-V2 border at right angles (small arrows). The V1-V2 border is best seen at the far right in this section, indicated by a single large arrow. In V2 a crude pattern of cytochrome oxidase stripes is present (curved arrows). The regular alternating pattern of thick, thin, and pale stripes shown in Figure 23-22 is not well visualized in this section. (From Horton JC: Phil Trans R Soc Lond B 304:199, 1984.[64])

of oval patches, most distinct in layers II and III, but visible in all cortical layers except IVC and IVA of macaque striate cortex (Fig. 23-25).[56,64,69] These patches are also present in human striate cortex.[67] Each patch is actually a cross-section of a vertical cylinder running through the cortical layers. The patches have been termed "blobs" because of their indistinct borders. They constitute zones of increased metabolic activity in striate cortex and can be labeled with special stains for many other enzymes besides cytochrome oxidase.

In macaque striate cortex cytochrome oxidase blobs are aligned in long rows spaced about 400 μm apart, like beads on a necklace (Fig. 23-25). After enucleation of one eye, the cytochrome oxidase blobs in every other row turn pale and shrink, reflecting a drop in their metabolic activity.[64,69] This result demonstrates that each row of cytochrome oxidase blobs fits in register with an ocular dominance stripe in layer IVC. While this experiment proves that blobs have a regular relationship with the columnar systems in striate cortex, the blobs are clearly much smaller than the modules originally envisaged by Hubel and Wiesel.[82] Their modules, defined as cortical domains of minimum size with nonoverlapping aggregate receptive fields, correspond to an ensemble of at least a dozen cytochrome oxidase blobs in layers II and III. This discrepancy underscores the fact that the iterative structure of striate cortex can be expressed in terms of either a physiologic concept (module) or an anatomic entity (blob). Whatever definition one prefers, it is remarkable that a sheet of tissue like striate cortex, engaged in processing sensory information from a seamless exterior surface like the visual field, should be carved into distinct repeating units.

The cytochrome oxidase blobs in the upper cortical layers receive a direct input from the lateral geniculate body.[64,95] In squirrel monkeys this projection appears to originate from a group of geniculate cells clustered into several distinct laminae intercalated between the parvocellular and the magnocellular laminae.[45,160] In macaque monkeys these intercalated layers are so small and fragmented it seems doubtful that they can account for the entire geniculate projection to the blobs. An alternative is that cells within parvocellular or magnocellular laminae project to the blobs. Input might derive either from a special subclass of cells projecting only to the blobs or from collaterals of axons projecting to layer IVC. More experiments are required to settle this issue. At any rate, the direct geniculate input to the blobs is relatively sparse compared with the massive intracortical projection contributed by stellate cells in layer IVCβ. It is likely, therefore, that the receptive field properties of cells situated within blobs are shaped more by intracortical input from layer IVCβ than by input from the geniculate body.

Hubel and Wiesel[78] originally claimed that the upper layers of macaque striate cortex contain only complex cells with oriented receptive fields. Dissenting reports of cells with unoriented or circularly symmetric fields were ignored because they ran counter to the prevailing model explaining how cortical receptive fields are generated (see Figs. 23-20 and 23-21). After the discovery of the blobs, extensive physiologic recordings were repeated in layers II and III and nests of cells with special receptive field properties were found within the cytochrome oxidase blobs.[96] The receptive field properties of these cells are radically different from those of complex, oriented cells situated in the interblob regions. Cells within cytochrome blobs have circularly symmetric receptive field organization and therefore lack any orientation selectivity. Moreover, about 70% of these nonoriented units give special responses to colored stimuli. Most of these color-coded cells resemble the four types of cells described previously in the macaque lateral geniculate body.[106,150] One new cell type has been discovered, called a modified Type II cell.[150] It has a color opponent center like a standard type II cell, plus an opponent surround that receives mixed cone input. The cell's response is reduced by colored spots larger than the field center or by annuli of any color. Modified type II cells are thought to provide a high-resolution channel for information about color contrast.

Microcircuitry of primate striate cortex

Our ultimate goal is to understand vision in cellular terms, by describing the properties and projections of every type of neuron involved in visual processing. The extraordinary increase in the complexity of striate cortex moving up the evolutionary ladder compounds the difficulty of this task. Humans are endowed with a striate cortex containing a diversity of cell types and connections unrivaled by any subprimate. Certain features like the stria of Gennari and the cytochrome oxidase blobs appear well developed only in primates.[64] Despite progress in identifying the basic components of the cellular microcircuit in primate striate cortex, any account is limited by serious gaps in our knowledge and the daunting intricacy of this tissue.

A cortical module is comprised of a few million cells. Each cortical module receives input from only a few thousand geniculate fibers.[24] The ratio of cortical cells to geniculate afferents ($\sim 10^6/10^3$) indicates that after relatively direct transmission through the lateral geniculate body, the retinal signal activates a cortical unit containing approximately a thousandfold more processing elements. Each parvocellular fiber makes several thousand synapses upon spiny stellate cells within a zone in layer IVCβ spanning about 200 μm.[13,47] The exact number of stellate cells contacted by an individual geniculate fiber is uncertain, because many synapses are made upon the same spiny stellate cell. About

15% of the stellate cells in layer IVCβ are inhibitory interneurons with aspinous dendrites and a positive immunoreaction for γ-aminobutyric acid (GABA).[100]

In cats geniculate cells with center-surround fields synapse in layer IV upon stellate cells with simple receptive fields. Surprisingly, in primates the expected jump in the hierarchy from center-surround to simple receptive field does not occur with the transition from geniculate to cortex. The spiny stellate cells in layer IVCβ in macaque striate cortex have circularly symmetric receptive fields. Their receptive fields have not been well studied but many cells appear similar to color-coded cells found in the parvocellular laminae of the lateral geniculate body.[78,96]

Stellate cells in layer IVCβ project most heavily to layer III.[99] It is unknown whether the blobs and the interblob regions in layer III receive inputs from separate subpopulations of cells in layer IVCβ. This seems likely given the striking differences in receptive field properties reported for cells in these two separate cortical domains. The majority of cells in the blobs have circularly symmetric receptive fields and color-selective responses. The interblob regions also contain color-coded cells, but their fields are oriented and complex. Their receipt of direct input from center-surround spiny stellate cells in layer IVCβ, without an intermediate tier of simple cells, appears to violate the Hubel & Wiesel model (see Figs. 23-20 and 23-21). How color-coded cells within the blobs and the interblob regions of layers II and III differ in their contribution to color perception is currently a matter of intense interest. Their roles are likely to be different because they maintain carefully segregated projections to V2, the next cortical target (see Fig. 23-22).

Magnocellular geniculate fibers arborize over a terminal field in layer IVCα six times greater in surface area than the terminal fields of parvocellular afferents in layer IVCβ.[13,47] The wider coverage of magnocellular units compensates for the fact that they are greatly outnumbered by parvocellular units. Each magnocellular fiber makes thousands of synapses with an indeterminate number of spiny stellate cells in layer IVCα. Information about the receptive field properties of cells receiving magno input is scant. Most cells in layer IVAα are simple, oriented, and not color-coded.[12,96] They send the bulk of their output to cells in layer IVB.[99,100] Cells in layer IVB have receptive field properties similar to those of cells in layer IVCα, except that a much greater proportion of layer IVB units are strongly direction selective.[96] Cells in layer IVB send their projection to a number of extrastriate targets, including V2 and MT.

Both magno and parvo geniculate fibers send collaterals to pyramidal neurons in layer VI. These pyramidal neurons also receive geniculate input via apical dendrites branching in layer IVC. Layer VI pyramidal cells send axon collaterals back to layer IVC, setting up a reverberating intracortical circuit of unknown function.[100] The pyramidal cells in layer VI are also believed to give rise to the major reciprocal projection to the lateral geniculate body.[52] Layer V, which receives input from layers II, III, and IVB, contains cells projecting to a number of other important subcortical targets, including the pulvinar and the superior colliculus.

In summary, striate cortex receives segregated input from two distinct geniculate cell channels, magno and parvo. The parvo input goes via layer $IVC\beta$ to layers II and III to supply cells within blobs and between blobs. Blob cells and interblob cells project to separate targets in the next visual area, V2. The magno input proceeds independently from layer $IVC\alpha$ via layer IVB to V2 and MT. The layers superficial to layer IVC give rise to the main extrastriate projections while the layers deep to IVC connect back to subcortical areas.

EXTRASTRIATE VISUAL CORTEX

According to the classical view, the striate cortex performs a basic analysis of geniculate input and then transmits some critical essence to higher peristriate cortical areas for further interpretation. Visual perception is thought to be enshrined in two visual association areas surrounding striate cortex, which Brodmann called area 18 and area 19.[19] In sections stained for Nissl substance these areas look quite uniform and even skilled anatomists have trouble distinguishing between them. Their apparent homogeneity in tissue sections prepared with routine neuroanatomical techniques camouflages a remarkable landscape of functional visual areas (Fig. 23-26). Recent studies in monkeys using physiologic recordings and anatomic tracers have revealed that areas 18 and 19 together contain at least five distinct cortical areas devoted to visual processing: V2, V3, V3A, V4, and V5. Other visual areas within and beyond areas 18 and 19 remain to be completely mapped and characterized. So far 25 cortical areas predominately or exclusively engaged in vision have been identified in the macaque monkey. An additional seven regions are classified as visual as-

sociation areas based upon their connections with other known visual areas, making a grand total of 32 visual areas interconnected by 305 separate pathways.[43] In the context of this maze of extrastriate visual areas, "area 18" and "area 19" are not meaningful labels, because they do not correspond to any single area or ensemble of areas.

The 32 visual areas in the macaque monkey occupy about 55% of the neocortex, implying that visual processing consumes a large amount of cortical tissue compared with other functions like audition or somesthesia.[43] The striate cortex constitutes the largest single cortical area, averaging 1200 mm^2 or about 12% of the neocortex. V2, just slightly smaller than V1, is the second largest cortical area. Together, V1 and V2 account for about 20% of the entire surface area of the neocortex. Progress in mapping the boundaries and connections of the various extrastriate cortical areas has far outstripped our ability to determine their contribution to visual function. In this discussion we will touch upon a few of the best understood extrastriate visual areas and speculate briefly about their role in vision.

Extrastriate visual cortex receives a weak thalamic input directly from the lateral geniculate body and the pulvinar. However, the vast bulk of the thalamic projection terminates exclusively in striate cortex. After completion of initial processing in striate cortex, visual information is transmitted to areas V2, V3, V4, and V5. Projections unite corresponding retinotopic points in the visual field representation in each of these cortical areas.

V2 and V3

The boundaries of V2 and V3 were mapped originally by cutting the splenium of the corpus callosum to disrupt axons that travel between the left and right hemispheres.[30,169] Transcallosal fibers unite the two visual hemifields by connecting neurons in each occipital lobe located along the representation of the vertical meridian in V1, V2, and V3. The distribution of degenerating terminals proved that the representation of the vertical meridian in V2 is shared along the common border with V1 (Fig. 23-27). The representation of the horizontal meridian in V2 splits within a few degrees of fixation to wrap around the outside of V2 along the border shared with V3.[3] The outer border of V3 contains a second representation of the vertical meridian.

V1, V2, and V3 are arranged to permit an orderly topographic representation of the visual

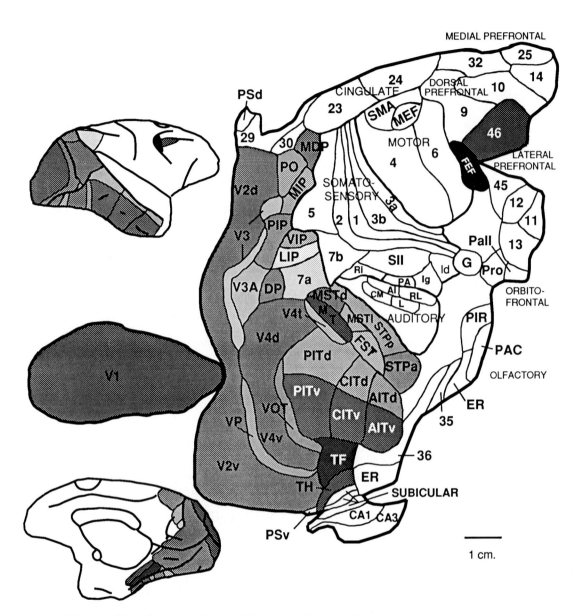

FIG. 23-26 Two-dimensional map of the cerebral cortex of the right hemisphere in the macaque monkey. The 32 separate cortical areas involved with visual processing are indicated with shading. A relieving cut has been made between V1 and V2 to minimize distortion in this flat representation of the brain surface. The total surface area of neocortex in this monkey hemisphere is 9940 mm², of which 5385 mm² (55%) is occupied by visual or visual association cortex. Some cortical areas are identified by the old Brodmann designations and other areas are identified by a modern alphabet soup of initials. (From Felleman DJ, Van Essen DC: Cerebral Cortex, 1:1, 1991.[43])

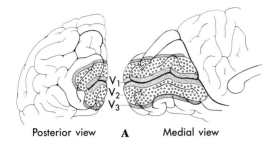

Posterior view   **A**   Medial view

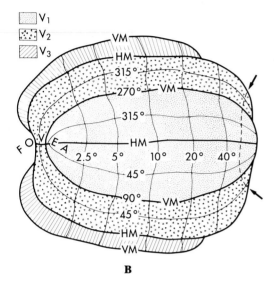

B

FIG. 23-27 A, Schematic diagram of the left occipital lobe of the human brain showing the arrangement of V1, V2, and V3 along the calcarine sulcus. The relative position and size of these different cortical visual areas varies widely among individuals. **B,** Flattened representation of the cortical areas shown in **A,** with coordinates of the right visual hemifield indicated directly on the maps (see Fig. 23-6,*D* for key to visual field coordinates). Note that the horizontal meridian in V2 splits within a few degrees of fixation to wrap around the outside of V2, dividing V2 into dorsal and ventral halves representing the lower and upper quadrants of vision respectively. The vertical meridian is shared between V1 and V2, and reduplicated along the outer border of V3. Ventral V3 is called VP (ventral posterior area) by some authors.

hemifield in each area while contact is maximized between adjacent cortical areas (Fig. 23-27). The brain appears to achieve the best compromise betwen the competing exigencies of retinotopy and contiguity by dividing V2 and V3 into dorsal and ventral halves that wrap around V1. As a result the inferior and superior visual field quadrants are mapped in a retinotopic fashion in V2 and V3, but are discontinuous across the representation of the horizontal meridian. V3 is actually divided completely into separate dorsal and ventral halves, representing the lower and upper contralateral quadrants of vision respectively (Fig. 23-27). Dorsal V3 and ventral V3 differ in their anatomical connections and physiological properties. Consequently, some investigators define ventral V3 as a separate cortical area called the ventral posterior area (VP, Fig. 23-26).[21,156]

The cytochrome oxidase stain reveals an array of coarse parallel stripes in V2 (see Fig. 23-22).[64,95,146] This pattern looks quite different from the fine mosaic of patches or blobs visible in V1. The stripes in V2 appear alternately thick and thin, and extend across the full width of V2 from the V1-V2 border to the V2-V3 border. The thin stripes receive input from V1 cells located within the cytochrome oxidase blobs in layers II, III.[96] The thick stripes receive input from V1 cells scattered throughout layer IVB.[97] The pale interstripe zones that separate the thin and thick stripes of intense cytochrome oxidase activity get their input from V1 cells located between the blobs in layers II, III (see Fig. 23-22).[96]

The receptive field properties of cells in V2 have been correlated with the stripelike pattern of cytochrome oxidase activity.[36,73] Unoriented, color opponent units are plentiful in the thin stripes. These cells are similar in many respects to cells within the cytochrome oxidase blobs in V1. The thick stripes contain rather few color-coded units, but instead, a high proportion of oriented, direction-selective cells. Most of these cells are selective for binocular disparity, suggesting that they may contribute to stereoscopic depth perception (Chapter 24). The pale interstripes are filled with oriented, complex cells that are not direction selective. Many of these units are color-coded and end-stopped.

These findings indicate that V2 is subdivided into separate domains comprised of cells with distinct receptive field properties. These domains also differ in terms of their cytochrome oxidase activity and their inputs from V1. Apparently the functional segregation evident in V1 is maintained at the level of V2. The subsequent pattern of connections between V2 and other extrastriate areas suggests that this division of labor is perpetuated at even higher levels of cortical processing (see Fig. 23-22).

V4

Approximately 20 years ago Zeki[170] discovered a cortical area in the lunate sulcus of the macaque monkey that contains a preponderance of neurons with selective responses to stimuli of different wavelength. This region, christened as V4, has come to be known as the "color area" in extrastriate cortex (see Fig. 23-26).[167] It receives a small direct input from V1 but derives most of its input from the color-coded cells located within the thin dark cytochrome oxidase stripes in V2.[36,139] Input may also be received from cells within the pale interstripes in V2. Most neurons in V4 have complex, oriented, and end-stopped receptive fields.[35,172] Only a minority of units are direction selective. The most distinctive characteristic of neurons in V4 is that they respond better to an optimal colored stimulus than to a white light.[131] In V1 a preference for colored stimuli is shared by a relatively low percentage of complex cells.

V5 (middle temporal area)

In their anatomic studies of the owl monkey Allman and Kaas[2] noticed a distinct cytoarchitectonic area in the middle temporal (MT) area defined by a very high content of myelin. Recording from this extrastriate area, they quickly established that it contains a representation of the contralateral visual hemifield. Zeki later recorded from an equivalent area in the macaque monkey, which he called V5. He reported that neurons in V5 were exquisitely sensitive to stimulus motion.[171] Some units responded well to a light spot, bar, or slit moved briskly in a preferred direction and gave no response to an opposite, null direction. For these cells the stimulus shape mattered little as long as the direction of movement was correct. Other units required a properly oriented slit or bar moved in a certain direction. These oriented

units resembled complex cells in V1, except that receptive fields of V5 units were much larger and invariably direction selective. Cells in V5 with common direction preference showed an intriguing tendency to cluster within columns together. Few V5 units showed any wavelength selectivity.

V5 receives a direct projection from layer IVB in V1 and from the thick cytochrome oxidase stripes in V2.[36,139,151] Both these afferent regions are populated with direction-selective units that presumably account for the directional selectivity of neurons in V5. Directional selectivity of cells is such a singular feature of V5 that it has been called the "motion area" in extrastriate cortex. V5 is thought to govern smooth pursuit mechanisms and perception of visual motion. Lesions placed in V5 selectively interfere with the ability of a macaque monkey to discriminate net direction of motion in a dynamic random dot display.[114] However, recovery of function occurs within a matter of weeks, suggesting that other cortical areas can take over the task of mediating motion perception. An alternative explanation is that the V5 lesions are less permanent than one might infer from inspection of histologic sections.

Functional specialization

The parcellation of extrastriate cortex into dozens of separate visual areas, far beyond anything contemplated by Brodmann's division of the occipital lobe into areas 17, 18, and 19, tempts one to endorse the view that different areas may serve specific aspects of visual perception. This concept has received some support from clinical studies with patients suffering lesions of the occipital lobe. Bilateral injury to the fusiform and lingual gyri has been reported to cause a disturbance in the perception of colors.[104] However, the deficit is not entirely selective, inasmuch as these patients often have other deficits consisting of a superior altitudinal field cut and trouble recognizing familiar faces or objects. V4 has not yet been identified in the human brain, so it is unclear whether V4 (or perhaps a different color area) has been damaged in these patients.

Selective impairment of motion perception has also been reported from lesions of the occipital lobes. Most of the evidence derives from a single, well studied patient with large bilateral lesions in the putative cortical motion area.[173] The lesions may have damaged the equivalent of V5 or the middle temporal area (MT). This is a matter of speculation, because the precise location of this area in the human brain is still unknown.

Clinical experience thus upholds the notion of selective impairment of visual function, although it is puzzling how rarely such patients are encountered in actual practice. Strokes and tumors tend to produce large, unselective lesions that show no respect for the boundaries of cortical areas. Nevertheless, by chance alone one might expect to encounter patients more frequently with lesions in discrete cortical areas causing selective functional deficits. Either visual parameters are less tightly compartmentalized than some researchers argue or else current methods used by physicians to screen patients for selective deficits are inadequate.

Segregation of function is implied by the anatomy and physiology of the visual pathway.[98,168] The color-opponent parvo channel projects to layer $IVC\beta$ of striate cortex and then divides to supply blobs and interblobs in the upper layers. Blobs and interblobs project to separate V2 domains. In V2 the thin stripes project to V4; the pale stripes may also project to V4. Thus V4 is fed by the parvo channel and richly endowed with color-coded cells. It seems reasonable therefore to consider V4 a "color" area, but one must recall that color information is also processed in other cortical areas (at least V1 and V2), and that V4 almost certainly handles other visual parameters such as form and texture. Interconnections between V4 and MT suggest considerable sharing of cortical function.[151] Moreover, color perception is only partially impaired after lesions in V4.[58] In the final analysis the issue of whether V4 merits the sobriquet of "color area" becomes a matter of definition and semantics.

The broad-band magno channel projects via layer $IVC\alpha$ to layer IVB. Filtering magno input through layer $IVC\alpha$ generates noncolor-coded, oriented, directional units that project to V5 and to the thick stripes in V2. The thick stripes in V2 also project to V5. These circuits, dominated by the magno channel, clearly play an important role in the detection of motion. Recent evidence suggests that other cortical areas adjacent to V5 are also involved in motion perception.[43]

The color-opponent and broad-band channels are most sharply segregated at the level of the lateral geniculate body. A clever approach to isolating their relative contributions to visual function involves making selective parvo or magno lesions in the lateral geniculate body of a monkey and then testing visual performance.[105,135] Such experiments show that parvo

lesions severely impair the perception of color, texture, pattern, and shape. Contrast sensitivity is greatly reduced for high spatial frequencies but only mildly reduced for low spatial frequencies. A major deficit in stereopsis is also produced, a finding that is quite surprising in view of reports that disparity-sensitive cells in V2 are concentrated in thick bands supplied by the magno system. After lesions of the magno geniculate layers, the most serious deficits appear in motion and flicker perception, particularly with low-contrast stimuli. The fast conducting, phasic magno units apparently are specialized to handle these aspects of perception.

In the past few decades new information about the central visual pathways has accumulated at an accelerating rate. Despite this rapid progress, our knowledge of most visual cortical areas is still rudimentary. More experiments and further data are required before we can explain vision in biological terms. Until then, the impulse to construct overly speculative models should probably be resisted.

VISUAL DEPRIVATION

Amblyopia is a fairly common disease affecting between 1 and 2% of the American population. It can be defined as a condition caused by abnormal visual experience during childhood resulting in unilateral or bilateral decrease in acuity that cannot be explained by a disorder of the eye itself. Often amblyopia is precipitated by some type of ocular anomaly—congenital cataract is the archetypical example—but even after removal of the media opacity and prescription of the proper refractive correction, the vision remains poor. Without an ocular explanation for the low acuity, ophthalmologists have speculated that amblyopia is caused by anomalous wiring of the eye's central connections in the brain. This view has been confirmed in dramatic fashion by elegant studies involving kittens and baby monkeys conducted by investigators working in a number of laboratories. In this section we shall review the normal development of the central visual pathways and then consider the pathologic effects of visual deprivation.

Intrauterine development

Data pertaining to the prenatal development of the central visual pathways in humans are limited by practical difficulties in obtaining adequately fixed specimens and the fact that powerful experimental techniques suitable for animal studies cannot be used to investigate human necropsy tissue. In the human retina most of the ganglion cells are generated between the eighth and fifteenth weeks of gestation.[103] The ganglion cell population reaches a plateau of 2.2 to 2.5 million by week 18 and remains at that level until the thirtieth week of gestation.[122,127] After week 30, the ganglion cell population falls drastically during a period of rapid cell death that lasts for about 6 to 8 weeks. Thereafter cell death continues at a low rate through birth and into the first few postnatal months. The ganglion cell population is reduced to a final count of about 1 million. The loss of more than a million supernumerary optic axons may serve to refine the topography and specificity of the retinogeniculate projection by eliminating inappropriate connections.[125]

In fetal macaque monkeys the neurons of the lateral geniculate nucleus are born between embryonic (E) days E36 to E43 according to ^{3}H-thymidine labeling studies.[124] Pregnancy in macaques lasts only 165 days compared with 280 days in humans. Adjusting for the difference in the length of pregnancy, macaque embryonic days E36 to E43 correspond roughly with human embryonic weeks 8 to 11. Assuming that the lateral geniculate body in humans is generated at an equivalent stage of pregnancy, the neurons of the human lateral geniculate are born between gestational weeks 8 and 11. By week 10 the first retinal ganglion cell fibers begin to invade the primordial human lateral geniculate nucleus. In the macaque, Rakic has shown that initially the inputs from each eye intermingle to occupy the entire lateral geniculate body.[124] The segregation of ocular inputs occurs on a parallel timetable with the development of lamination. Retinal afferents prune back their axon terminals so that synaptic connections are preserved only within appropriate geniculate laminae. In the human fetus the geniculate laminae emerge between weeks 22 and 25.[61] By inference the segregation of afferents from each retina occurs during this period.

In the macaque monkey the cells destined to comprise striate cortex are born between days E43 and E102.[124] This period corresponds to weeks 10 to 25 in the human fetus. In macaques the geniculate afferents begin to innervate striate cortex by E110, a time equivalent to gestational week 26 in humans. Injection of anatomic tracers reveals that initially the geniculate afferents representing each eye overlap extensively in layer IVC. The segregation of inputs into ocular dominance columns transpires during the last few weeks of pregnancy and is almost complete at birth.[124] The development of the ocular dominance columns is difficult to study in monkeys, because it requires injecting the fetus with intraocular tracers. Column development is easier to study in cats, because the feline visual system is relatively more immature at birth, so injections can be made postnatally.[90,91] At age 15 days (a week after the kitten's eyes open) intraocular injection of ^{3}H-proline shows a uniform band of label in layer IV (Fig. 23-28). Over the next few months the ocular dominance columns gradually emerge as label becomes restricted to distinct clumps in layer IV. The dark gaps are filled with unlabeled geniculate afferents that belong to the other eye.

The maturation of the ocular dominance columns requires thousands of left eye and right eye geniculate afferents to gradually disentangle their overlapping axon terminals in striate cortex. In a 17-day-old kitten a single geniculocortical fiber arborizes over a uniform area in layer IV that spans several millimeters (Fig. 23-29A).[90] At this stage in development the ocular dominance columns in cats have not quite begun to segregate (Fig. 23-28). In an adult animal the terminals of a single geniculocortical afferent appear clustered into several discrete regions that correspond to the ocular dominance columns (Fig. 23-29B).[44] The gaps between clumps of labeled axon terminals are filled with unlabeled afferents serving the other eye. These studies provide convincing evidence that individual geniculate fibers remodel their terminal arbors to generate the ocular dominance columns in layer IV.

Newborn function

Any parent can testify that the visually guided behavior of human newborns is quite primitive. This observation implies that visual acuity is still rather poor at birth. A number of methods are available to test vision quantitatively in babies.[15] These techniques rely either upon visual evoked potentials, optokinetic nystagmus, or preferential looking by an infant toward a patterned visual stimulus. Each technique exploits a different approach to measure acuity, but all three techniques agree fairly well that visual acuity is only about 20/400 at birth. Visual acuity quickly improves to a level of 20/20 within the first few years of life. This rapid refinement in visual acuity is paralleled by maturation of mechanisms that control accommodation, stereopsis, smooth pursuit, and saccadic eye movements.[15,46]

The continued development of visual function after birth is accompanied by major anatomic changes that occur simultaneously at all levels of the central visual pathways. The

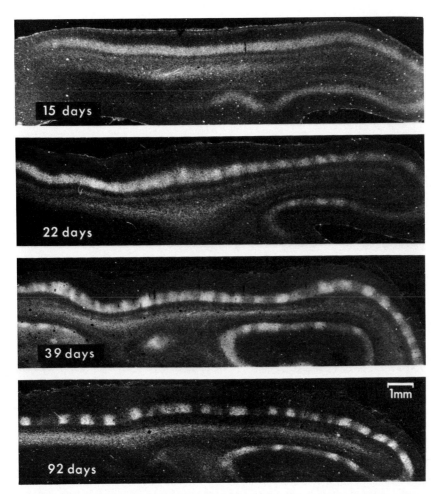

FIG. 23-28 Postnatal development of ocular dominance columns in the cat as shown by transneuronal transport of [³H]proline injected into one eye. These are darkfield autoradiographs of striate cortex from four different animals ipsilateral to the injected eye. At 15 days the afferents are spread uniformly along layer IV, completely intermingled with the unlabeled afferents serving the contralateral eye. At later ages the afferents progressively aggregate into ocular dominance columns. The gaps are occupied by unlabeled afferents serving the other eye. (From LeVay S, Stryker MP, Shatz CJ: J Comp Neurol 179:223, 1978.[91])

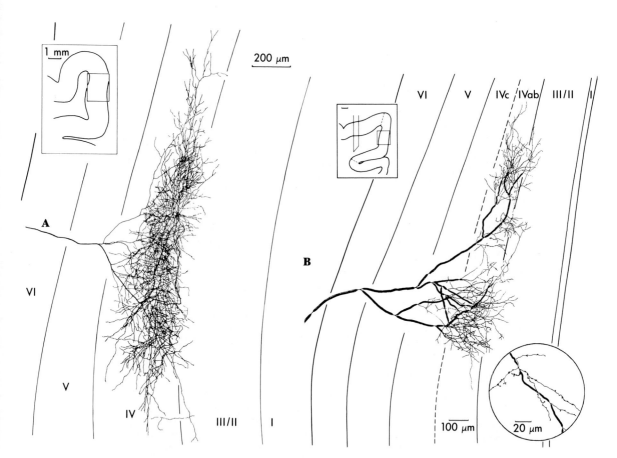

FIG. 23-29 **A**, Arborization of a single geniculocortical afferent in striate cortex of a 17-day-old kitten, just prior to the beginning of ocular dominance column segregation. This reconstruction was made from 25 serial sections of an axon impregnated with the Golgi method. The axon arborizes uniformly over a disc-shaped area 2 mm in diameter. The entire arborization is unmyelinated. (From LeVay S, Stryker MP: Soc Neurosci Symp 4:83, 1979.[90]) **B**, Arborization of a large geniculocortical afferent in an adult cat. The axon was filled with horseradish peroxidase and reconstructed from 16 serial sections. In its overall form and laminar distribution this axon resembles the one from the young kitten in **A**. However, the terminals are grouped into several discrete clumps that correspond to the ocular dominance columns belonging to one eye. The arborization has also acquired a myelin coat. (From Ferster D, LeVay S: J Comp Neurol 182:923, 1978.[44])

human macula is immature at birth.[1] The fovea is still covered by multiple cell layers and only sparsely packed with cones. During the first year of life the photoreceptors redistribute within the retina and peak foveal cone density increases by fivefold to achieve the concentration found in adult retina.[116] In newborns the white matter of the visual pathways is only scantily clad with myelin.[101] For the first two years after birth the myelin sheaths enlarge rapidly. Myelination continues at a slower rate throughout the first decade of life. At birth, neurons of the lateral geniculate body are only 60% of their average adult size.[59] Their volume gradually increases until the age of 2 years. In striate cortex refinement of synaptic connections continues for many years after birth. The density of dendritic spines and synapses reaches a peak at 8 months of age.[16,85] Subsequently the level declines by 40% over a period of several years to attain the final adult level.

The role of activity

The visual system begins to form in utero before visual experience can exert any possible influence. The continued development of the central visual pathways after birth suggests a potential for postnatal activity to shape the maturing visual system. To define the relative importance of prenatal factors versus postnatal factors in visual development, Wiesel and Hubel[164] recorded from newborn macaque monkeys that were born by Cesarian section and delivered to the laboratory with their eyes closed. They found that newborn monkeys have precisely oriented simple cells and complex cells similar to units found in adult animals. The striate cortex of these visually naive animals contains orderly sequences of orientation columns and ocular dominance columns virtually indistinguishable from those of adult monkeys. These physiologic findings are consistent with anatomic studies showing that by the end of gestation the cytochrome oxidase blobs, ocular dominance columns, and the cortical laminae are all well developed in fetal monkeys.[64,92,124] Apparently the basic elements of the cortical module are generated before birth, according to instructions that are innately programmed.

Surprisingly, physiologic activity in the fetus plays a vital role in the development of normal anatomic connections in the visual system. In utero, mammalian retinal ganglion cells discharge spontaneous action potentials in the absence of any visual stimulation.[50] Abolishing these action potentials with tetrodotoxin, a sodium channel blocker, prevents the normal prenatal segregation of retinogeniculate axons into appropriate geniculate laminae.[137] Intraocular administration of tetrodotoxin also blocks the formation of ocular dominance columns in striate cortex.[143] These experiments indicate that although the functional architecture of the visual system is ordained by genetics, the specificity and refinement of connections are molded by physiologic activity occurring in the fetus.

Eyelid suture

If a newborn monkey is reared in the dark or with both eyes sutured closed, cells in striate cortex eventually develop bizarre receptive field properties. The cells lose sharp orientation tuning and normal binocular responses. Some cells become oblivious to visual stimulation and can be detected only by virtue of their erratic spontaneous activity. The remaining units give sluggish and unpredictable responses to visual stimulation. After a long period of deprivation, if the monkey is introduced to a normal visual environment (or the eyelids are reopened), the animal is left profoundly blind with minimal potential for recovery. Cells in striate cortex do not recover normal response properties.

These laboratory observations demonstrate that patterned visual stimulation is required for a critical period after birth to preserve and promote normal visual function. In ophthalmology an analogy can be drawn with the newborn baby suffering dense, bilateral, congenital lens opacities. In this clinical situation the cataracts must be removed soon after birth to avoid permanent visual loss from bilateral amblyopia. Cataract extraction delayed beyond the critical period will not allow the child the chance to enjoy normal visual function.

After the postnatal critical period has elapsed, the visual system becomes impervious to the deleterious effects of sensory deprivation. For example, if a monkey is visually deprived as an adult by suturing closed both eyelids, there is no effect upon the properties of cells in striate cortex. In adult patients, form deprivation induced by slowly advancing cataracts does not impair visual function in a permanent manner. After successful removal of the cataracts, the patient experiences full restoration of sight.

LeVay, Hubel, and Wiesel[83,92] tested the consequences of monocular visual deprivation by suturing closed one eye in baby macaque monkeys. This procedure reduces retinal illumination by several log units and eliminates all patterned vision but does not injure the eye in any way. The occluded eye usually develops axial myopia but no other significant abnormality en-

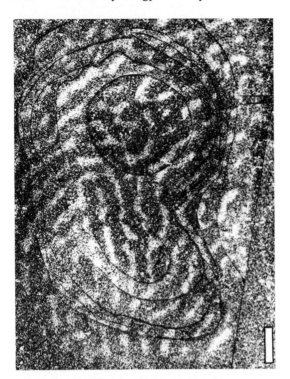

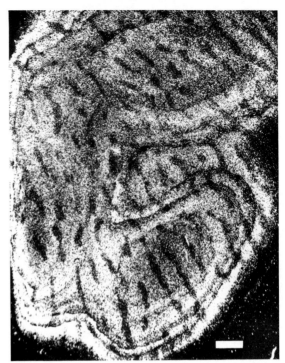

FIG. 23-30 Autoradiographic montage of sections through layer IVC from a monkey whose right eye was closed at 3 weeks of age. The right eye was injected with [³H]proline at 6 months of age. The labeled ocular dominance columns of the deprived right eye appear markedly shrunken but their periodicity is normal. (From Hubel DH, Wiesel TN, LeVay S: Phil Trans R Soc Lond B 278:377, 1978.[83])

FIG. 23-31 The counterpart to Figure 23-30: an autoradiographic montage of sections from a monkey whose right eye was closed at 5.5 weeks of age. The left eye was injected at 20 months of age. The labeled ocular dominance columns of the left eye appear extra wide because they have expanded to occupy cortical territory that normally would belong to the right eye. The gaps in label correspond to the withered right eye dominance columns. Scale bar = 1 mm. (From LeVay S, et al: J Comp Neurol 191:1, 1980.[92])

sues.[126] In the lateral geniculate body the cells in deprived laminae become slightly shrunken compared with the cells in normal laminae. Although cells within deprived laminae are shrunken, they have normal center-surround receptive fields and respond briskly to visual stimulation.[162] These findings imply that a defect at the level of the lateral geniculate body is unlikely to account for amblyopia. Interestingly, deprived cells located within the temporal crescent representation of the lateral geniculate body contralateral to the sutured eye do not show any atrophy.[53] Presumably no atrophy develops because cells of the deprived eye face no competition from cells of the normal eye in this portion of the lateral geniculate body.

Monocular visual deprivation produces a radical alteration in the ocular dominance columns in striate cortex. The ocular dominance

columns of the closed eye appear severely narrowed when labeled with a radioactive tracer (Fig. 23-30).[83,92] The mechanism underlying this striking change in the anatomy of striate cortex is not completely understood. According to the most popular theory, in the developing cortex the two eyes compete for synaptic contacts upon stellate cells in layer IVC. Monocular eyelid suture imposes a severe handicap in this contest. As a result, the deprived eye loses many of the connections already formed at birth with postsynaptic cortical targets. This leads to excessive pruning of the terminal arbors of geniculate cells driven by the deprived eye. In turn, the ocular dominance columns of the deprived eye begin to shrink. The open eye profits by sprouting of terminal arbors beyond their usual boundaries to occupy territory relinquished by the deprived eye. This effect can be shown by injecting a tracer into the open eye of a monocularly deprived monkey. Expanded columns of label alternate with thin gaps in label, although the overall configuration and periodicity of the columns is unaffected (Fig. 23-31). If correct, this explanation accounts for the shrinkage of cell somas previously observed in deprived laminae of the lateral geniculate body. Deprived cells are smaller, because they are required to sustain a reduced arbor of axon terminals in layer IVC of striate cortex.[53]

The abnormality in the ocular dominance columns induced by monocular deprivation has a marked physiologic correlate. In normal monkeys most cells in striate cortex are binocular, although many respond better to stimulation via one eye or the other. In a monkey raised with one eye closed most cells in striate cortex respond exclusively to stimulation through the normal open eye (Fig. 23-32).[92] It should be noted that the acuity of the normal eye does not improve beyond 20/20. The benefit derived by invading the cortical territory of the deprived eye is unclear.

The critical period

If one eye is closed in an adult macaque monkey, rather than a baby monkey, no alteration is produced in the morphology of the ocular dominance columns (Fig. 23-33).[92] This holds true even if the animal is subjected to years of monocular deprivation. Electrode recordings in striate cortex of monkeys visually deprived as adults reveal a normal distribution of ocular preference (Fig. 23-34).[92] The conclusion from performing eyelid closure in different animals at various ages is that macaque monkeys are vulnerable to the effects of eyelid suture for only a

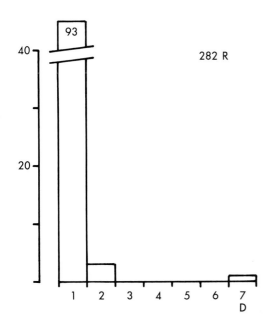

FIG. 23-32 Histogram showing the ocular dominance preference of 97 cells outside layer IVC recorded in electrode penetrations through striate cortex of the monkey illustrated in Figure 23-31. Number of cells is indicated on the ordinate. The abscissa is divided into 7 categories. Cells in category 1 responded exclusively to the left eye while cells in category 7 responded exclusively to the right eye. Categories 2 to 5 correspond to intermediate ocular dominance values. Virtually all the cells in this experiment preferred stimulation of the normal left eye. (From LeVay S, et al: J Comp Neurol 191:1, 1980.[92])

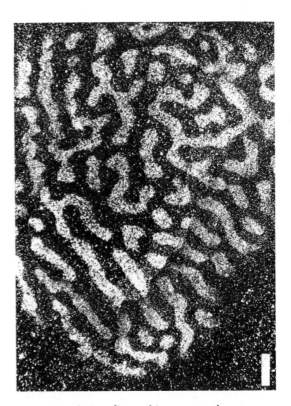

FIG. 23-33 Autoradiographic montage from a monkey whose right eye was closed when it was an adult. After more than a year of monocular visual deprivation, the left eye was injected with [³H]proline. The ocular dominance columns appear normal, indicating that monocular deprivation initiated after expiration of the critical period does not alter the ocular dominance columns. Scale bar = 1 mm. (From LeVay S, et al: J Comp Neurol 191:1, 1980.[92])

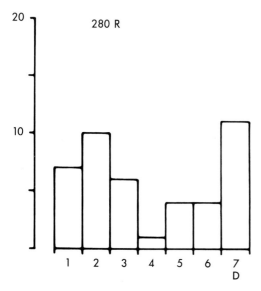

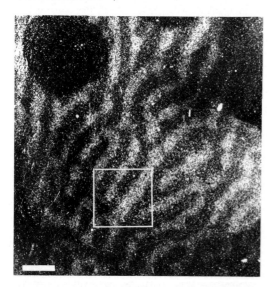

FIG. 23-34   Histogram showing the ocular dominance preference of 43 cells recorded outside layer IVC in striate cortex of the monkey illustrated in Figure 23-33. The influence of the two eyes was about equal, as in a normal animal. (From LeVay S, et al: J Comp Neurol 191:1, 1980.[92])

FIG. 23-35   Autoradiographic montage from a monkey whose right eye was closed from 3 days to 6 weeks of age. This procedure shrinks the ocular dominance columns of the right eye as shown in Figure 23-30. However, at 6 weeks of age the right eye was opened and the left eye was closed ("reverse" suture—equivalent to visually rehabilitating the right eye and patching the left eye). At 6 months of age the right eye was injected with radioactive tracer. The ocular dominance columns appear virtually normal, indicating anatomic recovery from the effects of early deprivation. Scale bar = 1 mm. (From LeVay S, et al: J Comp Neurol 191:1, 1980.[92])

few months after birth.[83,92] This period is defined as the "critical period." In the macaque monkey the closure of one eye any time during the critical period, even for just a week, can result in the shrinkage of ocular dominance columns and the loss of the deprived eye's ability to drive cells in striate cortex.

The critical period corresponds to a time when the wiring of striate cortex is still malleable and hence vulnerable to the effects of visual deprivation. During the critical period the deleterious effects of eyelid closure can also be corrected by "reverse" eyelid suture. Figure 23-35 shows the ocular dominance columns in a monkey raised with the right eye closed from 3 days to 6 weeks of age.[92] At 6 weeks the eyelid suture was reversed by opening the right eye and closing the left eye. The ocular dominance columns were labeled at 6 months of age by injecting the right eye with radioactive tracer. The ocular dominance columns appear practically normal, which indicates that anatomic recovery of the initially shrunken right eye columns was induced by opening the right eye and penalizing the left eye. Figure 23-36 shows the ocular dominance columns in a monkey whose right eye was closed at 7 days of age.[92] At 1 year the right

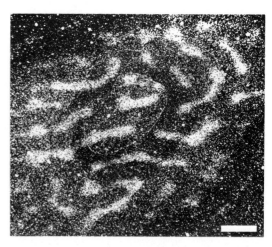

FIG. 23-36   Autoradiograph montage from a monkey whose right eye was closed at 7 days of age. At 1 year of age the right eye was opened and the left eye was closed. Several years later the right eye was injected with [3H]proline. Despite the "reverse" suture procedure, the ocular dominance columns of the right eye have remained severely narrowed. This experiment indicates that reverse suture initiated after the critical period has expired does not permit anatomic recovery from the effects of early deprivation. Scale bar = 1 mm. (From LeVay S, et al: J Comp Neurol 191:1, 1980.[92])

eye was reopened and the left eye was closed. Several years later the right eye was injected with [³H]proline to label the ocular dominance columns. The columns belonging to the initially deprived right eye show persistent shrinkage. This experiment indicates that reexpansion of deprived eye columns does not occur if reverse suture is carried out beyond the critical period. It may explain in part why patching in a child to improve vision in an amblyopic eye is fruitless if instigated after the end of the critical period.

Clinical implications

Eyelid suture in the baby macaque monkey is a good model for amblyopia *ex anopsia*—the severe form of amblyopia that develops when the retina is deprived of patterned visual stimulation. In children this condition can be caused by any dense opacity of the ocular media. The most common etiologies are unilateral ptosis and cataract. The work of LeVay, Hubel, and Wiesel offers new insight into the pathologic basis of amblyopia. Their studies provide a strong rationale for early intervention in patients to correct any factor that might cause amblyopia. Experiments in animals demonstrate that penalizing the normal eye by reverse suture can restore the ocular dominance columns in striate cortex to their normal appearance but treatment must be initiated before the end of the critical period to be effective. In humans, patching of the normal eye is the mainstay of treatment for amblyopia. Recent clinical experience suggests that good visual function can be achieved in children with congenital monocular cataract.[8] Effective therapy requires early surgical removal of the offending cataract, appropriate refractive correction, and vigorous patching of the normal eye. The lens opacity must be evaluated by an experienced ophthalmologist to determine whether it is severe enough to warrant cataract surgery.

The critical period in humans has been defined by documenting the visual outcome in children after surgical removal of congenital cataracts performed at different ages.[4,153] These studies indicate that the human critical period extends for at least several years after birth. This finding is consonant with the fact that the human visual system is less well developed at birth than the macaque visual system. The duration of the critical period may also vary according to the etiology of the amblyopia.

Although eyelid suture in monkeys is a good model for amblyopia ex anopsia, in clinical practice only a minority of cases of amblyopia are caused by media opacity. Other common etiologies in children include strabismus, anisometropia, nystagmus, and extreme refractive error. These conditions are more difficult to simulate with reliable animal models. Strabismus can be created artificially in monkeys by sectioning an extraocular muscle.[5,162] After this procedure, some animals switch ocular fixation constantly and thereby maintain normal acuity in each eye. In such animals physiologic recordings in striate cortex reveal cells with normal receptive fields and equal numbers of cells responsive to stimulation of either eye. However, the cortex is bereft of binocular cells. A similar picture can be created by raising an animal with alternate daily occlusion of one eye using a translucent contact lens.[76] The selective loss of stereopsis with normal acuity in each eye can be viewed as a special form of amblyopia due to a breakdown of binocular connections in striate cortex.

After cutting one extraocular muscle, some monkeys do not alternate fixation but instead fixate constantly with the same eye.[5,162] The deviating eye invariably develops amblyopia. Few cells in striate cortex can be driven by stimulation of the amblyopic eye. The anatomy of the ocular dominance columns in these monkeys has not been studied. From the physiology it would be reasonable to imagine that the ocular dominance columns belonging to the amblyopic eye are shrunken. However, this assumption has not been tested and caution must be exercised in generalizing from one model of amblyopia to another. It is quite possible that different mechanisms may be operating in amblyopia ex anopsia, strabismic amblyopia, and other forms of amblyopia. Further study of the various types of human amblyopia and correlation with animal models are required before we can fully explain the biological basis of this important cause of visual loss.

The implications of laboratory work on the pathologic basis of amblyopia reach far beyond clinical ophthalmology. Suturing the eyelids closed in a baby monkey causes no harm to the eye. Nonetheless, depriving the retina of patterned visual stimulation produces an anomaly in the wiring of striate cortex. It is remarkable that sensory deprivation alone is sufficient to alter the normal anatomy of the visual cortex. It seems plausible that other areas of cerebral cortex in the developing child, areas that have nothing to do with vision, may also depend upon sensory stimulation to form the proper anatomic circuits for normal adult function. This notion underscores the importance of providing children with an adequate and healthy sensory environment.

REFERENCES

1. Abramov I, Gordon J, Hendrickson A, et al: The retina of the newborn human infant, Science 217:265, 1982.
2. Allman JM, Kaas JH: A representation of the visual field in the caudal third of the middle temporal gyrus of the owl monkey *(Aotus trivirgatus)*, Brain Res 31:85, 1971.
3. Allman JM, Kaas JH: The organization of the second visual area (V II) in the owl monkey: a second order transformation of the visual hemifield, Brain Res 76:247, 1974.
4. Awaya S, Sugawara M, Miyake S, et al: Form vision deprivation amblyopia and the results of its treatment—with special reference to the critical period, Jpn J Ophthalmol 24:241, 1980.
5. Baker FH, Grigg P, von Noorden GK: Effects of visual deprivation and strabismus on the response of neurons in the visual cortex of the monkey, including studies on the striate and prestriate cortex in the normal animal, Brain Res 66:185, 1974.
6. Baker FH, Malpeli JG: Effects of cryogenic blockade of visual cortex on the responses of lateral geniculate neurons in the monkey, Exp Brain Res 29:433, 1977.
7. Bell RA, Thompson HS: Relative afferent pupillary defect in optic tract hemianopias, Am J Ophthalmol 85:538, 1978.
8. Beller R, Hoyt CS, Marg E, et al: Good visual function after neonatal surgery for congenital cataracts, Am J Ophthalmol 91:559, 1981.
9. Bender DB: Retinotopic organization of macaque pulvinar, J Neurophysiol 46:672, 1981.
10. Bender MB, Strauss I: Defects in visual field of one eye only in patients with a lesion of one optic radiation, Arch Ophthalmol 17:764, 1937.
11. Benevento LA, Rezak M: The cortical projections of the inferior pulvinar and adjacent lateral pulvinar in the rhesus monkey *(Macaca mulatta)*: an autoradiographic study, Brain Res 108:1, 1976.
12. Blasdel GG, Fitzpatrick D: Physiological organization of layer 4 in macaque striate cortex, J Neurosci 4:880, 1984.
13. Blasdel GG, Lund JS: Termination of afferent axons in macaque striate cortex, J Neurosci 3:1389, 1983.
14. Blasdel GG, Salama G: Voltage-sensitive dyes reveal a modular organization in monkey striate cortex, Nature 321:579, 1986.
15. Booth RG, Dobson V, Teller DY: Postnatal development of vision in human and nonhuman primates, Ann Rev Neurosci 8:495, 1985.
16. Boothe RG, Greenough WT, Lund JS, et al: A quantitative investigation of neurons in visual cortex (area 17) of *Macaca nemestrina* monkeys, J Comp Neurol 186:473, 1979.
17. Bowling DB, Michael CR: Projection patterns of single physiologically characterized optic tract fibres in cat, Nature 286:899, 1980.
18. Boycott BB, Wässle H: The morphological types of ganglion cells of the domestic cat's retina, J Physiol (Lond) 240:397, 1974.
19. Brodmann K: Vergleichende Lokalisationslehre der Grosshirnrinde, Leipzig, Johann Ambrosius Barth, 1909.
20. Bunt, AH, Minkler DS: Foveal sparing: new anatomical evidence for bilateral representation of the central retina, Arch Ophthalmol 95:1445, 1977.
21. Burkhalter A, Felleman DJ, Newsome WT, et al: Anatomical and physiological asymmetries related to visual areas V3 and VP in macaque extrastriate cortex, Vision Res 26:63, 1986.
22. Campos-Ortega JA, Hayhow WR, Cluver RE: A note on the problem of retinal projections to the inferior pulvinar of primates, Brain Res 22:126, 1970.
23. Clark WE Le Gros: Anatomical basis of colour vision, Nature 146:558, 1940.
24. Clark WE Le Gros: The laminar organization and cell content of the lateral geniculate body in the monkey, J Anat (Lond) 75:419, 1941.
25. Clark WE Le Gros, Sunderland S: Structural changes in the isolated visual cortex, J Anat (Lond) 73:563, 1939.
26. Cleland BG, Dubin MW, Levick WR: Simultaneous recording of input and output of lateral geniculate neurones, Nature (New Biol) 231:191, 1971.
27. Conley M, Fitzpatrick D: Morphology of retinogeniculate axons in the macaque, Vis Neurosci 2:287, 1989.
28. Cooper HM, Magnin M: A common mammalian plan of accessory optic system organization revealed in all primates, Nature 324:457, 1986.
29. Cowan WM: Centrifugal fibres to the avian retina, British Medical Bulletin 26:112, 1970.
30. Cragg BG: The topography of the afferent projections in the circumstriate visual cortex of the monkey studied by the Nauta method, Vision Res 9:733, 1969.
31. Curcio CA, Allen KA: Topography of ganglion cells in human retina, J Comp Neurol 300:5, 1990.
32. Cynader M, Berman N: Receptive-field organization of monkey superior colliculus, J Neurophysiol 35:187, 1972.
33. Daniel PM, Whitteridge D: The representation of the visual field on the cerebral cortex in monkeys, J Physiol (Lond) 159:203, 1961.
34. de Monasterio FM: Properties of concentrically organized X and Y ganglion cells of macaque retina, J Neurophysiol 41:1394, 1978.
35. Desimone R, Schein SJ: Visual properties of neurons in area V4 of the macaque: sensitivity to stimulus form, J Neurophysiol 57:835, 1987.
36. DeYoe EA, Van Essen DC: Segregation of efferent connections and receptive field properties in visual area V2 of the macaque, Nature 317:58, 1985.
37. Dow BM, Vautin RG, Bauer R: The mapping of visual space onto foveal striate cortex in the macaque monkey, J Neurosci 5:890, 1985.
38. Dreher B: Hypercomplex cells in the cat's striate cortex, Invest Ophthalmol 11:355, 1972.
39. Dreher B, Fukada Y, Rodieck RW: Identification, classification and anatomical segregation of cells with X-like and Y-like properties in the lateral geniculate nucleus of old-world primates, J Physiol (Lond) 258:433, 1976.
40. Ellis CJK: Afferent pupillary defect in pineal region tumour, J Neurol Neurosurg and Psychiatry 47:739, 1984.
41. Enroth-Cugell C, Robson JG: The contrast sensitivity

of retinal ganglion cells of the cat, J Physiol (Lond) 187:517, 1966.

42. Falconer MA, Wilson JL: Visual field changes following anterior temporal lobectomy: their significance in relation to "Meyer's loop" of the optic radiation, Brain 81:1, 1958.

43. Felleman DJ, Van Essen DC: Distributed hierarchical processing in primate cerebral cortex, Cerebral Cortex 1:1, 1991.

44. Ferster D, LeVay S: The axonal arborizations of lateral geniculate neurons in the striate cortex of the cat, J Comp Neurol 182:923, 1978.

45. Fitzpatrick D, Itoh K, Diamond IT: The laminar organization of the lateral geniculate body and the striate cortex in the squirrel monkey (Saimiri sciureus), J Neurosci 3:673, 1983.

46. Fox R, Aslin RN, Shea SL, et al: Stereopsis in human infants, Science 207:323, 1980.

47. Freund TF, Martin KAC, Soltesz I, et al: Arborisation pattern and postsynaptic targets of physiologically identified thalamocortical afferents in striate cortex of the macaque monkey, J Comp Neurol 289:315, 1989.

48. Fukuda Y: Receptive field organization of cat optic nerve fibers with special reference to conduction velocity, Vision Res 11:209, 1971.

49. Fukuda Y, Sawai H, Watanabe M, et al: Nasotemporal overlap of crossed and uncrossed retinal ganglion cell projections in the Japanese monkey (Macaca fuscata), J Neurosci 9:2353, 1989.

50. Galli L, Maffei L: Spontaneous impulse activity of rat retinal ganglion cells in prenatal life, Science 242:90, 1988.

51. Gilbert CD: Laminar differences in receptive field properties of cells in cat primary visual cortex, J Physiol (Lond) 268:391, 1977.

52. Gilbert CD, Kelly JP: The projections of cells in different layers of the cat's visual cortex, J Comp Neurol 163:81, 1975.

53. Guillery RW, Stelzner DJ: The differential effects of unilateral lid closure upon the monocular and binocular segments of the dorsal lateral geniculate nucleus in the cat, J Comp Neurol 139:413, 1970.

54. Hamos JE, Van Horn SC, Raczkowski D, et al: Synaptic circuits involving an individual retinogeniculate axon in the cat, J Comp Neurol 259:165, 1987.

55. Harrington DO, Drake MV: The visual fields: text and atlas of clinical perimetry, 6th ed, St Louis, CV Mosby, 1990.

56. Hendrickson AE, Hunt SP, Wu JY: Immunocytochemical localization of glutamic acid decarboxylase in monkey striate cortex, Nature 292:605, 1981.

57. Hendrickson AE, Wilson ME, Toyne MJ: The distribution of optic nerve fibers in Macaca mulatta, Brain Res 23:425, 1970.

58. Heywood CA, Cowey A: On the role of cortical area V4 in the discrimination of hue and pattern in macaque monkeys, J Neurosci 7:2601, 1987.

59. Hickey TL: Postnatal development of human lateral geniculate nucleus: relationship to a critical period for the visual system, Science 198:836, 1977.

60. Hickey TL, Guillery RW: Variability of laminar patterns in the human lateral geniculate nucleus, J Comp Neurol 183:221, 1979.

61. Hitchcock PF, Hickey TL: Prenatal development of the human lateral geniculate nucleus, J Comp Neurol 194:395, 1980.

62. Hoffmann KP, Distler C: Quantitative analysis of visual receptive fields of neurons in nucleus of the optic tract and dorsal terminal nucleus of the accessory optic tract in macaque monkey, J Neurophysiol 62:416, 1989.

63. Holmes G, Lister WT: Disturbances of vision from cerebral lesions with special reference to the cortical representation of the macula, Brain 39:34, 1916.

64. Horton JC: Cytochrome oxidase patches: a new cytoarchitectonic feature of monkey visual cortex, Phil Trans R Soc Lond B 304:199, 1984.

65. Horton JC, Dagi LR, McCrane EP, et al: Arrangement of ocular dominance columns in human visual cortex, Arch Ophthalmol 108:1025, 1990.

66. Horton JC, Greenwood MM, Hubel DH: Non-retinotopic arrangement of fibres in cat optic nerve, Nature 282:720, 1979.

67. Horton JC, Hedley-Whyte ET: Mapping of cytochrome oxidase patches and ocular dominance columns in human visual cortex, Phil Trans R Soc Lond B304:255, 1984.

68. Horton JC, Hoyt WF: The representation of the visual field in human striate cortex: a revision of the classic Holmes map, Arch Ophthalmol 109:816, 1991.

69. Horton JC, Hubel DH: Regular patchy distribution of cytochrome oxidase staining in primary visual cortex of macaque monkey, Nature 292:762, 1981.

70. Hoyt WF, Luis O: Visual fiber anatomy in the infrageniculate pathway of the primate, Arch Ophthalmol 68:94, 1962.

71. Hoyt WF, Rios-Montenegro EN, Behrens MM, et al: Homonymous hemioptic hypoplasia, Br J Ophthalmol 56:537, 1972.

72. Hubel DH, LeVay S, Wiesel TN: Mode of termination of retinotectal fibers in macaque monkey: an autoradiographic study, Brain Res 96:25, 1975.

73. Hubel DH, Livingstone MS: Segregation of form, color, and stereopsis in primate area 18, J Neurosci 7:3378, 1987.

74. Hubel DH, Wiesel TN: Integrative action in the cat's lateral geniculate body, J Physiol (Lond) 155:385, 1961.

75. Hubel DH, Wiesel TN: Receptive fields, binocular interaction and functional architecture in the cat's visual cortex, J Physiol (Lond) 160:106, 1962.

76. Hubel DH, Wiesel TN: Binocular interaction in striate cortex of kittens reared with artificial squint, J Neurophysiol 28:1041, 1965.

77. Hubel DH, Wiesel TN: Receptive fields and functional architecture in two non-striate visual areas (18 and 19) of the cat, J Neurophysiol 28:229, 1965.

78. Hubel DH, Wiesel TN: Receptive fields and functional architecture of monkey striate cortex, J Physiol (Lond) 195:215, 1968.

79. Hubel DH, Wiesel TN: Laminar and columnar distribution of geniculocortical fibers in the macaque monkey, J Comp Neurol 146:421, 1972.

80. Hubel DH, Wiesel TN: Sequence regularity and geometry of orientation columns in the monkey striate cortex, J Comp Neurol 158:267, 1974.

81. Hubel DH, Wiesel TN: Uniformity of monkey striate cortex: a parallel relationship between field size, scatter, and magnification factor, J Comp Neurol 158:295, 1974.

82. Hubel DH, Wiesel TN: Functional architecture of macaque monkey visual cortex, Proc R Soc Lond B198:1, 1977.

83. Hubel DH, Wiesel TN, LeVay S: Plasticity of ocular dominance columns in monkey striate cortex, Phil Trans R Soc Lond B278:377, 1977.

84. Hubel DH, Wiesel TN, Stryker MP: Anatomical demonstration of orientation columns in macaque monkey, J Comp Neurol 177:361, 1978.

85. Huttenlocher PR, de Courten C, Garey LJ, et al: Synaptogenesis in human visual cortex—evidence for synapse elimination during normal development, Neuroscience Letters 33:247, 1982.

86. Inouye T: Die Sehstörungen bei Schussverletzungen der kortikalen Sehsphäre, Leipzig, W Engelmann, 1909.

87. Kennedy C, Des Rosiers MH, Sakurada O, et al: Metabolic mapping of the primary visual system of the monkey by means of the autoradiographic [^{14}C] deoxyglucose technique, Proc Natl Acad Sci 73:4230, 1976.

88. Kuffler SW: Neurons in the retina: organization, inhibition, and excitation problems, Cold Spring Harbor Symp Quant Biol, XVII:281, 1952.

89. LeVay S, Connolly M, Houde J, et al: The complete pattern of ocular dominance stripes in the striate cortex and visual field of the macaque monkey, J Neurosci 5:486, 1985.

90. LeVay S, Stryker MP: The development of ocular dominance columns in the cat, Soc Neurosci Symp 4:83, 1979.

91. LeVay S, Stryker MP, Shatz CJ: Ocular dominance columns and their development in layer IV of the cat's visual cortex: a quantitative study, J Comp Neurol 179:223, 1978.

92. LeVay S, Wiesel TN, Hubel DH: The development of ocular dominance columns in normal and visually deprived monkeys, J Comp Neurol 191:1, 1980.

93. Leventhal AG, Ault SJ, Vitek DJ: The nasotemporal division in primate retina: the neural bases of macular sparing and splitting, Science 240:66, 1988.

94. Leventhal AG, Rodieck RW, Dreher B: Retinal ganglion cell classes in the old world monkey: morphology and central projections, Science 213:1139, 1981.

95. Livingstone MS, Hubel DH: Thalamic inputs to cytochrome oxidase-rich regions in monkey visual cortex, Proc Natl Acad Sci 79:6098, 1982.

96. Livingstone MS, Hubel DH: Anatomy and physiology of a color system in the primate visual cortex, J Neurosci 4:309, 1984.

97. Livingstone MS, Hubel DH: Connections between layer 4B of area 17 and thick cytochrome oxidase stripes of area 18 in the squirrel monkey, J Neurosci 7:3371, 1987.

98. Livingstone MS, Hubel DH: Segregation of form, color, movement, and depth: anatomy, physiology, and perception, Science 240:740, 1988.

99. Lund JS: Organization of neurons in the visual cortex, area 17, of the monkey (Macaca mulatta), J Comp Neurol 147:455, 1973.

100. Lund JS: Anatomical organization of macaque monkey striate visual cortex, Ann Rev Neurosci 11:253, 1988.

101. Magoon EH, Robb RM: Development of myelin in human optic nerve and tract, Arch Ophthalmol 99:655, 1981.

102. Malpeli JG, Baker FH: The representation of the visual field in the lateral geniculate nucleus of Macaca mulatta, J Comp Neurol 161:569, 1975.

103. Mann I: The development of the human eye, 4th ed, New York, Grune and Stratton, 1964.

104. Meadows JC: Disturbed perception of colours associated with localized cerebral lesions, Brain 97:615, 1974.

105. Merigan WH: Chromatic and achromatic vision of macaques: role of the P pathway, J Neurosci 9:776, 1989.

106. Michael CR: Columnar organization of color cells in monkey's striate cortex, J Neurophysiol 46:587, 1981.

107. Michael CR: Retinal afferent arborization patterns, dendritic field orientations, and the segregation of function in the lateral geniculate nucleus of the monkey, Proc Natl Acad Sci 85:4914, 1988.

108. Miller NR: Walsh and Hoyt's clinical neuroophthalmology, 4th ed, Baltimore, Williams and Wilkins, 1982.

109. Minckler DS: The organization of nerve fiber bundles in the primate optic nerve head, Arch Ophthalmol 98:1630, 1980.

110. Minkowski M: Über den Verlauf, die Endigung und die zentrale Repräsentation von gekreuzten und ungekreuzten Sehnervenfasern bei einigen Säugetieren und beim Menschen, Schweiz Arch f Neurol u Psychiat 6:201, 1920.

111. Moore RY: Retinohypothalamic projection in mammals: a comparative study, Brain Res 49:403, 1973.

112. Nagel-Leiby S, Bender DB, Butter CM: Effects of kainic acid and radiofrequency lesions of the pulvinar on visual discrimination in the monkey, Brain Res 300:295, 1984.

113. Naito J: Retinogeniculate projection fibers in the monkey optic nerve: a demonstration of the fiber pathways by retrograde axonal transport of WGA-HRP, J Comp Neurol 284:174, 1989.

114. Newsome WT, Pare EB: A selective impairment of motion perception following lesions of the middle temporal visual area (MT), J Neurosci 8:2201, 1988.

115. Ogden TE: Nerve fiber layer of the macaque retina: retinotopic organization, Invest Ophthalmol Vis Sci 24:85, 1983.

116. Packer O, Hendrickson AE, Curcio CA: Development redistribution of photoreceptors across the Macaca nemestrina (pigtail macaque) retina, J Comp Neurol 298:472, 1990.

117. Perry VH, Cowey A: The morphological correlates of X- and Y-like retinal ganglion cells in the retina of monkeys, Exp Brain Res 43:226, 1981.

118. Perry VH, Oehler R, Cowey A: Retinal ganglion cells that project to the dorsal lateral geniculate nucleus in the macaque monkey, Neurosci 12:1101, 1984.

119. Plant GT, Perry VH: The anatomical basis of the caecocentral scotoma, Brain 113:1441, 1991.

120. Pollack JG, Hickey TL: The distribution of retino-collicular axon terminals in rhesus monkey, J Comp Neurol 185:587, 1979.

121. Polyak S: The vertebrate visual system, Chicago, University of Chicago Press, 1957.

122. Provis JM, Van Driel D, Billson FA, et al: Development of the human retina: patterns of cell distribution and redistribution in the ganglion cell layer, J Comp Neurol 233:429, 1985.

123. Radius RL, Anderson DR: The course of axons through the retina and optic nerve head, Arch Ophthalmol 97:1154, 1979.

124. Rakic P: Prenatal development of the visual system in rhesus monkey, Phil Trans R Soc Lond B278:245, 1977.

125. Rakic P, Riley KP: Overproduction and elimination of retinal axons in the fetal rhesus monkey, Science 219:1441, 1983.

126. Raviola E, Wiesel TN: An animal model of myopia, N Engl J Med 312:1609, 1985.

127. Rhodes RH: A light microscopic study of the developing human neural retina, Am J Anat 154:195, 1979.

128. Robinson DA: Eye movements evoked by collicular stimulation in the alert monkey, Vision Res 12:1795, 1972.

129. Sadun AA, Johnson BM, Schaechter J: Neuroanatomy of the human visual system: Part III, Three retinal projections to the hypothalamus, Neuro-ophthalmol 6:371, 1986.

130. Schaechter J, Sadun AA: A second hypothalamic nucleus receiving retinal input in man: the paraventricular nucleus, Brain Res 340:243, 1985.

131. Schein SJ, Desimone R: Spectral properties of V4 neurons in the macaque, J Neurosci 10:3369, 1990.

132. Schiff D, Cohen B, Buttner-Ennever J, et al: Effects of lesions of the nucleus of the optic tract on optokinetic nystagmus and after-nystagmus in the monkey, Exp Brain Res 79:225, 1990.

133. Schiller PH, Malpeli JG: Functional specificity of lateral geniculate nucleus laminae of the rhesus monkey, J Neurophysiol 41:788, 1978.

134. Schiller PH, Stryker M: Single-unit recording and stimulation in superior colliculus of the alert rhesus monkey, J Neurophysiol 35:915, 1972.

135. Schiller PH, Logothetis NK, Charles ER: Functions of the colour-opponent and broad-band channels of the visual system, Nature 343:68, 1990.

136. Shapley R, Kaplan E, Soodak R: Spatial summation and contrast sensitivity of X and Y cells in the lateral geniculate nucleus of the macaque, Nature 292:543, 1981.

137. Shatz CJ, Stryker MP: Prenatal tetrodotoxin infusion blocks segregation of retinogeniculate afferents, Science 242:87, 1988.

138. Sherman SM, Wilson JR, Kaas JH, et al: X- and Y-cells in the dorsal lateral geniculate nucleus of the owl monkey (Aotus trivirgatus), Science 192:475, 1976.

139. Shipp S, Zeki S: Segregation of pathways leading from area V2 to areas V4 and V5 of macaque monkey visual cortex, Nature 315:322, 1985.

140. Smith CG, Richardson WFG: The course and distribution of the arteries supplying the visual (striate) cortex, Am J Ophthalmol 61:1391, 1966.

141. Spalding JMK: Wounds of the visual pathway, Part II, The striate cortex, J Neurol Neurosurg Psychiat 15:169, 1952.

142. Stone J, Leicester J, Sherman SM: The naso-temporal division of the monkey's retina, J Comp Neurol 150:333, 1973.

143. Stryker MP, Harris WA: Binocular impulse blockade prevents the formation of ocular dominance columns in cat visual cortex, J Neurosci 6:2117, 1986.

144. Teuber HL, Battersby WS, Bender MB: Visual field defects after penetrating missile wounds of the brain, Cambridge, Harvard University Press, 1960.

145. Tigges J, O'Steen WK: Termination of retinofugal fibers in squirrel monkey: a re-investigation using autoradiographic methods, Brain Res 79:489, 1974.

146. Tootell RBH, Silverman MS, De Valois RL, et al: Functional organization of the second cortical visual area in primates, Science 220:737, 1983.

147. Tootell RBH, Switkes E, Silverman MS, et al: Functional anatomy of macaque striate cortex, II, Retinotopic organization, J Neurosci 8:1531, 1988.

148. Traquair HM: An introduction to clinical perimetry, 5th ed, St Louis, CV Mosby, 1948.

149. Ts'o DY, Frostig RD, Lieke EE, et al: Functional organization of primate visual cortex revealed by high resolution optical imaging, Science 249:417, 1990.

150. Ts'o DY, Gilbert CD: The organization of chromatic and spatial interactions in the primate striate cortex, J Neurosci 8:1712, 1988.

151. Ungerleider LG, Desimone R: Cortical connections of visual area MT in the macaque, J Comp Neurol 248:190, 1986.

152. Unsöld R, Hoyt WF: Band atrophy of the optic nerve, Arch Ophthalmol 98:1637, 1980.

153. Vaegan, Taylor D: Critical period for deprivation amblyopia in children, Trans Ophthalmol Soc UK 99:432, 1979.

154. Van Buren JM, Baldwin M: The architecture of the optic radiation in the temporal lobe of man, Brain 81:15, 1958.

155. Van Essen DC, Newsome WT, Maunsell JHR: The visual field representation in striate cortex of the macaque monkey: asymmetries, anisotropies, and individual variability, Vision Res 24:429, 1984.

156. Van Essen DC, Newsome WT, Maunsell JHR, et al: The projections from striate cortex (V1) to areas V2 and V3 in the macaque monkey: asymmetries, areal boundaries, and patchy connections, J Comp Neurol 244:451, 1986.

157. Vrabec F: The temporal raphe of the human retina, Am J Ophthalmol 62:926, 1966.

158. Walls GL: The lateral geniculate nucleus and visual histophysiology, The University of California Publications in Physiology, vol 9, Berkeley and Los Angeles, University of California Press, 1953.

159. Watanabe M, Rodieck RW: Parasol and midget ganglion cells of the primate retina, J Comp Neurol 289:434, 1989.

160. Weber JT, Huerta MF, Kaas JH, et al: The projections of the lateral geniculate nucleus of the squirrel monkey: studies of the interlaminar zones and the S layers, J Comp Neurol 213:135, 1983.

161. Wentworth HA: Variations of the normal blind spot

with special reference to the formulation of a diagnostic scale, Am J Ophthalmol 14:889, 1931.

162. Wiesel TN: Postnatal development of the visual cortex and the influence of environment, Nature 299:583, 1982.

163. Wiesel TN, Hubel DH: Spatial and chromatic interactions in the lateral geniculate body of the rhesus monkey, J Neurophysiol 29:1115, 1966.

164. Wiesel TN, Hubel DH: Ordered arrangement of orientation columns in monkeys lacking visual experience, J Comp Neurol 158:307, 1974.

165. Wilbrand HL: Schema des verlaufs der sehnervenfasern durch das chiasma, Z Augenheilk 59:135, 1926.

166. Wong-Riley M: Changes in the visual system of monocularly sutured or enucleated cats demonstrable with cytochrome oxidase histochemistry, Brain Res 171:11, 1979.

167. Zeki SM: A century of cerebral achromatopsia, Brain 113:1721, 1990.

168. Zeki SM, Shipp S: The functional logic of cortical connections, Nature 335:311, 1988.

169. Zeki SM: Representation of central visual fields in prestriate cortex of monkey, Brain Res 14:271, 1969.

170. Zeki SM: Colour coding in rhesus monkey prestriate cortex, Brain Res 53:422, 1973.

171. Zeki SM: Functional organization of a visual area in the posterior bank of the superior temporal sulcus of the rhesus monkey, J Physiol (Lond) 236:549, 1974.

172. Zeki SM: Uniformity and diversity of structure and function in rhesus monkey prestriate visual cortex, J Physiol (Lond) 277:273, 1978.

173. Zihl J, Von Cramon D, Mai N: Selective disturbance of movement vision after bilateral brain damage, Brain 106:313, 1983.

Binocular Vision

LAWRENCE TYCHSEN, M.D.

Binocular vision is seeing with two eyes simultaneously. Normal binocular vision implies fusion, the blending of sight from the two eyes to form a single percept. Normal binocular vision also implies the most acute kind of depth perception—stereopsis—based on the horizontal separation of the two eyes in the skull.

The greatest conceptual change in the field of binocular vision has been the dichotomization of visual processing into parvocellular and magnocellular streams, a concept introduced almost simultaneously by several teams studying visual processing in animals a decade ago.[201,238,319,349,383,413] The notion of parallel streams has now been used to explain two different kinds of stereopsis in humans and two different types of visual drive to the vergence motoneurons controlling binocular eye alignment. Only recently has interest turned to postnatal development of these streams and the way in which maldevelopments explain the two major classes of pathologic binocularity: amblyopia and strabismus.

In the sections that follow, the psychophysics of fusion and stereopsis in normal adult humans is discussed first, followed by a discussion of underlying neural mechanisms in human and monkey. This is followed by a section on normal variations in stereopsis and vergence eye movement. Using the normal adult as a reference, the discussion then proceeds to binocular development in infancy and the maldevelopments of strabismus and amblyopia. The final section of the chapter deals with information of relevance to primates that has been gathered from studies of binocular vision in other animals.

NORMAL ADULT PSYCHOPHYSICS
Binocular correspondence

When viewed monocularly, a stimulus projects an image to a region on the retina that is to the right, left, above, or below the foveola. The stimulus is said to have a specific oculocentric* visual direction. When viewed binocularly, the stimulus will project to either corresponding or noncorresponding regions on the two retinas. As shown in Figure 24-1,*A*, corresponding regions on the two retinas are the same horizontal and vertical distance from the two foveolas, i.e., they have identical visual directions.

The geometric horopter

The notion of binocular correspondence and noncorrespondence was recognized by Euclid and by Leonardo da Vinci, but it was not until 1613 that Aguilonius used the term "horopter"

This work was supported by a Career Development Award from Research to Prevent Blindness Inc., by the Knight's Templar Eye Research Foundation, and by a Biomedical Research Support Grant from the N.I.H.

*When viewing binocularly the nomenclature changes to "egocentric," because perceptually the binocular visual direction appears to emanate from the head, midway between the two eyes.

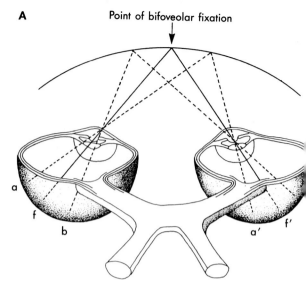

FIG. 24-1 A, Eccentric stimuli that project to corresponding regions on retina of left and right eye. *Solid line* depicts the point of binocular foveolar fixation. The distances af = a'f' (and bf = b'f'), hence the stimuli project to corresponding retinal regions. **B,** Fundus of right eye in human. Histologic definition of terms foveolar, foveal, and macula: the foveola contains photoreceptors but no ganglion cells; the fovea (= L. a depression) is an area in which the retina is reduced to half its normal thickness; the outer boundary of the perifovea (or macula = L. spot) is demarcated by transition to a single layer of ganglion cells. "Posterior pole" or "central retina" are ill-defined clinical terms, generally synonymous with macula.

af = a'f' = Correspondence = No disparity
bf = b'f' = Correspondence = No disparity

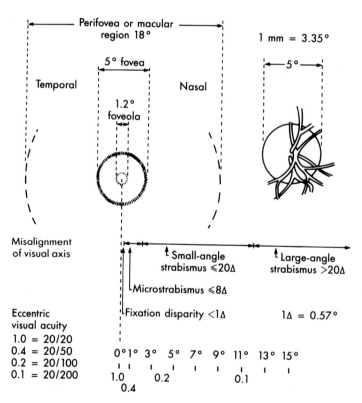

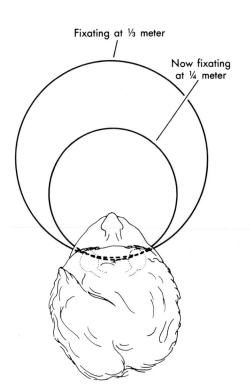

FIG. 24-2 Change in diameter of geometric (Vieth-Müller) horopter with change in fixation distance.

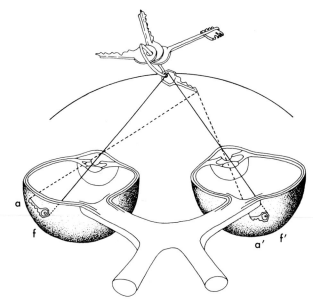

af > a'f' = Noncorrespondence = Disparity

FIG. 24-3 Horizontal disparity caused by horizontal separation of eyes in the skull. The solid lines depict the point of bifoveolar fixation. Each eye has a slightly different view of the key. Part of the key lies nearer than the horopter. Hence that part of the image falls on noncorresponding regions of the retinae in the two eyes (af > a'f').

(the "horizon of vision").[3] Aguilonius introduced the horopter to postulate the existence of a set of binocularly corresponding points. He defined the set of points geometrically as lying on a circle in the horizontal plane of the head that passed through the optical centers (nodal points) of the two eyes and the momentary point of fixation. When the point of fixation was near, the circle was small. When the point of fixation was far, the circle was large (Fig. 24-2). The geometric horopter of Aguilonius was reintroduced by Vieth in 1818[387] and further refined by Müller in 1840,[249] hence the geometric Vieth-Müller horopter.

Horizontal disparity and the longitudinal horopter

The two eyes are separated horizontally but not vertically in the skull, so that each eye has a slightly horizontally different view of the world. Wheatstone, in 1838, was the first to formally demonstrate that stimuli lying in front of or behind the horopter cause horizontal image disparity, and that this disparity serves as a powerful cue for depth perception[403] (Fig. 24-3). Once the concept of binocular disparity had been introduced the horopter could be defined

as the locus of stimulus points having zero binocular disparity.

The horopter can be plotted perceptually by requiring observers to adjust a set of vertical sticks ("a picket fence") located left and right along the frontoparallel plane, until all the sticks appear to be equally far away (Fig. 24-4). The task is performed while the observer steadily fixates on only one reference stick located at zero eccentricity straight ahead. Because of the resemblance of the set of sticks to the vertical lines that mark longitude on a globe, the perceptual horopter plotted in this way is known as the longitudinal horopter. Several famous visual psychophysicists after Wheatstone used the longitudinal horopter as a tool to quantify depth perception in great detail, notably Hering,[141] Hillebrand,[145] and Ogle.[267]

The longitudinal (Hering-Hillebrand) horopter is slightly flatter (has a greater radius of curvature) then the geometric (Vieth-Müller) horopter. The deviation of the perceptual from the geometric horopter is known as the Hering-Hillebrand deviation. The deviation is now felt

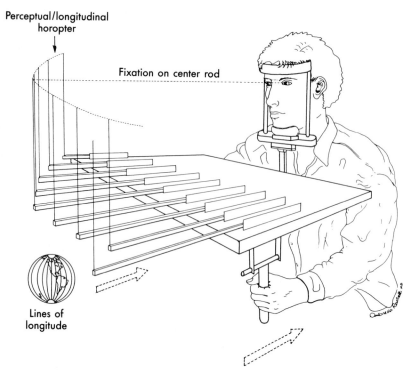

FIG. 24-4 Apparatus for plotting perceptual (longitudinal) horopter. The subject steadily fixates the center rod and then moves the other rods back and forth in peripheral vision until they appear equidistant. The subject has completed the task for all but the most eccentric rod in the left visual field. *Inset:* lines of longitude on a globe.

to be due to both neural and optical factors[269,373]: the nasal hemi-retinae at any given eccentricity contain more photoreceptors per unit area than the temporal hemi-retinae, producing a deviation in horopter mapping in the visual cortex. Optical distortions of off-axis rays passing through the lens of the eye also play a role.* Figure 24-5 shows how the horopter curve flattens as the fixation point recedes from the observer.

Fusion and Diplopia

If a stimulus is moved off the horopter to a location in front or behind, it will stimulate horizontally disparate (noncorresponding) regions on the two retinas. If this disparity is small, the stimulus will continue to be perceived as a single image, albeit an image in depth. The range of horizontal disparities within which the stimulus will continue to be perceived as single is known classically as Panum's fusional area (L. *fusio* = a melting together).[275] As depicted in Figure

*See "Development of the Horopter and Panum's Area in Early Infancy," p. 806.

24-6, outside Panum's area the stimulus is seen as two separate images, one for each eye. This perception of a single real stimulus as doubled is diplopia.

The reader can plot his own Panum's area by performing the following exercise. Hold a pencil vertically in your right hand a foot from your nose in the midline of your head. Position the index finger of your left hand 4 inches to the left of the pencil, so that the pencil and finger are parallel. Keep the pencil stationary, binocularly fixate the pencil tip, and move your left hand directly toward and away from you. The left index finger will be seen in peripheral vision to become diplopic several inches in front of and behind the pencil, as the finger travels from in front of Panum's area, through Panum's area, and out behind Panum's area.

Panum's fusional area varies according to the spatial and temporal properties of the stimulus

Panum's area is narrowest at the fixation point and becomes broader in the periphery at a rate of 1 to 2 arc min per degree of visual field

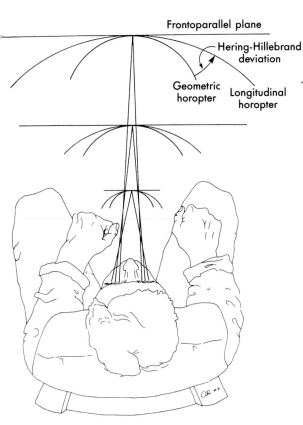

FIG. 24-5   The horopters at three different distances of binocular fixation. The horopters flatten as the point of fixation recedes. The difference between the geometric (Vieth-Müller) and perceptual (longitudinal) horopter is the "Hering-Hillebrand deviation."

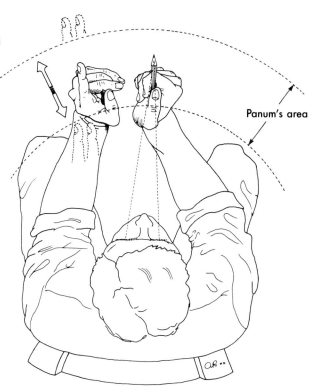

FIG. 24-6   When the finger is within Panum's area, it is seen as single but when moved outside Panum's area, it is seen in diplopia. See text for description.

eccentricity[269] (Fig. 24-7). Tyler has pointed out that the increase in spatial extent of Panum's area in the peripheral visual field serves three useful purposes.[373,376] First, increasing size of Panum's area matches increasing coarseness of peripheral vision. Receptive field size increases and visual acuity decreases as a function of eccentricity. Second, increasing the thickness of Panum's area prevents bothersome peripheral diplopia when fixating flat targets held at close range. The edges of this page, for example, are not diplopic when the reader fixates a word at page center. Third, increasing the extent of Panum's area peripherally makes cyclofusion possible despite cyclovergence errors of as much as 2 degrees between the two eyes.

Panum's area is not a fixed size. Systematic study of Panum's area in humans has shown that large, blurred, slowly changing images remain fused over a much greater range than small, sharply focused, rapidly changing images.

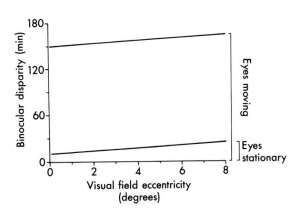

FIG. 24-7   Increase in width of Panum's area with increase in visual field eccentricity. Targets with disparities below the lines are seen as single, those above the lines as diplopic. Panum's area is narrower during steady fixation and wider when the eyes and/or head are freely moving. Replotted using data of Ogle (1962).

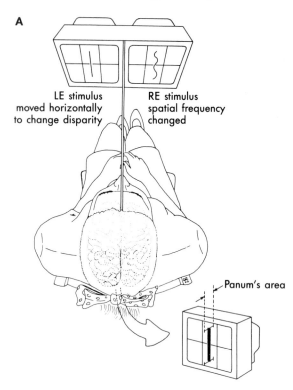

FIG. 24-8 Width of Panum's area varies with the spatial and temporal frequencies of the fusion stimuli. **A,** The observer views dichoptically (a separate stimulus is seen by each eye). The spatial frequency (waviness) of the image seen by the right eye can be varied, and the two stimuli can be moved closer together or further apart to cause crossed or uncrossed disparity. The grid lines maintain a stable vergence angle. Within Panum's area the stimuli are seen as a slightly fuzzy, single line. Outside Panum's area two separate lines would be seen (not shown). **B,** As spatial frequency of the right eye stimulus is increased by 2 log units (from .03 to 3 cycles-per-degree), the width of Panum's area narrows by 2 log units (from 200 to 2 arc min). **C,** The observer dichoptically views two lines oscillating left and right in pendular (sinusoidal) motion; both move nasally (into crossed disparity) then temporally (into uncrossed disparity). **D,** As the temporal frequency of the oscillation increases (in cycles-per-second), Panum's area narrows. Replotted using data of Tyler (1983).

The data of Figure 24-8, *B* show the results of an experiment in which an observer was required to fuse images that differed in spatial frequency under conditions of dichoptic viewing (separate images seen by each eye). The stimulus seen by one eye was a straight vertical line. The stimulus seen by the other eye was a vertical line that could be varied in sinusoidal waviness (spatial frequency). When the sinusoidal waves were of very low frequency (the equivalent of a blurred image), the lines could be separated by a large horizontal disparity and still be fused into a single image, i.e., Panum's area was thick. Panum's area became progressively thinner,

i.e., the observer was more prone to report diplopia, as the spatial frequency (waviness) was increased.[372]

Analogous changes in the extent of Panum's area are observed when the temporal frequency (the equivalent of velocity) of the stimulus is changed (Fig. 24-8,*D*). In this experiment the observer dichoptically viewed two lines separated by a horizontal disparity. When fused, the lines appeared to be a single line oscillating forward and back in depth. Panum's area proved to be thick for low-frequency (slow-velocity) image oscillation but became progressively thin-

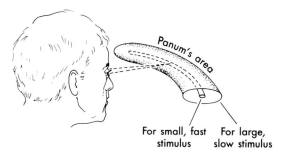

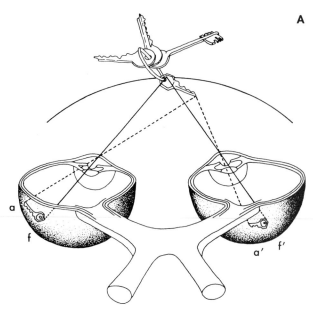

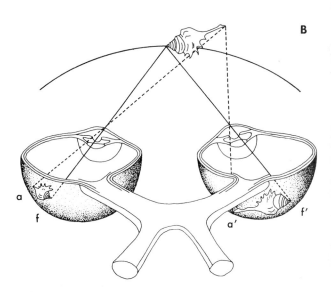

af > a'f' = Noncorrespondence = Disparity

FIG. 24-9 Change in size of Panum's area with a change in the spatiotemporal properties of the fusion stimuli. The inner-boundary Panum's area is for stimuli having a spatial frequency of 2 c/deg and a temporal frequency of 5 c/sec. Outer-boundary Panum's area is for stimuli 0.125 c/deg and 0.1 c/sec. Drawn using data of Schor and Tyler (1981).

ner as the temporal frequency of image oscillation increased.[373,377]

To explore the spatiotemporal tuning properties of Panum's area a human observer can be tested using dichoptic stimuli that combine both spatial and temporal changes, i.e., each line's spatial frequency (waviness) can be changed, and at the same time the two lines can be moved toward and away from each other so as to appear in fusion as though they were a single stimulus oscillating forward and back in depth.[330] The results of this experiment are shown in Figure 24-9. Panum's area for stimuli that are fuzzy and slow moving (low spatial and temporal frequency) is 20 times wider than it is for stimuli that are sharply focused and rapidly moving. Thus the notion that Panum's area is a fixed property of a given retinal region must be abandoned in favor of the notion that Panum's area expands and contracts depending on the size, sharpness, and speed of the stimulus.[330,373]

Stereopsis (disparity sensitivity)

Because the eyes are separated about 6.5 cm in the horizontal plane of the head, each eye has a slightly horizontally disparate view of the world. Stereopsis is the ability to use horizontal disparity cues to construct a percept of solid depth (Gr. *stereos* = solid). An observer who possesses stereopsis is able to construct a three-dimensional percept from two two-dimensional retinal images.

An object confined to the horopter is seen as flat because it projects to corresponding retinal regions, causing zero horizontal disparity. Nonzero disparities giving rise to stereoscopic depth are divided into crossed and uncrossed. Figures 24-10, *A* and 24-11 show that crossed dispari-

af < a'f' = Noncorrespondence = Disparity

FIG. 24-10 Binocular disparity caused by stimuli lying nearer ("crossed") or further ("uncrossed") than the horopter. **A,** The stimulus is nearer than the horopter; hence its image falls more temporalward on the retina of the left eye than the right eye. A greater temporalward shift is seen as crossed disparity. **B,** The stimulus is farther than the horopter; its image falls more nasalward on the retina of the right eye. A greater nasalward shift is seen as uncrossed disparity. Compare with Figure 24-1,*A*.

ties are created by objects in front of the horopter (near objects). The disparity is termed "crossed" because the monocular image of the object when viewed by the right eye is displaced to the left, whereas that viewed by the left eye is displaced to the right. When an object is located behind the horopter (a far object), it gives rise to an uncrossed disparity (Fig. 24-10, *B*). In this case the monocular image of the object viewed by the right eye is displaced to the right, whereas that viewed by the left eye is displaced to the left. The reader can demonstrate this for himself by holding two fingers at different distances from the head (Fig. 24-11). When the more distant finger is fixated binocularly, the nearer finger is seen in crossed disparity. With the right eye viewing monocularly (the left eye is momentarily shut) the image of the nearer finger is displaced to the left. With the left eye viewing monocularly, the image of the nearer finger will be displaced to the right. The exercise is then repeated with the nearer finger serving as the point of binocular fixation, causing the more distant finger to be seen in uncrossed disparity.

Crossed disparities are characterized by greater temporalward image shifts, and uncrossed by greater nasalward shifts (see Fig. 24-10).[376] This does not mean that crossed disparity images must fall on temporal hemi-retinae and uncrossed on nasal hemi-retinae, which is true only for the very limited case of an object that happens to lie directly on a line bisecting the visual axes. All that is required is that there be a greater *relative* temporalward or nasalward shift of one of the retinal images. Clinical demonstration of this principle is found in patients who have a complete hemianopia (e.g., from a lesion of the visual pathways posterior to the optic chiasm.) Stereopsis within the intact hemifield in such patients is normal, yet they are obviously able to use only one nasal and one temporal hemi-retina.[363,364]

As shown in Figure 24-12, binocular disparity is measured as the difference between angle "a" and "b" (or if more convenient to measure, between "c" and "d"). Stereoacuity, or the stereoscopic threshold, is the smallest binocular disparity that can be reliably detected. Like measurement of other psychophysical thresholds, the stereoscopic threshold is assessed on a statistical basis. Reliable detection is usually considered to be the point at which 75 percent of judgments are correct.[60] Stereoacuity is reported in seconds of arc, minutes of arc, or degrees.*

The ranges of stereopsis, fusion, and depth perception

Figure 24-13 shows thresholds and ranges for stereopsis, fusion, and depth perception as a function of binocular disparity for targets located near the foveola (0° eccentricity). The ranges vary depending on whether the target is

---

*1 degree = 60 arc minutes, 1 arc minute = 60 arc seconds. Thus 1 degree of binocular disparity = 3600 arc seconds.

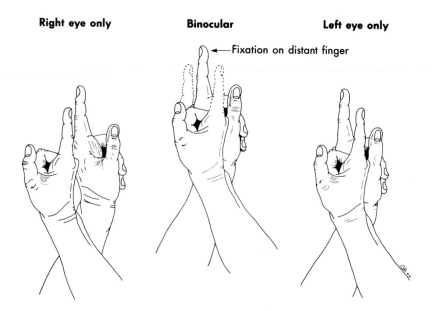

Right eye only　　　　**Binocular**　　　　**Left eye only**

←—Fixation on distant finger

FIG. 24-11　Stimuli nearer than the horopter are seen in crossed disparity, and further than the horopter in uncrossed disparity. See text for description.

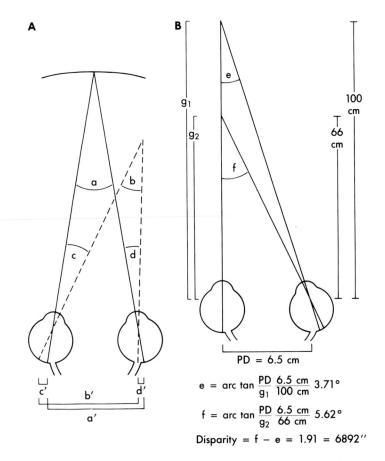

$$e = \arctan \frac{PD}{g_1} \quad \frac{6.5 \text{ cm}}{100 \text{ cm}} \quad 3.71°$$

$$f = \arctan \frac{PD}{g_2} \quad \frac{6.5 \text{ cm}}{66 \text{ cm}} \quad 5.62°$$

Disparity $= f - e = 1.91 = 6892''$

FIG. 24-12 Measuring binocular disparity by comparing the angles subtended by two stimuli at different distances from the observer. **A,** The disparity can be measured as (angle b − angle a) or, alternatively (angle c − angle d). The shift on the retina c′ corresponds to angle c, and the shift d′ to angle d. Similarly, a′ corresponds to the distance subtended by angle a, and b′ to that subtended by angle b. **B,** Trigonometry used to calculate an unknown binocular disparity. The problem is simplified by aligning the stimuli on a parasagittal line in front of either eye. A ruler is used to find distances g_1, g_2, and the interpupillary distance of the observer (PD), all in cm. Angles e and f are the arc tangents of the ratios shown. The disparity is the difference between angles e and f.

stationary or moving, and whether the eyes are stationary or moving. The stereoacuity threshold for static targets is in the range of 2 to 10 arc sec.[150,409] For targets in motion toward and away from the observer the threshold increases to about 40 arc sec.[371] Panum's limit, or the largest disparity that can still be fused into the percept of a single object in depth, varies according to the spatiotemporal properties of the target from 1.5 to 20 arc minutes when the eyes are held steady.[330] In the graph Panum's limit is plotted as 10 arc minutes, or the midpoint of the range obtained in these recent experiments. The value of 10 arc minutes also coincides with the values obtained in the classical experiments of Ogle

using a longitudinal horopter apparatus.[269] When the eyes are moving during natural head motion, Panum's area can expand sevenfold, up to a width of about 150 arc min (2.5 degrees).[347]

Note in Figure 24-13 perception of depth is actually maximal at the point at which binocular disparity is so large that the images cannot be fused and are seen as doubled.[317] Although it has been common to refer to this as diplopic stereopsis, this is terminologically confusing in that the doubled images obviously lack the perceptual quality of three-dimensional solidity that characterizes stereopsis. It would perhaps be better to simply say that binocular disparity can still be used as a cue to depth in the range in

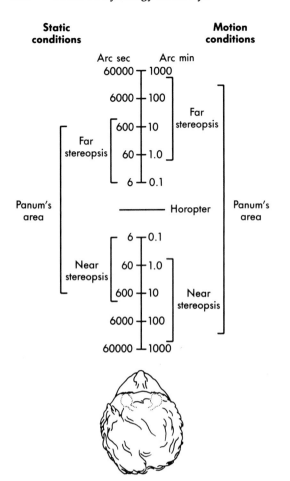

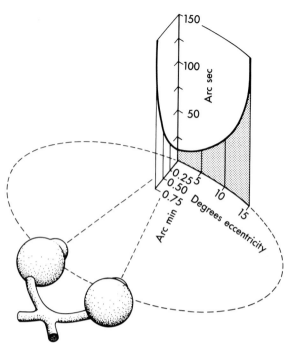

FIG. 24-14 Degradation of stereopsis (increasing threshold) with increasing lateral eccentricity from the foveola, and increasing anterior-posterior distance from the horopter. Plotted using data of Ogle (1950) and Blakemore (1970).

FIG. 24-13 Thresholds and ranges of stereopsis under static vs. motion conditions. Static here means the observer kept the eyes steadily fixating and the head still. Motion means eyes and/or head moving, which would also cause some retinal image motion. Note that stereopsis is present outside Panum's area and the maximum raw sense of depth in human occurs at about 20 arc min disparity (in the diplopic range under static viewing conditions). Sense of depth falls rapidly to zero beyond 600 arc min.

which images are seen in diplopia. The perception of depth is maximal for these diplopic images up to a disparity of 30 to 120 arc minutes (0.5 to 2 degrees). For larger disparities perception grossly underestimates actual depth, falling to a perception of no depth when image disparity reaches about 480 to 600 arc min (8 to 10 degrees).

Stereoacuity is maximal about 0.25 degrees off dead center in the foveola,[147] and diminishes exponentially with increasing eccentricity along the x-axis.[268] Stereopsis is nil beyond 15 degrees

eccentricity (Fig. 24-14). Stereoacuity diminishes in similar exponential fashion when the target is moved in front of or behind the horopter along the y-axis.[40] In the y-axis experiments the task was to discern differences in disparity between targets in front of or behind the horopter. Targets were presented in 100 msec exposures to preclude vergence and hence a shift in the location of the horopter.

Stereopsis without monocular form or motion cues
Monocular depth perception
During natural viewing a variety of depth cues are available that do not involve binocular disparity.[138,269,308] A catalog of these monocular cues to depth are shown in Figure 24-15 and are discussed briefly here to emphasize the point that binocular disparity is only one aspect of depth perception. Monocular form and motion processing alone provide robust cues to depth in natural viewing situations.

1. Apparent size: because we know that real objects do not change in size (size con-

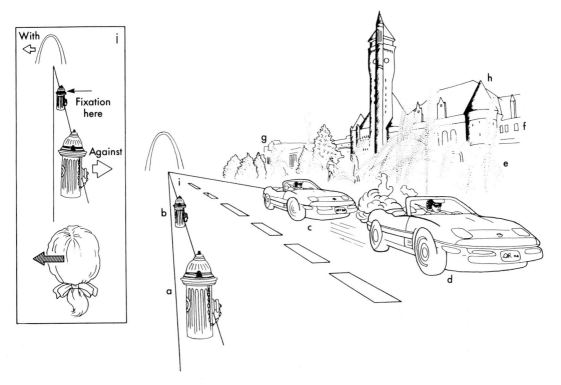

FIG. 24-15 Multiple monocular cues to depth in a view of Union Station, St. Louis. Letters mark individual cues: a,b = apparent size; c,d = looming; e,f = interposition; g = aerial perspective; h = shading; i = geometric perspective; c,d = relative velocity and velocity flow. *Inset:* j = motion parallax: fixation is at an intermediate distance and the head is translated to the left. Near objects move against head motion (rightward) and far objects with head motion (leftward), analogous to crossed and uncrossed disparity.

stancy), small retinal images are interpreted as distant objects and large retinal images are interpreted as near objects. Objects progressively increase in size as they move toward us (looming).

2. Interposition: relatively nearer objects tend to conceal or overlay more distant objects.

3. Aerial perspective: water vapor, dust, and smoke in the atmosphere scatter light and make distant objects indistinct and relatively color-desaturated.

4. Shading: light falling on solid objects causes shadows to be cast, and on curved surfaces causes a gradation in the intensity of the shadow. That the brighter of two objects is interpreted as nearer can also be considered a cue derived from shading.

5. Geometric perspective: physically parallel lines converge toward a vanishing point at the horizon, e.g., railroad tracks. Detail decreases and crowding of objects increases toward the horizon.

6. Relative velocity: the image velocity of a moving target in the distance is lower than the image velocity of the same moving target when it is nearby (assuming the real velocity in space remains the same). The image velocities of moving objects steadily increase as they approach and pass behind us (velocity flow), e.g., approaching and passing a road sign in an automobile.

7. Motion parallax: translations of the head cause the images of near objects to move opposite the head and the images of far objects to move with the head, assuming the fixation point is at an intermediate distance. Relative velocity is also available as a cue during motion parallax: the "against" motion is higher velocity than the "with" motion.

These cues are well known to artists. They are commonly employed in video games and television graphics to create an illusion of three-dimensionality. The masterful combination of these cues made the early animated movies of Walt Disney revolutionary for their time, e.g., the wonderful forest scenes of Snow White and the Seven Dwarfs. That these monocular cues serve as powerful inputs to perception for real depth is attested to by the skill of certain one-eyed individuals in performing tasks that are believed to require precise degrees of stereopsis. Highly competent one-eyed aviators and one-eyed surgeons are examples.

Random dot stereopsis

Use of the leaf room was an early effort to separate binocular disparity cues from monocular cues.[169] The leaf room was for all practical purposes the first random dot stereogram: a depth stimulus containing no monocularly visible cues (Fig. 24-16).

This room is a cubical box about 2 meters on an edge, open at one end, with the walls vertical and the floor and ceiling level. To the inside surfaces of the room are stapled many artificial vines that literally cover these surfaces. The leaves are adjusted individually so that they stand out from the surface in a random orientation. Under good illumination the rough edges of the leaves and their haphazard orientation provide many contours to stimulate stereopsis. The cubical shape of the room is readily perceived in binocular vision, but the perspective features are weak. Indeed, with continued monocular observation (one eye occluded) the room appears to lose its cubical shape entirely; the corners tend to blend with the walls into a uniform shapeless concavity covered with leaves. The cubical appearance of the room in stereoscopic vision is easy for the observer to describe.[269]

The leaf room experiments provided compelling evidence that binocular disparity was the necessary and sufficient cue for stereopsis.

The first random dot stimuli made for dichoptic viewing were created by Aschenbrenner in 1954.[7] Julesz,[177] in 1960, provided a major in-novation by having a computer draw a matrix composed of thousands of black and white dots on a gray background (Fig. 24-17). The computer randomly chose whether to make an individual dot black or white, and then created an exact duplicate of the entire matrix, one for each eye. A central region of dots, matched dot-to-dot in the two stimuli, was then shifted horizontally. This left a vertical row of blank spaces at one border of the shifted region, which the computer then filled in by the same randomizing process.[178,308]

When viewed monocularly, the random dot stimuli had no evident form, texture, or depth, but when viewed in a stereoscope a vivid perception of depth was evoked, with the shifted region popping out or receding, depending upon whether the shift created crossed or uncrossed disparity. The shape of the shifted region can only emerge by matching of disparity cues at the level of striate cortex lamina IVB and higher, since this is the first level in the central nervous system at which monocular inputs combine. Julesz used computer-generated random dot stimuli to test a number of classical visual illusions.[178] If the illusion persists when presented in a random dot stereogram, it has to have arisen in the visual cortex, not the eye. Random dot stereopsis thus serves as a benchmark for determining the level in the visual pathway at which perceptions are generated. Julesz termed this level of stereoscopic perception "cyclopean," since it could only arise from complete blending of images from the two eyes.[178*] "Non-cyclopean" stereopsis employs monocularly visible cues.

---

*Cyclops was the one-eyed monster of Homer's *Odyssey*. Julesz uses the term "cyclopean" in a way different from that first used by Hering. Hering's (1868) "cyclopean" meant egocentric visual direction (a ray emanating from the head), since under binocular conditions we view the world as though from a single eye in the midline of the head.

Monocular

Binocular

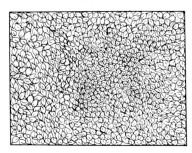 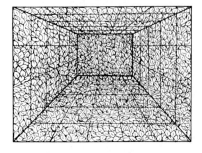

FIG. 24-16   The leaf room: the earliest "random dot" test of stereopsis. See text for description.

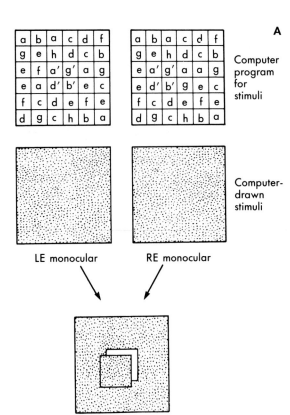

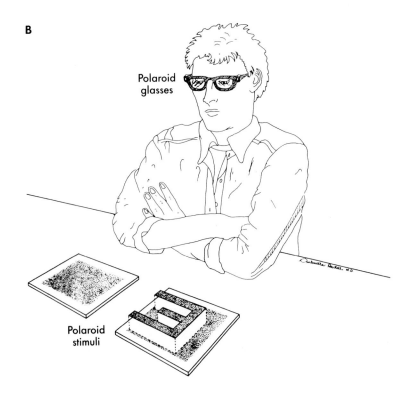

FIG. 24-17 Modern computer-generated random-dot stereograms for clinical testing. **A,** The computer algorithm shifts a subset of pixels horizontally to create a horizontal disparity. Viewed monocularly, the stimuli lack any figure emerging from the random dot background, but when viewed with normal binocular vision a vivid square emerges. **B,** A ''catch'' stimulus on the subject's right and a random-dot E stimulus on the subject's left, consisting of a sandwich of two monocular, polarized stimuli. The subject wears glasses polarized in an orientation identical to that of the stimuli to detect the disparity of the ''E'' pixels.

In 1950 Ogle had postulated two kinds of stereopsis.[268] The first kind was "quantitative," and was devoted to processing small disparities. The second was "qualitative," and was devoted to processing large disparities. His experiments showed that small-disparity stereopsis required continuous exposure of test stimuli and steady fixation. On the other hand, large-disparity stereopsis was unimpaired by brief stimulus exposures and scanning eye movements.[271]

The data from these studies suggest that for a true, quantitative, and patent sense of depth the simultaneous stimulation of horizontally associated disparate retinal elements is necessary. A more vague qualitative perception of depth, also arising from inferred disparate images, may provide the observer with an experience only of "farther" or "nearer" than the point of fixation. The experiments show further that the qualitative sense of depth is enhanced by momentary stimuli, but depressed with continuously visible disparate stimuli. Eye movements also may enhance this aspect of depth perception.[269]

Ogle's dichotomization of stereopsis into two classes, one small and one large disparity, was taken up by Julesz and Spivack in 1967 in their designation of "global" and "local" stereopsis.[178,180] "Global stereopsis" was a slow neural process requiring the combination of many disparity matches across the foveal visual field. The buildup eventually gave rise to the perception of a well-defined object at a precise depth. "Local stereopsis" was a quicker process. It required disparity matches at only a few foveal locations and produced a cruder percept of object shape and a cruder percept of near or far. Although not articulated precisely, Julesz implies that "global" vs. "local" is equivalent to "cyclopean" vs. "non-cyclopean."* Global matching presumably occurs at a higher hierarchical level in visual cortex than local stereopsis and requires more neuronal connections.

Parvocellular and magnocellular streams

Division of the human visual pathway into two major streams is based on neurophysiologic and neuroanatomic work in the macaque monkey and owl monkey.[81,238,382,383,384] These neuron streams are defined histologically by layering of the lateral geniculate nucleus into parvocellular and magnocellular laminae, and by layering of the striate cortex into parvo- and magno-recipient laminae. Figure 24-18 shows schematically how the parvocellular and magnocellular streams differ, and how processing in the parvocellular stream can be further segregated into two substreams, a parvo-blob and parvo-

*For a lengthier discussion of this distinction, see Tyler[373,374]

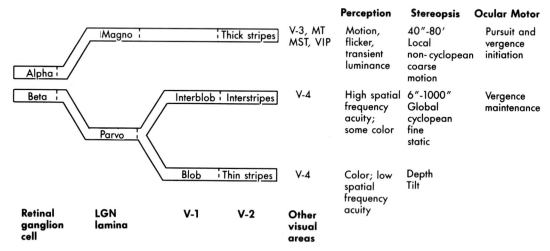

				Perception	Stereopsis	Ocular Motor
	Magno		Thick stripes	V-3, MT MST, VIP	Motion, flicker, transient luminance	40"-80' Local non-cyclopean coarse motion	Pursuit and vergence initiation
Alpha						
Beta		Interblob	Interstripes	V-4	High spatial frequency acuity; some color	6"-1000" Global cyclopean fine static	Vergence maintenance
	Parvo					
		Blob	Thin stripes	V-4	Color; low spatial frequency acuity	Depth Tilt	
Retinal ganglion cell	LGN lamina	V-1	V-2	Other visual areas			

FIG. 24-18 Parallel visual pathways or streams for general visual perception, stereopsis, and eye movement. Postulated input of signals for vergence initiation and maintenance are listed. V1 = striate cortex, primary visual area, or area 17 in old Brodmann scheme; V2 and other extrastriate areas are subdivisions of Brodmann areas 18,19, and more anterior regions of tempero-parietal cortex. Depth tilt is a crude depth sensation caused by differences in the spatial frequency of stimuli seen by the two eyes, as discussed in Tyler (1983).

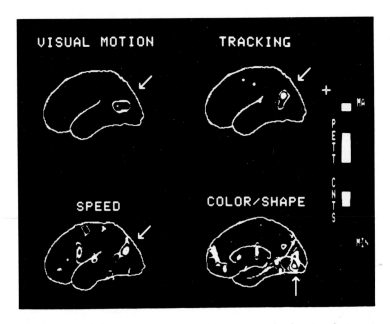

FIG. 24-19 Sagittal blood-flow images of normal human cerebral cortex during visual tasks. The bright areas indicate high metabolic activity. Motion/tracking/speed ("magno") regions of extrastriate cortex lie dorsal to color/shape ("parvo") regions. Tasks in various trials were: to discriminate direction of motion; to smoothly pursue a target; to judge target speed (20 to 30 deg/sec); or to discriminate differences in shape or color between successive stimuli displayed on a video monitor. Sagittal reconstruction from positron emission transverse tomograms (PETT). CNTS = counts. Time per scan = 40 sec. Courtesy of Dr. Steven E. Petersen, Washington University School of Medicine.

interblob stream. Blobs are clusters of cells in the striate cortex that stain darkly for cytochrome oxidase, an intracellular enzyme indicative of high metabolic activity.[212,407] The parvo-interblob stream appears to be involved in fine spatial acuity and the parvo-blob in color discrimination. Studies using noninvasive probes, e.g., MRI, PET scanning (Fig. 24-19), evoked potentials, eye movement recording, and psychophysics, have now shown that human cortex is organized into highly similar streams.[59] For the purposes of the discussion that follows it will be assumed that monkey and human anatomic and physiologic data are interchangeable. The most striking difference between macaque and human cortex is sheer size; the human cortex has ten times the surface area of the macaque, and the human occipital lobe is about five times larger than that of macaque.[22,382]

Taking inspiration from the work of Ogle and that of Julesz and Spivack, Tyler has divided stereopsis into two categories of disparity processing: fine-global-static stereopsis and coarse-local-motion stereopsis.[373,374] The former is particularly suited to seeing random dot stereo-

grams that are stationary, and the latter is suitable for seeing nonrandom dot stereotargets (targets that contain monocularly visible form cues) that move or rapidly change. Tyler proposes that this psychophysical division is due to the division of disparity processing in parvocellular and magnocellular neurons. The division is not absolute, but is meant rather to emphasize the "optimal tuning properties" of the two neuron populations.

Table 24-1 summarizes the findings of a large number of human and monkey experiments that justify this division of stereopsis into fine-parvocellular and coarse-magnocellular components. Major distinctions are discussed below. The data is from human unless indicated otherwise.

Properties of static stereopsis

1. Disparity range: static stereopsis operates within a binocular horizontal disparity range of 2 to 20 arc min (2 to 1200 arc sec, or less than 0.33 degrees).[269,373,374]
2. Latency: evoked potential studies indicate

TABLE 24-1 Components of Fine-Parvocellular (Static) and Coarse-Magnocellular (Motion) Stereopsis

	Static stereopsis	Motion stereopsis
Disparity	2″–1200″ (0–.33 deg)	40″–36,000″ (0.1–10 deg)
Latency	250 msec	130 msec
Retinotopic location	foveal; 0–5 deg eccentric	parafoveal
Temporal frequency	500 msec–3,000 msec, i.e., below 2 Hz	less than 333 msec, i.e., above 3 Hz
Spatial frequency	sensitivity increases toward higher frequencies, i.e., above 3 c/deg	broad range, extends very low, i.e., 0.1 c/deg
Color sensitivity	sensitive; persists with chromatic equiluminance	insensitive; impaired with red-green equiluminance

that static stereopsis has a latency of about 250 msec.[179,200,257]

3. Retinotopic location: it is best for targets located on the fovea.[269,377]

4. Temporal frequency range: it is best when targets remain stationary for at least 500 msec (when the temporal frequency of target change is below 2 Hz).[271,374,377] Static stereopsis improves with exposure time up to a maximum of 3 sec,[269,271] suggesting linear summation or integration over time.

5. Spatial frequency range: static stereopsis increases as the spatial frequency of the target increases.[331] Static stereopsis shows position sensitivity, i.e., it is enhanced when a stationary reference is available to define the horopter.[309,377]

6. Color effects: static stereopsis persists in the presence of chromatic equiluminance, i.e., neurons that process static stereopsis are color sensitive.[375]

Neuroanatomy and physiology of static stereopsis

Retinal ganglion cells of the parvocellular stream (beta cells) are concentrated in the fovea and decrease in number systematically toward the peripheral retina.[78,320,323] They have small dendritic field diameters (Fig. 24-20). Neurons of the parvo-interblob stream in monkey respond to high spatial frequency and static visual targets, and chemical lesions of parvocellular layers of the LGN severely impair fine random dot stereopsis in trained monkey.[324,325] Discrimination of coarse dot stereograms is less severely affected. The parvocellular recipient lamina of area V1 is layer IVCβ.[216] Here, as in the LGN, the inputs are strictly monocular, from the nasal hemi-retina of the contralateral eye and the temporal hemi-retina of the ipsilateral eye.[155,157] The paired right eye and left eye monocular cells of layer IVC beta converge on binocular cells of layer IVA, which then send afferents to binoc-

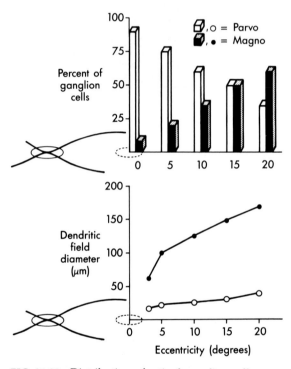

FIG. 24-20 Distribution of retinal ganglion cells as a function of eccentricity from the foveola. Viewed as if looking at flattened left fundus. *Top:* Parvocellular pathway ganglion cells (beta cells) tend to dominate in the fovea, and magnocellular (alpha cells) dominate at the boundary of the perifovea and beyond. Magnocellular cells outnumber parvo in the periphery, but also diminish beyond 20 deg (not shown). *Bottom:* Dendritic field diameter, an indirect measure of receptive field size, is much larger for magnocellular pathway cells. Plotted using human data of Rodieck et al. (1985); and macaque data of de Monasterio and Gouras (1975); Schiller and Malpeli (1977).

ular laminae II, III, and V. Thus lamina IVA of V1 is the first level of binocularity in the central nervous system for the parvocellular pathway.

Four types of binocular neurons in area V1 of

monkey are sensitive to small disparities on or near the horopter and are therefore likely candidates for static stereopsis neurons.[288-290,374] They have reciprocal push-pull sensitivities that allow definition of the plane of fixation (the horopter) and targets just in front of or behind it. The sensitivity ranges for these neurons are shown in Figure 24-21.

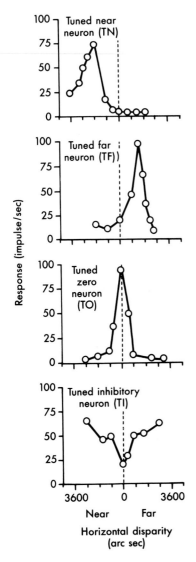

FIG. 24-21 Neurons sensitive to horizontal binocular disparity in area V1 of macaque. These four types of sharply tuned neurons are found in roughly equal proportion in V1, and have also been identified in areas V2 and V3. Stimuli used were vertically oriented bars presented under conditions of dichoptic viewing. Single unit recordings from alert monkeys trained to maintain vergence on an accommodative target. Redrawn using data of Poggio and Fischer (1977) and Poggio et al. (1988).

1. Tuned zero (T0) neurons respond maximally to targets on the horopter (targets having zero to 180 arc sec of crossed or uncrossed disparity) and are inhibited by targets in front of or behind the horopter.
2. Tuned near (TN) neurons respond maximally to targets 900 to 1800 arc sec in front of the horopter (crossed disparity), and are inhibited by targets nearer or farther than this narrow band of disparities.
3. Tuned far (TF) neurons are the mirror image of the TN neurons, responding maximally to targets 900 to 1800 arc sec behind the horopter (uncrossed disparity) and displaying inhibition for nearer or farther targets.
4. Tuned inhibitory (TI) neurons are the mirror image of the T0 neurons. TI cells would signal movement off the plane of fixation, as they remain quiet when targets are on the horopter but begin to fire when the fixated target is 0 to 180 arc sec off the horopter.

The available evidence indicates that neurons of each type are irregularly distributed throughout the layers of V1. It is methodologically difficult to test disparity sensitivity for a large number of neurons at one specific cortical sublamina. For that reason it is not clear whether parvocellular lamina IVA and the interblob regions of laminae II, III, and V contain a greater number of T0, TN, TF, or TI neurons (as would be expected). No difference in disparity sensitivity has been found between neurons possessing what Hubel and Wiesel[289] designated as "simple" and "complex" properties.

Properties of motion stereopsis

1. Disparity range: motion stereopsis operates over a broader disparity range than static stereopsis (from 40 to 36,000 arc sec or 0.1 to 10 degrees).[267,374] Motion stereopsis thus overlaps static stereopsis from 40 to 1200 arc sec, but operates alone from 1200 to 36,000 arc sec (beyond 20 arc min or 0.33 degrees); 600 to 1200 arc sec is the boundary of Panum's area at the fovea in normal humans under conditions of stationary gaze (Fig. 24-13). With the head and eyes moving, the boundary increases to 9000 arc sec (2.5 degrees).[347] Thus in this motion mode stereoscopic targets with disparities greater than 1200 arc sec would not be seen in diplopia.
2. Latency: evoked potential studies indicate that motion stereopsis has a latency of about 130 msec, or one half that of static stereopsis.[257,311]

3. Retinotopic location: target locations off the fovea impair motion stereopsis less than static stereopsis,[269,309,377] indicating that motion stereopsis plays a dominant role in stereopsis at extrafoveal locations. The relative superiority of motion stereopsis at extrafoveal locations is true for targets located to the right or left of fixation (x axis)[269,377] and in front of or behind the horopter (y axis).[309]

4. Temporal frequency range: optimal for targets that move or change at a rate of up to 3 to 10 cycles per second or more (3 to 10 Hz).[258,374,377]

5. Spatial frequency range: about 10 times more sensitive than static stereopsis system for low spatial frequency (0.1 cycle per degree) moving targets.[331]

6. Color effects: little if any color sensitivity; disparity sensitivity decreases eight- to tenfold for colored targets having equal red-green luminances.[375]

Neuroanatomy and physiology of motion stereopsis

Magnocellular ganglion cells (alpha cells) are relatively sparse in the foveola and increase in number systematically toward the near periphery.[78,320,323] They have large dendritic field diameters (see Fig. 24-20). Neurons of the magnocellular stream in monkey respond optimally to low spatial frequency, moving visual targets, and chemical lesions of magnocellular layers of monkey LGN severely impair responses to target motion and target flicker. The chemical lesions do not impair static stereopsis.[324,325] The magnocellular recipient lamina of area V1 is IVCα.[216] The LGN inputs to IVCα are monocular from the right or left eye.[155,157] The paired right eye and left eye monocular cells of lamina IVCα converge on binocular cells of layer IVB and VI. Thus IVB and VI are the first level of binocularity in the magnocellular pathway. Lamina IVB and VI of area V1 contain the highest proportion of binocular neurons showing strong responses to visual motion.[99,134] These neurons are highly sensitive to luminance contrast and targets of low to middle range spatial frequency.[134]

Two types of binocular neurons in area V1 of monkey have receptive field properties that make them sensitive to large disparities and they are therefore leading candidates for motion stereopsis neurons.[288-290,373] As noted earlier, it is not clear at present that they are present in higher concentration specifically in laminae IVB and VI. The two types have reciprocal sensitivities, as shown in Figure 24-22.

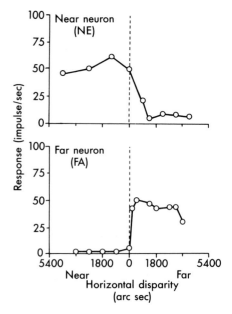

FIG. 24-22 Two other types of neurons sensitive to horizontal binocular disparity in macaque area V1. Tuning is much flatter than that of cells shown in Figure 24-21. Similar cells have been identified in areas V2 and V3. Plotted using data of Poggio et al. (1988).

1. Near (NE) neurons respond maximally to targets 450 to 7200 arc sec (0.125-2 degrees) in front of the horopter (crossed disparity) and are inhibited by all targets behind the horopter (all uncrossed disparities).

2. Far (FA) neurons are the mirror image of the NE neurons, responding maximally to targets 450 to 7200 arc sec behind the horopter and displaying inhibition for all targets in front of the horopter.

Ninety-seven percent of cells in foveal and parafoveal striate cortex of macaque are binocular.[288] Approximately 50 percent are sensitive to horizontal disparity. Within this 50 percent the six different types of disparity sensitive neurons are about equally represented, so that roughly 8 percent of the cells in V1 are T0, 8 percent TN, 8 percent NE, etc. The remaining 50 percent respond to all disparities and are designated flat (FL).

Binocular correlation sensitivity, rivalry, and suppression

The two essential neural steps necessary for stereopsis are: (1) the identification of two images belonging to the same object in space, the "matching" or "correspondence" problem, and

(2) the detection of disparity between the corresponding images. The two neural tasks are, in a certain sense, incompatible, since one seeks similarities and the other small differences.[220,228,287]

About 50 percent of the neurons in V1 are sensitive to similarities in the shape, contrast, and texture of the targets seen by the two eyes.[289] This is termed binocular correlation and is tested using correlograms (Fig. 24-23). Note how correlograms differ from stereograms.* Binocular uncorrelation in a correlogram refers to random mismatches at multiple locations in a two-dimensional dot pattern presented to the right and left eye. Binocular disparity in a stereogram refers to a precise horizontal shift of a subset of dots that are otherwise perfectly correlated in the two eyes. A stereogram is a correlogram of a special type: the only uncorrelation being a precise horizontal shift of a subset of dots.

Correlation responses of binocular neurons provide the neural basis for fusion. Suppression of responses to uncorrelated images provides the neural basis for avoiding confusion. When the right eye receptive field and the left eye receptive field of a binocular disparity neuron are not activated by a single target located in depth at the binocular neuron's preferred disparity, the receptive fields could still be stimulated by two different targets, one for each receptive field, nearer or farther than that disparity. The two targets would have different shapes and contours; they would be binocularly uncorrelated (Fig. 24-24). During this kind of image uncorrelation, suppression of T0 neurons would avoid visual confusion. On the other hand, activation of NE, FA, and TI neurons for small amounts of image uncorrelation would be useful for fusion of slightly different-appearing images within Panum's area. This is compatible with what has been found in recording from binocular neurons in monkey cortex: all T0 neurons are suppressed by image uncorrelation, while most TI, NE, and FA neurons are activated.[289] A substantial number of FL neurons (flat neurons) are also correlation sensitive. These FL neurons could encode two-dimensional fusion.

Rivalry is the psychophysical term used for

___
*The two terms are sometimes used in confusing ways. Julesz[178] defines stereograms as a special subclass of correlograms, but then uses the terms almost interchangeably. Poggio et al.[289] uses the term "stereopairs" for a strictly flat, 2-D pair of correlograms composed of random dots.

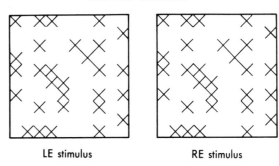

Binocular correlation

LE stimulus   RE stimulus

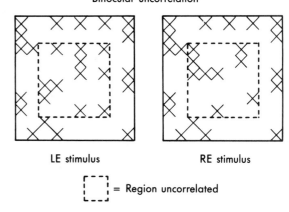

Binocular uncorrelation

LE stimulus   RE stimulus

[⬚] = Region uncorrelated

FIG. 24-23 Correlation and uncorrelation of binocular images. Correlated images allow fusion, and uncorrelated images cause rivalry, confusion, diplopia, or suppression. Uncorrelation can occur when the visual axis of one eye is blocked, when the eyes are misaligned, or when one eye is defocused.

the visual confusion caused when uncorrelated images simultaneously stimulate corresponding regions on the two foveas.[39,111,112] During rivalry, patches of the visual field are dominated by one image or the other and the patches fluctuate from moment to moment (Fig. 24-25). Rivalry is uncomfortable and confusing. Suppression of rivalry is important under normal conditions whenever some object passing close to the head momentarily blocks the visual axis of one eye, e.g., movements of the arm or hand during work or play. Rivalry (or confusion) is rarely a clinical complaint in patients who suddenly acquire pathologic eye misalignment, because one of the foveal images is quickly suppressed. The perceptual system then attends to the foveal image from one eye and the same image at a noncorresponding region on the retina of the other eye, giving rise to diplopia (the perception

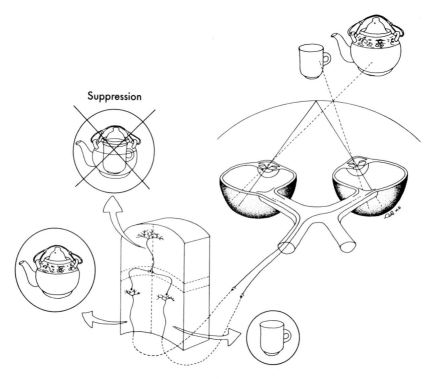

FIG. 24-24 Need for suppression of binocular neuron to avoid visual confusion or rivalry. A neuron in lamina IV B of the left visual cortex has a binocular receptive field tuned for zero disparity (i.e., on the horopter). No stimulus is present at the preferred binocular disparity. The monocular receptive fields are occupied by uncorrelated stimuli that lie beyond the horopter.

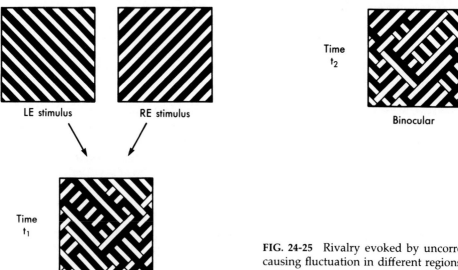

FIG. 24-25 Rivalry evoked by uncorrelated stimuli, causing fluctuation in different regions of the visual field from moment to moment. The sensation is unpleasant.

of the same object at two locations in space). Diplopia is bothersome but far less confusing than rivalry (the perception of two different objects at the same location in space).

Image uncorrelation that impairs fusion and stereopsis can be caused in a variety of ways. Monocular blur (anisometropia) impairs stereopsis when the blur is sufficient to degrade the acuity of one eye to a level of 6/12 (20/40).[86,121,214] Experimental anisometropia is produced by placing plus lenses before one eye. Similar impairments of stereopsis are produced by a difference in image size between the two eyes (aniseikonia). Differences in retinal illuminance, or pupil size, have very little effect on static stereopis as long as the illuminance difference does not exceed 1 log unit.[214] Small differences in retinal illuminance have major effects on motion stereopsis, as discussed in a later section ("Pulfrich illusion").

Binocular neurons in extrastriate areas

There is a systematic increase in the proportion of neurons sensitive to binocular disparity as one progresses from area V1 to V2 to V3 in monkey: 50 percent, 66 percent, and 80 percent respectively.[289] A trend is also evident for increasing preferred disparity and increasing receptive field eccentricity: V1 neurons prefer fine disparities and have receptive fields congregated within 5 degrees of the foveola, V2 neurons preferring intermediate disparities at intermediate eccentricities, and V3 preferring coarse disparities at extrafoveal eccentricities (Fig. 24-26).

As shown in Figure 24-27, V1 sends both parvo-interblob and magnocellular projections to V2, consistent with the finding that V2 contains a high proportion of both color selective and motion sensitive cells.[53,80,213,382] Thus the intermediate disparity sensitivities, color selectivity, and motion sensitivity of V2 neurons suggest that V2 plays a role in both static and motion stereopsis.

V1 sends magnocellular projections to V3.[52,382] V3 contains a high proportion of motion sensitive, but few, if any, color selective cells. Thus it is likely that V3 participates mainly in motion stereopsis.

V1 sends a major magnocellular projection to *visual area MT*,[222,378] an area in macaque and human that is thought to be highly specialized for motion perception and eye movement (Figs. 24-19 and 24-29).[211,254,255,366] About 50 percent of the cells in visual area MT are disparity sensitive.[224] Another 30 percent are binocular but

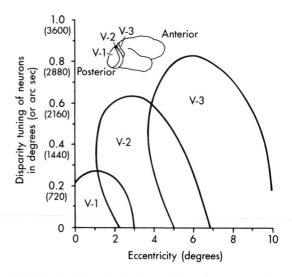

FIG. 24-26   Disparity tuning of binocular neurons increases in coarseness from area V1 to V3 of macaque. Receptive field eccentricity from the foveola also increases. Curved lines indicate region within which the majority of neurons from each visual area fell. Ordinate plotted in both degrees and arc sec. Drawn using data of Poggio et al. (1988).

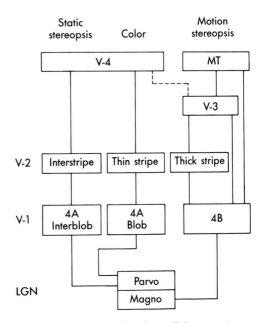

FIG. 24-27   Hierarchical and parallel processing connections, for static and motion stereopsis, between visual area V1 (striate cortex) and extrastriate visual areas. Modification of connection scheme of Van Essen (1985).

lack disparity sensitivity (FL or flat neurons). Each type of disparity sensitive cell found in V1 has been found in MT, the major difference being coarser disparity tuning of MT neurons and twice the number of near cells (TN and NE) as compared to far cells (TF and FA). Both MT, V1, and V2 have been shown to have "opposed movement" cells, selective for opposite directions of movement in the two eyes.[290,412] These cells would be suitable for signaling motion toward and away from the head (Fig. 24-28). All cells tested in macaque MT prefer frontoparallel motion, albeit not always at zero disparity. A population of such cells tuned for zero disparity, combined with opposite motion cells, could account for perception of motion in depth.[382] Adult humans who have acquired lesions of the extrastriate area homologous to monkey visual area MT have been shown to have deficits in the perception of motion in depth.[414]

The majority of cells in MT are selective for velocities of about 32 degress/sec, which is 10 times higher than the average preferred velocity of V1 cells (1 to 4 degrees/sec).[99,223,382] The combination of fine-disparity tuning and low-velocity tuning in V1 justify speculation that the mo-

tion stereopsis neurons of this area provide the signals for fine vergence movements within Panum's area, whereas the coarser-disparity and higher-velocity tuning of the motion stereopsis neurons in MT provide the signals for rapid vergence to a new fixation plane, well beyond Panum's area (Fig. 24-29). The possible role of area MT in the ocular motor anomalies of humans who have onset of strabismus in infancy are addressed in a later section.[360,367]

Neurophysiologic studies in behaving monkeys, along with lesion studies in monkeys and humans, implicate posterior parietal cortex (areas 7a, LIP, VIP) in directing visual attention for fixation, smooth pursuit, and saccades.[246,357] The cells in this area are thought to encode complex spatial relationships. Gnadt and Mays[119] found visual and motor cells in this area, and in an area contiguous with area MT (area MST), that discharge for vergence eye movement in behaving monkey. The visual cells encode binocular disparity for vergence and for smooth pursuit in depth. The motor cells encode both vergence velocity and velocity of lens accommodation.

Extrastriate area V4 in monkey receives input

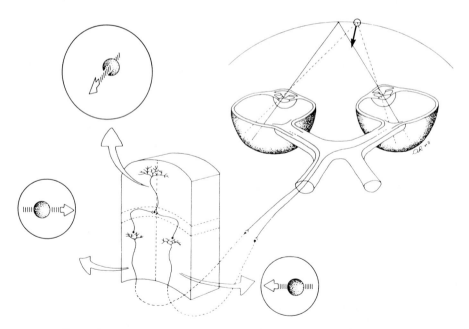

FIG. 24-28   Binocular opponent-motion or "looming" cell in left visual cortex, area V1, V3, or MT. Motion of ball toward the head is conveyed as nasally directed 2-D motion, from the monocular receptive field of the nasal retina in right eye, and temporal retina in left eye. Monocular direction-selective neurons are depicted in lamina IV C α, and binocular motion neuron in lamina IV B.

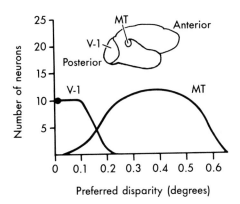

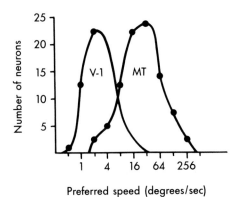

FIG. 24-29 Tuning properties of neuron populations in area V1 vs. MT suggest that V1 is suited for vergence maintenance near the horopter and MT for vergence initiation and pursuit to a new horopter. The preferred disparity of V1 neurons is $4\times$ to $10\times$ narrower than MT, and the preferred stimulus speed is $8\times$ to $30\times$ slower. Plotted using data of Fischer et al. (1981); Maunsell and Van Essen (1983); Van Essen (1985).

from parvo-blob (color selective) and parvo-interblob (orientation selective, i.e., form vision) cells of V1. The parvo-interblob cells are believed to be responsible for the disparity selectivity demonstrated in many cells of V4 in monkey.[96] A patient with an acquired lesion in an area of extrastriate cortex homologous to monkey area V4, had a deficit in color and form vision but no deficit in stereopsis.[318] Presumably, the lesion had produced greater damage to parvo-blob than to parvo-interblob cells. Acquired lesions of the right cerebral cortex in adult patients tend to degrade stereopsis more than lesions of the left cortex.[133] The degradation is greater for random-dot stereopsis than for monocular-cue stereopsis.

Role of the optic chiasm and corpus callosum in fusion and stereopsis

Visual input to both cerebral hemispheres is not necessary for fusion or stereopsis. Humans with complete hemianopia due to lesions of striate cortex have visual input into only one cerebral hemisphere, yet they have normal fusion and normal random dot stereopsis.[358,363] The hemidecussation of fibers at the optic chiasm allows pairing of inputs within the hemisphere, from corresponding regions on the nasal retina of the contralateral eye and the temporal retina of the ipsilateral eye. Thus callosal transfer is unnecessary for calculation of binocular disparity or fusion of correlated images within a hemifield.

Callosal transfer of position information may be necessary for processing of binocular disparity[26,38,40,101,240] if a target is located (a) exactly at the vertical meridian of the visual field or (b) off the vertical meridian at perfectly symmetric locations in the two nasal or two temporal hemifields* (Fig. 24-30). But even here 2 degrees of overlap in the distribution of contralaterally and ipsilaterally projecting retinal ganglion cells would provide up to 7200 arc sec of disparity information without callosal transfer.† One to two degrees of overlap has been documented anatomically in normal adult monkeys.[48,204] There is no anatomic data on the degree of overlap in human. If 2 degrees of overlap is present in human, callosal transfer for disparity judgments would only be necessary for targets located on the vertical meridian at disparities in the diplopic range, i.e., more than 7200 arc sec in front of or behind the horopter.

Humans who have split their optic chiasm (e.g., as a result of a motor vehicle accident) suffer complete loss of binocular correspondence, due to loss of visual information from both temporal hemifields. Loss of correspondence precludes fusion, causing wandering misalignment of the visual axes (the "hemifield slide phenomenon"). The patient's perception is a panoramic view that is disjointed along the vertical midline[100,190,251] (Fig. 24-31). Testing for stere-

---

*That is, the target in space would be located on a line perfectly bisecting the visual axes.

†Fibers from ganglion cells straddling the vertical meridian of the retina do not segregate perfectly at the optic chiasm in normal monkey (Bunt et al.,[48] Leventhal et al.[204]). Perfect segregation would produce no nasotemporal overlap. Overlap occurs when ganglion cells nasal to the foveola send their fibers to the ipsilateral, rather than the contralateral, LGN. The same appears to be true, mutatis mutandis, for some fibers from temporal retina. This overlap is much greater in nonprimates.

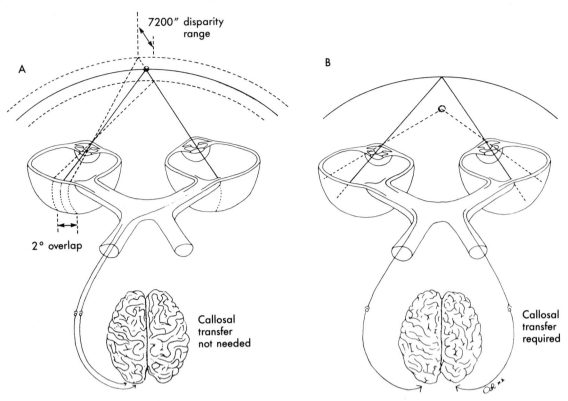

FIG. 24-30 Nasotemporal overlap and issue of callosal transfer for stereopsis. **A,** Retinal ganglion cells in macaque do not segregate perfectly at the optic chiasm, resulting in about 2 deg of overlap at the vertical meridian of the visual field. This degree of overlap would permit pairing of any left eye receptive field within the 2 deg swath, with a receptive field from the right eye foveola. Thus up to 7200″ of stereopsis is possible without any callosal transfer of visual information from the right hemisphere. **B,** If a stimulus is situated on a line bisecting the visual axes, and lies more than 7200″ from the horopter, the stimulus will excite eccentric receptive fields in both cerebral hemispheres. In this case, pairing of monocular receptive fields for stereopsis could only occur via transfer across the corpus callosum.

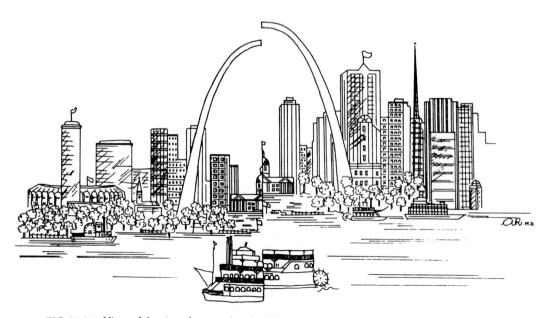

FIG. 24-31 View of the river front and arch, St. Louis, as seen by a patient whose optic chiasm has been split. A transecting lesion of the chiasm eliminates any possibility of binocular correspondence; there are no temporal visual field regions to pair with the preserved nasal visual field regions in each cerebral hemisphere. This causes wandering misalignment of the intact hemi-fields, and, classically, a vertical step-off of all objects in the midline ("hemi-field slide phenomenon").

opsis in a patient with a split optic chiasm was reported by Blakemore.[40] Targets positioned in a tachistoscope, at symmetric regions 0.5 to 7 degrees eccentric in the intact nasal visual field of each eye elicited a gross perception of near disparity. Since each nasal field projects only to the ipsilateral cerebral hemisphere, Blakemore concluded that the judgment of near disparity could only have arisen from callosal transfer of position information.

Support for the notion that callosal transfer is necessary for disparity judgment of targets on the vertical meridian has also been provided by testing of stereopsis and vergence eye movements in a patient who had the callosum surgically sectioned.[240,402] Stereopsis and evoked vergence eye movements were normal when the target was located off the vertical meridian in either visual hemifield, but both were deficient when the target was located on the vertical meridian.

Normal variations in human stereopsis

The idea that binocular disparity was processed by different populations of neurons in human visual cortex was first provided by psychophysical studies that revealed systematic variations in stereopsis in large numbers of normal subjects. Richards[315,316] tested static stereopsis in some 150 subjects in a college community by requiring subjects to judge whether briefly exposed, large-disparity, stereoscopic targets (0.5 to 4 degrees or 1800 to 14,400 arc sec) were in front of, on, or behind the fixation plane. Plotting percentage of correct responses as a function of disparity produced response curves like those shown in Figure 24-32. The majority of subjects responded as in Figure 24-32,A displaying the highest proportion of correct judgments for disparities near the horopter. The anomalous response shown in Figure 24-32,B was typical of subjects who appeared to have a relative deficit of uncrossed disparity neurons, since their responses to uncrossed disparity targets fell to chance level (33 percent). The anomalous response pattern shown in Figure 24-32,C was also encountered, which appeared to represent a relative deficit in crossed-disparity neurons. A large-disparity stereoanomaly of one kind or another was found in 30 percent of the subjects tested.

The surprising finding that deficits in sensitivity to crossed or uncrossed disparities could occur in normal humans was replicated by Jones,[176] who tested judgments of large disparities presented in brief exposures of 200 msec. Jones recorded binocular eye movements during

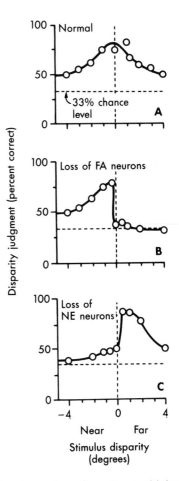

FIG. 24-32 Anomalous disparity sensitivity in clinically normal humans. **A,** Symmetric sensitivity to crossed and uncrossed static disparities, most acute around zero disparity. **B,** Anomalous insensitivity to uncrossed disparities, suggesting absence of FA neurons (cf. Figure 24-22). **C,** Anomalous insensitivity to crossed disparities, suggesting absence of NE neurons. Dichoptic stimuli were presented in exposures of 100 msec to preclude vergence. Each graph shows the responses of one subject to a three-alternative forced-choice paradigm: near, zero, or far. Plotted from data of Richards (1971).

testing, and documented that each of his subjects had normal static stereopsis, to a level of 20 arc sec, when they were allowed to continuously view a standard clinical stereogram. By this careful methodology, Jones was able to rule out microstrabismus or amblyopia as causes of large-disparity stereoanomaly in his subjects. Jones' data clearly supported the contention that small-disparity, static stereopsis was normal in many humans who displayed striking anomalies of large-disparity, transient stereopsis. Thus the static and motion stereo systems in humans, as in macaque, appeared to use different populations of disparity detector neurons.

Explicit testing for anomalies of stereomotion sensitivity in normal humans was first reported by Regan et al.[310] The central 60 degrees of the visual field was tested using a 1 × 0.2 degree target that oscillated 180 arc sec in depth. In each of the five subjects tested, small islands in the visual field were found in which one or several of the following anomalous responses was reported: (a) attentuation of the motion-in-depth perception after only a few cycles of oscillation, (b) diplopia because of a focal constriction of Panum's area for stereomotion, (c) the target appeared stationary or only flickering, (d) the target appeared to be moving flat laterally in the frontoparallel plane, or (e) the target appeared to be orbiting elliptically in depth at that location rather than straight anterior-posterior. Stereomotion scotomata existed for crossed disparities, but not for uncrossed, or vice versa, and these areas retained disparity sensitivity for static targets. Stereomotion scotomata were present in 80 percent of normal subjects and varied from only 2 degrees in diameter up to an entire visual field quadrant (Fig. 24-33). The results of Regan et al.'s study provide further support for the notion that static and motion stereopsis are processed by different populations of neurons, some sensitive to crossed and others to uncrossed disparities.

Normal variations of human vergence

Movements that rotate the eyes in opposite directions are termed *vergence*. Vergence movements shift the location of the horopter nearer or further from the head, by shifting the location in space at which the visual axes converge (the vergence angle, which is large for near targets and small for distant targets) (Fig. 24-34). What has become clear conceptually is that the function of vergence is to bring the fixated target into a general range within which stereopsis operates best. Precise vergence movements are not essential for stereopsis, and vergence itself is a very poor depth cue.

In 1894 Hillebrand[146] showed, by carefully controlled experiments, that the change in vergence angle associated with fixation of near vs. distant targets acts as an ineffective depth cue. A summary of recent work in primates leads to the same conclusion: spindle afferents of the trigeminal nerve from extraocular muscle do not convey useful proprioceptive information encoding vergence angle[105,106] (for review see Carpenter[54]). Evidence also suggests that primates do not keep an accurate copy of the innervation command sent to vergence motoneurons ("efferent copy") in order to increase the accuracy of depth judgments. For example, when the task is to manually match one distant target to another using vergence angle as the primary cue, humans underestimate the true depth by 50 to 75%.[106]

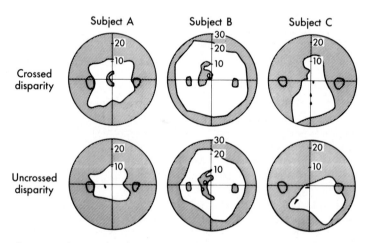

FIG. 24-33 Scotomas for motion stereopsis in three clinically normal humans. The areal extent of sensitivity to crossed disparities *(top)* is slightly greater than that to uncrossed disparities *(bottom)*. White areas indicate regions of normal stereomotion sensitivity. Physiologic blind spots are shown at 15 deg eccentricity in each hemi-field. Stimuli were 1 × 0.2 deg bars, viewed dichoptically, oscillating horizontally at 0.5 c/sec through a disparity range of 0' to 30' (similar to the method shown in Figure 24-8,C). Redrawn using the data of Regan et al. (1986).

Vergence

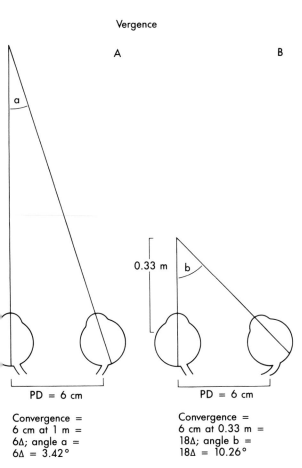

A   B

a

0.33 m   b

PD = 6 cm   PD = 6 cm

Convergence =   Convergence =
6 cm at 1 m =   6 cm at 0.33 m =
6Δ; angle a =   18Δ; angle b =
6Δ = 3.42°   18Δ = 10.26°

FIG. 24-34 Measurement of vergence in prism diopters, degrees, or meter angles. **A,** One prism diopter (Δ) is defined as that power of prism that deviates a light ray 1 cm at 1 m. Therefore, convergence to a stimulus located 1 m away, with an interpupillary distance (PD) of 6 cm = 6Δ of convergence. One prism diopter also = .57°, so that 6Δ of convergence = 3.42°. **B,** With the same 6 cm PD, convergence to a stimulus at .33 m = 6/.33 = 18/1, and 18Δ = 10.26°. Meter-angles: a meter-angle of convergence = 1/distance of stimulus in meters, so that (A) = 1/1 = 1 meter-angle, and (B) = 1/.33 = 3 meter-angles of convergence. Meter-angles are convenient because the amount of convergence in m-a will equal the amount of accommodation required in lens diopters. Alternatively, the convergence angle in degrees needed in (A) or (B) could be calculated by finding the arc tangent of "a" or "b" (as used to find angular disparity in Figure 24-12).

Vergence is not necessary for the operation of stereoscopic perception. The first demonstration that stereopsis could occur without vergence was reported by Dove in 1841.[87] He used an electric spark to present stereoscopic targets in exposures on the order of several microseconds in duration, well below the reaction time of vergence in humans (average vergence latency in humans = 125 msec).[93] Fender and Julesz[97] nullified vergence by stabilizing images on the two retinas and found that robust stereopsis was maintained up to a disparity of 1 to 2 degrees when disparity was increased at a rate of 2 min/sec.

Learning of a precise vergence angle was initially postulated as the mechanism for shortened perception times when subjects were reexposed to a random dot stereogram they had viewed previously.[178] The role of vergence was rejected by a subsequent study showing that the learning was attributable to memory of the overall structure of the dot pattern (which facilitated the complex, global matching process.[305])

Errors of static vergence are common in humans with normal stereopsis.[174,328] When the subject believes he or she is accurately fixating a target with both eyes, only one eye is actually on target. The other is deviated in a convergent or divergent direction 1 to 5 arc min. This normal vergence error was termed *fixation disparity* by Ogle.[270] When the error is 25 times larger (120 to 240 arc min or 4 to 8 prism diopters) and the subject has subnormal stereopsis, the nomenclature changes to pathologic "heterotropic microstrabismus."* Fixation disparity should not be confused with binocular disparity: fixation disparity is a misalignment of the visual axes; binocular disparity is noncorrespondence of the retinal regions stimulated by a target located off the horopter. Short-term and long-term fixation disparities can be induced in normal humans when they are required to view through wedge prisms. Schor has developed a quantitative model to account for such vergence adaptations, composed of both fast and slow vergence pathways.[326,328]

---

*Strabismus is misalignment of the visual axes that exceeds normal fixation disparity range. Strabismus is divided into heterophoria and heterotropia. Heterophoric strabismus is misalignment of the visual axes under conditions of monocular viewing. Heterotropic strabismus is misalignment under conditions of binocular viewing. The prefix *eso-* means convergent misalignment, and *exo-*, divergent. Fixation disparity is a tiny, normal heterotropia.

The effect of fixation disparity on the horopter and Panum's area is predictable: (1) the horopter, and hence the zone of greatest stereoscopic sensitivity, moves forward or back to the actual point of intersection of the visual axes (Fig. 24-35), and (2) the width of Panum's area increases correlatively with the size of the fixation disparity.[328] The direction and magnitude of fixation disparity is also roughly related to the direction and magnitude of heterophoria: esophoria often accompanies convergent fixation disparity, and exophoria divergent fixation disparity (Fig. 24-36).[174] The relation suggests that visuomotor imbalances in many normal humans keep the eyes away from the perfect angle of convergence. Under binocular conditions this is measured as fixation disparity, and under monocular conditions heterophoria. Stereoacu-

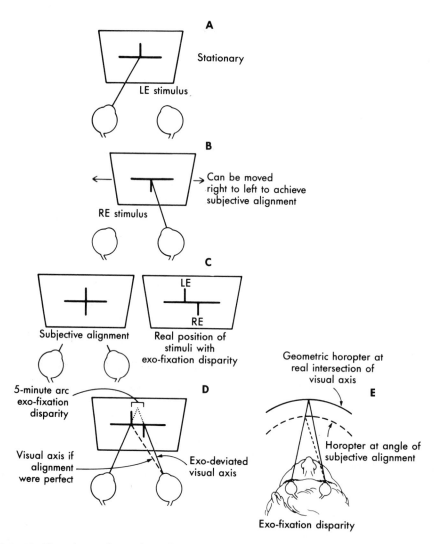

FIG. 24-35 Experimental set-up used to measure fixation disparity in normal humans. The left eye (A) sees only a horizontal and upward line, and the right eye (B) only a horizontal and downward line (i.e., dichoptic viewing using polaroid or red-green stimuli and glasses). With both eyes open (C), the right eye stimulus is moved horizontally to subjectively align the upward and downward lines. The difference between the subjective alignment of the lines and real alignment is the fixation disparity. The disparity may be exo (divergent) or eso (convergent). Note that an exo-fixation disparity causes the subjective horopter to be displaced anterior to the geometric (Vieth-Müller) horopter. Method used by Ogle, and by Jampolsky et al.

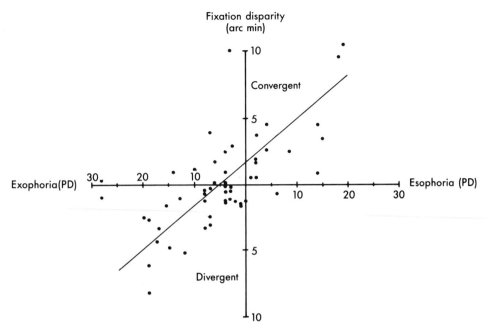

FIG. 24-36 Relationship between fixation disparity and physiologic heterophoria in normal humans. Humans with exophorias tend to have divergent fixation disparities, and humans with esophorias tend to have convergent fixation disparities. Phorias measured fixating an accommodative target at .33 m. Redrawn using the data of Jampolsky et al. (1957).

ity measured clinically is normal. It is not clear whether subtle imbalances in populations of crossed or uncrossed disparity neurons provide the visual drive for maintaining fixation disparity. This issue is taken up in a later section under the topic of pathologic microstrabismus.

The most convincing evidence that vergence precision is unnecessary for fusion and stereopsis was reported in a series of elegant experiments conducted by Steinman, Collewijn, and Erkelens.[56,57,92,93,346,347] Using binocular magnetic search coil recordings they studied changes in vergence (dynamic vergence) during smooth pursuit and saccadic eye movements as the head was oscillated naturally. They found that vigorous head shaking induced vergence errors of up to 2.5 degrees but these errors did not disrupt fusion or stereopsis.[346,347] They also found that superficially conjugate saccadic eye movements were in fact disconjugate. Because nasally directed saccades lag temporally directed saccades, transient vergence errors are the rule. Thus, Hering's law of equal innervation holds only at a gross level of observation. The law is routinely violated when precise recordings are made of vergence during natural eye movement. These transient errors of vergence produce crossed horizontal disparities of up to 2.5

degrees each time the eyes make a 15 degree saccade.[56] The errors may serve to enhance stereopsis by continually causing non-zero disparities.

Binocular disparity is the major visual input driving vergence.[92,401,402] Accommodation provides much weaker input.* Given that disparity is the dominant input, one would predict that humans who have deficits in one population of disparity neurons would tend to have deficits in one direction of dynamic vergence. Figure 24-37 shows the results of an experiment by Jones that specifically tested this hypothesis.[176] Step changes in target disparity of 0.6 to 4 degrees were presented to subjects who were known to have relative insensitivities to crossed or uncrossed disparities based on previous psychophysical testing. The eye movement task was to initiate vergence to a briefly exposed target at its new position, in front of or behind the horopter. Convergence initiation deficits were found in subjects who had insensitivity to crossed dis-

---

*In 1893 Maddox[217] described four components driving vergence: fusional (disparity) vergence, accommodative vergence, proximal (awareness of near) vergence, and tonic (resting) vergence. Maddox postulated that the components were additive.

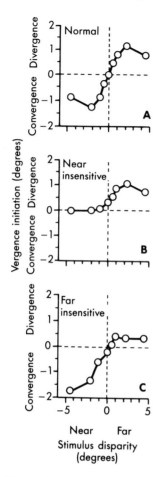

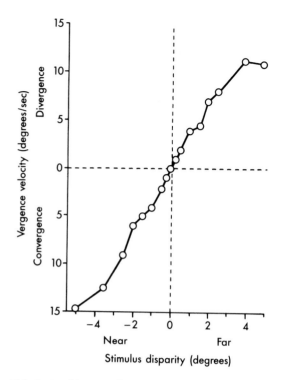

FIG. 24-37 Correlation between anomalous vergence initiation and anomalous disparity sensitivity in clinically normal humans. Stimuli were presented dichoptically in 125 msec exposures, and the task was to change vergence to the location of the target. **A,** Subject with symmetric disparity sensitivity and vergence initiation for near and far disparities. **B,** Subject with insensitivity to near disparities and correlative vergence deficit. **C,** Subject with insensitivity to far disparities and correlative vergence deficit. The subjects had normal visual acuity and no microstrabismus. Eye movements were recorded using infrared oculography. Plotted from data of Jones (1977).

FIG. 24-38 Linear relationship between velocity of vergence initiation and the binocular disparity of the stimulus in normal human. Stimuli were presented dichoptically in individual trials. The stimuli created a step-change in disparity under closed-loop (i.e., vergence could ultimately reduce the disparity to zero) or open-loop (i.e., uncorrectable) conditions. Plotted using data of Rashbass and Westheimer (1961).

parities, and divergence initiation deficits were found in subjects who were insensitive to uncrossed disparities. The correlation between disparity insensitivity and vergence non-initiation suggests that the neurons of the visual cortex that are sensitive to large disparities (FA and NE neurons) provide the major input for vergence initiation. Vergence velocity is about 4 degrees/sec/degree of disparity for step changes in disparity up to 5 degrees[307] (Fig. 24-38). Vergence velocity falls to zero as disparities approach 8 to 10 degrees,[92] consistent with the falloff of disparity sensitivity in FA and NE cells of monkey cortex,[289] and the fall off of psychophysical disparity sensitivity in human,[317] at such large disparities.

NORMAL DEVELOPMENT OF BINOCULAR VISION
Development of fusion and stereopsis in infancy[27]

Early studies of human infants used observation of the infant's response to a visual cliff, to impending collision of objects, or to skill in reaching to infer perception of depth.[45,397] Although these studies verified in a general way that depth perception improved systematically as a function of postnatal age, they could not tease apart improvements due to stereopsis from improvements due to attention or motor skill. Moreover, these studies used physical objects as stimuli in natural settings filled with monocular and binocular depth cues.

Recent studies have enhanced our understanding of binocular development by limiting stimulus cues to binocular correlation or binocular disparity. Much of this human work has been motivated by insights derived from physiologic and anatomic study of monkey visual cortex. That work has in turn inspired ophthalmologists and optometrists to intervene earlier and earlier in infancy with therapies designed to avert maldevelopment.

Studies of the development of infant stereopsis have generally used forced choice preferential looking paradigms.[13,15,28,137] The infant is shown a pair of matched stereograms side by side. One stereogram contains binocular disparity and the other does not. If the infant can appreciate the disparity, he gazes at the disparate stereogram consistently in repeated trials (Fig. 24-39). An observer, who is unaware of which stereogram contains the disparity in any given trial, records the gaze preference. If the infant's preference for the disparate stereogram reaches statistical significance over a number of trials, the infant can be said to have developed stereopsis.

Variations of this paradigm have used eye movements recorded by electro-oculography to document fixation preference, or left-right movement of stereograms on a video screen to elicit smooth pursuit.[5,199] As an alternative, the visually evoked response can be recorded when a video stimulus containing binocular disparities is alternated with an image containing no disparities. Time-locked changes in voltage over the occipital cortex indicate sensitivity to binocular disparity.[282]

Most studies have used disparities of 0.5 to 1 degree (30 to 60 arc min) to document that onset of stereopsis in normal human infants occurs abruptly at age 3 to 5 months (Fig. 24-40).[29,110,282] Females, on average, demonstrate stereopsis 4 weeks earlier than males.[125] Sensitivity to crossed disparities appears, on average, 3 weeks earlier than sensitivity to uncrossed disparities.[28,137]

The abrupt onset of stereopsis at age 3 to 5 months cannot be ascribed to retinal photoreceptor immaturity and hence, poor visual acuity. As shown in Figure 24-41,A, visual acuity changes remarkably little during and after the period of stereopsis onset.[27,30] Moreover, resolution of the immature fovea is sufficient to process disparities much finer than 1 degree. Likewise, the abrupt onset of stereopsis cannot be attributed to immature, imprecise vergence eye

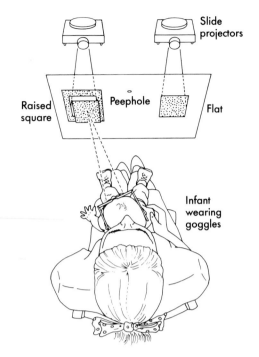

FIG. 24-39   Preferential looking method used to measure stereoacuity (or visual acuity) in infant human and monkey. The infant, wearing polaroid goggles, shifts eye and head position in the direction of the more compelling of two polaroid random-dot targets. In the trial shown only the left stimulus contains a center region of crossed binocular disparity. Stimuli are randomized left-right from trial to trial. Bar stereograms can be substituted for random-dot stimuli. Gratings can be substituted (without goggles) for testing of visual acuity, and printed card stimuli (e.g., Teller acuity cards) can be substituted for the projectors and slides.

movements. As we have seen, imprecision of dynamic vergence of as much as 2.5 degrees does not impair stereopsis in normal adults. To specifically rule out vergence error as a cause of stereo-insensitivity, Birch et al.[29] tested stereopsis in infants using stimuli composed of multiple vertical black bars spaced more than 1 degree apart. The stimulus thus contained multiple fusion loci with an approximate upper disparity limit that would compensate for as much as 12 degrees of vergence error (21 prism diopters). Despite this huge tolerance for vergence error, normal infants displayed no stereopsis before age 3 to 5 months.

In testing infants' responses to binocular disparity, it is important to rule out the possibility that infants are merely displaying a curious preference for targets that are binocularly un-

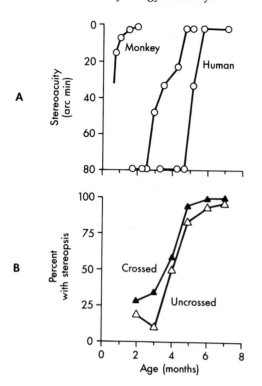

FIG. 24-40   Onset of stereopsis in normal infants occurs abruptly at age 3 to 5 months. **A,** Random-dot stereoacuity measured using the preferential looking technique in two human infants and one monkey infant. The monkey data can be superimposed on the human by changing one week in monkey to one month in human. **B,** Development of crossed disparity sensitivity occurs earlier than uncrossed. Ordinate is percentage of a group of approximately 100 human infants. Redrawn using human data of Birch et al. (1982,1985) and Birch (1992). Monkey data from Tychsen, Quick, and Boothe (1991).

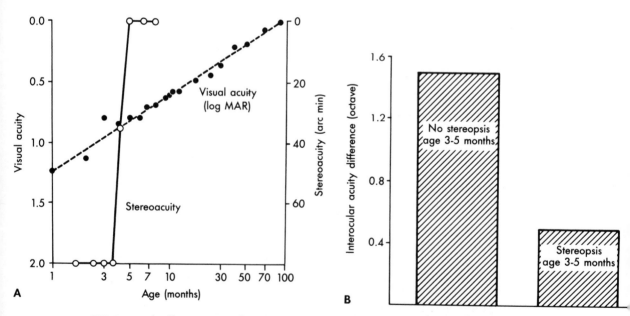

FIG. 24-41   **A,** Abrupt onset of stereopsis cannot be explained by improvement in visual acuity. Grating visual acuity (in a group of approximately 100 human infants) and random-dot stereoacuity (in a representative infant) measured using the preferential looking technique. MAR = minimum angle of resolution, which is 1/Snellen fraction: e.g. 1/[20/20] = 1, log 1 = 0; 1/[20/200] = 10, log 10 = 1. **B,** Normal human infants who have small interocular acuity differences show stereopsis, but those who have large differences do not show stereopsis at age 3 to 5 months. See footnote (p. 806) for explanation of octave units. Redrawn using data of Birch and Swanson (1991) and Birch (1992).

correlated. If infants were in fact responding merely to uncorrelation, one would expect infants to respond similarly to vertical and horizontal disparities, since either kind of disparate stimulus has a subtle region of uncorrelation—the shifted region—in the image seen by the right vs. the left eye. If on the other hand, infants were truly responding to a compelling percept of stereoscopic depth, one would expect them to show preferences for horizontal disparities but no preferences for vertical disparities, since only horizontal disparities give rise to stereopsis. In fact, infants who prefer horizontal disparity either show no preference, or avoidance, of the disparate stimulus when the disparity is vertical.[28,110]* Moreover, only infants who

---

*Adult humans and monkeys show avoidance or aversion to binocularly uncorrelated stimuli, because uncorrelated stimuli cause rivalry. At age 3 to 5 months, but not before, human and monkey infants exhibit aversion. Onset of aversion to rivalrous stimuli is thus a useful indicator of onset of binocular fusion. Lack of rivalry in young infants strongly implies that they lack two-dimensional fusion.

prefer horizontally disparate stimuli display reaching behaviors compatible with stereopsis.

In the first 1 to 3 months of life infants do not alternately suppress each eye but instead superimpose images. At age 3 months they begin to show binocular fusion in the form of rivalry aversion.[125,336] Between 3 and 6 months their sensitivity to stereoscopic disparities systematically improves. Thus the time course of postnatal development of fusion and stereopsis in human infants parallels the hierarchical ranking of clinical binocular function proposed by Worth in 1903.[410] Worth ranked binocular function at three distinct ascending levels: simultaneous perception of binocular images as the lowest, fusion of images as intermediate, and stereopsis as the highest.

Interpupillary distance changes from an average of 4 cm in the neonate to 6.5 cm in the adult.[95] The greatest change takes place in the first year of life. Greater interpupillary distance causes greater angular disparity and increased stereoacuity, all else being equal (Fig. 24-42,*B*). Growth in interpupillary distance may be one

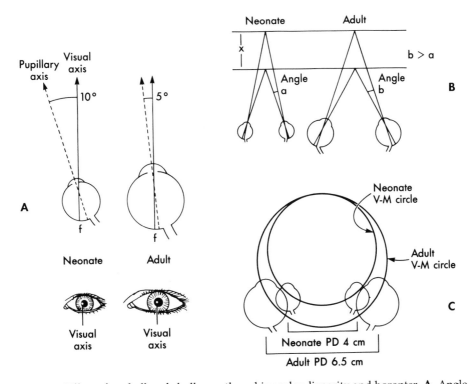

FIG. 24-42 Effect of eyeball and skull growth on binocular disparity and horopter. **A,** Angle kappa (difference between pupillary and visual axis) at birth is on average twice the magnitude it is in adulthood. **B,** Narrower interpupillary distance makes for smaller binocular disparity for any given depth displacement at any fixation distance. **C,** For any given fixation distance, the narrow interpupillary distance of the neonate makes the geometric horopter more tightly curved than in the adult. As discussed by Schor (1992).

factor contributing to the emergence of stereopsis in infancy.

By 6 months of age the average human infant attains a stereoacuity of 60 arc sec (.016 degree).[28] The improvement is rapid, as shown by the data of two human infants in Figure 24-40,A. From age 3 months to 6 months, stereopsis improved in these infants at an average rate of 600 arc sec per week. Infant macaque monkeys show a remarkably similar time course for onset and maturation of stereopsis.[265] The time courses for maturation of several visual functions (e.g., grating acuity, contrast sensitivity) in infant monkeys have been related to human by adjusting the age scales by a factor of four.[41] That is, "months" for human development is converted to "weeks" for monkey development. When this adjustment is made, the data for maturation of stereopsis in infant monkey can be superimposed on the human data of Figure 24-40,A.

Development of the horopter and Panum's area in early infancy

Development of the horopter and vergence is also influenced by dramatic changes in eyeball size and orbital position during infancy.[329] Axial length increases from an average of 17 mm in the neonate to 24 mm in adults, which alters angle kappa* from 10 degrees in the neonate eye to 5 degrees in the adult eye (see Fig. 24-42,A). The large angle kappa in neonates leads to greater prismatic distortion by the infant lens. The prismatic distortion for eccentric targets flattens the infant horopter, away from the Vieth-Müller circle, toward the frontoparallel plane (the Hering-Hillebrand deviation), much more than in adults. However, the smaller separation of the eyes in the neonatal skull produces a smaller, more tightly curved Vieth-Müller circle (see Fig. 24-42,C). Thus the Hering-Hillebrand deviation toward flatness is larger, but the Vieth-Müller circle itself is much more curved; the two factors effectively cancel each other out.

Based on the vergence response of infants to horizontal disparities of 2.5 and 5 degrees (produced by wedge prism) Aslin concluded that Panum's area in infants less than 6 months old was much larger than in infants age 6 to 12 months.[8]

Binocular vs. monocular visual acuity in infants

Binocular visual acuity exceeds monocular visual acuity at about age 6 months.[15,36] The mechanism for this improvement is explained as "probability summation," based on the engineering notion that two detectors are better than one. Probability summation holds only if: (a) both detectors provide similar input and (b) the inputs are independent.

Psychophysical data from infant humans and anatomic data from infant human and monkey, indicate that although neither of these criteria are met in the first months of life, both criteria are met by age 6 months. Interocular grating acuity differences of about 1 octave* are common in normal infants before age 3 to 5 months.[31] Lack of independence of the input of the right and left eye in laminae II and III of the striate cortex is evident as a lack of segregation into distinct columns (or blobs) of right and left eye dominance at birth.[156,404] Over the first 6 postnatal months, interocular acuity differences diminish and ocular dominance columns emerge, providing the necessary conditions for probability summation. As a separate issue, one would predict that disappearance of acuity differences in infants would correlate with the emergence of stereopsis, since stereopsis in normal adults is known to be impaired by differences in the quality of the images presented to the two eyes. The data of Figure 24-41,B shows that infants who have acquired stereopsis by age 3 to 5 months have interocular acuity differences that are on average threefold (from 1.5 to 0.5 octaves) lower than infants who have not.

Development of binocular motion processing in infancy

Magnocellular neurons appear earlier in development than parvocellular neurons[303,304] and the magnocellular pathway at birth is biased so as to respond preferentially to targets that move in a temporal-to-nasal direction in the visual field[11] (for review see Tychsen[360,362]). Under conditions of monocular viewing, the preference is evident as robust smooth pursuit or optokinetic nystagmus evoked by a target that moves nasally with respect to the fixating eye[14,252] (Fig. 24-43). The human or monkey infant either ig-

---

*The line of sight, or visual axis, passes nasalward through the pupil to form an angle with the pupillary axis. This angle measured at the major nodal point of the eye (posterior lens) is known as angle kappa. Measured at the the first nodal point of the eye it is angle alpha, and at the pupil, angle lamda.

---

*One octave is a doubling of the frequency. In the case of gratings composed of vertical black and white bars, one black bar and one white bar = 1 cycle of luminance change. An octave is a doubling of the number of bar pairs for each degree of visual angle subtended, e.g., the infant's right eye might resolve only a 2 cycle/degree grating but the left eye a 4 cycle/degree grating.

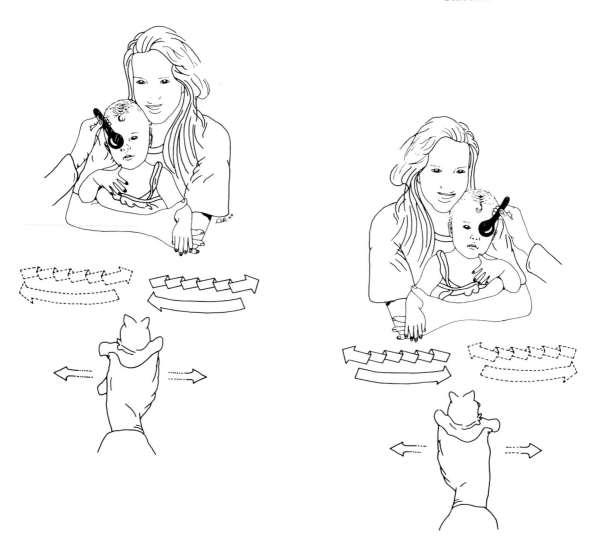

FIG. 24-43 Asymmetry of horizontal smooth pursuit evident during monocular viewing. When a handheld toy is moved from temporal-to-nasal before the fixating eye, pursuit is smooth. Pursuit is absent or cogwheel when the target moves nasal-to-temporal. The movements of the two eyes are conjugate, and the direction of the asymmetry reverses instantaneously with a change of fixating eye, so that the direction of robust pursuit is always for nasally directed targets in the visual field. The asymmetry is seen best by moving the target at a brisk pace. The asymmetry indicates immaturity of binocular motion processing connections in visual cortex. Dashed lines = conjugate movements of the eye under the cover.

nores or tracks poorly a target that moves temporally with respect to the fixating eye. The nasal preference is due to biases in visual, *not* motor pathways; eye rotations evoked by head rotation in the dark are symmetric.[98,274,365]

A nasal bias of motion processing under conditions of monocular viewing can be demonstrated in the majority of normal adult humans by filling the entire foveal visual field with a very low-contrast, low-spatial-frequency, high-

temporal-frequency stimulus.* The subject's perception is that the flickering stimulus is moving nasally at a low velocity.[358] The perception is accompanied by a nasally directed, conjugate, pursuit movement of the eyes (latent nystagmus, see below). This nystagmus is much easier to evoke in patients who have a history of early-

*For example, light stroboscopically flashed through an eye shield of translucent plexiglass.

onset strabismus.[381] Wang and Norcia have demonstrated that the nystagmus and perception of nasal motion can also be evoked by a vertically oriented sine-wave grating, with a spatial frequency less than 4 cycles/degrees, that reverses at a rate exceeding 6 Hertz.[399] Norcia and coworkers[262–264] have shown that correlative biases favoring nasally directed motion are apparent in the VEP recorded over the occipital lobes of very young normal infants, older infants who have infantile esotropia, and adults with a history of infantile esotropia.

The nasally directed bias of visual pursuit is replaced by symmetric naso-temporal pursuit if an infant develops normal binocularity by age 3 to 5 months.[11,252] The motion VEP asymmetry disappears in parallel with the pursuit asymmetry.*[262–264] Onset of binocularity is evident as aversion to nonfusable stimuli[125]; attraction to stereoscopic targets[29,110,282]; and vergence movements made to eliminate the binocular disparity produced when a horizontal prism is held before one eye.[8]

Development of vergence and binocular eye alignment

During this same period normal infants begin to establish stable alignment of the visual axes. Before age 3 to 5 months the majority of infants display, from minute to minute, variable angles of divergent eye misalignment and disconjugate eye movement.[6,8,256,313,342]

A relative weakness of convergence appears to be the major factor contributing to divergence of the visual axes in early infancy. Binocular eye position at rest (e.g., in coma or under deep anesthesia) is approximately 20 degrees exotropic in adults, or 10 degrees divergent from parallel for each eye. The position of rest is estimated to be twice as divergent in neonates.[1] Only a small part of this is attributable to the greater divergence of the orbital axes in the neonate (each orbit diverges an average of 25 degrees from the midsaggital plane in the neonate and 22.5 degrees in the adult).[95] Vergence in neonates is unstable, wavering between under- and overconvergence. Errors of underconvergence are more common.[10] Vergence becomes remarkably accurate by age 6 months, implying substantial development of input to the motoneurons encoding convergence.

Figure 24-44 is a graph drawn from the data of Archer et al.,[6] which plots alignment of the eyes as a function of postnatal age for 3316 healthy infants examined serially over the first 9 months of life. Onset of eye alignment occurred between postnatal months 2 and 6 for the majority of infants, as indicated by the steep negative slope of the upper curve during this interval. These observations support the notion that establishment of binocular connections in visual cortex, during a "window" spanning the third to fifth month of postnatal life, provide the necessary signals not only for eye alignment, but also for conjugate eye movement, and symmetric naso-temporal pursuit.[360]

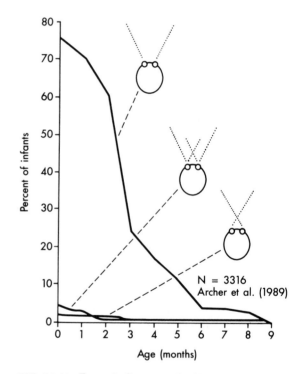

FIG. 24-44 Eye misalignment in 3316 normal full-term human infants as a function of postnatal age. The majority of infants have transient divergent misalignment in the neonatal period. A smaller proportion vary between divergent and convergent or are predominantly convergent. Decreasing proportions along the y-axis with time indicate onset of eye alignment in most infants was established by age 3 to 5 months. None of the infants who had early convergent misalignment developed infantile esotropia, but several did who had early divergent misalignment. Replotted from the data of Archer et al. (1989).

---

*Pursuit for low-velocity stimuli becomes symmetric earlier than pursuit for higher-velocity stimuli, and the motion VEP for low-temporal frequency stimuli becomes symmetric earlier than the motion VEP for high-frequency stimuli.

Neural mechanisms of normal binocular development

Lateral geniculate nucleus (LGN)

LGN neurons in monkey and human become segregated sandwichlike in alternating ipsilaterally and contralaterally innervated laminae of the lateral geniculate nucleus between gestational days 100 and 150.[405] The majority of the first-generated geniculate neurons come to lie in magnocellular laminae.[303] The LGN is functionally monocular throughout life in that no individual neurons receive binocular input.[323a] The "binocular segment" of the LGN refers anatomically to the postero-dorsal five-sixths, which receive segregated inputs from the ipsilateral and the contralateral eye[218] (Fig. 24-45). The "monocular segment" refers to the antero-ventral one-sixth, which contains neurons receiving input from only the contralateral eye (the extreme temporal visual field). In both human[335] and monkey infant[303] there is a "nasal bias" in the binocular segment of the LGN: neurons in laminae 1, 4, and 6, which are driven by the contralateral nasal hemiretina, establish connections earlier and outnumber (by an average of 7 percent) those in laminae 2,3, and 5 driven by the ipsilateral temporal hemiretina (Fig. 24-46). The "nasal bias" may have important functional consequences on development of binocularity in the cortex (see below).

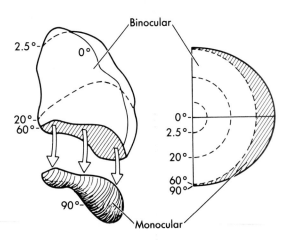

FIG. 24-45 Left lateral geniculate nucleus as viewed from below and anterior, binocular *(above)* and monocular *(below)* portions. Most antero-ventro-medial one sixth of LGN in primate is monocular, receiving input from eccentric nasal retinal ganglion cells. These cells subserve the monocular temporal crescent, extending from approximately 60° to 90° in the hemi-field contralateral to the LGN. Horizontal lines on LGN are iso-azimuth lines, and the vertical line is 0° iso-elevation line. Monocular portion is sandwich of laminae 1 and 6 (not shown). Drawn using data of Malpeli and Baker (1975).

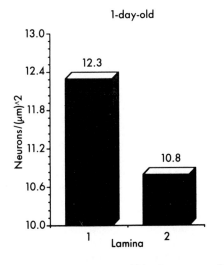

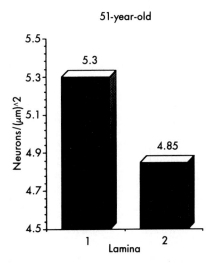

FIG. 24-46 Naso-temporal bias in magnocellular laminae of normal human LGN. Lamina 1 receives input from contralateral nasal hemiretina and lamina 2 from ipsilateral temporal hemiretina. Nasal density exceeds temporal density by an average of 7%. LGN doubles in size from birth to adulthood but number of neurons remains constant, hence cell density decreases by 50%. Unpublished data from Tychsen and Burkhalter.

Striate cortex

In neonatal monkey, geniculate afferents from each eye are intermixed throughout layer IV so that terminal arbors are distributed over a much wider area than in the mature animal.[203] Segregation of afferents proceeds rapidly under conditions of normal binocular experience, resulting in the formation of alternating columns of cells driven predominantly, but not exclusviely, by the right or left eye* (Fig. 24-47). Formation

---

*Ocular dominance columns are made visible by either injecting anterograde tracer into one eye, e.g., [³H] proline or alternatively, by ablating one eye using lid closure or enucleation, followed by labeling of cortex with a stain for metabolic activity, e.g., cytochrome oxidase.

of dominance columns proceeds by competition.[156,404] Under normal conditions, the zones at the edge of columns are binocular in that they are occupied by about equal numbers of afferents from the right and left eye. In normal monkey dominance columns are complete by 2 months after birth, which coincides with the period of rapid maturation of stereopsis. Nascent dominance columns are apparent in human infants at birth and are mature by age 6 months (A.Burkhalter, unpublished data). A "nasal bias" is apparent in dominance column width even in adulthood; columns driven by the contralateral eye are larger than columns driven by the ipsilateral eye. [203a]

Lateral connections in lamina IVB (the stria of Gennari) of the human neonate are remarkably

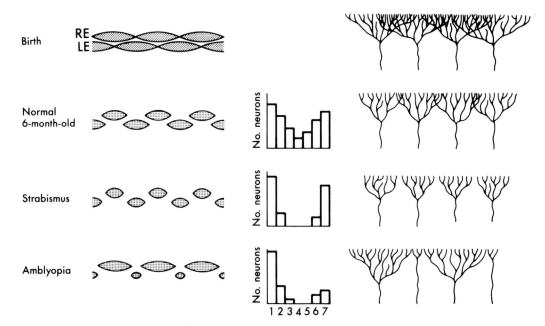

FIG. 24-47   Anatomic and physiologic maturation of ocular dominance in lamina IV of left primary visual cortex in normal and deprived monkeys. *Birth:* Broad overlap of afferents from LGN to lamina 4, hence little dominance by right vs. left eye. *Normal 6 month old:* Regression of overlapping afferents from both eyes with distinct areas of monocular dominance. Bar graph shows the classical U-shaped distribution obtained by single cell recordings from the visual cortex. About half the cells are driven predominantly by the contralateral right eye and the other half by the ipsilateral left eye. A small number are driven equally by the two eyes. 1 = driven only by contralateral eye; 7 = driven only by ipsilateral eye; 2 to 6 = driven binocularly. *Strabismus:* Effect of artificial eye misalignment in the neonatal period upon ocular dominance. Monkey alternated fixation (no amblyopia) and lacked fusion. Lack of binocularity is evident as exaggereated segregation into dominance columns. Bar graph shows results of single cell recordings obtained from this animal after age 1 year. Almost all neurons are driven exclusively by the right or left eye. *Amblyopia:* Effect of suturing the left eyelid shut shortly after birth. Dominance columns of the normal right eye are much wider than those of the amblyopic left eye. Bar graph shows markedly skewed ocular dominance. Drawn using data of Hubel, Wiesel, and LeVay (1977) and Wiesel (1982).

extensive compared to connections of neurons in other laminae.[50,51] Lamina IVB is a second-order magnocellular layer containing large numbers of binocular disparity-sensitive[289] and binocular motion-sensitive[134] neurons. the relative maturity of these connections at birth may account for the rapid onset of several magnocellular functions in early human life: human infants develop adultlike, motion-evoked VEPs and high contrast sensitivity,[261] robust OKN/pursuit[11] and vergence eye movements,[8] and large-disparity stereopsis[27] by 3 to 5 months of age.

Acute spatial vision appears to be mediated by parvocellular neurons,[323-325] which do not achieve adultlike dendritic morphology in human LGN until age 8 or 9 months.[72] During the same interval, the visual cortex undergoes its most rapid increase in volume. Synaptogenesis peaks in human infant visual cortex at age 8 to 10 months,[159,160] Synaptic density then declines to reach adult levels at approximately age 10. The time course of parvocellular synapse formation and synapse elimination coincides with the two phases of visual acuity development in the human (Fig. 24-48): an initial rapid rise in visual acuity to age 10 months, followed by a much more gradual improvement to age 10 years. The time course of the second phase correlates with the clinical observation that occlusion therapy for amblyopia is ineffective after age 9.

Extrastriate cortex

No detailed information is available regarding the time course of binocular development of extrastriate regions. Since these regions are known to receive major projections from striate cortex,[222,382] e.g., the projection from lamina IVB to area MT in macaque, and from IVA to V4, it is reasonable to postulate that maturation of these regions lags that in striate cortex. Indirect evidence supporting this conclusion is available from behavioral and evoked potential studies of human and monkey infants. Motion-VEPs in human infants can initially be driven only by relatively low frequencies of stimulus jitter,[262,263] corresponding to a system tuned to relatively low velocities, i.e., motion-sensitive cells in striate cortex. Between age 6 and 12 months the response to much higher rates of jitter matures, suggesting that areas responsive to higher stimulus velocities have come on line, e.g., area MT. Correlative improvement in the speed of pursuit eye movement is seen in human infants.[9,127,358] Young infants only pursue at relatively low stimulus velocities, but older infants will pursue

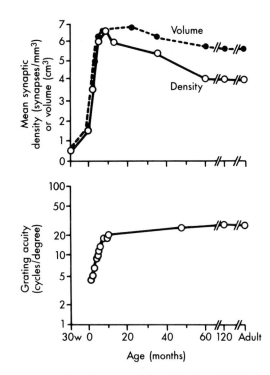

FIG. 24-48 Two phases to the critical period for development of primary visual cortex and visual acuity in human. *Top:* Synaptic density and cortical volume rapidly increase from birth to age 10 months, then slowly decline to reach adult levels by age 9. Plotted from data of Huttenlocher (1984). *Bottom:* Two phases of development of visual acuity as measured using grating spatial-sweep VEP technique. Plotted from data of Orel-Bixler (1989).

much higher velocities. In analogous fashion progressive improvements in fine spatial acuity and color sensitivity may be ascribed to maturation of extrastriate area V4.

MALDEVELOPMENT OF BINOCULAR VISION: STRABISMUS AND AMBLYOPIA

Developmental abnormalities of binocular vision fall into one of two major classes: *strabismus,** a misalignment of the visual axes (Gr. *strabismos* = to twist or squint), and *amblyopia,* developmentally poor visual acuity (Gr. *amblys* = dull + *opsis* = eye). Humans and monkeys may have strabismus alone, amblyopia alone, or both strabismus and amblyopia. Human and monkey laboratory work has shown that amblyopia and strabismus affect magnocellular

---

*Discussion here is limited to primary forms of nonparalytic strabismus. Paralytic strabismus (e.g., aplasia or palsy of cranial nerves) is rare in childhood; for a review see Tychsen.[360]

and parvocellular pathways in the brain differently. For example, optical defocus in infant monkeys produces major deficits in parvocellular visual cortex neurons normally responsive to high spatial frequency stimuli.[247] Strabismus is associated with major abnormalities in magnocellular neurons normally responsive to specific directions of stimulus motion.[132,367,368] Subnormal fusion and stereopsis are the major binocular psychophysical deficits caused by amblyopia and strabismus. Early onset strabismus is also associated with deficits in binocular motion processing.[70,360,367]

In this section the clinical features and psychophysical characteristics of the major subtypes of strabismus and amblyopia are outlined along with discussion of what is known about underlying neural mechanisms. The distribution of the major strabismus subtypes is shown in Figure 24-49. Esotropic strabismus is more common than exotropic. A substantial proportion of cases of esotropia have onset in infancy and have large constant angles of deviation. The largest proportion of cases of exotropia have onset after infancy and are only intermittent. For this reason, it is not surprising that early onset esotropia is associated much more frequently with major deficits in stereopsis and binocular motion processing.

Critical periods for development of spatial acuity, stereopsis, and binocular motion processing

Evidence from psychophysical,[27] evoked potential,[260] eye movement,[128,360] and neuroanatomic studies of human[159,160] and monkey infants[155] have shown two phases to the sensitive or *critical period** of visual development: (1) a rapid infantile phase, spanning birth to age 6 to 10 months for human, and (2) a much slower postinfantile phase, spanning age 10 months to age 9 years (see Fig. 24-48). If visual functions are divided along parvocellular and magnocellular lines, a conclusion emerging from the available data would be that the infantile phase of the critical period begins and ends earlier for magnocellular functions such as large-disparity stereopsis and pursuit motion processing, and begins and ends later for parvocellular functions like fine spatial acuity (Fig. 24-50). Normal infants show disparity sensitivity[27] and symmetric pursuit by age 5 months,[360,362] but do not show fine spatial acuity until age 10 months.[260] Infants who have surgery for congenital cataract at age

----

*A period of time, early in life, during which the visual system shows lability to deprivation and reversal of deprivation. The term "critical period" was coined by D.H. Hubel and T.N. Wiesel.

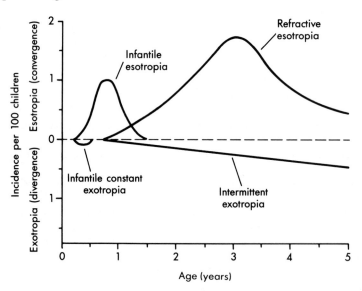

FIG. 24-49 Frequency of major subtypes of developmental strabismus in humans. Infantile esotropia is of major importance because it is associated with permanent deficits in stereopsis and binocular motion processing, and often requires multiple surgical procedures to achieve stable eye alignment. Refractive esotropia (partially accommodative or accommodative) is often cured with spectacles and/or one surgery. Intermittent exotropia is often cured with one surgery. Constant infantile exotropia is distinctly rare. Estimated by pooling data of Crone and Velzeboer (1956), Fletcher and Silverman (1966), Graham (1974), Lang (1984), and that of the author.

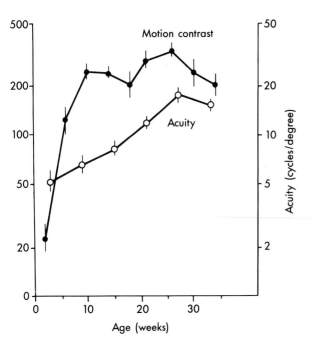

FIG. 24-50 Earlier development of adult-like motion contrast sensitivity, and later development of visual acuity, in normal human infants. Measured by sweep VEP technique. Plotted using data of Norcia et al. (1988).

3 months retain asymmetric pursuit, but they may attain excellent spatial acuity. Infants who develop strabismus at age 3 months may show stereoblindness at age 4 months, but do not show deficits in spatial acuity until age 6 to 8 months.

The post-infantile phase of the critical period begins at age 6 to 10 months and persists neuroanatomically and clinically until age 9. The clinical evidence for this is responsiveness to occlusion therapy for amblyopia, and the neuroanatomic evidence is synapse elimination in striate cortex. It is evident from cases of amblyopia detected in infancy, but treated suboptimally, that amblyopia causes progressive spatial acuity loss in humans up to age 9. At approximately age 9 the degree of loss is static. As expected from the difference in speed of development in the infantile and post-infantile phases, the speed at which spatial acuity loss progresses in childhood is proportional to the child's age: the younger the child, the faster the progression. The speed of reversal of the acuity loss is likewise proportional to the child's age, with infants responding rapidly and dramatically to occlusion therapy.

STRABISMUS
Infantile esotropia complex

In the developmental "window" spanning the first 3 to 5 months of postnatal life, 98 percent of human infants develop normal binocularity in the form of aligned eyes, stereoscopic vision, and symmetric smooth pursuit.[360,362] The other 2 percent fail to develop normal binocularity and begin to show a fascinating constellation of perceptual and ocular motor abnormalities: (1) strabismus, the overwhelming majority being esotropic; (2) deficits in stereopsis; (3) asymmetry of smooth pursuit and motion misperception for moving targets; (4) latent fixation nystagmus and motion misperception for stationary targets; (5) face turn and abduction deficit, and (6) vertical deviation.

Esotropic strabismus. Eye alignment is a visually guided process that takes place months after birth. The physiologic eye misalignments seen in normal infants in early infancy systematically decrease in frequency so that accurate alignment is achieved in most infants by the age of 3 to 5 months[6,8,256,313,342] (see Fig. 24-44). Onset of esotropia occurs during or after this period, implying that there is a finite window of time within which visual connections for alignment must be established or strabismus will result. The term "infantile esotropia" has supplanted "congenital esotropia" to more accurately connote that the esotropia does not appear until several months after birth. The magnitude of the esotropia when it does appear is usually, but not invariably, large (e.g., 15 degrees or more). About one half of infants who develop esotropia alternate fixation and have normal visual acuity in both eyes,[33,82] i.e., no amblyopia for stationary targets such as sine-wave gratings.

Deficits in stereopsis. Stereopsis is normal in esotropic infants until the age of 4 months, after which time esotropic infants become stereoblind (Fig. 24-51).[33] Stereopsis is tested in esotropic infants by optically realigning the visual axes using wedge prisms. Stereopsis can be restored in a substantial number of esotropic infants by early surgical realignment (see below).

Pursuit asymmetry. Infants who fail to develop eye alignment and stereopsis have asymmetric horizontal pursuit similar to that seen in normal infants before the age of 3 months (see Fig. 24-43).[14,253,360,365] Infants who have the asymmetry appear as though they had "motion amblyopia" for temporally directed targets, despite the fact that visual acuity for stationary targets is normal in both eyes. Under conditions of monocular viewing, pursuit is robust for nasally directed target motion and absent or weak for temporally directed target motion.[76,365] The direction of defective pursuit changes instantaneously with a change of fixating eye, eye rota-

tions in the dark are normal, and the rotations of the two eyes are conjugate, ruling out an abnormality of the pursuit motor pathways, cranial nerves, or extraocular muscles.

The asymmetry suggests a delay in binocular development specific to the visual motion pathway when it persists beyond the age of 6 months, and it is pathologic when it persists beyond the age of 12 months.[76,365] Judgment of horizontal target velocity, independent of eye movement, is also asymmetric, with nasally directed targets being judged as moving as much as 40 percent faster than temporally directed targets (Fig. 24-52).[367] The pursuit and perceptual asymmetries persist into adulthood in individuals who had onset of strabismus in infancy, independent of whether the strabismus is surgically corrected.[365,367] The asymmetries serve as markers of an arrest of development of the visual motion pathways in the first months of life.

The pursuit asymmetry is also apparent in humans[11,210,226,327] and monkeys[343] who have infantile onset unilateral amblyopia. The critical factor causing maldeveloped motion processing in these cases would appear to be disruption of binocularity during the critical period, and not the deprivation itself. Onset of amblyopia or strabismus after infancy is not associated with pursuit asymmetries.[341,365]

Nonprimates who have been monocularly deprived,[148,385] or who have had their visual cortex removed,[408] show analogous tracking biases. They retain the ability to track nasally directed optokinetic targets, but show no response to temporally directed targets. Hoffman[148] hypothesized that temporally directed tracking in these animals was lost because such tracking involved an indirect, ontogenetically and phylogenetically more recent, cortical pathway, which was easily disrupted by deprivation. Nasally directed tracking was retained because it involved only direct subcortical inputs from retina to brainstem-pretectum, which were resistant to deprivation.

Is it valid to use Hoffman's hypothesis to explain the nasally directed bias of pursuit in strabismic or amblyopic humans? The answer would appear to be yes and no. There is ample evidence to support the argument that in the infant human, visual cortex neurons mediating temporally directed motion processing develop later, are fewer in number, and are more susceptible to deprivation. Thus, extending this part of Hoffman's hypothesis to humans appears to be reasonable. However, extending the second part of the hypothesis, that one direction of motion processing is mediated by a subcortical pathway

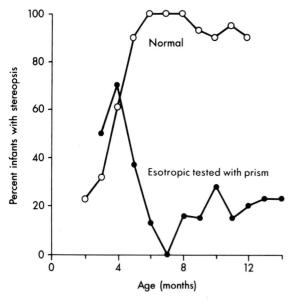

FIG. 24-51 Stereoblindness in human infants who develop esotropia. Sensitivity to binocular disparity is lost rapidly if the eyes remain misaligned after age 4 months. Esotropic infants were tested with prisms to optically realign the eyes and a bar stereogram was used that permitted fusion over an error range of 25Δ. Few of the esotropic infants studied developed esotropia before age 4 months. Each group (normal vs. esotropic) contained over 50 infants. Plotted using the data of Birch and Stager (1985).

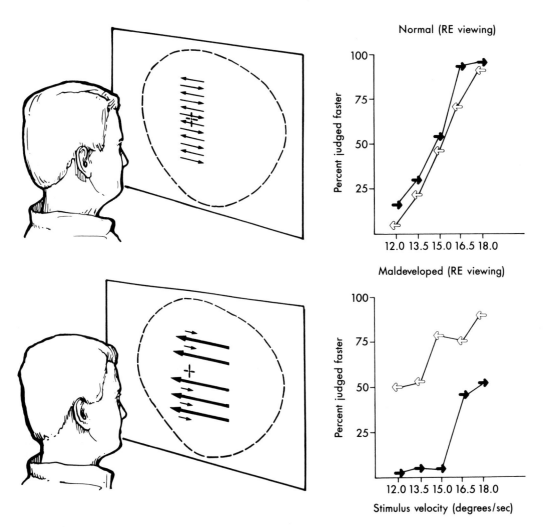

FIG. 24-52 Judgment of stimulus velocity during steady fixation in a normal human vs. a human who has nasally biased motion processing. *Top,* Cartoon showing sensitivity to motion is symmetric for nasally vs. temporally directed targets. Graph shows results of experiment in which a target moved at constant speed, horizontally, across the foveal visual field in exposures brief enough to preclude pursuit eye movement. Viewing was monocular through the right eye. Target speed and direction for any given trial was randomized from 12 to 18 deg/sec with a mean of 15 deg/sec. The subject's task was to judge whether an individual trial was "faster" or "slower" than a subjective mean of all of the trials seen up to that point in the session. Responses are plotted as percentage judged faster at each stimulus velocity; nasally directed stimulus motion (*white arrows*) vs. temporally directed motion (*black arrows*). The normal subject judges nasally vs. temporally directed targets to be moving at the same speeds. Higher velocities of stimulus motion are judged as "faster" than slower velocities. *Bottom,* Human who failed to develop normal binocular vision during the critical period has retained immature bias favoring nasally directed motion (as depicted by larger arrows). Data in graph show that he consistently judges nasally directed stimuli to be moving "faster" than temporally directed stimuli, despite the fact that the stimuli actually moved at the same speed. Technique of McKee and Welch (1985); data from Tychsen (1992).

and the other by a cortical pathway appears to be less valid for several reasons.

First, the naso-temporal motion asymmetry in the human infants is present at the level of striate cortex in that evoked potentials recorded over the occipital lobes in very young human infants show responses biased for nasally directed motion.[132,263,264] Second, humans who have nasally directed biases in pursuit have correlative biases in velocity perception.[359,367] It would be difficult to explain velocity perception biases on the basis of subcortical pathways. Third, subcortical inputs for optokinetic tracking in nonprimates cannot be equated with inputs for motion processing and foveal pursuit in human and monkey. Nonprimates lack well-developed foveas or smooth pursuit. Primates have well-developed foveas and exquisite pursuit, and show profound, permanent deficits in pursuit after loss of the visual cortex.[357,369,411] Moreover, the deficits in strabismic humans are most pronounced for the initiation of pursuit,[367] and recordings from pretectal nuclei (nucleus of the optic tract) in monkey indicate that the subcortical pathway in primates is not involved in initiation or maintenance of pursuit.[182,250]

Latent fixation nystagmus. Infants who fail to develop eye alignment and stereopsis display a fixation nystagmus that is analogous to the pursuit asymmetry.[74,75,365] When attempting to foveate a small stationary target, the eyes drift nasally with respect to the fixating eye (the velocity of the slow drift, and the number of corrective fast-phase jerks, is accentuated by covering the deviated eye, hence the term "latent"). The nystagmus is detectable as a series of small jerks that are temporally directed with respect to the fixating eye (Fig. 24-53). The nystagmus may be difficult to detect if the examiner cannot get the infant to attentively fixate a small target.

As with the pursuit asymmetry, the direction of the nystagmus reverses instantaneously with a change of fixating eye, the direction of the slow drift is always nasally directed with respect to the fixating eye, and the movements of the two eyes are conjugate (i.e., when fixating with the right eye both eyes drift leftward and jerk rightward). The nystagmus persists into adulthood despite surgical correction of the strabismus and thus suggests, like the pursuit asymmetry, maldevelopment of the visual motion pathways.[360,365,367]

Studies in which moving images are stabilized on the retina have revealed a possible visual mechanism for latent nystagmus: individuals who have the nystagmus appear to see

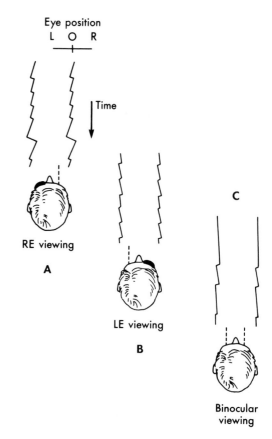

FIG. 24-53 Latent fixation nystagmus in human who had interruption of binocular development during the critical period. **A,** Viewing a stationary target with the right eye, the left eye is occluded. The eyes drift conjugately to the left, in a nasal direction with respect to the fixating eye. Corrective fast-phase jerks are made to the right. **B,** Viewing with the left eye, the direction of slow-phase drift reverses so that it is again nasally directed with respect to the fixating eye. Note that the velocity of the drift is different when viewing with the left vs. right eye. **C,** When viewing binocularly the velocity of the drift is slow and the nystagmus is less conspicuous.

stationary targets as though they were moving nasally at low velocities.[367] This motion misperception likely stems from the same maldevelopment of the visual motion neurons that causes the pursuit asymmetry. Because of the misperception, the pursuit system appears to always be "switched-on" for nasal pursuit. The inappropriate pursuit takes the eyes off the target, visual acuity is degraded, and a saccadic refixation occurs. The cycle is repeated incessantly because of the chronic motion misperception. Cognitive adaptation to this misperception takes place early in life, as indicated by lack of awareness of the misperception and absence of illusory movement of the visual world (oscillopsia).

The velocity under conditions of binocular viewing is intermediate between the oppositely directed velocities recorded under conditions of monocular viewing (e.g., -1.0 degree/sec when the left eye is occluded, $+1.5$ degree when the right eye is occluded $= +0.5$ degree/sec when neither eye is occluded). This summation of visual motion signals from the two eyes under binocular conditions occurs despite the fact that at a cognitive level the patient may suppress visual inputs from the nonfixating eye (e.g., using red-green or polarized glasses). In total darkness the nystagmus velocity decreases to an average of 30 percent of that recorded when fixating in light. Persistence of the nystagmus in total darkness does not indicate that it is "motor" in origin. Chronic visual drive can produce long-term adaptations in motor neurons that persist when the visual drive is temporarily removed.[231,362,367]

The velocity of latent nystagmus varies from individual to individual, as does the magnitude of infantile esotropia. Infants with high-velocity latent nystagmus (greater than 1.5 degree/sec) often have large, variable angles of esotropia.[74,390] They appear to use convergence to mechanically dampen the nystagmus velocity and improve visual acuity ("nystagmus compensation syndrome").

The prevalence of latent nystagmus in infantile esotropia probably approaches 100 percent, but no large-scale studies using quantitative recordings have been done. Gross clinical observation indicates a prevalence exceeding 50 percent.[197] Small-scale studies using eye movement recording indicate prevalences above 95 percent.[73,365,367] Although latent nystagmus is most commonly associated with infantile esotropia, it can occur as the result of *any* visual lesion that interrupts binocular development in the first 6 months of life, e.g., monocular cataract, infantile glaucoma, corneal leukoma, marked anisometropia, and infantile constant exotropia or hypertropia. Latent nystagmus and the pursuit asymmetry occur rarely in individuals who have no strabismus or amblyopia ("primary maldevelopment of the visual motion pathway.").[359] The primary maldevelopment has a prevalence approaching 5 percent in children with Down's syndrome and in first-degree nonstrabismic relatives within pedigrees in which multiple individuals have classical infantile esotropia.[360] These observations suggest that genetic factors

play an important role in development of binocular motion processing.

Face turn and abduction deficit

Infants with latent fixation nystagmus and the pursuit asymmetry prefer to view targets by placing the eye at a nasal position in the orbit.[168,360] This is achieved by turning the face toward the fixating eye (Fig. 24-54). Eye movement recordings indicate that with the fixating eye in the nasal orbit the nystagmus velocity decreases an average of 25 percent.[75,358] The reduced nystagmus velocity improves visual acuity.

Infants who have esotropia may appear as though they have limited abduction.[360] The abduction deficit, if moderate, can be overcome with vigorous rotation of the head (doll's head maneuver or vestibulo-ocular reflex). Marked degrees of abduction deficit will often not be overcome with rotation. The clinical notion that the abduction deficit is due to chronic contracture of the medial recti is reasonable given the fact that alternate patching of the eyes over several days in such patients considerably improves abduction.

Vertical deviation

The ocular motor abnormalities of infantile esotropia are not limited to horizontal movements. Dissociated vertical deviation (DVD) is a maldevelopment of vertical vergence characterized by an upward-directed slow movement of the nonfixating eye. The hallmark of the deviation is that it violates Hering's law of equal innervation: the fixating eye does not move, or moves minimally, while the eye with the DVD is moving up under cover and down when uncovered as much as 10 degrees. The prevalence of DVD in infantile esotropia is 70 to 88 percent.[139,348,365,367] DVD is bilateral but of different magnitude in the two eyes.

Studies of visual motion processing in individuals who have DVD have revealed vertical asymmetries analogous to those found horizontally.[367] The cortical motion neurons in individuals who have DVD appear to be more sensitive to upward-directed motion, measured as better pursuit of upward-directed moving targets and misperception of downward target velocities. The preference for upward-directed motion is similar to that seen transiently in healthy young infants[129] before the onset of normal binocularity. A bias favoring upward motion has been reported in the cells of visual area MT[223] and in the visual motion cells of the pretectum in normal monkeys.[250]

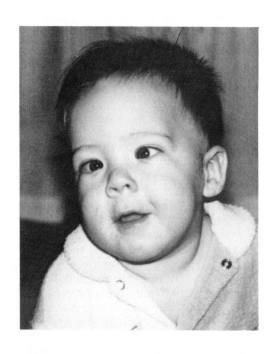

FIG. 24-54 Infants with latent nystagmus and the pursuit asymmetry prefer to view targets by placing the eye at a nasal position in the orbit. This is achieved by turning the face toward the fixating eye, which reduces nystagmus velocity an average of 25%. Alternating face turn implies near equal acuity in the two eyes. A consistent face turn in one direction often indicates amblyopia in the eye that is opposite the direction of the face turn (the left eye in an infant with a right face turn).

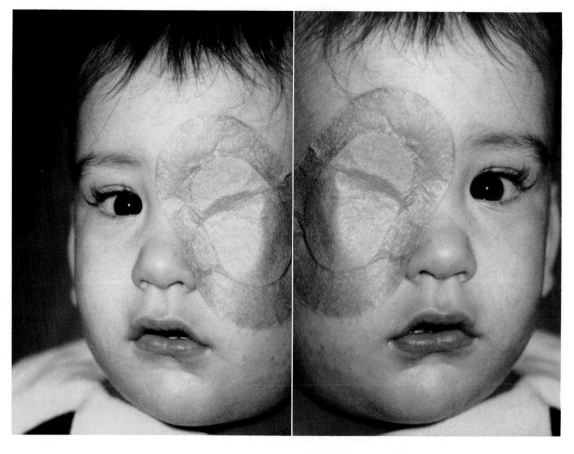

Neural mechanisms of infantile esotropia

Esotropia represents over 90 percent of all strabismus that appears in infancy, and over 75 percent of all primary strabismus that appears before the age of 6 years (Fig. 24-49).[66,101a,122a,360] Esotropia occurs in monkey infants at the same prevalence observed in humans[185,186] and the complex of ocular motor behaviors in the esotropic monkey has been shown to be remarkably similar to that in the esotropic human.[221] It is therefore reasonable to devote major attention to the mechanism of infantile esotropia, as it can be considered the paradigmatic form of developmental strabismus in primates.

Infantile esotropia has been viewed by and large as an ill-defined congenital problem of the ocular muscles, analogous to the experimental strabismus produced by sectioning of eye muscles in animals. The cause of infantile esotropia is unknown, however, and converging lines of evidence suggest that maldevelopment of the visual pathways may be the primary deficit. Implicit in this paradigm is the notion that eye alignment is not established at birth and that eye alignment is a visually guided process that takes place during a critical period of ocular motor development months after birth. Viewed from this perspective, esotropia is a problem in visually guided motor learning.

Codevelopment of motion processing, stereopsis, and eye alignment

Stereopsis, visual motion processing, and eye alignment codevelop during similar critical periods: normal human and monkey infants are born stereoblind; they have nasal biases for pursuit and OKN eye movement; and they display unstable eye alignment.[70,360,362] Stereopsis, symmetric naso-temporal pursuit, and normal eye alignment emerge together at age 3 to 5 months. The available evidence indicates that these three binocular functions (stereopsis, motion processing, and vergence) are interdependent. Normal binocularity depends upon the development of each, and interrupting the development of any one function appears to interrupt the development of the others, in a vicious cycle of maldevelopment (Fig. 24-55). For example, artificial

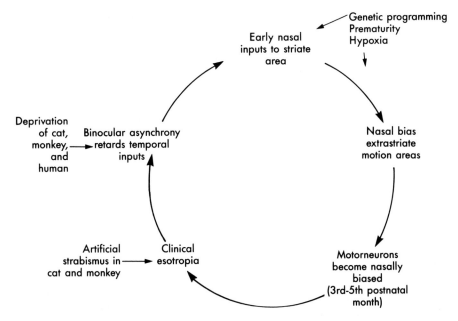

FIG. 24-55 A vicious cycle in which nasal biases of motion processing precipitate eye misalignment, and eye misalignment disrupts development of binocularity, further aggravating the motion bias. The nasal bias of motion processing is both cause and effect. *Upper right,* Inborn and environmental insults to the visual pathways delay development, which prevents resolution of the nasal bias in the primary visual area, eventually biasing development of MT, and, in turn, vergence motoneurons. *Lower left,* Artificial strabismus produces a nasal bias by causing image uncorrelation. The uncorrelation causes synchrony and, via Hebbian mechanisms, a failure to develop binocularity. If severe and of early onset, amblyopia (monocular deprivation) produces the same result. As discussed in Tychsen and Lisberger (1986) and Tychsen (1992).

esotropia in the infant monkey leads to permanent stereoblindness[404,651] and permanent nasal biases of pursuit.[398] Monocular pattern deprivation also leads to a permanent nasal bias of pursuit,[210,226] stereoblindness, and a high prevalence of infantile esotropia.[300]

Naso-temporal development of cortical motion pathway neurons

A logical place to begin thinking about the neural conjunction of this development is at lamina IV of striate cortex. The first-order neurons of lamina IVC in the striate cortex of monkey are known to be strictly segregated in nasal vs. temporal columns,[202] with a neonatal bias favoring nasal inputs.[335] These neurons converge on binocular neurons of lamina IVB,[155] which play a major role in disparity sensitivity and motion processing[134,289,382] (Fig. 24-56). The binocular neurons of lamina IVB provide the major projection to extrastriate area MT,[215,222] which is in turn known to provide a major signal driving eye movements.[211,255] Following this line of reasoning, normal development of disparity sensitivity, symmetric development of motion processing, and unbiased signals for pursuit and vergence, would require normal development of IVB and IVB-like neurons in striate cortex. The critical factor in this development would be anatomically balanced and physiologically synchronous nasal and temporal axon input to IVB, which, stated another way, would be simultaneous, equal, right eye and left eye input. Any one of a number of postulated perturbations (e.g., monocular deprivation, artificial strabismus, striate cortex hypoxia, or genetic influences on axon sprouting) could retard symmetric naso-temporal input to IVB neurons. The retarded development would be manifested

chiefly as a prolonged bias favoring nasally directed motion. Tychsen and Lisberger[367] have postulated a mechanism for esotropia based on this motion bias, as depicted in the vicious cycle of Figure 24-55 and as outlined below. The vicious cycle incorporates the old paradigm, "strabismus causes maldevelopment of the visual cortex," into a new paradigm, "maldevelopment of the visual cortex can also cause strabismus."

Most studies on strabismic animals have described combined effects of strabismus and amblyopia. Few studies have documented the neurophysiologic and neuroanatomic abnormalities that accompany infantile strabismus in primates who have equal visual acuity in both eyes. What is known is summarized briefly here.

Retina and LGN

Monkeys who alternate fixation and have esotropia induced by prism goggles have no neuroanatomic abnormalities of the LGN.[62,63*]

Striate cortex

Infantile strabismus induced by prism rearing or muscle sectioning in monkeys is accompanied by a marked deficit in binocularly driven striate

---

*It would also be difficult to ascribe human infantile esotropia to an albino-like abnormality of the optic chiasm, in which retinal ganglion cells normally projecting to the ipsilateral LGN decussate inappropriately to project to the contralateral LGN (Guillery, 1979; Guillery, 1986; Leventhal, Vitek, & Creel, 1985). Humans with classical infantile esotropia lack the funduscopic abnormalities, acuity deficits, and pendular nystagmus seen in albinos, and do not show the abnormal lateralization of the VEP that typifies albinism (Apkarian, Reits, & Spekreijse, 1984; Hoyt & Caltrider, 1984).

FIG. 24-56 Inputs and intrinsic-extrinsic connections of motion-pathway neurons in visual cortex of newborn primate. Neurons from LGN laminae 1 and 2 provide input to monocular direction-selective neurons of lamina IVC alpha in area V1. These monocular cells converge on first binocular neurons in magnocellular pathway, lamina IVB. Neurons of IVB provide major extrinsic projection to visual areas V3/MT. These areas in turn provide signals to pursuit and vergence premotor neurons. Not shown: extrinsic projection of IVC or monocular IVB neurons to V3/MT for opponent motion (looming cells).

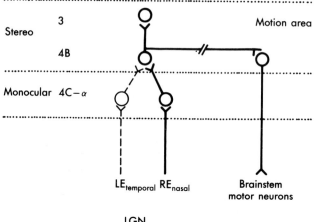

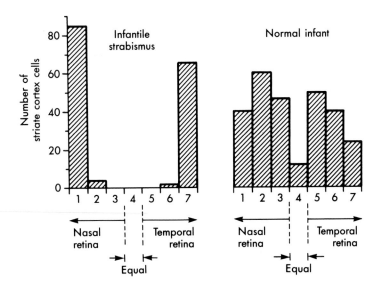

FIG. 24-57 Frequency histograms showing absence of binocularly driven neurons in infantile esotropic as compared to normal monkey. Neurons recorded from lamina IV of primary visual cortex (area V1). Artificial strabismus was created by lateral rectus muscle sectioning in the first weeks of life. Esotropic monkey alternated fixation (no amblyopia) and lacked fusion. Note small bias favoring nasally driven neurons. Fewer neurons overall were sampled in normal infant, therefore ordinate of normal (21-day-old) monkey graph has been adjusted to facilitate comparison with young adult esotrope. Plotted from data of Wiesel (1982) and Wiesel and Hubel (1974).

cells. The most profound abnormalities have been recorded in the normally binocular laminae II, III, V, and VI.[62,63,65,404] A nasal bias is observed in that a greater number of striate cells are monocularly driven by the eye contralateral to the sampled cerebral hemisphere (see Fig. 24-57 and compare Figs. 24-46 and 24-47). The neurophysiologic deficit in binocular responsiveness is accompanied by stereoblindness and lack of fusion during behavioral testing.[65,404] Spatial acuity and contrast sensitivity of striate neurons driven by nonamblyopic eyes of strabismic macaque are normal.[90]

Extrastriate cortex

There are no neurophysiologic studies of directional sensitivity or binocular responsiveness in extrastriate neurons in strabismic macaque. Studies of pursuit eye movement in naturally esotropic macaque,[221] and in macaque with artificial infantile esotropia,[398] indicate strong biases favoring nasally directed motion. The inference drawn from these biases of pursuit is that esotropic macaques have biases favoring nasally directed motion in the neurons of area MT and MST. The significance of the motion bias, as a factor promoting esotropia, is discussed below.

Visual motion pathway mechanism for esotropia

From birth to age 3 months the visual axes are moderately, divergently misaligned (see Fig. 24-44),[6,256,342] and eye rotations evoked by head rotation are symmetric and full.[98,274] During this early period in which the motor pathways are unstable but symmetric, the visual motion pathway is nasally biased: under conditions of monocular viewing VEP[263,264] and OKN testing[11,252] show strong responses to nasally directed target motion, but weak or absent responses to temporally directed target motion. In 98 percent of infants the nasal pursuit bias is replaced by symmetric naso-temporal pursuit and stable eye alignment emerges (Fig. 24-58). In the remaining 2 percent of infants the nasal motion bias persists and 9 in 10 of these infants develop esotropia.[360] These observations suggest that visual motion signals play a role in establishing normal eye alignment.

Over the first three months of life, the nasally directed bias of motion processing in each eye would provide a chronic visual signal driving the eyes from a position of divergence to a position of more normal eye alignment. At the same time, emerging sensitivity to binocular disparity would provide a negative feedback loop

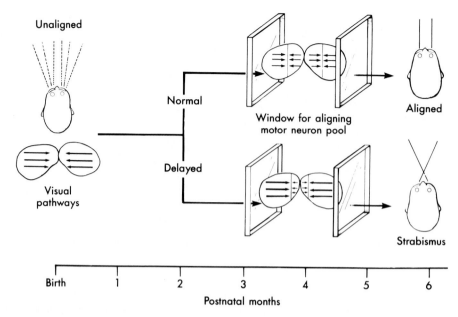

FIG. 24-58   Development of the visual motion pathway and eye alignment during the first 6 months of life. *Left,* At birth motion sensitivity when viewing monocularly with either eye is heavily weighted in favor of nasally directed motion. The directional bias is present across the visual field and is not hemi-retinal. Eye alignment in the first months of life is unstable, varying between exo-deviated and eso-deviated. *Middle,* 98% of infants (normal) outgrow the nasal bias and develop symmetric motion sensitivity. A small centripetal bias is apparent in the motion pathways, favoring horizontal stimulus motion toward the vertical meridian in each hemi-field. Onset of stable eye alignment occurs in the majority of infants within a developmental window spanning the third to fifth month postnatally. Approximately 2% of infants (about 1% of whom are full-term and another 1% premature or complicated pregnancies) suffer developmental delay of the visual motion pathway, and enter the alignment "window" with signals strongly biased for nasally directed motion. Many of these infants begin to manifest the constellation of ocular motor findings that typify infantile strabismus.

to help calibrate vergence motoneurons (to maintain convergence within Panum's area). In this schema eye alignment is dependent upon motion and disparity signals of the correct magnitude being present to vergence neurons at the appropriate time. If the nasal motion bias is too great or the disparity signal too weak esotropic strabismus eventually ensues.

The notion that a chronic motion bias can promote a convergent adaptation of immature motor pathways is supported by several lines of reasoning. Ocular motor adaptation to visual motion inputs is well documented in adult monkeys and humans.[57,77a,117,120,232] Asymmetric motion has been produced by wearing magnifying, minifying, or reversing-prism lenses, or by exposure to a scene that always moves in one direction.[231] Vergence can be adapted to produce a convergence bias that persists for hours in normal viewing conditions[57,273]; and pursuit pathways can be adapted to produce a nystagmus that persists for hours in total darkness.[231] Ver-

gence and pursuit adaptations would be expected to be more pronounced were the visual stimulation applied during a labile period of early ocular motor development. The notion that development of vergence is also guided by binocular disparity is supported by the finding that infant monkeys reared under conditions of alternating monocular viewing fail to develop stable vergence eye movements, and remain stereoblind.[368]

The visual motion mechanism is appealing because it can parsimoniously account for a number of otherwise unrelated phenomena: (1) the time of onset, direction, and magnitude of the strabismus, (2) the other ocular motor signs that accompany the strabismus, e.g., latent fixation nystagmus, pursuit asymmetry, and abduction deficit, (3) the associated motion misperceptions, and (4) recurrence of the strabismus despite optimal, initial, surgical correction. The mechanism is also appealing because it is consistent with current knowledge of

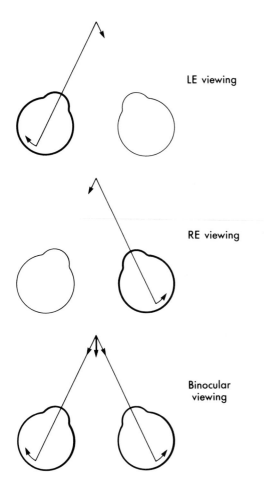

LE viewing

RE viewing

Binocular
viewing

FIG. 24-59   Nasally directed 2-D motion in each eye is equivalent to binocular opponent motion toward the head. See also Figure 24-28.

the visual signals necessary to drive vergence to moving targets. Counterphase binocular motion signals used to drive vergence are assumed to arise from simpler in-phase motion signals used to drive conjugate eye movements.* Counterphase frontoparallel motion is known to evoke vergence in humans.[310] Recordings from extrastriate cortex[119] and from premotor convergence neurons[229] in behaving monkey have shown that vergence is driven by disparity and motion signals.

Under conditions of binocular viewing, a bias for nasally directed visual motion in each eye would be interpreted as a target moving on a collision course toward the head, commanding initiation of convergence (Figs. 24-59 and 24-

*Counterphase motion is motion oppositely directed in the two eyes, e.g., rightward motion in the left eye and leftward motion in the right eye. In-phase motion is rightward motion in both eyes.

28). The schematic of Figure 24-60 depicts the vergence premotor neuron pool as a crosslink matrix driven by disparity and motion signals. Disparity and motion pathways drive individual vergence neurons with unequal weight. The vergence pool is calibrated by negative feedback loops. Failure to develop robust disparity sensitivity and temporally directed motion sensitivity allows the system to run open loop toward esotropia.

Alternative mechanisms for infantile esotropia

It is important to consider other postulated mechanisms for infantile esotropia, and to help clarify thinking I have attempted to bring hypotheses predating 1980 into a modern frame of reference by couching them in current physiologic terminology. Little was known about the neural development of fusion, stereopsis, and vergence at the time many of these hypotheses were framed, forcing arbitrary translation decisions on my part. Perhaps the biggest terminologic problem is that caused by vagaries associated with the clinical term "fusion." By "fusion" did the author mean the blending of images from the two eyes to form the percept of a single object (the definition used psychophysically and the definition used in this chapter), or did the author mean vergence movements made to align the visual axis of each eye on a stimulus?

Historical hypotheses regarding the mechanism of infantile esotropia suffer from two general weaknesses. As noted above, the first is lack of anatomic or physiologic specificity. To say that esotropia is caused by an excess of tonic convergence is a meaningless tautology, since it does not explain the origin of the excess. A second general weakness is a lack of comprehensiveness: a failure to account for the timing, constellation of ocular motor signs, perceptual deficits, and predicted response to treatment. While it might be reasonable to postulate that the esotropia itself is due to a primary myopathy of the eye muscles, this cannot account for sudden emergence of the esotropia 3 months after birth, for nystagmus and conjugate asymmetries of pursuit, for deficits in motion processing, or for the high prevalence in infants who suffer delayed development of cerebral cortex.

Nature vs. nurture

Historical viewpoints on the cause of infantile esotropia can be divided along a nature-nurture axis (Fig. 24-61). Worth[410] was a strong "nature" proponent, postulating an inborn irreversible defect of fusion. Although he did not specify a location in the central nervous system for the

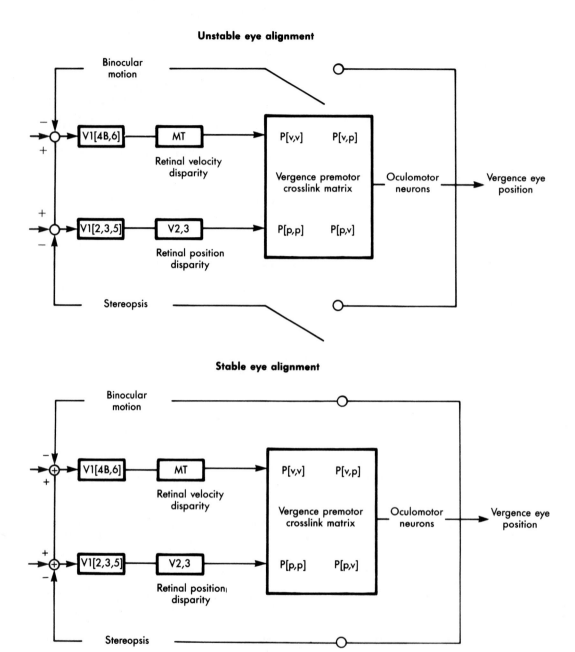

FIG. 24-60   The vergence premotor neuron pool as a crosslink matrix driven by motion and disparity inputs. Before age 3 to 5 months, image disparity and binocular motion feedback loops are open, motion input is nasally biased, and vergence is unstable (the visual axes are eso- or exo-deviated and eye movements are often disconjugate). At age 3 to 5 months binocular motion and stereopsis emerge and eye alignment is stable. P = premotor neuron; v,v = neuron driven exclusively by image velocity (motion) inputs; v,p = neuron driven predominantly by image velocity with some image position (disparity) inputs; p,p = neurons driven exclusively by disparity inputs; p,v = neuron driven predominantly by disparity inputs with some image velocity inputs.

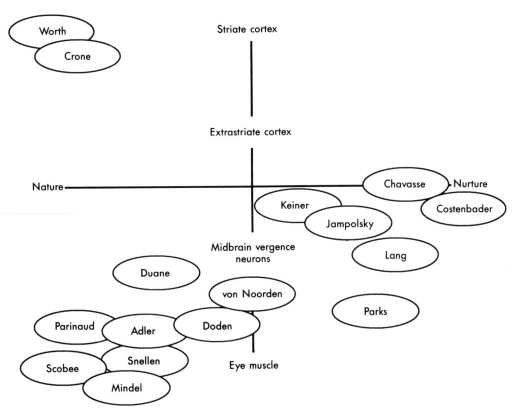

FIG. 24-61   Historical notions of the cause of infantile strabismus, arrayed along prenatal vs. postnatal and visual pathway vs. motor pathway axes. See text for discussion. Earliest authors are to rear of more recent authors. The list of authors is not exhaustive, but includes almost all those who proposed a mechanism for infantile esotropia in their writings. Excluded are those who did not address specifically the topic of nonrefractive infantile esotropia.

congenital defect, it is reasonable to translate this as a congenital defect of disparity-sensitive neurons in the striate cortex. Crone[67] postulated in similar fashion a primary dysfunction in the development of binocular sensitivity.

The leading proponent of a "nurture" hypothesis was Chavasse.[55] Chavasse contended that the neural components necessary for normal binocular fusion were present in strabismic individuals at birth, but the development of fusion postnatally was impeded by abnormalities of optical input (e.g., monocular cataract) or muscular output (e.g., a cranial nerve palsy). Chavasse couched his argument in Pavlovian terminology, binocular vision being a reflex conditioned in the early postnatal period. A key point in Chavasse's argument was that the strabismic patient could develop normal binocularity if the input or output impediments were removed by early therapy. Costenbader[61] and Parks,[278] as consistent advocates of early surgery

to restore eye alignment, subscribe to the outline of the nurture hypothesis.

Visual pathways vs. motor pathways

Opposing viewpoints on the origins of infantile esotropia are also arrayed along a visual-motor axis. Worth[410] and Crone,[67] in arguing for a congenital deficit in binocularity, can be positioned at the visual cortex end of this axis. The majority of other hypotheses fall into a vague middle ground between visual cortex and muscle. Snellen,[340] Scobee,[332] and Mindel[236,237] define the muscle end of the axis.

Keiner[184] postulated a defect of cortical binocularity compounded by direct subcortical "light tonus" inputs. Keiner claimed that at birth illumination of the temporal retina drove the eyes nasalward. Keiner's writing repeatedly touched on the topics of unstable infant vergence, a vague nasally directed bias, and what can be interpreted as a defect of disparity sensitivity. Keiner firmly believed that esotropia developed postnatally: "All children are born with a potentiality to squint and an almost total dissociation of the two eyes. Congenital squint does not exist; strabismus cannot occur until the light stimulus is able—in connection with the stage of development of the reflex paths—to produce a motor effect."[183]

Jampolsky's[173] "bilateral monocular esotropia" hypothesis is thematically related to the thinking of Keiner.

I offer the hypothesis that very early neonatal visual influences may be responsible for motor misalignment and anomalous motor development. Light stimulus in the premature insufficiently developed eyes (with yet incompletely resolved media diffusors in the vitreous and lens) fulfills the essential overall diffusion stimulus criterion—the chain of exaggerated monocular and binocular dominances with altered muscle tonus.

According to this model, the diffuse light excites a primitive brainstem motor reflex, driven by the nasal hemi-retinae, which evokes bilateral monocular adduction movements. Lang's[197] hypothesis similarly cites subcortical light inputs as the mechanism for infantile esotropia. The subcortical inputs cause "fixation on the nasal side of both foveas, and the eyes assume a convergent position. Only with development does fixation return to the fovea, but it has a tendency to slide over to the nasal retinal half." Lang postulates that delay in myelination of the optic nerves may be a factor, as well as "difficulty in coordination between ocular and vestibular influences."

The notion of a primary defect of vergence motoneurons, "excessive tonic convergence," has attracted the largest number of proponents. Duane[89] ascribed the esotropia to an excess of subcortical "convergence tonus" unopposed by cortical influences. Parinaud[276] and Adler[2] pointed to a primary anomaly of convergence innervation, which produced, over time, secondary changes in the medial rectus muscle attachments. Parks[278] noted that the mechanism for the excessive convergence was unknown. Von Noorden[391] has proposed that

a delay in the development or a permanent defect of motor . . . vergences in a sensorially normal infant causes esotropia during the vulnerable first three months of visual immaturity under the influence of factors that destabilize the oculomotor equilibrium. These factors are uncorrected hypermetropia and anisometropia already mentioned by Worth, excessive tonic convergence, an abnormally high AC/A ratio, or anomalies of the neural integrators for vergence movements . . .

Doden[85] implicated an unspecified lower brainstem vestibulo-ocular mechanism for esotropia, based on the observation that strabismus was highly associated with fixation nystagmus.

Snellen[340] believed the primary defect to be partial muscle paralysis. Similarly, Scobee[332] argued that infantile esotropia was caused by inborn defects of the extraocular muscles and their tendinous attachments. Mindel[236] appears to share some of the views of both Snellen and Scobee. Mindel postulates that the cause of esotropia is a relative excess of en grappe acetylcholine receptors on the medial rectus muscles. A secondary increase in such receptors would be expected following chronic excitation of the muscles from any cause. Mindel implies a primary excess.

Non-infantile esotropia: accommodative abnormalities and comparative surgical success

There are major differences between children who develop strabismus during, as opposed to after, infancy. Strabismus with onset after infancy is not associated with the constellation of ocular motor and motion processing abnormalities outlined above. Other important differences are the presence of refractive errors and improved response to extraocular muscle surgery.

Infants who develop esotropia generally lack significant refractive errors, whereas children who develop esotropia after the age of 12 months typically have hyperopic refractive errors exceeding 3 diopters.[280,392] The refractive error forces these children to accommodate to see targets clearly even at optical infinity. A disproportionately large number of these children also have exuberant convergence for fixation of near targets. Because accommodation and convergence are neurally linked, excessive accommodative demand in these cases is postulated to precipitate the esotropia.* These accommodative esotropias are often correctable with hyperopic and bifocal spectacles alone. When spectacles do not fully correct the esotropia, strabismus surgery is performed, which can achieve long-term eye alignment, with fusion and stereopsis, in 80 to 90 percent of cases.[295] This success rate is considerably higher than

---

*Excessive convergence per unit of accommodation is the historical mechanism proposed for accommodative esotropia. Although there is no direct physiologic support for this notion in human, adult monkeys who have acute experimental lesions of the medial longitudinal fasciculus have been shown to have pathologically high accommodative-convergence gain (large AC/A ratio).[115]

that achieved by surgical treatment of infantile esotropia. Success rates for long-term restoration of stereopsis are approximately 50 percent, and for long-term eye alignment after one surgery, 63 percent in esotropic infants who have surgery before age 12 months.[35] The probability of restoring fusion and stereopsis decreases systematically the longer surgical realignment is delayed beyond age 12 months.[61,391]

Amblyopia cannot explain the difference in outcome between these two populations (infantile vs. non-infantile), since: (1) amblyopia is corrected with occlusion therapy before surgery, and (2) visual acuity develops normally after surgery.[35] The difference is more likely related to the degree to which connections for normal binocular motion processing and stereopsis were established before onset of strabismus. Infants who develop strabismus have arrested development of motion processing and arrested development of stereopsis during the critical period for development of both of those binocular functions, whereas children who develop esotropia after infancy have enjoyed an early period of normal binocular development.

Psychophysical testing,[35] evoked potential studies,[262] and eye movement recordings[361] of esotropic infants suggest that early surgical realignment restores both parvocellular and magnocellular visual functions. Random dot stereopsis can be restored, motion-stimulus VEPs become more normal, and pursuit eye movements show more normal naso-temporal symmetry.

Anomalous binocular correspondence and micro-esotropia

Any patient who has a heterotropic strabismus and fuses images from the two eyes under natural viewing conditions has anomalous binocular correspondence.*[21,49,102,171] Anomalous connections in the visual cortex allow receptive fields in the two eyes to be paired over distances that are normally too far apart for such pairing. The anomalous correspondence provides a new horopter for fusion and for stereopsis. As one would expect, the fusion and stereopsis at the anomalous horopter are not as good as normal.

Large angles of heterotropia would require anomalous connections over vast distances in the visual cortex. For this reason, anomalous correspondence is much more common on a statistical basis in patients with small angles of heterotropia, classically, microstrabismus.[174,277] Mi-

crostrabismus is a cosmetically inconspicuous heterotropia of less than 4 degrees (8 prism diopters).† The overwhelming majority of such cases are micro-esotropias. The patient consistently prefers to fixate with only one eye and there is usually a small degree of amblyopia in the deviated eye.

The two characteristic psychophysical findings in micro-esotropia are: (1) a foveal suppression scotoma of the deviated eye that is present only under conditions of binocular viewing and (2) preserved stereopsis for large-disparity targets (Fig. 24-62). The boundaries and depth of

† A heterophoria larger than the heterotropia may be apparent under conditions of monocular viewing.

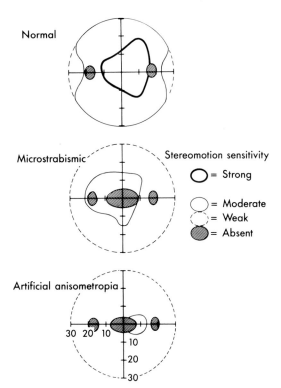

FIG. 24-62 Scotomas for motion-in-depth caused by microstrabismus or by artificial anisometropia. *Normal:* Regions within central 30° of visual field showing strong, moderate, and weak stereomotion sensitivity in normal subject. Physiologic blind spots are present at 15° eccentric in either hemifield. *Microstrabismic:* Shows stereomotion blindness in the form of an oval-shaped central scotoma. This subject had amblyopia of 20/80 in the deviated eye, and a larger scotoma than that seen in other microstrabismics who had less amblyopia. *Artificial anisometropia:* Image uncorrelation caused by blurring one eye with a +5.0 diopter lens produces a scotoma in the normal human. Stimuli were 2.5° × 2.5° squares oscillating from 0° to 2.5° crossed disparity. Drawn using data of Sireteanu et al. (1981).

---

*The term "anomolous retinal correspondence" is used synonymously in the older clinical literature. "Retinal" is misleading in that the mechanism is cortical.

FIG. 24-63 Anomalous binocular correspondence in strabismus. **A,** The left eye has a microesotropia of 2° ~ 4Δ. **B,** *Normal,* A slab of the right visual cortex showing afferent input from the right and left eye onto monocular neurons. The paired afferents and monocular neurons encode corresponding regions on the right temporal and left nasal hemiretinae. Foveolar pairs = 0° eccentric. Cortical magnification devotes more cortical territory to the foveola, and progressively less to eccentric regions of the visual field. **B,** *Strabismic,* The misalignment of the eyes is accompanied by anomalous pairing of retinal regions. Axons from the monocular neurons of lamina IVC alpha must sprout laterally to pair 0° RE with 2° LE, 2° RE with 4° LE, and so on. Anomalous pairing is more difficult, and hence weaker, in foveolar cortex: cortical magnification requires that the sprouting axon travel a greater distance laterally. Anomalous correspondence is depicted here in area V1, but could occur even more easily in extrastriate areas V2, V3, or MT where receptive fields are larger and cortical magnification is less.

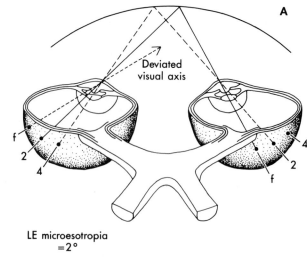

LE microesotropia
=2°

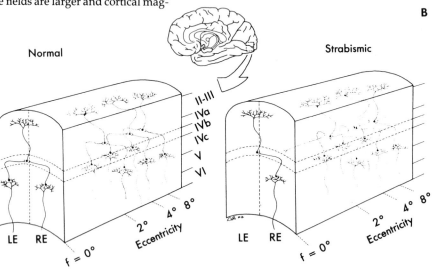

the foveal suppression scotoma have been plotted using dichoptic viewing (e.g., red-green or polarized glasses).[338,339] The scotoma is horizontally oval and its diameter approximates the angle of heterotropia. Since disparities greater than about 0.3 degrees lie outside Panum's area under static viewing conditions, and the heterotropia is 2 to 4 degrees, a scotoma is necessary to avoid diplopia. It is likely that the reason the scotoma is confined to the fovea is that foveal receptive fields have the smallest tolerance for error. Increased receptive field size off the fovea allows greater latitude for fusion, provided the anomalous visual cortex connections are able to pair a foveal receptive field from the normal eye with a nonfoveal receptive field from the deviated eye.

The larger receptive field size at nonfoveal locations would be expected to correlate with expanded width of Panum's area and degraded stereopsis. Panum's area in microstrabismus can exceed 1 degree of visual angle, at least three times the width found in normal subjects fixating a static target with the eyes steady.[369a] Stereoscopic sensitivities are seldom better than 100 arc sec, and are more typically on the order of 400 arc sec (normal is clinically defined as 20 to 40 arc sec).[277]

Figure 24-63 shows anomalous receptive field pairing in the striate cortex (area V1). Alternatively, anomalous correspondence could be achieved by anomalous pairing of the much larger binocular receptive fields in extrastriate areas V2, V3, or MT. In monkey MT extensive regions of the peripheral visual field are connected by callosal inputs.[225]

The cause of microstrabismus is unknown. Primary motor error is an unappealing explanation,[245] since it cannot explain why the angle of misalignment is so consistently maintained in these patients at 2 to 4 degrees convergent. One clue may lie in the fact that microstrabismus is often accompanied by unequal refractive errors and hence interocular acuity differences early in development. As we have seen, interocular acuity differences appear to interfere with development of stereopsis in early infancy, and uncrossed disparity neurons emerge psychophysically later in stereoscopic development. Arrested development of uncrossed disparity neurons early in life would require a convergent fixation disparity to provide an uncrossed disparity error signal large enough to stabilize vergence. The foveal suppression scotoma in this model would be secondary and adaptive: the fixation disparity needed for stable vergence would exceed the binocular correlation limits of foveal fusion neurons (e.g., FL neurons in foveolar macaque area V1 having small receptive fields). Exceeding the correlation limits would necessitate suppression to avoid bothersome diplopia.

The model is appealing in that it can account for the fact that infants who had large-angle esotropia consistently develop micro-esotropia following surgery.[280,391] Arrested development of uncrossed disparity neurons early in infancy would force them to maintain a disparity error signal to stabilize vergence, despite perfect surgical realignment. The model also accounts for the response of microstrabismic patients to wedge prisms (prism adaptation). The prism does not eliminate the disparity in such patients. Rather, the patient changes the angle of vergence by an amount equal to the prism so as to reestablish fixation disparity.*[277] The range over which prism-induced disparity elicits appropriate vergence movements is known clinically as "fusional vergence amplitude." This range is typically normal or near normal in microstrabismus.

Anomalous correspondence in micro-esotropia (and larger angles of strabismus) supplants but does not obliterate normal correspondence. When fusional cues are few (i.e., a point target in an otherwise empty visual field), correspondence may revert to normally paired receptive fields of the two foveas, evoking diplopia. Eye movement or target motion make anomalous correspondence less susceptible to disruption, suggesting that anomalous connections may principally involve magnocellular neurons.[358,369a]

As would be expected on the basis of decreased cortical plasticity, adult patients who acquire strabismus as the result of nerve palsies or orbital disorders have a much more limited capacity for developing "secondary" anomalous correspondence, even if the heterotropia barely exceeds the width of Panum's area. Their diplopia is often relieved only by surgical or optical realignment of the visual axes.[172,195,293] When perfect realignment cannot be achieved, partial suppression of the diplopic image usually occurs over a period of months to years.

Intermittent exotropia

Exotropic strabismus in the vast majority of human cases is intermittent, so that brief periods of heterotropia are interspersed among longer periods each day in which the visual axes are aligned.[281] The periods of eye alignment provide for more normal binocular visual experience than is the case in most types of esotropic strabismus. It is the intermittency of the heterotropia that accounts for preservation of stereopsis and a much reduced prevalence of amblyopia in these cases, not the fact that the visual axes are divergently rather than convergently deviated.

This point is underscored by the high prevalence of visual loss in cases of constant infantile exotropia. Cases of constant exotropia in infancy are rare: at least ten times less common than cases of esotropia.[281,360] Moreover, the majority of infants who have constant exotropia have structural anomalies of the ocular fundus, optic nerve, or brain, suggesting that there is not a unifying explanation for the strabismus in such cases beyond the categorization that they generally have gross structural lesions impeding the development of binocularity.[360] Much more commonly, infants who are clinically evaluated for exotropia prove to have early-onset intermittent exotropia, or, in those under 3 to 5 months old, the normal transient exodeviation of early infancy.

The visual axes are more likely to remain aligned in patients with intermittent exotropia when they are viewing near targets. The visual drive for eye alignment may be more robust in this circumstance because near targets occupy a larger portion of the visual field and provide more disparity cues, or because the linkage between accommodation and vergence aids dis-

---

*If 4 diopters of base-out wedge prism are placed in front of one eye of a patient who has a 4 diopter micro-esotropia, the patient adapts by converging to a new vergence angle of 8 diopters.

parity-driven convergence.* Intermittent exotropia can deteriorate such that the heterotropic state predominates or becomes constant. The probability that strabismus surgery will be able to produce long-term restoration of eye alignment and stereopsis in such cases is high, typically 85 percent or better.[314,333] The high surgical success in these cases, as in many cases of noninfantile, or accommodative esotropia, is attributed to the fact that fusion, stereopsis, and binocular motion processing developed relatively normally during infancy.

AMBLYOPIA

Amblyopia is failure to develop normal visual acuity because of abnormal early visual experience. Amblyopia implies normal structural visual pathways, which distinguishes amblyopia from visual loss due to abnormalities such as retinal detachment, stroke, or tumor. In the older literature the term "functional amblyopia" was used because visual loss due to a structural lesion was occasionally called "organic amblyopia."

Three categories of amblyopia

Amblyopia is caused by abnormal visual input. The abnormal input is grouped into one of three categories of risk, ranked from the most to the least severe: (1) pattern deprivation, (2) optical defocus, and (3) strabismus.[41] A "dose-response" relationship exists between the severity of input deprivation (age at blur onset, degree of blur, duration of blur) and the severity of amblyopia suffered. Amblyopia is generally unilateral. In a minority of cases both eyes may be affected, e.g., excessive refractive error in each eye or bilateral infantile cataracts.

Pattern deprivation amblyopia

Infants at high risk for amblyopia are those who experience early pattern deprivation. The most common cause of pattern deprivation is a dense infantile cataract, which acts to scatter light, thereby removing low and high spatial frequency information from the retinal image and markedly lowering image contrast. Similar deprivation is caused by dense corneal opacities or

complete blepharoptosis. Lid suturing in monkey mimics complete ptosis in human.

Pattern deprivation in the first 3 postnatal months produces profound and permanent reductions in spatial acuity, typically to the level of legal blindness.[16-20] Deprivation during this period is highly correlated with later development of sensory deprivation nystagmus* in bilateral cases, and later development of strabismus in both unilateral and bilateral cases.[300,360] Deprivation in the human before the age of 30 months for a period of at least 3 months leads to a visual acuity of less than 20/200.[243,380] Deprivation commencing between the ages of 30 months and 8 years differs only in that vision is reduced at a slower rate and is more likely to respond to subsequent occlusion therapy. Clinical reports over the last decade have shown that if surgery and optical correction are performed in the first 3 months of life, good visual acuity can be preserved (e.g., acuity of 20/50 or better) even in the face of a dense unilateral cataract.[32,34,88,118,194,279] Delay of surgery beyond the third postnatal month greatly decreases the probability that acuity will be better than 20/200 and greatly increases the risk of sensory deprivation nystagmus.

In monkeys the effects of monocular pattern deprivation, and the sensitive periods for its effects upon spatial vision, are remarkably similar to those found in human infants.[42,116,298,299,395] Monkeys reared with monocular lid suture, or uncorrected aphakia, instituted during the first 12 weeks of life, have extremely poor visual acuity, to the level of finger counting, and exhibit a high incidence of nystagmus and strabismus in the deprived eye.[300] Clinical estimates regarding the optimal timing for surgical and optical correction have been refined by carefully controlled studies in aphakic monkeys.[43,406] The two critical factors in these studies have been, first, intervention before the equivalent of the fourth month of postnatal human life, and second, maintenance of a high-percentage occlusion regimen in the dominant eye (greater than 75 percent but less than 90 percent of waking hours). Occlusion exceeding 90 percent causes acuity deficits in the normal eye. Monkey studies have reinforced the point that even when optically corrected following cataract removal, aphakes are focused at a fixed distance, and

---

*The neural mechanism for intermittent exotropia is unknown. There is no evidence to date of a primary vergence motor abnormality; accommodative convergence gain is typically within the normal to high normal range.[58] A visual mechanism would be divergence evoked by a relative excess of uncrossed disparity neurons, but there is no physiologic data to support this notion.

---

*Sensory deprivation nystagmus is rhythmic oscillation of the eyes appearing 2 to 4 months after birth. For a review of sensory deprivation nystagmus and other types of infantile ("congenital") nystagmus see Tychsen.[360]

therefore continue to be at risk for optical defocus amblyopia.

Optical defocus amblyopia

Less drastic amblyopia is produced by optical defocus. Optical defocus is generally the result of refractive errors, which selectively remove high spatial frequencies from the retinal image. Low frequencies are relatively preserved. For spherical errors, the loss affects contours of all orientations. For astigmatic errors, the loss is more severe at a specific orientation.[126,239] Acuity differences in the two eyes typically begin to appear between the fourth and sixth postnatal month. The differences diminish systematically for onset of defocus after 3 years of age.[243]

Anisometropic defocus (a difference in refractive error between the two eyes) is most likely to produce amblyopia in the more hyperopic eye, except in cases of high axial myopia, in which case the more myopic eye is at greatest risk. The prevalence of amblyopia increases with increasing amounts of anisometropia. Studies of anisometropic patients found an amblyopia prevalence of 100 percent in hyperopes with 4.0 diopters of anisometropia and myopes with 6.0 diopters of anisometropia. The prevalence was still 50 percent for hyperopes with 2.5 diopters and myopes with 4.0 diopters. The data also suggest that the depth of the amblyopia increases with the magnitude of the refractive error.[192,351]

Small-scale studies of humans have shown benefits from optical correction in anisometropic amblyopes detected at age 3 to 5 years.[227,242,243] For example, acuity deficits in uncorrected high hyperopes age 30 weeks to 3 years were eliminated when they were tested after a period of optical correction. Although optical correction alone may produce improvements in monocular amblyopia, the most rapid and complete return of spatial acuity is achieved when optical correction is supplemented by occlusion of the dominant eye.

Does optical correction of large refractive errors in infancy prevent amblyopia? Two studies from the United Kingdom, the first led by Ingram[163–165] and the second by Atkinson,[12] have attempted to answer this question by assessing the value of proactive treatment. In the Ingram et al. study, 186 children were examined at age 1, at age 3½ and at age 5. Fifteen and a half percent were found to have significant hyperopia, astigmatism, or anisometropia at age 1. Seventy-three percent of these children developed amblyopia by age 3½, as compared to 3 percent of those with normal refractions. The subgroup at greatest risk were infants found to have +3.50 diopters or more of meridional hyperopia, 48 percent of whom became amblyopic. Ingram proactively treated some of these infants and did not find a clear indication that early spectacle wear significantly altered the risk of developing amblyopia.

The study of Atkinson[12] examined 3166 infants at age 6 months and again at age 15 to 18 months. Infants found to have significant refractive errors were followed to age 4. More than 9 percent of infants were found to have a refractive error greater than +2.5 diopters of hyperopia or astigmatism. These infants were proactively treated with spectacles. Compliance with spectacle wear (defined as spectacle wear greater than or equal to 50 percent of waking hours) was just over 60 percent. Seventy percent of untreated (noncompliant) infants with refractive error became amblyopic, compared to 25 percent in the treated (compliant) group, a nearly threefold reduction in amblyopia prevalence. Factors important in reconciling the Ingram and Atkinson studies may be the larger scale of the Atkinson study and Atkinson's use of a compliance measure in analysis of the data. Both the Ingram and Atkinson studies indicate that screening for refractive errors is a useful tool for predicting amblyopia. The Atkinson study provides support for the notion that early intervention substantially reduces amblyopia risk.

Strabismic amblyopia

Strabismus often occurs in conjunction with amblyopia. The direction of the causality in individual cases is difficult to unravel. Existing data strongly imply that both directions occur. Strabismus causes abnormal input by depriving the visual cortex of the synchronous firing provided by simultaneous correlated images from the two retinal foveas. The uncorrelation evokes binocular rivalry and suppression of one eye's inputs at the level of the striate cortex.[156,404] Another factor that may contribute to this inhibition is optical defocus of the deviated eye: when the dominant eye is focused on the object of interest, the deviated eye is aligned with some other point in space, which may be optically too near or too distant to produce a sharp image.[162] Either of these uncorrelation mechanisms can produce asynchrony in the discharge pattern at striate lamina IVA or IVB, forcing inhibition of one set of signals. If the patient adopts the strategy of alternating fixation, then the input of each eye is uninhibited 50 percent of the time, thereby averting amblyopia.

Clinical observation of strabismic infants suggests a prevalence of amblyopia of 40 percent at the time the strabismus is documented by a visit to an optometrist or ophthalmologist.[61] Grating acuity studies of infant patients indicate slightly lower[33,82] and evoked potential study slightly higher prevalences,[71] respectively. One grating acuity study indicated onset of strabismic amblyopia after age 5 to 8 months.[33] The evoked potential study indicated a general delay in development of spatial acuity in both eyes.[71] Preferential looking and visually evoked potential studies have shown that the spatial acuity difference between eyes of strabismic infants and young children can be manipulated rapidly and dramatically with occlusion therapy.[35,266,355]

Psychophysical deficits in amblyopic foveal visual field

Humans who develop amblyopia from any cause have deficits in optotype acuity and grating acuity when viewing through the amblyopic eye. Amblyopic eyes also have deficits in contrast sensitivity when measured at high, but not low, spatial frequencies.[47,142,205] These deficits are limited to the foveal visual field, as testing of acuity at eccentricities beyond 10 degrees is equal to that found in normals.[144]

Foveal vision in amblyopes resembles peripheral vision in normals, suggesting that the major deficit in amblyopia is inappropriately large receptive fields (spatial summation) in the foveal visual cortex.[24,104,143,206,233] Inappropriately large receptive fields would explain the loss of contrast sensitivity at high spatial frequencies, with preservation at low spatial frequencies. Inappropriately large receptive fields would also explain spatial uncertainty in amblyopia,[25,208] deficits in judging line offset for vernier* acuity, and difficulties separating closely spaced targets (contour interaction or "crowding effects") (Fig. 24-64). The "crowding effect" causes optotype-equivalent acuity (i.e., vernier acuity) to be much worse than grating acuity. Strabismic patients who develop amblyopia are especially prone to exhibit "crowding effects."[103,124,207,312] The greater loss of vernier acuity in strabismic amblyopia has been used to argue that strabismic amblyopia is fundamentally different from optical defocus amblyopia.

---

*After Paul Vernier (b.1580), French mathematician = minute measurement on the graduated scale of a technical instrument. The scale uses nonius lines. "Nonius" is named for Pedro Nunez (b.1492), Portugese mathematician. Vernier improved on the instrument scaling of Nunez.

Kiorpes and Movshon[188] have shown that monkeys reared under conditions of profound unilateral optical defocus suffer deficits in vernier acuity as severe as those seen in monkeys with strabismic amblyopia. Kiorpes and Movshon contend that distinctions between optical defocus and strabismic amblyopia in humans may be merely a matter of severity, with strabismus generally causing greater image uncorrelation than moderate defocus.[188,247] Support for this notion has been found in a large-scale, collaborative laboratory study of adult human amblyopes jointly conducted at the Smith-Kettlewell Eye Research Institute, the University of California at Berkeley, and New York University.[154] Preliminary findings from this study indicate that amblyopes cluster into two major groups: a group characterized by severe deficits in spatial (contrast and vernier) acuity and a group characterized by severe deficits in motion processing for pursuit eye movement. Roughly equal numbers of deprivation, optical defocus, and strabismic amblyopes have been found to fall into the two groups. Thus the traditional classification of amblyopia by etiology, as outlined above, may in the future yield to a dichotomization based on severity of form or motion pathway deficits.

Luminance sensitivity and pupillary responses in amblyopia

Humans with normal binocular vision show summation of luminance inputs for pupillary constriction. The pupils are larger when a light is shined in only one eye and about 30 percent smaller when a light is shined in both eyes.[337] Amblyopic humans often lack binocular summation, but the response is inconsistent from patient to patient, even when rigorously quantified using videopupillography in a Ganzfeld bowl. The binocular summation response tends to decrease with decreasing levels of fusion and stereopsis (Fig. 24-65). Eighty percent of amblyopic humans also have a tiny relative afferent pupillary defect (0.3 log units or less) in the amblyopic eye.[292] Presence or absence of a pupillary defect, and magnitude of a pupillary defect, do not correlate with visual acuity.

The inconsistencies in binocular summation and afferent defects are consistent with the neurophysiologic finding that neural deficits in amblyopia are cortical and not retinal. Pupillary response abnormalities in amblyopia most likely reflect impairment of efferents from cortex to pretectum that indirectly modulate retinal input rather than impairment of retinal ganglion cell input itself.

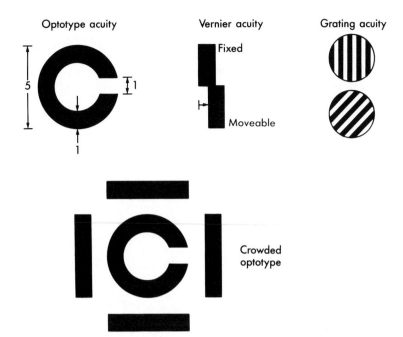

FIG. 24-64 Various methods for measuring visual acuity in amblyopia. *Optotype:* May be Snellen alphabet letter or Landolt ring. Task is to identify letter or correctly name orientation of gap in ring, e.g., right, left, up, or down. *Vernier:* Vernier acuity requires detection of offset in lines. Vernier acuity in normal humans is better than would be predicted by cone spacing in the foveola, hence the synonym "hyperacuity." *Grating:* Acuity task usually requires adult subject to identify correct orientation of grating. However, preferential looking task in infant requires only that infant distinguish grating stimulus from a homogeneous gray stimulus of equal luminance. *Crowding:* Surrounding contours often degrade optotype acuity in strabismic amblyopes more than in anisometropic amblyopes. The same effect is achieved clinically by showing a line of letters rather than an individual letter.

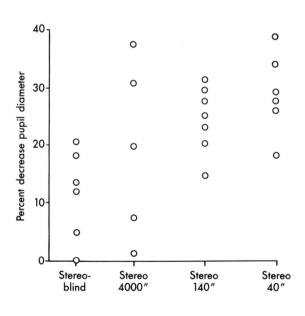

FIG. 24-65 Binocular luminance summation measured as pupillary diameter in humans with various degrees of binocularity. Normal humans have about a 30% decrease in pupil diameter from monocular to binocular viewing conditions. The effect is weaker in those who lack stereopsis. Stereoacuity was measured with contour stereograms; those labeled 4000″ were sensitive to a static stereogram or to a motion-indepth stimulus. Plotted using data of Sireteanu (1987).

Pulfrich illusion in strabismus and amblyopia; synchrony of inputs for accurate motion stereopsis

A difference in stimulus intensity between the two eyes produces a difference in signal conduction time to the visual cortex: the signal from the brighter eye arrives at the cortex sooner than the signal from the dimmer eye. The cortex can interpret this as a difference in time or space. For example, if simultaneous flashes are presented separately to the two eyes (dichoptically), it will appear that the flash to the dimmer eye occurred later. In the case of pendular motion in the frontal plane darkening one eye by a filter or by damage to the optic nerve makes the object appear to follow an elliptical path in depth (Fig. 24-66). This spatial illusion was described by Pulfrich in 1922[296] and numerous investigators have since adapted it to clinically detect visual conduction delays (for review see Tychsen[370]). Conduction is delayed an average of 1.5 msec per 0.1 log unit decrease in stimulus intensity to one eye. Delay measured using the Pulfrich illusion correlates well with that measured using visually evoked potentials.

The Pulfrich stereo-illusion illustrates that temporal synchrony of signals from the two eyes is critical for accurate perception of motion-in-depth. When tested using an electronic Pulfrich device, subjects with normal stereopsis can discern binocular asynchronies on the order of 1 msec. Micro-esotropic patients with subnormal stereopsis have asynchrony thresholds that are on average threefold higher.[370]

Some patients who have optical defocus or strabismic amblyopia are able to appreciate the Pulfrich illusion spontaneously.[356] In these cases it would appear that conduction of signals from the amblyopic eye is delayed by a tiny amount, either in geniculostriate neurons or within the cortex itself.

Occlusion and defocusing therapy for amblyopia

All amblyopia therapy that has been shown to be effective entails: (1) restoring a sharp image to the nondominant eye, by optical correction, surgery, or both and (2) temporarily shutting down the dominant eye, by occlusion or by defocusing. Effective amblyopia therapy allows the nondominant eye to develop stronger synaptic inputs to the striate cortex. Clinical observation indicates that in humans these inputs remain modifiable up to age 9.[297,301] Individual patients have been reported who appear to have gained vision by therapy beyond age 9,[272] but for the majority of amblyopic children the visual

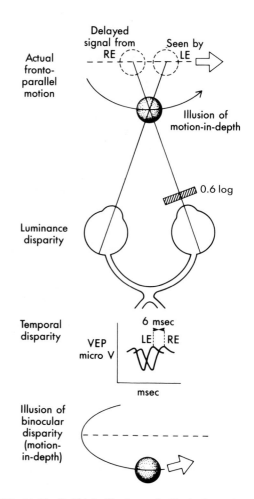

FIG. 24-66 Pulfrich illusion of elliptical motion in depth. The target (at the top) actually moves horizontally back and forth in the frontoparallel plane, but only one half cycle of pendular motion is shown here. A neutral density filter is placed before one eye, which causes a conduction delay in the right optic nerve, as shown by the latency delay in the VEP (1 msec per 0.1 log unit of filter density). The temporal disparity between the eyes causes a percept of binocular motion disparity (elliptical motion in depth). The disparity is seen as crossed when the target travels toward the dimmed eye (rightward), and uncrossed when the target travels away from the dimmed eye (leftward). Any object in frontoparallel motion can be used to elicit the illusion, including dynamic noise ("snow") on an otherwise blank television screen.

gains achieved beyond this age are so small as to make therapy impractical.

Occlusion of the dominant eye obliterates all pattern vision from that eye, ensuring total reliance on the amblyopic eye. A physiologic benefit of occlusion is that it produces the most marked decrease in neural signals from the dominant eye, as demonstrated by recordings from the visual cortex in animals.[156,248,404] Partial inhibition is produced by defocusing the image using plus lenses or by paralyzing accommodation using atropine eyedrops or ointment.[247] Occlusion and defocussing are the only methods proven to be clinically effective in treating amblyopia. The value of eye movement exercises, or methods designed to stimulate or suppress vision using flashing lights or high-contrast rotating patterns, was not confirmed in controlled studies (for review see Mehdorn et al.[230]).

Neuroanatomic and neurophysiologic abnormalities in amblyopia

Several general conclusions emerge from neuroanatomic and neurophysiologic study of experimental amblyopia in monkey. First, major abnormalities are found more consistently in parvocellular as opposed to magnocellular neurons. Second, vulnerability to deprivation is greatest for neurons driven by the temporal hemiretina (ipsilaterally projecting inputs) and least for neurons driven by the nasal hemiretina. Third, the effects of deprivation can be accounted for on the basis of competitive suppression, not simple disuse (image uncorrelation is a major factor in suppression). Fourth, the neural abnormalities caused by deprivation become magnified as one hierarchically ascends the visual pathways (major deficits are only observed at the level of the visual cortex). And finally, the effects of deprivation can be reversed more readily the higher a neuron is in the hierarchy.

Retina and LGN

Retinal ganglion cells are anatomically and physiologically normal in amblyopia, as is the electroretinogram.[170,241,395] LGN cells in amblyopia show no physiologic deficits; receptive field size and spatial resolution are normal.[155,247]

Monocular *pattern deprivation* in the monkey produced by lid suture or uncorrected aphakia causes minor cell shrinkage in both parvocellular and magnocellular layers of the LGN.[203,393] The cell shrinkage is limited to those laminae receiving input from the deprived eye. The combined parvo-magno LGN effect is consistent with deficits for both high and low spatial frequency stimuli, in physiologic recordings from striate cortex,[203,393] and in behavioral testing.[42,298] *Optical defocus* in monkey causes cell shrinkage limited to the deprived parvocellular lamina.[140] The parvocellular shrinkage correlates with behavioral losses limited to high spatial frequency stimuli.[187] There is only a single case report of

LGN findings associated with anisometropic amblyopia in humans: a small but statistically significant amount of cell shrinkage was observed in parvocellular lamina receiving input from the temporal hemiretina of the amblyopic eye.[394] *Strabismic* amblyopia causes cell shrinkage in parvocellular laminae of the esotropic monkey.[64] The reduction in cell size of LGN neurons is due mainly to a reduction in the striate cortex area occupied by that cell's axons (and correlative expansion of the area occupied by axons from the normal eye, a competitive mechanism). Direct deprivation, i.e., disuse, may play a minor role since cell shrinkage is also observed in the monocular segment of the LGN.[140] Cortical axons from this area of the LGN would not be subject to competitive suppression.

Striate cortex

Pattern deprivation produced by monocular lid suture in the infant monkey causes a decrease in the width of the ocular dominance columns driven by the deprived eye.[155,203] The change in width reflects the fact that cortical cells that should have been driven by the deprived eye shifted allegiance so that the overwhelming majority are driven by the dominant eye (see Fig. 24-47). In the monocularly aphakic monkey, dominance column width varies systematically as a function of the degree of deprivation.[406] Monkeys who are optically corrected using a contact lens within a few weeks of lensectomy, and who are then raised under conditions of 90 percent occlusion of the normal eye, attain normal spatial acuity and have normal width of the ocular dominance columns driven by the aphakic eye. Column width and acuity for the deprived eye decreases systematically as percentage occlusion of the normal eye decreases from 90 percent to 10 percent.

Pattern deprivation devastates binocularity so that very few cells can be driven by both eyes.[155,203] The responses of the few cells driven by the deprived eye are so poor that spatial resolution cannot be reliably tested. Effects are most clearly seen in lamina IV. The sensitive period for altering differences in column width extends longer in laminae II and III than it does in lamina IV, reinforcing the point that first-order cortical neurons have shorter sensitive periods than higher-order neurons.

Optical defocus amblyopia produced by atropinization causes less drastic narrowing of ocular dominance columns.[140] The narrowing is limited to parvocellular neurons, e.g., lamina IVA. Spatial responses of these cells were poor for high-frequency but normal for low-frequency stimuli[247] (Fig. 24-67), correlating with deficits measured by VEP and by behavioral discrimination paradigms.[187] Binocular responses were also spatial frequency dependent: many more cells could be driven binocularly using low spatial frequency stimuli than could be driven using high spatial frequency stimuli. *Meridional* amblyopia, produced by artificial astigmatism, causes spatial frequency deficits in those cortical cells having preferred orientations at the axis of the induced astigmatism.[189,404] *Strabismic* amblyopia (in monkeys who do not alternate fixation) produces qualitatively similar but quantitatively more severe deficits than those produced by moderate optical defocus.[90,247] This

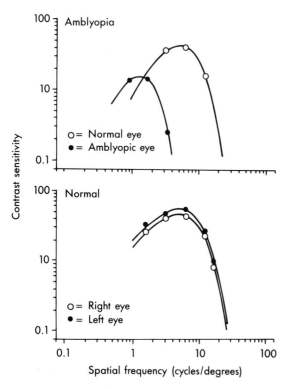

FIG. 24-67 Loss of sensitivity to high, but not low, spatial frequencies in monkey with anisometropic amblyopia. *Normal monkey:* Peak sensitivity occurs at 3 to 5 c/deg and acuity cutoff is about 30 c/deg (i.e., 20/20) in both eyes. *Amblyopic monkey:* Loss of sensitivity is apparent at mid to high spatial frequencies in amblyopic eye, but not at spatial frequencies below 2 c/deg. Measurements are highly similar to those obtained in humans with anisometropic amblyopia. Anisometropic amblyopia was produced by chronic atropine instillation in one eye from birth. Contrast sensitivity measured by preferential looking and VEP technique. Plotted using data of Kiorpes et al. (1987).

suggests that the extreme image uncorrelation caused by eye misalignment leads to extreme inhibition, whereas the moderate image uncorrelation caused by defocus leads to moderate inhibition.

Extrastriate cortex

No systematic studies have been conducted on the effects of amblyogenic deprivations in extrastriate cortex. However, a number of isolated observations on individual animals allow some preliminary conclusions. *Pattern deprivation* causes physiologic shifts in ocular dominance of extrastriate areas V2 and V3, similar to that found in striate cortex.[23] Parietal cortex neurons, which are normally responsive to visual and somatic stimuli, lose their visual responsiveness following bilateral pattern deprivation.[161] *Optical defocus* produces spatial acuity deficits in area V4 similar to those produced in striate cortex.[247] Optical defocus also causes a loss of normal binocularity in V4 with few cells able to be driven by the deprived eye. Positron emission tomograms of human adults who have optical defocus and strabismic amblyopia have shown greater cerebral glucose utilization in extrastriate and striate cortex contralateral to the viewing eye.[77] This cerebral asymmetry is consistent with the finding in the amblyopic monkey that vulnerability to deprivation is greatest for neurons driven by the temporal hemiretina (ipsilaterally projecting inputs) and least for neurons driven by the nasal hemiretina (contralateral inputs).[140,203]

Competition vs. disuse

The historical notion of disuse as a mechanism for amblyopia was embodied in the clinical term "amblyopia ex anopsia" ("blunt vision from absence of vision").[55] In amblyopia ex anopsia the implication was that disuse caused an arrest of axon growth, as opposed to the notion that competition between weak and strong led to suppression of weak axon growth by the strong.[404] If disuse were an important mechanism in amblyopia, one would expect a marked loss of responsiveness from cortical cells when both eyes are closed early in the critical period. Such deprivation for the first month of life in monkey (the equivalent of 4 months in human) does not produce functional abnormalities in monocular responses of cortical cells: the cells remain briskly responsive and retain normal orientation selectivity.[404]

The clinical condition most often cited to support a mechanism of disuse is unilateral optical defocus amblyopia of a mild degree. In some children the amblyopia is corrected by spectacle wear alone. If the mechanism was active suppression, why should merely restoring a focused image end the suppression? The obvious reply is that restoring image sharpness eliminates binocular image uncorrelation and asynchronous discharge, and hence the need for binocular suppression. However the mechanism of disuse or arrest cannot be dismissed entirely: in the unilaterally amblyopic monkey minor amounts of cell shrinkage are found in LGN neurons, sending input to strictly monocular areas of the striate cortex.[140] Binocular competition cannot account for shrinkage of these cells.

That competitive inhibition is a major mechanism in amblyopia is supported by several findings. First, the effects of deprivation on LGN cell size are most conspicuous in the binocular segment, corresponding to cortical areas in which LGN axons from the two eyes commingle.[140,404] Second, pattern deprivation amblyopia in monkey produced by monocular lid suture is not reversed if the lid is merely opened. The dominant eye must be occluded by reverse lid suturing to affect a change in LGN cell size, spatial resolution of striate cortex cells, or ocular dominance column width.[203] Third, competitive inhibition is orientation and spatial frequency specific. A monkey raised in an environment of vertical stripes, with one eyelid sutured, showed equal responsiveness of both eyes to horizontal stripes, but responsiveness to vertical stripes only in cells driven by the open eye.[404] Cells selective for horizontal orientation were equally deprived (and therefore uninhibited), but cells selective for vertical orientation were monocularly deprived, causing inequality and inhibition. Similarly, monkeys raised with unilateral optical defocus show normal binocular responsiveness for low spatial frequency stimuli but typical monocular deprivation effects for high frequencies.[247] The blur did not significantly degrade low spatial frequencies and thus did not evoke inhibition for cells responsive to low frequencies.

The neural mechanism for binocular suppression is usually explained along the lines proposed by Hebb in 1949.[136,404] Hebb postulated that learning at any site in the central nervous system proceeded by a process of synapse sustenance or elimination, which was in turn based on correlations in firing pattern between presynaptic and postsynaptic neurons. In the visual cortex, for example, right eye and left eye inputs converge on a binocular cell. The binocular cell will tend to be driven by the dominant eye. If the firing pattern of the nondominant eye repeatedly fails to correlate with the firing pattern of the binocular cell, the nondominant synapses are not sustained and wither away.

Prevalence of binocular vision disorders

Amblyopia and strabismus are two of the most prevalent health problems among children in the western hemisphere, and during the first four decades of life amblyopia is responsible for loss of vision in more persons than all other ocular disease and trauma combined.[94,321,322,379,388] Amblyopia affects 5 in every 100 U.S. citizens, or some 12 million persons in a population of 245 million.[321] One half of these persons are estimated to have severely impaired vision (visual acuity equal to or worse than 20/80 when tested using optotypes) in one eye.[388] In the United States amblyopia and strabismus account for over 1.2 million medical office visits and for over 90,000 surgical operations each year.

The best estimate of the prevalence of amblyopia and strabismus in the United States is the Rand Health Insurance Experiment reported in 1985.[321] A total of 1141 children 5 and 6 years old were examined using standardized techniques in six sites, chosen to represent four census regions of the country and an urban-rural mix. Five percent of children had amblyopia of two lines or more when tested with letter charts. Four percent of children had strabismus under conditions of binocular viewing (heterotropia) and 6.7 percent under conditions of monocular viewing (heterophoria). These figures closely approximate the estimates by the National Center for Health Statistics compiled in 1972.[379]

The prevalence of strabismus and amblyopia is substantially higher in low-birth-weight and premature infants[153,191,196,219,386] and in infants who suffer perinatal hypoxia.[123,191] Infants born at less than 1500 grams have a prevalence of amblyopia and strabismus 7 times that of normal-weight, term infants.[191] Infants born at less than 2500 grams have a prevalence of strabismus 4 times that of normal-weight infants.[153] The risk of strabismus increases roughly 4 percent for each 100 gram decrease in birth weight below 2500 grams.[130]

The increased risk of strabismus in these infants is most likely due to maldevelopment of binocular connections in the visual cortex. The occipital lobes in newborns are especially vulnerable to damage from hypoxia.[363,389] Premature infants frequently suffer ischemic injury to the optic radiations near the occipital trigone. Full-term infants are prone to hypotensive injury to the dorsal motion processing area of extrastriate cortex, since this area represents the watershed zone for all three major cerebral vessels. Striate cortex in humans has the highest neuron-to-glia ratio of the entire cerebrum[22,159,160] and the highest regional cerebral consumption of glucose.[286]

Maternal smoking, drug use, and alcohol abuse are associated with increases in amblyopia or strabismus risk equivalent to those seen with prematurity or hypoxia.[130,235,306]

Genetic factors also play a role. Longitudinal studies show prevalences four to sixfold higher in infants born to a parent who has amblyopia or strabismus.[334,344,400] Primary maldevelopment of binocular motion processing has been documented in blood relatives of strabismics[359] and in children with trisomy 21.[360]

Infant vision screening for amblyopia and strabismus

Amblyopia and strabismus stigmatize children and adults by depriving them of the many advantages bestowed by normal binocular vision. Normal binocular vision makes school, work-related, and recreational tasks easier to perform, with cumulative benefit over a lifetime of activities. Binocular vision is a requirement for a variety of visually demanding career fields. Normal vision in each eye reduces the likelihood of strabismus, avoiding the detrimental effects and the costs associated with its correction. Normal vision in each eye substantially lowers the risk of visual loss from ocular injury, thus reducing the tremendous costs imposed on individuals and society by legal blindness. Normal vision frees individuals from the psychological burden and loss of self-esteem often associated with physical disability. Taken together, these benefits would appear to readily justify the expenses and inconveniences of programs aimed at early detection and treatment.

For mass screening to be effective in any disease, five criteria must be met.[107] First, the disease should be an important health problem and have a high prevalence. Second, the disease should have a recognizable latent period. Third, efficacious treatment should be available for patients with recognized disease. Fourth, the screening test used should be simple to administer, accurate, reliable, and acceptable. And finally, the costs of case-finding should be low.

The first three criteria are immediately met in that amblyopia and strabismus are much more easily and successfully treated when caught early in life and are in many cases avoidable.

The second two criteria may possibly be met by a newer screening test discussed below, especially when applied to infants in high-risk groups. The screening test chosen for these infants must be capable of detecting each of the three major risk factors: opacities of the ocular media, refractive errors, and strabismus. An effective test would also meet each of the following requirements: (1) it would involve little testing time, (2) it could take place in any setting, e.g., clinic, day care center, mobile van, or pediatrician's office, (3) it could be performed by a technician with minimal training, and (4) it would use simple, inexpensive equipment.

The only current screening methodology that fulfills most of these criteria is photorefraction[46,69,114,131,135,151,152,244] (Fig. 24-68,A). Other screening methods, e.g., acuity card procedures or VEP, fail to meet several criteria. The acuity card procedure is a useful method for quantifying visual acuity in preverbal children[83,84,352-354] but it is time-consuming to perform, is somewhat expensive, requires a skilled examiner, and needs dedicated space.[91,345] The visually evoked potential obtained using the Norcia-Tyler rapid-sweep technique has proven to be a remarkably sensitive and accurate research tool for measurement of form and motion pathway development in young infants (Fig. 24-68,B).[259] However, it is impractical at present for testing large numbers of infants: expensive and complex equipment is required; a highly skilled operator is needed; set up time is on the order of 30 minutes per infant; and wire electrodes must be pasted to the head.

Photorefraction[46,69,114,131,135,151,152,244] is photography of the light reflected from the ocular fundus by a coaxial or nearly coaxial flash source (similar to the "cat eye" reflex so bothersome in family photos). The time required is that needed to take two flash photographs.*[131] Photorefraction allows estimation of spherical and astigmatic refractive errors from −6 to +6 diopters; provides a Bruckner reflex for detection of strabismus; and provides a red reflex for detection of media opacities. Several studies have shown that photorefraction is an effective screening tool in preschool and schoolage children.[114,135,244] Two large-scale studies to date have demonstrated its efficacy in testing of infants.[12,152a]

---

*Sensitivity and specificity when the pupils are undilated is approximately 85 percent. Both can be improved if a mydriatic is used, the trade-off being increased testing time.

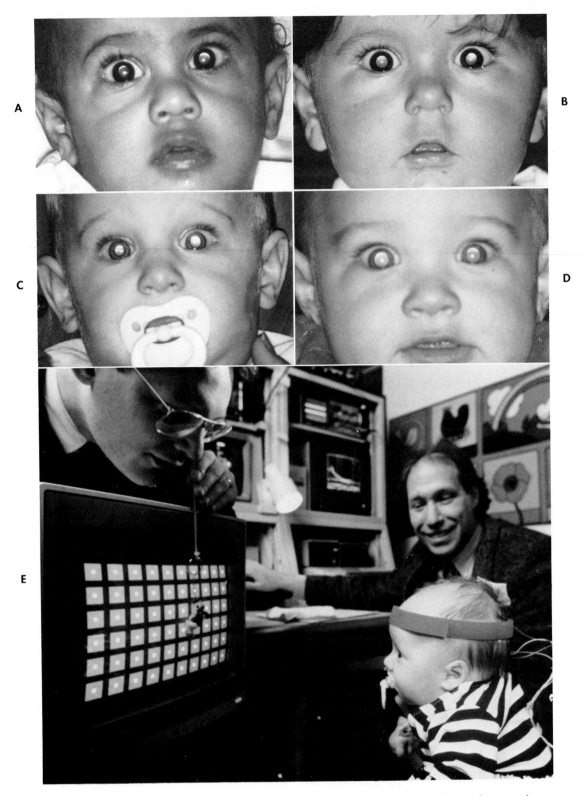

FIG. 24-68 Infant vision screening using photorefraction and VEP. **A–C,** Photorefraction of three infants detected to have anisometropia, with greater spherical or cylindric hyperopia in their left eyes. Note that the reflected-light crescents are larger in the upper pupil of their left eyes as compared to right eyes. **D,** Emmetropic infant with symmetric reflected-light crescents. Size of crescents can be used to quantify magnitude and sign of refractive error. **E,** Spatial-sweep VEP. The squares on the monitor sweep from large to small in a trial that lasts 10 sec. Courtesy of Drs. A. M. Norcia and R. D. Hamer, Smith-Kettlewell Eye Research Institute.

BINOCULAR VISION IN OTHER ANIMALS

Up to this point, human and monkey data have been emphasized to the exclusion of other species. Emphasis on human and monkey is justified, not only because of limitations of space, but also because the monkey visual system has been shown to be most similar to the human system in its psychophysical, neuroanatomic, and physiologic properties. Only monkeys and humans have a highly developed fovea centralis with opponent color organization, smooth-pursuit eye movements, robust vergence, and a large binocular visual field for exquisite stereopsis. The magnocellular and parvocellular organization of visual streams appears to be highly similar in humans and monkeys. Developmental studies have demonstrated that the prevalence of amblyopia and strabismus is similar in the two species, and that the naturally occuring strabismus of the monkey mimics in all important respects the strabismus of human infants.

Development of binocular vision in cat

In the same way that our understanding of human binocular vision has been made possible only through detailed study of the monkey, so our understanding of the monkey has been enhanced by a large body of work devoted to exploration of the visual cortex of other species, notably the cat. In 1982 Hubel and Wiesel[156,404] were awarded the Nobel Prize for describing the hierarchical organization of striate cortex, the effects of deprivation on ocular dominance, and the concept of the critical period. All of Hubel and Wiesel's early work was done in the cat. As detailed in the previous edition of this chapter, Bishop and Pettigrew's[37] work in the cat provided the first detailed descriptions of disparity-sensitive neurons.

Three current areas of work in the cat are of special relevance to clinicians and neuroscientists interested in the development of binocular vision: activity-dependent formation of ocular dominance columns, the effects of deprivation on the topography of callosal connections, and the role of neurotransmitters in regulating plasticity of inputs to the striate cortex.

Ocular dominance columns

An elegant series of experiments performed in the cat by Stryker and coworkers[234,350] have shown that the formation of ocular dominance columns during the critical period is dependent on synchronous firing of inputs from each eye at the level of the striate cortex. Injection of the agent tetrodotoxin into the vitreous cavity turns off neural activity. Unilateral injection produces effects similar to monocular deprivation: an abnormally small number of cortical cells continue to be driven by the injected eye. Bilateral injection produces effects similar to binocular deprivation: the cells fail to segregate into columns. Miller, Keller, and Stryker[234] have produced a computational neural network model of ocular dominance column formation.

Topography of hemi-visual field connections

Van Sluyters and colleagues[44] have shown that the callosal fibers that join the midlines of the two hemi-visual fields are abnormally distributed in cats made artificially strabismic. These fibers were initially thought to be widespread at birth, interdigitating a broad strip along the vertical meridians of the fields.[166,167] Strabismic animals appeared to have retained the neonatal distribution, presumably because the loss of binocularity caused by strabismus interfered with postnatal "pruning" of exuberant fibers.[166,167] However, Van Sluyters et al.[44] have shown, using more extensive sampling methods, that the callosal distribution in strabismic animals is, if anything, narrower than that in normal adult animals.

Neuropharmacology of visual plasticity

Neuropharmacologic regulation of the critical period has become an area of intense scrutiny by two teams, one in Germany headed by Singer, and the other in St. Louis headed by Daw. NMDA (N-methyl-D-aspartate) receptors appear to play a key role in controlling visual cortex plasticity. The extent of that role is as yet unclear. The amino acid glutamate is the transmitter that carries the visual signals. NMDA receptors accentuate these signals and thereby solidify synapses that are being formed.[68] NMDA receptors on postsynaptic membranes in cat striate cortex decrease in number during the period in which afferents from the geniculate are segregating to form dominance columns.[109] The antagonist APV blocks NMDA receptors and blocks the dominance shifts caused by monocular deprivation.[193] Unfortunately, APV cannot be used to prevent amblyopia, as APV also blocks maturation of receptive field properties for the normal eye.

The glutamate-NMDA mechanism directly involves visual signals. Acetylcholine, serotonin, and noradrenaline inputs to the visual cortex from the pons and basal forebrain do not carry visual signals.[108,181] For this reason the

NMDA mechanism would appear to play a primary role in the regulation of visual plasticity. The other inputs may play a subsidiary role, modulating visual activity under different conditions of arousal.[108] Two recent studies in amblyopic adult humans have shown improvements in optotype acuity and contrast sensitivity, and decreases in the area of suppression scotomas, for a few hours following single-dose administration of a precursor of dopamine and norepinephrine.[122,198]

Binocular vision and evolution

Darwin posited that the great diversity of life on this planet was: (1) the result of random forces, and (2) continuous, one species begetting another. Because evolutionary theory cannot explain discontinuities, several vision scientists have made efforts to show a systematic progression in the development of binocular vision, from lower species to primates.[4,67,291,283–285,396] What is noteworthy in these efforts is the paucity of data (credible transitional forms) currently available to sustain such an argument. Darwin himself was concerned by this; the sudden and inexplicable appearance of two elegantly engineered eyes was an embarrassment to his theory.[79,175,302]

Having two eyes affords obvious advantages.[376] First, two eyes laterally placed provide a panoramic, nearly 360-degree view of the world (Fig. 24-69). Second, where the fields overlap, there is the advantage of summation in the detection of faint targets (increased signal-to-noise ratio). Third, a second eye provides a backup if one is injured. Fourth, if the two eyes are mobile, convergence could be used as a crude gauge of depth. And finally, two eyes can provide stereopsis. Julesz[178] contends that one of the main advantages of stereopsis is the ability to see objects camouflaged in monocular view (camouflage breaking).

Stereopsis is made possible by overlap of the visual fields of frontally placed eyes, along with semidecussation of retinal fibers to provide the necessary binocular interaction in higher centers. Although these characteristics are most apparent in primates, and carnivores such as the cat, stereopsis is present in some other vertebrates below the level of mammal.

Lower vertebrates

There is behavioral evidence for stereopsis in toads.[55a] Two avian species with stereopsis are the owl[283,284] and the falcon.[113] Physiologic recording experiments have shown neurons sen-

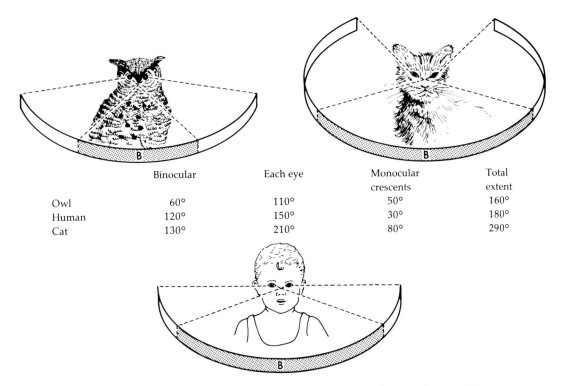

	Binocular	Each eye	Monocular crescents	Total extent
Owl	60°	110°	50°	160°
Human	120°	150°	30°	180°
Cat	130°	210°	80°	290°

FIG. 24-69 Portions of visual field that are binocular vs. monocular in owl, cat, and human. Drawn using data from various sources cited in Walls (1942).

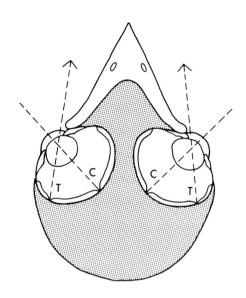

FIG. 24-70   Bifoveate bird (e.g., swallow). Each fovea on the temporal retina provides a narrow zone of binocular vision directly ahead; each fovea on the central retina provides panoramic lateral vision. Redrawn using data of Pettigrew (1986).

sitive to binocular disparity in the avian Wulst, the analog of mammalian striate cortex. Several avian species possess two foveae in each eye, one located on the central retina and the other on the temporal retina (Fig. 24-70) Pettigrew[285] has hypothesized that the central fovea projects to the optic tectum and is used for monocular tracking eye movements, while the temporal foveae project to the Wulst and are used for limited, conjugate, binocular eye movements. Despite complete decussation at the chiasm, binocularity is provided to the Wulst by fibers that cross back through the avian supraoptic decussation. Thus stereopsis in these birds is achieved through a double decussation mechanism entirely different from the partial decussation mechanism used in mammals. It is difficult to imagine that both mechanisms could arrise from a common ancestor if topographic organization was to be maintained.

A second difficulty encountered in attempting to show a continuous progression of binocular vision from lower to higher vertebrates is the lack of correlation between functional binocularity and binocular overlap of the visual field. The swift and the oilbird are two avian species possessing substantial field overlap but no evidence of functional binocular vision.[285]

A third difficulty encountered in attempting to show a continuous progression of binocular vision is the position of the eyes in the head. As pointed out by Walls:

Many a careless writer has stated that phylogenetically, from "fish to man," there has been a gradual migration of the eyes from a position back-to-back to one in which the two lines of sight are forward and parallel. Actually, a complete series of eye positions can be arranged wholly within the fish group, another such series within the birds, and a third within the mammals. Scattered species elsewhere have the lines of sight parallel, but directed upward rather than forward.[396]

Higher vertebrates

A credible evolutionary schema for binocular vision will be difficult to construct in mammals, since binocular vision has been demonstrated in every mammal so far studied, including the rabbit. The normal ocular motor posture of the rabbit is markedly divergent. However, when feeding, rabbits exhibit limited convergence and have neurons in the visual cortex subserving a narrow region of functional binocular vision.[158]

A curious feature of the binocular visual pathway of cat, as well as ungulates like sheep and goats, is a shift in the location of the vertical meridian of the visual field from Y, to X, to W ganglion cells (Fig. 24-71). The chiasmal decussation of Y cell fibers places the Y cell meridian 2 degrees into the temporal retina, the X cell meridian 1 degree into the temporal retina, and the W cell meridian directly through the area centralis.[209] The monocular result is that the contralateral cerebral hemisphere contains a substantial representation of the ipsilateral as well as contralateral visual field. The binocular result is that the Y cell meridians align at a point in space nearest the animal, with the X cell meridians more distant, and the W cell meridians most distant. Based on these differences in the vertical meridia, Levick has hypothesized that the different ganglion cell populations in the cat subserve binocular vision at different depths in

Retina of right eye

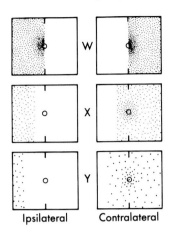 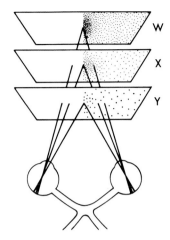

Ipsilateral   Contralateral

FIG. 24-71   Nasotemporal decussation pattern for different classes of ganglion cells in cat. W-cells decussate at the area centralis; X-cells a few degrees temporal; and Y-cells several degrees temporal. When viewing binocularly, the vertical meridia for these three classes of ganglion cells therefore intersect at three different depth planes, or horopters, with Y-cells responding to the most convergent disparities. Drawn using data of Levick (1977) and Pettigrew (1986).

space, with the Y cells subserving the most convergent disparities.[209]

Bishop suggested that the short snout and more frontally placed eyes of primates provided evolutionary impetus for eye-hand coordination. He hypothesized that "... evolution of binocular vision was undoubtedly a major factor in bringing manual skills to their highest level of performance in the human. Under normal viewing conditions the quality of stereoscopic vision improves as the objects regarded are brought closer to the eyes, up to a point where the ability to focus begins to fall off."[37] Bishop goes on to acknowledge, however, the difficulties with this hypothesis in that "... stereoscopic perception no longer seems to have the important place it is widely held to have had in the evolution of our species. For us, stereopsis can be replaced to a very large extent by higher order secondary cues to depth that are operative in monocular, as well as binocular, vision." In similar fashion, Previc[294] has recently developed an "ecological hypothesis," in which he argues that motion stereopsis in the lower visual field of primates is intended mainly to aid grasping.

REFERENCES

1. Abraham S: The basic position of rest—convergence and divergence, J Pediat Ophthalmol Strab 1:9, 1964.
2. Adler F: Pathologic physiology of convergent strabis-
mus: motor aspects of the non-accommodative type, Arch Ophthalmol 33:362, 1945.
3. Aguilonius F: Opticorum libri sex, Antwerp, Plantin, 1613.
4. Allman J: Evolution of the visual system in the early primates, in Sprague JM, ed: Progress in psychobiology and physiological Psychology, vol 7, New York & San Francisco, Academic Press, 1977, pp 1-53.
4a. Apkarian P, Reits D, Spekeijse H: Component specificity in albino VEP asymmetry; maturation of the visual anomaly, Exp Brain Res 53:285, 1984.
5. Archer SM, Helveston EM, Miller KK, et al: Stereopsis in normal infants and infants with congenital esotropia, Am J Ophthalmol 101:591, 1986.
6. Archer SM, Sondhi N, Helveston EM: Strabismus in infancy, Ophthalmol 96:133, 1989.
7. Aschenbrenner C: Problems in getting information into and out of air photographs, Photogramm Eng 20:398, 1954.
8. Aslin RN: Development of binocular fixation in human infants, in Fisher DF, Monty RA, Senders J, eds: Eye movements: cognition and visual perception, Hillsdale, NJ, Erlbaum, 1977, pp 31-51.
9. Aslin RN: Development of smooth pursuit in human infants, in Fisher DF, Monty RA, Senders J, eds: Eye movements: cognition and visual perception, Hillsdale, NJ: Erlbaum, 1981.
10. Aslin RN, Dumais S: Binocular vision in infants: a review and a theoretical framework, Adv Child Dev Behav 15:53, 1980.
11. Atkinson J: Development of optokinetic nystagmus in the human infant and monkey infant: an analogue to development in kittens, in Freeman RD, ed: Develop-

ment neurobiology of vision, New York, Plenum, 1979, pp 277-287.

12. Atkinson J: The Cambridge infant photorefraction screening programme: prediction and prevention of strabismus and amblyopia, in Simon K, ed: Infant vision: basic and clinical research, New York, Oxford University Press, 1992 (in press).

13. Atkinson J, Braddick O: Stereoscopic discrimination in infants, Perception 5:29, 1976.

14. Atkinson J, Braddick O: Development of optokinetic nystagmus in the human infant and monkey infant, in Fisher DF, Monty RA, Senders JW, eds: Eye movements: cognition and visual perception, Hillsdale, NJ, Erlbaum, 1981, pp 53-64.

15. Atkinson J, Braddick O, Pimm-Smith E: 'Preferential looking' for monocular and binocular testing of infants, Br J Ophthalmol 66:264, 1982.

16. Awaya S: Stimulus vision deprivation amblyopia in humans, Strab 31, 1978.

17. Awaya S: Studies of form vision deprivation amblyopia, Acta Soc Ophthalmol Jpn 91:519, 1987.

18. Awaya S, Miyake S: Form vision deprivation amblyopia: further observations, Graefe's Arch Clin Exp Ophthalmol 226:132, 1988.

19. Awaya S, Miyake Y, Imaizumi Y, et al: Amblyopia in man, suggestive of stimulus deprivation amblyopia, Jpn J Ophthalmol 17:69, 1973.

20. Awaya S, Sugawara M, Miyake S, et al: Form vision deprivation amblyopia and the results of its treatment—with special reference to the critical period, Jpn J Ophthalmol 24:241, 1980.

21. Bagolini B: Anomalous correspondence: definition and diagnostic methods, Doc Ophthalmologica 23:346, 1967.

22. Bailey P, von Bonin G: The isocortex of man, Urbana, University of Illinois Press, 1951.

23. Baker FA, Grigg P, von Noorden GK: The effects of visual deprivation and strabismus on the responses of neurons in the visual cortex of the monkey including studies on the striate and prestriate cortex in the normal animal, Brain Res 66:185, 1974.

24. Bedell H, Flom M: Monocular spatial distortion in strabismic amblyopia, Invest Ophthalmol Vis Sci 20:263, 1981.

25. Bedell HE, Flom MC, Barbeito R: Spatial aberrations and acuity in strabismus and amblyopia, Invest Ophthalmol Vis Sci 26:909, 1985.

26. Berlucchi G: Anatomical and physiological aspects of visual functions of corpus callosum, Brain Res 37:371, 1972.

27. Birch E: Stereopsis in infants and its developmental relationship to visual acuity, in Simons K, ed: Infant vision: basic and clinical research, New York, Oxford University Press, 1992 (in press).

28. Birch EE, Gwiazda J, Held R: Stereoacuity development for crossed and uncrossed disparities in human infants, Vision Res 22:507, 1982.

29. Birch EE, Gwiazda J, Held R: The development of vergence does not account for the onset of stereopsis, Perception 12:331, 1983.

30. Birch EE, Hale LA: Criteria for monocular acuity deficit in infancy and early childhood, Invest Ophthalmol Vis Sci 29:636, 1988.

31. Birch EE, Shimojo S, Held R: Preferential-looking assessment of fusion and stereopsis in infants aged 1 to 6 months, Invest Ophthalmol Vis Sci 26:366, 1985.

32. Birch EE, Stager D, Wright W: Grating acuity development after early surgery for congenital unilateral cataract, Arch Ophthalmol 104:1783, 1986.

33. Birch EE, Stager DR: Monocular acuity and stereopsis in infantile esotropia, Invest Ophthalmol Vis Sci 26:1624, 1985.

34. Birch EE, Stager DR: Prevalence of good visual acuity following surgery for congenital unilateral cataract, Arch Ophthalmol 106:40, 1988.

35. Birch EE, Stager DR, Berry P, et al: Prospective assessment of acuity and stereopsis in amblyopic infantile esotropes following early surgery, Invest Ophthalmol Vis Sci 31:758, 1990.

36. Birch EE, Swanson WH: Probability summation of grating acuity in the human infant, Invest Ophthalmol Vis Sci, 1991 (in press).

37. Bishop PO: Binocular vision, in Moses RA, Hart WM, eds: Adler's physiology of the eye: clinical application, 8th ed, St. Louis, CV Mosby, 1987, pp 619-689.

38. Bishop PO, Henry GH: Spatial vision, Ann Rev Psychol 22:119, 1971.

39. Blake R, Fox R: Binocular rivalry suppression: insensitive to spatial frequency and orientation change, Vision Res 14:687, 1974.

40. Blakemore C: The range and scope of binocular depth discrimination in man, J Physiol 211:599, 1970.

41. Boothe RG, Dobson V, Teller DY: Postnatal development of vision in human and nonhuman primates, Ann Rev Neurosci 8:495, 1985.

42. Booth RG, Gammon JA, Tigges M, et al: Behavioral measurements of acuity obtained from aphakic monkeys raised with extended wear soft contact lenses, Invest Ophthalmol Vis Sci 25(Suppl):216, 1984.

43. Boothe RG, Tigges M, Wilson J, et al: Monkey model of treatments for infantile aphakic amblyopia, Invest Ophthalmol Vis Sci 31(Suppl):279, 1990.

44. Bourdet C, Van Sluyters RC: Visual callosal development in strabismic cats, Soc Neurosci Abstr 15:1338, 1989.

45. Bower TGR: Object perception in infants, Perception 1:15, 1972.

46. Braddick O, Atkinson J, Wattam-Bell J: Videorefraction, immediate measures of refractive state in subjects of all ages, Perception 17:(Abstr):418, 1988.

47. Bradley A, Freeman R: Contrast sensitivity in anisometropic amblyopia, Invest Ophthalmol Vis Sci 21:467, 1981.

48. Bunt A, Minckler DS, Johanson GW: Demonstration of bilateral projection of the central retina of the monkey with horseradish peroxidase neuronography, J Comp Neurol 171:619, 1977.

49. Burian H: Anomalous retinal correspondence: its essence and its significance in diagnosis and treatment, Am J Ophthalmol 34:547, 1951.

50. Burkhalter A, Bernardo K: Development of local connections in human visual cortex, Soc Neurosci Abstr 15:2, 1989.

51. Burkhalter A, Bernardo K, Charles V: Postnatal development of intracortical connections in human visual cortex, Soc Neurosci Abstr 16:1129, 1990.

52. Burkhalter A, Felleman DJ, Newsome WT, et al: Anatomical and physiological asymmetries related to visual areas V3 and VP in macaque extrastriate cortex, Vision Res 26:63, 1986.

53. Burkhalter A, Van Essen DC: The connections of the ventral posterior area (VP) in the macaque monkey, Soc Neurosci Abstr 9:153, 1983.

54. Carpenter RHS: Movements of the eyes 2nd ed, London, Pion Limited, 1988.

55. Chavasse F: Worth's squint or the binocular reflexes and the treatment of strabismus, 7th ed, London, Bailliere Tindall and Cox, 1939.

55a. Collett T: Stereopsis in toads, Nature 267:349, 1977.

56. Collewijn H, Erkelens CJ, Steinman RM: Binocular coordination of human horizontal saccadic eye movements, J Physiol (Lond) 404:157, 1988.

57. Collewijn H, Martins A, Steinman RM: Natural retinal image motion: origin and change, Ann N Y Acad Sci 374:312, 1981.

58. Cooper J, Ciuffreda K, Kruger P: Stimulus and response AC/A ratios in intermittent exotropia of the divergence excess type, Br J Ophthalmol 66:398, 1982.

59. Corbetta M, Miezin FM, Dobmeyer S, et al: Selective and divided attention during visual discrimination of shape, color, and speed: functional anatomy by positron emission tomography, J Neurosci 11:2383, 1991.

60. Cornsweet TN: Visual perception, New York, Academic Press, 1970.

61. Costenbader FD: Infantile esotropia, Tr Am Ophthal Soc 59:397, 1961.

62. Crawford MLJ, von Noorden GK: Optically induced comitant strabismus in monkeys, Invest Ophthalmol Vis Sci 19:1105, 1980a.

63. Crawford MLJ, von Noorden GK: Concomitant strabismus and cortical eye dominance in young rhesus monkeys, Trans Ophthalmol Soc UK 99:369, 1980b.

64. Crawford MLJ, von Noorden GK: The effects of short-term experimental strabismus on the visual system in macaca mulatta, Invest Ophthalmol Vis Sci 18:496, 1979.

65. Crawford MLJ, von Noorden GK, Meharg LS, et al: Binocular neurons and binocular function in monkeys and children, Invest Ophthalmol Vis Sci 24:491, 1983.

66. Crone FA, Velzeboer CMJ: Statistics on strabismus in the Amsterdam youth, Arch Ophthalmol 55:455, 1956.

67. Crone R: Diplopia, Amsterdam, Excerpta Medica, 1973.

68. Daw NW, Fox K: Function of NMDA receptors in the developing visual cortex, in Lam DM, Shatz CJ, eds: Development of the visual system, Cambridge, MIT Press, 1991, pp 243-252.

69. Day SH, Norcia AM: Photographic detection of amblyogenic factors, Ophthalmol 93:25, 1983.

70. Day SH, Norcia AM: Infantile esotropia and the developing visual system, Ped Ophthalmol 3:281, 1990.

71. Day SH, Orel-Bixler DA, Norcia AM: Abnormal acuity development in infantile esotropia, Invest Ophthalmol Vis Sci 29:327, 1988.

72. de Courten C, Leuba G, Huttenlocher PR, et al: Volumetric, neuronal and synaptic development of human primary visual cortex, Neurosci Lett 10(Suppl):S135, 1982.

73. Dell'Osso LF, Traccis S, Abel LA: Strabismus: a necessary condition for latent and manifest latent nystagmus, Neuro-ophthalmology 3:247, 1983.

74. Dell'Osso LF, Ellenberger C, Abel LA, et al: The nystagmus blockage syndrome: congenital nystagmus, manifest latent nystagmus, or both? Invest Ophthalmol Vis Sci 24:1580, 1983.

75. Dell'Osso LF, Schmidt D, Daroff RB: Latent, manifest latent, and congenital nystagmus, Arch Ophthalmol 97:1877, 1979.

76. Demer JL, von Noorden GK: Optokinetic asymmetry in esotropia, J Ped Ophthal & Strab 25:286, 1988.

77. Demer JL, von Noorden GK, Volkow ND, et al: Imaging of cerebral blood flow and metabolism in amblyopia by positron emission tomography, Am J Ophthalmol 105:337, 1988.

77a. Demer LJ, Porter FI, Goldberg J, et al: Adaptation to telescopic spectacles; vestibulo-ocular reflex plasticity, Invest Ophthalmol Vis Sci 30:159, 1989.

78. DeMonasterio FM, Gouras P: Functional properties of ganglion cells of the rhesus monkey retina, J Physiol 251:167, 1975.

79. Denton M: Evolution: a theory in crisis, Bethesda, MD, Adler & Adler, 1985.

80. DeYoe EA, Van Essen DC: Clustering of physiological properties in macaque V2 correlates with cytochrome oxidase and efferent cell stripes, Invest Ophthalmol Vis Sci 26(Suppl):9, 1985.

81. DeYoe EA, Van Essen DC: Concurrent processing streams in monkey visual cortex, Trends Neurosci 11:219, 1988.

82. Dickey CF, Metz HS, Steward SA, et al: The diagnosis of amblyopia in cross-fixation, J Ped Ophthalmol Strabis 28:171, 1991.

83. Dobson V: Visual acuity testing in infants: from the laboratory to the clinic, in Simons K, ed: Infant vision: basic and clinical research, New York, Oxford University Press, 1992 (in press).

84. Dobson V, McDonald MA, Kohl P, et al: Visual acuity screening of infants and young children with the acuity card procedure, J Am Optom Assoc 27:284, 1986.

85. Doden W, Adams W: Elektronystagmographische Ergebnisse der Prufung des optischvestibularen Systems bei Schielenden, Ber Zusammenkunft Dtsch Ophthalmol Ges 60:316, 1957.

86. Donzis PB, Rappazzo JA, Burde RM, et al: Effect of binocular variations of Snellen's visual acuity on Titmus stereoacuity, Arch Ophthalmol 101:930, 1983.

87. Dove HW: Uber stereoskopie, Ann Phys 110:494, 1841.

88. Drummond GT, Scott WE, Keech RV: Management of monocular congenital cataracts, Arch Ophthalmol 107:45, 1989.

89. Duane A: A new classification of the motor anomalies of the eyes, New York, JH Vaio Co, 1897.

90. Eggers H, Gizzi M, Movshon J: Spatial properties of striate cortical neurons in esotropic macaques, Invest Ophthalmol Visual Sci 25(Suppl):278, 1984.

91. Ellis GS, Hartmann EE, Love A, et al: Teller acuity cards versus clinical judgement in the diagnosis of amblyopia with strabismus, Ophthalmol 95:788, 1988.

92. Erkelens CJ, Steinman RM, Collewijn H: Gaze shifts

between real targets differing in distance and direction, Proc R Soc Lond (Biol) 236:441, 1989b.

93. Erkelens CJ, Van der Steen J, Steinman RM, et al: Ocular vergence under natural conditions, I, Continuous changes of target distance along the median plane, Proc R Soc Lond (Biol) 236:417, 1989a.

94. Evens L, Kuypers C: Frequence de l'amblyope en Belgique, Bull Soc Belge Ophthalmol 147:445, 1967.

95. Feingold M, Bossert W: Normal values for selected physical parameters: an aid to syndrome delineation, in Bergsman D, ed: Birth defects: original article series, vol 10, New York, The National Foundation/March of Dimes, 1974.

96. Felleman DJ, Van Essen DC: Distributed hierarchical processing in the primate cerebral cortex, Cerebral Cortex 1:1, 1991.

97. Fender D, Julesz B: Extension of Panum's fusional area in binocularly stabilized vision, J Opt Soc Am 57:819, 1967.

98. Finocchio DV, Preston KL, Fuchs AF: A quantitative analysis of the development of the vestibulo-ocular reflex and visual-vestibular interactions in human infants, Invest Ophthalmol Vis Sci 19(Suppl):83, 1990.

99. Fischer B, Boch R, Bach M: Stimulus versus eye movements: comparison of neural activity in the striate and prelunate visual cortex (A17 and A19) of trained rhesus monkey, Exp Brain Res 43:69, 1981.

100. Fisher N, Flom M, Jampolsky A: Traumatic bitemporal hemianopsia, Part II, Binocular cooperation, Am J Ophthalmol 65:558, 1968.

101. Fisher NF: The optic chiasm and the corpus callosum: their relationship to binocular vision in humans, J Ped Ophthalmol Strab 23:126, 1986.

101a. Fletcher MC, Silverman SJ: Strabismus, Am J Ophthalmol 61:86, 1966.

102. Flom M, Weymouth F: Retinal correspondence and the horopter in anomalous correspondence, Nature 189:34, 1961.

103. Flom M, Weymouth F, Kahnerman D: Visual resolution and contour interaction, J Opt Soc Am 53:1026, 1963.

104. Flynn J: Spatial summation in amblyopia, Arch Ophthalmol 78:470, 1967.

105. Foley FM: Primary distance perception, in Held R, Leibowitz HW, Teuber HL, eds: Handbook of sensory physiology, vol VII, Perception, Berlin, Springer-Verlag, 1978.

106. Foley FM: Effect of distance information and range on two indices of perceived distance, Perception 6:449, 1977.

107. Foltz A, Kelsey JL: The annual pap test: a dubious policy success, Health and Society 56:426, 1978.

108. Foote S, Morrison J: Postnatal development of laminar innervation patterns by monoaminergic fibers in monkey (macaca fascicularis) primary visual cortex, J Neurosci 4:2667, 1984.

109. Fox K, Sato H, Daw N: The location and function of NMDA receptors in cat and kitten visual cortex, J Neurosci 9:2443, 1989.

110. Fox R, Aslin RN, Shea SL, et al: Stereopsis in human infants, Science 207:323, 1980.

111. Fox R, Check R: Binocular fusion: a test of the suppression theory, Percept Psychophys 1:331, 1966.

112. Fox R, Check R: Detection of motion during binocular rivalry suppression, J Exp Psychol 78:388, 1968.

113. Fox R, Lehmkuhle S, Bush R: Stereopsis in the falcon, Science 197:79, 1976.

114. Freedman HL, Preston K: Photorefractive screening for amblyogenic factors in children, Ophthalmol 95(Suppl):132, 1989.

115. Gamlin PDR, Gnadt JW, Mays LE: Lidocaine-induced unilateral internuclear ophthalmoplegia: effects on convergence and conjugate eye movements, J Neurophysiol 62:82, 1989.

116. Gammon J, O'Dell C, Quick M, et al: Visual function in monkeys modeling infantile aphakia-amblyopia treatment, Invest Ophthalmol Vis Sci 29(Suppl):75, 1988.

117. Gauthier G, Robinson D: Adaptation of the human vestibulo-ocular reflex to magnifying lenses, Brain Res 92:331, 1975.

118. Gelbert SS, Hoyt CS, Jastrebski G, et al: Long-term visual results in bilateral congenital cataracts, Am J Ophthalmol 93:615, 1982.

119. Gnadt J, Mays L: Posterior parietal cortex, the oculomotor near response and spatial coding in 3-D space, Soc Neurosci Abstr 15:786, 1989.

120. Gonshor A, Melvill Jones G: Extreme vestibulo-ocular adaptation induced by prolonged optical reversal of vision, J Physiol 256:381, 1976.

121. Goodwin RT, Romano PE: Stereoacuity degradation by experimental and real monocular and binocular amblyopia, Invest Ophthalmol Vis Sci 26:917, 1985.

122. Gottlob I, Strangler-Zuschrott E: Effect of levodopa on contrast sensitivity and scotomas in human amblyopia, Invest Ophthalmol Vis Sci 31:776, 1990.

122a. Graham PA: Epidemiology of strabismus, Br J Ophthalmol 58:224, 1974.

123. Groenendaal F, van Hof-van Duin J, et al: Effects of perinatal hypoxia on visual development during the first year of (corrected) age: Early Hum Dev 20:267, 1989.

124. Gstalder R, Green D: Laser interferometric acuity in amblyopia, J Pediatric Ophthalmol Strab 8:251, 1971.

124a. Guillery R: Normal and abnormal visual pathways, Trans Ophthalmol Soc UK 99:352, 1979.

124b. Guillery R: Neural abnormalities of albinos, TINS 9:364, 1986.

125. Gwiazda J, Bauer JAJ, Held R: Binocular function in human infants: correlation of stereoptic and fusion-rivalry discriminations, J Pediatr Ophthalmol Strab 26:128, 1989.

126. Gwiazda J, Scheiman M, Held R: Anisotropic resolution in children's vision, Vision Res 24:527, 1984.

127. Hainline L: Oculomotor control in human infants, in Groner R, McConkie GW, Menz C, eds: Eye movements and human information processing, Amsterdam, Elsevier-North Holland, 1985.

128. Hainline L: Conjugate eye movements in infants, in Simons K, ed: Infant vision: basic and clinical research, New York, Oxford University Press, 1992 (in press).

129. Hainline L, Lemerise E, Abramov I, et al: Orientational asymmetries in small-field optokinetic nystagmus in human infants, Behav Brain Res 13:217, 1984.

130. Hakim R, Tielsch J, Canner J, et al: Prenatal and fetal risk factors for childhood strabismus, Invest Ophthalmol Vis Sci 30:107, 1989.

131. Hamer RD, Hsu-Wignes C, Wesemann I, et al: Refractive error screening with a polaroid photoretinoscope, Invest Ophthalmol Vis Sci 29(Suppl):76, 1988.

132. Hamer RD, Norcia AM, Orel-Bixler D, et al: Cortical responses to nasalward and temporalward motion are asymmetric in early but not late-onset strabismus, Invest Ophthalmol Vis Sci 31(Suppl):289, 1990.

133. Hamsher K: Stereopsis and unilateral brain disease, Invest Ophthalmol Vis Sci 17:336, 1978.

134. Hawken MJ, Parker AJ, Lund JS: Laminar organization and contrast sensitivity of direction-selective cells in the striate cortex of the old world monkey, J Neurosci 8:3541, 1988.

135. Hay S: Retinal reflex photometry as a screening device for amblyopia and preamblyopic states in children, South Med J 76:309, 1983.

136. Hebb D: The organization of behavior, New York, Wiley, 1949.

137. Held R, Birch EE, Gwiazda J: Stereoacuity in human infants, Proc Natl Acad Sci USA 77:5572, 1980.

138. Helmholtz S: Helmholtz's treatise on physiological optics, vol 3, 3rd ed, Southall SPC, ed, New York, Optical Soc America, 1925.

139. Helveston EM: Dissociated vertical deviation—a clinical and laboratory study, Trans Am Ophthalmol Soc 78:734, 1981.

140. Hendrickson A, Movshon J, Eggers H, et al: Effects of early unilateral blur on the macaque's visual system, II, Anatomical observations, J Neurosci 7:1327, 1987.

141. Hering E: The theory of binocular vision (1868), New York, Plenum Press, 1977.

142. Hess R: Contrast sensitivity assessment of functional amblyopia in humans, Trans Ophthalmol Soc UK 99:391, 1979.

143. Hess R, Campbell F, Greenhalgh T: On the neural abnormality in human amblyopia: neural aberrations and neural sensitivity loss, Pfluegers Arch 377:201, 1978.

144. Hess R, Jacobs R: A preliminary report of acuity and contour interactions across the amblyopes visual field, Vision Res 19:1403, 1979.

145. Hillebrand F: Die stabilitat der Raumwerte auf der Netzhaut, Z Psychol 5:1, 1893.

146. Hillebrand F: Der Verhaltnis von Akkommodation und Konvergenz zur Tiefenlokalisation, Z Psychol Physiol Sinnesorg 7:97, 1894.

147. Hirsch M, Weymouth F: Distance discrimination, II, Effect on threshold of lateral separation of the test objects, Arch Ophthalmol 39:224, 1948.

148. Hoffmann K: Optokinetic nystagmus and single-cell responses in the nucleus tractus opticus after early monocular deprivation in the cat, in Freeman RD, ed: Developmental neurobiology of vision, New York and London, Plenum Press, 1979, pp 63–72.

149. Horton JC, Hedley-Whyte ET: Mapping of cytochrome oxidase patches and ocular dominance columns in human visual cortex, Phil Trans R Soc Lond 304:255, 1984.

150. Howard H: A test for the judgement of distance, Am J Ophthalmol 2:656, 1919.

151. Howland H, Atkinson J, Braddick O, et al: Infant astigmatism measured by photorefraction, Science 212:331, 1978.

152. Howland H, Braddick O, Atkinson J, et al: Optics of photorefraction: orthogonal and isotropic methods, J Opt Soc Am 73:1701, 1983.

152a. Howland H, Sayles N: Photorefractive characterization of focussing ability of infants and young children, Invest Ophthalmol Vis Sci 28:1005, 1987.

153. Hoyt CS: The long-term visual effects of short-term binocular occlusion of at-risk neonates, Arch Ophthalmol 98:1967, 1980.

153a. Hoyt CS, Caltrider N: Hemispheric visually-evoked responses in congenital esotropia, J Pediat Ophthalmol Strabis 21:19, 1984.

154. Hsu-Winges C, McKee SP, Schor CM, et al: The classification of amblyopia on the basis of laboratory and clinical measurements, Invest Ophthalmol Vis Sci 32(Suppl):960, 1991.

155. Hubel DH, Wiesel TN, LeVay S: Plasticity of ocular dominance columns in monkey striate cortex, Philos Trans R Soc London Ser B 278:377, 1977.

156. Hubel DH: Exploration of the primary visual cortex, 1955–78, Nature 299:515, 1982.

157. Hubel DH, Wiesel TN: Laminar and columnar distribution of geniculo-cortical fibers in macaque monkeys, J Comp Neurol 146:421, 1972.

158. Hughes A, Vaney D: The organization of binocular cortex in the primary visual area of the rabbit, J Comp Neurol 204:151, 1982.

159. Huttenlocher PR, de Courten C, Garey L, et al: Synaptogenesis in human visual cortex: evidence for synapse elimination during normal development, Neurosci Lett 33:247, 1982.

160. Huttenlocher PR: Synapse elimination and plasticity in developing human cerebral cortex, Am J Ment Def 88:488, 1984.

161. Hyvarinen J, Hyvarinen L, Linnankoski I: Modification of parietal association cortex and functional blindness after binocular deprivation in young monkeys, Exp Brain Res 42:1, 1981.

162. Ikeda H: Is amblyopia a peripheral defect? Trans Ophthalmol Soc UK 99:347, 1979.

163. Ingram R, Traynar M, Walker C, et al: Screening for refractive errors at age 1 year: a pilot study, Br J Ophthalmol 63:243, 1979.

164. Ingram R, Walker C, Wilson J, et al: A first attempt to prevent amblyopia and squint by spectacle correction of abnormal refractions from age 1 year, Br J Ophthalmol 69:851, 1985.

165. Ingram R, Walker C, Wilson J, et al: Prediction of amblyopia and squint by means of refraction at age 1 year, Br J Ophthalmol 70:12, 1986.

166. Innocenti G, Clarke S: The organization of immature callosal connections, J Comp Neurol 230:287, 1984.

167. Innocenti G, Frost D, Illes J: Maturation of visual callosal connections in visually deprived kittens: a challenging critical period, J Neurosci 5:255, 1985.

168. Isenberg S, Yee R: The ETHAN syndrome, Ann Ophthalmol 18:358, 1986.

169. Ittelson WH: The Ames demonstrations in perception, Princeton: Princeton University Press, 1952.

170. Jacobson S, Sandberg M, Effron M, et al: Foveal cone electroretinograms in strabismic amblyopia, Trans Ophthal Soc UK 99:353, 1979.

171. Jampolsky A: Retinal correspondence in patients with small degree strabismus, Arch Ophthalmol 45:18, 1951.

172. Jampolsky A: Characteristics of suppression in strabismus, Arch Ophthalmol 54:683, 1955.

173. Jampolsky A: Unequal visual inputs and strabismus management: a comparison of human and animal strabismus, in Helveston EM, Jampolsky A, Knapp P, eds: Symposium on strabismus: transactions of the New Orleans Academy of Ophthalmology, St Louis, CV Mosby, 1978, pp 358–492.

174. Jampolsky A, Flom B, Freid A: Fixation disparity in relation to heterophoria, Am J Ophthalmol 43:97, 1957.

175. Johnson P: Darwin on trial, Washington, DC, Regnery Gateway, 1991.

176. Jones R: Anomalies of disparity detection in the human visual system, J Physiol (Lond) 264:621, 1977.

177. Julesz B: Binocular depth perception of computer-generated patterns, Bell System Tech J 39:1125, 1960.

178. Julesz B: Foundations of cyclopean perception, Chicago, University of Chicago Press, 1971.

179. Julesz B, Krofli WJ, Petrig B: Large evoked-potentials to dynamic random-dot correlograms and stereograms permit quick determination of stereopsis, Proc Nat Acad Sci 71:2348, 1980.

180. Julesz B, Spivack G: Stereopsis based on vernier acuity cues alone, Science 157:563, 1967.

181. Kasamatsu T, Pettigrew J, Ary M: Cortical recovery from the effects of monocular deprivation: acceleration with norepinephrine and suppression with 6-hydroxydopamine, J Neurophysiol 45:254, 1981.

182. Kato I, Harada K, Hasegawa T, et al: Role of the nucleus of the optic tract in monkeys in relation to optokinetic nystagmus, Brain Res 364:12, 1986.

183. Keiner GBJ: New viewpoints on the origin of squint: a clinical and statistical study on its nature, cause and therapy, the Hague, Martinus Nijhoff, 1951.

184. Keiner GBJ: Physiology and pathology of the optomotor reflexes, Am J Ophthalmol 42:233, 1956.

185. Kiorpes L, Boothe RG, Carlson M, et al: Frequency of naturally occurring strabismus in monkeys, J Ped Ophthalmol Strabismus 22:60, 1985.

186. Kiorpes L, Boothe RG: Naturally occurring strabismus in monkeys (Macaca nemestrina), Invest Ophthalmol Vis Sci 20:257, 1981.

187. Kiorpes L, Boothe RG, Hendrickson AE, et al: Effects of early unilateral blur on the macaque's visual system, I, Behavioral observations, J Neurosci 7:1318, 1987.

188. Kiorpes L, Movshon A: Vernier acuity and spatial contrast sensitivity in monkeys with experimentally induced strabismus or anisometropia, Invest Ophthalmol Vis Sci 30(Suppl):327, 1989.

189. Kiorpes L, Thorell L, Boothe RG: Response properties of cortical cells in monkeys with experimentally produced meridional amblyopia, Invest Ophthalmol Vis Sci 18(Suppl):194, 1979.

190. Kirkham TH: The ocular symptomatology of pituitary tumors, Proc R Soc Med 65:517, 1972.

191. Kitchen W, Rickards A, Ryan MM, et al: A longitudinal study of very low-birthweight infants, II, Results of controlled trial of intensive care and incidence of handicaps, Develop Med Child Neurol 21:582, 1979.

192. Kivlin J, Flynn J: Therapy of anisometropic amblyopia, J Ped Ophthalmol Strab 18:47, 1981.

193. Kleinschmidt A, Bear M, Singer W: Blockade of "NMDA" receptors disrupts experience-dependent plasticity of kitten striate cortex, Science 238:355, 1987.

194. Kushner BJ: Visual results after surgery for monocular juvenile cataracts of undetermined onset, Am J Ophthalmol 102:468, 1986.

195. Kushner BJ: Postoperative binocularity in adults with long standing strabismus: is surgery cosmetic only? Am Orthopt J 40:64, 1990.

196. Kushner BJ: Strabismus and amblyopia associated with regressed retinopathy of prematurity, Arch Ophthalmol 100:256, 1982.

197. Lang J: Strabismus, Thorofare, NJ: Slack, 1984.

198. Leguire LE, Rogers GL, Bremer D, et al: Levodopa treatment for childhood amblyopia, Invest Ophthalmol Vis Sci 32(Suppl):820, 1991.

199. Leguire LE, Rogers GL, Fellows RR: Toward a clinical test of stereopsis in human infants, Invest Ophthalmol Vis Sci 24(Suppl):34, 1983.

200. Lehmann D, Skrandies W, Lindenmaier CL: Sustained cortical potentials evoked in humans by binocularly correlated, uncorrelated and disparate dynamic random-dot stimuli, Neurosci Lett 10:129, 1978.

201. Lennie P: Parallel visual pathways: a review, Vision Res 20:561, 1980.

202. LeVay S, Hubel DH, Wiesel TN: The pattern of ocular dominance columns in macaque visual cortex revealed by a reduced silver stain, J Comp Neurol 159:559, 1975.

203. LeVay S, Wiesel TN, Hubel DH: The development of ocular dominance columns in normal and visually deprived monkeys, J Comp Neurol 191:1, 1980.

203a. LeVay S, Connolly M, Houde J, et al: The complete pattern of ocular dominance stripes in the striate cortex and visual field of the macaque monkey, J Neurosci 5:486, 1985.

203b. Leventhal A, Vitek D, Creel D: Abnormal visual pathways in normal pigmented cats that are heterozygous for albinism, Science 229:1395, 1985.

204. Leventhal AG, Ault SJ, Vitek DJ: The nasotemporal division in primate retina: the neural bases of macular sparing and splitting, Science 240:66, 1988.

205. Levi DM, Harwerth RS: Spatio-temporal interactions in anisometropic and strabismic amblyopia, Invest Ophthalmol Vis Sci 16:90, 1977.

206. Levi DM, Harwerth RS: Psychophysical mechanisms in humans with amblyopia, AM J Opt Physiol Opt 59:936, 1982.

207. Levi DM, Klein SA: Differences in vernier discrimination for gratings between strabismic and anisometropic amblyopes, Invest Ophthalmol Vis Sci 23:398, 1982.

208. Levi DM, Klein SA, Yap YL: Positional uncertainty in peripheral and amblyopic vision, Vision Res 27:581, 1987.

209. Levick W: Participation of brisk-transient retinal ganglion cells in binocular vision—an hypothesis, Proc Aust Physiol Pharmacol Soc 8:9, 1977.

210. Lewis TL, Maurer D, Brent HP: Optokinetic nystagmus in normal and visually deprived children: implications for cortical development, Can J Psychol 43:121, 1989.

211. Lisberger SG, Morris EJ, Tychsen L: Visual motion processing and sensory-motor integration for smooth pursuit eye movements, Ann Rev Neurosci 10:97, 1987.

212. Livingstone MS, Hubel DH: Thalamic inputs to cyto-

chrome oxidase-rich regions in monkey visual cortex, Proc Natl Acad Sci USA 79:6098, 1982.

213. Livingstone MS, Hubel DH: Anatomy and physiology of a color system in the primate visual cortex, J Neurosci 4:309, 1984.

214. Lovasik JV, Szymkiw M: Effects of aniseikonia, anisometropia, accommodation, retinal illuminance, and pupil size on stereopsis, Invest Ophthalmol Vis Sci 26:741, 1985.

215. Lund JS, Lund R, Hendrickson A, et al: The origin of efferent pathways from the primary visual cortex, area 17, of the macaque monkey as shown by retrograde transport of horseradish peroxidase, J Comp Neurol 164:287, 1975.

216. Lund JS: Intrinsic organization of the primate visual cortex, area 17, as seen in Golgi preparations, in Schmitt FO, Worden FG, Adelman G, et al, eds: The organization of the cerebral cortex, Cambridge, MIT Press, 1981, pp 105-124.

217. Maddox E: The clinical use of prisms; and the decentering of lenses, Bristol, John Wright & Sons, 1893.

218. Malpeli J, Baker F: The representation of the visual field in the lateral geniculate nucleus of Macaca mulatta, J Comp Neurol 161:569, 1975.

219. Manning K, Fulton A, Hansen R, et al: Preferential looking vision testing: application to evaluation of high-risk, prematurely born infants and children, J Pediatr Ophthalmol Strabismus 19:286, 1982.

220. Marr D, Poggio T: A computational theory of human stereo vision, Proc R Soc Lond Ser B 204:301, 1979.

221. Matsumoto B, MacDonald R, Tychsen L: Constellation of ocular motor findings in naturally-strabismic macaque: animal model for human infantile strabismus, Invest Ophthalmol Vis Sci 32(Suppl):820, 1991.

222. Maunsell JHR, Van Essen DC: The connections of the middle temporal visual area (MT) and their relationship to a cortical hierarchy in the macaque monkey, J Neurosci 3:2563, 1983.

223. Maunsell JHR, Van Essen DC: Functional properties of neurons in middle temporal visual area of the macaque monkey, I, Selectivity for stimulus direction, speed, and orientation, J Neurophysiol 49:1127, 1983.

224. Maunsell JHR, Van Essen DC: Functional properties of neurons in middle temporal visual area of the macaque monkey, II, Binocular interactions and sensitivity to binocular disparity, J Neurophys 49:1148, 1983.

225. Maunsell JHR, Van Essen DC: Topographic organization of the middle temporal visual area in the macaque monkey: representational biases and the relationship to callosal connections and myeloarchitectonic boundaries, J Comp Neurol 266:535, 1987.

226. Maurer D, Lewis T, Brent H: Peripheral vision and optokinetic nystagmus in children with unilateral congenital cataract, Behav Brain Res 10:151, 1983.

227. Mayer D, Fulton A, Hansen R: Preferential looking acuity obtained with a staircase procedure in pediatric patients, Invest Ophthalmol Visual Sci 23:538, 1982.

228. Mayhew J, Longuet-Higgins H: A computational model of binocular depth perception, Nature 297:376, 1982.

229. Mays LE, Porter JD, Gamlin PDR, et al: Neural control of vergence eye movements: neurons encoding vergence velocity, J Neurophysiol 56:1007, 1986.

229a. McKee SP, Welch L: Sequential recruitment in the discrimination of velocity, J Opt Soc Am AZ:243, 1985.

230. Mehdorn E, Mattheus S, Schuppe A, et al: Treatment for amblyopia with rotating gratings and subsequent occlusion: a controlled study, Int Ophthalmol 3:361, 1981.

231. Miles F: Effects of a continuously moving environment on the rhesus monkey's ocular stability in the dark, Soc Neurosci Abstr 2:273, 1976.

232. Miles FA, Lisberger SG: Plasticity in the vestibulo-ocular reflex: a new hypothesis, Ann Rev Neurosci 4:273, 1981.

233. Miller E: The nature and cause of impaired vision in the amblyopic eye of a squinter, Am J Optom Arch Am Acad Optom 31:615, 1954.

234. Miller K, Keller J, Stryker M: Ocular dominance column development: analysis and simulation, Science 245:605, 1989.

235. Miller M, Israel J, Cuttone J: Fetal alcohol syndrome, J Pediatr Ophthalmol Strabismus 18:6, 1981.

236. Mindel JS, Raab EL, Eisenkraft JB, et al: Succinyldicholine-induced return of the eyes to the basic deviation: a motion picture study, Ophthalmol 12:1288, 1980.

237. Mindel JS, Eisenkraft JB, Raab EL, et al: Succinyldicholine and the basic ocular deviation, Am J Ophthalmol 95:315, 1983.

238. Mishkin M, Ungerleider LG, Macko KA: Object vision and spatial vision: two cortical pathways, Trends Neurosci 6:414, 1983.

239. Mitchell D, Freeman R, Millodot M, et al: Meridional amblyopia: evidence for modification of the human visual system by early visual experience, Vision Res 13:535, 1973.

240. Mitchell DE, Blakemore C: Binocular depth perception and the corpus callosum, Vision Res 10:49, 1970.

241. Miyake Y, Awaya S: Stimulus deprivation amblyopia: simultaneous recording of local macular electroretinogram and visual evoked response, Arch Ophthalmol 102:998, 1984.

242. Mohindra I, Jacobson SG, Held R: Binocular visual form deprivation in human infants, Documenta Ophthalmol 55:237, 1983.

243. Mohindra I, Jacobson SG, Thomas J, et al: Development of amblyopia in infants, Trans Ophthal Soc UK 99:344, 1979.

244. Morgan K, Johnson W: Clinical evaluation of a commercial photorefractor, Arch Ophthalmol 105:1528, 1987.

245. Morgan MW: Anomalous correspondence interpreted as a motor phenomenon, Am J Optom Arch Am Acad Optom 38:131, 1961.

246. Mountcastle VB, Motter BC, Steinmetz MA, et al: Looking and seeing: the visual functions of the parietal lobe, in Edelman WE, Gall WE, Cowan WM, eds: Dynamic aspects of neocortical function, New York, Wiley, 1984, pp 159-193.

247. Movshon JA, Eggers HM, Gizzi MS: Effects of early unilateral blur on the macaque's visual system, III, Physiological observations, J Neurosci 7:1340, 1987.

248. Movshon JA, Van Sluyters RC: Visual neural development, Ann Rev Psychol 32:477, 1981.

249. Muller J: Vom Gesichtsinn, in Handbuch der Physiol-

ogie des Menschen fur Vorlesungen, Coblenz: Holscher, 1840.

250. Mustari MJ, Fuchs AF: Discharge patterns of neurons in the pretectal nucleus of the optic tract (NOT) in the behaving primate, J Neurophysiol 64:77, 1990.

251. Nachtigaller H, Hoyt WF: Storungen des Seheindruckes bei bitemporaler Hemianopsie und Verschiebung der Sehachsen, Klin Monatsbl Augenheilkd 156:821, 1970.

252. Naegele J, Held R: The postnatal development of monocular optokinetic nystagmus in infants, Vision Res 22:341, 1982.

253. Naegele J, Held R: Development of optokinetic nystagmus and effects of abnormal visual experience during infancy, in Heim A, Jeannerod M, eds: Spatially oriented behavior, New York: Springer-Verlag, 1983, pp 155-174.

254. Newsome WT, Pare EB: A selective impairment of motion perception following lesions of the middle temporal visual area MT, J Neurosci 8:2201, 1988.

255. Newsome WT, Wurtz RH, Dursteler M, et al: Deficits in visual motion processing following ibotenic acid lesions of the middle temporal visual area of the macaque monkey, J Neurosci 5:825, 1985.

256. Nixon RB, Helveston EM, Miller K, et al: Incidence of strabismus in neonates, Am J Ophthalmol 100:798, 1985.

257. Norcia AM, Sutter E, Tyler C: Electrophysiological evidence for the existence of coarse and fine disparity mechanisms in human vision, Vision Res 25:1603, 1985.

258. Norcia AM, Tyler C: Temporal frequency limits for stereoscopic apparent motion processes, Vision Res 24:395, 1984.

259. Norcia AM, Tyler C: Infant VEP acuity measurements: analysis of individual differences and measurement errors, Encephalog Clin Neurophysiol 61:359, 1985.

260. Norcia AM, Tyler C: Spatial frequency sweep VEP: visual acuity during the first year of life, Vision Res 25:1399, 1985.

261. Norcia AM, Tyler C, Hamer R: High visual contrast sensitivity in the young human infants, Invest Ophthalmol Vis Sci 29:44, 1988.

262. Norcia AM, Garcia H, Humphry R, et al: Anomalous motion VEPs in infants and in infantile esotropia, Invest Ophthalmol Vis Sci 32:436, 1991.

263. Norcia AM, Hamer RD, Orel-Bixler D: Temporal tuning of the motion VEP in infants, Invest Ophthalmol Vis Sci 31(Supp):10, 1990.

264. Norcia AM, Humphrey R, Garcia H, et al: Anomalous motion VEPS in infants and in infantile esotropia, Invest Ophthalmol Vis Sci 30(Supp):327, 1989.

265. O'Dell CD, Quick MW, Boothe RG: The development of stereoacuity in infant rhesus monkeys, Invest Ophthalmol Vis Sci 32:1044, 1991.

266. Odom J, Hoyt CM, Marg E: Eye patching and visual evoked potential acuity in children four months to eight years old, Am J Optomet Physiol Opt 59:706, 1982.

267. Ogle KN: Analytical treatment of the longitudinal horopter, J Opt Soc Am 22:665, 1932.

268. Ogle KN: Researches in binocular vision, Philadelphia, WB Saunders, 1950.

269. Ogle KN: The optical space sense, Part II, in Davson H, ed: The eye, vol 4, New York, Academic Press, 1962, pp 211-417.

270. Ogle KN, Mussey F, Prangen AH: Fixation disparity and the fusional processes in binocular single vision, Am J Ophthalmol 32:1069, 1949.

271. Ogle KN, Weil MP: Stereoscopic vision and the duration of the stimulus, Arch Ophthalmol 59:4, 1958.

272. Oliver M, Neumann R, Chiamovitch Y, et al: Compliance and results of treatment for amblyopia in children more than 8 years old, Am J Ophthalmol 102:340, 1986.

273. Oohira A, Zee DS, Das S: Disconjugate ocular motor adaptation in rhesus monkeys, Invest Ophthalmol Vis Sci 30(Suppl):133, 1989.

273a. Orel-Bixler DA: Subjective and VEP measures of acuity in normal and amblyopic adults and children, Unpublished doctoral dissertation, University of California, Berkeley, 1989.

274. Ornitz E, Atwell C, Walter D: The maturation of the vestibular nystagmus in infancy and childhood, Acta Otolaryngol 88:244, 1979.

275. Panum PL: Physiologische Untersuchungen uber das Sehen mit zwei Augen, Kiel, Schwering, 1858.

276. Parinaud H: Le strabisme et son traitement, Paris, Gaston Doin, 1899.

277. Parks M: The monofixation syndrome, Trans New Orleans Acad Ophthalmol 121, 1971.

278. Parks M: Ocular motility and strabismus, Hagerstown, MD, Harper and Row, 1975.

279. Parks M: Visual results in aphakic children, Am J Ophthalmol 94:441, 1982.

280. Parks M, Wheeler M: Concomitant esodeviations, Chapter 12, in Duane T, Jaeger E, eds: Clinical ophthalmology, vol 1, Philadelphia, Harper and Row, 1987.

281. Parks M, Mitchell P: Concomitant exodeviations, Chapter 13, in Duane T, Jaeger E, eds: Clinical ophthalmology, vol 1, Philadelphia, Harper and Row, 1987.

282. Petrig B, Julesz B, Kropfl W, et al: Development of stereopsis and cortical binocularity in human infants: electrophysiological evidence, Science 213:1402, 1981.

283. Pettigrew JD: Comparison of the retinotopic organization of the visual Wulst in nocturnal and diurnal raptors, with a note on the evolution of frontal vision, in Cool S, Smith E, eds: Frontiers of visual science, New York, Springer-Verlag, 1979, pp 328-335.

284. Pettigrew JD: Binocular visual processing in the owl's telencephalon, Proc R Soc Lond, Ser B 204:435, 1979.

285. Pettigrew JD: The evolution of binocular vision, in Pettigrew JD, Sanderson KJ, Levick WR, eds: Visual neuroscience. Cambridge: Cambridge University Press, 1986, 208–222.

286. Phelps M, Mazziotta J, Kuhl D, et al: Tomographic mapping of human cerebral metabolism: visual stimulation and deprivation, Neurology 31:517, 1981.

287. Poggio GF, Poggio T: The analysis of stereopsis, Ann Rev Neurosci 7:379, 1984.

288. Poggio GF, Fischer B: Binocular interaction and depth sensitivity in striate and prestriate cortex of behaving rhesus monkey, J Neurophysiol 40:1392, 1977.

289. Poggio GF, Gonzalez F, Krause F: Stereoscopic mech-

anisms on monkey visual cortex: binocular correlation and disparity selectivity, J Neurosci 8:4531, 1988.

290. Poggio GF, Talbot WH: Mechanisms of static and dynamic stereopsis in foveal cortex of the rhesus monkey, J Physiol 315:469, 1981.

291. Polyak S: The vertebrate visual system, Chicago: University of Chicago Press, 1957.

292. Portnoy JZ, Thompson HS, Lennarson L, et al: Pupillary defects in amblyopia, Am J Ophthalmol 96:609, 1983.

293. Pratt-Johnson J, Tillson G: Intractable diplopia after vision restoration in unilateral cataract, Am J Ophthalmol 107:23, 1989.

294. Previc F: Functional specialization in the lower and upper visual field in humans: its ecological origins and neurophysiological implications, Behav Brain Sci 13:519, 1990.

295. Prism Adaptation Study Research Group: Efficacy of prism adaptation in the surgical management of acquired esotropia, Arch Ophthalmol 108:1248, 1990.

296. Pulfrich C: Die Stereoskopie im Dienste der Isochromen und heterochromen Photometrie, Naturwissenschaften 10:533, 1922.

297. Quality of Care Committee Pediatric Panel: Preferred practice pattern: amblyopia, American Academy of Ophthalmology 1992 (in press).

298. Quick MW, O'Dell CD, Boothe RG: Long-term grating and optotype acuity in a primate model of aphakia, Invest Ophthalmol Vis Sci 30:376, 1989.

299. Quick MW, O'Dell CD, Gammon JA, et al: Assessment of spatial vision in monkeys with experimentally induced aphakia, Soc Neurosci Abstr 13:1243, 1987.

300. Quick MW, Tigges M, Gammon JA, et al: Early abnormal visual experience induces strabismus in infant monkeys, Invest Ophthalmol Vis Sci 30:1012, 1989.

301. Rabinowicz M: Amblyopia, Chapter 11, in Harley R, ed: Pediatric ophthalmology, vol 1, 2nd ed, Philadelphia, WB Saunders, 1983, pp 293–342.

302. Rachels J: Created from animals: the moral implications of Darwinism, New York, Oxford University Press, 1990.

303. Rakic P: Genesis of the dorsal lateral geniculate nucleus in the rhesus monkey: site and time of origin, kinetics of proliferation, routes of migration and pattern of distribution of neurons, J Comp Neurol 176:23, 1977.

304. Rakic P: Prenatal development of the visual system in rhesus monkey, Phil Trans R Soc Lond B 278:245, 1977.

305. Ramachandran VS: Learning-like phenomena in stereopsis, Nature 262:382, 1976.

306. Rantakallio P, Krause U, Krause K: The use of the ophthalmological services during the preschool age, ocular findings and family background, J Pediatr Ophthalmol Strabismus 15:253, 1978.

307. Rashbass C, Westheimer G: Disjunctive eye movements, J Physiol 159:339, 1961.

308. Reading RW: Binocular vision: foundations and applications, Boston, Butterworth, 1983.

309. Regan D, Beverley KI: Some dynamic features of depth perception, Vision Res 13:2369, 1973.

310. Regan D, Erkelens CJ, Collewijn H: Visual field defects for vergence eye movements and for stereomotion perception, Invest Ophthalmol Vis Sci 27:806, 1986.

311. Regan D, Spekreijse H: Electrophysiological correlate of binocular depth perception in man, Nature 255:92, 1970.

312. Rentschler I, Hilz R, Brettel H: Spatial tuning properties in human amblyopia cannot explain the loss of optotype acuity, Behav Brain Res 1:433, 1980.

313. Rethy I: Development of the simultaneous fixation from the divergent anatomic eye-position of the neonate, J Pediatr Ophthalmol 6:92, 1969.

314. Richard J, Parks M: Intermittent exotropia: surgical results in different age groups, Ophthalmol 90:1172, 1983.

315. Richards W: Stereopsis and stereoblindness, Exp Brain Res 10:380, 1970.

316. Richards W: Anomalous stereoscopic depth perception, J Opt Soc Am 61:410, 1971.

317. Richards W, Kaye MG: Local versus global stereopsis: two mechanisms? Vision Res 14:1345, 1974.

318. Rizzo M, Blake R, Nawrot M: Human brain damage mimicking a V-4 lesion, Invest Ophthalmol Vis Sci 32(Suppl):1117, 1991.

319. Rockland K, Pandya D: Laminar origins and terminations of cortical connections of the occipital lobe in the rhesus monkey, Brain Res 179:3, 1979.

320. Rodieck RW, Binmoeller KF, Dineen J: Parasol and midget ganglion cells of the human retina, J Comp Neurol 233:115, 1985.

321. Rubenstein R, Lohr K, Brook R, et al: Measurement of physiological health for children, vol 4, Vision impairments, Santa Monica: Rand Corporation, 1985 Rand Health Insurance Experiment Series.

322. Sachsenweger R: Problems of organic lesions in functional amblyopia, in Arruga A, ed: International strabismus symposium, Basel and New York, S Karger, 1966.

323. Schiller PH, Malpeli JG: Properties and tectal projections of monkey retinal ganglion cells, J Neurophysiol 40:428, 1977.

323a. Schiller PH, Malpeli JG: Functional specificity of lateral geniculate nucleus laminae of the rhesus monkey, J Neurophysiol 41:788, 1978.

324. Schiller PH, Logothetis NK: The color-opponent and broad-band channels of the primate visual system, Trends Neurosci 13:392, 1990.

325. Schiller PH, Logothetis NK, Charles ER: Functions of color-opponent and broad-band channels of the visual system, Nature 343:68, 1990.

326. Schor CM: The relationship between fusional vergence eye movements and fixation disparity, Vision Res 19:1359, 1979.

327. Schor CM, Levi D: Disturbances of small-field horizontal and vertical optokinetic nystagmus in amblyopia, Invest Ophthalmol Vis Sci 19:668, 1980.

328. Schor CM: Fixation disparity and vergence adaptation, in Schor CM, Ciuffreda KJ, eds: Vergence eye movements: basis and clinical aspects, Boston, Butterworth, 1983, pp 465-516.

329. Schor CM: Sensory-motor adaptation and the development of the horopter, in Simons K, ed: Infant vision: basic and clinical research, New York, Oxford University Press, 1992 (in press).

330. Schor CM, Tyler CW: Spatio-temporal properties of Panum's fusional area, Vision Res 21:683, 1981.

331. Schor CM, Wood I, Ogawa J: Spatial tuning of static and dynamic local stereopsis, Vision Res 24:573, 1984.

332. Scobee R: Anatomic factors in the etiology of heterotropia, Am J Ophthalmol 31:781, 1948.

333. Scott WE, Keech R, Mash J: The postoperative results and stability of exodeviations, Arch Ophthalmol 99:1814, 1981.

334. See L, Tielsch J, Hakim R: Familial aggregation of childhood strabismus, Invest Ophthalmol Vis Sci 31:607, 1990.

335. Segal W, MacDonald R, Burkhalter A, et al: Topographic variation of magnocellular neurons in normal human lateral geniculate nucleus: temporal and lower field visual biases, Invest Ophthalmol Vis Sci 32(Suppl):1116, 1991.

336. Shimojo S, Bauer JA Jr, O'Connell KM, et al: Prestereoptic binocular vision in infants, Vision Res 26:501, 1986.

337. Sireteanu R: Binocular luminance summation in humans with defective binocular vision, Invest Ophthalmol Vis Sci 28:349, 1987.

338. Sireteanu R, Fronius M: Naso-temporal asymmetries in amblyopic vision: consequences of long-term interocular suppression, Vision Res 21:1055, 1981.

339. Sireteanu R, Fronius M, Singer W: Binocular interaction in the peripheral visual field of humans with strabismic and anisometropic amblyopia, Vision Res 21:1065, 1981.

340. Snellen H: Die Ursache des Strabismus Convergens Concomitans, Arch Ophthalmol 24:433, 1913.

341. Sokol S, Peli E, Moskowitz A, et al: Pursuit eye movements in late-onset esotropia, J Ped Ophthalmol Strabismus, 1990 (in press).

342. Sondhi N, Archer S, Helveston E: The development of normal ocular alignment, J Ped Ophthalmol Strabismus 25:210, 1988.

343. Sparks D, Mays L, Gurski M, et al: Long and short-term monocular deprivation in the rhesus monkey: effects on visual fields and optokinetic nystagmus, J Neurosci 6:1771, 1986.

344. Spivey B: Strabismus: factors in anticipating its occurrence, Aust J Ophthalmol 8:5, 1980.

345. Stager D: Teller acuity cards versus clinical judgement: discussion, Ophthalmol 95:791, 1988.

346. Steinman RM, Collewijn H: Binocular retinal image motion during active head rotation, Vision Res 20:415, 1980.

347. Steinman RM, Levinson JZ, Collewijn H, et al: Vision in the presence of known natural retinal image motion, J Opt Soc Am A 2:226, 1985.

348. Stewart S, Scott W: The age of onset of dissociated vertical deviation (DVD), Am Orthop J 41:85, 1991.

349. Stone J, Dreher B, Leventhal AG: Hierarchical and parallel mechanisms in the organization of visual cortex, Brain Res Rev 1:345, 1979.

350. Stryker M, Harris W: Binocular impulse blockade prevents the formation of ocular dominance columns in cat visual cortex, J Neurosci 6:2117, 1986.

351. Tanlanai T, Goss D: Prevalence of monocular amblyopia among anisometropes, Am J Optom Physiol Opt 56:704, 1979.

352. Teller D: The forced-choice preferential looking procedure: a psychophysical technique for use with human infants, Infant Beh Dev 2:135, 1979.

353. Teller D: Teller acuity card manual, Dayton, OH, Vistech, Inc, 1990.

354. Teller D, McDonald M, Preston K, et al: Assessment of visual acuity in infants and children: the acuity card procedure, Dev Med Child Neurol 28:779, 1986.

355. Thomas J, Mohindra I, Held R: Strabismic amblyopia in infants, Am J Optomet Physiol Opt 56:197, 1979.

356. Tredici T, von Noorden G: The Pulfrich effect in anisometropic amblyopia and strabismus, Am J Ophthalmol 98:499, 1984.

357. Tusa RJ, Herdman SJ, Mishkin M: Ocular motor deficits in retinotopic and craniotopic space in monkeys with unilateral striate and corpus callosum lesions, Soc Neurosci Abstr 14:796, 1988.

358. Tychsen L: Unpublished data.

359. Tychsen L: Primary maldevelopment of visual motion pathway in humans, Invest Ophthalmol Vis Sci 30(Suppl):302, 1989.

360. Tychsen L: Pediatric ocular motility disorders of neuro-ophthalmic significance, in Shults WT, ed: Ophthalmology clinics of North America, vol 4, Philadelphia: WB Saunders, 1991, pp 615-643.

361. Tychsen L: Improvements in smooth pursuit and fixational eye movements after strabismus surgery in infants, Ophthalmol 98(Suppl):94, 1991.

362. Tychsen L: Motion sensitivity and the origins of infantile strabismus, in Simons K, ed: Infant vision: basic and clinical research, New York, Oxford University Press, 1992 (in press).

363. Tychsen L, Hoyt WF: Occipital lobe dysplasia, Arch Ophthalmol 103:680, 1985.

364. Tychsen L, Hoyt WF: Relative afferent pupillary defect in congenital occipital hemianopia, Am J Ophthalmol 100:345, 1985.

365. Tychsen L, Hurtig RR, Scott WE: Pursuit is impaired but the vestibulo-ocular reflex is normal in infantile strabismus, Arch Ophthalmol 103:536, 1985.

366. Tychsen L, Lisberger SG: Visual motion processing for the initiation of smooth-pursuit eye movement in humans, J Neurophysiol 56:953, 1986.

367. Tychsen L, Lisberger SG: Maldevelopment of visual motion processing in humans who had strabismus with onset in infancy, J Neurosci 2495, 1986.

368. Tychsen L, Quick MW, Boothe RG: Alternating monocular input from birth causes stereoblindness, motion processing asymmetries, and strabismus in infant macaque, Invest Ophthalmol Vis Sci 32(Suppl):1044, 1991.

369. Tychsen L, Rizzo M, Hurtig RR, et al: Visual motion processing in humans after loss of striate cortex, Soc Neurosci Abstr 14:796, 1988.

369a. Tychsen, L: Microstrabismics who have normal visual acuity perform well as jet aircraft pilots, Ophthalmol 96(Suppl):132, 1989.

370. Tychsen L, Thompson HS: An electronically-induced Pulfrich illusion as a measure of visual delay and stereopsis, Doc Ophthal Proc Series 37:453, 1983.

371. Tyler CW: Stereoscopic depth movement: two eyes less sensitive than one, Science 174:958, 1971.

372. Tyler CW: Stereoscopic vision: cortical limitations a disparity scaling effect, Science 181:276, 1973.

373. Tyler CW: Sensory processing of binocular disparity,

in Schor CM, Cuiffreda KJ, eds: Vergence eye movements: basic and clinical aspects, Boston, Butterworth, 1983, pp 199–296.

374. Tyler CW: A stereoscopic view of visual processing streams, Vision Res 30:1877, 1990.

375. Tyler CW, Cavanagh P: Purely chromatic stereomotion perception, Invest Ophthalmol Vis Sci 30:324, 1989.

376. Tyler CW, Scott AB: Binocular vision, in Records RE, ed: Physiology of the human eye and visual system, Hagerstown, MD: Harper & Row, 1979, pp 643–671.

377. Tyler CW, Torres J: Frequency response characteristics for sinusoidal movement in the fovea and periphery, Perception Psychophys 12:232, 1972.

378. Ungerleider LG, Mishkin M: The striate projection zone in the superior temporal sulcus of Macaca mulatta: location and topographic organization, J Comp Neurol 188:347, 1979.

379. US Department of Health, Education, and Welfare: Eye examination findings among children, National Health Survey 11:1, 1972.

380. Vaegan TD: Critical period for deprivation amblyopia in children, Trans Ophthal Soc UK 99:432, 1979.

381. van Dalen JTW: Flash-induced nystagmus: its relation to latent nystagmus, Jpn J Ophthalmol 25:370, 1981.

382. Van Essen DC: Functional organization of primate visual cortex, in Peters A, Jones E, eds: Cerebral cortex, New York, Plenum, 1985, pp 259–329.

383. Van Essen DC, Maunsell JHR: Hierarchical organization and functional streams in the visual cortex, Trends Neurosci 6:370, 1983.

384. Van Essen DC, Zeki SM: The topographic organization of rhesus monkey prestriate cortex, J Physiol 277:193, 1978.

385. van Hof-van Duin J: Direction-preference of optokinetic responses in monocularly tested normal kittens and light-deprived cats, Arch Ital Biol 116:471, 1978.

386. van Hof-van Duin J, Evenhuis-van Launen A, et al: Effects of very low birth weight (VLBW) on visual development during the first year term, Early Hum Dev 20:255, 1989.

387. Vieth G: Ueber die Richtung der Augen, Ann Phys 48:233, 1818.

388. Vision problems in the US, Data analysis: definitions, data sources, detailed data tables, analysis, interpretation, New York, Nat Soc to Prevent Blindness, 1980, vol publication P-10.

389. Volpe JJ: Hypoxic-ischemic encephalopathy: neuropathology and pathogenesis, in Volpe J, ed: Neurology of the newborn, vol 22, 2nd ed, Philadelphia, WB Saunders, 1987, pp 209-235.

390. von Noorden GK: The nystagmus compensation (blockage) syndrome, Am J Ophthalmol 95:748, 1976.

391. von Noorden GK: Current concepts of infantile esotropia, XLIV Edward Jackson Memorial Lecture, Am J Ophthalmol 105:1, 1988.

392. von Noorden GK: Binocular vision and ocular motility: theory and management of strabismus, 4th ed, St Louis, CV Mosby, 1990.

393. von Noorden GK, Crawford M: Form deprivation without light deprivation produces the visual deprivation syndrome in Macaca mulatta, Brain Res 129:37, 1977.

394. von Noorden GK, Crawford J, Levacy R: The lateral geniculate nucleus in human anisometropic amblyopia, Invest Ophthalmol Vis Sci 24:788, 1983.

395. von Noorden GK, Dowling J, Ferguson D: Experimental amblyopia in monkeys, I, Behavioral studies of stimulus deprivation amblyopia, Arch Ophthalmol 84:206, 1970.

396. Walls G: The vertebrate eye and its adaptive radiation, New York & London: Hafner Publishing, 1942.

397. Walters CP, Walk RD: Visual placing by human infants, J Exp Child Psychol 18:34, 1974.

398. Walton P, Lisberger SG: Binocular misalignment in infancy causes directional asymmetries in pursuit, Invest Ophthalmol Vis Sci 30(Suppl):304, 1989.

399. Wang AH, Norcia AM: Reversing gratings are perceived as drifting nasally when viewed monocularly by patients with early onset esotropia, Unpublished data, 1991.

400. Wattam-Bell J, Braddick O, Atkinson J: Measures of infant binocularity in a group at risk for strabismus, Clin Vis Sci 1:327, 1987.

401. Westheimer G, Mitchell AM: Eye movement responses to convergent stimuli, Arch Ophthalmol 55:848, 1956.

402. Westheimer G, Mitchell DE: The sensory stimulus for disjunctive eye movements, Vision Res 9:749, 1969.

403. Wheatstone C: Some remarkable phenomena of binocular vision, Phil Trans R Soc 128:371, 1838.

404. Wiesel TN: Postnatal development of the visual cortex and the influence of environment, Nature 299:583, 1982.

404a. Wiesel TN, Hubel DH: Ordered arrangement of orientation columns in monkeys lacking visual experience, J Comp Neurol 158:307, 1974.

405. Williams RW, Rakic P: Elimination of neurons from the rhesus monkey's lateral geniculate nucleus during development, J Comp Neurol 272:424, 1988.

406. Wilson J, Tigges M, Boothe R, et al: Correlations between anatomy, physiology, and behavior for monocular infantile aphakia, Invest Ophthalmol Vis Sci 32(Suppl):819, 1991.

407. Wong-Riley M: Changes in the visual system of monocularly sutured or enucleated cats demonstrable with cytochrome oxidase histochemistry, Brain Res 171:11, 1979.

408. Wood C, Spear P, Braun J: Direction-specific deficits in horizontal optokinetic nystagmus following removal of visual cortex in the cat, Brain Res 60:231, 1973.

409. Woodburn L: The effect of a constant visual angle upon the binocular discrimination of depth differences, Am J Psychol 46:273, 1934.

410. Worth C: Squint: its causes, pathology, and treatment, Philadelphia, Blakiston, 1903.

411. Zee DS, Tusa R, Herdman S, et al: Effects of occipital lobectomy upon eye movements in primate, J Neurophysiol 58:883, 1987.

412. Zeki SM: Cells responding to changing image size and disparity in the cortex of the rhesus monkey, J Physiol 242:549, 1974.

413. Zeki SM: Functional specialization in the visual cortex of the rhesus monkey, Nature 274:423, 1978.

414. Zihl J, Von Cramon D, Mai N: Selective disturbance of movement vision after bilateral brain damage, Brain 106:313, 1983.

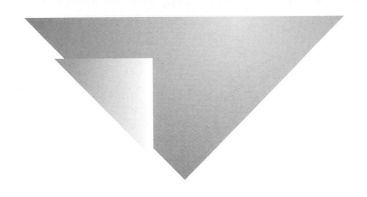

Index

Italic indicates references to illustrations, tables, diagrams.